CONTRIBUTORS.

BARR, DAVID P., A.B., M.D., LL.D., F.A.C.P.

BLOOMFIELD, ARTHUR L., A.B., M.D., F.A.C.P.

BROWN, GEORGE E., M.D., F.A.C.P.

CHESNEY, ALAN M., A.B., M.D.

COOKE, ROBERT A., A.M., M.D., F.A.C.P.

CRAIG, CHARLES F., M.A., M.D., F.A.C.P.

FAUST, ERNEST CARROLL, A.B., M.A., Ph.D.

KINSELLA, RALPH A., A.M., M.D., F.A.C.P.

KRUMBHAAR, EDWARD B., Ph.D., M.D., F.A.C.P.

LEMANN, ISAAC IVAN, B.A., M.D., F.A.C.P.

McCANN, WILLIAM SHARP, A.B., M.D., F.A.C.P.

MEANS, JAMES H., A.B., M.D., F.A.C.P.

MILLER, JAMES ALEXANDER, A.M., M.D., Sc.D., F.A.C.P.

MITCHELL, A. GRAEME, M.D.

MUSSER, JOHN H., B.S., M.D., F.A.C.P.

PEPPER, O. H. PERRY, B.S., M.D., F.A.C.P.

PINCOFFS, MAURICE C., S.B., M.D., F.A.C.P.

REIMANN, HOBART A., M.D.

SMITH, FRED M., B.S., M.D., F.A.C.P.

STRECKER, EDWARD A., A.M., M.D., F.A.C.P.

STURGIS, CYRUS C., B.S., M.D., F.A.C.P.

SYDENSTRICKER, VIRGIL PRESTON, A.M., M.D., F.A.C.P.

TORREY, ROBERT GRANT, M.D., F.A.C.P.

VAN VALZAH, ROBERT, B.A., M.D., F.A.C.P.

WILDER, RUSSELL M., Ph.D., M.D.

WILSON, GEORGE, M.D.

INTERNAL MEDICINE

ITS THEORY AND PRACTICE

IN CONTRIBUTIONS BY AMERICAN AUTHORS

EDITED BY

JOHN H. MUSSER, B.S., M.D., F.A.C.P.

PROFESSOR OF MEDICINE IN THE TULANE UNIVERSITY OF LOUISIANA SCHOOL OF
MEDICINE; SENIOR VISITING PHYSICIAN TO THE CHARITY HOSPITAL,
NEW ORLEANS, LOUISIANA

SECOND EDITION, THOROUGHLY REVISED

ILLUSTRATED

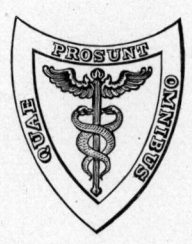

LEA & FEBIGER
PHILADELPHIA

PRINTED IN U. S. A.

PREFACE.

In this second edition the same general principles have been followed in the preparation of the text as in the first edition. The contributing authors have presented their material in a manner similar to that which they have found most satisfactory in the instruction and teaching of students. After all, in a broad sense, a scientific book is a textbook, and if certain methods of teaching have been found efficacious by practical experience they should prove valuable in the preparation of a textbook. The group of authors, twenty-six in number, are all teachers of medicine in prominent medical schools. They have been selected because of their particular interest in, and knowledge of, the group of diseases or disorders about which they write. Their information has been obtained by experimental and extensive clinical observations so that they are recognized as being authorities in this or that special branch of internal medicine.

Extensive revision has been made in most of the sections. The extent of these revisions is such that a complete survey of all the changes made would occupy an undue amount of space. The revisions and additions have to do very largely with the developments of the last two years that are recognized as being new but well established. This statement applies particularly to the more important features of the etiology and of disturbed physiology of disease and especially to the newer drugs that have proved efficacious in treatment. Most extensive changes have been in the section on diseases of the lung which has been largely rewritten. New material has been included on bacillary dysentery in the section devoted to bacillary diseases. A section on the classification of arthropods involved in disease dealing with ticks, mites and various other insects has been incorporated. Diseases of the lymphatic vessels has been added, as has tuberculosis of the kidneys and urinary tract. For the purpose of greater compactness disorders of the liver, bile passages, pancreas and peritoneum have been merged with the chapter on diseases of the gastro-intestinal tract. It is for this purpose only that these chapters have been combined as one chapter, *Diseases of the Alimentary Tract*.

There has been some slight change in the classification of disease. Sprue has been listed among the deficiency diseases; milk sickness in the intoxications. Criticism might be made of the classification of some of the other diseases. It might seem at first glance to be inappropriate not to place diphtheria and tuberculosis among the other bacillary diseases but it is obvious why such a classification is followed. The former disease is essentially within the province of the pediatrician, the latter disease is cared for usually by the phthisiologist whose primary interest is in diseases of the lung. Criticism might be made also of the classification of some of the blood diseases, but it would seem proper to put there those diseases in which the outstanding expression is chiefly in the blood picture.

As in the first edition, the main headings and special features only have been indexed. It has seemed a needless waste of space to index subheads, such as definition, history, etiology, incidence, pathology, pathologic-physiology, symptoms, prognosis and treatment when they appear in black-face type in regular sequence which can be seen at a glance when the reader turns to the page on which appears the disease indexed.

Again the editor wishes to express his gratitude and thanks to the authors who have contributed to this second edition. They have been helpful in their suggestions, they have coöperated expeditiously and heartily in the revision, and in every way they have made the prompt appearance of this second edition possible. The editor also wishes to thank Miss Sarah Magill and Mrs. Gusse Patten who have read proof assiduously and assisted in innumerable ways in the preparation of this volume; also Messrs. Lea & Febiger who have been courteous and helpful at all times.

JOHN H. MUSSER, M.D.

1430 TULANE AVENUE
  NEW ORLEANS, LA.

LIST OF CONTRIBUTORS.

DAVID P. BARR, A.B., M.D., LL.D., F.A.C.P.,
Busch Professor of Medicine in the Washington University School of Medicine, St. Louis, Mo.

ARTHUR L. BLOOMFIELD, A.B., M.D., F.A.C.P.,
Professor of Medicine in the Stanford University School of Medicine, San Francisco, Calif.

GEORGE E. BROWN, M.D., F.A.C.P.,
Head of Section in Division of Medicine, The Mayo Clinic; Associate Professor of Medicine, The Mayo Foundation for Medical Education and Research, Graduate School, University of Minnesota, Rochester, Minn.

ALAN M. CHESNEY, A.B., M.D.,
Associate Professor of Medicine and Dean of the Johns Hopkins University School of Medicine, Baltimore, Md.

ROBERT A. COOKE, A.M., M.D., F.A.C.P.,
Assistant Professor of Clinical Medicine in the Cornell University Medical College, New York City.

CHARLES F. CRAIG, M.A., M.D., F.A.C.P., F.A.C.S.,
Colonel, United States Army, Retired. D.S.M., Professor of Tropical Medicine and Head of Department of Tropical Medicine in the Tulane University of Louisiana School of Medicine, New Orleans, La.

ERNEST CARROLL FAUST, A.B., M.A., Ph.D.,
Professor of Parasitology in the Tulane University of Louisiana School of Medicine, New Orleans, La.

RALPH A. KINSELLA, A.M., M.D., F.A.C.P.,
Professor of Internal Medicine and Director of the Department in the St. Louis University School of Medicine, St. Louis, Mo.

EDWARD B. KRUMBHAAR, Ph.D., M.D., F.A.C.P.,
Professor of Pathology in the University of Pennsylvania School of Medicine, Philadelphia, Pa.

ISAAC IVAN LEMANN, B.A., M.D., F.A.C.P.,
Professor of Clinical Medicine in the Tulane University of Louisiana School of Medicine, New Orleans, La.

WILLIAM SHARP McCANN, A.B., M.D., F.A.C.P.,
Charles A. Dewey Professor of Medicine in the University of Rochester School of Medicine and Dentistry, Rochester, N. Y.

J. H. MEANS, A.B., M.D., F.A.C.P.,
Jackson Professor of Clinical Medicine in the Harvard Medical School; Chief of the Medical Service of the Massachusetts General Hospital, Boston, Mass.

JAMES ALEXANDER MILLER, A.M., M.D., Sc.D., F.A.C.P.,
Professor of Clinical Medicine in the Columbia University School of Medicine, New York City.

A. GRAEME MITCHELL, M.D.,
B. K. Rachford Professor of Pediatrics in the University of Cincinnati College of Medicine, Cincinnati, Ohio.

JOHN H. MUSSER, B.S., M.D., F.A.C.P.,
  Professor of Medicine in the Tulane University of Louisiana School of Medicine, New Orleans, La.

O. H. PERRY PEPPER, B.S., M.D., F.A.C.P.,
  Professor of Medicine in the University of Pennsylvania School of Medicine, Philadelphia, Pa.

MAURICE C. PINCOFFS, S.B., M.D., F.A.C.P.,
  Professor of Medicine in the University of Maryland School of Medicine, Baltimore, Md.

HOBART A. REIMANN, M.D.,
  Associate Professor of Medicine in the University of Minnesota, Minneapolis, Minn.

FRED M. SMITH, B.S., M.D., F.A.C.P.,
  Professor and Head of the Department of Theory and Practice of Medicine in the State University of Iowa, Iowa City, Iowa.

EDWARD A. STRECKER, A.M., M.D., Sc.D., F.A.C.P.,
  Professor of Psychiatry and Head of Department of Psychiatry, School of Medicine, University of Pennsylvania, Philadelphia, Pa.

CYRUS C. STURGIS, B.S., M.D., F.A.C.P.,
  Professor of Internal Medicine in the University of Michigan Medical School; Director, Thomas Henry Simpson Memorial Institute for Medical Research; Director, Department of Internal Medicine, University Hospital, Ann Arbor, Mich.

VIRGIL PRESTON SYDENSTRICKER, A.M., M.D., F.A.C.P.,
  Professor of Medicine in the University of Georgia School of Medicine, Augusta, Ga.

ROBERT GRANT TORREY, M.D., F.A.C.P.,
  Professor of the Principles and Practice of Medicine and Clinical Medicine in the Women's Medical College, Philadelphia, Pa.

ROBERT VAN VALZAH, B.A., M.D., F.A.C.P.,
  Professor of Medicine in the University of Wisconsin Medical School, Madison, Wis.

RUSSELL M. WILDER, Ph.D., M.D.,
  Professor of Medicine, and Chief of the Department of Medicine in The Mayo Foundation, University of Minnesota, Rochester, Minn.

GEORGE WILSON, M.D.,
  Professor of Clinical Neurology at the School of Medicine of the University of Pennsylvania; Professor of Clinical Neurology at the Woman's Medical College of Pennsylvania; Neurologist to the Philadelphia General, the Abington and the Bryn Mawr Hospitals, Philadelphia, Pa.

CONTENTS.

PART I.

INFECTIOUS DISEASE.

CHAPTER I.

THE BACILLARY DISEASES.

By HOBART A. REIMANN, M.D.

Introduction 13
The Typhoid-Colon-Dysentery Group 23
    Typhoid 23
    Paratyphoid Bacillus Infections 41
    Colon Bacillus Infections 41
    Bacillary Dysentery, Acute and Chronic 43
Undulant Fever 51
Leprosy 64
Tetanus 69
Tularemia 76
Plague 82
Anthrax 87
Influenza 92
Glanders 103
Cholera 107

CHAPTER II.

THE COCCAL DISEASES.

By RALPH A. KINSELLA, M.D.

General Considerations 113
Staphylococcal Infections 117
    Septicemia 118
    Pneumonia 118
Streptococcal Infections 119
    Non-hemolytic Streptococcus 120
    Focal Infections 120
    Hemolytic Streptococcus 122
Special Streptococcal Infections 124
    Streptococcal Sore Throat 124
    Wound Infections 125
    Septicemia 126
    Erysipelas 127
    Bronchopneumonia 129
    Empyema 132
Pneumococcal Infection 133
    Lobar Pneumonia 137
Cerebrospinal Fever 148
Gonococcal Infections 154
    Gonorrheal Rheumatism 155

CHAPTER III.

THE VIRUS DISEASES.

By O. H. PERRY PEPPER, M.D.

Introduction 159
Smallpox 163

Cowpox 170
Vaccination 171
Rabies 172
Yellow Fever 176
Dengue 180
Pappataci Fever 183
Infectious Cold 185
Psittacosis 186
Foot-and-mouth Disease 188

CHAPTER IV.

DISEASES DUE TO RICKETTSIÆ.

By ROBERT VAN VALZAH, M.D.

Typhus Fever 190
Rocky Mountain Spotted Fever 197
Trench Fever 200
Tsutsugamushi Disease 202

CHAPTER V.

DISEASES DUE TO SPIROCHETES.

By ALAN M. CHESNEY, M.D.

Syphilis 204
Yaws 228
Rat-bite Fever 229
Relapsing Fever 229
Epidemic Jaundice 230

CHAPTER VI.

THE PROTOZOAL DISEASES.

By CHARLES F. CRAIG, M.D.

Amebiasis 232
Intestinal Flagellate Infestations 242
The Leishmaniases 243
    Kala-azar 244
    Oriental Sore 248
    Espundia 249
The Trypanosomiases 251
    African Sleeping Sickness 251
    Chagas Disease 254
Coccidiosis 256
The Malarial Fevers 257
Sarcosporidiosis 273
Balantidiasis 273

CHAPTER VII.

THE METAZOAL DISEASES.

By ERNEST CARROLL FAUST, PH.D.

Introduction 276
General Classification of Helminthic Diseases 278
Nematode Infections 279
    Ancylostomiasis 279
    Trichocephaliasis 283
    Ascariasis 283
    Oxyuriasis 285
    Strongyloidosis 286
    Trichinosis 287
    Filariasis 288

Cestode or Tapeworm Infections 290
   Teniasis 290
   Echinococcosis (Hydatid Cyst) 291
   Hymenolepiasis 292
   Dipylidiiasis 293
   Diphyllobothriasis 293
   Sparganosis 294
Trematode or Fluke Infections 294
   Intestinal Distomiasis 295
   Liver Distomiasis 296
   Pulmonary Distomiasis 297
   Schistosomiasis 298
General Classification of Arthropods Involved in Disease 302
   Ticks, Mites, Spiders and Scorpions 302
   Blood-sucking Insects 304
   Filth and Myiasis-producing Insects 306
   Nettling, Vesicating and Stinging Insects 307

CHAPTER VIII.

THE CONTAGIOUS DISEASES OF CHILDHOOD.

By A. GRAEME MITCHELL, M.D.

Diphtheria 309
Scarlet Fever (Scarlatina) 314
Pertussis (Whooping Cough) 322
Measles 325
Varicella 329
Mumps 332
Roseola Infantum (Exanthema Subitum) 334
Fourth Disease and Fifth Disease 334
Rubella 334

CHAPTER IX.

DISEASES OF DOUBTFUL ETIOLOGY.

By VIRGIL PRESTON SYDENSTRICKER, M.D.

Rheumatic Fever 336
Infectious Mononucleosis 345
Infectious Jaundice 347
Ephemeral Fever (Febricula) 349
Miliary Fever 349
Ainhum 350
Gangosa 351

CHAPTER X.

THE FUNGUS DISEASES (NON-BACTERIAL).

By ISAAC IVAN LEMANN, M.D.

Introduction 352
Integument and Skeleton 353
Special Organs 354
Internal Fungus Disease 354
Respiratory Tract 355
Gastro-intestinal Tract 355
Central Nervous System 356
Genito-urinary System 356

PART II.

SYSTEMIC DISEASES.

CHAPTER XI.

DISEASES OF THE HEART.

By FRED M. SMITH, M.D.

General Discussion of Diseases of the Heart 359
    Etiologic Types 359
    Symptoms 361
Rheumatic Heart Disease 365
Bacterial Endocarditis 371
    Acute Bacterial Endocarditis 371
    Subacute Bacterial Endocarditis 371
Arteriosclerotic Heart Disease (Hypertensive Heart Disease) 375
Angina Pectoris 380
Coronary Occlusion 386
Syphilitic Heart Disease 391
Thyrotoxic Heart Disease 394
Congenital Heart Disease 396
Pericarditis 400
    Acute Fibrinous Pericarditis 401
    Pericarditis with Effusion 402
    Adherent Pericardium (Chronic Adhesive Pericarditis) 406
Chronic Valvular Heart Disease 408
    Mitral Valve Disease 409
    Aortic Valve Disease 415
    Tricuspid Valve Disease 421
    Pulmonary Valve Disease 422
Diseases of the Myocardium 424
    Myocarditis 424
    Other Forms of Myocardial Involvement 427
Functional Disorders of the Heart 427
    Cardiac Neuroses 427
    Irritable Heart (Effort Syndrome, Neuro-circulatory Asthenia) . . . 428
Disorders of the Heart Beat 430
    Normal Cardiac Mechanism 430
    Disturbance in Rate 431
    Disorders of the Heart Beat Due to Disturbance in Conduction—Heart
        Block 434
    Disorders of Heart Beat Due to Abnormal Impulse Formation . . . 437
Treatment of Congestive Heart Failure 448

CHAPTER XII.

DISEASES OF THE BLOOD-VESSELS.

By GEORGE E. BROWN, M.D.

Structures and Mechanism of Disturbances in General 455
The Arteries 457
    Functional or Vasomotor Disturbances 457
    Vasoconstricting Disturbances 457
    Vasodilating Disturbances 460
        Normal Blood Pressure 462
    Vasoconstricting Disturbances (Hypertension; Hyperpiesia; High Blood
        Pressure) 463
    Vasodilating Disturbances (Hypotension; Low Blood Pressure) . . . 479
    Organic Disturbances, Localized Forms 481
        Generalized Forms and Forms Affecting Special Systems (Arterio-
            sclerosis; Atheromatosis or Atherosclerosis 493

Arteriovenous Fistula (Arteriovenous Aneurysm; Cirsoid Aneurysm; Pulsating Venous Aneurysm) 497
Diseases of the Veins 499
Diseases of the Peripheral Lymphatic Vessels (Lymphedema) 502

CHAPTER XIII.

DISEASES OF THE URINARY TRACT.

By WILLIAM SHARP McCANN, M.D.

General Symptomatology in Relation to Pathologic Physiology 505
Nephritis or Bright's Disease 525
Hemorrhagic Bright's Disease 526
Degenerative Bright's Disease; The Nephroses 539
Arteriosclerotic Bright's Disease 550
Infarcts of the Kidney 553
Chronic Passive Congestion of the Kidneys 554
Renal Pain 555
Hydronephrosis and Pyonephrosis 555
Nephrolithiasis 557
Bacterial Infections of the Kidneys and Urinary Passages 558
    Non-tuberculous Infections 558
    Abscess of the Kidney 558
    Pyelitis and Pyelonephritis 559
    Tuberculosis of Kidneys and Urinary Tract 562
Tumors of the Kidney 563
Polycystic Kidneys 563

CHAPTER XIV.

DISEASES OF THE ALIMENTARY TRACT.

By ARTHUR L. BLOOMFIELD, M.D.

The Mouth, Pharynx and Tonsils 565
    Medical Aspects of Dental Disease—Focal Infection 568
    Vincent's Angina 569
    Syphilis of the Mouth and Pharynx 571
    Neoplasms of the Buccal-pharyngeal Structures 572
    Acute Tonsillitis 572
    Chronic Tonsillitis 574
    Tuberculosis of the Tonsils 575
The Esophagus 576
    Spasm of the Esophagus 577
    Cancer of the Esophagus 581
The Stomach 583
    The Classifications of Disorders of the Stomach 583
    Diagnosis of Disorders of the Stomach 585
    Indigestion 591
    Gastritis 598
    Gastric and Duodenal Ulcer 600
    Cancer of the Stomach 617
    Other Tumors of the Stomach 623
    Syphilis of the Stomach 623
    Deformities, Displacements and Anomalies of the Stomach 624
The Intestine 624
    Intestinal Neuroses 625
    Constipation 028
    Diarrhea 631
    Intestinal Obstruction 634
    Appendicitis 638
    Ulcerative Colitis 641
    Tuberculosis of the Intestine 644
    Tumors of the Bowel 645
    Cancer of the Colon 646
    Anomalies and Deformities of the Intestine 651

The Rectum 652
 Infections of the Rectum 652
 Tumors of the Rectum 653
 Hemorrhoids 654
Diseases of the Liver 655
 Jaundice (Icterus) 656
 Hepatitis (Non-suppurative) 658
 Suppurative Hepatitis (Abscess of Liver) 667
 Syphilis of the Liver 668
 Neoplasms of the Liver 669
 Anomalies of Form and Position of the Liver 671
Diseases of the Gall-bladder and Bile Ducts 672
 Cholangitis 672
 Cholecystitis 673
 Cancer of the Gall-bladder and Bile Ducts 674
 Cholelithiasis (Gall Stones) 675
 Stenosis and Congenital Obliteration of the Bile Passages . . . 679
Diseases of the Pancreas 679
 Pancreatitis 680
 Cancer of the Pancreas 681
 Cysts of the Pancreas 682
 Pancreatic Calculi 683
Diseases of the Peritoneum 683
 Acute General Peritonitis 684
 Localized Peritonitis (Abscess)—Acute and Chronic 685
 Chronic Adhesive Peritonitis 686
 Tumors of the Peritoneum 687

CHAPTER XV.

DISEASES OF THE RESPIRATORY TRACT.

By JAMES ALEXANDER MILLER, M.D.

Functional Pathology of Pulmonary Disease 688
Pulmonary Atelectasis 699
Emphysema 703
Pulmonary Fibroses, Pneumoconiosis, Pulmonary Arteriosclerosis . . 707
 Pneumoconiosis (Occupational Fibroses) 712
 Pulmonary Arteriosclerosis 716
Bronchiectasis and Cystic Disease of the Lung 717
Infections of the Upper Respiratory Tract 721
Abscess of the Lung 729
Gangrene of the Lung 734
Pulmonary Tuberculosis 734
Syphilis of the Lung 775
Mycotic Diseases of the Lung 777
Hydatid Disease of the Lung 780
Tumors of the Lung and Pleura 781
The Pleura 786
 Pleurisies 786
Hydrothorax 794
Pneumothorax 794
The Mediastinum 797
 Tumors of the Mediastinum 799
 Inflammatory Processes of the Mediastinum 800
The Diaphragm 801
 Organic Diseases of the Diaphragm 803

CHAPTER XVI.

DISEASES OF THE ENDOCRINE GLANDS.

By J. H. MEANS, M.D.

Introduction 806
The Thyroid Gland 809
 Endemic Goiter 812

The Thyroid Gland—
  Sporadic Colloid Goiter 814
  Nodular Goiter 814
  Exophthalmic Goiter 815
  The Heart in Thyrotoxicosis 820
  Myxedema 821
  Cretinism 825
  Malignant Disease of the Thyroid Gland 826
  Thyroiditis 827
  Developmental Anomalies of the Thyroid Gland 828
  Hypometabolism without Myxedema 829
  The Thyroid Problems of Pregnancy 830
The Parathyroid Glands 830
  Hypoparathyroidism 831
  Hyperparathyroidism 833
The Adrenal Glands 835
  Addison's Disease 837
  Hyperfunction of the Adrenal Medulla 840
  Hyperfunction of the Adrenal Cortex 841
  Other Diseases of the Adrenal Glands 842
The Pituitary Glands 842
  Acromegaly 845
  Gigantism 847
  Simmonds' Disease 847
  Hypophyseal Dwarfism 848
  Fröhlich's Syndrome 849
  Cushing's Syndrome 850
The Pancreas 850
The Female Gonads 851
  Hyperfunctional States 852
  Hypofunctional States 852
  Amenorrhea 853
  Functional Uterine Bleeding 853
The Male Gonads 853
  Hyperfunctional States 854
  Hypofunctional States 854
The Pineal Body 854
The Thymus Body 855

CHAPTER XVII.

DISEASES OF THE BLOOD.

By CYRUS C. STURGIS, M.D.

Introduction 856
Chronic Secondary Anemia (Chronic Microcytic Anemia) 859
Idiopathic Microcytic Anemia 861
Pernicious Anemia 863
Aplastic Anemia 870
Chronic Hemolytic Jaundice 871
Chlorosis 872
Sickle-cell Anemia 873
Purpura 874
Hemophilia 878
Leukemia 880
Agranulocytic Angina 886
Hodgkin's Disease 888
Splenic Anemia 890
Polycythemia Rubra Vera (Erythremia) 891

CHAPTER XVIII.

DISEASES OF THE SPLEEN AND THE RETICULO-ENDOTHELIAL SYSTEM.

By EDWARD B. KRUMBHAAR, M.D.

The Spleen 894
  Diagnosis of Splenomegaly 894

The Spleen—
    Anomalies 895
    Atrophy 895
    Movable Spleens (Floating Spleen, Lien Mobile) 895
    Congestion and Aucte Splenic Tumor 896
    Abscess 896
    Infarction and Necrosis 896
    Amyloid Degeneration (Waxy Degeneration, Lardaceous Disease) . . 896
    Thrombosis of the Splenic Vein 897
    Cirrhotic Splenomegaly 897
    Chronic Infectious Splenomegalies 897
    Syphilis of the Spleen 897
    Tuberculosis of the Spleen 897
    Malaria of the Spleen 898
    Cysts 898
    Neoplasms 898
The Reticulo-endothelial System 899
    Aleukemic Reticulosis (Reticulo-endotheliosis) 900
    Gaucher's Disease (Large Cell Splenomegaly) 900
    Niemann-Pick's Disease (Lipoid Histocytosis) 901
    Hand-Christian's Syndrome 902
    Xanthomatosis 902

CHAPTER XIX.

DISEASES OF THE LOCOMOTOR SYSTEM.

By ROBERT GRANT TORREY, M.D.

The Joints 904
    Chronic Arthritis 904
    Arthritis Deformans 908
    Spondylitis Deformans 919
    Acute Arthritis 919
The Bursæ 919
    Bursitis 919
The Bones 920
    Congenital Defects of the Bone Structure 920
    Bone Defects Not Congenital 921
    Neoplastic Bone Disease 922
The Muscles 923
    Diseases of the Voluntary Muscles 923
Fibrositis 926

PART III.

DISEASES OF NUTRITION—ALLERGY—METABOLISM— PHYSICAL AND CHEMICAL AGENTS.

CHAPTER XX.

DISEASES OF NUTRITION.

By JOHN H. MUSSER, M.D.

Deficiency Diseases 929
    Avitaminoses 929
Beri-beri 936
Scurvy 940
Rickets 944
Pellagra 949
Sprue 953

CHAPTER XXI.

DISEASES OF ALLERGY.

By ROBERT A. COOKE, M.D.

Allergy 959
Asthma 968
Allergic Coryza (Hay Fever) 974
Serum Sickness 980
Serum Shock 981
Urticaria and Angioneurotic Edema 982
Other Allergies 983

CHAPTER XXII.

DISEASES OF METABOLISM.

By RUSSELL M. WILDER, M.D.

Gout 985
Diabetes Mellitus 992
Hyperinsulinism 1011
Acidosis 1012
Alkalosis 1014
Obesity 1015
Lipomatosis 1019
Diabetes Insipidus 1021
Hemochromatosis 1023
Ochronosis 1024

CHAPTER XXIII.

DISEASES DUE TO PHYSICAL AND TOXIC AGENTS.

By DAVID P. BARR, M.D.

Diseases Due to Physical Agents 1026
    Heat Exhaustion and Heat Stroke 1026
    Caisson Disease 1028
    Mountain Sickness 1030
    Electric Shock 1031
    Radio-active Substances 1033
The Intoxications 1034
    Alcoholism 1034
    Opium Habit 1039
    Cocainism 1041
    Food Poisoning 1042
    Snake Venom Poisoning 1047

CHAPTER XXIV.

DISEASES DUE TO CHEMICAL AGENTS.

By MAURICE C. PINCOFFS, M.D.

Carbon Monoxide Poisoning 1049
Lead Poisoning 1054
Arsenic Poisoning 1061
Mercury Poisoning 1064
Benzene Poisoning 1067

PART IV.

DISEASES OF THE NERVOUS SYSTEM.

CHAPTER XXV.

DISEASES AND ABNORMALITIES OF THE MIND, INCLUDING THE NEUROSES.

By EDWARD A. STRECKER, M.D.

The Psychoses 1069
  Paresis 1077
  Senile Psychoses 1079
  Psychoses with Cerebral Arteriosclerosis 1081
  Epileptic Psychoses 1081
  Psychoses with Mental Deficiency 1083
  Psychoses with Cerebral Syphilis, Huntington's Chorea, Brain Tumor,
    Encephalitis and Other Brain and Nervous Diseases, Traumatic
    Psychoses 1084
The Toxic Psychoses 1085
  Exogenous Toxic Psychoses 1085
  Psychoses with Somatic Disease 1087
  Manic-depressive Psychoses 1087
  Involution Melancholia 1092
  Schizophrenia (Dementia Præcox) 1093
  Constitutional Psychopathic Inferiority 1096
The Neuroses 1097
  Hysteria 1099
  Neurasthenia 1099
  Psychasthenia 1100
  Anxiety Neurosis 1100
  Glossary 1107

CHAPTER XXVI.

ORGANIC DISEASES OF THE NERVOUS SYSTEM.

By GEORGE WILSON, M.D.

Introduction 1111
The Cranial Nerves 1115
The Reflexes 1125
The Motor System 1127
  Gaits 1131
  Tremor 1133
Sensation 1134
Cerebrospinal Fluid 1138
Pathologic States of the Nervous System Occurring During Pregnancy and
  the Puerperium 1143
Neurological Syndromes 1146
Neurosyphilis 1148
  General Paresis . . . . : . 1150
  Tabes Dorsalis 1154
The Spinal Cord 1158
  Compression of the Spinal Cord 1158
  Tumors of the Spinal Cord 1158
  Tumors of the Spine 1160
  Subdural Abscess of the Spinal Cord 1161
  Circumscribed Serous Meningitis 1162
  Tuberculous Spondylitis (Caries of the Spine, Pott's Disease) 1162
  Injuries to the Spinal Cord 1164
  Hematomyelia 1164
  Amyotrophic Lateral Sclerosis 1166
  Progressive Spinal Muscular Atrophy 1167

Combined Sclerosis Due to Pernicious Anemia (Postero-lateral Sclerosis) 1167
Syringomyelia 1169
Myelitis 1170
Hypertrophic Cervical Pachymeningitis 1172
Friedreich's Ataxia 1173
Disease of the Blood-vessels of the Spinal Cord 1174
Herpes Zoster (Zona or Shingles) 1174
Acute Anterior Poliomyelitis 1175
Multiple Sclerosis 1180
The Brain 1183
Focal Signs Due to Localized Cerebral Lesions 1183
Aphasia 1186
Disorders of Articulation 1188
Diseases of the Blood-vessels of the Brain 1189
Spontaneous Subarachnoid Hemorrhage 1194
Sinus Thrombosis 1195
Cerebral Aneurysm 1196
Brain Tumors 1197
Injuries of the Brain 1203
Disorders of the Central Nervous System Occurring at Birth 1207
Internal Hydrocephalus 1208
Infantile Hemiplegia 1210
Little's Disease 1210
Tay-Sachs' Disease 1210
Bulbar Palsy 1211
Pseudobulbar Palsy 1211
Myasthenia Gravis 1212
Paralysis Agitans 1213
Sydenham's Chorea 1216
Huntington's Chorea 1218
Progressive Lenticular Degeneration 1219
Epidemic Encephalitis 1220
Epilepsy 1224
Migraine 1234
The Peripheral Nervous System 1236
Neuritis 1236
Neuralgia 1247
Neurotic Progressive Muscular Atrophy 1249
Lesions of the Peripheral Nerves of the Extremities 1249
The Myopathies 1252

INTERNAL MEDICINE.

PART I.
INFECTIOUS DISEASES.

CHAPTER I.

THE BACILLARY DISEASES.

By HOBART A. REIMANN, M.D.

INTRODUCTION.
BACILLARY DISEASES.
  Typhoid Fever.
  Paratyphoid Bacillus Infections.
  Colon Bacillus Infections.
  Bacillary Dysentery.
  Undulant Fever.
  Leprosy.
  Tetanus.
  Tularemia.

BACILLARY DISEASES.—*Continued.*
  Plague.
  Anthrax.
  Influenza.
  Glanders.
  Cholera.
  Tuberculosis.[1]
  Diphtheria.
  Pertussis.

INTRODUCTION.

IT has been estimated that 50 per cent of the diseases with which we deal are caused primarily by the presence and growth of pathogenic microörganisms. This is a conservative estimate if the after effects of some primary infectious diseases as syphilis or rheumatic fever are considered, or if one includes the tropical fevers of infectious origin.

Before presenting a detailed description of infectious diseases there will be discussed briefly a few factors involved in the causation of these diseases; factors which influence the reaction of the host and others which apply to the invading organism. It is desirable to emphasize the intimate relationship existing between clinical medicine, bacteriology and immunology, and to realize that a rational view of infectious disease rests on a knowledge of underlying fundamental facts.

Many interrelated, complex factors are operative in the production of infectious disease. Four requisites may be listed and discussed: (1) a susceptible host; (2) virulent organisms; (3) a sufficient quantity of virulent organisms; (4) the means or the conditions operative to bring the invading organisms into contact with the host.

---

[1] Tuberculosis is presented in the section on Diseases of the Lungs, page 734; Diphtheria and Pertussis in The Contagious Diseases of Childhood, page 309.

1. **The Susceptible Host.**—The susceptible host is obviously important, for with absolute immunity infection does not occur. The human race, as a whole, appears to be relatively resistant to infection because of natural and acquired immunity which renders the invasion and growth of microörganisms difficult. Immunity, however, is relative and probably never absolute. It may be broken down by organisms of sufficient virulence or in sufficient quantities. Immunity varies greatly in different individuals, and in the same individual at different times. In every epidemic, no matter how severe, some individuals are more immune than others and escape infection. Similarly, under experimental conditions, all animals of a certain species are not equally susceptible to infection. *Natural immunity* may simply imply that the environment found in the host renders the existence of the invading organisms impossible and that the organisms cannot adapt themselves to the conditions and die out. *Acquired immunity* induced naturally or artificially is more or less specific in nature and involves physicochemical phenomena which are, for the most part, still obscure. The equilibrium established by the host in maintaining a healthy state by restricting the growth of microörganisms is indeed subtle and depends upon many factors of humoral and cellular immunity. For an adequate discussion of these factors, the student is referred to text-books on immunology.

Immunity or resistance to infection may be reduced by exposure to cold, by fatigue, trauma, shock, inanition, excesses of various sorts, and by various other conditions. It has been shown clinically and experimentally that individuals suffering from leukemia, kala-azar, influenza, diabetes and other chronic diseases have relatively less resistance and are more subject to infection than normal persons.

The rôle of allergic hypersensitivity in immunity is not well understood. It appears that hypersensitivity to bacterial substances or products may modify the reaction of the host to certain infections, particularly tuberculosis, rheumatic fever, lobar pneumonia and syphilis.

2. **Virulent Microörganisms.**—To be pathogenic, bacteria or viruses must possess what is called *virulence*. In one sense virulence implies the ability of a microörganism to overcome resistance, invade tissues, multiply and produce disease. Virulence under certain circumstances may merely imply that an organism finds suitable soil, so to speak, in which to grow. In another sense, virulence depends upon the potency of the poisonous substances elaborated by the invading bacteria. Of the myriads of bacteria which normally swarm in and on the human body, not all are virulent or pathogenic. Furthermore, certain pathogenic microörganisms are sometimes found living a harmless saprophytic existence in the body, as for example, type-specific pneumococci in the throat, or tetanus, typhoid and dysentery bacilli in the intestines. A healthy person harboring such organisms is a *carrier*. At any time, conditions may change, upset the equilibrium, and invasion and disease may follow. Pathogens may, at times, reside in tissues and still not cause disease, as is shown by the presence of the Welch bacillus or tetanus bacillus in otherwise symptomless ulcers. On the other hand, organisms ordinarily regarded as avirulent, like

the colon bacillus, may under certain conditions become invasive and cause disease.

Recent studies indicate the possibilities of symbiotic requirements for the development of certain diseases. Swine influenza appears to be due to a combination of a hemophilic bacillus and a filtrable virus. Experimental inoculations of bacilli alone or virus alone do not produce symptoms.

3. **Massive Infection.**—The third factor implies that the resistance of the host may be sufficient to cope with few virulent organisms whereas a massive infection may overcome immunity and cause disease. During the World War soldiers protected by vaccine rarely contracted typhoid fever. Typhoid fever occurred, however, in those who ingested grossly contaminated food or water containing great numbers of typhoid bacilli.

4. **Mode of Infection.**—Pathogenic microörganisms may be brought into contact with the host in many ways. The most important portals of entry are: (*a*) through the mouth and gastro-intestinal tract, as in typhoid fever or dysentery; (*b*) through the respiratory tract by the inhalation of the virus, as in measles, meningococcus meningitis or lobar pneumonia; (*c*) through the skin or exposed mucous membranes as in tularemia, undulant fever, gonorrhea or syphilis. Other infections are introduced by blood-sucking insects. As examples may be cited the rôle of fleas in regard to plague, ticks in rickettsial diseases, deer-flies in tularemia, mosquitoes in malaria and yellow fever, and the tsetse-fly in trypanosomiasis. Some infections like influenza may attack the host promptly after a single exposure; others like leprosy require prolonged contact before infection occurs. In certain diseases the clinical picture varies according to the portal of entry of the pathogens. When plague bacilli are introduced by insect bites, bubonic plague results; inhalation or droplet infection causes pneumonic plague. The portal of entry of certain diseases—kala-azar, poliomyelitis and others—is unknown.

Of increasing importance is the *relation of animal to human disease.* Heretofore, tuberculosis, smallpox, anthrax and glanders were chiefly considered in this regard. Recent studies have brought to light other infections which involve both man and animal. The infections may be transmitted directly to man, as in the case of undulant fever, streptococcus sore throat, tularemia, anthrax, glanders, psittacosis, rat-bite fever, or through an intermediary insect host, as in bubonic plague, typhus or spotted fever. Tularemia and plague may be transmitted both directly and indirectly.

In connection with the question of animal disease, human infestation due to higher forms of parasites such as the Trichina spiralis and tapeworm may also be considered. Food poisoning may be caused by the ingestion of uncooked meat derived from animals infected with bacilli of the colon-typhoid group.

The mode of action of pathogenic microörganisms in producing disease and the response of the host to infection are exceedingly complex and variable. Bacteria provoke disease in different ways. Certain forms exert their harmful effects by liberating extremely toxic, soluble substances called exotoxins (tetanus, botulinus and diphtheria bacilli). Certain toxins act by combining with vital nerve or muscle tissue or cause extensive capillary damage with hemorrhage. Others cause hemolysis or impair the hematopoietic centers. Some organisms like typhoid, dysentery and cholera bacilli give off poisons more slowly, after disintegrating (endotoxins). Anthrax bacilli, some believe, liberate no toxin, but cause death by overwhelming numbers in the circulation. Organisms like the tubercle or leprosy bacillus or the spirochetes of syphilis are able to grow and to produce extensive tissue changes over long periods of time.

Various organisms are *selective of their localization* in the body: meningococci usually select the meninges; pneumococci, the lungs; typhoid, dysentery and cholera bacilli, the intestines; Brucella melitensis, the genitalia of cattle; plague and tularemia bacilli, the lymphoid tissue; rickettsia and leishmania, the endothelium; rabies and encephalitis, the nervous tissue. In other words, living viruses adapt themselves, grow and multiply in environments apparently best fitted to support their existence.

The response of the host and the mechanism of recovery from infectious disease are, for the most part, obscure. In general, infections provoke or are accompanied by a rise in body temperature caused by disturbance of the heat-regulating mechanism in some unknown manner. The disturbance may be due to: (*a*) products of the growth of the invading bacteria; (*b*) the liberation of noxious substances from tissues damaged by infection or from disintegrating bacteria, or (*c*) a combination of factors. It has been suggested that fever is due to anaphylaxis, and that the incubation period represents the time required for sensitization to take place. Whatever the cause, the body temperature increases several degrees due to a derangement of the heat-regulating center supposedly in the region of the thalamus which regulates the dissipation of heat by controlling the peripheral vascular bed and sweat glands. Fever causes, or is associated with, an increase in the metabolism, sometimes to 30 or 40 per cent over the normal rate. It has been shown that more than 250 grams of body tissue may be consumed per day during high fever. Considerable body weight is lost unless a suitable diet is arranged. Weight loss is further augmented by diminished food intake due to anorexia, by profuse sweating, vomiting and diarrhea. Fever is accompanied by a change in the albumin-globulin ratio of the blood plasma. The fibrinogen and globulin fractions are increased relatively and absolutely. In lobar pneumonia, for example, the albumin-globulin ratio begins to change promptly after the onset and, in some cases, months elapse before normal equilibrium is regained. The change in the plasma proteins is paralleled by a decrease in the suspension stability of the blood, the significance of which is not yet clear. Malaise and various aches and pains often occur during fever. Albuminuria and febrile nephrosis commonly occur. The excretion of nitrogen in the urine is often increased during fever due to infection, while the elimination of inorganic compounds, particularly of chlorides, is diminished. In certain diseases a marked water retention occurs. The sugar-tolerance test during fever often shows a diabetic type of curve in normal individuals. In diabetics the sugar tolerance is actually depressed. Fever due to infection usually causes a temporary diminution in the number of blood platelets. The leukocytes are probably influenced by other factors in addition to fever; they are usually increased in number, but may remain unchanged as in typhus fever or may be diminished as in influenza, typhoid fever and kala-azar. There is frequently a transitory achlorhydria during fever. Tachycardia and tachypnea are present. It is doubtful whether acidosis ever occurs to such a degree that the hydrogen-ion concentration of the blood is actually changed. In some infections, lobar pneumonia for example, there is a tendency toward alkalosis. Fever in itself, unless high or prolonged, is not harmful. It is looked upon as an important factor in the defense mechanism of the host. Numerous studies indicate that high fever temperatures ($40°$ C.+) are unfavorable to the growth of bacteria and diminish the potency of toxins. Fever is associated with certain physico-chemical changes in the blood which favor agglutination of bacteria.

Various infections provoke different types of temperature reaction, known as *continued*, when the temperature at fever level does not vary more than $1°$ C. over a period of a few days, as in typhoid fever; *remittent*, when the daily variations exceed $1°$ C., as in a certain form of undulant fever; *intermittent* when periods of normal temperature alternate with bouts of fever, as in malaria or relapsing fever. Fever may rise abruptly to a high level and disappear just as abruptly as in malaria or sepsis or may last for days before declining abruptly (crisis) as in lobar pneumonia and typhus fever. It may, on the other hand, appear very gradually and diminish slowly (lysis) as in undulant fever or typhoid fever.

It is generally accepted that mouth temperature of $37°$ C. ($98.6°$ F.) is normal. Rectal temperature is $0.4°$ C. higher. Various influences may cause slight variations. Shock, collapse or hemorrhage may depress the level; exercise, menstruation, dehydration or an overheated environment may cause elevation.

The response of the host in regard to the elaboration of specific immunity is complex and is discussed at length in text-books on immunology. The subtle changes which develop in the host to render pathogens innocuous are obscure. It is not known whether organisms are killed directly by bactericidal or virucidal substances, by enzymes, by phagocytes or whether they simply die off for want of favorable growth conditions. According to some observers, agglutination is of especial importance in the successful disposal of bacteria. In tetanus and diphtheria the neutralization of toxin appears to be the decisive factor. Recovery from infectious disease in most cases does not appear to be due to loss of virulence or to a change in the causative organisms. In lobar pneumonia, for instance, virulent and apparently unchanged pneumococci may be found in the lung and in the blood stream before, during and after the crisis. Similar observations have been made in rickettsial diseases. In many diseases recovery appears to be due to changes in the host, not in the bacteria. The eventual outcome in regard to the life or health of the host depends upon the ability to

2

overcome the invaders by killing them directly, by neutralizing their harmful products, or by rendering the environment unsuitable for their existence.

The rôle played by hypersensitivity in the defense mechanism is not clear. In some diseases, particularly in tuberculosis and rheumatic fever, the response to infection is influenced by a hypersensitive state of tissues. It has also been shown experimentally that hypersensitive and normal tissues behave differently when subjected to infection. Hypersensitive tissue responds promptly with a marked inflammatory "exudative" reaction accompanied by an outpouring of fluid and cells into the tissues or into serous cavities. Non-hypersensitive tissue usually responds in a slower and less explosive manner. In the latter case the response has been termed "proliferative" and consists predominantly of the formation or aggregation of cells at the site of invasion.

Many new facts discovered in the field of immunology and bacteriology have necessitated radical changes in the rigid system and nomenclature developed by Ehrlich, and have opened the way for further progress. Research has been especially fruitful as a result of the application of physics and chemistry, particularly of colloid chemistry, to immunologic problems.

Much progress has been made recently in regard to diseases caused by filter-passing and invisible viruses, for example, the common cold, psittacosis, yellow fever and herpes, and in diseases caused by fungi. Researches on the obscure etiology of maladies like acute anterior poliomyelitis, epidemic encephalitis, influenza and Hodgkin's disease are in progress at present. Of particular interest are the new developments in bacteriology dealing with life cycles of bacteria, especially in regard to filterable stages in the life cycles of various known bacteria, like Mycobacterium tuberculosis. Suggestions made from time to time hint at a relationship of filterable forms of bacteria to Hodgkin's disease, measles, influenza and poliomyelitis. Proofs for such hypotheses are problems for the present and future.

Diagnosis.—Infectious disease was at one time classified largely by the character of the fever curve. Progress was made in differentiating diseases by Laennec's pioneer work in developing physical diagnosis, and a great advance in diagnostic methods occurred after the development of cellular pathology. Descriptive terms such as bronchitis, bronchopneumonia or lobular pneumonia gradually came into use. Anatomic diagnoses of this nature served their purpose until the Pasteur era. With the discovery of the constant association of bacteria of fixed and definite characteristics with disease in man, etiologic diagnosis became possible. At first it appeared as if simplification had been reached, that infectious diseases, for instance typhoid fever, could be considered as units. But further knowledge has split up supposed units into composites; typhoid must be differentiated from paratyphoid fevers, lobar pneumonia must be classified as Type I, II or III. Different varieties of typhus fever and dysentery exist. Nevertheless, even though complicated, it is chiefly by methods of positive etiologic diagnosis that progress in the prevention or treatment of disease is made. Consider for a moment the rational control and the diminution of typhoid fever and diphtheria since the identification of the respective causative bacilli. Contrast this with the lack of progress made in the treatment of respiratory infections, encephalitis and poliomyelitis, the etiology of which has only recently been sought. As a result of etiologic diagnostic methods, diseases heretofore unrecognized have been discovered—Rocky Mountain spotted fever, tularemia and undulant fever. Many of the new diagnostic methods involve the use of experimental animals, and are essentially laboratory problems, thus increasing the importance of the laboratory to clinical medicine.

Prophylaxis.—In general, preventive measures have been more efficacious than specific treatment in the control of infectious disease. It is safe to prophesy that many diseases will be reduced to unimportance by preventive measures long before specific therapy for them is developed. Typhoid fever, cholera and yellow fever have been greatly reduced by preventive measures, yet no advances have been made in their specific treatment.

Prophylaxis may be divided into several phases. The first concern is in regard to the patient himself, that is, the source of infection. Every effort should be made to destroy the causative organisms as they leave the host in secretions, excretions or otherwise. If this procedure could be made absolute, many infectious diseases would disappear. The second concern is to control the agencies whereby infections are transmitted from person to person. This is an enormous field to cover and includes the prevention of contamination or the sterilization of food, drink, air and the detection, control and elimination of human, animal and insect carriers of infection. The third problem is the protection of healthy individuals who become exposed to infection. This resolves itself into several endeavors: (*a*) avoiding contact with the source of infection or with carriers; (*b*) maintaining health and resistance by proper diet, exercise and rest, and (*c*) stimulating specific immunity by the use of vaccines or sera. Vaccines and toxins are administered for the purpose of stimulating the specific defense mechanism of the body (active immunity); immune and antitoxic serum is given because it already contains the desired antibodies (passive immunity).

Vaccines have proved of great value in the prevention of typhoid fever, rabies and smallpox; less effective for anthrax, cholera and plague. Antitoxic sera are valuable in preventing tetanus and diphtheria. The value of prophylactic vaccines for pneumonia, gonorrhea, tuberculosis and other conditions is still uncertain, and their use has not passed the experimental stage.

Treatment.—Considering the enormous amount of research, progress in the *specific treatment* of infectious disease has been relatively meager. The greatest success has been achieved in the *specific serotherapy* of a few diseases caused by toxin-forming bacteria by the injection of specific antitoxins, as in diphtheria. In other diseases like Type I lobar pneumonia, the mechanism of the beneficial effect resulting from serotherapy is unknown. Beneficial results are also obtained in the specific treatment of scarlet fever, erysipelas, anthrax, plague, cholera, dysentery and meningococcus meningitis, but only if specific immune serum is given in large doses early in the disease.

Vaccines have not proved of value in the treatment of any infectious disease, although studies are at present in progress regarding their use in the treatment of rheumatic fever, chronic arthritis, undulant fever and other infections. Investigation of the therapeutic value of *bacteriophages* has not as yet led to any conclusive results.

Chemotherapy of bacterial diseases has been disappointing. The value of various dyes and other medicaments given intravenously has not been proved. Certain advances have been made since the time of Ehrlich in the chemotherapy of infectious disease, but only in those caused by organisms biologically higher than bacteria. Arsenic preparations are specific for certain spirochetal diseases, antimony salts for leishmaniasis, and emetine for amebiasis. The value of chaulmoogra oil for leprosy is questioned by some. A new field for research has recently been opened by the demonstration of the specific effect of an enzyme on Type III pneumococci.

Our present method of treating many infectious diseases must rest on purely empirical grounds until the etiology of each disease in question is discovered and specific therapy is developed. At present the most that can be done in many cases is to place the patient in the most favorable circumstance for spontaneous recovery by building up or supporting his own defense mechanism. We can attempt to make the patient comfortable, to regulate diet and elimination, to prevent complications and, to a large extent, prevent the spread of infection to others.

Effect of Infectious Disease on Other Conditions.—It is well known that individuals suffering from senility, debility or chronic illness are more susceptible to infection than normal persons. Infections in such cases often end fatally. During diabetes, infections lower the sugar tolerance and insulin dosage must frequently be increased. In pernicious anemia, infection often depresses the red count further and lowers the efficacy of liver therapy. Tuberculosis is adversely affected by superimposed infections. Infection not related to the primary cause of chronic nephritis often causes an increased output of albumin which may return to the previous level without evidence of further change, but it often aggravates the kidney damage.

On the other hand, several examples may be cited to show the beneficial effect of infection or fever in certain conditions. Transient infections may stimulate the formation of red cells in certain cases of anemia. Paretics are often markedly improved by infection and fever resulting from malaria or rat-bite fever. Corneal ulcers respond favorably to fever therapy. Artificial fever produced by diathermy or foreign protein injection is widely employed in the treatment of arthritis and other conditions. Numerous other observations have been made on the apparent beneficial effect of acute infection on chronic disease. Several cases of nephrosis have been reported cured after an attack of some intercurrent infection.

Epidemiology. There are at present two main views regarding the mode of origin and spread of infectious or contagious disease. One view assumes that organisms lie dormant in an avirulent state in many individuals. Under certain conditions involving a reduction of resistance in the host, these organisms are enabled to acquire virulence and multiply. As the organism is passed from person to person, virulence gradually increases, step by step, until it reaches a point where it is able to invade individuals ordinarily resistant, and an epidemic results. The decline of an epidemic is explained by a similar step-like loss of virulence, as susceptible hosts become fewer and fewer.

There are certain facts indicating that augmentation of virulence alone cannot account for epidemics. It is well known from laboratory experience that the virulence of certain organisms can be increased to its maximum by only one or two animal passages, and cannot be further increased. One strain of avirulent pneumococcus in my experience was passed through 105 mice without augmentation of virulence. Similarly, strains of typhus and of spotted fever virus showed no change of virulence after passage through many guinea-pigs. Similar results are reported for Pasteurella tularensis and the virus of yellow fever.

The second view tends to minimize the importance of increase of virulence as a cause of epidemics and stresses changes in susceptibility of the population instead. It is assumed that virulence, when once established, fluctuates very little, if at all. Epidemics may originate from a single patient or from a carrier, who constitute the chief source of infection. Virulent organisms from these sources invade a susceptible individual, multiply, cause disease and become disseminated in *large numbers*. From these foci the organism spreads to others and, if virulent enough, and if the population is generally susceptible, large epidemics or pandemics occur.

It is probably safest not to generalize, but to consider each epidemic disease separately. There are, no doubt, some in which the virulence of the causative organisms is increased to a certain degree by passage, but after the maximal virulence is attained the dissemination of disease depends more upon host susceptibility than on fluctuations of virulence. In most cases a combination of these, and probably of many other factors (climate, war, famine, occupation), plays a rôle. The important point to bear in mind is that the source of most infection is to be found in the sick human being or animal or in healthy carriers.

Certain diseases, like influenza and pneumonic plague, become pandemic at long intervals and involve enormous numbers of people. Other diseases have a seasonal epidemicity, like lobar pneumonia, measles and typhoid fever, depending upon conditions favorable for transmission or reduction of host resistance by cold or by other mild infections. Still others assume epidemic proportions only under artificial conditions—tetanus after battles, tularemia during the hunting season and anthrax after unloading a cargo of infected hides. The last mentioned diseases further emphasize the importance of the transmission of virus and host susceptibility rather than changes in virulence.

Relative Incidence of Infectious Diseases.—The statistics gathered by the United States Public Health Service are the most comprehensive ones available for the United States. They are admittedly only approximate, since many infectious diseases are not reported, state laws in regard to the registration of infectious diseases vary, and diagnoses are often erroneous or concealed. Statistics from the United States army are, no doubt, more reliable because of better controlled conditions and uniformity in maintaining records.

A striking feature of the statistics covering a period of thirty years is the changing incidence of various diseases. Most noteworthy is the great reduction of typhoid fever, dysentery and tuberculosis—all diseases of established etiology and with definite measures for prophylaxis or therapy. Little or no change in the incidence of pneumonia has occurred. Typhus, Rocky Mountain spotted fever, tularemia and undulant fever are being recognized more and more frequently, which probably alone accounts for the apparent increase in the number of cases of these diseases. The reported incidence of certain diseases, for example influenza and measles, varies greatly from year to year. Others, like malaria, pneumonia or syphilis are fairly constant. According to the 1932 report of the United States Public Health Service, influenza topped the list with 569,000 cases; measles, 403,000; syphilis, 251,000; chicken-pox, 227,000; whooping cough, 214,000; scarlet fever, 210,000; mumps, 99,000; pneumonia, 92,000; tuberculosis, 77,000; malaria, 68,000; diphtheria, 59,000; small-pox, 11,000. Of special significance is the diminution of tuberculosis until the total is less than the reported number of cases of pneumonia. Twenty-six thousand cases of typhoid fever are reported, a number inexcusably high.

Statistics from the United States army show that during the recent years typhoid fever, diarrhea and dysentery caused less than 600 cases among 100,000 men per year as compared with 85,000 cases a century ago. Little decline has occurred in the prevalence of respiratory infections. During 1930, automobile accidents caused more deaths than infectious disease among the personnel.

The following tabulation is a report of the death-rate per 100,000 on an annual basis (1929) of the combined experience of 7 legal reserve life insurance companies.

Organic heart disease	140	Puerperal state	11
Pneumonia and respiratory infections	100	Meningitis	10
		Suicide	9
Tuberculosis	79	Diphtheria	7
Nephritis	72	Homicide	5
Cancer	72	Whooping cough	5
Accidents	60	Measles	2
Cerebral hemorrhage	48	Scarlet fever	2
Influenza	39	Typhoid fever	2
Diarrhea, enteritis	18	Other causes	191

It is not too rash to predict a reduction in the death-rate from pneumonia if the increased interest in the etiologic diagnosis is followed by the development of specific prophylaxis and treatment of respiratory infections. Death from organic heart disease and nephritis may possibly be reduced by the prevention and rational treatment of acute rheumatic fever and streptococcal infections. Little or no improvement is to be anticipated for cancer or influenza until further progress is made regarding their cause or control.

THE TYPHOID-COLON-DYSENTERY GROUP.

TYPHOID FEVER.

Definition.—Typhoid fever is an acute general infection caused by Bacillus typhosus, characterized by a gradual onset, a continuous high fever, a rose colored eruption appearing in crops, leukopenia, slow pulse, tympanites, splenomegaly and stupor. Pathologically there are hyperplasia and ulceration of lymphoid tissue, especially of Peyer's patches; bacteriemia; proliferative and regressive changes in other organs and tissues.

History.—Typhoid fever has been recognized for about two hundred years, although highly suggestive descriptions appeared even earlier. Prost in 1804 demonstrated the association of intestinal lesions with the disease. In 1837 Gerhard first clearly differentiated typhoid from typhus fever. Since then, typhoid fever has been recognized as a distinct entity. Bacillus typhosus was first isolated and associated with the disease in 1880 by Eberth. Several other diseases have been confused with typhoid fever (tularemia, undulant fever, kala-azar). It was not until the etiologic agent of each disease was discovered that differentiation was possible. Typhoid fever was once a disease of great importance, involving vast numbers in epidemic outbursts. It is now relatively uncommon and even rare in many localities.

Wright and Pfeiffer are credited with the first practical application of antityphoid vaccine.

Etiology.—Bacillus typhosus (Eberthella typhi) is a short, actively motile, non-spore-forming, Gram-negative bacillus. It grows aërobically on ordinary media. It is differentiated from colon bacilli by its inability to ferment lactose, and from paratyphoid bacilli by failure to produce gas from dextrose. Final differentiation is based on specific agglutination. It is killed by temperatures over 56° C., by prolonged drying or by exposure to sunlight. Under certain conditions, in ice, soil, and in excreta, it may live for months. Bacillus typhosus produces an endotoxin, but there is also evidence of the formation of an exotoxin.

Pathogenesis.—In the vast majority of cases, typhoid bacilli enter through the mouth. In resistant individuals the bacilli pass through the intestinal tract and are killed or excreted without invading the tissues. In susceptible individuals the bacilli invade the tissues and lymphatics of the small intestine and mesentery without any visible local lesion and are carried to the mesenteric lymph nodes. The mesenteric nodes become swollen before any visible change takes place in the intestinal mucosa. During this period of invasion, comprising the incubation period, which lasts from eight to fourteen days, there are often no symptoms. The actual onset dates from the time the bacilli break the barriers of immunity and are disseminated from the mesenteric lymph nodes. Bacilli from the mesenteric nodes are theoretically returned to Peyer's patches in the small intestine by reversal of the lymph flow and also enter the general circulation through the thoracic duct. This general distribution partly accounts for the numerous complications of the disease. The mesenteric lymph node—Peyer's patch complex constitutes the *primary focus*. From this focus bacilli are constantly fed to the lymphatics and blood stream. Fever continues until the focus disappears. In rare instances the primary focus may be found elsewhere in the body. *Relapses* are due to the reactivation of the primary focus or to lighting up of new foci. The symptoms of typhoid fever are largely due to tissue damage and to general intoxication resulting from the liberation of "typhotoxin." Local symptoms are due to the lodgment and growth of bacilli causing local toxic injury.

Distribution of Bacilli in the Body.—Bacilli are found in the blood in almost all cases, especially early in the disease. Bacilli appear in the feces later, as a result of ulceration of Peyer's patches or discharge from the biliary system. Bacilli are most numerous in the duodenum and jejunum. Very few are found from the cecum to the rectum, many having apparently died enroute. They have been isolated from practically every organ and tissue in the body and from areas of suppuration. Bacilli are excreted chiefly in the feces, urine and vomitus; less commonly in sputum, milk, seminal fluid and other secretions. Organisms usually disappear following recovery but may persist in excretions for long periods of time.

Epidemiology.—The typhoid fever patient and the healthy carrier of typhoid bacilli are the chief factors in the spread of the disease. The greatest progress in the reduction of the incidence of typhoid fever has been due to the proper isolation and treatment of these sources, the prevention of contamination of food and drink, and by prophylactic vaccination. It is noteworthy that although the incidence of the disease is vastly reduced, the case mortality-rate in the unvaccinated remains unchanged, indicating that no progress has been made in specific therapy.

As in other infections, not all individuals who are exposed to similar amounts of bacilli contract the disease. Some are naturally immune and some have become immunized by a previous attack or by vaccination. Immunity is only relative and it is probable that a massive dose of bacilli may break down resistance and infect all individuals.

Mode of Conveyance.—Water, ice, milk, food and flies are the chief factors of conveyance of bacilli from the source to the susceptible persons. Shellfish and oysters dredged from sewage-contaminated water are also dangerous. Dust is of lesser importance, especially if exposed to sunlight and prolonged drying. Direct contact with a patient or carrier may result in infection by way of finger to mouth, and in rare instances by other methods. The patient's bedding and clothing may be infectious for several days. "Flies, food and fingers" are all important conveyances.

Carriers are a special problem. At least 5 per cent of all recovered cases continue to excrete typhoid bacilli in feces or urine for long periods of time. Particularly dangerous are persons with mild infections who are able to remain at work, especially if they handle foodstuffs or beverages. Apparently normal individuals exist who harbor and excrete typhoid bacilli, although they have never had the disease. Various estimates indicate that from 4 to 32 per cent of typhoid fever cases can be traced to carriers. For a detailed description of methods to detect and treat carriers, reference should be made to the studies of Gay and Browning.

Incidence.—The incidence of typhoid fever in 1900 was 6 per 1000; in 1929, 0.2 per 1000. The mortality-rate from typhoid fever in 1900 in the United States was 0.57 per 1000; in 1909, 0.31 per 1000 and in 1916, 0.16 per 1000. The diminution between 1900 and 1909 is due to general improvement of sanitation. The use of prophylactic vaccination caused the accelerated diminution after 1909. The effect of vaccination is strikingly shown by United States army statistics. Between 1909 and 1912 when compulsory vaccination was begun, the mortality-rate dropped abruptly from 0.25 to 0.03 per 1000. During the Spanish American War the mortality from typhoid fever was 15 per 1000; in the World War, 0.05 per 1000.

The statistical incidence of typhoid fever has also been reduced by the discovery and recognition of other similar diseases which, no doubt, were often erroneously diagnosed as typhoid fever. Among these are undulant fever and tularemia. In certain localities undulant fever is, at present, of greater importance than typhoid fever.

Typhoid fever is a seasonal disease. The peak of incidence occurs in autumn, the minimum number in early summer. A secondary peak sometimes occurs in winter. Age, sex and race have but little influence on the incidence. Typhoid fever was more prevalent in the south Atlantic and Gulf coast states than elsewhere in the United States in recent years.

Pathology.—Specific proliferative and non-specific exudative and regressive reactions occur. The *specific lesions* consist of submiliary granulomata or lymphomata. They are composed chiefly of hyperplastic endothelial cells in the lymph nodules (Mallory) and are caused by the presence of typhoid bacilli and liberated toxins. The lesions are found best and most typically in the liver, spleen and lymph nodes, but are widespread in other tissues. When the granulomata are ill-defined or confluent the general tissue reaction is considered specific (Christeller). Not all observers admit the specificity of the lesions.

The *non-specific lesions* are exudative, regressive or degenerative and are the late stages of the specific changes.

The striking pathologic characteristic of typhoid fever is found in the small intestines. There is an inflammatory enlargement of the solitary lymph nodes and Peyer's patches. The lymphoid tissue proliferates and projects above the level of the surrounding membrane. In mild cases the process ceases at this stage, when regressive changes and recovery occur. If the disease progresses the process continues, and necrosis begins in the lymphoid tissue as a result of obstruction of blood-vessels by pressure of the newly-formed cells or by plugging of the blood-vessels. Long occluding thrombi are formed by proliferation of the endothelium in the lymph vessels and veins. Necrosis commences about the beginning of the *second week*. Erosion of blood-vessels with subsequent hemorrhage may occur at this time. Ulceration of the lymphoid tissue may extend outward and penetrate the muscular coat. Perforation of the intestinal wall and discharge into the peritoneal cavity may occur. As necrosis proceeds the nodes soften, break down and discharge into the lumen of the intestine, the base forming an ulcer. The ulcers may remain discrete or may increase in size until the entire intestinal wall is a mass of slough. The ulcers are found chiefly in the ileocecal region, seldom in the colon. They extend the long way of the bowel.

About the beginning of the *third week* the ulcers become covered with granulation tissue, the edges flatten out and the continuity of the epithelium is gradually restored. When ulceration has been extensive the floor of the ulcer is converted into a scar containing no glandular tissue. The mesenteric lymph nodes are congested and enlarged, often to walnut size. Occasionally suppuration of the nodes leads to rupture and discharge into the peritoneal cavity.

The liver is frequently large, flabby and in the state of parenchymatous degeneration. Specific nodules are commonly found in it. The spleen is nearly always enlarged throughout the illness. It is congested, hyperplastic and firm. When its maximum size is reached it becomes softer. Acute cholecystitis is occasionally noted. Ulceration of the bile ducts may occur. The kidneys may show cloudy swelling or specific acute inflammation. There is often a toxic, parenchymatous or fatty degeneration of the tubules and occasionally a mild glomerulonephritis. There may be a catarrhal cystitis. Orchitis and epididymitis may develop as sequelæ.

The myocardium may be the seat of fatty, hyaline or albuminous degeneration. Changes in blood-vessels similar to those in other acute infections occur, especially in the coronary arteries. Catarrhal inflammation of the large bronchi is common. Pneumonia may occur and may be caused by Bacillus typhosus, but usually by the organisms commonly found in the respiratory tract. Bacillus typhosus has been found in pus in empyema. Ulceration of the larynx is common. It is probably due to involvement of the local lymphoid tissue. Necrosis or abscess formation may result, causing lung abscess or gangrene. Meningitis and brain abscess occur. Suppurative inflammation may occur in almost any part of the body. Post-typhoid bone complications are relatively common. Zenker's degeneration of muscle tissue and deep abscesses may occur. Thrombophlebitis of the leg veins is frequent. In children, involvement of Peyer's patches is less common and less severe, accounting for the infrequency of perforation. The chief focus of infection in children is often in the mesenteric lymph nodes.

Congenital typhoid fever is transmitted from the mother to the fetus through the placenta.

Varieties.—All gradations of severity occur. Ambulatory cases may never be obliged to go to bed. Mild cases are confined to bed for a few days or a week; moderately severe cases for several weeks, and severe or protracted cases longer, running into months. In certain severe forms, patients at times continue to be ambulatory. Such cases, called "walking typhoid," are often fatal. Europeans often use the undesirable terms nephrotyphoid, pneumotyphoid, meningotyphoid, to designate typhoid fever characterized by certain predominant symptoms.

Typhoid fever in vaccinated individuals is a problem of increasing importance. As stated previously, immunity is only relative. A massive dose of ingested bacilli can break down artificial immunity established by vaccination, or some unrelated condition may temporarily diminish resistance to small doses. Other possibilities to account for infection in the vaccinated are: (*a*) the use of improperly prepared vaccine, (*b*) insufficient dosage of vaccine, (*c*) infection with strains other than those represented in the vaccine, and (*d*) gradual diminution of immunity after vaccination. There are, it appears, individuals in whom even a potent vaccine fails to stimulate immunity.

An unusual opportunity for the observation of typhoid fever in vaccinated soldiers presented itself during the World War. The clinical course of 270 cases did not vary from that in unprotected individuals. The average duration was twenty-seven days. Relapse occurred in 10 per cent and death in 11 per cent of cases. According to other observers, and in a few cases seen by the writer, the attacks of typhoid fever in the vaccinated were mild, often without fever or with a low, brief fever. Bronchitis is common.

Roseola and the diazo reaction are present in 20 per cent of cases. Complications are rare. Diagnosis is usually difficult because of the mildness of symptoms and of the difficulty in isolating bacilli from the blood in most cases (Schottmüller). Moreover, typhoid fever is not expected in vaccinated individuals. The mortality is less than 1 per cent.

Typhoid fever *in infants* is difficult to diagnose and probably occurs more frequently than is believed. The course in infants and children is even more variable than in adults. Clinical evidence may be lacking except for indications of a general blood infection. There may be no intestinal lesions. Nervous symptoms are usually dominant. The prognosis is grave. Among 22 congenital cases only 3 recovered. Among 105 cases in the first year of life, 28 recovered and 77 died (Weech). Blood culture offers the best method of diagnosis. The Widal reaction may not appear.

Paratyphoid Fever.—It has been customary to separate typhoid and paratyphoid fever into separate chapters. From a clinical viewpoint there is no more reason for this than to devote separate chapters to each type of pneumococcus pneumonia. It is sufficient in both cases to regard the infections as similar clinically, but as separate specific entities as regards prognosis, specific prophylaxis or therapy.

Infection due to Bacillus paratyphosus A (Salmonella typhi) and Bacillus paratyphosus B (Salmonella Schottmülleri), gained recognition and prominence during the World War. Many troops were vaccinated against Bacillus typhosus alone. Consequently, many cases of infection with Bacillus paratyphosus arose. In the American army the use of "triple typhoid" vaccine (typhoid, paratyphoid A and B) prevented these infections.

Clinically, typhoid and paratyphoid fever are often indistinguishable, although certain characteristics of paratyphoid fever may be mentioned. The incubation period is often shorter than that of typhoid fever, and the onset may be more abrupt, with a chill, abdominal pain and vomiting. The course is usually milder, with fewer complications and a lower mortality-rate. The temperature curve is more apt to approach the remittent type. Herpes is said to occur in from 5 to 10 per cent of cases. The rash may be morbilliform. Otherwise, in severe cases, the clinical picture is the same. The only certain method of differ-entiation is the isolation and identification of the causative organism. The demonstration of specific immune bodies in the blood alone is not reliable for differential diagnosis. The average mortality is low, varying from 1 to 8 per cent.

Symptoms.—Few acute infections exhibit such great variations in clinical course, symptoms and signs as typhoid fever. For convenience in discussion the course of the disease is arbitrarily separated into first, second, third and fourth weeks, corresponding roughly to the changes occurring in the intestine. During the first week there is invasion and swelling of the lymphoid tissue, in the second and third weeks necrosis and ulceration and in the fourth, healing. (Fig. 1.)

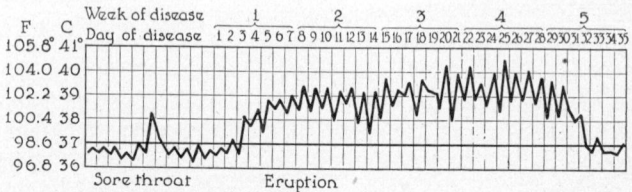

F_IG. 1.—Temperature curve of a typical case of typhoid fever observed from the begin-ning of illness (Jochmann-Hegler). Patient was a girl, aged eighteen years. Prodrome of sore throat. Severe epistaxis on third day of illness. Rose spots appeared on the eighth day and bacteriemia on the tenth.

For several days, in the beginning, the patient is aware of slight headache, a disinclination for work, malaise, vague aching pains, anorexia or restlessness. Sore throat and cough are occasionally present. These *prodromal symptoms* may be absent. The actual *onset*, subsequent to the dissemination of bacilli throughout the body, is sometimes difficult to date, but may be heralded by a chill or chilly sensations. There is almost always dull headache, anorexia and aching. Bronchitis is present in about 25 per cent of cases. Patients are often able to remain at work for several days until obliged to go to bed by the increasing severity of symptoms. Fever and prostra-tion increase proportionately. The pulse-rate is slow.

About the end of the *first week* the symptoms are well marked. The expression is dull and apathetic, the face is flushed, the eyes glassy and the skin hot and dry. Fever is high, the pulse slow, soft and dicrotic. There is severe headache, dizziness and prostration. The tongue is heavily coated, white or brownish, the tip and edges are reddened. The mouth becomes drier and sordes appear on the gums and lips in cases not properly cleansed. Nosebleed occurs in from 5 to 20 per cent of cases. Sweating is uncommon. Marked bronchitis at times obscures the diagnosis. Constipation is common. Diarrhea occurs at some time during the disease in less than one-third of all cases. Rose spots and splenic enlargement often appear about this time.

During the *second week* the fastigium is reached. Increasing stupor causes the patient to complain less. It is often difficult to establish contact. Responses to questions are sluggish or distorted. The eyes are half closed. Delirium is often present at this period, especially at night when attempts may be made to get out of bed. Restraint may be necessary to prevent serious accidents. The flushed face becomes slightly cyanotic. The lips and tongue are dry and the voice hoarse. The pulse is full, regular, slow and dicrotic. The blood pressure is diminished. A careful daily registration of blood pressure is important, since hemorrhage or perforation are often detected by abrupt changes in the pressure. Signs of bronchitis increase. The abdomen generally becomes more distended or tympanitic. The spleen is soft and definitely palpable. Urine and feces often are voided involuntarily. At the height of fever there may be complete stupor or muttering delirium with twitching of the muscles. Coöperation is poor, rendering feeding necessary. Serious complications are most apt to occur during the second and third weeks. In severe cases death results from toxemia, circulatory failure, exhaustion or from complications.

During the *third* or *fourth week* recovery commences. (Fig. 1.) The temperature curve shows increasing remissions. A decline of each successive peak becomes evident. The pulse becomes smaller and dicrotism disappears. Abnormal symptoms gradually disappear and convalescence begins.

In 8 to 11 per cent of patients *relapse* or *recrudescence* occurs after the temperature has been normal for a variable length of time. The term relapse implies a repetition of the disease with all its symptoms; a recrudescence implies only a short recurrence of fever. It is stated that relapses more frequently follow mild attacks of the disease. A relapse may be mild and brief, but may be more severe than the original attack. Relapses frequently occur without any known cause or provocation and probably result from a reinvasion of bacilli. There may be several relapses. Intestinal lesions are less marked; hemorrhage and perforation occur less often than in the primary attack.

Atypical Onset.—The symptoms and course may be so mild as to pass unrecognized. An abrupt onset may at first be confusing until other signs and symptoms appear. Onset with severe bronchitis, especially when accompanied by leukocytosis suggests pneumonia at first. Severe meningeal symptoms suggest meningitis. Occasionally, intense abdominal cramps, nausea, vomiting and tenderness are mistaken for some other acute abdominal accident. In the so-called "walking typhoid," hemorrhage from the bowel or perforation may be the first evidence of disease.

Special Symptoms.—The typical *fever* curve commences with a steplike rise, higher each succeeding day until the fastigium is reached in the second week. (Fig. 1.) It remains rather constant at a high level with slight daily remissions for another week or more, when gradually the remissions become more marked. There is then a tendency downward and each succeeding peak is slightly lower, until fever disappears. Less often the onset may be ushered in by an abrupt rise of fever. In certain cases the remissions may be extreme, describing the peaks of a "septic" type of curve. Recovery by lysis is the rule; crisis is rare. During the disease sudden changes in temperature frequently indicate complications. Hemorrhage often causes a sudden fall, and perforation either an abrupt rise or fall in temperature.

The persistence of fever indicates continued infection or the presence of some complication, sequela or a relapse. Severe chills may occur repeatedly in uncomplicated cases, but more often point to the onset of some complication.

Rose spots appear about the end of the first week, but may appear at any time thereafter. They are pale pink, slightly elevated, rounded spots, from 1 to 4 mm. in diameter. The color fades on pressure. They most often appear on the abdomen, chest or back; seldom on the limbs, neck or head. From 1 to 20 are frequently present at a time. A crop lasts from three to five days and disappears without leaving any trace. Other crops, characteristically, appear and disappear. Rose spots are caused by the lodgment of typhoid bacilli in lymph vessels of the skin. In severe cases the spots may become hemorrhagic.

Sudamina are common but herpes is rare. Temporary loss of hair sometimes occurs. Ridges appear in the nails. Sweating is uncommon unless caused by complications or medication.

Pulse.—The relative slowness of pulse-rate in relation to fever is one of the diagnostic features of typhoid fever. The pulse-rate may be 90 per minute while the temperature is 40° C. (104° F.). There are, of course, exceptions to the rule when the pulse-rate is rapid. Dicrotism is common. Bradycardia may persist into convalescence and probably signifies myocardial damage. Sudden increases of pulse-rate may indicate the onset of various complications. Electrocardiographic tracings often reveal a prolongation of the *P–R* interval.

Complications.—The general dissemination of the bacilli accounts for the frequency and multiplicity of complications which are characteristic of typhoid fever. Complications bear no relation to the severity of the disease. Many of the deaths in typhoid fever are due to complications.

Hemorrhage from the bowel occurs in from 5 to 8 per cent of cases and is a serious accident. The mortality is 25 per cent. It results from the erosion of blood-vessels in the ulcers, and may occur at any time after the second week, but most often in the third. The seriousness of the situation depends upon the amount of blood lost. As much as 2000 cc. may be lost. Repeated hemorrhages may occur. Occasionally, the first indication of bleeding is the passage of blood or a tarry stool. Warning symptoms are chilly sensations, pallor, coldness of the skin or a sensation of faintness. The pulse-rate increases and the temperature may dip downward. The blood pressure, erythrocyte count and hemoglobin percentage fall. Transient leukocytosis may occur. Pain is not present.

Perforation of the intestine at the site of ulceration is the most serious complication. It occurs in from 1 to 6 per cent of cases. It is commonest late in the second, in the third week or the fourth week when sloughing of the necrotic lymphoid tissue occurs. Perforation may occur during convalescence. Usually a single ulcer breaks through but multiple perforation may take place. The commonest site is in the lower ileum. Predisposing causes are gaseous distention of the intestines, hyperperistalsis, straining at stool or vomiting, or the passage of large, hard masses of feces.

The onset is sudden. It is characterized by sudden severe abdominal pain, often located in the right lower quadrant. Pain may be severe enough to arouse a patient from coma. Soon afterward, the signs and symptoms of acute general peritonitis develop. The abdomen becomes tense, tympanitic and distended. Nausea, vomiting or chills and rigors may occur. Muscle rigidity and a thready, rapid pulse follow. Free fluid may be demonstrable. Changes in the pulse-rate, temperature curve and leukocyte count are variable. They may be suddenly increased, diminished or unchanged. Any change should excite suspicion. In rare cases the onset of perforation is insidious with few early symptoms.

Perforation is often difficult to diagnose and may be simulated by acute cholecystitis, appendicitis, thrombosis of the iliac or mesenteric blood-vessels, rupture of a mesenteric lymph node, or even by acute pleuritis. Whenever suspicion of perforation arises, laparotomy should be performed promptly.

Perforation is almost always fatal and in certain reports accounts for about 11 per cent of deaths from typhoid fever. Of 23 cases of perforation in one series, 20 died and 3 that were operated upon recovered. The mortality of cases operated upon ranges from 30 to 80 per cent.

Cholecystitis occurs in about 2 per cent of cases. The onset may be gradual or sudden and is accompanied by the usual signs and symptoms of cholecystitis.

Typhoid fever is said to be a predisposing factor in the appearance of gall stones later in life and a cause of chronic cholecystitis.

Thrombosis of the veins may appear late in the disease and often during convalescence. It is probably due in part to local phlebitis and to an increase in the number of platelets. The symptoms and signs are frequently obscure and are overlooked, especially if the thrombus is situated in deeply located veins. Thrombosis occurs in about 2 per cent of cases. The femoral veins are most often involved. The onset is sometimes sudden with a chill, increase of fever and leukocytosis. There is pain or tenderness along the affected vein and, if superficially located, the involved vein can be felt as a cord. Edema of the area drained may follow.

Arterial thrombosis is rare and leads to gangrene in certain cases.

Parotitis, mastitis, thyroiditis, orchitis are less common as complications. The lesions may consist of typical typhoidal tissue infiltration or reactions with frank suppuration.

Myocarditis is unusual. It is manifested clinically by bradycardia, arrhythmia, signs of circulatory failure, lowered blood pressure, edema or cardiac dilatation. Pathologic changes can often be found in the smaller coronary arterioles with patchy focal degeneration in the myocardium.

Pneumonia is a serious complication. The frequency of bronchitis during typhoid fever predisposes to pneumonia. In rare instances the typhoid bacillus is the causative organism, but usually pneumococci, streptococci or a mixture of organisms are found. *Ulceration* of the larynx is seen quite commonly.

Febrile nephrosis is common. Mild glomerulonephritis is occasionally observed. Cystitis, pyelonephritis and pyelitis are not uncommon. *Rupture, abscess* and *infarct* of the spleen are rare. *Arthritis* is rare. *Osteitis, periostitis* and *osteomyelitis* are more often sequelæ. They may become manifest long after the disease is over. They are apt to become chronic and difficult to heal. The sites of predilection are in the clavicles, ribs and the long bones. The symptoms are tenderness, pain, swelling and redness. There is seldom much fever. "Typhoid spine," causing annoying backache, is an osteoarthritis of the vertebræ. Roentgen-ray examination is valuable in diagnosing bone involvement.

Complications of the *eye* and *ear* are uncommon. Deafness occurs occasionally. Otitis media occurs in 1 to 2 per cent of cases.

Nervous System.—Convulsions are rare. Multiple neuritis appears occasionally as a sequela. Local neuritis occurs during the illness and is characterized by intense pain with motor and sensory disturbances. Myelitis, meningitis and brain abscess are rare complications. Transient typhoid and post-typhoid psychoses occur in about 1 per cent of cases.

Clinical Pathology.—The *leukocytes* during the first few days are slightly increased in number. As the disease progresses they diminish until there are but 2000 to 4000 per c.mm. of blood. The number may increase following the appearance of certain complications. Lymphocytes frequently outnumber the neutrophil cells. The *erythrocytes*, as in other prolonged febrile diseases, are diminished, probably as a result of toxic influences on the bone-marrow and especially after hemorrhage. The hemoglobin diminishes accordingly. The *blood platelets* are diminished during the early febrile period and are increased over the normal level for a time during convalescence. The *globulins* are relatively increased and the sedimentation time of erythrocytes is diminished. The stools are variable. About 30 per cent are diarrheal. Occult blood is present in most cases. Gross blood is present when hemorrhage has occurred. The *urine* usually contains a trace of albumin and a few casts. *Bacilluria* is common. The *diazo reaction*, indicating severe illness with parenchymatous changes in various organs, is present.

The *Gruber-Widal reaction* refers to the presence of agglutinins in the patient's blood serum for known strains of Bacillus typhosus and paratyphosus A and B. Previous vaccination may account for the presence of agglutinins in low titer; it is important to bear in mind that other infectious processes can stimulate these agglutinins temporarily to a high titer. It is unfortunate for early diagnosis that during typhoid fever agglutinins seldom develop before the beginning of the second week. The reaction is absent in about 10 per cent of adult cases and in a higher percentage of infants. To be of clinical significance the titer should exceed 1 to 80. It sometimes reaches

1 to 20,000. The average ranges from 1 to 160, to 1 to 1280. The reaction may disappear within a few months after recovery, but often persists at a low titer for years.

Demonstrable *bacteriemia* is present in over 90 per cent of cases early in the disease and later in about 40 per cent. Stool cultures are positive for typhoid bacilli in 80 per cent of cases, especially after the third week.

Diagnosis.—The diagnosis of typhoid fever in well developed cases, or during epidemics, is comparatively easy. Early in the disease, in atypical or in mild cases when early diagnosis is so important, it is often impossible to differentiate typhoid fever clinically from certain other infections. Assistance must be sought in laboratory procedures. A clinical diagnosis is relatively certain in patients giving a history of drinking or eating contaminated material and in whom, after about two weeks' time, continuous and increasing malaise, headache, aching, prostration and bronchitis are noted. The steady, step-like rise of fever, a slow dicrotic pulse, together with the appearance of a palpable spleen, characteristic rose spots, intestinal hemorrhage and stupor should point to typhoid fever. Confirmatory evidence is furnished by the laboratory. Leukopenia and, later on, anemia are the rule. The isolation of bacilli of the typhoid group from the blood is the best early proof of diagnosis. Later, bacilli are recovered from the feces and urine or from various suppurating foci. The Gruber-Widal reaction appears in most cases after the first week. If a negative result is obtained at first, repeated trials should be made at three- or four-day intervals until agglutination appears. The diazo reaction in the urine is of importance to rule out other illness of less gravity than typhoid fever. Special methods are required to identify bacilli isolated from the blood, feces or urine.

Differential Diagnosis.—*Bacteriologic* and *immunologic* methods offer ultimate proof of diagnosis and differentiation from the diseases discussed below.

In mild *gastro-intestinal* upsets which occur under suspicious circumstances, the presence of leukocytosis, the absence of diazo reaction and the further course rules out typhoid fever. *Simple bronchitis* and *bronchopneumonia* are determined by a predominance and persistence of respiratory symptoms, a lower fever and leukocytosis. Because of the presence of leukopenia and of the severity of illness, *influenza* is less easy to differentiate. The presence of an epidemic of either disease is helpful in diagnosis. Influenza and typhoid may occur in the same patient. Cyanosis and the later course of the disease aid in diagnosis. *Meningitis* is ruled out by examining the spinal fluid. Specific typhoid meningitis may occur. Acute *appendicitis* and *cholecystitis* are accompanied by leukocytosis. The subsequent course is diagnostic. *Miliary tuberculosis* is indicated by a previous history of tuberculosis, hemoptysis or by a long period of failing health. The pulse-rate is rapid, cyanosis and dyspnea are present. Pulmonary râles and roentgen-ray evidence favor tuberculosis. Meningitic symptoms are common in tuberculosis. The diazo reaction is present in both conditions. *Subacute bacterial endocarditis* is differentiated by the recovery of strepto-

3

cocci from the blood, the development of heart murmurs, particularly if diastolic in time, the appearance of petechiæ, hematuria, embolic phenomena, leukocytosis and the absence of stupor. *Trinchinosis* is sometimes impossible to differentiate until the positive features of either disease become fully developed. In trichinosis there may be a history of eating undercooked meat, particularly pork or game. There is muscle tenderness, edema of the face, leukocytosis and especially eosinophilia. The demonstration of Trichina spiralis in the original supply of meat or in the muscle tissue of the patient proves a diagnosis. *Atypical malaria* may resemble typhoid fever except that the daily temperature variations are greater and the spleen larger. Diagnosis is established by the demonstration of plasmodia in the blood smear and by the response to quinine therapy. In *tularemia* there is often a history of handling wild rabbits or other game, and of an ulcer on the skin, except in the "typhoidal" type. Diagnosis is established by the demonstration of agglutinins for Bacillus tularensis in the blood or by the recovery of the organism from the blood or from the liver by cultural methods or by animal inoculation. *Undulant fever* is a prolonged fever, with occasional relapses, profuse sweating, joint pains and a remarkable feeling of well-being of the patient in spite of high fever. The demonstration of agglutinins for brucella in the blood stream or the recovery of the organism itself from the blood, feces or urine by cultural methods or by animal inoculation is diagnostic. A specific skin test for brucelliasis is used. *Typhus* and *Rocky Mountain spotted fever* have a more abrupt onset; there is often a history of louse, tick or flea bites. Slight leukocytosis may occur. Deafness, conjunctivitis and bronchitis are common. The spleen is less often palpable. The characteristic skin eruption, the presence of agglutinins for Bacillus proteus X 19 and the transmission of the virus to guinea-pigs are diagnostic factors. In typhus, biopsy of the skin lesions reveals specific diagnostic changes. *Kala-azar* is diagnosed by the presence of Leishman-Donovan bodies in the spleen or blood by means of smear or culture.

Prognosis.—The average duration of the febrile period in moderately severe and severe cases of typhoid fever is from three to five weeks. In mild cases it is less. In Curschmann's large series the duration of the febrile period was as follows:

Up to three weeks	57 per cent
Three to five weeks	31 per cent
More than five weeks	11 per cent

The febrile period may last for months in certain cases. The duration, measured from the onset of the disease to the end of convalescence, averaged fifty-five days.

The case mortality from typhoid fever thirty years ago averaged, according to different observers, from 14 to 20 per cent. The case mortality-rate in the United States in 1929, according to the statistics compiled by the Surgeon-General, is about 22 per cent. This figure is probably too high, since many mild cases are probably not reported. Statistics from the U. S. Army are better controlled and show a case mortality-rate of approximately 15 per cent. These figures show how little progress has been made in regard to therapy. It would seem that the death-rate should be lower since the more rational management of diet and of baths, but the figures do not show it. According to many observers, prophylactic vaccination in patients who later develop typhoid fever has a marked effect, reducing the mortality to about 1 per cent. Statistics from the U. S. Army show otherwise, revealing a mortality-rate of 11 per cent. The prognosis is grave in infants under one year, in the aged and in individuals with other chronic illness. The mortality-rate in children is about 6 per cent.

Toxemia and exhaustion are the chief causes of death; perforation is responsible for 11 to 15 per cent and hemorrhage for 10 per cent of the deaths from typhoid fever. Perforation is always fatal unless promptly repaired. Severe bacteriemia, hyperpyrexia, circulatory failure, meteorism, coma and the appearance of serious complications are ominous signs.

Prophylaxis.—*General Measures.*—The control of sources of infection is of prime importance. Patients and carriers should be strictly isolated. Mild cases should be promptly recognized. All excretions and secretions must be sterilized before disposal by mixing with suitable chemical disinfectants or by heat. Urine, vomitus, sputum and finely broken-up feces should be mixed with bichloride of mercury, 1 to 1000, with phenol preparations, 10 per cent formalin or 3 per cent bleaching powder and allowed to remain several hours before discarding. Sterilization by heat in special containers is satisfactory. All linen, clothing and utensils used by patients or carriers should be sterilized, preferably by steam in autoclaves or by soaking in antiseptics. The hands of attendants should be scrubbed with soap and 1 per cent cresol or immersed in a 1 to 1000 solution of bichloride of mercury after coming in contact with the patient or with materials contaminated by the patient.

Convalescents and carriers are dangerous as long as they excrete bacilli. Carriers must be prohibited from handling any kind of beverage or food, including ice.

Modern improvements in building and household comforts have greatly facilitated cleanliness and have eliminated depressing and unhygienic surroundings. Modern plumbing and sewage disposal have done much to reduce the incidence of typhoid fever. Care must be taken to insure an uncontaminated water supply. Uncertain water and food must be boiled before using. Milk is rendered safe by pasteurization, provided it is not contaminated thereafter. Flies should be eliminated by screens or by special chemical sprays. Oyster beds must be kept free from pollution. Sea foods should not be fished from polluted waters.

Personal Prophylaxis.—Water or food from uncertain sources should be avoided, unless first sterilized before ingestion. Bathing in polluted water is dangerous. It is wise for individuals exposed to typhoid fever to avoid fatigue and strain from overwork. Ample nutrition and rest are important to maintain resistance against infection. As little contact as possible should be made with the patient or with contaminated materials, and the hands should be washed after each exposure, especially before meals. Sterile gowns, masks and gloves are valuable measures when worn in the sick room.

Specific Immunization.—The use of antityphoid fever vaccine is based on the sound facts that specific immunity is conferred by an attack of the disease itself and by experiments in animals showing that the administration of a sublethal dose of typhoid bacilli protects against a subsequent massive inoculation. Until the existence of Bacillus paratyphosus A and B was discovered, vaccine was prepared with Bacillus typhosus alone. As a result, cases of paratyphoid fever occurred and until they were recognized as different specific infections, doubt was cast on the efficacy of the vaccine. After 1916, when paratyphoid organisms were added to the vaccine, paratyphoid fever also diminished. The desired results of prophylactic vaccination against typhoid fever are strikingly shown by statistics from the U. S. Army in Table 1.

TABLE 1.—DECREASE OF TYPHOID FEVER IN THE U. S. ARMY FOLLOWING THE INTRODUCTION OF VACCINATION.

		Cases per 100,000.
1901.	No vaccination	674
1905.	No vaccination	314
1909.	Voluntary vaccination	335
1911.	Partial compulsory vaccination	85
1913.	Compulsory vaccination	4

Between 1909 and 1912, when vaccination was introduced, the *mortality-rate* of typhoid fever in the army was reduced abruptly from 0.25 per 1000 to 0.03 per 1000. Similar though less striking improvement was noted in the civilian population, in which vaccination was not compulsory.

Method of Vaccination.—Although numerous variations exist, the most commonly used method which has given satisfactory results is as follows: vaccine is prepared so that each cubic centimeter of saline solution contains 1 billion killed typhoid bacilli and 750 million each of killed paratyphoid bacilli A and B. Injections are given subcutaneously in the deltoid region at seven- to ten-day intervals. The first dose is 0.5 cc.; the second and third, 1 cc. each. There is often transient soreness, redness and swelling at the site of injection and perhaps in the adjacent lymph nodes. Later, there is frequently slight fever, malaise, aching, anorexia and headache, which may last for a day after injection. More severe reactions are apt to occur when the vaccine has been accidentally introduced into a small vein. It is best to administer vaccine late in the day and to avoid undue fatigue for twenty-four hours thereafter. Adequate doses of aspirin, 0.6 gram (10 grains), or amidopyrine, 0.3 gram (5 grains), often lessen the unpleasant symptoms. Hypodermic injections of 0.5 cc. of adrenalin solution are used to control more severe reactions. Nothing can be done beforehand to avoid reactions, and reactions cannot be predicted. There is no rule. Some may be more severe than others or no after-effects at all may be noted.

Agglutinins appear in the blood after the second injection and reach their highest titer about two weeks after the third injection. The titer then diminishes rather rapidly at first and finally trails off very gradually. The titer may reach 1 to 20,000, but averages between 1 to 320 and 1 to 1280, and diminishes to 1 to 40, or 1 to 80. In some rare instances, agglutinins fail to appear at any time. Agglutinins at a low titer are sometimes demonstrable many months or years later. It is quite generally agreed that the presence of agglutinins does not guarantee the existence of immunity, but they are usually quite parallel and, at present, a measure of the agglutinin titer is the nearest artificial measure for immunity that we possess.

As stated previously, the immunity derived from vaccination is only relative and can be temporarily depressed by various agencies or can be broken down completely by massive infection. Vaccination should be repeated every three years, and oftener during epidemics or after undue exposure. As a general rule, it is wise for all healthy children and adults to be vaccinated, especially if contemplating a vacation trip to localities where the water or food supply is not controlled. Physicians, hospital attendants and laboratory workers especially should be immunized.

Vaccine, if given shortly before the onset of symptoms of typhoid fever, shortens the course of the disease; when given after the onset of symptoms it has no effect whatever. Recent studies have shown that vaccine given by mouth stimulates the production of agglutinins without any unpleasant reactions. The procedure is still in the experimental stage.

Contraindications to vaccination are the presence of other infections (tuberculosis) and chronic illness such as nephritis, hypertension or diabetes. The writer has vaccinated several diabetic and nephritic patients without harmful effect.

Treatment.—The treatment resolves itself into four main endeavors: (1) careful nursing, (2) proper nutrition, (3) prevention of the spread of infection to others, and (4) the detection and treatment of complications.

In spite of the vast amount of investigation nothing has as yet been discovered with which to combat typhoid fever specifically. Antityphoid vaccine given therapeutically is useless. Specific antiserum, antitoxin and convalescent serum have been thoroughly tried with but little or no success. Foreign protein shock therapy is not recommended, although a few reports indicate a decline of fever afterward. Too little is as yet known concerning bacteriophage for its use in therapy.

As soon as typhoid fever is suspected, the local health officers should be notified. The patient should be isolated and the attendants instructed in regard to hygienic measures, especially in the proper disposal of excreta, care of linen and utensils. Transfer to a hospital where proper facilities exist for such purposes is highly desirable. Close associates of the patient should be promptly vaccinated.

The patient's room should be light, airy and quiet. Window screens must be used to keep out flies. The mattress and pillows should be smooth and comfortable to avoid decubitus during a long illness. A rubber sheet is advisable to prevent soiling the mattress with excreta. The patient must be watched carefully at all times and gently restrained if necessary. Serious accidents and death have occurred during attempts to escape when delirious. The patient should be bathed regularly with tepid water and thoroughly dried. Alcohol rubs and dusting powders add to comfort.

Special attention is given to the mouth. Alkaline mouth washes or a 3 per cent solution of hydrogen peroxide, diluted with water, should be used once or twice daily. In uncoöperative patients a mouth swab may be used. The teeth and gums should be brushed twice daily. Cold cream or glycerin applied to the lips prevents drying and cracking. Oral hygiene is the best prophylaxis against serious stomatitis, parotitis, otitis media and even pneumonia.

Constipation is combated with small plain water or soap suds enemata. Liquid petrolatum, 15 cc. (½ ounce) by mouth, may be given. Mild laxatives are usually contraindicated, but may at times be used. Cathartics are dangerous and are apt to cause hemorrhage or perforation.

High temperature and delirium can often be reduced by tepid or cool sponging. As a rule, bathing should be continued only if agreeable to the patient or if objective symptoms are improved. Cold baths in tubs are exhausting and do more harm than good. Antipyretic drugs are no longer used.

Nutrition.—Plenty of water is allowed. In comatose patients salt solution should be given subcutaneously or intravenously. Since the metabolism during high fever is 30 to 40 per cent above that of normal individuals it is plain that in prolonged fever, emaciation rapidly results if the food intake is restricted. Many studies have shown that typhoid fever patients do well on liberal, well-selected, high caloric diets. A patient on a proper diet of about 3000 calories may maintain his normal weight and blood count throughout the illness. Adequate diets prevent constipation and thereby reduce the possibility of intestinal hemorrhage and perforation. Food should be attractively prepared and offered to a patient according to his taste. Frequent small feedings are desirable. The greatest bulk should be provided in the form of carbohydrates, with fats and proteins in proportion. Lactose is preferable to cane sugar. As much as 100 grams of lactose can be added to a glass of lemonade. Candy, jelly, strained honey and sweetened fruit juices also supply carbohydrates. Butter, cream and ice cream furnish fats. Eggs, milk, and finely chopped lean beef, poultry, or fish furnish proteins. Vegetable purées, baked or mashed potatoes, toast, or zwieback are permissible. Beverages may include ginger ale, fruit juices, carbonated water, wine, brandy or whisky. In comatose or uncoöperative patients it may be necessary to administer glucose solutions intravenously; 200 cc. of a 25 per cent solution may be given several times daily.

The following list represents a satisfactory 3000 calorie diet:

8 A.M.—Farina gruel: farina, ¾
cup; milk, ½ cup; cream,
¼ cup; salt.
Toast, 1 slice.
Butter, 1 tablespoonful.
10 A.M.—Cocoa, 1 cup.
12 NOON—Milk toast: milk, ½ cup;
cream, ¼ cup; toast, 1
slice.
Cream of pea soup, 1 cup.
Egg, 1.
Chocolate blanc - mange,
¾ cup.
Butter, 2 tablespoonfuls.

2 P.M.—Malted milk, 1 cup.
4 P.M.—Orangeade, 1 glass.
6 P.M.—Farina gruel, 1 cup.
Milk, ½ cup.
Toast, 1 slice.
Butter, 1¼ tablespoonful.
Egg, 1.
Cup custard, ⅓ cup.
8 P.M.—Chocolate egg-nog, 1 glass.

Medicinal Treatment.—Drugs are generally unnecessary unless special symptoms arise. Acetylsalicylic acid, 0.6 gram (10 grains), or amidopyrin, 0.3 gram (5 grains), sometimes relieves severe headache and aching. Various drugs of the barbital group or other mild hypnotics may be used judiciously for a short period of unusual restlessness, excitement or insomnia. Hyoscine or morphine should be reserved as last resorts for extreme excitement and mania.

Treatment of Special Symptoms and Complications.—Fever and toxemia are best treated by the maintenance of elimination through the kidney and bowels. Antipyretic drugs are contraindicated. Cool or tepid sponges reduce the fever a degree or more and lessen delirium. Lumbar puncture and drainage is advisable if the spinal fluid is under pressure.

Abdominal distention can often be avoided by providing a proper diet. When present, it is treated by altering the diet or by reducing the proportion of milk, sugar or protein. Experimentation is sometimes required before a suitable diet is arranged. An enema or the insertion of a rectal tube may be tried. Passage of a stomach tube or drinking carbonated water often relieves flatulence. Diarrhea is seldom troublesome and can usually be corrected by altering the diet. When severe or protracted, small doses of opium, 0.06 gram (1 grain), may be given with bismuth subnitrate, 1 to 2 grams (15 to 30 grains), or chalk mixture, 15 to 30 cc. (½ to 1 ounce).

Hemorrhage.—Absolute rest must be enforced. Food should be temporarily withheld, but water may be given in small amounts. Red cell counts, hemoglobin and blood-pressure determinations should be made at intervals. When reasonably certain that perforation has not occurred, morphine, 0.015 gram (¼ grain), may be given. It should be remembered that opiates favor tympanites, which is to be avoided. The patient should not exert himself to use a bed-pan but should pass the stool on a large pad. When bleeding has been profuse and the anemia profound, transfusion should be performed. It is questionable whether transfusion increases the danger of dislodgment of the clot formed to stop the hemorrhage, as is often claimed. The value of the administration of various coagulants is doubtful. *Calcium chloride,* 1 gram (15 grains), or *calcium lactate,* 5 grams (75 grains), is said to favor clotting. Feeding may be gradually resumed when indications of bleeding cease.

Perforation and *peritonitis* are surgical problems. Perforation demands repair as promptly as possible. Closure of the tear offers the only hope of recovery. Laparotomy is usually well tolerated. Experience has proved that it is better to operate and be mistaken than to wait and permit general peritonitis to follow. No case of perforation is too desperate to be operated upon.

Most cases of *cholecystitis* recover spontaneously. Surgical drainage may be required in rare severe cases. An ice-bag, hot-water bottle or narcotics are used to relieve pain. *Thrombosis* is treated by keeping the affected part quiet. Heat or sedatives give relief from pain. For *failing circulation or pneumonia*, oxygen should be administered and the patient kept warm with hot-water bottles or an electric pad if collapse threatens. The so-called cardiac stimulants are of questionable value in severe toxic conditions. Digitalis is recommended for patients with previous cardiac disease or if auricular fibrillation develops. The usual bradycardia during typhoid fever must be considered in administering digitalis.

Bed-sores which may develop in spite of the best of care in protracted cases should be treated by exposure to the air or by keeping them clean and dry with dusting powder. Ointments macerate the skin and should not be used.

Other complications such as suppurations or bone lesions require no specific care and should be treated in the usual manner.

Convalescence.—The danger of relapse, which occurs in about 10 per cent of cases, should be constantly borne in mind. Relapses and recrudescences are provoked by various indiscretions in diet or exercise. The speed of recuperation is so variable in different cases that each must be considered individually. The diet may be gradually increased, particularly after the tenth day of normal temperature. The patient may sit up for a short time after the end of the first week of convalescence. Gradually, in the following weeks, increasing exercise and walking are permitted. It is better to be over-cautious than over-confident. Perforation has occurred during convalescence. Complications and sequelæ, such as bone suppuration, psychoses and neuritis, are treated according to the usual manner. They may prolong convalescence distressingly and persist for many months.

A wise precaution is to require that three stool and urine samples, tested at intervals of several days, should not contain typhoid bacilli, lest the patient be discharged as a carrier. In certain localities this rule is enforced.

Carriers constitute an important problem. An individual is considered a carrier as long as he harbors or excretes typhoid bacilli. Carriers may or may not have had typhoid fever. From 9 to 50 per cent of typhoid fever patients become carriers. Most of these are temporary carriers from one to three months, while a small number, 3 or 4 per cent, become permanent carriers. The majority harbor the bacilli in the liver, gall-bladder and intestines and excrete them in the feces. Bacilli are often excreted intermittently in the urine. About 50 per cent of patients have bacilluria during convalescence for longer or shorter periods. Bacilli are also excreted from suppurating foci.

The treatment of carriers is unsatisfactory. Cholecystectomy is recommended only in cases where bacilli are present in the bile alone. This is obviously difficult to determine. Satisfactory results can never be assured. Frequent vaccination has been recommended. Intestinal or urinary "antiseptics" are useless. Of far greater importance, at present, is the education of carriers in regard to their dangerousness in spreading disease. Instruction should be given as to definite methods for the disinfection and disposal of excreta. Carriers should never be permitted to handle foodstuffs or beverages for others. Carriers willfully violating these rules or incapable of observing them may require confinement to institutions for supervision.

REFERENCES.

BROWNING, C. H.: Chronic Enteric Carriers and Their Treatment, Med. Res. Council, Spec. Rep. Series No. 179, 1933, London.
CHRISTELLER, E.: Der Typhus Abdominalis, Handb. d. spez. path. Anat. u. Hist., Berlin, 1928, **4**, pt. II, p. 500.
CURSCHMANN, H.: Typhoid and Typhus Fever, Nothnagel's Encyclopedia of Practical Medicine, Am. Ed., Philadelphia, 1901.
GAY, F. P.: Typhoid Fever, New York, 1918.
JORDAN, E. O.: Epidemiology of Paratyphoid Infection, Jour. Prevent. Med., 1929, **3**, 279.
Medical Department of the U. S. Army in the World War, vol. **9**, War Department, 1928.

PARATYPHOID BACILLUS INFECTIONS.

Bacillus paratyphosus A (Salmonella paratyphosus or typhi) and Bacillus paratyphosus B (Salmonella schottmülleri) are the causative agents of a disease clinically indistinguishable from typhoid fever. Certain characteristics of disease caused by these organisms are discussed on page 27. Kuttner has recently reported several cases of infection in children due to Salmonella cholera suis.

Other serologically distinct members of the large paratyphoid group, namely, Salmonella aërtrycke, Salmonella enteriditis and Salmonella cholera suis, are usually responsible for disease of an entirely different nature. These three types of bacilli are associated primarily with infections in animals. Human infection is practically always derived from the ingestion of meat obtained from sick animals. Other foods (shell fish, custards, ice cream) may also become contaminated with any of the paratyphoid group of bacilli and give rise to the condition known as "food" poisoning.

Epidemics of "meat" or "food" poisoning appear explosively when variable numbers of people consume contaminated food. The disease never spreads further unless others partake of the same contaminated supply. The mortality varies greatly in different outbreaks. Sometimes hundreds are poisoned without fatality, but in other epidemics the mortality is 10 per cent or more (see page 28).

Bacillus Coli Infections.—The colon bacillus which is constantly present in the normal gastro-intestinal tract may, under certain conditions, become invasive and cause disease. The bacillus may be associated with sepsis, pyemia, meningitis, peritonitis, pneumonia, cystitis, pyelitis, pyelonephritis, osteomyelitis, cholecystitis, arthritis and other conditions. The bacillus is carried to the site of infection *via* the blood stream or by direct local invasion of tissue. In most instances the portal of entry is in the urogenital, intestinal or biliary tracts, or from wound infections, especially about the buttocks. In new-born infants, sepsis due to Bacillus coli which gains entrance through the umbilical cord is known as Winkel's disease. Injury of any sort to the areas mentioned favors the invasion of the ever-present colon bacilli.

Colon Bacillus Septicemia.—Several recent studies (Barrington, Felty, Scott) show that colon bacilli are frequently recovered from the blood stream after instrumentation or operations on the urethra. In one study, colon bacilli were recovered from the blood in 6 out of 18 cases shortly after operation on the urethra; in another study, in 40 per cent of 82 cases. Blood stream invasion is usually transient unless the local injury is extensive. Spontaneous invasion may occur during severe pyelonephritis or puerperal infection, but in most instances infection occurs after surgical manipulation in an infected field, especially in the urethra, intestines or female genitalia. Women are most often involved during the child-bearing period, and men after the age of fifty years when prostatic obstruction appears.

The severity of the disease appears to depend more upon the extent of the local process than upon the blood stream invasion. The symptoms of infection are caused partly by the local process and partly by the bacteriemia or septicemia. The symptoms are often not characteristic. The onset may be sudden or gradual. Chills and sweats are common. Petechiæ, herpes and jaundice occur. Fever is often high, continuous, remittent or intermittent, averaging from 37.8° C. (100° F.) to 40° C. (104° F.). The course may last from two to ten days and terminates by lysis. Mild cases may show nothing but fever; fulminating cases may die within a day or two; protracted cases may last a month or more. The leukocytes vary greatly, from 3000 to 30,000. Moderate leukocytosis is the rule. Metastatic infections are common. Bronchopneumonia, pyelitis, endocarditis, pericarditis, meningitis and osteomyelitis have been observed.

The mortality-rate is difficult to determine, due to the occurrence of unrecognized cases and to the difficulty of deciding whether death is due to the septicemia or to some other primary condition if present. In Felty and Keefer's series the mortality was 32 per cent. There is no specific treatment. The intravenous injection of various dyes or antiseptics is of no value. More can be done as prophylaxis by reducing operative traumatization to a minimum, especially when working in contaminated fields.

Colon Bacillus Cystitis, Pyelitis and Pyelonephritis.—It is said that 90 per cent of these infections are due to colon bacilli. It is probable that the incidence is not so high and that in certain cases the colon bacillus is present as a secondary invader. Any trauma to the mucous membranes of the genito-urinary tract is apt to favor an invasion of colon bacilli. Cystitis may be due to instrumentation, the presence of foreign bodies, retention of urine from obstruction or to other causes, or it may be secondary to pyelitis.

Renal infection is usually hematogenous in origin. Less commonly infection from the lower urogenital tract ascends to the kidney through the lumen of the ureter, along the walls of the ureter or by way of the lymphatics around the ureter wall. A direct lymphatic communication between the ascending colon and the right kidney suggests another pathway of infection.

Other Colon Bacillus Infections.—Meningitis, cholecystitis and pneumonia are usually not diagnosed from an etiologic point of view except when special attempts are made to do so. Attempts to discover the etiologic agents should be made in every case. *Morgan bacilli* comprise an ill-defined group of organisms related to the colon-typhoid group. They have been occasionally associated with human disease. Diagnosis is made by identifying the organisms found in the blood, or in the stool, and by the presence of specific agglutinins in the serum.

REFERENCES.

FELTY, A. R., and KEEFER, C. S.: Bacillus Coli Sepsis, Jour. Am. Med. Assn., 1924, **82**, 1430.

JORDAN, E. O.: Food Poisoning and Food Borne Infection, Univ. Chicago Press, 1931.

SCOTT, W. W.: Blood-stream Infections in Urology, Jour. Urol., 1929, **21**, 527.

BACILLARY DYSENTERY, ACUTE AND CHRONIC.

The word "dysentery," which means bowel trouble, has been loosely applied to many diseases or conditions accompanied by diarrhea and abdominal pain. It is desirable, however, to use the word only as a suffix following the term which indicates the causative organism, as, for example, bacillary dysentery or amebic dysentery.

Definition.—Bacillary dysentery is an infection of the large intestine characterized by the frequent passage of stools composed of mucus, pus and blood, by abdominal pain and tenesmus and by general symptoms of toxemia. The disease may appear sporadically or in epidemics. Acute and chronic forms occur.

History.—Ulcerative diseases of the bowel were described by Hippocrates and Galen. Unfortunately, these early teachings were forgotten, and until comparatively recent times, various diarrheal diseases were classed as "dysentery." Many cases formerly called follicular enteritis, cholera infantum, summer diarrhea or infectious diarrhea of infants were undoubtedly bacillary dysentery. With the development of pathology the term became limited to diphtheritic or ulcerative diseases of the colon due to infection, heavy metal poisoning or uremia. When amebæ were found in the stools in 1875 it was believed for a time that the etiology was settled. In 1898, Shiga, while investigating an epidemic of dysentery in Japan, was unable to find amebæ. In a systematic study he demonstrated the causative agent to be a bacillus which was found in the stool and agglutinated specifically in the serum of the victims of the disease. Two years later Kruse isolated a similar organism in Germany. Flexner and Strong isolated bacilli not identical with, but clearly related to, the Shiga type. Thereafter different strains of dysentery bacilli have been encountered to which many names have been given.

Etiology.—Dysentery bacilli are morphologically similar to Bacillus typhosus. They are Gram-negative short rods rounded at the ends with a tendency to pleomorphism, non-motile and aërobic. Growth in artificial media occurs quite easily and is not particularly character-istic. As previously mentioned, many names have been given to various strains, different names being given to identical organisms in some cases. It is desirable that some uniform nomenclature be adopted similar to the Roman numeral system as applied, for example, to the different types of pneumococcus. For the general purposes of clini-cians it is sufficient to regard two general subdivisions, represented by the Shiga-Kruse type which do not ferment mannite and produce a powerful toxin, and by the Flexner-Strong-Hiss-Sonne varieties which ferment mannite and produce a less potent toxin. All strains evoke agglutinins which are fairly specific and can be identified by this means or by means of fermentation tests with various sugars. For a detailed description of the methods employed in differentiation the reader is referred to larger works on bacteriology.

The bacilli are easily killed by heat, chemicals, sunlight and drying. They may live in moist garden soil, clothing and ice for more than a month.

Pathogenesis.—Dysentery bacilli enter the body through the mouth. Other modes of entry are rare. They pass through the stomach and small intestine and apparently become invasive only in the colon. The organisms penetrate the mucosa, localize and produce the charac-teristic membranous and ulcerative lesions. Soluble toxic substances are elaborated locally and carried throughout the system by the blood stream. In this respect the nature of the disease is somewhat analogous to that of diphtheria.

Pathology.—The lesion is usually a superficial inflammation of the large intestine. In certain cases the ileum may be involved. All gradations of severity occur from simple inflammation to widespread necrosis and destruction of the mucous membrane and underlying tissues. The earliest lesions probably occur in the lymphoid follicles of the colon. The toxins cause the mucous membrane to become swollen and inflamed, resembling red velvet in appearance. The blood-vessels are engorged and the lymphatics are filled with leukocytes. At this period necrosis of the epithelium is indicated by the appearance of small flecks here and there. The necrotic tissue forms a false mem-brane. Patches of the membrane slough off, leaving shallow, irregular, discrete or confluent ulcers; in extreme cases, an entirely denuded surface. Bacilli may be found in the membrane, the mucosa or sub-mucosa. Ulcers are seldom deep enough to perforate the bowel wall. The bowel wall in the region involved often becomes greatly thickened and, in rare cases, gangrenous. In chronic dysentery, the wall may become fibrosed and stenotic. Numerous irregular ulcers may be found in the lower portions of the large bowel.

Healing commences from points of regeneration in the follicles of Lieberkühn. The mucous membrane in most cases may be fully restored to normal, but if the process has been too severe no secreting cells may regenerate, and extensive scar formation and possible stricture result.

Pathologic changes in other organs are usually unimportant. The mesenteric lymph nodes are often swollen and hyperemic, the kidneys may be congested and there may be hemorrhages into the adrenals. The spleen is seldom enlarged. Specific pyelonephritis and liver abscess have been observed.

Dysentery bacilli are present in the early stage in the intestinal contents, especially in the flakes of mucus, in the ulcerated bowel wall and less often in the mesenteric lymph nodes; occasionally in the blood stream, spleen, biliary system and kidneys (Posselt).

Epidemiology.—Bacillary dysentery is widely distributed throughout the world, but is more prevalent in tropical climates than elsewhere. In the United States it appears that bacilli of the mannite fermenting group (Flexner, Sonne) are responsible for most of the cases, but Shiga's variety is occasionally encountered. The epidemiology of dysentery is much the same as that of typhoid fever. Sporadic cases occasionally occur. Epidemics are usually small and limited to the environment of the source. Numerous small epidemics occur in camps, boarding schools, hospitals and other resident institutions. As in other infectious diseases, the healthy carrier and the ambulatory patient are dangerous as disseminators of infection. In a recent study in New Orleans, Browne found 9 of 100 normal individuals to be carriers of dysentery bacilli, 1 harboring the Shiga type. The infection is conveyed by contaminated food or drink, by direct contact and by flies. Water-borne and dust-borne infection is uncommon because the bacillus is not especially resistant to unfavorable environments. It is therefore comparatively easy to prevent the spread of infection. The disease is generally more prevalent in the summer and autumn. Debilitation, poor hygiene, exhaustion, coarse irritating food and starvation predispose individuals to infection. It is largely a disease of the poorer classes.

The *incubation period* is short, varying from one to eight days, depending upon the susceptibility or resistance of the host, the size of the inoculum and the virulence of the bacilli. Prodromal symptoms of general malaise, headache, anorexia and nausea may be present.

Symptoms.—All gradations of severity of symptoms occur regardless of the type of infecting organism. Usually, bacilli of the Shiga type cause the most profound illness. The mildest infections may be manifested merely by a day or two of diarrhea with little or no constitutional disturbance. Severe fulminating infections may end fatally in several days. Contrary to general opinion in localities where dysentery is uncommon, the disease may produce grave illness.

In the typical case of moderate severity, the onset is sudden with colicky abdominal pains, constant desire to defecate and tenesmus. The stools at first may be formed, but soon become diarrheal and contain mucus and streaks of blood. The passages increase in frequency until 20 or 30 or more occur in twenty-four hours. The griping pain becomes distressing. Prolapse of the rectum may occur. At the height of the illness the patient appears very ill. The stools may be composed entirely of pus, mucus and blood. Due to the rapid loss of water, thirst, oliguria and dehydration occur. In rare cases constipation occurs. The tongue is heavily coated. Aching pains, vomiting and dysuria are present at times. The temperature rises at the onset to 38° C. (100.4° F.) or higher, and is often not in proportion to the severity of the attack. The pulse is frequent. There is abdominal tenderness, headache, drowsiness and occasionally cough. As recovery commences after two or more weeks, the stools diminish in number and become fecal, discomfort diminishes and the temperature declines. Undue exertion or too rapid increase of diet often causes relapses. Spontaneous relapses may recur. The patient may recover completely or may pass into the chronic stage, especially if proper treatment is neglected. In fatal cases the stools may become serous and lessen in frequency as the patient becomes weaker. Circulatory collapse manifested by a weak, thready pulse, fall in blood pressure and temperature develops. Death may be due to complications.

In infants and children the symptoms are usually more severe due to the more serious effects of the toxemia and especially of dehydration and ketosis. The onset is marked by fever, irritability, feeding difficulties, vomiting or convulsions followed by drowsiness and apathy. Fever is high and emaciation rapid. The stools are numerous and are composed of muco-pus and blood. In non-fatal cases recovery often occurs within two or three weeks.

Atypical Cases.—Many sporadic cases characterized by a day or two of indisposition, diarrhea and little or no fever are unrecognized as bacillary dysentery. Such cases frequently predominate in epidemics of dysentery. This form is probably the one most frequently encountered in northern United States. The terms para-, pseudo- or meta-dysentery should not be applied to these cases since they are actually true bacillary dysentery probably due to the less pathogenic strains or to more resistant hosts. The fulminating type with sudden onset, early collapse and rice-water stools occurs. The symptoms resemble those of cholera. Death may occur in a few days.

In recent years numerous small epidemics due to "Sonne" dysentery bacilli have been reported from various parts of the temperate zones, usually among children. The disease is usually mild, but a few fatal cases are recorded. The signs and symptoms are like those just described.

Complications and Sequelæ.—Complications and sequelæ are often limited to the severe Shiga type of infection. The toxin liberated at the site of infection in the bowel may cause a number of neurologic complications of which peripheral neuritis is the commonest. Polyneuritis and paraplegia have been noted. The occurrence of acute exudative *arthritis* has been ascribed by some to the toxin, by others to allergy, but the actual cause or relationship to dysentery is unknown. It is an uncommon complication. The large joints are usually affected and become swollen, painful, and contain an effusion of sterile, turbid, gelatinous fluid. Arthritis often develops after the acute period of dysentery is over and may persist for months. It may be accompanied by fever. The pain is sometimes relieved by aspiration, but it is often uninfluenced by analgesic drugs. Healing ultimately occurs without deformity. Patients may seek medical aid for the arthritis after an attack of dysentery so mild as to pass almost unnoted. In patients receiving antidysentery serum, the arthritis of serum disease may occur. Conjunctivitis, iridocyclitis, parotitis and urethritis are rarer complications; otitis media occurs in infants. Stenosis of the bowel, or perforation and peritonitis have been noted.

Laboratory Observations.—The typical stool is pathognostic. It is composed of mucus, pus and blood in varying proportions. Gross hemorrhage is uncommon. Microscopically there are many polymorphonuclear leukocytes in varying degrees of degeneration, large macrophages and erythrocytes. Dysentery bacilli can often be cultivated in the early stages. Leukocytosis of 12,000 to 15,000 is the rule. Leukopenia or normal counts may occur. The polymorphonuclear cells predominate. The hemoglobin and red cells may be slightly increased due to dehydration, but fall in number as the disease progresses. Severe anemia is common in the chronic form. Specific agglutinins appear in the serum after the first week. The urine may be reduced in amount due to water loss. Traces of albumin are common.

Diagnosis.—Diagnosis in the epidemic form usually presents no difficulties. The sporadic cases especially if mild are often unrecognized. Few other conditions are characterized by the stools as described in the preceding paragraph. A presumptive diagnosis can be made from the acute febrile onset, frequent mucopurulent bloody stools, abdominal cramps and tenesmus. Efforts should be directed to establish etiologic diagnosis by isolating and identifying the organism from the stools. Bacilli may be cultivated from the stools, especially from flecks of mucus, early in the disease in 50 to 60 per cent of cases if repeated attempts are made. The chances of isolating the bacilli rapidly diminish after the first few days. Positive cultures can be obtained later in 80 per cent of cases by swabbing the ulcerated areas during sigmoidoscopy and transferring the material directly to fresh media. Care must be taken to avoid injury with the sigmoidoscope. For methods of identification of the bacilli, the reader is referred to more detailed treatises. Determination of the serum agglutinins should be made only by experienced individuals. Agglutinins are of great value in diagnosis, since they are highly specific and occur in practically all cases of dysentery and are absent in other diseases. The titer seldom exceeds 1 to 1000.

Sigmoidoscopy is painful and frequently impossible in acute cases, but if possible it is valuable as a diagnostic method. The bowel wall appears as described in the paragraph on pathology.

Differential Diagnosis.—Amebic dysentery resembles the bacillary form in certain respects, especially when the latter has become chronic. The history of intermittent attacks of diarrhea without much impairment of health is more characteristic of the amebic form in which toxic symptoms are seldom present. Large shallow ulcers with overhanging margins may be seen with the sigmoidoscope. The mucous membrane between the ulcers appears to be generally normal as contrasted with the bacillary form in which the whole membrane is inflamed in addition to the presence of the shallow ulcers. The stools

of amebic dysentery are liquid, reddish-brown and contain comparatively few polymorphonuclear leukocytes. The presence of Ameba
histolytica establishes the diagnosis. In certain indefinite cases, a
favorable response to emetine suggests amebic infection. Amebic liver
abscess is a frequent complication.

Various parasitic conditions, balantidiasis, distomiasis, giardiasis and
others are apt to be confusing, but can often be recognized by identifying the respective organisms in the stools. Mixed infections with
any form may occur. In *cholera* the stools are usually watery and
profuse; prostration and dehydration are more marked. Vibrios can
be found in the stools. *Typhoid fever* is seldom confusing. Typhoid
fever and bacillary dysentery may coexist. Other diseases of the
colon—intussusception, neoplasm, tuberculosis and syphilis—must be
excluded. Drastic cathartics, certain heavy metal poisons or "food
poisons" (botulinus, salmonella, staphylococcus) cause severe entero-
colitis with blood and mucus. Differentiation is made by the history
and more or less typical course of the respective conditions, or by the
bacteriologic or serologic identification of dysentery.

Prognosis.—The disease may cause invalidism lasting from a few
days to several months. Untreated cases and patients who neglect
proper measures often develop chronic dysentery. The mortality-
rate varies greatly depending upon the virulence of the organism, the
resistance or susceptibility of the host, the age of the host, the presence
of other diseases or complications and the character of treatment.
The death-rate for infants and the aged is considerably higher. Generally the mortality is about 2 per cent in the acute forms. It may
vary from 0.4 per cent to 25 per cent in certain epidemics, and among
infants may be as high as 30 or 40 per cent. Specific serotherapy is
said to reduce the mortality-rate in Shiga infections by 50 per cent.

Prophylaxis.—Under normal circumstances it is comparatively easy
to avoid bacillary dysentery by observation of the simplest rules of
hygiene, especially regarding the prevention of contamination or the
sterilization of food and drink. Under adverse conditions of war,
famine or other disaster such procedures are often impossible to follow.
Prophylactic vaccine administered either parenterally or by mouth
has not proved to be of value. Carriers must be prohibited from
handling food or drink and must be educated regarding the proper
disposal of stools. Stools from patients must be sterilized or protected
from flies and other vermin.

Treatment.—The treatment is directed toward (a) complete rest
with careful nursing, maintenance of nutrition, replacement of fluid
loss and relief of distress, (b) specific serotherapy and (c) proper disposal of excreta to avoid spreading the infection to others. Complete
bed rest is of greatest importance and often suffices to relieve all symptoms in mild cases. Patients should not be permitted to leave the
bed until the fever has disappeared and the stools are normal for
several days in mild cases and longer in severe ones. Numerous
relapses and certain chronic cases can be attributed to undue exertion
before complete recovery has occurred. To obtain relaxation and
sleep, barbitals may be used. Occasionally patients who become

exhausted from repeated bowel movements, straining and pain, require hypodermic injection of morphine; for children, paregoric may be used. The buttocks should be kept scrupulously clean. The anus and surrounding skin often become irritated from the repeated passage of stools. Applications of soothing ointments, or suppositories containing tannic acid or cocaine often relieve pain. In certain patients, rectal injections of warm saline or starch solutions are agreeable. Rectal instillations of 100 to 200 cc. of 0.5 per cent iodoöxyquinoline sulfonic acid ("chiniofon," "yatren") to be retained fifteen or twenty minutes once a day have been recommended. Heat applied to the abdomen by an electric pad or other means often gives comfort. If vomiting is present in the early stages, food may be withheld for a day. Diet may be gradually resumed in the form of thin gruels or jellies and increased until a diet similar to the one described on page 39 is given. Breast-feeding or protein milk is recommended for infants under two years of age. In all cases it is highly essential to provide fluid to replace that lost by the frequent passage of stools. It is preferably given by mouth in the absence of nausea, in the form of water, fruit juices, tea or milk. It may be necessary to inject normal physiologic saline solution intravenously every eight or twelve hours in amounts varying from 100 cc. to 1500 cc., according to the size of the patient and his requirements. Transfusions of blood, when necessary, are often strikingly beneficial.

As paradoxical as it may seem, the administration of 4 to 8 cc. of a saturated solution of sodium sulphate every hour or two during the first twenty-four or thirty-six hours until free watery stools are passed often provides relief from pain and tenesmus. Care must be observed, especially in children, to avoid dehydration. It should not be used in infants or in severe cases. Patients exhibiting signs of collapse must be kept warm with hot-water bottles and should be given fluids intravenously.

Specific serotherapy is of greatest value when given in large doses intravenously early in the course of severe acute infection caused by the Shiga group of bacilli. It is of less value in infections due to strains of the mannite fermenting group. The difficulties probably lie in the multiplicity of strains; unless the antiserum contains a sufficient concentration of specific homologous antibodies against the strain causing the infection it is useless. It appears to be desirable, when possible, to prepare antidysentery serum with the strains prevalent in a locality where the serum is to be used. When serum is to be given, the patient must be tested for serum sensitivity in the usual manner. If not hypersensitive, 40 to 120 cc. of serum, depending upon the size of the patient, should be given intravenously, repeating the dose every eight or twelve hours for a day or two until the temperature returns to normal and the diarrhea ceases. If no beneficial effect is derived from 4 or 5 doses it is useless to give more. The suggestion has been made to administer serum per rectum for the purpose of neutralizing the toxin and destroying the bacilli directly. Needless to say, it is necessary to determine the type of infecting organism and to administer serum containing specific antibodies against the strain. Unfortunately,

4

the bacteriologic work involved often requires a day or two of valuable time. Bacteriophage has not proved to be of value.

Chronic Bacillary Dysentery.—Chronic bacillary dysentery varies so much from the initial acute stage in its symptoms as to justify separate discussion. Rogers arbitrarily regards dysentery lasting more than a month as chronic. The acute form may gradually merge into the chronic form; the patient may recover from his first acute infection and have several relapses before the chronic form begins; or there may be but little evidence of an acute stage, the chronic form commencing insidiously and continuing as such. Patients who neglect treatment and convalescence from an acute attack, or those becoming ill under circumstances (war, famine) which preclude treatment, are especially liable to develop the chronic form. About 5 per cent of all acute cases eventually become chronic. Either the mannite-fermenting or non-mannite-fermenting strains give rise to the chronic dysentery. Occasionally both are found in the same patient.

Symptoms.—The symptoms of more or less constant loose stools containing pus and mucus, slight fever, abdominal pain, emaciation, anorexia and subnormal health may persist for months or years in various grades of severity. Acute exacerbations may punctuate the course and hemorrhages may occur. Occasionally there are no subjective or objective symptoms except for pus in the stool. The ulcers often become secondarily infected with other organisms. Severe anemia may occur which resembles the anemia of sprue or of the pernicious type. Stricture or perforation of the bowel may occur. Death occurs from exhaustion, toxemia or complications.

Diagnosis.—Diagnosis is greatly facilitated by sigmoidoscopy. The lesions are usually found in the lower half of the large intestine. The mucosa shows varying grades of inflammation, roughening or granulation. The mucosa is thickened and mucus exudes from the surface. The majority of cases show irregular ulcers varying in size from a millimeter to a centimeter in the rectum or sigmoid. The ulcers are shallow with sharply defined flat edges. Stool cultures are frequently negative, but dysentery bacilli can often be cultivated from scrapings made directly from the ulcers and immediately plated on suitable warm culture media.

Chronic bacillary dysentery is rather easily differentiated from amebic dysentery if the causative organisms can be isolated in either case, or by the nature of the discrete ulcers with undermined edges in an otherwise normal mucous membrane in the amebic form and the response to emetine. Chronic non-specific ulcerative colitis is often indistinguishable from chronic dysentery. Syphilis, tuberculosis and malignancy must be considered. Sigmoidoscopy and roentgen-ray study often render diagnosis possible.

Treatment.—Treatment is tedious and must often be prolonged for months. The general symptomatic treatment is the same as that described on page 48. Smyly recommends 3 or 4 injections daily of Dakin's solution beginning with 300 to 500 cc. of a 20 per cent solution and increasing the strength and the amount injected. Special drugs such as chiniofon by mouth and by enema have also been used. Bacteriophage therapy has not passed the experimental stage. Serum and vaccine therapy are useless. The anemia is corrected with diet and iron or liver therapy. The author has noted striking improvement from single large blood transfusions. It is helpful to control therapy and to observe the progress of the lesions by frequent sigmoidoscopy.

Surgical intervention, cecostomy, appendicostomy and ileostomy have not proved to be worth the risk in most patients.

REFERENCES.

DAVISON, W. C.: A Bacteriological and Clinical Consideration of Bacillary Dysentery in Adults and Children, Medicine, 1922, **1**, 391–477.

LENZ, O., and PRIGGE, R.: Dysenterie, Handb. d. path. Micro., 1931, **3**, 1377–1584.

NELSON, R. L.: Sonne Dysentery, Am. Jour. Dis. Child., 1931, **41**, 15–25.

SOULE, M. H.: Bacteriologic and Serologic Study of Eighty-nine Cases of Dysentery, Jour. Lab. and Clin. Med., 1933, **18**, 549–565.

SMYLY, H. J.: The Diagnosis and Treatment of Chronic Dysentery, Trans. Roy. Soc. Trop. Med. and Hyg., 1930, **24**, 39–66.

UNDULANT FEVER.

Synonyms.—Brucelliasis; Malta, Mediterranean or Gibraltar fever; Febris melitensis; Mittelmeer fieber; Bang's disease.

Definition.—Undulant fever is a specific generalized infection caused by Brucella melitensis, characterized by an insidious onset, a prolonged remittent or undulatory type of fever, weakness, profuse sweating, loss of weight, anemia, splenomegaly, constipation, a low mortality-rate and a prolonged convalescence.

History.—Undulant fever was apparently a disease of antiquity. Hippocrates described fevers which included all the features of undulant fever. Numerous writers in the eighteenth and nineteenth centuries have reported fevers which appear to have been undulant fever. After 1800, British medical officers in Malta, especially Chartres, repeatedly described it and called attention to its increasing prevalence. In 1886 Bruce discovered the causative organism in the spleen, which was named Micrococcus melitensis at that time. Wright and Semple devised the specific agglutination test as an aid in diagnosis, in 1897.

A search by Hardy has revealed that a syndrome similar in all respects to undulant fever was described by numerous physicians in America after the Civil War. It was probably often classified as atypical typhoid fever, typho-malarial fever or fever of unknown origin. Malta fever, as such, was first recognized in the United States by Musser and Sailer in 1898, among men returned from the tropics. The first indigenous case was described in 1904 by Craig who suggested, at the time, that many cases were probably mistaken for typhoid fever. Other cases were subsequently reported from the goat-raising districts in the southwestern states. The first human case of undulant fever in the United States proved to be due to Brucella melitensis variety abortus, was reported by Keefer in 1924. Since then the disease has rapidly gained prominence.

The term "Malta" fever was replaced in 1897 by the term "undulant" fever. Although the latter removes the geographic restriction it is not altogether satisfactory, since the disease, as seen in the United States is not always characterized by a typical undulating type of fever.

Almost parallel with the early studies of Malta fever, Bang (1897) discovered and studied the etiologic agent of contagious abortion in cattle, known thereafter as Bacillus abortus. Similar studies were made by Theobald Smith. Although the similarities between Bacillus abortus and Micrococcus melitensis were striking, it was not until twenty years later that Evans demonstrated their morphologic and cultural identity. Since then they have been classified together as Brucella melitensis, variety melitensis, abortus or suis, depending upon their origin from goats, cattle or swine, respectively.

Etiology.—The brucellæ are small (0.3 to 0.5 by 0.6 to 1.5 microns), non-capsulated, non-motile, Gram-negative organisms. Pleomorphism is constant, coccoid forms often predominating in animal tissue and bacillary forms on artificial media. Growth is slow. On agar, small translucent colonies appear after forty-eight to seventy-two hours. In broth, growth rarely occurs before the fourth, and occasionally not until the tenth day, or later. The brucellæ do not ferment sugars. They are pathogenic for man, monkeys, cattle, sheep, goats, swine, horses, guinea-pigs, chickens, dogs and probably for other species.

As indicated previously, three types of brucella are recognized, caprine, bovine and porcine, depending upon their source. According to Theobald Smith the bovine and caprine types have been adapted to their respective hosts by a long series of passages; the porcine type may be a recent adaptation from the bovine type, infecting swine as a result of close contact with cattle.

Several tests have been employed to differentiate the three varieties, none of which is constantly reliable. The strains are so closely related serologically that slight differences between the melitensis (goat) and abortus (cattle) varieties can be shown only by agglutinin absorption. Occasionally the bovine type demands an atmosphere containing CO_2 for growth, a characteristic not shown by the other types. The porcine type is said to be more virulent than the bovine type. The technic of differentiation is still in the experimental stage. Little is known of the caprine strain, although it has been under observation the longest.

Sources of Infection.—Goats, sheep, horses, cattle and swine are the reservoirs of infection. The latter two are apparently of greatest importance in the United States, although goats constitute a source in the southwestern area. In cattle the infection is chronic, residing primarily in the pregnant uterus and mammary glands or in the male genitalia. Organisms can readily be demonstrated in the tissues and are often located intracellularly. In goats the infection is more generalized. Infected animals usually exhibit no signs of illness aside from abortions and premature births. There is often a mucopurulent vaginal discharge heavily loaded with organisms. Little is as yet known regarding the infection in hogs. Large numbers of bacteria are shed in goat's milk and urine, fewer in cows' milk. In horses, Brucellæ have been isolated from fistulas commonly known as fistulous withers or poll evil.

Mode of Infection.—The ingestion of raw milk or milk products containing brucella is the most obvious method of infection of humans. This is especially true regarding goats' milk. Other modes of infection exist. The possibility of direct infection by contact with infected exudates, urine and feces is highly probable, since Hardy demonstrated that the unabraded skin of the guinea-pig may be a portal of entry. Infections are not infrequent among meat packing-house employees. Spengler reports several cases of primary skin infection. Cattle can be infected by placing a small amount of culture in the con-

junctival sac. Otero reports that human volunteers have contracted
the disease by inoculation through abraded skin. Person to person
infection is unknown.

Pathogenesis.—It has been suggested that the pathogenesis is
similar to that of typhoid fever, although but few facts are thus far
known to substantiate this theory. The portal of entry is either in the
gastro-intestinal tract or in the skin or mucous membranes. It is
possible that, as in typhoid fever, there is first a generalized distribution of organisms *via* the lymphatics and blood stream, resulting
in the clinical picture of a general infection with later localization in
various sites. There is often a bacteriemia. Ulcers have been found
in the small intestine, and the mesenteric lymph nodes are often hyperplastic and contain brucellæ. Brucellæ have been found in the gall-
bladder, kidneys, liver, spleen and lymph nodes, and have been isolated
from the feces and urine. It has been suggested that the gall-bladder,
as in typhoid fever, may serve as a focus of infection and is responsible
for relapses, chronic disease or the "carrier" state.

Pathology.—Since undulant fever has so recently been given wide
consideration, and since the mortality-rate is low, few pathologic studies are available. The findings in general are variable, but are somewhat similar to those observed in animals.

The spleen and liver are almost always enlarged and soft. There
is congestion and hyperplasia of the lymph nodes and occasionally
congestion or ulceration of the intestinal mucosa. Fatal cases of
Malta fever with intestinal hemorrhages have been reported. Histologically, in Gregerson's case, the lymph follicles of the spleen were
sparse and hypoplastic. There was marked hyperplasia of the pulp
and an increased amount of blood in the sinuses. The liver showed
small round-cell perivascular infiltrations around the portal vessels
and small foci of granulation tissue containing lymphocytes and plasma
cells. Similar foci were present in the kidneys. Löffler found granulomata in the spleen resembling miliary tuberculosis, but no necrosis
or softening was observed. Exudative and sclerotic processes were
found in the spleen. Endophlebitis and thrombophlebitis of the larger
veins were present, resembling the changes found in typhoid fever.
There was nodular thickening and evidence of inflammation of the
capsule of the spleen. The liver showed endophlebitis and discrete
and confluent tubercle-like granulomata similar to those in the spleen.

Vegetative endocarditis and acute nephritis have been reported.
As yet no specific lesions have been described.

Epidemiology.—*Incidence.*—Undulant fever is a widespread disease
among humans and animals, occurring in many parts of the world,
either endemically or sporadically. It has been recognized on all
continents. In the United States, endemic foci of the caprine variety
exist in the southwestern states; elsewhere, the bovine or porcine
types predominate. Table 2 serves to give an impression of the
increasing number of recognized cases.

The increasing number does not indicate an increase in the incidence
of the disease, but the recognition and diagnosis of a hitherto obscure
and incorrectly diagnosed fever. The total number of cases is no doubt

much higher, but until all cases are recognized and until all State Departments of Health require the registration of cases of undulant fever, no accurate statistics will be available. Fig. 2 conveys an impression of the distribution of cases reported in 1929. It is noteworthy that most cases were recognized in Iowa and Ohio where the most thorough investigations have been conducted, notably by Hardy, Bierring and Simpson. In many localities brucella infections are more prevalent than typhoid fever.

TABLE 2.—CASES OF UNDULANT FEVER REPORTED IN THE UNITED STATES EXCLUSIVE
OF TEXAS, ARIZONA AND NEW MEXICO.

Year	Number reported
1922	1
1923	0
1924	2
1925	8
1926	42
1927	206
1928	635
1929	1301
1932	1502

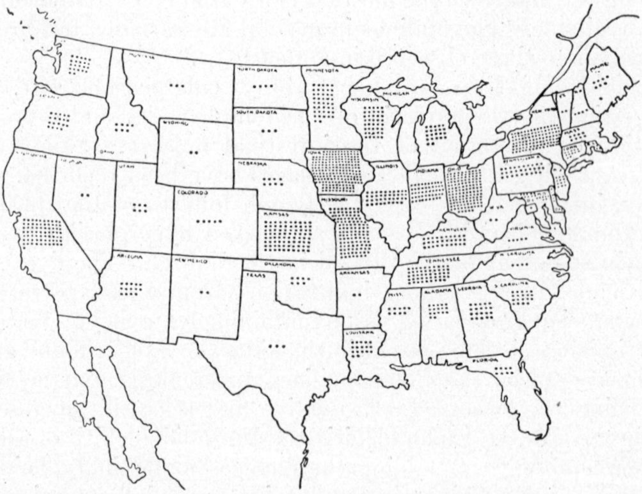

FIG. 2.—Distribution of cases of undulant fever reported in 1929. (Hardy.)

Age and Sex.—The greatest number of cases occur among young and middle-aged individuals, from fifteen to fifty years of age. Children, like young calves, are said to be relatively immune, although it is possible that many cases are unrecognized. A few cases have been reported in infants. Males are more commonly affected than females. Various figures indicate that, of the total number of cases, from 70 to 80 per cent occur in males, which strongly suggests some dependence upon occupational contact infection since both sexes appear to be equally susceptible otherwise.

Occupation.—It appears that farmers, stockmen and veterinarians who come in close contact with cattle and swine are subject to direct infection, but many cases occur among persons remote from cattle who apparently acquire infection by ingesting raw milk or milk products. Packing-house employees and laboratory workers who handle infected tissues and cultures are especially liable to infection.

Seasonal Distribution.—Accurate information is as yet unavailable. Most of Hardy's cases occurred during the summer months.

Epidemiology in Cattle.—The actual incidence of infection among domestic animals is unknown. From serologic studies and from histories of abortion, it is evident that the disease is widespread. As high as 90 per cent of herds in some localities are said to be infected. Fitch has shown that 13 per cent of 30,000 cattle in Minnesota showed positive agglutination reactions. Simpson found 86 per cent of positive reactions among 103 cattle, including cows and bulls. Calves were all negative, indicating that infection rarely, if ever, exists in sexually immature cattle. The organism can be recovered from the milk of many cows which are serologically positive. Some cows excrete organisms throughout their lifetime. Carpenter and King have recovered organisms from the milk of several cows whose serum contained no agglutinins. Brucella abortus was found in 20 per cent of samples of unpasteurized milk supplied to 70 urban communities.

Hardy found that, of 611 hogs tested, 18 per cent showed positive agglutination reactions, 16 per cent doubtful reactions and 66 per cent were negative. Other studies have shown a much lower incidence of positive reactions in other parts of the country. Statistics regarding the evidence of infection in other domestic animals are not at present available, although positive serologic tests have been reported in mules, asses, dogs, cats and chickens. Monkeys, rabbits, guinea-pigs and mice are susceptible to experimental infection.

Symptoms.—In human volunteers, the *incubation period* varied between ten and fifteen days (Otero). The average period is from ten days to three weeks.

The *onset* is usually gradual; occasionally with an abrupt chill. Prodromal symptoms are similar to those found in any general infection—weakness, lassitude, chilliness, anorexia and general aching. Less common in the early period are night sweats, arthralgia, abdominal pain and dizziness. So gradually do the symptoms appear that it is often impossible to date the actual onset. Several weeks may elapse before medical aid is sought, during which time the patient is ambulatory. A frequent first concern of the patient is a suspicion of fever; next, he notices aches or pains, loss of weight, weakness and, in more uncommon instances, painful urination, cough and constipation. Cases may commence with sore throat and a "cold." Among 230 of Hardy's cases, the period of onset was less than one week in 12 per cent, one week in 17 per cent, two weeks in 24 per cent, one month in 26 per cent, six weeks in 8 per cent, two months or more in 13 per cent.

Clinical Varieties.—For convenience in discussion, several clinical forms are recognized:

1. Spengler emphasizes the importance of *latent infections* during which the organisms reside in the body without causing symptoms. He mentions several examples in which a long symptom-free period elapsed between the initial skin infection and the onset of undulant

fever. Amoss' demonstration of brucella in the gall-bladder furnishes additional evidence that Brucella may be found quiescent in certain foci.

2. About one-fourth of the cases are considered to be of the *ambulatory type*. This form is mild and frequently permits a patient to remain at work, if obliged to for economic reasons. Weakness, lack of endurance or irritability are usually the only symptoms.

3. The type characterized by *remittent fever* is the commonest variety seen in the United States and in northern Europe. It is due to the bovine or porcine types of Brucella. It is characterized by an insidious onset and a prolonged remittent fever, exhibiting in its rise and decline a single large wave lasting from six weeks to several months.

4. *Undulating waves* of fever, lasting for days or weeks and interrupted by periods of remission, are observed in about 15 per cent of the cases observed in the United States. The temperature during the periods of remission may or may not remain at the normal level. The undulations are due to relapses which were commonly observed in Malta, and for which the disease was named. Caprine infections are apparently characterized by this form of fever curve. They are usually more severe and are accompanied by joint effusions and neuritis.

5. Cases exhibiting either form of temperature curve which last a year or more may be regarded as *chronic*.

6. The malignant or fulminating type is, fortunately, rare. It is characterized by a sudden onset, evidence of an overwhelming infection and death within a few days.

Sample temperature curves are shown in Figs. 3 and 4.

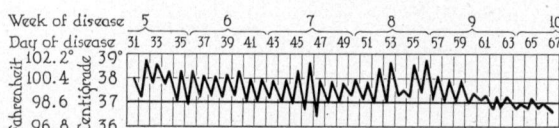

Fig. 3.—Remittent type of undulant fever. Male, aged twenty-five years, ill one month before observation. Gradual onset. Pulse-rate varied between 100 and 120. Agglutinin titer for Br. melitensis 1 to 1280 on the thirty-first day.

Atypical Forms.—When various isolated symptoms are outstanding and are considered alone, many other diseases are often suspected at first. Among them are acute orchitis, cystitis, appendicitis, rheumatic fever, bronchopneumonia and meningitis. It is only when the disease is considered as a whole that prominent symptoms are recognized as only a part of the general process.

General Symptoms.—In spite of a general opinion to the contrary, the clinical picture of a case of undulant fever is quite characteristic. A striking feature is that patients can often remain at work with considerable fever. They become vaguely aware of an afternoon or evening rise of temperature and begin to notice tiring, weakness and vague aching pains. Anorexia, constipation, chilliness or rigors often occur. Patients usually feel quite well in the morning when the temperature is normal. As the day progresses fever appears, and with it, chills followed by sweating. Later, when the disease has become established, profuse, drenching, nocturnal perspiration is a prominent feature. Many have noted a peculiar, sweetish, fetid odor of the perspiration. Even at this stage, the patient may not be incapacitated, although his fever may rise to 39.5° C. (103° F.). There may be no objective evidence of fever except by thermometer. There is often marked irritability, restlessness and insomnia. Delirium seldom occurs, and the stupor as seen in typhoid fever, practically never. Severe shaking rigors may occasionally recur throughout the illness. Backache, pain and stiffness of the joints, constipation and marked loss of weight are common. Hacking cough or bloody sputum are sometimes present.

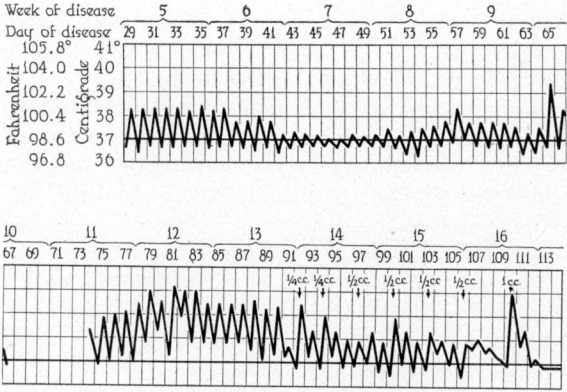

Fig. 4.—Remittent type with superimposed undulations lasting sixteen weeks. Male, aged twelve years. Onset with chills, fever, sweats and weakness two weeks after drinking raw milk. Leukocytes, 4400; 58 per cent lymphocytes; agglutination titer, 1 to 320 for Br. melitensis; skin test positive on the seventy-ninth day. Vaccine therapy commenced on the ninety-second day. Spike of fever on the one hundred and tenth day due to an overdose of vaccine. Effect of vaccine in causing defervescence was questionable since the trend of temperature was downward before beginning treatment.

The majority of patients are compelled to spend some time in bed. Rest usually gives great relief. After a period averaging from six weeks to four months, one-third of this time being spent in bed, the temperature gradually falls until it reaches normal. Overexertion or other indiscretions at this time favor relapse. In some instances, the disease persists for years, continuously or with remissions and relapses. Simpson noted a case of eight years' duration.

Special Symptoms.—Weakness, sweating and chilliness were the outstanding symptoms of Hardy's 300 cases, occurring in 100 per cent, 84 per cent and 77 per cent of the cases, respectively. Weakness, in the mild cases, was usually the sole symptom. It was usually greatest at the height of illness and persisted longest during convalescence. Sweating was absent only in the very mild and in the fatal cases. It occurred usually at night. The patient was awakened, but rested again after a change of linen. Occasionally several sweats occurred during the night and sometimes during sleep in the day time. Chilliness was frequently noted as long as a patient remained ambulatory, but disappeared when confined to bed. Ambulatory patients don additional clothing even in hot weather for comfort. True rigors occurred in one-third of the cases. They were common in severe cases.

Anorexia, noted in about 75 per cent of the cases, was variable, most marked in severe cases and absent in mild ones. Fever usually increased anorexia. A good appetite in spite of fever presaged an early recovery.

Nausea, vomiting and constipation were frequently noted, the latter most often. Intestinal hemorrhages are mentioned by European observers. Pain in the joints occurs in almost one-half of the cases and is the principle feature in about 10 per cent. Hydrarthrosis occurred in a number of Simpson's cases and Brucella was recovered from the joint fluid. Redness and severe pain, common in rheumatic fever, are not marked. Aching is transient and shifts from one joint to another. Headache is usually present in the early period. It occurs with fever and is most distressing in the afternoon and evening. General aching, muscle soreness, lumbar pain and stiffness of the neck frequently occur. Pains generally are aggravated by exercise and relieved by rest. Abdominal pain occurs in about one-third of cases. It is sometimes the chief complaint and has led to erroneous diagnoses of appendicitis or gall-bladder disease.

Nervous symptoms include insomnia, which occurs in about 50 per cent of patients, and irritability.

Both Kristenson and Hardy have noted occasional *bronchitis* with mucopurulent sputum, but Spengler emphasizes its absence. We have observed atypical *pneumonia* in 2 of our cases and bloody sputum in another. Hardy suggests that the inflammatory changes in the respiratory tract may be of a specific nature, since bronchopneumonia is often found in animals experimentally infected.

Special Signs.—*Fever.*—In the *remittent type* the morning temperature varies between normal and 39° C. (102° F.), the evening temperature between 38° C. and 40° C. (101° and 104° F.). (See Fig. 3.) It may reach 41° C. (106° F.). In the early period there is a tendency upward followed by more or less constant fluctuation from normal to a high level. Superimposed undulations may be observed (see Fig. 4). After a long single wave, the level lowers and terminates by lysis. The *undulatory* type is characterized by step-like increase until the fastigium is reached. The daily remissions are less marked. The temperature falls by lysis, reaches normal, and after a variable period rises again in another curve, constituting a relapse. Several such relapses may occur.

Nutritive Changes.—Weight loss is noted in most cases and especially in the severe ones. Most commonly, 9 to 14 kg. (20 to 30 pounds) are lost. Emaciation is avoided by bed rest and proper diet.

Physical Signs.—There is frequently a remarkable absence of any abnormal physical signs. Furthermore, there is a considerable variation in the appearance of patients. Many do not appear to be ill, even when confined to bed. Except for pallor and a fatigued appearance, they are comfortable, mentally alert and conversant. When the infection is severe patients may appear very ill indeed, but even then their mentality is usually clear.

The tongue is coated as in other fevers. Congestion of the pharyngeal mucosa occurs. In a small proportion of cases rāles are heard, indicating a mild bronchitis or atypical pneumonia. Abdominal tenderness is present in about 20 per cent of the cases. It may be diffuse or localized in the epigastrium, right upper or lower quadrants; seldom in the left side. The spleen is palpable after the first week in about 35 per cent, and the liver in about 4 per cent of the cases. Jaundice is rare. General lymph node swelling does not occur. Various joints may be swollen and tender. Simpson reports a skin eruption in 10 of 90 cases. The lesions were generalized small pink macules which could easily be confused, in certain cases, with the rose spots of typhoid fever, especially when prominent on the abdomen. In one of his cases, the eruption was maculo-papular. Spengler mentions several cases of bullous dermatitis.

The pulse-rate is often relatively slow in proportion to the fever. In a few cases the pulse-rate is rapid and increases with the temperature. A moderate decrease of blood pressure is common. Dicrotic pulse and auricular fibrillation are rare, but have been reported.

Laboratory Observations.—A mild secondary anemia is common. The erythrocytes average about 4 million per c.mm., and the hemoglobin varies from 60 to 80 per cent. Anemia is severe in caprine brucelliasis. Leukopenia or a normal total leukocyte count is the rule, even with high fever. The average number at the height of the disease is 4000 to 6000 per c.mm. The count may be as low as 2000, but seldom exceeds 10,000. Hegler found a leukocytosis in his cases. The neutrophil cells are chiefly reduced; the eosinophils are often absent. The lymphocytes and mononuclear cells are relatively or absolutely increased. In several cases the lymphocytosis approached 80 per cent of the total count. The sedimentation time of erythrocytes is usually normal, which is exceptional among infectious diseases (Curschmann).

The urine shows no important changes other than a slight increase of albumin. The diazo reaction is frequently positive and persists throughout the illness. The cerebrospinal fluid shows no abnormalities.

Agglutinins for Brucella in the blood may appear as early as the fifth day, but in most cases not until the second week; in some cases, not until the fourth week and, occasionally, not at all. To be significant, the titer should be 1 to 80 or higher. Titers of 1 to 40 are doubtful. In most cases the titer averages from 1 to 160 to 1 to 1280 during the third or fourth week. Occasionally it reaches 1 to 20,000. After recovery, agglutinins tend, in general, to disappear rapidly. Agglutinins may persist at a low level for years.

Occasionally, *non-specific agglutinins* may appear in the blood during undulant fever, notably those for Bacillus tularensis and for bacilli of the typhoid group. Brucella agglutinins are frequently found in healthy individuals known to drink milk contaminated with Brucella. The presence of agglutinins in such cases is explained by a previous attack of undulant fever, or by subclinical or latent infections. Normal individuals not exposed to infection do not develop specific agglutinins. Brucella can be recovered from the blood, feces and urine, and has been found in the pus in localized infections. Brucella was recovered from the blood of 7 of 10 patients by Simpson when special attempts were made.

Complications.—The following conditions are probably all due to Brucella and may therefore be regarded as part of the disease itself rather than complications. Several cases of specific endocarditis have been reported. It occurs in less than 1 per cent of all cases. It is diagnosed by the appearance of a diastolic murmur or by the appearance of embolic phenomena and petechiæ, and by the recovery of Brucella from the blood stream. In de la Chappele's case the aortic valves were completely destroyed.

As in animals, Brucella may have a predilection for the genital organs. Orchitis, suppurative prostatitis and epididymitis occur in about 5 per cent of cases. These complications may appear at any time during the disease and often dominate the clinical picture.

Abortion has been observed in 7 women. Carpenter has recovered Brucella from a four-month fetus. Mastitis occurred in 3 per cent of non-lactating adult females in Hardy's series. Menstrual pain may be increased during the illness.

Baker reported a striking case of hydrarthrosis in which joint effusions appeared and disappeared at seven-day intervals regularly for months. Brucella was isolated from the knee joint. Suppuration of joints has occurred during caprine infections. Jenson has observed osteomyelitis of the spine. Specific meningitis has been observed.

Bronchopneumonia occurred in 2 cases and pulmonary abscess in one of Hardy's cases. Pneumonia was an outstanding feature in 2 of our cases. Interesting skin complications are discussed by Spengler. Three cases developed bullous dermatitis (erythema brucellum) after contact with infected cows. There was a latent period between the dermatitis and the onset of undulant fever in each case, varying from five months to two years. The eruption is said to be common among veterinarians. It appears shortly after contact with infected material, lasts a few hours and is attended by intense inflammation and itching. It is regarded as an allergic reaction.

Sequelæ.—By means of a questionnaire, Hardy has ascertained that prolonged disability is the most serious feature from an economic standpoint. Weakness and undue tiring, stiff joints, anorexia, aching and even fever were reported. Mental depression and nervous irritability were also mentioned. Leavell and Amoss report a case of cholecystitis. Brucella were isolated from the gall-bladder and bile after operation. The spleen and liver may remain enlarged for a considerable time.

Convalescence is often prolonged and characterized by various symptoms.

Diagnosis.—The recognition of typical cases of undulant fever, by one familiar with the disease, is not difficult. Undulant fever should be considered in all cases of prolonged fever of obscure origin. It is important not to focus too much attention on isolated symptoms, but to consider the clinical picture as a whole. It is of some assistance to inquire as to the occupation of the patient, since certain classes come into closer contact with infection than others, as do veterinarians, farmers and packing house employees. On the other hand, anyone may be infected upon consuming contaminated milk, butter or cheese. Clinical diagnosis rests upon the appearance of symptoms and signs already described. Whenever a suspicion of undulant fever is raised, efforts should be made to confirm or disprove a diagnosis by laboratory methods.

The *agglutination test* is usually of value; 4 or 5 cc. of blood should be collected in a sterile tube, allowed to clot, and sent to the nearest laboratory equipped to perform the test. In the case of a negative result, several successive samples should be tested. A routine procedure in some laboratories is to make tests for brucella agglutinins in the blood received for the Widal test in which the latter test is negative. A number of cases of undulant fever have been discovered in this way. The presence of anemia, leukopenia and a relative lymphocytosis is suggestive but may occur in other similar illnesses. The normal sedimentation time of the blood may serve to differentiate brucelliasis from other infections in which the time is usually shortened.

Blood cultures are of great value but require special care and considerable time. Several cultures from the same patient are often required before a positive result is obtained.

Urine or exudates from areas of suppuration for culture should be collected with as little contamination as possible, centrifuged and inoculated on solid media, or preferably, injected into a guinea-pig. Brucella may be recovered from the stool by special methods. Bruce obtained organisms for diagnosis by means of spleen puncture.

Animal Inoculation.—Guinea-pigs can be inoculated intraperitoneally with 2 or 3 cc. of whole blood or of milk to be tested. Crushed tissue, sputum, urine or feces must be injected subcutaneously into the groin. After four weeks a Brucella agglutination test may be performed on blood obtained from the guinea-pig's heart. Clinically, disease is manifest by weight loss, enlarged joints and swollen testes. Proof is obtained at necropsy after six or eight weeks by the presence of small, whitish foci of necrosis in the liver, spleen or lymph nodes; by demonstrating the organisms in the tissues or by positive cultures on solid media from lungs, liver, spleen, kidneys, testicles or lymph nodes. Unfortunately, although it is reliable, considerable time is consumed by this method.

Skin Test.—A number of investigators have found the skin test to be of value. A simple procedure is to inject 0.05 cc. of a very light killed suspension of Brucella intracutaneously. A positive reaction appears in twelve to forty-eight hours, characterized, first by an area of redness and heat the size of a nickel, later by an area of induration or by a local granulomatous lesion or abscess. Healing occurs in ten to thirty days, leaving a scar which may persist for months. The test is said to be specific, but should be used in conjunction with the other tests just described. It is of most diagnostic value when strongly positive. Negative or doubtfully positive tests are often unreliable and confusing. The reaction is regarded as a cutaneous, hypersensitive phenomenon.

Differential Diagnosis.—The absence of any special pathognomonic signs or symptoms, together with the previous lack of information and consideration, has served to confuse undulant fever with several other common infections. The most commonly considered diseases are mentioned below.

Typhoid fever is characterized by a more rapid onset, stupor, prostration, sustained high fever, tympanites, dicrotic pulse and no sweating. Positive blood and stool cultures and a positive Widal test prove the diagnosis. Because of the absence of distinctive signs, many obscure fevers are commonly and erroneously called *influenza* or intestinal influenza, for want of a better term. Undulant fever has frequently been designated as such, although there are no resemblances between influenza and undulant fever, aside from general aching and leukopenia. *Tuberculosis* may cause confusion. Both diseases commence insidiously and are characterized by weakness, weight loss, anorexia, night sweats and leukopenia.

Subacute bacterial endocarditis also offers difficulties in differential diagnosis. The early course of both infections is similar. Anemia, weight loss, joint pain, remittent fever and splenomegaly occur in both. *Malaria* is recognized by the presence of plasmodia in the blood or by response of the fever to quinine. In *acute rheumatic fever*, the joints are more seriously disturbed. They are red and hot and the pain is relieved by salicylates. Rheumatic fever commences more abruptly and there is leukocytosis. *Pyogenic* infections are usually accompanied by leukocytosis. *Tularemia* of the typhoidal type may give rise to confusion, especially if cross-agglutination occurs, as it sometimes does. Specific agglutination, history of exposure to wild rabbits or to other game and the clinical course assist in diagnosis.

Abdominal pain and tenderness occasionally suggest *acute appendicitis* or *cholecystitis;* more often a chronic or subacute form is suspected. A consideration of the whole clinical picture, together with leukopenia and positive immunologic findings, indicates undulant fever. It must be remembered that a weak agglutination titer may be present in an individual actually ill with appendicitis or cholecystitis of different origin. *Gonorrhea* was suspected in several males with undulant fever, whose outstanding symptoms were those of orchitis and vesiculitis.

Prognosis.—The average duration is three months. A case lasting seven days and one of eight years' duration have been reported. The duration of the disease in 212 patients, measured from the time the patient found it difficult to continue his regular work until he was symptom-free and able to resume it, was as follows:

19 per cent	1 month or less
27 "	1 month to 10 weeks
34 "	3 to 4 months
11 "	5 to 6 months
9 "	Over 6 months

The time spent in bed was as follows:

26 per cent	Less than 1 week
8 "	1 to 2 weeks
33 "	2 weeks to 1 month
24 "	1 month to 10 weeks
9 "	More than 10 weeks

The *mortality* ranges from 2 to 4 per cent and may increase to 14 per cent in epidemics. In many cases the fatal outcome has been attributed partly to the presence of other preceding illness. Caprine and porcine varieties of brucelliasis have a higher mortality than the bovine type. A high agglutination titer in some cases appears to be of favorable import. Returning appetite in spite of high fever may foretell an early recovery. Low fever with a low agglutination titer may presage a prolonged course.

Prophylaxis.—At present this concerns itself with the prevention of human contact with infected milk and animals. The first factor is comparatively simple to attack. Uncontaminated or pasteurized milk should be used. This precaution prevents transmission of infection to individuals at a distance. The question of human carriers of the disease has been raised, but is as yet unproved.

The problem of contact infection is vastly more difficult to approach considering the widespread prevalence of the disease in domestic animals. Precautions should be taken by individuals obliged to handle or come in contact with animals. Gloves may prevent infection. Great care should be taken in handling animals which have recently aborted. The foregoing suggestions apply chiefly to farmers, live stock dealers and veterinarians. Packing house employees, and laboratory workers who come in direct contact with infected tissues should avoid abrasions or wounds in the hands. Gloves again are of value. Special care must be exerted in handling living cultures.

Prophylactic vaccination with killed cultures of Brucella does not promise to be of value. Experimental attempts at immunization have not been successful.

The ultimate eradication of undulant fever depends upon the success attained in ridding domestic animals of the infection. This, obviously, is a veterinary problem of great magnitude and will take many years to accomplish.

Treatment.—The patient should be isolated and health authorities notified as soon as a diagnosis is made. Stools, urine and other excretions or secretions must be sterilized before disposal. Rest in bed, an adequate and agreeable diet to prevent emaciation and anemia, plenty of fluid, and the treatment of various special symptoms constitute the important procedure of therapy at present. Antipyretics, as such, should not be used, but substances like amidopyrine or aspirin may be used temporarily, in sufficiently large doses for the control of marked headache, backache, joint or other pains. Cool compresses or an ice-bag often give comfort. For high fever, a tepid or cool sponge followed by an alcohol rub is often pleasant for the patient. Bed rest, warm blankets and hot-water bottles are agreeable during periods of chilliness. Luminal or other hypnotics may be used judiciously when insomnia or nervousness are especially disturbing. Undue exercise or exertion are to be avoided since they often precipitate a relapse. Mild laxatives or mineral oil may be used to keep the bowels open. The addition of cooked fruits and vegetables to the diet is also desirable.

Special complications should be treated in the usual manner.

Treatment with specific antiserum is in the experimental stage.

Intravenous injections of various substances, including arsphenamine, colloidal metals, mercurochrome, as in most other infections, have no specific value.

The injection of a suspension of heat-killed Brucella at three-day intervals is looked upon favorably by some, but its use is still in the experimental stage. The temperature curve of a case thus treated is shown in Fig. 4.

The injection of non-specific foreign protein, according to some observers, has apparently shortened the course of the illness, but one hesitates to recommend its use except in an experimental way.

REFERENCES.

HARDY, A. V., JORDAN, C. F., BORTS, I. H., and HARDY, G. C.: Undulant Fever, Bull. 158, Nat. Inst. of Health, 1930, U. S. Treas. Dept. (bibliography).
SIMPSON, W. M.: Undulant Fever, Brucelliasis, Ann. Int. Med., 1930, 4, 238.
SMITH, T.: Undulant Fever, Medicine, 1929, 8, 193.
SPENGLER, G.: Wien. Arch. f. inn. Med., 1929, 19, 145 (bibliography of European literature).
WOHLWILL, F.: Zur pathologischen Anatomie der Bangerkrankung des Menschen, Virchow's Arch. f. path. Anat. u. Phys., 1932, 286, 141.

LEPROSY.

Definition.—Leprosy is a chronic, generalized, specific, infectious and contagious disease caused by Mycobacterium lepræ, characterized by granulomatous infiltration into the skin, mucous membranes, peripheral nerves and viscera.

History.—Leprosy is one of the oldest of diseases. The Egyptians recognized it before 1500 B.C. Leprosy is mentioned in the Bible. The disease was probably introduced into Europe from the Orient by Roman soldiers. Infection was reintroduced by returning Crusaders. Leprosy was once widespread in Europe but now exists in only a few foci. The New World probably became infected by wanderers and immigrants from endemic areas, chiefly from Africa, China and Norway.

The discovery of the lepra bacillus was first reported by Hansen in 1879. The use of chaulmoogra oil for treatment was practised by East Indians and Chinese for centuries. Mouart introduced it into modern therapeutics in 1854. Hansen observed its use for several years but dropped it as ineffectual. In recent years, with improvements in its preparation and administration, it has again come into wide use.

Incidence.—At present, the chief centers of leprosy are in tropical Africa, South America, India and China. Lesser centers exist in Russia, Turkey, Greece, Spain, Norway and Iceland. Leprosy is, in fact, widespread and has appeared in almost all portions of the world from the Arctic zone to the tropics. Rogers estimates that 3 million lepers exist.

In the United States the chief foci are in Louisiana and California. A national leprosarium exists in Louisiana. The focus among Norwegian settlers in Minnesota fifty years ago has disappeared. Sporadic cases occasionally appear in the large cities. There were 361 lepers in the National Leprosarium in Louisiana in 1934. Of 999 patients admitted since its opening, 672 were native born. Approximately 1200 lepers exist in continental United States (1926).

Almost all statistics show a predominance of infected males, usually from 66 to 74 per cent. Race, occupation, social status and climate have no bearing on the incidence. The average age of first infection is about twenty years; the age of onset in the American series is about thirty years. Infants and the aged are seldom afflicted. Close contact over a prolonged period is necessary to establish infection. The patient is the only source of infection. Theories regarding the soil as a source have not been generally accepted. Rogers found that of 700 patients, 80 per cent had lived in the same house with a leper, and about 30 per cent had shared the same bed with one before developing the disease. On the other hand, only 3 to 5 per cent of individuals thus exposed became infected. In another study it was shown that of 100 lepers, there were 64 instances in which only one member of a family was affected, but in 36 other cases leprosy occurred in 83 additional relatives. There appears to be a strong familial predilection or tendency to contract leprosy. In some families certain branches have been practically exterminated. Physicians and attendants exercising reasonable prophylaxis rarely acquire the disease.

Etiology.—Although Koch's postulates have never been satisfactorily fulfilled in regard to the cultivation of leprosy bacilli on artificial media and the reproduction of disease in animals or humans, it is generally accepted that the Mycobacterium lepræ is the causative agent. The lepra bacillus is closely related to the tubercle bacillus, which it resembles morphologically. It is somewhat plumper and does not display "beading." It is acid-fast and stains with difficulty with the usual dyes. In leprous tissue and exudates, bacilli are often found in such great numbers that stained sections appear pink to the unaided eye. Although many attempts have been made to cultivate the leprosy bacillus, the results have usually been negative. Many investigators have succeeded in isolating rapidly growing actinomyces or diphtheroids from leprous material, and from the soil in leprous areas, but their interpretation as etiologic agents is not generally accepted.

Attempts to transfer infection from human to human have been reported, but with unconvincing results. Natural infections probably result from the entrance of bacilli through the skin or mucous membrane. The frequent early involvement of the lower extremities has suggested to some the possibility of infection derived from the soil. It is most commonly believed, however, that the patient is the only source of infection. Bacilli are widely distributed in the bodies of lepers. They are found in large numbers in the skin lesions, peripheral nerves, liver, spleen, lymph nodes, kidneys and endothelium, often within "lepra cells." Bacilli appear in the blood at times during fever, and are found with great regularity in the nasal secretions or scrapings of many patients. The saliva and other secretions and excretions serve as a vehicle for the exit of bacilli from the body. Lepers are regarded as dangerous only if they are "open" cases, cases in which there are discharging ulcers or in whom lepra bacilli can be demonstrated in excised tissues, scrapings or in secretions or excretions. Old "healed" cases like those of healed tuberculosis are no menace and need not live in strict isolation. It must be borne in mind, however, that appar-

5

ently healed cases or even individuals who have never shown any evidence of the disease, may harbor bacilli. Such instances are considered as *latent infections*, in which the disease may flare up at any time.

Pathology.—Lepra bacilli may invade any tissue or organ in the body, but, like the spirochete of syphilis, have a predilection for skin and nerve tissue. In this respect, the biologic behavior is in contrast with that of the closely related tubercle bacillus which seldom invades skin or nerve tissue.

The chief pathologic reactions are granulomatous and inflammatory. The formation of granulomata (lepromata) dominate the picture of nodular or skin leprosy. They are pea- to walnut-size fibrous infiltrations of the skin and mucous membrane. They are composed chiefly of epithelioid cells, giant cells, plasma cells, lymphocytes and fibroblasts. Certain large mononuclear cells contain many lepra bacilli within large vacuoles, and are called *lepra cells*. Miliary lepromata are found scattered throughout the viscera. The lymph nodes are usually enlarged. Ulceration of the skin frequently follows trauma or involvement of the blood or nerve supply. The ulcers may heal and result in extensive and deforming scar formation.

In the neural or anesthetic form of leprosy, bacilli and granulation tissue are found in the perineurium and nerve substance. Nodular and fusiform swellings of the nerve trunk appear. Degeneration of the axis cylinders, anesthesia, atrophy, palsy and trophic ulcers result.

The inflammatory reaction occurs chiefly as a perivascular infiltration leading to thickening of the blood-vessel walls.

Symptoms.—The *incubation period* is difficult to determine in many cases. Long exposure is required for infection, and latent infection may persist for years. Furthermore, the onset may be so insidious that early symptoms are often disregarded. Estimates extend from a few months to thirty or more years. Rogers states that the incubation period did not exceed five years in 80 per cent of cases.

Initial manifestations are often the appearance of one or more spots on the body; less often the formation of a few nodules or of swelling of the extremities. Rhinitis, muscle contractions, fever or unexplained ulcerations are occasionally the first evidence of infection. The initial symptoms are uncharacteristic and are usually mistaken for more common conditions. In 28 per cent of cases of one series, the first lesion appeared on the face; in 20 per cent on the legs and feet. Patients may notice malaise, fever, somnolence, headache, anemia and vague aches for a long period of time. Definite evidence of leprosy occurs when the skin lesions become typical. Repeated eruptions of sharply defined reddish or violaceous patches occur which become brownish. The eruptions are often accompanied by fever. As the patches increase in size the centers are apt to become white and depigmented. The patches are infiltrated, hyperesthetic and later become anesthetic. Pale depigmented areas may also be present. Differentiation into the nodular (skin) or anesthetic (nerve) types gradually occurs. In the American series the skin type comprised 39 per cent of cases, the nerve type 11 per cent and the mixed type 50 per cent of cases. Pure types of either kind seldom exist. A predominance of one type or the other leads to respective classification. Change from one type to the other is occasionally observed.

The *cutaneous (nodular) type* is characterized by the development of subcutaneous nodular infiltrations which often appear in the sites of the first skin eruption. Long periods of time may elapse between the skin eruption and the development of the nodules. The nodules most commonly involve the face, back of the hands and feet, but rarely the scalp. Loss of facial hair and beard occurs. As the nodules enlarge the skin becomes deeply furrowed; the ear lobes, lips and nose become thickened, tending to cause resemblance to a lion's face. The nodules appear in crops and are accompanied by leprous fever. Some may disappear, while others continue to increase in size and cause great deformity. The infiltration may spread to other parts of the body surface. The general appearance of the skin is unhealthy. It is often dusky or "muddy," dry or scaling. The nails are often striated. Ulcerations occur rather easily. Ulcers may heal, but often penetrate deeply and spread, causing appalling mutilation. Various digits may drop off. Nodular infiltrations and ulceration of the mucous membrane lead to hoarseness and aphonia. Destruction of the cornea and conjunctiva results in blindness. Perforation of the nasal septum occurs.

The process may last as long as twenty years, during which time the general health may be fairly good. Most often the accompanying fever and "toxemia" cause malaise, anemia and cachexia. Patients often die of secondary infections, such as tuberculosis and pneumonia, and often from nephritis. Spontaneous recoveries have apparently occurred, but such reports must always be accepted with caution, bearing in mind that leprosy bacilli may be harbored in internal organs for years without producing symptoms. Furthermore, remission and exacerbation commonly occur.

The *neural (anesthetic) type* of leprosy is characterized by an onset which is even more insidious than that of the skin type. The nervous symptoms may appear very gradually and are most often accompanied by the development of round or irregular varicolored skin plaques, more or less symmetrically distributed on the extensor surfaces of the extremities and on the back. The macules or plaques may coalesce and heal in the areas first involved. The involved areas are first hyperesthetic, later anesthetic. Pruritus and neuralgic pains occur. At this period the nerve trunks are usually tender and later the superficial nerves can often be palpated as thickened nodular cords. Anesthesia often commences peripherally and extends centripetally. Anesthesia may be complete. Burns and other traumata often incite the formation of ulcers which tend to become deep and mutilating. Secretory and trophic disorders are common. Trophic ulcers of the soles of the feet are common. Atrophy of muscles occurs, often affecting the muscles of the hand. The contracture leads to the characteristic "claw" hand. Gangrene or ulceration of the extremities or other portions of the body cause horrible deformity.

Mixed forms of leprosy are represented by combinations of the skin and nerve type. At a recent conference in Manila (1931) it was decided to drop the term "mixed," since it served no useful purpose.

Of the other portions of the body, the genital organs are most often implicated. Lymph nodes are often swollen. Fetid bronchitis and bronchopneumonia are frequently seen. The spleen is occasionally enlarged. There is usually a secondary anemia present; a normal, slightly increased or decreased number of leukocytes and often an eosinophilia. Bacilliemia occurs during febrile periods.

Diagnosis.—Early diagnosis, when recognition is most important, is often impossible. Unless leprosy is in mind, many other common diseases are considered first, until the characteristic changes appear. When leprosy is suspected or when patients come from endemic centers, they must be stripped and examined in a good light to detect early skin manifestations. When nodules or ulcers are present, diagnosis is confirmed if lepra bacilli are found in bits of excised tissue or in aspirated or discharged exudates. Bacilli can often be found in the nasal secretions or scrapings. Lepra bacilli must, of course, be differentiated from other acid-fast bacilli. Lepers often exhibit delayed but marked hypersensitive reactions to tuberculin. The Wassermann reaction is occasionally positive in non-syphilitic lepers. Outspoken, advanced cases with typical skin lesions are easily recognized by the mottled, pink, violet-brown or depigmented patches. Patches of anesthesia and nodular infiltration of the ear lobes, nose and lips, atrophy of muscles, mutilation, thickening and tenderness of nerve trunks are important diagnostic features.

Differential Diagnosis.—Syphilis and tuberculosis are probably the most important diseases to be considered. Early syphilis is proved by the demonstration of Treponema pallidum; late syphilis by the Wassermann reaction. Tuberculosis is diagnosed by isolating and identifying the Mycobacterium tuberculosis. A good discussion of the differentiation of leprosy from other common skin diseases is given by Hopkins and Denney.

Prognosis.—The average duration, in one series of cases, computed from the onset of symptoms until death occurred, was about fourteen years.

The prognosis in modern times is more hopeful than in the past. In America the mortality has declined from 126 per 1000 thirty years ago to about 72 per 1000 at present. The decrease is largely due to improvement in institutional treatment and in the earlier recognition of cases. The number of patients discharged as "cured" or arrested cases from various leprosaria appears to be increasing. In the American series, paroles were granted after repeated physical and bacteriologic examinations had been negative for eighteen months. Relapses after such careful precautions were reduced from 30 to 3 per cent. The effect of chemotherapy on prognosis is as yet uncertain.

Of 107 deaths, only 18 per cent were directly due to leprosy; the remainder succumbed to pneumonia, tuberculosis, nephritis, septicemia following gangrene, cardiovascular disease and other secondary accidents or suicides.

Treatment.—"Open" cases must be strictly isolated. Secretions and excretions must be disposed of so as to avoid infecting others. Physicians and attendants should avoid intimate or prolonged contact with lepers. Reasonable care such as that practised in the management of pulmonary tuberculosis usually prevents contagion. Arrested cases may be paroled after prolonged observation, but must still be kept under supervision lest relapse occur. Intelligent and humane isolation or segregation has done much to remove the tendency to conceal the disease. More early cases now present themselves for observation and treatment.

Patients are best treated in leprosaria where efforts are made to improve the patients' general health. Cleanliness, adequate diet and symptomatic treatment are most important. Physiotherapy, psychotherapy and rehabilitation accomplish much in improving the outlook on life. Frequent hot baths and a change of climate are often helpful.

Specific Therapy.—Chaulmoogra oil and its various derivatives and modifications are recommended by some observers, but are considered as remedies of unproved value by others. The oil is given by mouth in capsules in doses beginning with 0.3 to 0.6 cc. (5 to 10 minims) increasing to 4 to 8 cc. (1 to 2 drams), if tolerated. It is often irritating to the stomach. Intramuscularly, a mixture of chaulmoogra oil with camphorated oil and resorcin is injected in 0.3 to 3 cc. doses, twice a week. Various esters of the oil have been prepared and are less painful and irritating when injected. The oil is absorbed slowly. The best results are obtained in early cases. Various other methods of chemotherapy are discussed by Rogers.

Roentgen-ray or light treatments have, at times, a favorable influence on the skin lesions. Complications require appropriate medical, orthopedic or surgical treatment, as the case may be.

REFERENCES.

DENNEY, O. E., HOPKINS, R., and JOHANSEN, F. A.: Recoveries from Leprosy, Am. Jour. Trop. Med., 1930, **10**, 83.
DEYCKE, G.: Die Lepra, Spez. Pathol. u. Therap. d. inn. Krankh., Kraus, Brugsch, Berlin, 1919, **2**, 469.
HOPKINS, R., and DENNEY, O. E.: Statistical Study of 700 Cases, U. S. Pub. Health Rep., 1929, **44**, 695; Jour. Am. Med. Assn., 1929, **92**, 191.
———— Comments on Some of the Characteristics of Nodular Leprosy, Internat. Clin., 1931, **2**, 117.
ROGERS, L.: Treatment and Prophylaxis of Leprosy, Edinburgh Med. Jour., 1930, **37**, 1.
ROGERS, L., and MUIR, E.: Leprosy, John Wright and Sons, Bristol, 1925.
WALKER, E. L.: Some New Aspects on the Etiology and Endemiology of Leprosy, Jour. Prevent. Med., 1929, **3**, 167.

TETANUS.

Definition.—Tetanus is an acute infectious disease of the central nervous system caused by Clostridium tetani, characterized by hyperirritability of the motor nerve centers and tonic contractions of the musculature due to the action of tetanus toxin.

History.—Tetanus was described by Hippocrates, who gave a general rule for prognosis of the disease which is still valid. The infectious nature was first suspected by Giesinger and Strümpell about 1865, after tetanus had been produced in rabbits by the inoculation of material obtained from a patient. Nicolaier in 1885 produced tetanus by injecting garden soil into experimental animals and was the first to observe the specific organisms. A year later Rosenbach demonstrated tetanus bacilli in the wound secretion of a patient. Kitasato, by employing anaërobic technic, first cultivated the bacillus in 1887.

Etiology.—Clostridium tetani is a slender bacillus with slightly rounded ends. It is easily stained with the usual dyes and is classified as a Gram-positive bacillus although it is occasionally decolorized by alcohol. Motility is slight and is due to numerous delicate flagella. There are several characteristic features: (*a*) the production of end-spores in old cultures causing the typical drum-stick appearance, (*b*) the preference of anaërobic conditions for growth, and (*c*) the formation of a soluble toxin. The spores are very resistant to weak disinfectants and survive heating to 60° or 70° C., but are killed by five minutes' exposure to live steam and by direct sunlight. Bacilli may remain viable under certain conditions for years. They are often difficult or impossible to find in wounds. Growth takes place readily in slightly alkaline meat-infusion broth under anaërobic conditions. Gelatin is liquefied. The presence of carbohydrates enhances growth. Acid is formed in carbohydrate media.

Tetanus toxin (tetanospasmin) is one of the most powerful poisons known. An antitoxin can be produced artificially which neutralizes free toxin, both *in vitro* and *in vivo*. The toxin has an affinity for nervous tissue, and when once absorbed by protoplasm cannot be neutralized by antitoxin. Behring and Kitasato showed that animals could be rendered immune to tetanus toxin by previous repeated injection of small doses.

Pathogenesis.—The tetanus bacillus or spores may gain entrance into the body through any wound, however slight, but because of the special growth requirements and of the defensive mechanism of the host, growth may fail to occur. Tetanus bacilli may be present in a wound and the patient may not develop the disease. In certain cases the bacilli encounter favorable conditions for multiplication and disease follows. The presence of injured, devitalized or necrotic tissue, fragments of metal, wood, clothing or soil imbedded in the wound, and the presence of secondary infection provide media desirable for growth. Other factors influencing the occurrence of tetanus are the degree of susceptibility or resistance of the host and the number of bacilli or spores introduced. Certain types of wounds especially favor the development of tetanus. The most important are deep, penetrating, perforating, lacerating or crushing wounds in which particles of foreign matter containing tetanus bacilli or spores are carried deeply into the tissues and remain there. The presence of devitalized tissue and the exclusion of air furnish conditions suitable for growth. Once growth becomes established, bacilli multiply and liberate soluble exotoxin. Multiplication usually takes place locally at the site of entrance, but bacilli may be transported elsewhere, and have been found in the spinal fluid. A definite period of time elapses between the time of infection and the appearance of symptoms. Abel has questioned the theories current for years that the toxin reaches the central nervous system by way of the nerves or their lymphatics. He presents convincing evidence that the toxin is transported solely by the blood stream. The central nervous system is the chief site of action because of the apparent affinity of the toxin for nerve tissue. Some believe that the toxin acts directly on the lower motor neurones, on the hind-brain and cord, and may cause death from respiratory failure during a convulsion, due to spasm of the glottis, diaphragm and intercostal muscles. There is also a general increase of reflex sensitivity.

Pathology.—There are no characteristic pathologic findings in tetanus. Parenchymatous degeneration and hyperemia of the brain and other organs may be present. Slight perivascular infiltration and nerve cell changes have been described. The primary site of infection may be inflamed and contain tetanus bacilli or may be entirely healed.

Epidemiology.—Although the soil of many parts of the world contains tetanus spores, tetanus is a comparatively rare and sporadic disease. The natural habitat of the bacillus appears to be in the intestinal tract of cattle, horses and man. Studies have shown that one out of four individuals carries tetanus bacilli in his intestine. It is surprising, then, that tetanus does not occur more frequently. Soil fertilized with manure is most apt to be infected; the soil of deserts or forests is less likely to be contaminated with tetanus spores. It was at one time believed that the soil of certain limited localities was especially heavily infected, but this is probably due to the richly fertilized soil in these localities. The frequency of tetanus during the World War in the highly cultivated fields of northern France and the rarity of tetanus in the Boer War, which was fought on uncultivated soil, are cases in point. Small epidemics of tetanus frequently break out after battles and after fêtes celebrated with explosives and firearms. Sporadic cases occur following burns, frost-bite, bee sting, varicose ulcers, bed sores, fractures, surgical operations, intramuscular injections, otitis media, infected teeth and in wounds soiled with feces. Contaminated cat-gut and vaccine have been responsible for some cases. Vaccination wounds tightly covered with court-plaster or other dressings have been followed by tetanus. Tetanus neonatorum resulting from unhygienic management of the umbilical cord is a frequent condition in the tropics.

Incidence.—In the United States, 1488 deaths from tetanus occurred in 1922. The incidence in recent years has no doubt been reduced somewhat due to a number of causes, chiefly to the use of prophylactic treatment, the disappearance of horses and manure from city streets and the diminution of Fourth of July accidents. The greatest number of cases occurs during the summer months. Tetanus is more common in the tropics than elsewhere. Although males and females are equally susceptible, many more cases occur in males (3 or 4 to 1) due to the greater risk of exposure to wounds and infection. The disease is commonest between the ages of ten to twenty years.

The value of prophylactic antitoxin in diminishing the incidence is strikingly shown in army statistics. During the Civil War, 2 per 1000 of wounds were followed by tetanus; in the World War when prophylaxis was enforced, only 0.014 per 1000 of battle injuries later developed tetanus.

Clinical Varieties.—Superfluous classification is sometimes made according to the mode of infection, such as traumatic, postoperative, puerperal, visceral or tetanus neonatorum. In certain cases, "localized" tetanus occurs.

Local tetanus is an unusual condition which may develop when prophylactic antitoxin has failed to give complete protection. The effects of the toxin are limited to the muscles near the primary wound. There is local pain, increase of reflexes and tonic spasm of the involved muscles. Symptoms may persist for weeks or months (chronic tetanus).

Symptoms.—The *incubation period* usually lasts seven days. It may be as short as one day or may last for several weeks or months. The incubation time is markedly prolonged by the injection of antitoxin after the injury. During the World War the incubation period averaged twelve days before antitoxin was used and fifty days after prophylactic injection was enforced.

Prodromal symptoms may occur; there is often a sense of drawing pain in the wound with twitching of adjacent muscles, and restlessness, insomnia, irritability, headache, chilliness and fever may take place. In children recurrent convulsions have been noted. Early symptoms are sometimes masked by the severity of the primary wound or by secondary infection. Diagnosis at this early stage is of great importance if specific therapy is to be given.

The *onset* is usually characterized by stiffness of the muscles of the jaw and neck. It becomes more and more difficult to open the mouth, bend the head or to swallow. Presently the jaws may be clamped shut (trismus) and the neck becomes rigid. Attempts to take food or drink often precipitate or intensify the spasms. Due to the contraction of the facial muscles the corners of the mouth are drawn back and the eyebrows raised, causing the typical grinning expression (risus sardonicus). The abdominal muscles and later other muscle groups become involved. Occasionally, in severe cases, the disease reaches its height in twenty-four hours. Involvement of the lumbar, abdominal and thoracic muscles produces straight rigidity or arching of the back (opisthotonos). Arching to the side or forward is less common. Spasms and convulsive seizures are exceedingly severe and painful. Muscles are occasionally ruptured. Spasms occur spontaneously or may be precipitated by various stimuli such as sudden noises, jars or even by currents of air or sudden bright lights. Three to 40 spasms per hour may occur. Most of the reflexes are exaggerated. Involvement of the thoracic muscles may interfere with respiration. Spasm of the glottis may cause deep cyanosis and asphyxia. Retention of urine and feces may be caused by muscle spasm. The convulsions are agonizing and exhausting. They are followed by profuse sweating, dyspnea, tachycardia and collapse. Seizures are prevented only by sleep, coma or during narcosis. Fever of a moderate grade is often present, but it may be absent. Fatal hyperpyrexia may occur. The mentality remains clear throughout the illness, which adds to the distress. A coated tongue and constipation are the rule. Death is due to exhaustion, to asphyxia or to complications.

There is usually a polymorphonuclear leukocytosis, ranging from 10,000 to 15,000. The spinal fluid remains normal until intraspinal therapy is begun when leukocytes and globulin appear.

Complications.—The embarrassment of respiration during the convulsion, together with the aspiration of secretions during narcosis, often results in bronchitis or bronchopneumonia. Rupture of muscles with hemorrhage occasionally occurs. As sequelæ, various groups of muscles may be slightly stiff or shortened for years thereafter. Neuritis and insomnia occur. Relapse which may prove fatal may occur.

Diagnosis.—Diagnosis in outspoken cases is simple. The history of a wound followed after a period of time by trismus, convulsive seizures and opisthotonos leaves little room for doubt. In certain cases when the onset is gradual, the spasm and pain in the muscles of the neck and jaw may be mistaken for sore throat or tonsillitis, abscess of a tooth, inflammation of the tongue or other regional inflammatory processes. Arthritis of the mandibula or of cervical vertebræ may be suspected. Rigidity of the neck may suggest meningitis. The latter is ruled out by the absence of headache, herpes, pupillary changes, vomiting and an undisturbed sensorium. Absence of changes in the cerebrospinal fluid is conclusive.

In certain cases of tetanus the spasms evoked by attempts to drink or eat closely resemble the behavior during hydrophobia. In hydrophobia there is usually a history of being bitten by a rabid animal and, as a rule, only the muscles of deglutition are involved.

Strychnine poisoning greatly resembles tetanus. The attacks, however, are usually more sudden and affect the extremities first. The convulsions are separated by intervals of complete relaxation. Death or recovery occurs soon. A history of taking the poison, or the demonstration of strychnine in the stomach contents is diagnostic.

Tetany is easily ruled out by the characteristic spasms of the extremities and by the history of antecedent disorder. Hysterical contractions may be confusing for a time until their nature is determined.

Bacteriologic diagnosis is often difficult or impossible. In a few cases bacilli may be demonstrated in the primary wound. Anaërobic cultures made from wounds are usually contaminated with other bacteria. Such mixed growths should be heated to 70° C. for several minutes to kill off the contaminants, and leave tetanus spores unharmed. Further transfers are then made to dextrose-agar and cultivated anaërobically or injected subcutaneously, together with powdered glass or pumice, into mice. Death from tetanus occurs in two or three days.

Prognosis.—The prognosis in general is serious. It has been known for centuries that the longer the incubation period, the better the chances for recovery. In this respect prophylactic antitoxin which delays the onset or entirely prevents the disease, has been of great value. According to Bruce, antitoxin administered within four days after the injury reduced the mortality to 20 per cent among the few cases in which tetanus finally developed. Cases receiving several prophylactic injections showed a mortality-rate of 7 per cent. It is probably impossible to lower the general death-rate below 5 or 10 per cent since many cases succumb to secondary infection (Ghon and Roman), shock of the accident, pneumonia or hemorrhage.

The prognosis is influenced also by the duration of the disease; the longer the patient lives the better his chance for recovery. In Hill's large series the average mortality during the first five days was over 80 per cent; from the fifth to the tenth day 74 per cent. Beyond this time it was about 34 per cent. In cases lasting twenty days the mortality was 6 per cent. The nature of the wound has a bearing on prognosis; in Calvin and Goldberg's series of 183 cases the case mortality from gunshot and powder wounds was 95 per cent, while that from lacerating wounds was 44 per cent. Cases of tetanus following wounds of the head in their series, contrary to previous belief, were no more fatal than those of other parts of the body.

Opinion is still divided in regard to the effect of specific antitoxin therapy on the prognosis. The majority of recent observers feel that serum therapy has been disappointing and has not influenced the mortality-rate according to the statistics of large numbers of cases.

Unfavorable portents are the early appearance of severe symptoms, severe trismus, spasm of the glottis, respiratory or circulatory failure and high fever. The presence of large, infected wounds or other diseases adds to the gravity of the illness. Tetanus is more fatal in infants and children than in adults.

Prophylaxis.—Prophylaxis is of utmost importance in tetanus. All wounds acquired in localities in which the soil is likely to be infected, *i. e.*, farm-yards, gardens, fields, stables and highways should be treated as potential foci of tetanus. Gunshot and powder wounds appear to be especially dangerous. The wound should be opened, necrotic tissue and foreign bodies should be removed. A weak solution of tincture of iodine, hydrogen peroxide or Dakin's solution may be used to irrigate the area. Caustics or cautery are contraindicated and the wound should not be covered with air-tight dressings. As soon after the injury as possible, tetanus antitoxin (1500 U.S.A. units) should be injected subcutaneously. Injections should be repeated at weekly intervals until the wound is healed. Some have recommended the injection of antitoxin into the wound as well. Of recent years it has been recommended to add Bacillus perfringens (gas bacillus) antitoxin to the vaccine.

The incubation period of tetanus in cases receiving prophylactic antitoxin was increased from eleven to fifty days. The beneficial effects were strikingly shown in statistics from the British army during the World War. Before 1915 antitoxin was not generally used. After this time prophylaxis was enforced. The results are shown in the following table:

Percentage mortality of cases of tetanus in the World War:

1914	55 per cent
1915	56 "
1916	37 "
1917	20 "

Educational propaganda carried on by the American Medical Association against the use of explosives in celebrating Independence Day and other fêtes has done much to reduce the incidence of tetanus.

Treatment.—After the development of tetanus the patient should be placed in a darkened, quiet room. All sudden and loud noises or vibrations are prohibited. The patient is best moved, washed or otherwise manipulated during induced narcosis. The primary wound, if present, should be treated as described under prophylaxis. Taylor recommends complete excision of the wound whenever possible or complete exposure and search for foreign bodies under general anesthesia even if the wound appears to be healed. Feeding and the administration of fluids is sometimes difficult, especially if trismus is marked. A narrow stomach-tube may be passed through the nose or through the spaces of missing teeth, if necessary. Food and fluid may be introduced in this manner after making certain that the end of the tube is in the stomach. It may be necessary to administer fluid subcutaneously or intravenously, 500 to 1000 cc. of warm physiologic saline solution being injected slowly, several times a day, and 200 cc. of a 25 per cent solution of dextrose may also be given in this way several times daily for nutrition. Catheterization of the bladder and the administration of enemas are often required. Patients must be constantly watched to prevent injury during convulsions and to guard against death from asphyxia. Patients must be kept warm and covered.

In mild cases sedatives may suffice to control the irritable reflexes. Bromides in large doses, or luminal, 0.18 to 0.3 gm. (3 to 5 grains), are recommended. Care must be exercised in the use of drugs which are followed by toxic or cumulative effects, when given over a period of time. Many other depressant drugs have been used: chloral, chlorbutanol, hyoscine, morphine and chloroform. The ideal anesthetic is one whose effect is protracted, which is rapidly eliminated and which produces no harmful effects on other organs. The danger of aspiration pneumonia exists with any form of anesthesia.

The intravenous or intraspinous injection of a 25 per cent solution of magnesium sulphate, 1 cc. for each 10 kg. (22 pounds) of body weight, has been used in some cases with success. Injections are given several times a day intravenously, or once a day intraspinally. The danger from respiratory failure is considerable and can be corrected when threatened by the intravenous injection of 3 to 5 cc. of a 5 per cent solution of calcium chloride.

Tribromethanol ("avertin") and sodium isoamylethyl barbiturate ("sodium amytal") are the most satisfactory sedatives thus far employed. Doses of either drug can be regulated so as to keep the patient under moderate narcosis continuously. From 60 to 80 mg. of "avertin" per kg. of body weight may be injected per rectum several times daily or less often if desirable. The chief danger is a fall in blood pressure and respiratory failure. "Sodium amytal," 0.4 to 0.6 gram (6 to 9 grains) by mouth may be given at suitable intervals. In certain cases it may be necessary to administer the drug intramuscularly.

Specific Therapy.—The effect of antitoxin in the treatment of tetanus has been disappointing to some, but its use is strongly supported by others. Some recommend intravenous injection alone and others favor intraspinal treatment, or a combination of intravenous and intraspinal therapy.

The rational use of antitoxin is based on its ability to neutralize toxin formed by the growth of bacilli. Unfortunately, the toxin becomes fixed to nerve protoplasm from which it cannot be dislocated by antitoxin. Nevertheless, the favorable results of experiments on monkeys by Sherrington, in which treatment by the intraspinal route proved most efficacious and the clinical benefit occasionally observed after specific therapy, justify the continued use of serum and should stimulate efforts to produce a better antitoxin.

Method of Serotherapy.—If serum is to be given, the patient should be tested for sensitivity to horse serum and desensitized if necessary. Serum, to have any beneficial effect, must be given early in the disease. It is usually wisest to administer serum while the patient is anesthetized. For short periods of anesthesia, chloroform has been often used. Twenty thousand units are given at a time, every six or eight hours intraspinally, intravenously or intramuscularly. From numerous studies it would seem unnecessary to administer more than 60,000 units unless the case is protracted, when the dose may be repeated.

REFERENCES.

ABEL, J. J.: On Poisons and Disease and Some Experiments with Toxin of the Bacillus Tetani, Science, 1934, **79**, 121.
CALVIN, J. K., and GOLDBERG, A. H.: The Prognosis of Tetanus, Jour. Am. Med. Assn., 1930, **94**, 1977.
HILL, E. W.: Tetanus, Arch. Int. Med., 1911, **8**, 747.
TAYLOR, F. W.: Study of the Treatment in Acute Tetanus, Jour. Am. Med. Assn., 1934, **102**, 895.

TULAREMIA.

Synonyms.—Deer-fly fever; Rabbit fever; Francis' disease.

Definition.—Tularemia is an acute infectious disease, primarily of animals but transmissible to man, caused by Pasteurella tularensis, often characterized by the development of a primary ulcer and by the formation of tubercle-like necrotic foci in the liver, spleen and lymph nodes.

History.—The disease is known to have occurred among market-men for at least thirty years, as "rabbit fever." In 1907 Martin, in a personal letter, described 5 cases, in 3 of which the eye was involved. The first published report was made by Pearse, in 1911, who called the disease "deer-fly fever." The causative agent was discovered during researches on plague in California by McCoy and Chapin of the U. S. Public Health Service, and reported in 1912. They discovered a "plague-like" disease among squirrels in Tulare County and called the etiologic organism Bacterium tularense. Human infection with Pasteurella tularensis was described by Wherry in 1912, and by Vail in 1914. Francis, in 1919, recognized the identity of the organism causing the "plague-like disease of rodents" and "deer-fly fever," named the disease tularemia, and paved the way for its widespread recognition.

Etiology.—Pasteurella tularensis (Bacterium tularense) is closely related to organisms causing plague and to a rare condition known as pseudotuberculosis. It is a Gram-negative pleomorphic organism which grows slowly on blood-glucose-cystin agar or on coagulated egg-yolk. No growth occurs on plain agar or in broth. Coccoid, bacillary and bipolar-staining forms occur. It is not motile and forms no spores. The organisms are killed at 56° C. for ten minutes, by 0.1 per cent formalin in twenty-four hours and by 1 per cent tricresol in two minutes. Pasteurella tularensis remains viable and virulent in frozen rabbits for three weeks and in bedbugs for twenty-six days. The organisms are virulent for mice, guinea-pigs and rabbits; produce areas of focal necrosis in the liver, spleen or lymph nodes and cause death within a week.

Epidemiology.—Among *animals*, wild rabbits appear to be most commonly involved although many other rodents have been found to be infected. Green found tularemia to be most prevalent among rabbits during the average ten-year cycle when the rabbit population is at its height. The disease is probably a factor in causing the periodic decimation of wild rabbits, and in causing epizoötics among other species. Sheep, coyotes, cats, quail and grouse have also been found to be infected. Tularemia is transmitted from animal to animal by means of deer-flies, wood-ticks, rabbit-ticks, fleas and lice; from anima to bird and from bird to bird by the rabbit-tick. Animals ingesting infected flesh are apt to become infected or to become temporary carriers. No other specific organism has been found to invade so many different species of animals and birds. Horses, cattle, dogs and chickens are immune.

Tularemia in *man* is derived from at least three sources; (a) directly from the tissues of infected animals, (b) through the agency of blood-sucking insects which have previously fed on infected animals or birds, and (c) from laboratory infections. Less common sources are the bites of infected or carrier animals, the ingestion of partially cooked infected flesh, and by the inhalation of viable bacilli (droplet infection). Tularemia is an occupational disease affecting chiefly market-men, hunters and housewives who handle game, veterinarians and laboratory workers. Man to man infection is rare, but must be recognized as a possibility since one case has been reported.

Incidence.—Up to 1924, only 15 cases had been reported. Due to recognition, and not to the spread of the disease, thousands of cases have been reported since then. In 1932, 945 cases and 41 deaths were reported in the United States. Without doubt, many more undiagnosed cases occur. Tularemia has been recognized in almost every state in the Union, and in Canada. In Japan, tularemia was formerly called Ohara's disease. More than 1000 cases occurred in Russia in 1929 as a result of floods and subsequent human contact with the water vole, a rodent. Tularemia exists in Scandinavia and in Spain. With the increased interest in the disease and the perfection of diagnostic methods, it will, no doubt, be found to be widespread throughout the temperate zone.

The seasonal incidence depends upon the locality. West of the Mississippi River in areas infested with ticks and deer-flies, infections are more apt to occur during the warm months. In the eastern states the incidence increases after the opening of the hunting season, when contact with infected rabbits is afforded. Most of the cases occur in November and December.

Both sexes are equally susceptible. Adult males are most frequently infected due to greater chances for exposure.

Pathogenesis.—In man the organisms are introduced by blood-sucking insects, by applying cultures or infected tissues to abrasions or cuts, or to the unbroken skin or mucous membranes, and probably by inhalation. Frequently, infection is carried by contaminated fingers to the conjunctiva, where the primary ulcer occurs. Mme. Ohara was experimentally infected by rubbing rabbit tissue into the unbroken skin of her hand. The organisms multiply locally, enter the lymphatics and are carried to the regional lymph nodes, which become enlarged. Sudden and severe constitutional symptoms usually develop with the lymph node involvement. In some cases, organisms pass through the unbroken skin and cause no primary ulcer; enlarged lymph nodes and constitutional symptoms are the first manifestation of infection. In other cases no lymph node involvement is evident.

Bacteria pass the lymph node barrier, enter the blood stream and are distributed generally. Due to their predilection for lymphoid tissue they tend to localize in the lymph nodes, liver, spleen and lungs, where granulomatous lesions are produced. Pasteurella tularensis can be easily recovered from the blood, liver and spleen of experimental animals, and with more difficulty from the human blood and tissues. They have been isolated from the spinal fluid. The pathogenesis of tularemia is similar to that of plague.

Pathology.—The characteristic pathologic features are the ulcer at the site of infection and the areas of focal necrosis in the lymph nodes, spleen, liver and lungs. The lesions in man are granulomatous in nature and identical with those in animals. The liver and spleen are usually enlarged and studded with discrete or confluent, pin-head sized whitish spots—tubercles. The presence of numerous grayish-white flecks in the liver and spleen is at first suggestive of miliary tuberculosis. The cut surfaces show similar changes; the centers of the larger nodules are necrotic, softened and depressed. In some cases one or the other organ may be free from macroscopic nodules. Similar changes are often found in various lymph nodes, especially in those receiving drainage from the primary ulcer.

Histologically, submiliary areas of focal necrosis are found similar in nature to the macroscopic lesions. They are composed of collections of epithelioid cells, proliferated reticulo-endothelial cells and multi-nucleated cells. Typical giant cells of the Langhans type are rarely found. Karyorrhexis and necrosis are found in the center of the nodules, especially in the large ones. Pasteurella tularensis in clumps and in vast numbers can often be demonstrated in animal tissue, and with more difficulty in human tissue, when stained with Nile-blue sulphate (Foshay). The organisms may be found inside the nodules or in the surrounding tissue. They are found located both intra-cellularly and extracellularly.

The primary ulcer shows unspecific diffuse necrosis, nuclear fragmentation and polymorphonuclear cell infiltration. Lymphangitis and suppuration of the regional lymphatics and lymph nodes occasionally occur. The lungs frequently contain nodules of focal necrosis or patches of pneumonia. The tracheobronchial lymph nodes are fre-

quently enlarged. General peritonitis, pleurisy with effusion, ulcerations in the cecum, meningitis and encephalitis have been observed.

Symptoms.—The incubation period usually lasts from two to four
days after infection, but varies from one to twelve days. The onset
is usually abrupt. The patient may be stricken while at work or during
sleep. Severe headache, high fever, chills, sweating, prostration, aching
pains in the back and limbs, vomiting, abdominal cramps and delirium
may occur. Sore throat and aching of the eyeballs are rather common.

Although tularemia usually runs a fairly uniform clinical course
and can be considered as a unity, Francis recognizes several forms,
classified according to the site of the primary ulcer or its absence;
namely, *ulceroglandular* or *oculoglandular; glandular,* if the regional
lymph nodes are palpable without primary ulcer; and *typhoidal* when
neither lymph nodes nor ulcer are evident. The relative frequency
of types under this classification of 540 cases is as follows:

Ulceroglandular	455
Oculoglandular	32
Glandular	25
Typhoidal	28
	540

Except for the presence and location of the ulcer, the clinical features
are similar in all forms. Marked involvement of any special system
or organ may cause a predominance of certain symptoms as, for
example, those of arthralgia, meningitis or pneumonia.

A day or two after the onset of the constitutional symptoms, pain,
swelling and tenderness in the regional lymph nodes is noted in patients
who develop an ulcer. Pain, swelling and the formation of a papule
take place next at the site of infection, which up to this time has been
unnoticed or healed. The papule usually suppurates and leaves an
ulcer about ½ inch in diameter with raised edges and a punched-out
appearance. The lesion heals slowly and is replaced by scar tissue.
Lymphangitis and later suppuration of the lymph channels may occur.
The regional lymph nodes, most often the epitrochlear and axillary,
suppurate in about one-half of the cases. Subcutaneous nodules are
frequently seen proximal to the primary lesion. In certain cases, the
epitrochlear or axillary lymph nodes alone are involved without a
primary ulcer. The lymph nodes are frequently as large as walnuts
or eggs. The overlying skin is often reddened.

Similar changes are noted when the ulcer is located in the conjunctiva. In the early stage, irritation, lachrymation and edema are present.
A papule or ulcer develops, usually on the lower lid, accompanied by
swelling of the pre-auricular, parotid, submaxillary or cervical lymph
nodes. Small ulcers may appear on both lids. Blindness rarely results.

Constitutional reaction occurs when the lymphatics become involved
or else constitutes the only symptoms in those cases in which both
ulcer and lymphadenopathy are absent. The symptoms are a continuation or aggravation of those which develop at the onset, namely,
headache, fever, chills, sweats, prostration, vomiting, tachycardia,
abdominal pains and, in addition, epistaxis and cough.

The severity of the attack varies considerably. Some individuals, when obliged to, are able to continue work, but the majority are forced to bed where they remain for two or three weeks, as a rule. Mild and unrecognized ambulatory cases no doubt occur. Fulminating cases occur and have probably been frequently undiagnosed.

In certain patients evidence of bronchitis and pneumonia is manifested by pain in the chest, cough and bloody sputum. Specific meningitis and peritonitis occur. Severe shifting joint pains and neuralgia are at times distressing.

Signs.—Fever rises abruptly and may reach 104° F. (40° C.) or more. The fever curve may remain at a high level with but slight fluctuation or may exhibit marked daily remissions. A distinct period of remission of fever and symptoms may occur after one, two or three days of initial fever, lasts one, two or three days, and is followed by a secondary rise of high temperature. (Fig. 5.)

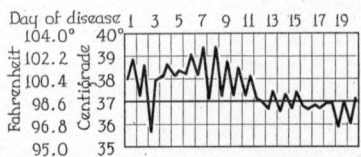

Fig. 5.—Temperature chart, typhoid type of tularemia. Male, aged thirty years, laboratory attendant. Onset marked by weakness, stiff joints, pain on deep inspiration, chill, fever and sweating. The later course was marked by weakness, aching of the eyeballs, blurred vision, neuralgic pains, backache, soreness of the abdomen, chilliness and epistaxis. Coughing occurred on the seventh and eighth days. The remission of fever on the third day was accompanied by a temporary relaxation of symptoms; the patient returned to work for a few hours but was soon forced to return to bed. Agglutination titer on the third day, 0; ninth day, 80; sixteenth day, 1280; twenty-third day, 320; forty-second day, 320. (Parker and Spencer.)

Skin eruptions are observed in about 5 per cent of cases. They are manifested in numerous ways, as macules, papules, vesicles, pustules or a combination of these types of eruption. The involved areas may desquamate later. The spleen is frequently palpable. Leukocytosis up to 15,000 is the rule.

Prognosis.—Confinement to bed for ten days to three weeks is the rule. Often a much longer time is required. Recovery is often very slow, especially in the more severe cases. *Convalescence* usually requires three or four months and occasionally is prolonged to a year. Lymphatic suppuration may occur at any time during convalescence and has been observed as long as two years after the original attack. Other sequelæ are rare. Relapses and recrudescences are common and are often precipitated by physical or other strain. They may appear months after the original attack and are usually mild. It is said that one attack confers lasting immunity.

Death occurs, according to the available statistics, in from 4 to 11 per cent of cases. Death is caused by overwhelming infection, pneumonia, peritonitis or meningitis. Fulminating cases may die in four days. Death has occurred as long as five months after the onset.

Complications.—Pneumonia, meningitis, pleurisy and peritonitis may be regarded as complications, but are more properly considered as part of the disease itself.

Diagnosis.—The abrupt onset of a severe infection in an individual who has handled game or cultures of Pasteurella tularensis or who has been bitten by ticks or flies, especially if an ulcer develops accompanied by a bubo, points to a diagnosis of tularemia. The absence of an ulcer or bubo renders recognition more difficult. The short period of remission after the first rise of fever is sometimes helpful.

Positive diagnosis can be established by *laboratory methods*. Agglutinins for Pasteurella tularensis in the blood serum appear during the second week and increase rapidly in titer. The titer may reach 1 to 1280 during the third week. Titers less than 1 to 80 are not significant. Agglutinins may be demonstrable in the serum years after an attack, longer than after most other diseases. Cross-agglutination with organisms of the brucella group is occasionally encountered and is confusing, but when this does occur, the titer for Pasteurella tularensis is usually higher. A skin test developed by Foshay is said to be strictly specific and positive reactions appear as early as the fourth day. Chemically treated bacilli are injected intradermally. In thirty-six hours a local reaction appears. Patients may react positively as long as fourteen months after recovery. The most certain method of diagnosis is the recovery of Pasteurella tularensis. This is most easily accomplished by inoculating guinea-pigs or rabbits intraperitoneally with pus from the ulcer or suppurating lymph nodes, 1 or 2 cc. of freshly drawn blood or with tissue from the liver or spleen obtained at necropsy. Animals die within a week if viable organisms are injected. At necropsy the usual spotted appearance of the liver or spleen is found and the organism can be recovered from the blood or tissues in pure culture. Occasionally, the areas of necrosis are minute and can only be recognized in stained sections under the microscope. Bacilli can often be demonstrated in smears or in sections from the liver or spleen. Infected tissue rubbed into the skin of another animal will cause infection.

Organisms can sometimes be cultivated on fresh blood-glucose-cystin agar directly from the patient's pus or blood, and identified according to the characteristics mentioned under etiology.

In studies of diseases of rodents it is necessary to differentiate Pasteurella tularensis from Pasteurella pestis and pseudotuberculosis which are occasionally encountered.

Differential Diagnosis.—Tularemia has been most frequently confused with typhoid fever, influenza, septicemia, tuberculosis, undulant fever and sporotrichosis. *Typhoid fever* can be ruled out by the absence of the Widal reaction and of typhoid bacilli in the blood or excreta, by the absence of leukopenia, typical course and complications. *Influenza* is often accompanied by respiratory infection and leukopenia. The *septicemias* are eliminated from consideration by the absence of organisms in the blood and by the clinical course. *Undulant fever* may be considered because of the occasional cross-agglutination of organisms of the brucella group during tularemia. *Tuberculosis* and *sporotrichosis* are recognized by demonstrating the respective etiologic agents.

Prevention.—Cooking infected meat renders it harmless. Rubber gloves should be worn when handling game or cultures. Laboratory

6

workers should be protected by gloves, goggles and mask when manipulating cultures, infected animals or insects. Hunters should avoid unnecessary contact with the blood or flesh of killed animals. Sick animals or those easily caught are to be suspected and disposed of by burying or burning. No prophylactic vaccine has, as yet, been developed. Experiments by the author indicate that vaccination of mice with killed cultures prolongs life several days, but does not prevent death.

Treatment.—Rest in bed is of greatest importance; the treatment otherwise is symptomatic. Immune serum has been used with encouraging results in regard to shortening the illness, but the study has not progressed beyond the experimental stage. Sixty-nine cases have been treated with serum prepared by Foshay; clinical improvement occurred in many of the treated patients. Enlarged lymph nodes should not be incised unless on the point of rupturing spontaneously. Hot packs often relieve the pain.

Care should be taken during convalescence to avoid undue strain which is apt to precipitate relapse.

REFERENCES.

FOSHAY, L.: Tularemia Treated by a New Specific Antiserum, Am. Jour. Med. Sci., 1934, **187**, 235.
FRANCIS E.: Symptoms, Diagnosis and Pathology of Tularemia, Jour. Am. Med. Assn., 1928, **91**, 1155.
GUNDRY, L. P., and WARNER, C. G.: Fatal Tularemia, Ann. Int. Med., 1934, **7**, 837.
PARKER, R. R., and SPENCER, R. R.: Six Additional Cases of Laboratory Infection of Tularemia in Man, U. S. Pub. Health Rep., July 2, 1926, p. 1341.
SIMPSON, W. M.: Tularemia, Paul B. Hoeber, Inc., New York, 1929 (bibliography).

PLAGUE.

Definition.—Plague is an acute, infectious and contagious disease of high mortality for rodents and man, caused by Pasteurella pestis and appearing in the bubonic, pneumonic or septicemic form.

History.—Plague has been recognized for three thousand years. It has repeatedly swept over parts of the world, decimating or depopulating vast areas in great pandemics.

The most recent great pandemic occurred in Manchuria in 1910 and 1911, killing over 50,000. One hundred cases were observed in Paris in 1920. Small epidemics occurred in Manchuria and Mongolia in 1928, 1929 and 1930. A severe outbreak occurred in Shansi in the summer of 1931.

In America plague was first discovered in San Francisco in 1900, when 22 fatal cases occurred. In the following years up to 1908 over 90 deaths were caused by plague. Cases have appeared in New Orleans, Florida and Texas. In 1925 there were 40 cases with 35 deaths in Los Angeles. Three cases and 2 deaths occurred in California in 1928.

Pasteurella pestis was discovered independently by Yersin and Kitasato in 1894. Haffkine prepared the first vaccine in 1897. The transmission of the disease from rats to humans by means of fleas was demonstrated by Simonds in 1898.

Etiology.—Pasteurella pestis is a pleomorphic organism which appears in bacillary, coccoid or intermediate form. It is Gram-negative, bipolar staining, non-motile and does not form spores. It grows well on the usual laboratory media. Under unfavorable cultural conditions, as on 3 per cent salt agar, large, vacuolated, pale staining "involution" forms appear. The organism is virulent for most rodents when infected by inoculation, inhalation or by application of the organisms to the unbroken skin. Bacilli exist for varying periods in fleas, lice and bedbugs. Pasteurella pestis is often found in enormous numbers in stained sections of infected tissue. No true toxin has been discovered. Presumably an endotoxin is formed and liberated.

The plague bacillus when protected from sunlight, heat or drying may survive for years with undiminished virulence. It is killed by a few hours' exposure to sunlight, within an hour in dry heat at 100° C., and within a few minutes by moist heat at 100° C. The bacillus may remain viable for a year in frozen corpses, for six days in clothing, and for five months in the feces of fleas and lice. Exposed in rooms, they usually die in two days. The rate of death is proportional to the temperature.

Epidemiology.—Plague is endemic in many widely scattered areas of the world. The chief centers are in northeastern Asia, Tibet, India, Arabia and central Africa. Lesser foci have appeared in South America and Europe. The disease is propagated in rodents, chiefly in rats. In California, ground squirrels are carriers. Rodents are chronic carriers of plague and may suffer no perceptible ill effects. At times, epizoötics break out, killing vast numbers. The infection is spread from animal to animal by means of fleas. Animals, therefore, constitute a perennial source of infection. Epizoötics among rodents commonly precede human epidemics. The infection is transmitted to humans by means of fleas or is contracted directly from tissues by individuals who hunt and dress infected animals.

In the beginning of an epidemic in humans, the disease occurs as the *bubonic form* which spreads to others gradually. In a certain number of patients the lungs become involved in a secondary pneumonic process. When this takes place the sputum becomes loaded with plague bacilli, which are disseminated in invisible droplets of sputum during coughing. This is the starting point of the highly contagious *pneumonic form*. Everyone within range of such a patient may become infected. The pneumonic form, therefore, in contrast with the bubonic form, spreads with appalling speed and soon becomes pandemic. The bubonic form may occur at any season; the pneumonic form is rampant chiefly in the cold months when bacilli survive longest in the sputum droplets. Both forms are usually encountered in epidemics.

The disease is spread to adjacent territories by infected persons, by carriers attempting escape from plague centers or by infected rodents disseminated by improper attempts at extermination. Opportunities for the spread of both forms of the disease are favored by poverty and overcrowding, and by the presence of rodents and vermin. Plague has been carried to remote portions of the world by rats, transported chiefly by ocean ships.

All races are susceptible to plague. Both sexes are equally susceptible, although males are more frequently affected than females due to greater opportunities for exposure. Infants are least involved, children more often, and adults from the ages of twenty to sixty years most often.

Pathogenesis.—The bacillus entering the body through the skin gives rise to the *primary bubonic form*. Bacilli are taken up by the lymphatics and carried to the nearest lymph nodes, usually the femoral, inguinal or axillary. Inflammation and swelling of these lymph nodes, forming the first bubo, constitutes the primary focus (Albrecht and Ghon). The process may cease here and recovery ensue, but most often it spreads further. From the primary focus, bacilli are disseminated to other lymphatics and are poured into the blood stream, causing generalized infection. In certain fulminating cases, infection becomes generalized immediately without any lymph node reaction.

As mentioned above, the lungs may become secondarily involved. The sputum becomes loaded with bacilli which are broadcast by coughing. Others are then infected by inhalation. True primary pneumonic plague occurs only by inhalation.

In some cases of plague, primary septicemia probably results from the direct invasion of bacilli through the membranes of the mouth or throat. Death occurs before any lymph node swelling is evident.

Pathology.—Rigor mortis sets in promptly. Cyanosis, lividity and hemorrhagic spots are commonly seen. The general pathology is characterized by hemorrhagic inflammation wherever the bacilli are localized. The primary bubo is composed of a group of swollen, inflamed lymph nodes, which on section appear yellowish and speckled with small hemorrhages. The adjacent tissue may be adherent and similarly involved. Later, as necrosis proceeds, the nodes break down and form large abscesses which rupture externally. The mesenteric, bronchial and other lymph nodes may be similarly but less intensely involved. Ecchymoses are found in the muscles, pericardium, pleura, peritoneum and less often in the small intestine, gall-bladder and kidneys. Hemorrhage in the dura, purulent meningitis or edema of the brain occurs. The spleen and liver are enlarged, dark red and contain areas of focal necrosis. Inflammation of the upper air passages and ulceration of the tonsils are common. Edema of the lungs is usually present, especially in the later stages.

Microscopically, bacilli are found in vast numbers in the lesions, in extravasations and in the blood. There is parenchymatous and fatty degeneration of the myocardium, spleen, liver and kidneys. Abscess formation occurs in cases that live long enough.

Pneumonic plague is characterized by specific changes in the lung. The lungs are dark red, voluminous, edematous and rich in blood. The distribution of the pneumonic patches varies greatly. Usually both lungs are involved.

Bronchitis is the rule. The bronchi or bronchioli contain frothy, hemorrhagic mucus. The trachea, larynx, pharynx and tonsils are often secondarily involved. There is often pleuritis with serosanguineous or gelatinous fluid in the pleural cavity.

Elsewhere in the body secondary changes occur like those in the bubonic form, except that superficial bubos are absent.

Symptoms.—*Bubonic Form.*—The incubation period is short—from two to five days. During this time there may be vague aches and pains. Pain occurs at the site of the swelling lymph nodes, which soon appear as the primary bubo. A day or two later other superficial lymph nodes may swell. Inguinal bubos occur in about 60 per cent, axillary bubos in 20 per cent, and neck bubos in 12 per cent of cases.

The *onset* is often sudden with a rapid rise of fever, frequently as high as 105.8° F. (41° C.) and a chill or chilly sensations. Headache, vertigo, sweating and tachycardia are common. Epistaxis and diarrhea occur. Conjunctivitis and photophobia are common. The facial expression may be anxious or apathetic. Unusual restlessness and a tendency to leave the bed are often observed. Delirium and coma occur. The pulse increases in rate and becomes weaker. Death often is caused by circulatory failure manifested by cyanosis, dyspnea and edema of the lungs.

In cases that recover, the temperature begins to decline after a week or more. Unless suppuration has occurred, the bubos slowly disappear, evidence of toxemia lessens and convalescence begins. Secondary infections frequently are the cause of death.

Physical examination reveals extremely ill patients. Hemorrhages into the skin caused the disease to be named the "black death." The skin is hot and dry, the face is often bloated in appearance and the conjunctivæ are reddened. The pulse is weak and the rate rapid. Bubos appear as irregular, localized, firm, tender masses which become boggy as necrosis progresses. The spleen is palpable in about 60 per cent of cases.

In the septicemic form the resistance to plague is so slight that overwhelming infection and death occur within a day or two, before any lymph node swelling occurs. In *ambulatory* cases, fever may be slight or absent, but typical bubos containing plague bacilli are present. Cases are often unrecognized or purposely concealed to avoid detention and quarantine.

Pneumonic Plague.—The onset occurs so soon after infection that prodromes are seldom noted. The onset is sudden, often with a rigor or chilly sensations. Symptoms of general sepsis and profound toxemia rapidly appear. The temperature rises abruptly. Headache, nausea, vertigo, tachycardia and dyspnea appear. The pulse soon becomes weaker. There is often a sense of oppression in the chest. The face is flushed and bloated, and the conjunctivæ suffused. Prostration is profound. Cough, dyspnea and cyanosis usually appear within twenty-four hours. The sputum is mucoid at first but rapidly becomes thinner, bright red and contains myriads of plague bacilli. Patients are too intensely ill to complain much about various other symptoms. Air hunger is the chief difficulty.

Laboratory Observations.—The urine shows the usual febrile changes. The leukocyte count varies greatly. A leukocytosis from 20,000 to 60,000 with a relative lymphocytosis is usually present in the bubonic form. In the septicemic and pneumonic forms leukopenia is reported. Bacilli can be demonstrated in blood smears in 50 to 75 per cent of cases. Bacteriemia is always present in the septicemic and pneumonic forms, and less often in the bubonic form. The sputum in pneumonic plague is thin, mucoid, bloody and loaded with plague bacilli. The urine, feces and other secretions or excretions often contain bacilli.

Diagnosis.—In epidemics the diagnosis is easy. The first case or cases of plague appearing in unsuspected areas are apt to be unrecognized until too late to prevent wide dissemination of infection. The death of large numbers of rodents should excite suspicion. The appearance of bubos in patients taken suddenly and severely ill is the first indicative sign. The conjunctival reddening, tachycardia, hemorrhages into the skin, prostration and nervous symptoms are helpful in diagnosis but appear in other illnesses. Positive diagnosis is made by demonstrating plague bacilli in material aspirated from bubos, in blood smears or by blood cultures. For further identification the organism may be injected into rats or guinea-pigs.

In the pneumonic form the diagnosis is made by the sudden onset of an overwhelming infection soon followed by evidence of pneumonia, and by the presence of plague bacilli in the sputum, often in almost pure culture.

Differential Diagnosis.—Few other diseases are apt to be confused with plague. The most important ones are lobar pneumonia, influenza and typhus fever. Typhoid fever is less apt to be confusing. Differentiation is made chiefly by the severity of the symptoms, and demonstration of plague bacilli. Herpes, present in pneumonia, influenza and typhus is never present in plague. Plague-like bacilli recovered from rodents must be differentiated from Pasteurella tularensis and Pasteurella pseudotuberculosis.

Prognosis.— *Duration.*—In general, bubonic plague lasts from four to eight days. Individuals surviving a week have a fair chance for recovery. The pneumonic and septicemic forms are practically always fatal within a few days. In bubonic plague the mortality ranges from 30 to 90 per cent in the different epidemics. Prognosis is better in infants and children. Prophylactic vaccination is said to diminish both the morbidity- and mortality-rates.

Prophylaxis.— *General Measures.*—Rats and other rodents which constitute the sources of infection must be exterminated. The snap-trap is the best means for rapidly reducing the numbers. Other methods involve fumigation with hydrocyanic acid gas or sulphur dioxide, starvation, destruction of nesting places by fire, and rat-proofing buildings. Ships should be periodically fumigated, especially if ports have been touched where plague is endemic. Hawser shields prevent ingress and egress of rats to and from ships at the wharf. Fleas which convey the infection from rodents to man are simultaneously eliminated with the destruction of rodents.

A strict blockade should be established around a plague center. All individuals leaving a plague area ought to be quarantined for at least two weeks to insure the detection and detention of incipient or mild cases.

The sick should be isolated as far as possible in specially requisitioned buildings. Excreta, clothing and other articles should be sterilized. Dead bodies must be promptly cremated or buried in deep trenches.

Personal Prophylaxis.—Attendants in plague areas or all who come in contact with plague patients must be protected by wearing insect-proof clothing. Long white gowns, gloves, boots, complete hood with a thick breathing mask and a celluloid shield for vision are most effective for protection against the pneumonic form.

Immune serum given prophylactically is said to prolong the incubation period, lessen the severity of the illness and favor recovery in the bubonic form. The immunity after an injection probably lasts about two weeks. Haffkine's vaccine, according to some observers, is of value in lessening both the morbidity and mortality.

Treatment.—Intravenous injection of 100 cc. doses of antiplague serum at intervals of six to eight hours is recommended by some. Many other remedies, drugs and charms have been used throughout history.

The management of cases resolves itself to the maintenance of proper nutrition and fluid intake. Fluids or sugar solution may be given intravenously if necessary. Strict bed rest is imperative. Oxygen may be used to lessen the load on the circulatory system. Tepid or cold sponges lessen the fever and delirium. Sedatives or hypnotics may be used in allaying restlessness. Resort to morphine may be necessary for the mentally disturbed cases. Cold packs or ice-bags relieve the pain in the bubos and headache. Incision and drainage of pus from bubos may be necessary.

REFERENCES.

ALBRECHT, H., and GHON, A.: Über die Beulenpest in Bombay, K. Akad. d. Wissensch., **66**, 1898, 1900, Vienna.
DIEUDONNÉ, A., and OTTO, R.: Handb. der path. Mikroorg., Kolle, Kraus and Uhlenhuth, 1928, **4**, 179.
WU, L. T.: Treatise on Pneumonic Plague, League of Nations, 1926.

ANTHRAX.

Synonyms.—Malignant pustule; Woolsorters' disease; Milzbrand; Charbon.

Definition.—Anthrax is an acute, specific, contagious and infectious disease, primarily of herbivorous animals, but transmissible to man by way of the skin or mucous membranes of the respiratory or digestive tract.

History.—Anthrax was recognized in antiquity. It was first accurately described by Maret in 1752. In 1823, Barthelmy proved its transmissibility by inoculation experiments. Pollender first saw the bacilli in blood smears in 1849, and Davaine in 1863 suggested and proved the etiologic relationship of the bacilli to the disease. Koch's first important publication in 1876 was a report of the cultivation of the anthrax bacillus and a description of the spores.

Subsequent research in anthrax was chiefly devoted to the development of specific vaccine and immune serum, notably by Pasteur, Sclavo, Marchoux and Sobernheim.

Etiology.—Bacillus anthracis is a relatively large, Gram-positive, non-motile rod, 5 to 10 microns long and 1 to 3 microns wide. Growth takes place readily on artificial media, forming long tangles of threads —the so-called "doll's-hair" growth. Characteristics of the bacillus are the sharpness of its corners and its growth in long chains, with an oblong or elliptical chink between each bacillus, giving the appearance of a bamboo rod. Oval, refractile, centrally located spores form during growth on artificial media in the presence of oxygen. Spores do not form in the animal body, but capsules are developed. As the bacillus ages, it undergoes degeneration and loses its ability to retain stains. The bacillus is virulent for guinea-pigs, mice and rabbits.

The spores of anthrax bacilli are extremely resistant and may live for years in a dried state. They are killed by dry heat after three hours at 140° C., by steam at 100° C. in five or ten minutes and by boiling for ten minutes. Spores may resist a 5 per cent solution of phenol for forty minutes. A 1 to 2000 solution of bichloride of mercury kills them in forty minutes and sunlight in six to twelve hours.

Pathogenesis.—Cattle, sheep, hogs and horses may become infected by direct contact with sick animals or by grazing in pastures contaminated by feces or the carcasses of animals dead from anthrax. Blood-sucking insects may transmit the disease. In man, direct or indirect infection may occur; directly, by contact with the exudate from the pustule on an animal or human or indirectly by contact with substances harboring bacilli or spores, chiefly hides, wool and fur. Inhalation of dust containing bacilli or spores may result in pulmonary anthrax. Ingestion of meat from an animal with anthrax may cause infection in the gastro-intestinal tract. Bacilli or spores may gain entrance through abrasions or may penetrate the unbroken skin or mucous membrane.

The mode of action of the anthrax bacillus is unknown. It has been suggested that death is caused chiefly by the mechanical blockage of blood-vessels in vital organs by the enormous numbers of bacilli during bacteriemia.

Pathology.—Cutaneous anthrax is characterized by the formation of a single, primary carbuncle. The central eschar is composed of degenerated epithelial cells and necrotic cuticular tissue. The surrounding tissues are infiltrated, hemorrhagic and edematous, often containing a mucinous substance called anthracomucin. Areas of gangrene may form. Anthrax bacilli are frequently, but not always, demonstrable in the lesion, especially in the deeper portions. Other organisms may be present as secondary invaders. Bacilli enter the lymphatics, produce lymphangitis and lodge in the adjacent lymph nodes which become swollen and hemorrhagic.

In pulmonary anthrax there is usually bronchitis and diffuse hemorrhagic infiltration of the lungs with necrosis of the epithelium. Areas of gangrene may be present. Pleurisy and hemorrhagic mediastinitis occur. The bronchial lymph nodes are usually swollen and hemorrhagic.

Gastro-intestinal anthrax is characterized by localized areas of necrosis or "carbuncles" in the mesentery of the small and large bowel. Ulceration with perforation and peritonitis occurs. Peritonitis is common.

Other organs are secondarily involved. The spleen is usually large and soft. The kidney shows acute nephritis or nephrosis. There are hemorrhages in the cortex and in the glomeruli; the renal capillaries may be plugged with bacilli and there is degeneration of the epithelium. Hemorrhagic meningitis occurs.

Incidence.—Anthrax is primarily a disease of animals. It has been responsible for vast epizoötics in which thousands of cattle, sheep and horses have been destroyed. It is much less common now, but outbreaks still occur, especially in Siberia. In the United States, 162 cases of human anthrax were reported during 1929. It is likely that more unreported or unrecognized cases occur.

Anthrax is largely an occupational disease. Individuals handling hides, furs, bristle, hair, wool, horn and bone are most often affected. Stockmen, butchers, tanners and veterinarians are exposed to infection. A number of cases in New York were caused by the use of cheap, unsterilized shaving brushes.

Symptoms.—Cutaneous anthrax usually occurs on the exposed surfaces of the body which become inoculated by contact with infected material. The head, face, and neck are involved in 85 per cent of cases, the arms in 12 per cent and the legs and trunk in 3 per cent. After an incubation period of from one to seven days, usually two to three days, prickling or intense itching and redness are noted at the site of infection. Very soon a small uncharacteristic papule or vesicle appears which rapidly enlarges to form a large carbuncle. At the same time the surrounding tissue becomes markedly inflamed and edematous. When the face or neck is involved the edema often closes the eyes or spreads down to the chest. Within twelve to eighteen hours the center of the pustule becomes necrotic and forms an irregular, depressed brown or black hard eschar. The characteristic black color of the eschar gives the disease its name—anthrax = coal (Greek). Secondary vesicles or pustules may form on the rim of the eschar. A purulent or hemorrhagic fluid exudes from the site. The regional lymphatics are inflamed and the lymph nodes are swollen.

In certain cases an eschar does not form, the lesion remains a diffuse, rapidly spreading inflammation. Occasionally, secondary pustules occur elsewhere in or on the body, either as the result of scratching in bacilli or as blood-borne infections. About the sixth or eighth day in cases that recover, the carbuncle becomes more demarcated, the mass softens and sloughs, the edema disappears and the lymph nodes return to normal. A scar usually remains.

Constitutional symptoms are often remarkably absent during the early stages, even in the presence of bacteriemia. The eschar itself is painless and the pain in the edematous tissue is not severe, as a rule. There may be irregular fever which reaches high levels or no fever at all. Malaise and anorexia are present. In severe cases, vomiting, prostration, severe headache, high fever and circulatory failure occur. Collapse and profuse sweating precede death or there may be delirium or coma. Patients sometimes appear to be in good condition when they are apparently suddenly overwhelmed and die within a few minutes or hours. Bacteriemia is almost invariably present in fatal cases.

Pulmonary anthrax may commence suddenly with a chill and high fever and signs of severe pulmonary inflammation. More often, the onset is gradual, suggesting bronchitis or mild bronchopneumonia. Cough, sputum which may contain anthrax bacilli, headache, malaise and a sense of oppression in the chest are present. The later stages are often characterized by a sudden change for the worse. Dyspnea, cyanosis, cough, bloody or foamy sputum and pleuritic pain occur. Death occurs on the second or third day. Recoveries have been reported.

Gastro-intestinal anthrax is rare. Solowieff reports an epidemic of 30 cases caused by the ingestion of contaminated meat. Peritonitis was found at necropsy in 20 of the 22 cases examined. Only 8 of these exhibited symptoms or signs of peritonitis during the illness. In certain cases the symptoms were referable chiefly to the site of localization; in the appendix, in various portions of the small or large intestine or at the site of obstruction of the bowel. In others, symptoms were indefinite, with a feeling of being unwell, chilliness, headache, vomiting or constipation, less often a hemorrhagic diarrhea. Death occurred in from two to five days; one lived for eleven days. Death was preceded by bacteriemia, peritonitis, delirium or coma.

In all forms of anthrax, metastatic infection may occur. Hemorrhagic meningitis and acute nephritis or nephrosis are occasionally noted.

Diagnosis.—In the early stages of cutaneous anthrax when prompt treatment is of value, diagnosis is often difficult. Later, after the eschar forms, the diagnosis is comparatively easy. The blackness and painlessness of the eschar and the unusual well-being of the patient with so large a pustule are characteristic. Leukocytosis is the rule. Demonstration of the causative organism in wound scrapings or in the exudate by smear, cultural or by animal inoculation methods, is conclusive evidence. Frequently, few or no bacilli can be isolated, especially in cases seen late and who recover. Repeated blood cultures should be made. In some cases bacilli may be seen in blood smears. The isolated bacilli should be inoculated subcutaneously into mice or guinea-pigs. Anthrax bacilli kill these animals in from forty-eight to seventy-two hours.

Pulmonary anthrax is often unrecognized clinically. An important point in diagnosis is the occupation of the patient. Individuals exposed to dust from animal hair, wool, feathers and grain most often contract the disease. The condition is usually classified clinically as bronchitis or bronchopneumonia unless anthrax is suspected. Confirmatory evidence can only be obtained by isolating the bacilli from the sputum, from pleural fluid or by lung puncture and aspiration. The diagnosis is most often made at necropsy.

Gastro-intestinal anthrax also occurs chiefly in individuals exposed to animal products. Intestinal anthrax may occur secondarily to skin anthrax. Unless an epidemic is present there is usually nothing to suggest anthrax, and the diagnosis is usually made at necropsy.

Prognosis.—The average mortality in 28,331 collected untreated cases was about 19 per cent. In the United States the mortality was about 10 per cent among 162 cases, treated and untreated, occurring during 1929.

Various methods of therapy apparently have a favorable effect in reducing the death-rate. In various groups of cases treated with immune serum, arsphenamine or with beef serum or peptone, the mortality percentage is sometimes as low as 4 per cent.

In cutaneous anthrax it is said that the prognosis is better when the infection is localized on the extremities or trunk. Some claim that infections on the neck are worse than those on the eyelid. In Solowieff's series of 30 cases of intestinal anthrax, 26 died. The mortality-rate from the pulmonary form varies from 50 to 87 per cent. The presence of a bacteriemia is of bad prognostic import.

Prophylaxis.—Infected animals should be immediately destroyed by cremation or buried deeply. Vaccination of animals exposed to infection with living, attenuated strains of anthrax bacilli is said to produce immunity. Industries concerned with the manipulation of animal products should protect its employees from inhaling dust. Hides coming from endemic centers of anthrax (Russia, China, South America) frequently cause anthrax infection, but as yet no satisfactory method of sterilization of hides or furs has been developed. Individuals obliged to handle such material should be advised how to minimize the risk of infection. Hides carried on the shoulder should not brush against the neck or face. Gloves afford protection. Cheap bristle brushes should be sterilized before using.

Treatment.—General supportive measures and bed-rest are necessary. The carbuncle should be covered with sterile, moist dressings to absorb the exudate. All soiled dressings or material must be sterilized and disposed of so as not to infect others. Incision, excision, cautery, or the application or injection of antiseptic substances around or into the carbuncle are distinctly contraindicated. The spread of infection and the precipitation of bacteriemia often result from meddling with the primary focus.

The best method of therapy appears to be the prompt use of large doses of *immune serum*. Even immune serum is not entirely satisfactory, as evidenced by the frequent announcement of different new methods of therapy. In cases without bacteriemia, 3 to 8 intravenous injections of 50 to 100 cc. of a potent serum at six- to eight-hour intervals are recommended. All patients must first be tested for hypersensitivity to horse serum and desensitized if necessary. In septicemic cases 100 to 150 cc. may be injected every three or four hours until the blood becomes sterile.

Becker, in 1911, introduced the use of *salvarsan*. He and others after him published enthusiastic accounts of its efficacy. Pijper especially states that salvarsan is of greatest value. Graf reported the treatment of 50 cases with this drug with only 2 deaths. The usual dose of *neoarsphenamine* employed is 0.45 to 0.6 gram daily, for several days. One patient treated by the author received 0.6, 0.9, and 0.9 gram during three days and recovered without ill effects. The use of the drug is still in the experimental stage and many more cases will have to be treated before its worth can be evaluated.

REFERENCES.

JOCHMANN, HEGLER: Milzbrand, Lehrbuch der Infektionskrankheiten, Berlin, 1924, p. 977.
REGAN, J. C.: The Advantage of Serum Therapy as Shown by a Comparison of Various Methods of Treatment of Anthrax, Am. Jour. Med. Sci., 1921, **162**, 406.

INFLUENZA.

Synonym.—Grippe. The term *influenza* was derived from *influenze di freddo*, "influence of the cold." *Grippe* is derived from the French, implying "to attack," "to catch."

Definition.—Influenza is an acute infectious and contagious disease occurring in pandemic, epidemic or endemic form, characterized by sudden onset with fever, aching and prostration, often accompanied by involvement of the respiratory, nervous or gastro-intestinal systems and marked tendency to develop pneumonia.

History.—Many epidemics and pandemics of influenza are recorded in history. The first authentic pandemic occurred about 1580, commencing in the Orient and spreading over North America and most of Europe. Thereafter, epidemics of more or less widespread distribution and severity have occurred at approximately ten-year intervals. Severe pandemics are recorded in 1781, 1832, 1847, 1889 and in 1918, corresponding roughly with each new generation. The recurrence of influenza at such widely spaced intervals has caused each generation of physicians to consider it a "new disease" until its true nature had again become recognized. Extensive historic studies of influenza have been made by Hirsch and Leichtenstern.

The last pandemic commenced in the spring of 1918. Its first appearance in Spain is responsible for the term "Spanish" influenza. The disease spread with rapidity over the rest of Europe and reached its first peak of incidence in July. The prevailing war conditions created favorable circumstances for a rapid dissemination throughout the world. America and England were chiefly involved in the second and most severe wave which occurred in October. A third wave appeared in the spring of 1919, and a fourth early in 1920. The latter, in certain places, was very severe. Estimates place the number of deaths following influenza during 1918 and 1919 in the United States at over 500,000; in the world, 6 million.

Etiology.—The cause of influenza has not been definitely determined. The weight of evidence is in favor of the influenza bacillus of Pfeiffer, Hemophilus influenzæ, as the cause, and for this reason influenza may be included among bacillary diseases until further work shows otherwise. The factors, as listed by Zinsser, supporting the influenza bacillus as the primary cause are: (1) the frequent presence of these bacilli in the throats of early cases (in from 60 to 100 per cent in certain series); (2) the frequency with which the organisms occur in complicating conditions; (3) their disappearance in normal and diseased respiratory tracts with the abatement of epidemics; (4) the demonstration of a powerful poison derived from cultures of bacilli, and (5) the experimental production of an influenza-like respiratory disease in monkeys by the injection of cultures of the bacilli.

Factors cited against the contention of influenza bacilli as the causal agency are: (1) the frequent failure to isolate the bacilli from early cases; (2) the presence of bacilli in normal individuals; (3) their presence in conditions other than influenza; (4) the antigenic multiplicity of strains isolated during an epidemic; (5) the lack of protection following vaccination with the bacilli; (6) the infrequency of bacteriemia in early cases; (7) negative results of numerous investigators in attempts to produce the disease experimentally in man, and (8) the production of influenza-like symptoms in humans by the application of filtered nasal secretions obtained from influenza patients. Most of these negative factors are inconclusive. The failure to isolate bacilli from certain cases is of little importance and can probably be explained by improper technic. Histologic studies have revealed influenza-like bacilli in tissues in a high percentage of cases whether they had been cultivated or not. The presence of bacilli in normal individuals finds an analogy in the case of the pneumococcus, streptococcus or tetanus bacillus, any of which may be found in normal individuals. The protection tests with vaccines thus far reported are inconclusive. The experimental production of influenza-like symptoms with filtrates of nasal secretions is important and bears further investigation.

Until new methods are developed for the classification of virulent and non-virulent strains of influenza bacilli, and until more knowledge is at hand in regard to fluctuation of immunity or resistance of the host, the final proof will not be forthcoming. A number of other difficulties hinder and confuse research on the problem: (1) the difficulty of diagnosing the earliest stages of uncomplicated influenza; (2) the unexpectedness of epidemics and the demoralization of research personnel with illness and overwork during an epidemic at a time when studies are vital; (3) the presence of many other organisms in the respiratory tract.

Other agents which, during the present state of uncertainty, must be considered in the causation of influenza are: (a) a new group of anaërobic, filter-passing bacteria, Bacterium pneumosintes. (b) An invisible and filtrable virus or the filtrable form of some known bacterium, especially of the streptococcus group, has been implicated by some observers. Numerous reports of the production of an influenza-like disease in man and in animals by the inoculation or instillation of filtrates of influenza material are available. Most significant are the recent experiments of Shope who showed that swine influenza is caused by the combined action of a filtrable virus and Hemophilus influenzæ suis. Subsequently Smith, Andrewes and Laidlaw isolated a virus from human cases of influenza which was indistinguishable from the virus isolated by Shope.

Hemophilus influenzæ was described by Pfeiffer in 1892. It is a small bacillus, 0.5 micron long by 0.3 micron in width. The bacilli often occur in groups, rarely in chains. They are non-motile, do not form spores, are Gram-negative, and stain best with 10 per cent fuchsin solution, or with Löffler's methylene blue. Influenza bacilli require hemoglobin for growth *in vitro*. On blood agar at 37° C., colonies appear after eighteen hours as very small, discrete, transparent, shiny droplets. There appears to be a variety of strains. Strains vary greatly in virulence; the same strain may vary in virulence and agglutinability at different times, so that with present methods no satisfactory classification has been devised. Considerable progress has been made, however, by the recent studies of Pittman. The bacilli are easily killed by heat, drying and by disinfectants. They die within two hours in dried sputum. Under proper cultural conditions the production of a powerful poison can be demonstrated.

Epidemiology.—No disease spreads with such rapidity as influenza. No other disease descends with such suddenness and becomes so widespread and destructive of life, and in none are the known methods of control or prevention more useless. Until the etiologic agent is determined, many problems of epidemiology will remain obscure. Certain facts are thoroughly established: (*a*) occurrence of influenza in pandemic waves; (*b*) origin from a definite focus or foci; (*c*) great speed of dissemination; (*d*) sudden mass infection; (*e*) rapid decline after lasting a few weeks in one locality; (*f*) independence of climatic conditions, age, sex or occupation; (*g*) general mass susceptibility; (*h*) enormous morbidity with but slight mortality, and (*i*) high death-rate from complications.

Pandemics are usually characterized by several distinct waves separated by months or a year. During the first wave, although many people are attacked, the disease is usually mild, as in the first wave of the pandemic in the spring of 1918. During the second wave the height of severity was reached. The morbidity-rate was as great or greater than during the first wave, but the mortality was markedly increased due to the frequent development of pneumonia. The third and fourth outbreaks were relatively less severe.

Several explanations are at hand to account for the epidemic periodicity. It is assumed that influenza is always with us, that is, it exists permanently as an endemic disease in mild form in many parts of the world. In the past, many believed that pandemics originated in the Orient. During the last pandemic several simultaneous points of origin appear to have existed. To explain the sudden mass infection the assumption is that a population comprised chiefly of non-immune individuals has gradually arisen. If, in such a population, a virulent strain of influenza virus is introduced, dissemination is inevitable. Dissemination is facilitated if *droplet infection* be the mode of transmission and if the *portal of entry* be the respiratory tract, as appears to be the case in influenza. The infection is probably spread directly from person to person by talking, coughing or sneezing. In this manner infection is spread as fast as man travels. The most susceptible individuals are attacked first. Those who survive are endowed with a low immunity of short duration. The epidemic in one locality lasts as long as susceptibles exist and then dies out. Subsequent epidemic waves involve susceptibles who have previously escaped or those in whom immunity has disappeared. When no more susceptibles are left the virus presumably dies out or becomes dormant.

Healthy carriers probably exist. Influenza is known to be infectious during the incubation period. Carriers and mild cases are the greatest menaces in the spread of infection.

It is noteworthy that the mortality is usually low during the first explosive wave of a pandemic, before secondary invading bacteria become established and rampant. The next wave is apt to be highly fatal, as it was in 1918, chiefly due to pulmonary infection with strep-

tococci, staphylococci and pneumococci. Subsequent waves appear
and disappear more slowly and are usually less serious.

Another factor, aside from host susceptibility, is fluctuation in virulence of the infecting organisms. Some have assumed that certain
conditions favor the acquisition or enhancement of virulence of organisms which hitherto were avirulent, residing as saprophytes in carriers.
It is true that rapid passage from person to person seems to enhance
virulence, but it does not appear to be increased beyond a certain
fixed level. It is logical to consider that both factors discussed, namely,
increase in susceptibility of the host and increase in virulence of the
virus, together with other obscure factors, determine the beginning and
spread of pandemics.

The duration of an outbreak of influenza in a community is comparatively short—from three to six weeks. The first and second
waves are apt to be more explosive than succeeding ones which develop
and disappear more slowly. In the interpandemic periods minor
epidemics undoubtedly occur.

Incidence.—Statistics in regard to the incidence of influenza are
notoriously unreliable, especially during interpandemic periods. It
is even difficult to secure accurate statistics during a pandemic. It is
common practice among many physicians to consider any indisposition,
from a slight "cold" to severe pneumonia, as "influenza." It is not
necessary to consider that fatal bronchopneumonia in adults must be
due primarily to influenza, since Cole has shown that primary bronchopneumonia frequently occurs. Errors in diagnosis are unavoidable
as long as the diagnosis rests upon clinical rather than etiologic criteria.
Minor outbreaks of influenza have been recognized by some in 1920,
1926, 1928–1929 and in 1932. In practically all minor outbreaks, the
peak of incidence occurs during the winter months when "colds" and
other respiratory diseases are common. True influenza is notoriously
independent of season. Many diagnoses of "influenza" must be
accepted with doubt.

In 1918 about one-third of the population had influenza. The attack-
rate was greatest in children between the ages of five and nine years.

Pathology.—Because of the mildness of typical influenza there are
usually no characteristic pathologic features aside from catarrhal
changes in the mucous membranes of the respiratory tract and possibly
a general hemorrhagic tendency. Simple hyperemia or catarrh of the
intestinal tract and non-specific hemorrhagic encephalitis may occur.
Gross pathologic changes are almost always the result of secondary
infection. Changes due to complications are discussed later.

Symptoms.—Typical cases of uncomplicated influenza are often
termed "three-day fever." (Fig. 6.) In many individuals the attack
may be so mild as to pass unrecognized. The majority of patients are
forced to spend several days in bed. Others may be indisposed with a
day or two of fever, followed by perspiration and rapid convalescence.

Prodromal symptoms are rare. After a short incubation period of
twelve to seventy-two hours (usually twenty-four to forty-eight hours)
the disease commences abruptly. The onset is almost always sudden,
with chilliness or rigor, and is soon followed by fever. Severe head-

ache, usually frontal, vertigo, pains in the back, limbs and in the eye-balls, and anorexia are prominent symptoms. Conjunctivitis occurs. Prostration, quite out of proportion to other symptoms, is a striking feature. Fever may rise to 104° F. (40° C.) or more and persist from two to five days. The respiration and pulse-rate are usually increased but often not in proportion to the fever. (Fig. 7.) There is often constipation and temporary suppression of urine. Epistaxis is uncommon, but has been reported as frequent in certain epidemics. Gastrointestinal symptoms are commonest in children. A heavily coated tongue, anorexia, vomiting and diarrhea may occur.

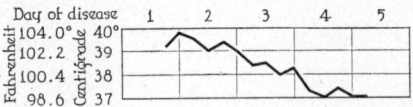

Fig. 6.—Temperature curve of a typical uncomplicated case of influenza. Onset with chilly sensations, aching of the legs and back. Prostration required rest in bed for six days. Recovery uneventful.

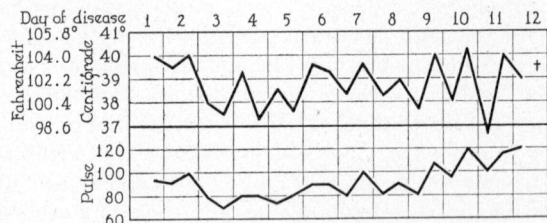

Fig. 7.—Temperature curve of a case of influenza complicated by atypical pneumonia which proved fatal. Note the relatively slow pulse during the early period of influenza and the increasing tachycardia and irregular temperature curve after the sixth day during the pneumonia.

Involvement of the respiratory tract occurs so frequently as to be regarded as belonging to the picture of typical influenza. It has not been determined whether the involvement is caused by the specific organism of influenza or by secondary invaders. At any rate, the majority of patients, 75 per cent according to Leichtenstern, develop coryza, rhinitis, pharyngitis, laryngitis, tracheitis, bronchitis or pneumonia. Any portion of the respiratory tract may be involved without implicating the others.

The absence of respiratory symptoms in many patients should be emphasized, since it is the general tendency of most physicians to consider inflammation of the respiratory tract essential for the diagnosis of influenza, which is not the case.

Physical Signs.—The patient appears apathetic, the face is usually suffused and the conjunctivæ often reddened. Herpes labialis is uncommon. The tongue is dry and coated. The pharynx is usually reddened. Lymph node swelling is absent and the spleen is seldom palpable. No abnormalities are detected in the heart. There may be signs of rhinitis. Severe cases frequently show a peculiar cyanosis of the lips, ears and fingers which is often described as ashy, violaceous or heliotrope. It is probably of toxic origin. Blotchy erythema occurs at times.

Special Forms.—According to the prominence of symptoms referable to certain systems, several forms of influenza are frequently mentioned, although such classification is superfluous.

After the respiratory tract, the nervous system is most frequently affected. The predominance of *nervous symptoms* was said to be greater in the pandemic of 1889 than in 1918. Many cases without catarrhal symptoms suffered profound prostration, insomnia, mental depression, intense headache and severe general aching pains. Delirium and mania were less common.

A diagnosis of *gastro-intestinal influenza* should be made with great caution. There exists an unfortunate common tendency among the profession and the laity to designate any unexplained gastro-intestinal disturbance, accompanied by fever and malaise, as "stomach flu."

In most epidemics of influenza a few patients develop predominating gastro-intestinal symptoms. The symptoms vary from simple anorexia and constipation to vomiting, severe abdominal pain and diarrhea. Gastro-intestinal influenza can only be regarded as influenza in which gastro-intestinal symptoms dominate the picture.

The *course* of uncomplicated influenza is short, seldom lasting more than five days, in the great majority of cases two or three days.

Convalescence is usually prompt, but may be protracted by mental depression, malaise, neuralgia, insomnia, weakness or by various gastro-intestinal disturbances.

Relapses are quite frequent. The temperature may drop to normal on the first or second day and the patient may feel better, then all of the symptoms recur. It has been observed that if, for example, the nervous symptoms predominate during the original attack, other symptoms may predominate during the relapse. The relapse is often more severe and more apt to be complicated by other infections.

Complications.—It is generally recognized that patients suffering from influenza are peculiarly liable to secondary infection with other organisms. Presumably the "toxins" liberated by the causative agent of influenza are responsible for a reduction of local tissue resistance, or a general lowering of resistance. Very likely a number of factors are involved. It is also noteworthy that, as a rule, complications are less common during the first wave of a pandemic than during later ones. This is probably due to the establishment of foci of other virulent organisms in certain individuals. From these sources, virulent organisms are disseminated and infect the mass of individuals in whom the soil has been prepared, so to speak, by influenza. This explanation is supported by the fact that in different localities the variety of secondary invaders takes on a local character. For example, in 1918, in certain localities streptococci predominated in the complicating lesions; in others, pneumococci, staphylococci or influenza bacilli. Other factors also play a rôle. It has been observed that soldiers with influenza who were cared for under comfortable conditions were much less apt to contract complications than soldiers taken ill during

7

combat operations. In other words, stress, strain, fatigue, hardship and exposure increase the chances for the development of complications.

Pneumonia.—Pneumonia is the most dreaded of all complications of influenza. During 1918 it occurred in about 6 per cent of cases. Pneumonia may develop at any time during the initial attack of influenza, but most frequently follows the disease. The earlier it appears, the more fatal it is apt to be. Patients dying from influenza almost invariably show physical signs and postmortem evidence of pneumonia. Typical lobar pneumonia seldom occurs. It is almost always of the atypical "bronchopneumonia" type. The lesions often commence with an acute, rapidly progressing, hemorrhagic bronchitis. Both lungs are usually involved with discrete or confluent areas of inflammation.

The *pathology* is largely dependent upon the causative organism. Considerable confusion and misunderstanding occurred in 1918 before pneumonia was classified on an etiologic rather than on an anatomic basis. The organisms commonly associated with atypical pneumonia are the Streptococcus hemolyticus, staphylococcus, influenza bacillus and the pneumococcus of Types III to XXXII. Table 3, given by Cole, shows the relative incidence of various types of bacteria causing atypical pneumonia during influenza observed in a New York hospital. It is noteworthy that the streptococcus so commonly encountered elsewhere was not found in his series of cases.

TABLE 3.

Bacterial incitant.	No. of cases.	Recovered.	Died.	Per cent mortality.
Pneumococcus	8	4	4	50
Streptococcus	0	0	0	0
Staphylococcus	13	4	9	69
Influenza bacilli	6	4	2	33
Mixed infection	50	38	12	24
Unknown	8	8	0	0
	85	58	27	31.7

These organisms may be found in the lung in pure culture or in various mixtures, depending upon the variety of bacteria prevailing in the environment as mentioned above.

Pneumonia due to the *streptococcus* is usually characterized by a diffuse inflammation of the bronchial tree and a lobular distribution throughout the lungs. The whole lung may be greatly inflamed and congested and drips with a thin sanguineous fluid when cut. Massive serous or serosanguineous pleural effusion or empyema commonly occurs (see page 129).

Staphylococcal pneumonia is characterized by a similar lobular distribution and by the formation of miliary abscesses. The abscesses become larger and coalesce if the patient lives long enough (see page 118).

The *symptoms* of pneumonia may commence at any time during influenza. The onset is usually late in the disease and is insidious. Less often the onset is early and fulminating with massive pulmonary edema, cyanosis and circulatory collapse. Cough, sputum, cyanosis and dyspnea gradually appear or, if already present, become worse.

The sputum soon assumes a hemorrhagic character. Bronchitis and pleurisy are common. In many cases, especially of streptococcal pneumonia, massive pleural effusion appears. The fluid is serous or bloody and rapidly reaccumulates after tapping. Cases that survive long enough may develop streptococcal empyema. In fatal cases death results from asphyxia, circulatory failure, toxemia or exhaustion.

The *physical signs* are variable. There is often a peculiar cyanotic pallor, described variously as heliotrope, plum or ashy, especially about the face and upper chest. Others have noted peculiar cherry-red color of the mucous membranes. The temperature, pulse-rate and respiration-rate increase (Fig. 7) and dyspnea may become marked. The fever curve is irregular. Signs of pulmonary involvement may be minimal with only a few crackling râles or may be those of massive consolidation, edema or hydrothorax. Leukocytosis is the rule.

Other Complications.—Nasal sinusitis and mastoiditis are common, otitis media less so. Various sorts of nervous complications arise— restlessness, insomnia, delirium, or transient psychoses. Peripheral neuritis, meningitis and myelitis occur. Of especial interest is a confusing condition usually called "postinfluenzal encephalitis." An increase in the number of cases of lethargic encephalitis has been noted after certain influenza epidemics. According to one view, the condition is directly related to influenza and probably caused by the same virus. Others feel that encephalitis lethargica is a distinct entity, accidentally accompanying influenza. A third opinion is that influenza increases the susceptibility to encephalitis lethargica. Until the etiologic agent of encephalitis lethargica is discovered, it will be difficult to differentiate it from the non-specific *hemorraghic encephalitis* which occurs during influenza as it does during other infectious diseases.

Gastro-intestinal disturbances including tympanites, hemorrhage from the bowel, enteritis and peritonitis may be considered as complications resulting from the effects of poisonous products of the causative organism.

Sequelæ.—*Lung abscess* or *bronchiectasis* may occur. *Nervous sequelæ* include peripheral neuritis, persistent asthenia, encephalitis, meningitis, myelitis and numerous psychoses which often clear up satisfactorily. Encephalitis occurring during influenza may be followed by paralysis agitans. Bradycardia has been observed.

Relation to Tuberculosis.—It is generally true that tuberculous patients are neither more nor less susceptible to influenza than normal individuals. No reliable data exist to show that influenza generally predisposes to tuberculosis in previously healthy individuals or that influenza tends to reactivate latent tuberculosis.

Influenza during *pregnancy* is said to be more dangerous than any other common infection, especially during the latter months. Abortion, miscarriage and premature labor are often induced. These accidents increase the mortality-rate considerably in pregnant women. In one series (Bland), the mortality among women whose pregnancy was interrupted was 57 per cent, in those not interrupted, 26 per cent.

Diagnosis.—Clinical criteria alone are available for diagnosis until the etiologic agent is proved. Excepting in pandemics or in epidemics, it may be difficult or impossible to differentiate influenza from the common cold or other common respiratory infections, especially if catarrhal symptoms are present. Typical influenza is characterized by the symptoms listed previously. Especially striking are the sudden onset, injected conjunctivæ, prostration, cyanosis and relatively slow pulse. The development of many similar cases at once and the frequency of catarrhal symptoms may be helpful. The leukocytes may be slightly increased at first but soon are diminished. A normal count or leukopenia with relative lymphocytosis is the rule. Leukocytosis generally heralds complications. The blood pressure is usually lowered. In cases in which fever persists longer than five days complications should be suspected and sought for.

It is recommended that the term *influenza* be used in its restricted sense alone and not applied indiscriminately as a blanket diagnosis for any obscure febrile disorder.

Prognosis.—Influenza is, in itself, seldom fatal. The percentage of deaths in the total number of cases during 1918, ranged from 0.8 per cent to 3.1 per cent. In a group of 130,000 cases, the case fatality-rate was 1.6 per cent. The frequency of complications renders it necessary, however, to regard every case of influenza seriously. The prognostic importance of pneumonia as a complication is illustrated in Table 4 prepared by Cole.

TABLE 4.

	No. of cases.	Recovered.	Died.	Per cent mortality.
Cases without lung signs . .	83	83	0	0
Cases with râles only . . .	37	37	0	0
Cases with signs of pulmonary involvement	85	58	27	31.7
	205	178	27	13.1

The death-rate of influenza complicated by pneumonia, or other conditions, varies from 20 to 60 per cent. The prognosis is graver when pneumonia is manifested at the onset of influenza, or when the pulmonary involvement is widespread. Other unfavorable signs are marked cyanosis, dyspnea and signs of circulatory failure. Sudden changes for the worse commonly occur during pneumonia. The prognosis is always serious in patients with other conditions, as chronic illness or pregnancy. Poor hygienic surroundings, poverty or war-time conditions are unfavorable influences.

Prophylaxis.—Until the etiologic agent of influenza is proved, prophylactic measures will rest entirely on the meager information available at present. Methods successful in controlling epidemics of other diseases failed when applied to influenza. It is known that the chief factor in the dissemination of influenza is the human carrier, that contagion is transmitted from person to person, directly or indirectly, and that the portal of entry is probably through the mucous membranes of the respiratory tract or conjunctiva.

If it were possible to determine the exact endemic centers of influenza, effective quarantine measures might be applied. But outbreaks are usually recognized too late, and in modern times, rapid transportation and free world intercourse preclude such measures. The only certain way of avoiding influenza during an epidemic is in complete isolation, preferably on a remote island or on a mountain top. Several communities thus situated escaped entirely during the last pandemic. Isolation must, of course, be absolute, and must be enforced before any healthy carriers are admitted. Under average circumstances, complete isolation is impossible to achieve.

General Control Measures.—Modern methods of communication make it possible to broadcast information in regard to the commencement and spread of an epidemic and permit certain preparations and precautions to be observed. It is wise to give wide publicity, by newspapers, radio or other means, to information in regard to the disease before or during an epidemic. Information should be given in regard to the proper quarantine of patients, the prevention of spread to others, and the reasons for various general prophylactic measures which may be adopted. This information given to the public would, to a large extent, prevent the bewilderment, terror and mass hysteria attendant to epidemics. Even in 1918 the wearing of amulets and charms was widely practised. Confidence was placed on bags of camphor or asafetida worn around the neck to prevent infection.

Theoretically, large gatherings of people should be discouraged, especially in country districts. The closing of schools, markets, theaters or churches in large cities may be desirable under certain circumstances, but had no apparent influence on the course of the pandemic of 1918, since many other possibilities of contact infection existed in public conveyances, stores, shops and the like.

Vaccination is a procedure of doubtful value considering that the cause of influenza is uncertain. Many studies designed to show beneficial effects of various vaccines were inadequately controlled. Carefully controlled observations have not revealed any evidence of protection afforded by vaccination (Zinsser). Vaccination with various organisms has no influence on the prevention of complications.

The wearing of face masks composed of several layers of 44 by 40 mesh gauze large enough to cover the nose and mouth are apparently effective in preventing influenza in individuals coming in contact with patients. The possibility of the conjunctiva serving as a portal of entry must also be considered, suggesting the use of goggles as well. In general, however, the inconvenience and discomfort of wearing face masks renders this measure impractical for general use.

Personal Prophylaxis.—Personal prophylaxis consists chiefly of avoiding contact with possible carriers or with patients. Individuals obliged to come in contact with patients should wear a face mask, goggles and gown. The hands must be thoroughly washed after each contact. Common drinking cups, utensils or towels are to be avoided. Fatigue, exposure to cold and wet, and all excesses predispose to infection. Moderate exercise in the open, comfort, good food and rest are recommended. The use of nasal sprays or gargles of various solutions and the inhalation of certain gases are not recommended for prophylaxis and may, in some instances, do harm.

Treatment.—As soon as a diagnosis is made, the case should be reported to the local health department. The patient should be immediately isolated. All persons apt to come in contact with him and all who have already been exposed to infection should be instructed as regards measures to prevent the spread of infection further, and how to avoid the disease personally.

The uncomplicated case of influenza is usually mild and requires little or no medication. Absolute rest in bed, warmth, fresh air, liberal diet and plenty of water are of greatest importance. The bowels should be kept open by a proper diet or, if necessary, by the occasional use of mild laxatives. For severe headache or aching pains, aspirin, 0.3 to 0.6 gram (5 to 10 grains); acetphenetidin, 0.18 to 0.3 gram (3 to 5 grains), or amidopyrine, 0.3 gram (5 grains) are useful and may be given several times, if necessary. An ice-bag to the head often affords comfort. Cough may be controlled by steam inhalations containing aromatic oils or resins (eucalyptol, benzoin) for agreeableness. Menthol cough lozenges are often useful. Codeine, 0.03 to 0.06 gram ($\frac{1}{2}$ to 1 grain) by mouth may be necessary. Cough syrups and the usual expectorants often cause nausea, disturb digestion, and are seldom used.

For restlessness or insomnia, luminal, 0.03 to 0.18 gram ($\frac{1}{2}$ to 3 grains), or sodium or potassium bromide, 1 gram (15 grains) may be given. Morphine is rarely required.

In severe cases with circulatory collapse, supportive measures are indicated. Heat should be applied to the body. Fluids may, if necessary, be given by rectum, subcutaneously or intravenously. Oxygen inhalations, preferably by use of the oxygen tent, are often of great value for the relief of dyspnea and cyanosis if the lungs are not already edematous.

Convalescence in bed of at least a week's duration in mild cases, and longer in severe cases, is advisable until the danger of complications is over. Change of scene is often valuable during convalescence, especially for patients mentally disturbed.

All efforts should be devoted to the prevention of complications, especially of pneumonia. Patients should be dressed warmly and protected from drafts. Attendants suffering from respiratory infections should be barred from the sick room. No visitors are to be permitted in the sick room.

Pneumonia is treated symptomatically. Absolute bed rest is essential. Warmth, fresh air, nutritious diet and maintenance of elimination are valuable in conserving the patient's resistive power. Hypnotics or narcotics may be useful in permitting rest and sleep. Oxygen is valuable in cyanosis or dyspnea, but ineffectual if the lungs are edematous. Cardiac stimulants as such are not recommended. If feeding is impossible, resort may be made to the intravenous injection of 200 cc. of a 25 per cent solution of dextrose several times daily. Cough is relieved by steam inhalations if the secretions are not already profuse and watery. For exhausting cough, codeine or morphine may be required to permit rest. Pleuritic pain is best relieved by the application of a many-tailed canton flannel binder, adjusted to suit the comfort of the patient. Adhesive tape should not be used. A hot-water bottle often gives relief. In certain intractable cases morphine is necessary. Abdominal distention is best avoided by regulating the diet from the beginning. When present, hot turpentine stupes or enemata may give relief. Pituitrin has been used.

Empyema requires special treatment according to the causative organism. In all forms of empyema, fluid is withdrawn with a needle at daily intervals or oftener if necessary. Surgical measures are required when the pus becomes too thick for aspiration. It is usually wisest to defer operation until the height of the illness has passed. Experience has shown that pneumococcus empyema is best treated by rib resection and free drainage after the acute stage has passed. In streptococcus empyema Graham recommends (*a*) careful avoidance of open pneumothorax in the acute pneumonic stage to obviate further respiratory embarrassment, (*b*) the prevention of a chronic empyema by the rapid sterilization and obliteration of the cavity, and (*c*) careful attention to the nutrition of the patient. Drainage during the acute stage may be secured by repeated aspiration or by use of the closed suction apparatus combined with the injection of Dakin's solution at frequent intervals.

The treatment of other complications is similar to that when these conditions occur alone and is discussed in appropriate sections.

REFERENCES.

COLE, R. I.: Acute Pulmonary Infections (bibliography), De Lamar Lectures, 1927–1928.

JORDAN, E. O.: Epidemic Influenza, A Survey (bibliography), Am. Med. Assn., Chicago, 1927.

LEICHTENSTERN, O.: Influenza, Nothnagel's Encyclopedia of Practical Medicine, American edition, Philadelphia, W. B. Saunders Company, 1905.

Pathology of the Acute Respiratory Diseases, The Med. Dept. of U. S. Army in the World War, 1929, vol. **12**, War Dept., Washington, D. C. (excellent illustrations).

ZINSSER, H.: Etiology and Epidemiology of Influenza, Medicine, 1922, **1**, 213.

GLANDERS.

Synonyms.—Farcy; Malleus; Rotz.

Definition.—Glanders is a highly fatal, specific, acute or chronic infectious and contagious disease, primarily of horses, but transmissible to man, caused by Pfeifferella mallei, and characterized by the formation of nodules in the skin, mucous membranes or viscera, which tend to ulcerate and suppurate.

In horses, the disease is known as *glanders* when localized in the nares and as *farcy* when the skin and subcutaneous tissues are involved. In man, the cutaneous form is commoner.

History.—Glanders was known by the ancients to exist in horses. Its communicability to man was recognized in the eighteenth century. There was considerable controversy over the contagiousness of the disease until 1882 when Löffler and Schütz obtained pure cultures of the causative organism.

Incidence.—Glanders was at one time a serious and widespread disease among horses, mules and asses in certain parts of the world. In England, for example, nearly 2000 cases occurred between 1887 and 1906. There were also 78 deaths from glanders among humans about this time. With the early recognition of the disease and its prompt isolation, glanders has been almost exterminated in the United States. No cases have been observed in Bellevue Hospital in New York City for over eight years, whereas previously 7 cases were admitted during a period of twenty years. Germany reported 100 cases, and France 27 cases in 1927. Glanders is apt to occur where large numbers of horses exist. The replacement of the horse by motor transportation has contributed to the disappearance of the disease.

Etiology.—Bacillus mallei is a small, non-motile, Gram-negative rod with rounded ends. The rods are usually straight, but may be slightly curved. In old cultures, coccoid and vacuolated forms appear. The bacillus is easily stained and easily decolorized. Stained bacilli show irregular patches of pale and deeply colored areas. The organisms grow readily on the usual laboratory media. Growth on potato is characteristic; within forty-eight hours, the surface is covered with a transparent yellowish or honey-like, mucoid layer which turns reddish-brown with age.

The bacillus is virulent for man, horses, asses, mules, cats and dogs, in which spontaneous infection may occur. Guinea-pigs and rabbits are susceptible when inoculated. The source of infection is in all cases the sick animal or man. Infection is transmitted by direct contact, or by contact with pus, tissue or dressings. The organism gains entry into the body presumably through lesions of skin, and nasal or oral mucous membrane. Gastro-intestinal infection has been suggested. The organism is a dangerous one with which to work and laboratory manipulations are hazardous.

Symptoms.—**Acute Form.**—Since the infection rapidly becomes generalized, the symptoms may be variable, depending upon the sites of localization of infection. The *incubation period* lasts from three to five days and may be accompanied by malaise, headache, chilliness or fever. The onset is characterized by an inflammatory reaction at the site of primary infection, consisting of an infiltration of the skin and an acute lymphangitis composed of epithelioid cells, leukocytes and bacilli. Abscesses form which soon become necrotic and suppurate. The regional lymphatics are usually involved in an extremely painful swelling. Acute pneumonia may be the first symptom. After three to seven days the infection becomes generalized and metastatic infections soon appear. Painful or painless bubos appear in distant areas, rapidly suppurate, discharge bloody pus and leave deep and extensive ulcers. A characteristic skin eruption sometimes appears between the sixth and twelfth day as discrete or confluent pustules in various parts of the skin and mucous membranes, often on the face. Abscesses occur in muscles and in the viscera, and especially in the mucous membranes of the nose and throat. Suppurative arthritis occurs. The fever is irregular and often of the "septic" type. The spleen and liver are usually enlarged. Prostration, diarrhea, bronchitis, bronchopneumonia and evidence of circulatory failure are characteristic. Death occurs in practically all cases.

Acute glanders is frequently primary in the nose, suggesting this region as the portal of entry. The first symptoms are rhinitis and the appearance of a small vesicle or pustule. The nasal discharge increases and becomes slimy, purulent and bloody. The lesion spreads until the lips, nose, pharynx, larynx, hard and soft palate, cheeks and gums are involved in an ulcerating, discharging mass of granulating tissue. Blindness results from conjunctival involvement. The submaxillary lymphoid tissue frequently suppurates. The process may be present without marked constitutional disturbance for a considerable period. Recovery is rare.

Chronic Form.—Certain individuals who contract the disease have apparently a certain degree of resistance. Instead of succumbing rapidly to an overwhelming infection, they are able to cope with the infection for a long period and, in some cases, overcome it. A few patients who survive an acute attack may become chronic cases. In other cases the chronic form commences insidiously. This form is characterized by some focus of infection from which bacilli are disseminated at intervals *via* the blood stream or lymphatics and involve adjacent or remote parts in metastatic infections. Long or short periods of remission may elapse between exacerbations. The symptoms are generally the same as in the acute form. Aching, severe joint pains, prostration and irregular fever appear. In some cases emaciation is out of proportion to the apparent mildness of the infection. Abscesses in various parts appear and spread. They are refractory to any form of treatment, but may heal during remissions with extensive scar formation. Various organs may be affected. Pulmonary, cerebral, and bone involvement occur. Periarticular tissue and joints are frequently involved and suppurate. The nasal passages are involved at some time during the course in most cases.

The course may last two or three years or more. Relapses are common. Latent infections are easily lighted up. Death occurs in at least 50 per cent of the cases, and is due to exhaustion, toxemia, acute exacerbation or to secondary infections.

Diagnosis.—Diagnosis is often extremely difficult. Glanders is a rare disease and unless it is in mind, many other diseases are first considered. The history of recent contact with an infected horse is most helpful. The appearance of multiple abscesses and ulcers with irregular, serpiginous, sharply demarcated but uninfiltrated margins, with a soft base covered with greenish, sticky or slimy exudate is an important diagnostic point. Glanders must be considered in cases in which ulcerative processes of mucous membranes resist treatment but heal spontaneously only to break out anew in the same or in adjacent areas. Further diagnostic points are: the rapidly progressive course in acute cases with exhaustion and prostration, a pyemic temperature curve, involvement of the joints and lymphatics and the slimy hemorrhagic character of the nasal discharge.

Laboratory procedures are most valuable in diagnosis. Although few specific organisms are present in exudates, and very frequently many other bacteria are present, they can sometimes be demonstrated in smears by staining with hot methylene blue. They are best isolated by inoculating male guinea-pigs intraperitoneally with small amounts of exudate or suspected cultures. Within one or two days a marked inflammatory reaction appears in the testes from which glanders bacilli are recovered. Guinea-pigs die ten days to six weeks after inoculation. Bacillus mallei can be identified by the character of its growth on potato and by agglutination with known antimalleus serum. Glanders bacilli can be cultivated from the blood and from joint exudate in most cases, especially late in the disease. The serum of patients and animals contains agglutinins for Bacillus mallei. The titer, to be significant, must be over 1 to 500, especially in horses.

Differential diagnosis may be difficult. Demonstration of the Bacillus mallei is the decisive factor in diagnosis. Syphilis,.tuberculosis and epithelioma are often considered for months or years in chronic cases before the true nature is discovered. Syphilis is ruled out by failure of specific therapy, by failure to demonstrate spirochetes in the lesions, and by the behavior and appearance of the lesions. Tuberculosis is ruled out by the absence of tubercle bacilli and by the subsequent course of the disease. Tuberculosis and glanders may coexist. Other infections which are likely to be confused with early glanders are typhoid fever, erysipelas, pyemia and suppurative polyarthritis. In the tropics, melioidosis and kala-azar may be confusing.

All acute cases, and at least 50 per cent of chronic cases, end fatally. The average duration of chronic cases is fourteen months. They may last five years.

Prophylaxis.—Animals infected with glanders must be promptly destroyed. Cremation or deep burial is recommended. The stable, all trappings and utensils, the feed and watering trough used by the infected animal must be sterilized. Other animals exposed to infection should be tested with mallein and, if reacting positively, should be destroyed. Great care must be exercised to prevent human or animal contact with infected exudates or tissues of animal or human origin and with living cultures. Prophylactic vaccine and serum are valueless. Suspicious ulcers or nodules should be excised promptly and the area cauterized. One attack of the disease does not confer immunity.

Treatment.—Strict isolation and disinfection of secretions, excretions and dressings are imperative. No specific treatment exists. Early excision and cauterization of skin lesions may prevent generalization of infection, but cases are rarely seen or diagnosed early enough. General symptomatic and supportive treatment is required. Antiseptic washes may be used to bathe ulcers and suppurating areas. Pain may be relieved by the application of heat or cold, by codeine or by morphine, if necessary. Pustules and abscesses, when well localized, may be opened and drained. Antiseptic solutions of phenol or Dakin's solution may be tried. In one patient with a chronic infection, who ultimately recovered, 82 operations were performed within a period of nearly five years.

REFERENCES.

FROTHINGHAM, C. L., and MCCLURE, C. W.: Glanders, Oxford Med., vol. **5**, p. 185.
GAIGER, S. H. (personal account): Proc. Roy. Soc. Med., 1929, **22**, 996.
LÜHRS, E.: Rotz, Handb. d. path. Mikro., Kolle, Kraus, Uhlenhuth, 1929, **6**, 1.
MENDELSON, R. W.: Glanders, Jour. Am. Med. Assn., 1929, **93**, 1379.
SAKAMOTO, K. J.: Diagnosis of Glanders, Jour. Immunol., 1930, **18**, 331.

CHOLERA.

Definition.—Cholera is a highly fatal, acute, specific, infectious and contagious disease of the gastro-intestinal tract, caused by Vibrio comma, characterized by profuse watery diarrhea, vomiting, muscle cramps, suppression of urine and collapse.

History.—Cholera has been endemic in lower Bengal, India, from time immemorial. From this source it has repeatedly spread and swept over large portions of the world. America was seriously involved in 1826, 1846 and in 1870. Minor epidemics have occurred from time to time in Europe, especially in Russia, where an endemic focus apparently exists. During the World War numerous limited outbreaks occurred in the Balkans and in Mesopotamia. In India and China, cholera ranks with plague in magnitude. Between February 8 and May 30, 1931, 45,000 cases were reported in India with 23,000 deaths, a mortality-rate of about 50 per cent.

Epidemiology.—Man is apparently the only source of the disease, and his excretions convey the infection to others, directly or indirectly. Individuals in contact with patients may become infected directly by contaminating the fingers and introducing vibrios into the mouth. The mouth and gastro-intestinal tract is probably the only portal of entry. Flies and cockroaches may convey infection from feces to food.

Uncooked vegetables fertilized by human feces or washed in contaminated water constitute another source. Probably the most important conveyance of infection is polluted drinking water. Contaminated streams spread infection to large numbers of people. Hamburg was infected in this manner in 1892. The Hamburg accident did much to direct general attention to the importance of pure water supply. An interesting and important observation in this connection is that cholera vibrios introduced into river water in localities previously free from cholera survive much longer than those placed in water which has been repeatedly or continuously contaminated with feces of cholera patients. The bactericidal or self-purifying property of the water of the large rivers of India was mentioned by Mark Twain. The phenomenon is now ascribed to the presence of bacteriophage in the water (d'Herelle).

Healthy carriers constitute a great problem in the control of cholera. No matter how strictly isolation and quarantine are enforced, healthy individuals who harbor virulent vibrios in their intestines often escape detection and carry infection to remote districts and may eventually be stricken themselves.

Etiology.—The cholera vibrio, or comma bacillus, was discovered by Koch, working in Egypt in 1883. The bacillus is very small, measuring about 2 microns long and 0.5 micron in thickness. It is often curved, especially in young cultures, and resembles a comma, from which it derives its name. Occasionally, distinct spiral forms are seen. The organism is actively motile due to a flagellum at one end which is often several times longer than the body. No spores are formed.

The bacillus is easily stained and is Gram-negative. Growth occurs aërobically on all of the usual media. An alkaline media is preferable to an acid one. Gelatin is liquefied. Growth is exceptionally luxuriant in alkaline peptone water (1 per cent peptone, 0.5 per cent sodium chloride), especially near the surface. In this medium, indol is formed which may be demonstrated by the "cholera-red" reaction, at one time believed to be a specific diagnostic test. Growth is best at 37° C. but may take place between 22° and 40° C. Bacilli remain viable after freezing in water for three to five days. They may live longer in water, milk, moist clothing and in food. Acidity, drying and sunlight are bactericidal. Boiling and chemical disinfectants destroy vibrios easily. Vibrios are susceptible to bacteriophage action.

Pathogenesis.—Cholera vibrios gain entrance into the body only through the mouth. Many are killed by the acidity of the stomach, but a certain number pass through unharmed into the intestine where a favorable alkaline peptone medium exists. The rapid multiplication of vibrios in the intestine with the probable liberation of toxins often causes diarrhea promptly. Soon afterward, the invasion of the epithelial lining commences, from which time the onset of the disease dates. Vibrios are often found deep in the crypts and may penetrate to the muscular wall. Hypothetically, the toxins liberated by death of the vibrios are absorbed by the lymphatics, enter the general circulation and produce "toxemia." Vibrios seldom, if ever, invade the blood stream. They are occasionally found in the gall-bladder, rarely elsewhere. Extensive inflammation and subepithelial edema of the intestinal lining results in the shedding of particles of tissue, which, together with flakes of mucus, appear in the stools giving them the characteristic "rice-water" appearance.

Pathology.—Rigor mortis appears early. Curious muscle contractions may occur after death. The body presents a livid and shrunken appearance. The tissues are unusually dark and dry. The spleen and liver are small. The serous surfaces are dry and sticky. A peculiar peach color is noticed in the intestinal serosa. Liquid and occasionally bloody fluid is present in the bowel. The membranes are pinkish, congested and soggy. Ulcerations due to secondary infection may be present.

Histologically, there is congestion and inflammation of the superficial epithelial layer. Subepithelial edema is present. Vibrios are present in great abundance in the liquid contents and in the epithelial layers and villi.

Symptoms.—The incubation period is short, from sixteen to twenty hours (measured in self-infected volunteers) to several days. The length of the incubation period was in inverse proportion to the size of the ingested inoculum. The incubation period may be symptomless or "premonitory diarrhea" may occur.

Several clinical forms of the disease are recognized:

(a) The *ambulatory type* (cholera-diarrhea) in which the diarrhea is always fecal in character and malaise is the chief symptom. The course is mild and the duration from four to ten days. Thirst, anorexia and a coated tongue may be present. This type occurs in most epidemics, and is commonest during the decline of an outbreak. Patients with this type of infection usually recover, but may rapidly become worse and pass into the more severe types.

(b) The *moderately severe type* (cholerine) is an exaggeration of the mild type. The diarrhea loses its fecal equality and becomes watery and copious. Vomiting, fever and tachycardia appear. The extremities become cold and the urine output diminishes due to excessive loss of water from the bowels or in the vomitus. Severe, agonizing muscle cramps appear, especially in the calves and thighs, and the voice becomes aphonic. Several days may elapse and the patient may recover or pass into the severe form.

(c) *Severe, algid* (cold) *type,* cholera gravis, and asphyxial cholera are terms indicating the occurrence of collapse. This form often comprises about one-half of the cases in an outbreak. It may commence abruptly or may be preceded by milder symptoms. The stools are of the rice-water type; 10 to 20 movements occur during a day. The passages may be painless, but are usually accompanied by severe tenesmus. Severe distressing vomiting appears, preventing retention of any food or water. Thirst becomes intense; hiccough is common. The tongue dries and is heavily coated. The body appears wasted, the face pinched and the eyeballs sunken. The skin looks wrinkled like a "washerwoman's hands." The extremities become clammy, cold and livid; cyanosis is marked. The circulation nearly comes to a standstill. Aphonia is present, due to dryness and weakness of the vocal cords. The surface temperature drops to subnormal levels, the internal temperature indicates fever. Dyspnea may be marked, the respiration-rate reaching 50 per minute. The heart sounds become feebler and the blood pressure falls. There is anuria.

Muscle cramps, especially of the legs, are exceedingly painful and distressing. Board-like contractions and even rupture occur. Contractions are said to be due to toxemia. Water depletion is apparently not the sole cause for cramps, as was once believed, for cholera with severe cramps occasionally occurs without excessive loss of fluid. A combination of factors is probably responsible. Studies of the rôle of tetany and the calcium metabolism have not come to the author's attention.

The mentality often remains clear. Restlessness and insomnia occur. Apathy, somnolence and coma precede death. Hyperesthesia may be distressing. The eyelids often remain partly open, causing dryness of the cornea. The severe type seldom lasts longer than a day or two. The circulation may fail during the first day.

Water depletion causes concentration of the blood. The red cells and leukocytes are increased, the latter sometimes to 60,000, but usually to about 20,000 per c.mm.

In certain cases which recover, the symptoms disappear with astonishing rapidity. The patient may sit up and smoke a day after being in an apparently moribund state. Recovery may be apparent for several days when a fatal relapse occurs.

The algid type is sometimes followed by a "reaction" during which the skin becomes warm, the diarrhea lessens, the hollows fill out, the pulse returns and urine is again secreted. These evidences of improvement are accompanied by higher fever, which may last a few hours and disappear or pass into the "typhoid" or comatose state. Complications such as pneumonia or enteritis occur. Death from exhaustion or uremia frequently occurs at this time. An urticarial, scarlatiniform or morbilliform skin eruption may appear, especially if the patient lives through the second week. An exanthema occurred in 8 per cent of the Hamburg cases. Nephrosis ending with uremic symptoms occasionally occurs.

(*d*) *Cholera sicca, siderans* or *fulminating cholera* is the most severe form. In this type the infection is overwhelming. The patient may be prostrated, collapse and die within a few hours after infection as from some violent poison, and before diarrhea and vomiting occur.

Complications.—Complications seldom occur. Bronchopneumonia and pulmonary congestion have been noted. Membranous inflammation of the bladder and vagina, parotitis, gangrene, jaundice, and secondary infections may occur. Cholera may coexist with typhoid fever or dysentery. *Sequelæ* such as mental depression, anemia, nephritis, and constipation have been observed.

Diagnosis.—Typical cases occurring during an epidemic are easily recognized. Sporadic cases or the first few cases of an epidemic, when detection is so important, are frequently missed. Strict isolation of the earliest cases may prevent an epidemic. The diagnostic features of cholera are the frequent, profuse, rice-water stools; clammy, shrunken, cold skin; collapse, cyanosis, suppression of urine, muscle cramps, aphonia and a high mortality. Mild cases may not show any of these striking symptoms and can be detected only by bacteriologic methods and history of exposure.

Diagnosis is confirmed by the demonstration of the comma vibrio in the stool in direct smears or by cultural methods. When the organisms are sparse, a small quantity of stool (1 cc.) may be inoculated into peptone water and incubated. Isolation of colonies can be accomplished in solid media. Further identification must be made by specific agglutination of the vibrios in cholera-immune serum in a dilution of at least 1 to 1000. Non-pathogenic vibrios are occasionally encountered which resemble the cholera vibrio, and can be differentiated by immunologic procedures. The Pfeiffer phenomenon or the disappearance of cholera vibrios when injected intraperitoneally into specifically immunized guinea-pigs is also of value in differentiation.

Differential Diagnosis.—Acute food poisoning may cause symptoms very similar to those of cholera. Such an outbreak is well localized, involves only those partaking of the contaminated food and never spreads farther. Arsenic, mercury, mushroom or methyl alcohol poisoning may all resemble cholera except that, in the case of cholera, diarrhea precedes vomiting. Malaria, bacillary dysentery, trichiniasis, lamblia infections, heat stroke and severe water deprivation may all cause symptoms resembling cholera.

Prophylaxis.—Since the patient is the chief source of infection, cholera is theoretically easy to control from an epidemiologic point of view. Were it not for the fact that healthy carriers exist, the strict isolation and quarantine of an infected center would suffice to prevent the spread of infection. A five-day period of quarantine of individuals leaving an infected locality suffices to detect most of the seriously infected persons. During an epidemic, travel should be restricted, public gatherings should be prohibited, and the water and food supply protected from contamination. Dejecta and articles soiled by patients must be disinfected. Recovered patients must be kept under supervision until their stools are free from cholera vibrios.

Personal Prophylaxis.—Personal prophylaxis consists chiefly in avoiding the introduction of infection into the mouth. The hands must be thoroughly washed after each contact with the sick or with infected materials. Hands must be washed especially before meals. Food and drink must come from uncontaminated sources or, better still, should be sterilized by cooking. A wise plan is to eat nothing but hot food. Fatigue or excess of any kind must be avoided.

Vaccination.—Haffkine's vaccine offers a limited degree of protection. Usually, subcutaneous injections of 4000 million and 8000 million attenuated vibrios at ten-day intervals are given. Local reactions may occur. The resulting immunity is short and uncertain, lasting at most three or four months. It is better to observe the rules of personal hygiene than to depend upon vaccination for protection.

Prognosis.—The average mortality is from 50 to 60 per cent. Some epidemics reveal a 25 per cent mortality, others, 70 per cent. Prompt recognition and treatment lowers the mortality-rate. The chances of recovery in children, in the aged and in those with chronic illness are poor. The approach to the algid state, the appearance of anuria and cyanosis are grave signs. The mortality in cases without anuria is about 5 per cent. Most of the deaths occur in the first two days; later, only one-fifth of the cases end fatally.

Treatment.—This should be directed toward (1) supporting the patient through a profound infection, (2) restoring the water lost, (3) combating "toxemia," and (4) the management of special symptoms.

1. The patient should be put to bed immediately and kept warm. Hot-water bottles, hot blankets, warm drinks or hot stupes to the abdomen may be used. Fluid should be freely given. A liquid diet is recommended.

2. If severe vomiting prevents the administration of fluid by mouth and the diarrhea renders proctoclysis useless, water must be given intravenously or subcutaneously. This procedure often produces striking improvement which sometimes leads to recovery. Hyperesthesia may render the treatment painful. From 1 to 2 liters of a normal physiologic saline solution may be given several times a day. The fluid should be warmed to about 40° C. and injected slowly. The use of hypertonic saline solution is strongly recommended by Rogers.

3. There is no specific treatment for the toxemia. Serums have not proved beneficial. The so-called intestinal antiseptics are useless. Some observers have recommended the use of calomel or castor oil to flush out the infection, but it must be remembered that the bacilli causing the toxemia are embedded deeply in the epithelium. The administration of large enemas of 2 liters or more of warm water containing 2 per cent tannic acid solution, several times daily have, according to some, caused improvement.

4. Hyperpyrexia is sometimes relieved by cold or tepid sponging or by cold-water enemas. Antipyretic drugs are contraindicated.

Collapse is combated by warmth and the restoration of fluid. Certain stimulants—caffeine, styrchnine, adrenalin, have been recommended. The painful muscle spasms are sometimes relieved by the administration of fluid. Injection of morphine may be necessary. Diarrhea may sometimes be controlled by the administration of bismuth subcarbonate or subnitrate. Carbonated water or ice often alleviate intense thirst.

Convalescence should be guarded carefully lest fatal relapse occur.

REFERENCES.

D'HERELLE, F., MALONE, R. H., and LAHIRI, M. N.: Studies on Asiatic Cholera, Ind. Med. Res. Memoirs, No. 14, February, 1930.

KHAN, S.: On the Carrier Problem of Cholera, Ind. J. Med. Res., 1929, **17**, 147.

KOLLE, W., and PRIGGE, R.: Cholera Asiatica, Handb. d. path. Mikro., 1928, **4**, 1, Kolle, Kraus, Uhlenhuth.

ROGERS, L.: Cholera and Its Treatment, 1907.

ZLATOGOROFF, S.: Die Cholera, Kraus-Brugsch, Spec. Path. u. Therap. inn. Krankh., Berlin, 1919, **2**, pt. I, 637.

CHAPTER II.

THE COCCAL DISEASES.

By RALPH A. KINSELLA, M.D.

GENERAL CONSIDERATIONS.
STAPHYLOCOCCAL INFECTIONS.
  Septicemia.
  Pneumonia.
STREPTOCOCCAL INFECTIONS.
  Non-hemolytic Streptococcus.
  Focal Infections.
  Hemolytic Streptococcus.
  Special Streptococcal Infections.
  Sore Throat.
  Wound Infections.

STREPTOCOCCAL INFECTIONS.—
  Continued.
  Septicemia.
  Erysipelas.
  Bronchopneumonia.
  Empyema.
PNEUMOCOCCAL INFECTIONS.
  Lobar Pneumonia.
MENINGOCOCCAL INFECTIONS.
  Cerebrospinal Fever.
GONOCOCCAL INFECTIONS.

Introduction.—Under the coccal infections are included infections by those cocci that are usually considered associated with disease. There are many other cocci which are found on normal tissue which are not known to have any connection with the production of infection. Coccal infections that will be treated in this chapter are those due to staphylococci, streptococci, pneumococci, gonococci, and meningococci.

Distribution.—The distribution of all of these organisms on normal tissue is worth considering. Each one of these organisms is prominently associated with a location in some particular part of the body with the exception of the gonococcus the location of which outside of disease is not known. In the naso-pharynx we have a number of Gram-negative diplococci which are relatively unimportant insofar as their association with infection is concerned. But among these relatively unimportant organisms is one, the meningococcus, which may be found in from 1 to 5 per cent of normal nasal mucous membranes, and which is extremely important in the production of a definite and highly infectious and dangerous disease. In the pharynx the most commonly found coccus is the non-hemolytic streptococcus and, in many persons, a type of pneumococcus which is usually classified as type IV. On the skin, of course, the staphylococcus is always available and this organism is also found in the mouth and in the intestinal tract. Besides being in the pharynx, streptococci are also found in the intestinal tract and may be recovered from normal feces.

It is an interesting thing that the more virulent types of cocci are not found commonly on normal tissues. Meningococci, for example, are rarely present in the naso-pharynx of normal individuals. Their existence fluctuates with the conditions of living and with the season of the year, being much more easily found under the conditions of crowding and in the months of the year when the ventilation of living quarters is naturally restricted, such as in the winter. Hemolytic

8

streptococci, while found frequently in normal throats, are not found in predominance in cultures except when the organism is associated with an existing infectious disease. The gonococcus is not found at any time on normal tissues. Of the various pneumococci the more virulent types such as types I, II and III are found with comparative infrequency in normal throats, while the less virulent types that are called type IV are found in well over 50 per cent of normal throats. There is, therefore, some inverse relationship between the frequency with which bacteria exist in the human body under normal conditions and the capacity of these bacteria to produce infection.

The locality of bacterial life in normal tissues is loosely associated with the atrium or point of entrance of these bacteria into the tissues when conditions permit. In streptococcal infections hemolytic streptococci are usually found in the throat except when introduced artificially through a wound in some other part of the body. In cerebrospinal fever, cultures are made of secretion from the naso-pharynx, where meningococci are almost always recovered.

Pathogenicity.—The cocci exhibit several varieties of activity. Some lead a purely saprophytic existence, as do non-hemolytic streptococci growing in vegetations on valves of the heart; some combine a tendency to grow actively in any tissue of the body with a capacity to produce toxins, such as the hemolytic streptococcus. The pneumococcus and meningococcus, while displaying a capacity to grow in many different kinds of tissue, still cling to tissues of selection or choice in their chief pathogenic activity—the lungs and meninges, respectively. The gonococcus is unique among the cocci in being introduced into the body only through a broken surface, usually urethral or conjunctival, and in having no normal habitat in the human body. There are no healthy carriers of gonococci as of all the other pathogenic cocci. Gonococci may cause all of the metastatic infections that are based on saprophytic activity such as the mere growing of the organism inside the body at a point away from its local infection.

In any coccal infection injury to tissue and virulence of the organism are important for the beginning of the invasion; and the organism with very low virulence will need greater tissue injury and the organism with very high virulence will need little tissue injury for the setting up of an infectious disease. How the organisms get into the body is a matter of discussion. It can be considered that infection begins either by direct implantation on an injured surface, thereby effecting the general reaction of the body from this local base; or, that these organisms gain access to the blood stream and inaugurate the disease by a bacteriemia which secondarily produces the infectious disease which is commonly associated with the coccus in question. This latter mechanism is supposed to operate in many if not all cases of cerebrospinal fever.

Many of the cocci of low virulence may have their virulence raised by passage from one patient to another so that as they progress they gain virulence to such an extent that they may be able to incite infection without preëxisting injury. For example, the staphylococcus is an organism which is almost always introduced through a wound and which produces the same characteristic effects in any locality, but the opinion has been expressed that under some conditions the staphylococcus may be so increased in its invasive activity that it may cause a primary infection of the lungs. During times of epidemics of measles the activity of hemolytic streptococci may be heightened so that pneumonic infection, usually a complication of measles, may be produced by the streptococcus alone without preceding measles. It should be borne in mind that what we refer to as previous injury to tissues may be due to the activity of filterable virus and in the future we may find it necessary to change our attitude towards the idea of enhanced bacterial virulence. A preceding injury, or an infection by virus, may always be necessary for what seems to be primary bacterial invasion. There is little evidence to show that the non-hemolytic streptococcus has inherent, highly invasive qualities which would permit it to become the primary factor under any circumstances.

Epidemiology.—With the exception of those infections which result from the inoculation of wounds or broken surfaces, the coccal infections are nearly always transmitted by infected droplets. Thus, the broken urethral surface may be infected by gonococcus; wounds by staphylococcus or hemolytic streptococcus; but sore throat, bronchopneumonia, lobar pneumonia and cerebrospinal fever are conveyed by infected droplets expelled from the respiratory passages of the patient.

Symptoms.—When any of the cocci gain entrance to the human body the same principles are followed for the production of infectious disease that prevail generally in bacterial infection. That is to say, there is a period of one to three or four days when the organism is apparently enjoying increasing growth, while the individual is exhibiting few or no symptoms. If he complains of slight symptoms these might be referred to as the prodromal symptoms of the infection and the entire period referred to as the incubation period of the infection. The infectious disease itself consists of those symptoms and signs which result from the reaction between the infecting organism and the tissue cells of the body. These reactions are represented by symptoms that are both general and local. The general symptoms are those common to almost all infectious diseases and consist of fever and prostration. The fever is to be looked upon as the result of increased heat-producing chemical reactions, with a concomitant lowering of the capacity to eliminate heat. Such greatly increased metabolism would naturally exhaust the resources of the tissues and directly lead to the symptom of prostration. This prostration is further aggravated in the usual case by headache and backache. If these were the only signs of the reaction of the body to the infectious organisms it would be difficult without the methods of bacteriology even to make a diagnosis of a special infection. But there are also local signs which give to the infection a particular name. These local signs usually are produced at the place where the organism is supposed to enter the body. For example, the throat may be inflamed and yield on culture the organisms which are infecting the tissues of the pharynx. The lungs may be involved and yield signs which lead to the diagnosis of lobar pneumonia or to the diagnosis of inflammation of the bronchi and its smaller branches. The meninges may be infected and lead to unmistakable evidence of the disease known as meningitis, and so on. Any part of the body may furnish the local signs of a coccal infection.

Leukocytosis.—The coccal infections uniformly produce leukocytosis. Leukocytosis is interesting not only as representing the reaction of the circulating blood but also as representing the local reaction in the tissues which the body makes to the coccal infections and, accordingly, this type of infection is usually known as a pyogenic infection. In a very definite way the leukocytic response is connected with the capacity of the individual to recover from the infectious disease. A failure to produce leukocytosis is regarded as a bad omen, and the production of vigorous leukocytosis is always regarded with satisfaction by the physician. Changes in the type of granulocytes are also regarded as important. Continuing increase in the number of "stab" leukocytes makes the same unfavorable impression as it does in other infections. The leukocytosis terminates with the infection and, therefore, seems directly connected with the mechanism of recovery. Recovery depends on many factors, none of which can be established as the most important. In a general way antibody formation as expressed by agglutinins and precipitins of the blood is looked upon as one of the important agencies in the production of recovery. Such antibodies may also be bactericidal antibodies. There may also be antitoxic antibodies.

Diagnosis.—The diagnosis of coccal infection, besides resting on certain definite clinical factors which will be discussed when particular diseases are considered, depends on bacteriologic diagnostic methods. There are many infections which we now poorly understand which will be better understood when complete methods are used for determining the bacteriology involved.

The diagnosis of any infection must be carried out rigidly by examining the local flora and also by blood culture. It is important to emphasize the value of examining the direct smear from an inflamed part, as many diagnoses may be made simply by examination of direct smears. It is practically the only method used in the diagnosis of gonococcal urethritis. Cultures are never necessary in this disease. The direct smear has an advantage over culture methods in that it usually shows the predominance of bacteria in the inflammation, whereas the culture may show that organism predominating which is able to grow the most rapidly on the particular culture medium that is used.

Treatment.—The treatment of the coccal infections follows the same general lines as the treatment of other infections. For some of the coccal infections there are successful antiserums as for meningococcal infection and for pneumococcal infection of type I. For infections by hemolytic streptococcus the attempt to produce successful antiserums has met with partial success. The serums devised by Amoss for the treatment of erysipelas and more recently for the treatment of streptococcal pneumonia have yet to establish their value. For the treatment of scarlet fever, which is commonly regarded as a streptococcal infection added to the factor of bacterial allergy, the use of the various commercial serums is usually favorably discussed. The serum employed for staphylococcic septicemia, while based on valid experimental evidence, has not proven of medical value. There are no vaccines or antigens which have been established as successful. Attempt was made by Cecil and Austin to establish the value of vaccination against lobar pneumonia, but the application of the results could be made only if large numbers of people could be studied. There are antigenic substances for the treatment of coccal infections under various names which represent the growth-products of both pneumococci and streptococci, but the use of which has not been reported as widely successful.

Non-specific therapy has been employed in the treatment of various streptococcal and staphylococcal infections, but seldom in the acute forms of the diseases and usually only in those rather vague chronic infections known as focal infections. The exact value of the febrile reactions following the injection of vaccines or products of growth is doubtful in most cases and when effective produces usually only a temporary result.

STAPHYLOCOCCAL INFECTIONS.

Bacteriology.—There are two main varieties of staphylococci, known as albus and aureus, and separated by the capacity of the latter to produce yellow pigment on solid media. There is also associated with some of the strains of Staphylococcus aureus a capacity to produce hemolysis both in blood-containing culture media and in the human body, and this hemolytic activity is associated with an increase in pathogenicity. The toxin of these strains of staphylococci has been studied by Parker, and experimental results pointed to a probable clinical value of a corresponding antitoxin in the treatment of severe infections with bacteriemia in humans. Such a favorable result, unfortunately, has not been obtained.

Distribution.—The staphylococci of both varieties are widely distributed on the human body: on the skin, and on the mucous surfaces of the gums and pharynx, and intestinal tract. In a general way this wide distribution speaks for a comparatively low invasive activity. The thought follows that the more commonly a bacterium occurs in the human body the less likely it is to incite primary disease.

Pathogenesis.—Accordingly, staphylococci usually need a considerable amount of injury to tissue before they may begin to live within the human tissues. They seldom acquire such virulence that they can be transmitted from person to person, and there is no epidemiology connected with staphylococcic infections. This tissue injury is usually of the nature of a wound, and the commonest staphylococcal infections, therefore, are wound infections. These infections may be attended by bacteriemia and there are then created symptoms of general infection; and signs pointing to the localization of staphylococci in various parts of the body. The body resists infection by staphylococci by means of leukocytosis and phagocytosis and, to some extent, perhaps, by means of antitoxin. The fully developed abscess represents the completed effort on the part of the body to resist localized staphylococcal infection. If this defense is penetrated, due either to the increased activity of the microörganisms or to the peculiar susceptibility of the host, then the signs of septicemia develop and the body may die of exhaustion following this experience. The susceptibility of the diabetic patient to staphylococcal infection is notorious. In some few instances it has been thought that the staphylococcus may acquire sufficient activity to be transmitted from person to person and to produce through such transmission a primary infection such as the staphylococcal pneumonia described by Chickering. However, there is no clear evidence even in such instances that the area infected was not previously prepared by some damage, such as a preceding respiratory infection of different origin.

Septicemia.—Staphylococcal bacteriemia is common and may exist without producing symptoms or signs. For example, a carbuncle may exist with little constitutional evidence in the presence of positive blood culture of staphylococcus. Mere occurrence of a positive blood culture does not always alter the prognosis unfavorably. Evidently there are other factors, such as the peculiar virulence of the organism itself, or the susceptibility of the patient at the moment, which permit bacteriemia to increase and to produce the symptoms of prostration and a febrile course. There is nothing characteristic of the course of staphylococcal septicemia. In the case of an extensive carbuncle the febrile course may be comparatively short, for example, eight to ten days, with temperature rising as high as 104° F., with numerous temporary remissions; or the course may be prolonged to six weeks as in staphylococcal endocarditis, with the same broken temperature chart showing many high peaks with occasional depressions to normal levels. Prostration, chills and sweats, and evidence of localization of the bacteria in various parts of the body, are the usual clinical signs of staphylococcal sepsis. Leukocytosis is the rule. Inflammation of the meninges or the joints or the heart valves or the kidneys may be reflected in rigidity of the neck with delirium, or painful red swelling in the neighborhood of joints, or increasingly rough murmurs, or red and white blood cells and staphylococci in the urine. Septic or metastatic pneumonia is a very common complication in fatal cases and betrays its presence through the increased respiratory effort and moist râles. In rare cases jaundice appears as a result of numerous abscesses in the liver. These localizations are common effects of staphylococcal bacteriemia. Localized infections occurring without known bacteriemia are found, as, for example, in cases of apparently primary osteomyelitis. In such instances local traumata such as sprains and abrasions may combine with upper respiratory infections to permit the entrance and deposit of staphylococci, although such factors may be impossible to recognize, at the time.

Pneumonia.—Besides the local manifestations of the infection, a special condition may exist in the lungs which has been described by Chickering as staphylococcal pneumonia. The cases described by this author were seen during the World War under conditions of epidemics, and it is not entirely certain that the staphylococci gained entrance to the lungs by means of their own inherent capacity to produce disease. This form of pneumonia would be expressed clinically by the picture usually described as that of bronchial pneumonia. That is to say, there would be symptoms and signs of urgent pulmonary distress without any evidence of consolidation. The sputum is yellow and contains great numbers of staphylococci. The roentgen-ray picture of the lungs is diagnostic and establishes the true state of affairs. These roentgen-ray pictures consist of multiple scattered shadows throughout both lungs, varying in size from a few millimeters to 2 cm. in diameter, and found at autopsy to be composed of small abscesses. In 416 cases of pneumonia at St. Mary's Hospital in St. Louis the condition has occurred once, when it existed as a complication of septicemia arising from a pelvic infection. Staphylococcal pneumonia is highly fatal.

Treatment.—The treatment of staphylococcal infections is successful with regard to the treatment of local infections and largely unsuccessful with regard to treatment of severe general infection. This does not mean that all cases of severe staphylococcal bacteriemia are fatal, but means that there is no method of treatment which brings about recovery with any degree of certainty. The treatment of local infection is entirely surgical. Without adequate drainage nothing can be accomplished by non-surgical procedures. Besides surgical methods the use of ultra-violet light has been employed in the more superficial forms of infection. In the treatment of the deeper infections the use of bacteriophage has been reported favorably from many sources. Attention must be paid to the general hygiene of the patient. He should be in a bright, well ventilated place. The diet should be of the high-caloric type. Since recovery depends on the native resources of the patient, these general measures are important. Transfusions of blood and glucose and the administration of solutions of gentian violet or mercurochrome have been used without definite success. Vaccines are inert. Antitoxic serums have not yet been developed to a point of assured usefulness.

Prophylaxis.—Prophylaxis against staphylococcic infections is largely a matter of cleanliness in handling wounds in order to prevent local and later, general infection.

STREPTOCOCCAL INFECTIONS.

Bacteriology.—There are two main varieties of streptococcus based on the classification offered by Schottmüller in 1903. According to this classification, one form of streptococcus is known by its capacity to produce hemolysis around a colony on blood agar and is then called a hemolytic streptococcus. If it fails to produce hemolysis it is called a non-hemolytic streptococcus. From the standpoint of infection the non-hemolytic streptococcus stands as a single group, although some of its members have the capacity to produce methemoglobin, which gives a green tint to the zone immediately surrounding the colony and leads to the expression "Streptococcus viridans." The other non-hemolytic strains which have no capacity to produce the green tint on blood agar are known as anhemolytic, or indifferent. A much more comprehensive study of the action of streptococci on blood agar has been offered by Brown, who refers to the alpha, beta and gamma types of hemolysis. The first of these corresponds to the green-producing type of non-hemolytic streptococcus; the second to the hemolytic variety; and the last to the anhemolytic or indifferent strains of non-hemolytic streptococcus.

Distribution.—Hemolytic streptococci are found comparatively rarely in normal bodies. They may be found in from 1 to 10 per cent of throat cultures from normal individuals, depending upon the methods of culture used; but all normal individuals yield cultures of non-hemolytic streptococci. Besides occurring in the throat these streptococci may also be found in the intestinal tract, and may be recovered from the feces, but here again the non-hemolytic variety is much more prevalent than the hemolytic type. According to fermentation reactions and immunologic tests there are numerous varieties in the non-hemolytic group, and as many as twenty variants may be found in a single normal throat. The non-hemolytic streptococcus has been isolated from the dust in rooms. It can also be recovered from the intestinal tract of animals. It is, therefore, an extremely ubiquitous type of bacterium.

Pathogenesis.—(a) **Non-hemolytic Streptococcus.**—In spite of the wide distribution of the non-hemolytic streptococcus, it is rarely reported in a local infection except in dental abscess. There is no doubt about the association of these organisms in the disease of subacute streptococcal endocarditis where the majority of cases yield blood cultures positive for non-hemolytic streptococcus. This disease will be discussed in a separate chapter. Although widely distributed on normal tissue—from which it might be inferred that the streptococcus was adapted to normal human tissue—and although rarely found in local infections such as abscesses, the organism has been described as having causal relationship with a great variety of diseases. Measles, chickenpox, poliomyelitis, herpes zoster, gastric ulcer, cholecystitis, appendicitis, peridental abscess, are among those disturbances which have been ascribed to infection by this type of streptococcus; but the acceptance of the idea of streptococcal origin of these diseases has not been widespread.

One reasonable attitude to assume toward the non-hemolytic streptococcus would be that this type of streptococcus resembles in pathogenicity the colon bacillus, seldom the producer of specific disease but capable of leading a parasitic existence when once introduced into the human body. Most of the infections which are ascribed to the activity of Streptococcus non-hemolyticus are of the type known as focal infections.

Focal Infections.—A focal infection is an infectious disease which is produced as a metastasis from an area in the body which has been previously infected. It perhaps might more properly be called a metastatic infection. The principle underlying the conception of focal infection is sound. There are numerous instances in which an infected area in the body may yield bacteria to the blood stream and thereby lead to the establishment, in remote parts of the body, of an infective process. Gonorrheal urethritis may lead to bacteriemia with the establishment of inflammation in the neighborhood of one or more joints. Chronic bronchial infections with bronchiectasis occasionally lead to the establishment of abscess in the brain. Any localized infection may, by means of bacteriemia, lead to the metastatic implantation of bacteria in remote parts of the body.

The development of the idea of focal infection dates from the work of Billings in 1912 and was based largely on the study of patients with chronic rheumatism. Subsequent bacteriologic studies ignored the possible etiologic activity of other bacteria, while stressing the finding of non-hemolytic streptococci in cultures from teeth, tonsils, sinuses and other local areas. In the more recent literature there has been renewed reporting of streptococci of the non-hemolytic and hemolytic varieties in joint fluid and blood of patients suffering from the form of chronic rheumatism loosely referred to as chronic infectious arthritis, or rheumatoid arthritis.

The application of this bacteriologic study to the therapy of chronic rheumatism has been ineffective. Recent reports by Clawson concerning the treatment of patients suffering from a form of chronic rheumatism by intravenous injections of hemolytic streptococci will be received with interest. We have been unable to obtain similar results in treating patients with rheumatoid arthritis, at the Arthritis Clinic of Desloge Hospital of St. Louis University. The rheumatism itself depends upon other factors as well as the factor of infection. The first of these is age. There are no focal infections of the nature of chronic arthritis in children or young adults which are referable to infected teeth, tonsils, or sinuses as the origin of those infections. Senescent changes in bones and joints themselves may be factors in permitting the localization of otherwise harmless bacterial invaders. The process of metastasis may also depend upon some factor other than the simple invasion of the blood stream. In animals, some organisms, such as the hemolytic streptococcus, may produce arthritis, at the first inoculation, but for the production of arthritis by non-hemolytic streptococcus, usually several inoculations must be made before localization in the joints takes place. So in the human it may be necessary for the infected focus, which is the source of the metastases, to have existed for some time before metastatic or focal infection may result. While admitting the validity of the principle of focal infection, the fact in any type of disease must be questioned unless based on accurate diagnostic methods. These methods usually fail to show a convincing cause for the average case of chronic rheumatism. Cultures of the blood and the joint fluid have been studied by several investigators and positive cultures of Streptococcus non-hemolyticus have been reported. One of the faults of such methods grows out of the time required for the development of these organisms in cultures. Periods of eight to twenty days have elapsed before these organisms have been recovered in culture media. This is in seeming contradiction to the fact that these organisms usually grow with great readiness on ordinary culture media. At the same time careful and competent investigators have obtained negative results.

The association of infected teeth or tonsils with focal infections such as chronic rheumatism is seldom based on secure evidence. The fact that non-hemolytic streptococci are found about the teeth does not in any way mean that these streptococci are responsible for the rheumatism that is being studied. The making of vaccines from such streptococci is invalid. Such vaccines are in no sense autogenous, since it is not known that these streptococci are the cause of the arthritis. The attitude toward infected foci should be that such foci should be drained or removed. This attitude would prevail even if there were no consideration of disease being produced at a distant part by a possible metastasis. There are undoubtedly instances in which actively infected local tissue may lead to the appearance of painful red areas in or about joints, and these should be regarded as focal infections even if the bacterial agent cannot be isolated. If the bacterial agent cannot be isolated, then the matter of treatment with vaccine is out of the question. The idea of focal infection is valid; the ideas of the bacteriology have not so far merited adoption.

For the *treatment* of such focal infections, non-specific reactions have been produced. This form of treatment is sometimes called "shock therapy." They might well be called "artificial fevers." Many agents have been used, such as proteose and sterile milk and killed typhoid bacilli. Of these the most widely used is the last named—the killed typhoid bacilli. Following the intravenous inoculation of an initial dose of 15 million typhoid-paratyphoid bacilli there is usually a chill, a rise in temperature as high as 102° F., headache, prostration, followed by a feeling of relief from the local arthritic manifestations for which the treatment was instituted. These interpolations of a reaction by the body in the presence of chronic infection rarely result in permanent relief from the chronic infection; just as the interpolation of some acute infection in the course of a chronic infection may result in the temporary alleviation of symptoms of the chronic disease, but rarely in its complete removal. Nevertheless this method of treatment is the most popular and, indeed, the most productive of results, even though these results are rarely lasting. Focal infection is included in the consideration of pathogenesis of non-hemolytic streptococcus, on account of the vast amount of argument in the literature.

(*b*) **Hemolytic Streptococcus.**—**Bacteriology.**—Just as the virulence of non-hemolytic streptococcus is questionable, the distribution of that organism widespread, and its connection with definite diseases unproven, so the virulence of hemolytic streptococcus is undoubted, its distribution much more limited, and its association with many definite diseases proven. The hemolytic streptococcus usually makes its entrance into the human body through an opening in the covering of the body. It has certain characteristic features of behavior wherever it makes its entrance, and there is a fairly constant reaction on the part of the body to the hemolytic streptococcus. In the earliest records hemolytic streptococcus was known chiefly as Streptococcus pyogenes, but with the use of blood agar the name was changed. It was known as pyogenes obviously because of its tendency to be associated with purulent inflammation.

Epidemiology.—Hemolytic streptococcal infections frequently arrange themselves in relation to other infections, notably to the "common cold." The virulence of hemolytic streptococcus is enhanced by the pre-existence of other diseases and apparently by the passage from one individual to another. The sources of infection are, first, direct contact, which is the least common source of infection; second, by the inhalation of infected droplets from the respiratory tract of a patient; third, by infected milk.

The second method is by far the most important, and those illnesses are most likely to produce contagion which are characterized by cough, such as respiratory infections. It has been shown that a patient without hemolytic streptococcus in his throat, entering a ward where coughing patients are present with hemolytic streptococcus in their throats, will, after twenty-four to forty-eight hours, acquire a rich culture of hemolytic streptococcus in the throat. Epidemics of streptococcal sore throat have been studied and shown to be produced by the drinking of infected milk. The milk becomes infected, according to the study of Brown, by the streptococcus gaining entrance into the milk by way of an infected udder.

Pathology.—When the hemolytic streptococcus comes in contact with the tissue, the immediate reaction is congestion and out-pouring of serum into the interstitial spaces, with the infiltration of such tissues by polymorphonuclear leukocytes and to some extent by monocytes. This reaction on the part of the body is attended by a fever, leukocytosis and prostration. The extent of the tissue reaction is comparatively small in the case of pharyngeal infection and comparatively large in the case of a phlegmon in an extremity. The extent of the reaction will determine the severity of the symptoms, the presence or absence of bacteriemia, the duration and, to a great extent, the outcome. It happens rarely that a small focus of infection may result fatally on account of the peculiar lack of resistance on the part of the patient at the moment.

The primary reaction on the part of the body may be followed at a later date by secondary responses which are characterized by purulent infiltration and abscesses. In some cases the body seems to remain in the primary reactive state which, if prolonged sufficiently, becomes exhausting and fatal.

Recovery takes place by drainage of the infected focus or by spontaneous localization of the process and neutralization of the toxins. The toxin production of various strains of hemolytic streptococcus is an important factor in such infections as scarlet fever and erysipelas, according to Dick, Dochez, and Amoss. It is likely that in any hemolytic streptococcal infection, particularly the infections attended by phlegmonous infiltration of the tissue, toxin formation is an important factor in the production of constitutional reaction.

Bacteriemia may occur in the course of any hemolytic streptococcal infection, and its mere presence is not necessarily a fatal omen.

Immunology.—Antitoxic serums have been prepared from the streptococcus of scarlet fever by Dick and Dochez, and from the streptococcus of erysipelas by Amoss. The success of the latter is not clearly established. There are no effective immune serums which are bactericidal or capable of limiting the growth activities of the streptococcus inside the human body. Experimentally it is impossible to produce effective active immunity by the use of vaccines and there is no successful treatment of infection in humans by vaccines. None of the infections by hemolytic streptococcus confers immunity except scarlet fever.

Prophylaxis.—In epidemics of respiratory infections and of measles, where the method of transmission is by droplets, the wearing of masks is essential for the protection of individuals coming in contact with patients. For avoiding contamination by direct contact the ordinary methods of isolation practised in hospitals are useful. For the prevention of milk-borne epidemics the prevention, of course, depends upon proper sanitary control of milk supply.

Treatment.—Whatever the particular character of the streptococcal infection, the same principle of treatment applies. First, an attempt is made to keep the infected area clean and, if possible drained. A conservative attitude is extremely important with regard to the institution of drainage in a given case. The early incision of phlegmonous areas often leads to disaster. The same principle applies to the surgery of mastoid infection. Incisions should be carefully limited to the purulent area. Patients with severe streptococcal infections lose weight with remarkable rapidity and in particular lose body-protein. Accordingly, a high protein, high caloric intake is extremely useful. This diet must naturally be in an acceptable form, which is usually fluid or semi-solid.

Special Streptococcal Infections.

Streptococcal Sore Throat.—Sore throat is one of the commonest streptococcal infections. It may be defined as acute streptococcal infection of the tissues of the pharynx occurring sporadically and in epidemics. The infection is found in individuals of both sexes and of all ages, but is most common in children and young adults.

Symptoms.—The onset is comparatively sudden, though not violent, and is characterized by the symptoms of malaise, increasing to prostration, fever, angina, and difficulty in swallowing. Inspection of the throat shows, in the first twelve hours, a diffuse vivid redness of the surface of the pharynx, tonsils and fauces, attended by swelling. During the following twenty-four hours the crypts of the tonsils frequently become plugged and the expression "follicular tonsillitis" is often applied to this phase. These whitish areas may become confluent and lead to the formation of a thin gray membrane which may cover the tonsil. During the third twenty-four hours there is, in favorable cases, a definite and marked regression of all of the signs. In other cases swelling increases in the tissues immediately behind and above the tonsil. The soft palate becomes involved, difficulty in swallowing is greatly increased, fever continues, and an abscess is established in the peritonsillar tissue. The spontaneous rupture of this abscess or its successful drainage by incision usually marks the beginning of recovery. The course of the disease lasts about three days in uncomplicated cases. The patient is usually unable to sleep the first night of the disease, pulse is rapid, fever varies in individual cases from 101° to 104° F. Leukocytosis of 14,000 to 18,000 is common, with a predominance of segmented forms.

Complications.—Peritonsillar abscess has already been referred to. Otitis media is not infrequently a sequel of streptococcal pharyngitis. Cervical adenitis is common in children. In rare cases this infection of the cervical tissue is attended by a continuation of the original phlegmonous reaction on the part of the body and a condition of cervical cellulitis known as "Ludwig's angina" may occur. Albuminuria occurs commonly during the course of the infection and glomerular nephritis may make its appearance after the infection has subsided. This type of nephritis has been studied by Longcope and has been shown to be related in duration to the persistence of hemolytic streptococcus in predominance in the throat of the individual. Purulent infiltrations, evidently metastatic infections, may occur in remote organs and be represented by pericarditis, arthritis and abscesses in muscles, which, like otitis media, are to be treated as local infections. In the course of epidemics of tonsillitis and sometimes in the absence of an epidemic, cases of apparently spontaneous peritonitis may develop. These occur chiefly in children and present themselves usually as cases of acute appendicitis. Operations usually are performed for appendicitis and reveal the widespread nature of the peritoneal infection. The death-rate in this form of spontaneous peritonitis is extremely high.

Prophylaxis.—Little can be said about the prophylaxis with regard to sporadic cases of sore throat. The usual attempts to keep the body in good condition by sufficient food, sleep, exercise, will probably result in freedom from infection in many instances.

Treatment.—If the body is put to rest in the early stages of a streptococcal infection the incidence of complications is extremely low. The principles of treatment outlined above apply to the treatment of sore throat. An attempt is made to clean the infected area. The use of antiseptic applications, the irrigation with hot salt solution and the cleaning of tonsillar crypts with diluted hydrogen peroxide are all popular measures. Feeding is important. The use of drugs is limited to the use of sedatives and antipyretics. A very popular combination is that of codeine with coal tar products.

Wound Infection.—There are three general types of wound infection commonly encountered in hospital practice: (1) the infection of wounds of the extremities or trunk, such as a laceration of the finger or foot; (2) the infection of the wounds of delivery which results in what is called "puerperal sepsis"; (3) postoperative infection, or the infection of operative wounds.

The first class is by far the most numerous. The features of all wound infections by hemolytic streptococci are the same as those discussed above. Frank formation of pus is comparatively a late feature and usually a favorable sign. Consideration of wound infection is important chiefly with regard to treatment. Conservatism is particularly important in the treatment. Incision should be delayed at least for three days after onset. The infection is apparently spread by too extensive incision.

Puerperal infection is remarkably fatal. In rare instances the infectious process is subdued and becomes pelvic cellulitis, which may last for weeks and even months before resolution occurs spontaneously. There is no surgical treatment for puerperal sepsis. The use of blood transfusion is purely supportive in its effect.

The intravenous inoculation of dyes, as well as the employment of antistreptococcal serums has little effect in the successful treatment of wound infection of any of the above types. The most important question usually is when to operate. An early operation may lead to a spread of the phlegmonous process and to an overwhelming septicemia. It is important to remember to feed all such patients a high protein, high caloric diet. The use of local applications is popular and useful. In the case of phlegmonous extremities the continuous bath of hot saline is the form of treatment most often used. Alcohol packs seem to have less value. Multiple incisions may be extremely harmful if performed too early.

Septicemia.—Any streptococcal infection may be attended by bacteriemia. This fact is not always of serious moment. We speak of septicemia when the patient presents a continuously high fever with evidence of marked exhaustion. When the exhaustion involves the mental processes the patient is often excited but, on the contrary, may be stuporous. In any event there is a definite disturbance of mental capacity. This appearance of the patient is usually included in the expression "toxic." We might, therefore, analyze the clinical features of septicemia as high fever and unusual exhaustion, both physical and mental. Bacteriemia is not essential to the diagnosis of septicemia, since patients may die with repeatedly negative blood cultures.

Temperature in streptococcal septicemia is of the remittent type, in mild cases lasting from three to seven days, in other cases longer. Fatal cases may be terminated in a week, or last several weeks. Outside the general symptoms of severe infection which characterize the clinical picture of septicemia, the symptoms of the patient relate entirely to the localization of the infection in various parts of the body. Thus a patient with streptococcal septicemia may display metastatic infections in the neighborhood of the joints, may develop meningitis, may develop purulent pericarditis, septic pneumonia and, most rarely, endocarditis. The result depends largely upon the extensiveness of the initial infection and the success with which the infection is met by local treatment.

In St. Mary's Hospital in the past nine years there have been 34 cases of streptococcal septicemia attended by bacteriemia. Of these, 6 recovered and 26 died. Of the patients that recovered, 5 were cases of otitis media in which it was possible to institute adequate surgical measures; 2 other cases of otitis media were fatal on account of an inaccessible jugular thrombosis. There were, at the same time, 19 patients with severe streptococcal infections without bacteriemia, of whom 3 died. Many forms of treatment were employed in caring for these patients, including transfusions, the use of anti-streptococcal serums, the use of various commercial antigens, the use of dyes intravenously, but no claims of merit can be made for any one of these agents.

Erysipelas.

Definition.—Erysipelas is an acute inflammation of the skin produced by infection with Streptococcus hemolyticus, is communicable and attended by the constitutional signs of general infection.

The connection of hemolytic streptococcus with erysipelas was first established by Fehleisen in 1883. Since that time new facts and methods of investigation have extended the understanding of this infection. There is apparently no particular strain of hemolytic streptoccus which alone is responsible for erysipelas, but the capacity to produce the disease may follow the inoculation of a minute area in the skin with any hemolytic streptococcus. It seems to be important that the point of inoculation be small so that in facial erysipelas the origin may be scarcely detectable.

Surgical erysipelas refers to the erysipelatous infection of postoperative or surgical wounds. In these conditions the erysipelas usually begins at one point along the edge of the wound and then spreads.

The degree of contagion is not pronounced and the usual hospital procedures employed for isolation of the patient are adequate to prevent the spread of the disease to other patients.

Pathogenesis.—There are evidently two factors concerned in the production of symptoms and signs, namely, the factor of bacterial growth and the factor of toxin. Early studies on local immunity to hemolytic streptococcus by Gay and Rhodes were extended by Amoss, who found that the erythematous reaction to the intradermal injection of hemolytic streptococcus was lessened on subsequent injection of the same organism; that is to say, that the site of the first injection seemed to acquire some immunity from a similar amount of reaction on subsequent injections. About the same time Birkhaug reported the isolation of a toxic principle from cultures of streptococcus obtained from erysipelas and for which he claimed the production of a successful antitoxic serum. Whatever the effects of serum manufactured for the treatment of erysipelas may be in neutralizing the symptoms of toxicity, they are apparently not potent in neutralizing the purely "growth" activity of the organism.

Pathology.—The upper layers of the skin are involved in a dense infiltration of serum and red blood cells, and this gives the external characteristics of hardness and redness to the lesion. At the periphery of the lesion microscopically there are numerous streptococci to be seen and this is the basis of the clinical practice of obtaining cultures of streptococci from the edge of the lesion, according to a method described by Amoss. The lymphatics are also filled with streptococci and mononuclear cells. Scattered throughout the entire area are leukocytes and there may be small islands of necrosis or pus.

Clinical Course.—The incubation period is probably the same as for scarlet fever or any other infection by hemolytic streptococci, namely, one to three days. The onset is abrupt, frequently attended by chill, rarely by vomiting, and by slight pain in the site of inoculation, whether at the corner of the nose, of the mouth, eye or ear. The general symptoms of acute infection, namely, aching through the body, headache and prostration, immediately follow. The fever rises to 101° to 103° F. and follows a remittent course, subsiding usually by lysis at the end of the seventh day. In this respect the fever chart also resembles that of scarlet fever. The leukocyte count is similar to that in streptococcal sore throat and scarlet fever and other streptococcal infections and varies between 12,000 and 20,000 as a rule.

The disease seems to be fairly self-limited and resembles the cycle of pneumococcal pneumonia in its duration except that the fever much more often falls by lysis than by crisis and the fever is more remittent than sustained. When the disease is unusually severe and prolonged beyond the seven-day period, secondary reactions such as abscess may develop within the infected area. There is a particular form of erysipelas called "migratory" in which, without the development of abscesses, the lesion spreads and at some time touches every portion of the body.

The Local Signs.—The affected area is hard, flat and the edge of the inflamed skin is abrupt, so that the palpating finger moving from the healthy to the diseased skin meets sudden hardness at the edge of the infected area. The inflammation spreads peripherally and tends to fade at its point of origin. The inflammation remains intense at any one point for from one to three days and the local and general symptoms together with the fever terminate with the cessation of the spread of the dermal inflammation. Blebs frequently appear in the protracted cases.

Complications.—Bacteriemia is uncommon during the course of erysipelas, but in certain cases, usually those complicated by the factor of old age or concurrent disease, there may be the signs of bacteriemia with local metastases so that endocarditis and pericarditis may develop, as well as pleurisy, meningitis, or arthritis. Pneumonic signs also may develop, based on pathologic lesions known as septic pneumonia.

Diagnosis.—Erysipelas has a marked clinical individuality which easily separates it from other local infections of the skin. It is to be differentiated chiefly from severe inflammations of the skin produced by staphylococcus, which usually arise at the site of some local injury. These staphylococcal infections are usually milder, have fewer constitutional signs and present a markedly different local appearance and do not have the sharp margin surrounding the inflamed area which erysipelas displays. Staphylococcal infections of the severe type spread more slowly and may be honeycombed with small abscesses.

Prognosis.—The death-rate from erysipelas is strikingly low. It is variously estimated at from 1 to 5 per cent. Death is brought about much more frequently as a result of lowered resistance due to old age, infancy or concurrent disease than by virulence of the infection itself.

Treatment.—*General.*—The patient is isolated according to the usual hospital standards or, if treated in the home, care is exercised to keep the utensils and bed clothing used by the patient from coming into contact with healthy persons. The treatment separates itself into the treatment with serum, and local treatment. The use of antistreptococcal serum manufactured for the treatment of erysipelas has not lived up to early anticipation. While in many cases the injection of serum at the edge of the infected area will stop the spread at that point, in other cases the inflammation will spread directly through such injections. If used, 50 to 100 cc. of serum, well diluted in normal salt solution, should be given intravenously every twelve hours until a favorable effect on the fever has been produced. Besides the use of serum, antipyretics may be employed for the reduction of temperature and the usual sponging may be used for the same purpose.

Local.—For many years it has been popular to cover the infected area with packs made from iced saturated solution of magnesium sulphate. Other solutions such as boric acid and even warm salt solution have been employed with apparently equally good results. Complications will demand special consideration.

Bronchopneumonia.

The term "bronchopneumonia" needs definition, since it is used frequently by clinicians to describe a variety of pulmonary infections. In the attitude of clinicians the term is used to describe severe pulmonary infection which has no sign of consolidation. Obviously bronchopneumonia refers to an acute inflammation of the lungs distributed chiefly throughout the small branches of the bronchial tree without producing massive filling of the alveolar spaces. The term "lobular pneumonia," which may mean an alveolar extension of a bronchopneumonic process, or fractional consolidation in a pneumococcal infection, is obviously not a clinical term but a diagnosis established at autopsy. In children, especially where signs of consolidation are not always easily detected, a diagnosis of bronchopneumonia may be made incorrectly when the diagnosis of lobar pneumonia should be made. It is extremely fortunate that the various types of pulmonary infection correspond fairly closely with the activity of certain bacteria so that lobar consolidation is almost always produced by pneumococcus and the pure type of bronchopneumonia is almost always produced by hemolytic streptococcus. The exceptions grow out of the fact that when the influence of climate, age of the patient and virulence of the organism is exerted, there may be infections produced which are so atypical as not to live up to the original definitions.

During the past seven years at St. Mary's (St. Louis University) Hospital in St. Louis, there have been 325 cases of lobar pneumonia with a death-rate of 33 per cent, and at the same time 91 cases listed as bronchopneumonia with a death-rate of 65 per cent. When the cases of bronchopneumonia were analyzed it was found that only 9 of the 91 supported the diagnosis, because the other cases included such cases as those of terminal infection, hypostatic congestion of the lung with infection, pneumonic evidences during the course of a fatal

9

septicemia and acute respiratory infections in persons having chronic bronchitis or asthma. In the case of many of the infants the diagnosis of bronchopneumonia was made by the clinician, while the roentgen-ray showed a definite area of consolidation. Obviously, the clinical diagnosis must be regarded as incorrect in the face of this type of evidence.

Definition.—True bronchopneumonia can be described as an infection of the bronchial tree by Streptococcus hemolyticus, characterized by the symptoms of severe general infection and urgent pulmonary embarrassment.

Pathogenesis.—During an epidemic of streptococcal infections the streptococcus is said to acquire a virulence which seems to be sufficient to initiate an attack of respiratory infection with bronchopneumonia. This state of affairs is unusual and in nearly all cases, true bronchopneumonia follows an attack of respiratory infection such as measles or some other virus infection. The etiology and epidemiology of this particular infection is well described by McCallum and Cole, reporting experiences obtained during the World War. In a few cases chronic bronchitis or asthma produces the dissemination of injury which invites the immediate spread of a later infection by hemolytic streptococcus, and thus leads to the production of the structural arrangement of the inflammation known as bronchopneumonia.

Bacteriology.—There is no particular strain of hemolytic streptococcus which is responsible for bronchopneumonia, but the strains isolated may be identified with those found in erysipelas, scarlet fever or other streptococcal infections.

Pathology.—The infection in most cases begins in the pharynx and extends to the alveoli. At this latter point the infection seems to spend itself. The tissues of the pharynx are reddened and swollen, and this fact frequently offers a useful differential point in distinguishing the case from that of lobar pneumonia. The covering of the trachea and bronchi is also thickened and red, and shows mucopurulent exudate on the surface. The bronchioles are filled with red blood cells and serum and mononuclear wandering cells. Fibrin is also prominent. The walls of the bronchioles are densely infiltrated with red blood cells and monocytes and show numerous streptococci as well. The expression "interstitial bronchopneumonia" arises from this last-described condition, that is to say, the dense infiltration of the walls of the bronchioles. Inflammatory reaction is not entirely confined to the bronchioles and bronchial walls but may extend into neighboring alveoli which become filled with the same type of exudate and fibrin, leading to the formation of islands of consolidated alveoli and producing a condition which might be called "lobular pneumonia." The infection spreads by the lymphatics carried by the interlobular septa, so that the structural framework of the lungs is thickened and on cut surface the cross-sections of bronchioles exude pus and stand out as small yellow points within a framework of thickened stroma. Infection may rapidly reach the pleural surface, and once this point is reached empyema results. In the early stages the pleural surface is highly congested, red blood cells are packed underneath the endothelial surface and serum rapidly exudes into the cavity, giving the pleural fluid in the early stages of empyema the appearance of nearly clear, reddish-brown fluid. Later, these signs of intense congestion pass over into signs of purulent inflammation and the pleural fluid correspondingly becomes more yellow and more thick.

Symptoms.—The incubation period is of little importance since the establishment of bronchopneumonia is usually a late development in the course of a streptococcal infection which began in the upper part of the respiratory tract in the neighborhood of the pharynx.

The onset of the disease is marked by coughing, prostration and, usually, pain in the chest. On account of the extensive involvement of the air passages *constant coughing* is usually a most striking feature of the disease, and this, added to dyspnea, makes the patient strikingly different from the patient with lobar pneumonia. The *sputum* also is characteristic. In the early days of the cough the sputum may be pink but soon becomes yellow and, in uncomplicated cases, never rusty. The appearance of rusty sputum is likely to mean complication by pneumococcal infection in the alveolar area. The temperature chart resembles that of erysipelas and scarlet fever with the exception that it is most often prolonged, due to the fact that this disease is much more virulent than other streptococcal infections, especially when occurring in epidemics. As it occurs in children following measles, in times of peace or in non-epidemic times, the disease is not necessarily severe, and the duration is usually limited to about seven days.

Physical Signs.—The marked dyspnea, the cough and the sputum have already been referred to. There is never the dulness on percussion that is found in cases of lobar consolidation. It may be impossible to determine the existence of any special dulness. There is seldom any true bronchial breathing to be heard on auscultation. On account of the interference with the passage of air through the small bronchioles, moist râles are prominent throughout the chest and may be heard even after the end of expiration. The heart is rapid, but signs of endo-carditis are remarkably rare. When empyema occurs, the physical signs change suddenly to conform with the signs of fluid.

Complications.—These are usually the complications that develop in the neighborhood of the pulmonary infection such as *empyema* or *pericarditis*. Of all complications, empyema is the most common and will be discussed separately. *Collapse* of the lung may follow the shutting off of the bronchioles by the exudate and the violent coughing effort may lead to *emphysematous* blebs which later rupture, producing *pneumothorax*. These accidents are found in only extremely severe infections. The remote complications are similar to the infections attending any streptococcal septicemia with positive blood culture. These are chiefly metastatic inflammation about joints or solitary abscesses in muscles. Nephritis is uncommon, although albuminuria is to be expected. Endocarditis occurs but is infrequent.

Diagnosis.—The diagnosis must depend not only on the evidence of severe pulmonary infection but chiefly on the bacteriology of the sputum. In these cases the sputum yields almost pure culture of hemolytic streptococcus. The roentgen-ray will eliminate the possibility of lobar pneumonia and other localized infections of the lung.

Prognosis.—The prognosis depends on the character of the disease which preceded the infection of the lungs. During epidemics of measles the lungs are extensively injured and subsequent streptococcal infections may be highly fatal. Such conditions have apparently never been encountered outside the time of war when the population was concentrated in barracks. In ordinary times the disease most frequently follows measles in children and as such is not highly fatal. No definite figures, therefore, can be given for the death-rate. Probably 5 to 10 per cent is the correct rate of mortality in civil life.

Treatment.—*Prophylaxis* is extremely important. It was shown during the World War that patients having negative throat cultures, coming into wards with coughing patients having throat cultures positive for hemolytic streptococcus, would rapidly become contaminated and in this way streptococcal bronchopneumonia was spread. Accordingly, a patient with hemolytic streptococcal bronchopneumonia should be rigidly isolated because the air in the neighborhood of such a patient will be charged with infected droplets. Persons coming into contact with such patients should wear masks and gowns. For the early medical treatment of streptococcal pulmonary infections, rest is the most important, and a high caloric diet is also necessary to prevent the waste which rapidly occurs in this disease. The drugs usually employed are the antipyretics and sedatives. The patients are greatly benefited by the use of the oxygen-tent.

The disease is usually self-limited and terminates in mild cases in seven days, following rather closely the course of scarlet fever and erysipelas. Cough may persist for several days after the temperature has become normal, and patients should be kept in bed for two weeks because streptococci remain in the sputum and in the throat in great numbers, and the possibility of later empyema is always present until recovery is complete. The treatment of empyema has been extensively described in the literature that accumulated during the World War.

Empyema.—While empyema of streptococcal origin is less common in hospital practice than that which complicates lobar pneumonia, it possesses certain clinical characteristics due to its venomous effect on the patient, and these merit emphasis. Such empyema is not as frequent a complication of the sporadic bronchopneumonias of childhood as it is of the pneumonic infections attending large epidemics of measles. But in any case, its mode of production is as described above.

Symptoms.—The onset is remarkably sudden. In an already sick individual the onset may escape special notice on the part of the physician. To the patient, however, *pain* is sharp on the affected side. The stage of dry pleuritis is short. Usually in twelve hours the pleural cavity is filled with fluid. This adds to the difficulty of aëration, and increases the dyspnea and cyanosis. If the effusion is on the left side the cardiac action is hampered and the pulse is accelerated. The patient feels the added burdens. The temperature chart is not especially changed in the first few days of empyema but becomes more remittent later. In fatal cases not complicated by ill-timed surgical treatment the fever becomes more sustained, the pulse-rate ascends to

130 or higher, the patient becomes delirious and exhaustion becomes complete. Such cases may terminate within two weeks. In more prolonged cases pus becomes pocketed in areas near the hilus and resists even surgical attempts to drain. Physical signs consist of flatness, absence of breath sounds and immobility of the affected side.

The fluid changes in appearance from a reddish brown, turbid but not opaque fluid in the early stage, to a frankly purulent fluid later. The finding of streptococci in the fluid is essential to the diagnosis. These are numerous early; infrequent later.

Prognosis.—Left to itself, without operation, streptococcal empyema will lead to pleural thickening in those cases which recover. Recovery depends on the degree of severity of the pulmonary infection and to a great extent on the wisdom displayed in deciding when to operate. Many of the reports of successful treatment do not contain accurate data concerning the bacteriology. The failure to distinguish between streptococcal and pneumococcal empyema leads to inaccurate conclusions regarding the validity of certain methods of treatment.

Treatment.—One of the important findings of the Empyema Commission, which studied empyema in the army base hospitals in this country during the World War, lay in the discovery that patients with this condition suffered a drastic loss of protein which it is essential to meet in order to protect the patient. Accordingly, a high-protein, high-caloric diet was found highly important. This must naturally be taken in liquid form, since the patients are usually too sick to chew.

Tapping, either with a needle and syringe or by means of a catheter placed in a small incision between the ribs, is important as an early measure of relief. Such procedures, while sometimes curative in pneumococcal empyema, are practically never sufficient for adequate drainage in the case of streptococcal empyema. In performing the maneuver of thoracentesis, it is well to bring the patient to the edge of the bed so that the needle may point upward in the postaxillary line in the seventh interspace. Thorough local anesthesia should be produced.

Thoracotomy and the resection of a portion of rib are the ultimate measures which must be used. It is important not to employ these methods before the appearance of the patient points to better organization of his resources. This is indicated chiefly by the change in the pleural fluid from the early thin, reddish-brown fluid filled with streptococci and red blood cells, to the later thick, yellow fluid with few streptococci, no red blood cells, and almost pure pus. Subsequent irrigation with normal saline or Dakin's solution is helpful. The reclamation of the lung is assisted by blowing exercises.

PNEUMOCOCCAL INFECTION.

Bacteriology.—The pneumococcus is a Gram-positive diplococcus, the opposite poles of which tend to be pointed. The diplococcus is usually alone, but may be found in short chains. It is soluble in bile. This feature of bile solubility is chiefly important in separating the pneumococcus from some strains of green-producing streptococcus. On blood agar the pneumococcus produces a green zone around its colony. It is extremely virulent for white mice, and this fact makes the mouse useful in diagnostic tests.

It presents a capsular envelope which is of vast importance in the immunology of pneumococcal infection, since it is in this capsule that a type-specific substance is to be found. Equipped with this capsule, the pneumococcus identifies its type, maintains its virulence and resists the phagocytic action of leukocytes; without this capsule the pneumococcus loses its type-identity, is stripped also of its virulence and is easily devoured by phagocytes. The study of this capsular substance by Avery and his associates represents one of the romances of modern bacteriology. Briefly stated, the features of this investigation include: (1) the discovery that the type-specific capsular substance was a polysaccharide; (2) the elucidation of the chemical conjugation between the carbohydrate and the protein fraction of the pneumococcus, as a result of which it is found that while the protein is antigenic, the carbohydrate determines the specificity of the antigenic property; (3) the finding that the carbohydrate is capable of inhibiting the action of protective antibodies.

Since this carbohydrate is so vital to the virulent activities of the pneumococcus, many attempts were made to find some enzyme which would act upon this particular polysaccharide, and after many years of effort Avery and his co-workers finally secured a bacillus of the soil which possessed an enzyme capable of acting upon the type-specific polysaccharide found in the pneumococcus capsules. This enzyme was found to have a protective action against pneumococcus injected simultaneously into white mice and, moreover, was effective when injected into white mice already infected with many times the lethal dose of pneumococcus. The strain that was studied in this work belonged to type III because of the larger supply of capsular substance available in that type. If it can be found that this enzyme can be brought into contact with the pneumococci in the lung in lobar pneumonia the mortality from this disease may be diminished considerably.

Since the work of Dochez and Gillespie it had been known that pneumococci may be grouped according to immunologic tests into three main types, known as types I, II and III. The remaining pneumococci were included in one group known as type IV. In recent years the fourth group of pneumococci has been subdivided. Pneumococci have been found, occurring with sufficient frequency to deserve individual marking. For convenience, these additional types are known as types V, VII, VIII, and so on. There is available, serum, both diagnostic and therapeutic for type VII. Laboratory reports will no longer read "type IV" but will indicate "not types I, II, III, VII," and so on. It is not likely that any important extension of typing will be made. It is not possible to distinguish types by cultural characteristics or microscopic appearances, except, perhaps, in the case of type III organisms, which are especially rich in capsular structure, frequently appear in chains and produce coarsely mucoid colonies on the surface of solid media.

Distribution of Pneumococci.—Occurrence of pneumococcus in the body under normal conditions has been studied and it is found that type I rarely occurs in a normal throat; type II may be found in from 1 to 3 per cent of normal throats; type III pneumococcus in 28 per cent and other types of pneumococcus in over 50 per cent. Accordingly, there must be many situations occurring in the upper respiratory passages which may readily invite infection by these last-named types of pneumonia. The rarely present pneumococci of types I and II produce more than 50 per cent of the cases of lobar pneumonia. This emphasizes the principle previously noted, that locally adapted bacteria are less invasive and *vice versa*.

Epidemiology.—The contaminated droplet, exhaled by the individual with a pneumococcal infection, forms the chief vehicle by which contagion is spread. The pneumococcus causing disease leaves the patient shortly after clinical recovery from infection. It has been shown that healthy individuals may acquire pneumococci from patients; no doubt by inhaling infected droplets. These normal individuals may thus become carriers. The dust in rooms of patients suffering from pneumonia has been shown to acquire a significant contamination with pneumococci corresponding to those found in the patients.

Immunology.—All pneumococci incite the formation of specific antibodies in the experimental animal. The serum of immunized animals will protect white mice against many times the lethal dose of fresh living broth culture. However, only in the case of type I anti-serum is the effect sufficiently pronounced to be of service in curing pneumococcal infections. There has accumulated, however, much clinical evidence to show that the anti-serum of type II or its concentrate is useful to a considerable degree, though not as effective as the serum against type I. There is not yet sufficient evidence to determine the value of type VII or VIII anti-serum. This curative effect is homologous; that is, type I serum will not be effective against type II or type III infection, and only type I anti-serum is effective against type I infections. Polyvalent serums, therefore, are not important.

Pathogenesis.—The virulence of pneumococci can be enhanced by passage through laboratory animals. So with human infections the virulence of pneumococci may be increased in times of epidemic respiratory infection. But the mere occurrence of pneumococci in a throat is probably insufficient for the production of infection. Other factors contributing to the injury of the host are important. Of these, the influence of epidemics of the "common cold" leads to situations in the respiratory tract inviting pneumococcal infection; and the debilitating effect of exposure to cold or of trauma is likewise important in making the individual susceptible. The infection, when it occurs, is probably most often the result of local implantation. The frequency, however, with which pneumococcal infections need preceding infections to prepare the field for invasion, suggests that the pathogenic properties of the pneumococcus are not of primary importance. The highest degree of pathogenicity exists in strains of types I and II.

Incubation Period.—No definite data are available concerning the time that elapses between the entrance of the pneumococcus and the production of symptoms. The fact that virulent pneumococci may be in the throats of normal individuals who are in contact with patients, without the production of infection, indicates the importance of preceding illness or injury in precipitating the onset of pneumococcal infection.

Pathology.—Two phases distinguish the reaction of tissues to pneumococcal infections. The first, as in streptococcal infection, consists in dense congestion which passes into a second purulent phase. In this second phase localizations of pus may occur, and these are sometimes spoken of as the complications. The purulent localization may be contiguous to the original infection as empyema is contiguous to pneumonia, or may be distant, blood-borne metastases, such as pneumococcal arthritis. The principal cellular response is represented by local and circulating polymorph leukocytosis.

Pneumococcal Otitis.—Otitis and meningitis are not uncommon complications attending injuries and infections in the neighborhood of the upper respiratory passage. Pneumococcal otitis media may complicate a primary infection of the throat which spreads to the middle ear, or it may exist as a secondary infection following primary streptococcal infection of the throat. The treatment of such a condition will follow the lines of the treatment of any case of purulent otitis media.

Pneumococcal Meningitis.—Pneumococcal meningitis may occur either as a metastasis in pneumococcal septicemia or as an extension from an infected sinus, or it may occur as an infection of a traumatized area such as would follow radical drainage of the sphenoid sinus. In times of epidemics of respiratory infections, rarely in other times, there may be cases of primary pneumococcal meningitis, that is to say, cases of pneumococcal meningitis without known preceding injury or infection and without the preëxistence of pneumococcal pneumonia. Of the various types of pneumococcal meningitis, those which seem to be primary are the most dangerous. In any case the disease begins as a severe frontal headache which, within twelve hours, increases in severity and leads to disturbances of the mental clearness of the patient. Delirium, therefore, is a very early symptom, and the patient is much more noisy and restless than in an infection by meningococcus. The spinal fluid is purulent, usually contains a considerable number of pneumococci, which may be identified by testing the supernatant spinal fluid, after centrifuging, with the various types of diagnostic serum. The treatment of pneumococcal meningitis, even where specific serum is available, is not satisfactory. Death usually occurs within three to four days following onset. Less virulent invasions have been reported in which lumbar laminectomy has been successful, and intraspinal injection of type I antipneumococcal serum should be used when the pneumococci are of the corresponding type. The injections should be carried out as in the treatment of cerebrospinal fever and should be repeated every eight hours until recovery is made probable.

Pneumococcal Arthritis.—Pneumococcal arthritis occurs rarely and when seen is usually in connection with lobar pneumonia. It appears in this situation to be a local metastasis of bacteriemia and, as such, is usually a feature of a fatal infection. Rarely it may occur without lobar pneumonia and may yield successfully to surgical treatment.

LOBAR PNEUMONIA.

It seems to be well established from the evidence obtained during the World War that streptococcal pneumonia is fairly typical both in its clinical manifestations and its pathologic appearance. It has been emphasized that hemolytic streptococcal infections involve the throat, pharynx and trachea and larger bronchi as well as the finest branches of the bronchial tree, so that the infection spreads up to the tissues of the pharynx and in this way presents a fairly definite arrangement. In the case of lobar pneumonia the infection seems to spare the upper reaches of the respiratory passage and to center chiefly in the lower extensions, namely, the alveolar spaces.

Definition.—Lobar pneumonia may, therefore, be defined as a pneumococcal infection of the lungs characterized by confluent inflammation of the alveolar area leading to consolidation of one or more lobes and further characterized by a very definite clinical course.

Frequency.—While we are in the habit of associating pneumococcal infections of the lower respiratory tract with lobar pneumonia, it is possible that less extensive invasions by pneumococci may occur in the respiratory tract. There are no adequate statistics to show how often cases of bronchitis, of ill-defined pneumonia and tracheitis may be in reality infections by pneumococci.

The expression "pneumonia" usually means lobar pneumonia. As such it constitutes an extremely frequent infection, since about 10 per cent of all the deaths are due to pneumonia in the general sense of this term. The death-rate due to lobar pneumonia differs in different countries and this difference is due to the difference in death-rate from bronchopneumonia. In other words, the attitude is slightly different toward the diagnosis of bronchopneumonia in the various countries where recording of mortality-rates is enforced. In those countries where a lower death-rate from lobar pneumonia is reported, a higher death-rate from bronchopneumonia is recorded. It is obvious that if the expression bronchopneumonia be limited to certain anatomically distributed infections, the lower percentage-rates of mortality due to lobar pneumonia will be corrected, as the higher rates due to bronchopneumonia will be corrected. Pneumonia is distributed chiefly through the temperate zones. It occurs, however, in other countries where statistics are maintained, but is infrequent in tropical countries where all coccal respiratory infections have a low rate of incidence. The incidence of lobar pneumonia is affected by the presence of other infections of the respiratory tract and epidemics of the "common cold" and of influenza cause a sharp rise in the number of cases of lobar pneumonia and its characteristic complications.

Etiology.—The pneumococcus was associated in a definite way with lobar pneumonia by Frankel in 1884 and conclusively by Weichselbaum in 1885, who isolated the organism from the blood and organs in cases of fatal pneumonia. The characteristics of the pneumococcus have already been discussed.

The first three groups of pneumococci, namely, types I, II, III, produce or are concerned with most of the clinical cases of lobar pneumonia and, while the clinical features of the disease are the same in all types, the possibility of successful treatment depends to a great extent on the prompt determination of the bacteriologic type of infection. These various types of pneumonia differ somewhat in virulence; and the death-rate, which of course is variable, depending upon local and climatic conditions, is highest in types II and III. Recent figures published by Cecil and Plummer show a mortality in 1000 cases of type II of lobar pneumonia of nearly 50 per cent. It is impossible to give final and definite figures concerning the virulence of any type of pneumonia, since the occurrence of lobar pneumonia depends not only on the virulence of the pneumococcus in question but also upon the local conditions surrounding the patient. These conditions are numerous.

Season.—The highest incidence and the highest death-rate from lobar pneumonia occur in the months of December, January, February and March. In a given year or in a given locality this arrangement may vary, as when the winter months are extremely mild and the greatest number of cases of lobar pneumonia may occur in March. The epidemics of "colds" and influenza-like infections that occur during the winter months usually determine the appearance of pneumonias. Another effect of season is to permit the occurrence of atypical forms of pneumococcal infections of the lungs. The greatest number of atypical pneumonias occurs in the months of September, October, April and May. During the same months typical pneumonia is extremely rare. By an atypical infection is meant a patchy alveolar inflammation which does not develop sufficiently to produce consolidation of an entire lobe.

Age.—The age factor is important. While pneumonia is very rare below the age of one year, it is extremely fatal at that time. Lobar pneumonia frequently occurs as a terminal infection of the lungs in old people. The highest incidence of the infection is between the second and the fifth decades.

Epidemics.—The existence of epidemics of respiratory diseases such as influenza often leads to the establishment of many cases of lobar pneumonia. During the World War the greatest incidence of lobar pneumonia occurred in connection with these related infections. During times of epidemic such pneumococcal infections of the lungs may occur in association with other coccal infections of the lungs, so that a given lung may show an area of alveolar consolidation and an area of streptococcal bronchopneumonia. Naturally these bacterial varieties and complications are associated with a confused clinical picture.

Exposure.—Exposure to cold and dampness, particularly to changing temperature and to hunger, are factors which make the human subject more susceptible to the production of pneumonia. The incidence of lobar pneumonia which has been receding in recent years may perhaps be associated with the development of better heating of living quarters.

Injuries to the Lungs.—Injuries to the lungs, as by foreign bodies or by trauma of the chest wall or by anesthesia, may invite the infection of the inflamed area by pneumococci, already in the upper respiratory tract of the host. The installation of nasal tubes used for feeding over a long period of time may lead to the irritation of the lower pharyngeal tissue, the aspiration of infected material from this tissue and the production thereby of an aspiration pneumonia, which in some cases may be a pneumococcal infection.

Sex.—Males are slightly more susceptible to lobar pneumonia than females and the death-rate is slightly higher.

Crowding.—The conditions of crowding are particularly important in the production of an epidemic of lobar pneumonia. Without this factor it has never been known that a pneumococcus can acquire virulence sufficient to spread the disease extensively. The greatest epidemics of lobar pneumonia have occurred during times of war and in construction camps where living quarters were small and crowded.

Pathogenesis.—Just as all of these factors are important in predisposing the patient for infection by pneumococcus, so the preparation of the lung field by forerunning respiratory infection in any case of lobar pneumonia is important; so that patients having lobar pneumonia in a considerable number of cases, over 40 per cent in the experience of the Rockefeller Hospital, give a history of a preceding coryza or bronchitis.

It is difficult to state whether or not this fact can be related in any way to allergy. As in many coccal infections the disease in question is not always established by the first contact between the human organism and the bacterial invader. It frequently happens that a period of days elapses before the typical infection is established. In most cases of lobar pneumonia in which preceding upper respiratory infection existed, the factor of allergy must be considered. That is to say, it is possible that in some instances the host acquired an altered behavior toward the pneumococcus by reason of the primary upper respiratory infection, which results in the later production of lobar pneumonia. On the other hand, the neglect of an early respiratory infection may lead to the increasing virulence of the infecting organism so that after a period of three to five days the pneumococcus may gain access to the tissue of the lung by reason of an advancing field of inflammation.

From the **experimental** standpoint Wadsworth, in 1904, was able to produce pneumonia-like infections in rabbits only after inoculating these rabbits intravenously with killed pneumococci. In 1912 Lamar and Melcher were able to produce pneumonia in dogs by the inoculation of large quantities of culture intratracheally; in 1920 Cecil and Blake reported the production of pneumonia in monkeys immediately following the intratracheal inoculation of small amounts of culture; in 1931 Robertson reported the production of lobar pneumonia in dogs following the intrabronchial inoculation of small amounts of semi-viscous cultures of pneumococci. These experiments seem to indicate that lobar pneumonia is, in the majority of cases, the effect of direct implantation of pneumococci, usually on previously damaged tissue, and perhaps made more possible by the altered behavior of an organism already damaged by a previous infection by the same or a different species of bacteria. From this it might be concluded that in some cases, at least, contact between the human host and the pneumococcus might readily and immediately lead to the production of lobar pneumonia, while in other cases a considerable amount of respiratory infection must be established before lobar pneumonia can be accomplished.

Epidemiology.—Lobar pneumonia is endemic everywhere. In spite of the fact that pneumococci occur in great numbers in the throats of normal individuals the disease is not easily spread to great numbers of people except under the conditions outlined above. It is extremely significant that while more than one-half of the pneumococci that occur in normal throats are of type IV and that types I and II are rarely found in normal throats, more than one-half of the cases of lobar pneumonia are produced by types I and II. This would immediately suggest the invasive superiority of types I and II and the comparatively weak invasive capacity of those types of pneumococci which occur in normal throats. That these pneumococci from lobar pneumonia may be spread to the throats of contacts is very well established. In the first place it has been found that a patient recovering from lobar pneumonia may harbor the particular pneumococci which caused his disease for from ten to thirty days following his recovery. The types which are more readily found following recovery are types II and III. Such patients may obviously be called carriers during this period. The carrier condition may be spread from these patients to normal individuals coming in contact with such patients. According to Stillman 13 per cent of 160 patients coming into contact with a patient carrying type I pneumococcus established the carrier condition in themselves, and 12 per cent of 149 healthy individuals coming in contact with patients carrying type II pneumococcus established the carrier condition. These facts definitely establish the communicability of lobar pneumonia and point definitely to the necessity for certain protective measures during the treatment of the disease.

Pathology.—The pathology of lobar pneumonia is characterized in all its stages by an apparent selection of the alveolar tissues for the production of the disease. For purposes of description the pathologic picture has been separated into the stage of congestion, red and gray hepatization and resolution. The physical composition of the lung in these various stages makes it easy to appreciate the reason for the physical signs which are characteristic of each stage, and which are to be found and emphasized by the clinician.

1. In the stage of congestion or engorgement the alveolar spaces are filled with red blood cells and a small number of leukocytes and a small amount of fibrin. The density of this infiltration is not great. The amount of air entering such a congested area is extremely small so that the transmission of the sounds of breathing is poor, but at the same time the air content of the area is sufficient to prevent marked dulness on percussion.

2. This stage passes immediately into a stage of more intense infiltration, particularly with leukocytes, and since the content of red blood cells is still great this stage is referred to as red hepatization. During this stage the amount of fibrin in the alveolus increases, the

lung becomes consolidated and, therefore, more easily transmits sound. No air enters the consolidated area and the sound that is transmitted comes directly from the trachea or main bronchus.

3. In the later stage of consolidation the red blood cells diminish and this robs the lung of its red appearance and leaves the color of leukocytes and fibrin predominant, and this stage is called the stage of gray hepatization. The same physical conditions prevail in the consolidated areas as far as the passage of air and the transmission of sound are concerned.

4. When the disease has run its course the elements—leukocytes, red blood cells, fibrin—which led to the consolidation of the lung disappear with surprising rapidity. This disappearance is largely due to the agency of absorption, since the quantity of sputum usually abates with the termination of the disease. This stage is referred to as the stage of resolution.

In all the stages, but particularly in the early stage, pneumococci are found in great numbers in the exudate.

Symptoms.—It is usual to describe the *onset* as being abrupt and without preceding illness, but many cases occur in which there is a history of preceding respiratory infection. Histories are not always taken with a view to determining this particular point, but in the experience of the Rockefeller Hospital, preceding respiratory infection occurred in slightly over 40 per cent of the cases. In a considerable number of patients the disease apparently begins without any preceding respiratory infection and an individual in good health may be stricken suddenly with the disease. In the aged and in debilitated patients lobar pneumonia may begin insidiously without announcing its arrival in the usual way. The disease begins almost invariably with a *chill*. This can usually be distinguished from simple chilliness which the patient may describe in other milder infections. It is more in the sense of rigor and may last from ten to thirty minutes. With the chill there is almost invariably *pain in the chest*, and the pain usually is felt in the position where the pneumonia is beginning. Least common is the symptom of vomiting. If *cough* has not already been present, it usually begins shortly after the chill.

Along with these initial symptoms are the symptoms of general infection such as prostration, aching of the body, fever and rapid pulse. After the disease has been present for twelve to twenty-four hours a *characteristic sputum* makes its appearance. *Dyspnea* soon follows upon the pain in the chest and the patient remains for a rather definite period of time in this condition of painful dyspnea, general prostration, with fever and cough. The disease terminates abruptly, and this abrupt termination is called the crisis. The crisis occurs most frequently at the end of seven days, but is occasionally deferred to the eighth or ninth day. The symptoms of infection involve so much of the body that it is necessary to consider almost every system, besides paying attention to the symptoms and signs that are peculiar to the condition in the lungs.

The Skin.—*Herpes* occurs about the lips and nares in a little less than one-half of the cases. The skin usually shows a flushed surface on one or both cheeks. There is no relationship between the side on which the lobar pneumonia exists and the side of the face which is flushed. *Jaundice* occurs in a small number of cases and often exists in connection with an enlarged liver and an area of tenderness in the region of the gall-bladder. The jaundice has no prognostic significance. Sweating is not common during the disease but may become prominent during empyema. Sweating is prominent when opiates are used.

The Circulation.—*Cyanosis* is common from the beginning of the disease. Cyanosis is associated with anoxemia, a feature described by Stadie. Cyanosis is most noticeable in the nail beds, lips and ears. The *pulse* is rapid from the start and remains so during the course of the disease, varying from 110 to 140. The pulse is surprisingly strong even in the last hours of a fatal case. The *blood pressure* is not much different from the blood pressure of the individual after recovery from the disease. The blood pressure for many years was thought to represent an index of the condition of the circulation, but more extensive clinical studies have shown that the study of the blood pressure in lobar pneumonia yields little of value to the treatment of the patient.

The Heart.—The heart is not greatly affected in lobar pneumonia, although it has been shown in the experience of Means and Porter, using a condition of bacillary pneumonia in dogs as a basis, that the blood of such animals is markedly toxic to the hearts of normal animals. Dilatation of the heart occurs near the end of the disease.

Gastro-intestinal System.—*Vomiting* at the onset has already been mentioned. Inability to take food on account of nausea may persist during the disease in a few patients. Hiccoughs are uncommon. *Abdominal distention* may be said to exist at some time in all cases and all of the time in most cases of lobar pneumonia. This distention is sometimes more noticeable on that side of the abdomen which corresponds with the side on which the pneumonia exists. The liver is usually slightly enlarged in lobar pneumonia. *Pain* may also be distributed to the abdomen and, when on the right side, may simulate acute appendicitis or acute infection of the gall-bladder.

The Kidneys.—There is constantly an albuminuria during the course of the disease. However, the renal capacity is not impaired and no consequent nephritis follows lobar pneumonia. Elevation of blood non-protein nitrogen is not uncommon and occurs in probably one-fourth of the cases, in patients past middle age.

Central Nervous System.—*Irritability*, which may be habitual in some patients, is accentuated in lobar pneumonia and sometimes offers an obstacle to recovery. *Delirium* occurs uncommonly in this disease and usually is related to the severity of the infection. *Meningismus* not infrequently attends the onset of pneumonia in children.

Respiratory System.— *Dyspnea* is a constant symptom in lobar pneumonia. Only in the aged is it less pronounced. In mild cases the respiratory rate varies between 28 and 32 per minute, while more severe cases may exhibit rates between 40 and 60 per minute. The necessity for rapid and shallow breathing in the presence of painful pleuritis leads to the production of a characteristic grunting type of breathing.

Pain in the affected side is extremely common. Pleuritis is common in lobar pneumonia and this explains the frequency with which pain occurs.

Cough is inevitable and exists in proportion to the extent of pulmonary involvement. Even in patients who do not expectorate, coughing is to be expected. The cough is short and interrupted on account of the pain which it incites. Cough is increased by edema of the lungs which attends terminal cardiac dilatation.

Physical Findings.—Sputum.—One of the first points of interest is the examination of the sputum of the individual. The sputum is typical in lobar pneumonia and makes its appearance in the first twelve hours of the disease as an extremely sticky, scanty, and bright red or rusty material which increases in amount. The feature of rustiness usually persists throughout the disease. It may be altered by the appearance of purulent components several days after the onset, but the most important change that has prognostic significance is the change in the direction of increased fluidity and redness. This change is usually the result of circulatory weakness in the lungs.

The Pharynx.—The pharynx in lobar pneumonia is frequently covered with flecks of sputum and may display a mild degree of redness and cyanosis due to coughing, but rarely appears to be itself infected.

The Chest.—*Inspection.*—One notices an increased respiratory movement, and this is seen to be more marked on the sound side. This inequality of the excursion of the two sides is also represented by the difference in the respiratory movement of the abdomen in the epigastric area, there being usually more rise and fall on the side of the healthy lung than on the affected side.

Percussion.—On percussion in the first twenty-four hours of the disease there may be very little difference in resonance of the two sides. As consolidation becomes established, however, the effect is represented by increasing dulness over the consolidated area.

Auscultation.—Auscultation in the early hours of the disease shows that breathing is usually diminished and accompanied by a few fine râles over the infected area. As consolidation becomes complete, bronchial breathing becomes more easily elicited until finally it can be heard nearly as plainly as though the stethoscope were placed over the trachea. In like manner the whispered voice is transmitted through the consolidated lung with remarkable clearness. Toward the end of the disease, râles are usually heard in the consolidated lung, and these are produced by the beginning resolution of the infected tissue. They have been referred to as "râles redux." When heard on the healthy side the râles are usually an evidence of weakness of the circulation of the lung and constitute an unfavorable sign.

Fever.—The fever chart in typical cases of lobar pneumonia presents striking and almost constant features. The fever is remarkably sustained throughout the course of the disease. There is no other infection that maintains the fever with such constancy as this pneumococcal infection of the lungs. In favorable cases the temperature begins to show remission on the fifth or sixth day, although these remissions are slight. In favorable cases the fever terminates within a period of twelve to eighteen hours after the beginning of defervescence, and this abrupt termination of the fever corresponds with the cessation in all of the other symptoms and signs, and constitutes the crisis of the disease. After the temperature has remained normal for twelve to twenty-four hours it frequently happens that there is a rise to 100° F. or even higher for twenty-four hours more and after this the temperature remains normal. This secondary fever may occur in the absence of complications such as empyema. In the aged and debilitated subjects the characteristic fever chart may be absent. Old people may have lobar pneumonia quietly with few symptoms and very little fever and yet come to a favorable conclusion. Very high fever may occur with a small amount of pulmonary consolidation, but usually there is a relationship between the extent of the involvement of the lungs and the degree of fever.

Leukocytosis.—One of the characteristics of pneumococcal pneumonia is presented by the high leukocyte count. The degree of leukocytosis is related to the seriousness of the disease and has a prognostic value. The death-rate is considerably higher in those patients who have a moderate or low leukocytosis than in those patients who display a marked increase in leukocytes. The count usually varies from 20,000 to 30,000 in the average adult, to 60,000 in occasional cases, particularly in children. No leukocytosis whatever may appear in patients who are weakened by disease or in the aged. In old people the absence of leukocytosis may occur in connection with a mild clinical course and may not have the same serious meaning that it would have in a robust adult. The leukocytes are increased as a result of the great increase in non-segmented forms. There is little effect on the red blood cells in lobar pneumonia because the disease does not last long enough to damage the hematopoietic tissues.

Bacteriemia.—There is a definite relation between the occurrence of a positive blood culture and the severity of the disease and the outcome. As a rule, patients having negative blood cultures have a much more favorable prognosis than those showing positive blood cultures. Patients who have many colonies per cubic centimeter are in greater danger of death than those having few colonies per cubic centimeter of blood. As a general rule, more than 25 colonies per cubic centimeter indicates a serious and most likely fatal infection.

Complications.—The most common complication is *empyema*. Suspicion is created by the return of the fever following the crisis and failure of the patient to appear as well as expected. The form of the temperature curve in empyema differs from the form of the curve in lobar pneumonia in that there are daily remissions and, as a rule, the peaks are not as high. The sputum and cough usually persist with the development of the empyema. In the first few days of pneumococcal empyema the fluid displays a thickness and yellowness which are not found in streptococcal empyema where the fluid is thin and reddish-brown in the first twenty-four hours. Pneumococci are usually found easily in the empyema fluid. They are present in greater numbers in the earliest stages. Empyema is to be distinguished from unresolved pneumonia, which is rare, and exists most frequently in the upper lobes where the lack of resolution is apparently dependent upon tuberculous activity. Empyema is further to be distinguished from abscess of the lung. The roentgen-ray is usually necessary to determine the nature of these secondary purulent affections. Aspiration is necessary to determine the character and bacteriology of the empyema fluid. Empyema occurs in between 3 to 5 per cent of cases.

Pericarditis occurs in less than 1 per cent of cases. It exists as a purulent inflammation and must be treated surgically.

Endocarditis may develop as the result of pneumococci in a bacteriemia becoming implanted on a valve damaged by sclerotic or atheromatous changes such as occur in people beyond middle age.

Phlebitis in the saphenous veins has been infrequently reported. At least three weeks of complete rest are essential before free movement is allowed.

Arthritis and *meningitis* are bacterial metastases and have been discussed as such.

Diagnosis.—The diagnosis of lobar pneumonia from the standpoint of its symptoms and physical signs is comparatively easy. The features which are most useful are the sudden onset, the chill, pain in the chest, the increased respiratory rate, rusty sputum and marked leukocytosis. The physical signs are undoubted when they occur, but in cases of incomplete consolidation these physical signs may not be easy to elicit. This is particularly true of lobar pneumonia in children. The use of the *roentgen-ray* is invaluable in certain cases in which the physical signs are not clear or in which no sputum is available.

It is extremely important to make a diagnosis of the type of pneumococcus which is concerned with the pneumonia. This is usually done by immediate collection of sputum which may be examined in one of several ways, chiefly by mouse inoculation. This method is by far the most valuable and most free from technical complications. The washed sputum is injected into the peritoneal cavity of the mouse and, after eighteen hours, or when the mouse dies, the peritoneal cavity is opened, washed with salt solution and the washings centrifuged at high speed. The supernatant fluid is tested with the three types of diagnostic serum. Lung puncture may be resorted to, and by this method a needle is inserted into the consolidated area and the 1 or 2 drops of bloody material so procured are planted in media or inoculated into the peritoneal cavity of a white mouse. Cultural methods of identifying types have been described by Avery. The method of typing described by Krumwiede is quick and simple, consisting essentially of boiling a specimen of sputum, centrifugalizing, and testing the supernatant fluid with diagnostic serums. The method of Neufeld, utilizing a microscopic effect of specific serum on the capsule of the pneumococcus, is convincing. The blood culture should be made in all cases on account of its prognostic value and also to check the value of injected antipneumococcal serum.

From streptococcal pneumonia, lobar pneumonia may be distinguished by the smaller amount of coughing, the rusty sputum and the sustained fever, and the higher leukocytosis. From tuberculous pneumonia, it is to be distinguished by the self-limited course, and the uniformity of the physical signs, and the higher leukocytosis.

10

Unfavorable Signs.—1. *Coughing.*—While coughing is usual in all cases, a persistent, frequent effort is debilitating and is a source of concern to the clinician. When coughing is frequent the amount of sputum is correspondingly copious.

2. *Excitement.*—Mental agitation also leads to an exhaustion of the patient. Like excessive coughing it not only damages the patient, but seems itself to be the product of an especially severe infection.

3. *Pain.*—Pain on breathing and coughing prevents sleep and usually exists as a result of unusually extensive pleurisy.

4. In the last days before the anticipated crisis the coloring of the sputum with blood, so that the sputum changes from rusty to bloody in appearance, usually is very unfavorable and represents congestion from circulatory weakness.

5. Râles in the unaffected lobe accompany the bloody sputum and speak for the same deficiency.

6. Positive blood culture has already been mentioned. It constitutes perhaps the most unfavorable evidence.

7. Absence of leukocytosis is usually reflected in the weakness of the patient, the more than usually rapid pulse and the tendency of the pneumonia to spread.

Favorable evidence consists in the absence of the above, and beginning of defervescence at the sixth day.

Treatment.—1. *Rest.*—The patient needs rest as early as possible. Many cases become fatal through failure of the patient or physician to recognize the disease. This results in protracted effort on the part of the patient. The semi-recumbent position is preferred by most patients. The room should be well ventilated and cool, but not necessarily cold. Most patients appreciate being placed in the open air, but this raises certain complications with regard to nursing. Besides bed rest it is extremely important to organize the environment of the patient so that no irritations or exciting influences may be at work.

2. *Serum.*—The serum treatment of lobar pneumonia is the most important advance in the cure of these patients. Type I infections are amenable to the use of type I antipneumococcus serum. The other types of infections have no corresponding treatment with serum, nor is type I serum of any value in the other types of pneumonia. Exhaustive studies of the usefulness of type I serum made by the workers in the Rockefeller Hospital and also in Bellevue Hospital indicate that where type I serum is employed within the first three days of the disease, the mortality will be reduced at least to one-half of the expected mortality. It has been shown that bacteriemia of the grade usually fatal can be removed in type I cases by appropriate use of serum. While the serum, or its concentrate, for type II pneumococcus is not so curative, extended studies indicate that there are a considerable number of instances in which such treatment is effective. Manufacturers are now supplying types I and II "antibody solution" in combination so that, pending a typing of the patient under consideration, treatment may be instituted without delay. In the experience of the author, although the effect of "antibody solution" is favorable, sudden improvement is not as frequent as with whole horse serum.

Before the patient receives serum he must receive an intradermal injection of horse serum or antipneumococcal serum for the purpose of detecting a possible allergy to horse serum. For this purpose a few cubic millimeters of horse serum diluted 1 to 20 are injected intradermally, and the area is watched for the formation of a wheal. If the patient is sensitive to horse serum he must be desensitized. By this process he receives 0.2 cc. of antipneumococcal serum subcutaneously and progressively doubled doses at one-half hour intervals thereafter, provided no general reaction follows. At the end of several such subcutaneous injections 0.1 cc. of serum is administered intravenously and the same doubling arrangement follows at one-half hour intervals until a satisfactory amount of serum has been administered. This amount is 50 cc. per dose and each dose is repeated after eight-hour intervals until the temperature remains normal. Whenever given in large doses this serum should be diluted with salt solution in proportions of 1 to 1.

3. *Drugs.*—Morphine is of particular value in bringing about the condition of rest and in allaying the cough, the pain, and the nervous manifestations of a patient. It is one of the most valuable drugs in the treatment of lobar pneumonia. Codeine is of equal value. Nausea may follow its use.

Stimulants, such as strychnine, camphor and whisky have little proven value in the treatment of lobar pneumonia.

Quinine derivatives, ethyl hydrocuprein, optochin, have been used in the treatment of lobar pneumonia and have an antipyretic effect, but have no effect on the bacteriemia or on the essential factors of the disease and do not alter the death-rate.

4. Next to the use of serum the use of oxygen is the most important measure for relieving the patient. The lowering of the pulse-rate and temperature, and the lessening of excitement are immediate effects of the use of oxygen as given in suitable tents. Inadequate equipment is of no value in using oxygen. However marked the beneficial effect may be on the symptoms, it is not certain that the use of oxygen prevents death in any given case.

5. *Diet.*—This should be nourishing and as rich in calories as compatible with the desire and capacity of the patient to take food. Alcohol, either as a drug or as a flavoring of food, seems of little importance.

6. Pneumothorax has been reported upon favorably by Stengel and by Blake in the United States. It is contraindicated in cases of bilateral infection and may be dangerous in children. It is essential to maintain a positive expiratory pressure.

7. Finally it is necessary for the clinician to see his patient at least three times a day in serious cases.

Treatment of Special Symptoms.—*Circulatory Weakness.*—In anticipation of later cardiac weakness, many consider it advisable to administer digitalis from the beginning of the disease so that the influence of the drug may be available before the crisis. Others believe the drug to have little value. Its use is not indicated in mild cases.

Abdominal Distention.—This feature persists throughout the disease and, while enemata are successful in producing release of flatus, the distention reaccumulates immediately. Gastric lavage and the use of carminatives are likewise of little avail. Distention is the effect of a severe infection but scarcely the cause of trouble. Besides enemata, turpentine stupes may be employed.

Fever.—Sponging is not used in pneumonia except in hot weather. Quinine and coal tar products are more effective in reducing excessively high temperatures, although the latter are not common or particularly distressing.

Treatment of Empyema.— *Tapping* is carried out preferably after information has been obtained from roentgen-ray pictures, because the clinical features may be simulated by abscess in the lung, which could not be reached by the aspirating needle. The character of the exudate should be noted. The fluid of pneumococcal empyema is usually of homogeneous fluidity and yellow. Many cases, with small amounts of exudate, will recover in the course of four to eight weeks without further interference. In such cases the temperature is usually normal in the morning and rises to 100° or 101° F. in the afternoon, and the leukocytosis hovers about 12,000 to 15,000 and gradually approaches the normal number. Where surgical procedures are indicated, the physical signs of fluid persist, and the fever and general symptoms speak for continuing, severe infection, and roentgen-ray studies reveal persistence of the effusion.

The clinical features of pneumococcal empyema are much less vehement than those of streptococcal empyema. In some cases, after empyema has existed for more than a week, a sudden attack of coughing results in the expectoration of fluid, purulent sputum—evidence that the empyematous pus has found its way into a bronchus. Such cases are of the kind that should have been treated surgically early.

Prophylaxis.—Lobar pneumonia is only mildly communicable, but persons with respiratory infection such as "colds" should not be in attendance upon a patient with pneumonia. Prophylactic vaccination in individual cases has little practical value.

CEREBROSPINAL FEVER.

Cerebrospinal fever is the term applied to an acute meningococcal infection which is characterized by purulent infiltration of the pia-arachnoid tissue of the brain and cord, and by symptoms arising from this involvement of the central nervous system. The term cerebrospinal fever is synonymous with the expressions "epidemic cerebrospinal meningitis" and "meningococcal meningitis," which were previously used.

Cerebrospinal fever exists throughout the year in endemic fashion, but is much more prevalent in the winter months or in those times of the year which necessitate living indoors and living in crowds. It occurs in all parts of the world. It was described in the United States in 1808; in New England, up to 1919, 85 epidemics had occurred, according to Hirsch. This tendency to occur in epidemics gave rise to the expression "epidemic cerebrospinal meningitis." During the World War extensive studies were made of the bacteriology and epidemiology of this disease and many questions previously unsettled were solved by this experience.

Etiology.—Bacteriology.—The meningococcus is the exciting agent of the disease. This is a Gram-negative diplococcus first described by Weichselbaum in 1887. It occurs as two round cocci in apposition and is distinct from the gonococcus, the apposing sides of which are concave. It is a member of a group of Gram-negative diplococci which are ordinarily found in the naso-pharynx. The meningococcus grows well on all serum-containing media and on media containing methemoglobin. For the isolation of meningococcus from the naso-pharynx, serum agar is a suitable medium in plate cultures. The meningococcus forms a uniformly turbid suspension in normal salt solution, and in this way differs from some of the other Gram-negative diplococci which occur in the naso-pharynx. Besides this feature, such suspensions in normal salt solution are precipitated by polyvalent antimeningococcal serum. In this way diagnosis is made of "meningococcus" in a given culture. Other members of the group of Gram-negative diplococci which occur in the naso-pharynx are Micrococcus catarrhalis, Micrococcus siccus and Micrococcus flavus. The two last named are described by adjectives which refer respectively to the dry and yellow appearance of the colonies, while the colonies of the meningococcus are gray. The meningococcus occurs in the throats of normal individuals in a percentage that varies with the seasons and conditions under which individuals live. A survey of nearly 10,000 contacts made during the World War showed that the meningococcus occurred in from 1 to 5 per cent of normal subjects, the variation being influenced by the weather. The higher percentages were obtained in the "shut-in" part of the season, the lower percentages occurring during the "open" weather.

There are different types of meningococci and each type produces in horses a corresponding antiserum which may not be effective against meningococcal infections due to other types of meningococci. This is of great importance in the treatment of the disease. Dopter has recognized three types of meningococcus: the normal strain, parameningococcus, and the intermediate strain. The English investigators, Gordon and Murray, have classified the meningococci into four types: type I, which corresponds to the parameningococcus of Dopter; type II to the normal meningococcus, and types III and IV to the intermediate strain. An antimeningococcal serum, to be of therapeutic value, must be made by the injection of horses with all of the types of the meningococcus family. Besides these three or four main types there are many intermediate variants, but the inclusion of these main types in the vaccine with which horses are inoculated is sufficient to give an antiserum which is curative for all types of the disease in man.

It has been noticed that epidemics differ not only in severity but in certain clinical characteristics, such as the prevalence of cutaneous eruptions, and some observers have thought that these differences were produced by the differing virulence of the various bacterial types.

Age.—The greatest number of cases occur in children below the age of ten years. Out of 3900 cases occurring in New York during

1905, 1906 and 1907, 66 per cent occurred under the age of ten years. During the World War, of course, the age incidence was higher on account of the fact that the age of the exposed subjects, the soldiers, was higher. The disease is uncommon over the age of fifty years.

Sex and Race.—The disease occurs somewhat more frequently in males than females, and negroes are more often affected than whites.

Other factors affecting the etiology are the condition of the patient previous to the development of the disease; preceding naso-pharyngeal infection may be part of the early stages of cerebrospinal fever, or there may be other forerunning infections which predispose to invasion by meningococcus. In the majority of cases of meningitis there is a history of preceding upper respiratory infection. Trauma—head injury—may be the predisposing cause. Nothing is known about the incubation period of cerebrospinal fever. However, there are sufficient observations to indicate that the period is very short, possibly two or three days in some cases.

Epidemiology.—The meningococcus, on account of its location in the upper respiratory passages, is obviously transmitted to other individuals by means of the droplet type of transmission. Although the evidence for direct contagion in times of epidemic is not impressive, numerous reports of such transmission, notably to physicians and nurses, are in the literature. Continued association with a patient seems to be necessary for transmission in many of the cases. Individuals developing the carrier condition as a result of contact with a patient, usually show negative cultures from the naso-pharynx in five to eight days. There is no special treatment of the naso-pharynx which will drive out the meningococcus in a shorter time. The number of carriers who develop meningitis is so small as to suggest that another factor—that of upper respiratory infection—may be necessary for the implantation or inoculation of meningococci.

Pathogenesis.—For laboratory animals the pathogenicity of meningococcus is almost negligible, when the organisms are injected intravenously or intraperitoneally. In monkeys the intraspinal injection of meningococci has produced purulent meningitis (Flexner).

The pathogenesis of the disease has excited a great deal of comment. There are three general theories. One is that the organism gains access to the cerebrospinal fluid through the lymphatics of the sphenoid and ethmoid sinuses, or along the olfactory nerve as it passes through the cribriform plate. This is the theory of direct extension. The second mechanism considered is a spread from the naso-pharynx along the lymphatics of the cervical roots, or from the intestinal tract along the lower dorsal roots, to the spinal cord. This idea is proposed to explain those rare cases which seem to show affection of the cord before involvement of the brain; and is really only a modified application of the theory of direct extension. The third theory regards the disease as beginning as a septicemia and later being represented as a metastasis of this septicemia in the cerebrospinal fluid and the pia-arachnoid tissue. Before the war the direct method of infection was the one usually thought to operate, but Herrick, from extended observations, reported many patients in whom positive blood cultures were obtained while the cerebrospinal fluid was sterile and in whom cerebrospinal meningitis later developed. There is no doubt that in many cases, and possibly the majority of cases, the disease begins as septicemia, which is presumed to derive from inflammation of the tissues of the nasopharynx. It is probable that both septicemia and direct extension operate together.

A fourth theory must be considered, namely, that a preceding virus infection of a neurotropic type prepares the field for infection, in those individuals who happen to be carriers.

Pathology.—The principal pathology concerns the localization of the disease around the brain and cord. This is represented as a two-phase reaction not unlike the reaction to pneumococcus and hemolytic streptococcus. In the first phase there is intense congestion of the arachnoid. Later, the second or purulent phase occurs with infiltrations of polymorph leukocytes about the blood-vessels. This purulent reaction frequently leads to obstructive collections of fibrin and pus and causes the complications, such as secondary abscesses in the brain or the blocking of the ventricles. The local situations thus created, such as pyocephalus or hydrocephalus, prolong the clinical disturbance and produce the sequelæ in the central nervous system.

Besides the disease of the meninges, there are changes throughout the body in cases of severe septicemia. These changes include hemorrhages in the skin and serous surfaces, swelling and softening of the spleen and of the lymphatics of the intestine.

Leukocytosis.—As representing the changes which take place in the tissues, the circulating blood invariably shows a marked increase in polymorphonuclear leukocytes. The usual count is between 20,000 and 30,000, but higher counts have been reported. Such high counts are not found in the mild and chronic case.

The Spinal Fluid.—In the first twelve hours, the spinal fluid may remain clear or show only a slight increase in lymphocytes. In a typical case, however, the fluid thereafter rapidly becomes turbid as a result of the accumulation of polymorph leukocytes. Meningococci are usually present in great numbers both inside and outside the leukocytes. In the beginning of the disease the spinal fluid flows freely under pressure, but later may be difficult to obtain by lumbar puncture owing to obstructive exudate higher in the canal.

Symptoms.—The *onset* of the meningitis is usually sudden. This onset may be preceded by a period of upper respiratory infection, but in some cases this period is not recognized by the physician or by the patient himself. The most important symptom at the time of onset is *headache*. The headache is peculiar in that it is persistent and does not yield to ordinary remedies. It disturbs the comfort of the patient in a very definite way. A *definite chill* is not uncommon. *Vomiting* occurs in most cases and frequently without nausea. Diarrhea and abdominal pain are less common. Nosebleed may be a symptom at the time of onset.

The *pulse* at first is fast, then retarded, but soon becomes accelerated again and remains rapid through the remainder of the disease. The *fever* is high (102° to 105° F.) throughout. The *respiration* is not disturbed in the beginning, but later may be of the interrupted type, and finally the patient may succumb to respiratory failure.

The Skin.—Of particular interest are the rashes which are found in this disease. These may be maculo-papular and resemble coarse rosé spots; or purpuric, and exist either as widely scattered small purple spots measuring a few millimeters in diameter; or as diffuse confluent purple blotching of the entire body. Herpes of the lips is a common sign.

The Kidneys.—Albuminuria is very common but is rarely accompanied by casts. Nephritis, however, does not occur.

The *central nervous system* is naturally involved in a striking way. Headache, which may not cloud the sensorium of the patient for twenty-four to forty-eight hours, soon produces a stuporous delirium. In this condition sphincter control may be lost. The delirium of the patient with cerebrospinal fever is much more pronounced than that found in tuberculous meningitis and much less pronounced than that found in pneumococcal meningitis. Muscular rigidity occurs throughout the body and in some localities gives rise to useful diagnostic signs.

Rigidity of the muscles of the neck gives rise to the so-called Kernig's sign. This sign is elicited when the thigh is placed at right angle to the axis of the trunk, and the leg then extended. The rigidity of the muscles is such that extension of the leg to the line of the thigh is impossible. This sign was described by Kernig in 1884, and is one of the most valuable features of physical examination of a patient suspected of having meningitis. Ankle clonus and patellar clonus are also commonly elicited. Strabismus and nystagmus are usually signs found only late in the disease. Other late signs are focal or general paralysis. Vasomotor instability is indicated in the so-called "tâche cerebrale." This is a response of the skin to light stroking with the tip of a pencil in which the irritated area becomes white and remains white. Normally the similar stroking of the skin produces a red line along the path of irritation. This sign is not of diagnostic importance. Patients who recover from cerebrospinal meningitis usually display a remarkable degree of *wasting*.

Unfortunately, cerebrospinal fever displays many clinical variations both as to character of onset, prominence of the various symptoms, and clinical course, but the above description applies to the average patient.

Clinical Variations.—Whether from a different pathogenesis, or from the effects of preceding infection in the naso-pharynx, cerebrospinal fever may present itself in a variety of clinical pictures.

1. *Fulminating Form.*—In this condition a previously healthy individual may be stricken suddenly with a headache. Fever appears at once and reddening of the conjunctiva is to be noted. This redness is due to extreme congestion of vessels suggesting impending petechiæ. The fulminating type of cerebrospinal fever is in reality a form of meningococcal septicemia which is so rapidly fatal that the signs of meningitis are not usually found. In this type of infection death may occur in from twelve to twenty-four hours after the first complaint of the patient. Physical examination fails to reveal any localization of

an infection, except congestion of the nasal mucosa, and sometimes the ear drums. The peculiar severity of the headache, however, and the fever should excite the suspicion of the physician. The only chance that such a patient has of recovery lies in the immediate use of extremely large doses of antimeningococcal serum. In these cases the blood culture is always positive and the purpuric rashes that occur in this type of infection are more extensive than are found in any other infectious process. The rash, however, may not occur until twelve hours after the onset.

2. The usual acute type has been described. There are variations of this type, so that a patient may present the picture of "hyperacute" meningitis in which all the signs of involvement of the central nervous system are accentuated, or there may be such mildness in the course that positive blood cultures are obtained in patients in whom only coryza and transitory meningitic phenomena are present.

3. Chronic cases are those abortive cases which remained untreated or, are the acute cases protracted on account of obstructive localizations of pus in the brain. These are the patients which display such devastating effects of wasting.

Diagnosis.—It may be very difficult to diagnose a case of cerebrospinal fever at the time of onset. This is particularly true in the so-called fulminating types where the signs of meningitis are absent and may never develop.

The particular symptoms and signs which the physician must recognize are the coryza, or history of coryza, the tenacious headache, the fever and leukocytosis. With increasing headache come neck rigidity and interference with mental calm and clearness. Spinal puncture will differentiate with certainty between the various types of meningitis. Lumbar puncture should not be undertaken in the absence of signs suggesting meningeal irritation. Blood cultures, routinely made in cases of fever, will bring to light those cases of the septicemic type without meningitis.

Treatment.—The treatment consists in the use of antimeningococcal serum. Since the disease is a septicemia as well as a localization in the arachnoid tissues, it is extremely important to use serum intravenously as well as intraspinally. Amoss and Eberson have found that the concentration of antimeningococcal serum in the spinal fluid of experimental monkeys is greater if the serum is injected by both routes than when injected by either route alone. The serum is administered intraspinally in quantities of 15 cc. after the withdrawal of a similar quantity of cerebrospinal fluid by lumbar puncture. The treatment is repeated every eight hours. Difficulty in obtaining cerebrospinal fluid may be encountered in later punctures due probably to the formation of local exudates in the lower spinal canal, so that irrigation with normal salt solution is a measure which may be employed to dilute and simplify the release of spinal fluid. Injections may also be made into the cisterna. The injections are continued until the fever returns to normal, or at least until the patient is pronounced recovering from the acute phases of the disease. This treatment, therefore, may be brief in some cases, lasting only a few days, and in others the injections may have to be continued, although some consider it unwise to use serum intraspinally for more than ten or twelve injections. The treatment is usually effective only when begun within the first three days of the disease, and most effective when begun within the first twenty-four hours. The commonest cause of death in acute cases is respiratory failure. The death-rate from the disease in the United States is over 50 per cent. In those cases which are treated early, the death-rate may be reduced to 15 per cent. However, no statistics are entirely reliable in this respect because a given epidemic may have cases that are fulminating which are incurable, or may have many cases, on the other hand, that are mild and easily cured, even with treatment instituted as late as the third day. If treatment is not begun within the first two days the death-rate is naturally much higher.

If one is fortunate enough to detect the diagnosis in those patients who have infections with positive blood cultures without meningitic signs, the intravenous use of serum will be found highly curative. For intravenous injection, 100 cc. of serum diluted with equal parts of normal saline solution should be employed twice a day until recovery is assured.

In all such cases the usual precautions should be taken to discover sensitiveness to serum and guard against allergic reactions. If, in chronic cases, it is advisable to resume the use of serum a week after a previous dose of serum, the factor of shock must be considered and the patient carefully given repeated doses of minute amounts until the danger is averted. The method of desensitization has been described in the section on Lobar Pneumonia.

The various complications which may occur would require surgical treatment in the case of abscess in the brain, or purulent arthritis, but many of the complications following cerebrospinal fever gradually disappear after months of convalescence. Deafness may be permanent. Blindness may occur as a result of a purulent infection in the orbit, and various local paralyses may resist treatment. The injection of antimeningococcal serum is to be considered in the treatment of any persistent complication, although its value is not great in this situation.

The *prophylaxis* consists, first, in making cultures of the throats of all contacts and in the isolation of carriers. Second, the persons coming in contact with patients, the nurses and physicians, should wear masks and gowns. The patient himself is isolated.

GONOCOCCAL INFECTIONS.

Clinical gonococcal infections are recognized chiefly as metastases or extensions from local infections of the urethra or other parts of the genital tract. It is not the part of this chapter to discuss gonococcal urethritis, since that is more properly treated as a specialty. The two chief metastases are gonococcal arthritis, or gonorrheal rheumatism, and gonococcal endocarditis. The chief extensions are into the Fallopian tubes in the female and into the seminal vesicles and prostate in the male.

Bacteriology.—The gonococcus itself is a Gram-negative diplococcus with a distinctive morphology due to the fact that the apposing sides of the cocci are flattened or concave, giving the contour of a biscuit. It has no capsule. It has no pathogenicity for laboratory animals. It is isolated with very little difficulty from local discharges by streaking these on so-called "burnt blood" agar. This is also sometimes referred to as "chocolate" medium on account of the color that is given by the heating of the blood. Many other media have been described, but this particular one is easily prepared and it also serves as a medium for preserving the strains that have been isolated. The gonococcus is subject to peculiar blighting influences sometimes not recognized while under artificial cultivation. They are easily killed by sterile water and all hypotonic solutions. Large quantities inoculated in the peritoneum of a white mouse produce no disturbances.

Pathogenesis.—The appearance of metastatic infections following urethritis is interesting. This metastasis does not occur immediately upon the establishment of the local infection. That is to say, it is extremely unusual to see a patient having gonorrheal rheumatism soon after gonococcal urethritis. Many days, usually months, elapse before such patients have rheumatism. This factor of delay in the appearance of the secondary infection may be regarded as a manifestation of bacterial allergy, but in reality the causes of such delay and secondary infection are not clearly understood. That the secondary infections are true metastases of gonococci streaming through the blood from the urethral source, to either the endocardial surfaces or the neighborhoods of joints, is undoubted, and gonococcal arthritis is a perfect type of focal infection.

The extension of a gonococcal infection to the Fallopian tubes may result in the symptoms of "acute surgical abdomen" and call for interesting differentiation from other acute events in the abdomen, such as appendicitis or painful infections of the urinary tract. Consideration must be given the tendency of the pain to radiate down to the inner side of the thigh in case of salpingitis and the coexistence of a purulent vaginal or cervical discharge containing gonococci. It is important to obtain smears from the cervix and from the opening of the urethra in such cases.

One of the most interesting features of gonococcal extensions into the seminal vesicles and prostate is the simulation of arthritis in one hip as a result of pain-radiation.

Gonorrheal Rheumatism.—The *onset* is invariably associated with a urethral discharge. In women this may be difficult to determine, and the diagnosis may depend on a clinical picture rather than a bacteriologic examination. If histories are written with a view to establishing the possible influence of an intercurrent acute event, it may be found, as it has happened in the experience of the writer in 11 cases, that some episode like an acute respiratory infection precedes the onset of rheumatism. The gonococcal urethritis is also activated by the respiratory infection, the streptococcal pharyngitis, or the trauma, and this may account for the ready access of gonococci to the blood stream. It may be assumed that this access to the blood stream is available to the gonococci during the initial urethritis when rheumatism is not produced. It is suggested that the sore throat so often found before an attack of acute rheumatic fever may play the same rôle in activating an infective process already in the body, but not able to involve the tissues of the heart and joints. It may be convenient to refer to the altered behavior of the body, permitting involvement of joints, as allergic, but the factors making up such allergy are scarcely understood.

Symptoms and Signs.—Leukocytosis of a moderate degree is the rule. There are no joints that are characteristically selected by gonococci to the exclusion of other joints. At one time it was thought that gonococcal arthritis showed a predilection for the sternoclavicular joint or for the vertebral joints. But the first of these is much more commonly affected in acute rheumatic fever and the other is more commonly affected in conditions that are not gonorrheal.

The joint manifestations may be separated into two main groups. The first of the two main types of gonorrheal rheumatism is one in which the joint shows diffuse tender swelling with marked fluctuation in the joint cavity due to its distention with fluid. This might be referred to as the "effusion type" of gonorrheal rheumatism. It is extremely easy to aspirate such joints and to withdraw a considerable quantity of fluid. The *joint fluid* so obtained is more turbid than joint fluid obtained in acute rheumatic fever, but it is not opaque enough to be termed pus. The cytology consists of an almost exclusive increase in polymorph leukocytes with fewer endothelial cells than in the fluid of acute rheumatic fever. In these cases in which effusion is readily aspirated cultures may be obtained with comparative frequency, but it usually takes at least one hour of searching to find gonococci microscopically in the direct smear.

The other type is strikingly different. The joint is enveloped in a diffuse, brawny and exquisitely tender inflammation. Such is the pain that the patient often prevents examination by pushing away the palpating hand. There is no fluctuation in such an inflammation. The place to aspirate is that in which the greatest amount of pink discoloration may be observed. This usually coincides with the point of greatest tenderness. When the needle is inserted, even to the point of being sure that it is in the joint cavity, fluid is seldom obtained, and yet the bloody pus expressed from the point of the needle may show gonococci in greater numbers than in the fluid taken from the "effusion" type.

The symptoms of these two types of rheumatism are different. The second, or infiltrative type, shows much more pain and tenderness and disability in the part. The duration of either type of rheumatism depends on the usually unknown factor of the extent of the focus and the success of the treatment.

Diagnosis.—The onset is not unlike the onset of acute rheumatic fever. Pains may be in several joints at the same time and these pains may migrate to other joints before localizing in one or at the most in two joints. The clinical picture is usually established when the infection localizes in one joint. It differs sharply in this respect from acute rheumatic fever, which does not delay in a single joint for more than three or four days, even though stiffness may persist for a long time afterward. This definite establishment of monarticular arthritis, whose features are obviously those of pyogenic infection, is characteristic of gonococcal arthritis. Fever occurs at the time of onset but is seldom as marked as in acute rheumatic fever. The finding of gonococci in the joint fluid is conclusive.

Treatment.—The treatment of the effusion type consists (1) in putting the joint at rest; (2) in aspirating the fluid; (3) in simple extension by means of a weight and pulley. If none of these measures are resorted to, there are many cases mild enough to recover without any special local treatment. Of those cases in which it is obvious that purulent infiltration penetrates the tissue around the tendons and around the synovial surfaces, it is obvious that unless this inflammation has an avenue of escape, scar tissue will replace the purulent infiltration, and so embrace the joint itself as to produce definite and troublesome ankylosis. Furthermore, such an inflammation, unless eradicated, will itself constitute a source of further metastases, and a condition of chronic gonorrheal rheumatism may result from neglect of this type of arthritis. In this second form of rheumatism or arthritis, immobilization by putting the joint in a cast may result in fixation of the joint, when it becomes ankylosed in an awkward position. Passive movement should be instituted as soon as possible in such cases. A successful form of treatment in this type of rheumatism is direct incision of the purulent area with subsequent drainage and irrigation, if necessary. Twenty-one cases of this type of rheumatism observed by the writer have been treated in this way with uniformly successful results and complete restoration of joint function in all but 2 cases. The use of vaccines and the use of non-protein shock therapy has not proven satisfactory. A study of 13 cases treated at St. Mary's Hospital, St. Louis, with injections of milk, has shown that recovery is not complete, and the hospital days were prolonged and the amount of disability was extensive. Most important in the treatment of gonorrheal rheumatism is the treatment of the local urethral infection or of its neighboring extensions into the seminal vesicles or prostate or tubes.

Gonococcal endocarditis is discussed elsewhere and gonococcal ophthalmia more properly belongs to a treatise on Ophthalmology.

REFERENCES.

Amoss, H. L.: Treatment of Recurrent Erysipelas, Ann. Int. Med., 1931, 5, 500.
Avery, O. T., and associates (see especially DuBos, Rene, and Avery, O. T.): Decomposition of the Capsular Polysaccharide of Pneumococcus Type III by a Bacterial Enzyme, Studies of Rockefeller Institute, 1931, vol. 79.
Brown, J. H.: The Use of Blood Agar for the Study of Streptococcus, Monograph of the Rockefeller Institute, 1919, No. 9.
Cecil, R. L., and Austin, H.: Prophylactic Inoculation Against Pneumococcus, Jour. Exp. Med., 1918, 28, 19.
Chickering, H. T.: Staphylococcus Pneumonia, Jour. Am. Med. Assn., 1919, 72, 617.
Cole, Rufus, and others: Acute Lobar Pneumonia, Prevention and Serum Treatment, Monograph of the Rockefeller Institute, 1917, No. 7.

HERRICK, W. W.:   Meningitis at Camp Jackson, Jour. Am. Med. Assn., 1918, **70**, 227.

KINSELLA, R. A.:   Recent Studies of Rheumatism, Jour. Lab. and Clin. Med., 1930, **15**, 1062.

LONGCOPE, W. T., O'BRIEN, D. P., and others: Relationship of Acute Infections to Glomerular Nephritis, Jour. Clin. Invest., 1927, **5**, 7.

McCALLUM, W. G.:   The Pathology of the Pneumonias in the U. S. Army Camps During the Winter of 1917–1918, Monograph of the Rockefeller Institute, 1919, No. 10.

PARKER, J. T.:   Production of Exotoxin in Certain Strains of Staphylococcus Aureus, Jour. Exp. Med., 1924, **40**, 761.

WEATHERBY, M., and CLAWSON, B. J.:   Intravenous Streptococcus Vaccine Therapy in Chronic Arthritis, Jour. Am. Med. Assn., 1932, **98**, 1974.

CHAPTER III.

THE VIRUS DISEASES.

By O. H. PERRY PEPPER, M.D.

INTRODUCTION.
SMALLPOX.
COWPOX AND VACCINATION.
RABIES.
YELLOW FEVER.

DENGUE.
PAPPATACI FEVER.
INFECTIOUS COLD.
PSITTACOSIS.
FOOT-AND-MOUTH DISEASE.

Introduction.—In this section will be considered those diseases which have automatically come to be grouped together for the reason that their etiologic agents are ultramicroscopic and are recoverable from the bacteria-free filtrate after passage through a porcelain filter. Other features will be mentioned shortly. Although the group may still be poorly defined it meets a need in classification and is an advance from the older heading "Diseases of Unknown Origin."

To this group of diseases the name Virus Diseases has been applied, often with the qualification "filterable." *Virus* in Latin means a poison, and in medicine it was at first used for any disease-producing agent. It has since come to be applied almost exclusively to those pathogenic agents that will pass a porcelain filter and are ultramicroscopic. Over a hundred diseases of bacteria, plants, insects, animals and man have been attributed to such viruses. Examples of the subdivisions include bacteriophage, the mosaic disease of tobacco and other plants, sacbrood of honey bees, foot-and-mouth disease of cloven-foot animals and man, and poliomyelitis of man and monkey.

The history of the present concept of the virus diseases begins with Pasteur's suggestion, while studying rabies, that there might be small, invisible microörganisms, but the first actual demonstration of a virus was that of the mosaic disease of tobacco by Iwanowsky in 1893. Since then, for various and not always very adequate reasons, a number of diseases of man have been placed in this class. The criteria for such classification include:

(*a*) **Filterability of the Virus.**—Passage through a porcelain filter is exhibited by the various viruses. That of vaccinia, however, passes only with the greatest difficulty, while certain bacteria, spirochetes and protozoa pass readily. This justifies the view expressed by Goodpasture that "filterability is not a sufficiently distinctive characteristic to cause a taxonomic separation of viruses from demonstrable microorganisms." Many factors enter into this problem, not only the size of the virus and the fineness of the filter but also the filtration pressure, the time and the very important question of adsorption. The material for filtration must usually be obtained by maceration and suspension of the tissue attacked by the virus in question (brain in poliomyelitis; body fluids in yellow fever alone). For study of a virus the resulting filtrate must not only contain the virus and be capable of initiating the disease process upon transmission but must be free of microorganisms by microscopic examination and culture. The matter is further confused by the evidence that various common microörganisms may exhibit filter passing phases.

(*b*) **Size of Virus.**—No accurate measure of any virus has been made, though many have been found to have a diameter of about 30 millimicra (10^{-6} mm.). Only those pathogenic agents which are ultramicroscopic truly belong in the virus group.

(*c*) **Formation of "Inclusion Bodies" in the Attacked Cells of the Host.**— Even though only about one-half of the usual list of virus diseases exhibit this phenomenon it has been considered of the greatest importance. In fact, this property alone has led some to include the Rickettsia among the virus diseases. Morphologically identical inclusion bodies are found in herpes, chickenpox and yellow fever, while the Guarnieri bodies of smallpox and the Negri bodies of rabies are distinctive. It is in the cells of the specific tissues attacked by the virus that the inclusion bodies occur, and it is from this same tissue that the virus is recovered. There is difference of opinion as to the actual nature of the inclusion bodies.

(*d*) **Cytotropism.**—This implies a tissue specificity in the relation of the virus to the cells of the host with a distinct reaction of the cells to the virus. In some instances active hyperplasia, in others disintegrative processes predominate; sometimes the latter follow a primary hyperplasia. Cytotropism is a characteristic of many but not all of the virus diseases. Measles and yellow fever do not meet the criterion; in yellow fever the virus is found in the fluids of the body. Rivers believes that the importance of cytotropism has been overemphasized, since vaccinia, herpes and chickenpox viruses attack both ectodermal and mesodermal cells. Most viruses prefer ectodermal tissues.

There are four diseases in which the virus seems to be distinctly neurotropic: poliomyelitis, rabies, encephalitis, and herpes, the latter exhibiting ectodermal tropism as well. There are different views concerning the occasional encephalitis which follows after vaccinia, measles and mumps. Possibly it is due to the specific virus of these several diseases. Others believe that it is caused by a latent encephalitis virus present in the patient and activated by the vaccination, for example. Ectodermal tropism is exhibited by the viruses of smallpox, measles, chickenpox and foot-and-mouth disease. It is interesting to note that at least four viruses appear in the saliva; those of rabies, herpes, mumps and foot-and-mouth disease; the first two being neurotropic, the last attacking only ectoderm. Furthermore, there is some evidence that the virus of herpes and that of chickenpox are identical.

(*e*) **Cultivation.**—The only exception to the rule that living specific tissue cells are necessary for *in vitro* cultivation of a virus is the so-called virus of pleuropneumonia of cattle, which may well be a microbe proper. Claims that vaccine virus can be cultivated in lifeless media have not been confirmed. By no means all of the filterable viruses have been cultivated.

(*f*) **Immunity.**—It is often stated that a virus disease confers lasting immunity, but Gye and others deny this, pointing out that foot-and-mouth disease fails to do so, and that just as great variability in immunity occurs in the virus disease group as in the bacterial.

Epidemiology.—The group of virus diseases presents the same problems in epidemiology as do the bacterial infections. Smallpox is highly contagious; poliomyelitis only slightly; rabies requires a tissue abrasion; foot-and-mouth disease enters by the respiratory or intestinal tract; yellow fever and dengue are carried by insect vectors.

Symptoms.—There is little or no similarity in the reaction of the human host to infection with the various viruses. Even viruses that are suspected of being closely related (herpes and encephalitis; dengue and yellow fever) are associated with very different symptom pictures. A number of the diseases exhibit a biphasic course, but not all. In

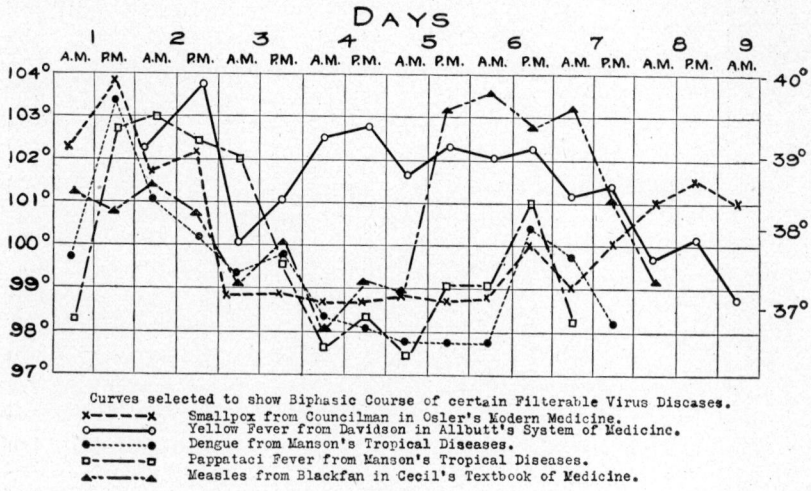

Curves selected to show Biphasic Course of certain Filterable Virus Diseases.
x———x Smallpox from Councilman in Osler's Modern Medicine.
o———o Yellow Fever from Davidson in Allbutt's System of Medicine.
●———● Dengue from Manson's Tropical Diseases.
□———□ Pappataci Fever from Manson's Tropical Diseases.
▲———▲ Measles from Blackfan in Cecil's Textbook of Medicine.

Fig. 8.

poliomyelitis this has been termed a "dromedary course," an amusing misnomer for it is the Bactrian camel, not the dromedary, that has two humps. Most of the virus diseases have no associated leukocytosis; only the four whose virus is neurotropic, and smallpox when the pustular stage with secondary infection is reached.

List of Virus Diseases.—In the past, the Rickettsia diseases (typhus, etc.), scarlet fever and Oroya fever have by some been included in the group of diseases due to filterable viruses, but today it seems best to exclude them. Mention of the virus of warts and *molluscum contagiosum* has been omitted as not pertinent to the present text. Those that remain are listed in the table on page 162 that presents the criteria justifying their inclusion. It will be seen how insufficient, in many instances, the data are. There is some evidence to suggest that perhaps influenza and whooping cough also belong in this group, but it is not yet conclusive.

11

TABLE 5.—CRITERIA FOR CLASSIFICATION OF DISEASES IN VIRUS DISEASE GROUP.

	Properties of virus.				Evidence in host.			
	Filterability.	Ultramicroscopic size.	Culture with tissue.	Transmissibility.	Inclusion bodies.	Cytotropism.	Immunity.	Comments.
Foot-and-mouth disease	Yes	Yes	Yes	Yes	Intranuclear	Ectodermal, disintegrative	Transient	Virus in saliva.
Smallpox	Yes with difficulty	Yes	Yes	Yes	Cytoplasmic and intranuclear, Guarnieri bodies, Paschen bodies	Ectodermal, first disintegrative, later proliferative	Yes	Evidence suggests close relationship or identity of the viruses of chickenpox and herpes.
Chickenpox	Little data			Yes	Intranuclear non-specific acidophil granules	Ectodermal, mesodermal, disintegrative	Yes	Virus of herpes in saliva.
Herpes	Yes	Yes	Yes	Yes	Intranuclear non-specific acidophil granules	Ectodermal, mesodermal, disintegrative	Transient	Experimental evidence confused by similarity of herpes virus and rabbit encephalitis virus.
Encephalitis group	Yes	Yes	?	?	None(?) (Reported in kidney in St. Louis epidemic, 1933)	Neurotropic	?	
Poliomyelitis	Yes	Yes	Yes	Yes	Intranuclear acidophil granules	Neurotropic, disintegrative	Yes	
Rabies	Yes	Yes	No(?)	Yes	Cytoplasmic Negri bodies	Neurotropic, disintegrative	Yes	Virus in saliva; transmissible only by local inoculation.
Measles	Yes	Yes	..	..	None	No (ectodermal?)	Yes	No data for rubella; neither surely virus diseases.
Yellow fever	Yes	Yes	No	Yes	Intranuclear non-specific acidophil granules in liver cells	No	Yes	In yellow fever virus found in body fluids.
Dengue	Yes	Yes	No	Yes	None	......	Transient	Viruses of yellow fever, dengue and pappataci fever possibly related.
Pappataci fever	Yes	Yes	Yes	Yes	None	No	Yes, transient	Virus in saliva.
Infectious cold	Yes	Yes	Yes	Yes	None	No	No(?)	Insufficient data.
Mumps	Yes	Yes	No	Yes	None	No	Yes	
Psittacosis	Yes	Yes	..	..	......	......	....	

In this present volume it has seemed best not to attempt to group all of the so-called virus diseases together. In the section on Contagious Diseases of Childhood will be found measles and German measles, chickenpox and mumps. Grouped with the organic diseases of the nervous system will be found poliomyelitis and the various forms of encephalitis and herpes. The discussion of the other members of the group of virus diseases follows this introduction.

REFERENCES.

A System of Bacteriology in Relation to Medicine, Volume **7**, Medical Research Council, London, 1930.

Filterable Viruses, edited by THOMAS M. RIVERS, Baltimore, Williams & Wilkins Company, 1928.

GOODPASTURE, E. W.: Etiological Problems in the Study of Filterable Virus Diseases, Harvey Lectures, 1929–1930.

D'HERELLE, FELIX: The Nature of the Ultrafilterable Viruses, Harvey Lectures, 1928–1929.

HURST, E. W.: The Occurrence of Intranuclear Inclusions in the Nerve Cells in Poliomyelitis, Jour. Path. and Bacteriol., 1931, **34**, 331.

MOMMSEN, H.: Relation Between Zoster and Chickenpox, Monatsschr. f. Kinderh., 1931, **50**, 11.

RIVERS, T. M., and WARD, S. M.: Further Observations on the Cultivation of Vaccine Virus in Lifeless Media, Jour. Exp. Med., 1933, **57**, 741.

SMALLPOX.

Synonyms.—Variola, from Latin *varus*, a pimple; German, *Blattern*.

Definition.—An acute infectious disease caused by a specific ultramicroscopic virus; preventable by vaccination and characterized by an abrupt onset, a cutaneous eruption and the development of specific "inclusion bodies" in the tissue cells.

History.—The startling pictures of smallpox and its epidemic occurrence make it possible to trace its history far into the past. In the early Christian epoch the Fathers of the church described the disease, and Marius, in 570 A.D., was the first to use the term variola. Rhazes (860–932), an Arabian physician, left a very remarkable description of the disease. In the tenth century, the Japanese isolated smallpox in special houses, and Gilbert (died in 1250) maintained its contagiousness only to have this denied later by the great Sydenham who, however, was the first to differentiate smallpox and measles.

The "pox" was pandemic in Europe in 1614 and occurred in New England throughout that century, reaching Pennsylvania in 1661. The name "pox" is derived from the Anglo-Saxon word "pocca," a pimple, and the prefix "small" served to exclude syphilis, the great pox. From the earliest times variolation or the intentional transmission of the disease in mild form had been practised. The Chinese placed old powdered crusts into the nostrils; the Brahmins applied crusts to the skin; the Persians ingested prepared crusts, while in Europe clear fluid from a vesicle was transferred by lancet.

By the eighteenth century it had been long noted that those who contracted cowpox did not take smallpox, and successful cowpox inoculation was done in England in 1774. Jenner, learning of the former fact from dairy maids, undertook the introduction of vaccination, and published his valuable results in 1798. In spite of the opposition of the inevitable noisy minority, vaccination has become universally employed with results approaching the miraculous. Only through negligence will the disease ever return to its former horrible prevalence and deadliness.

It was in 1892 that Guarnieri described and probably misinterpreted the specific inclusion bodies which bear his name.

Epidemiology.—Smallpox is so highly infectious that it spreads with the greatest certainty to all exposed and unvaccinated persons. From the latter days of the incubation period until the end of desquamation the disease is readily transmitted, at first chiefly by air-borne "droplet" infection, later by the scabs and scales. There is good evidence that the virus may be carried by articles and attendants; even the dead bodies of smallpox patients have been the frequent source of infection.

Before vaccination periodic epidemics were the rule. These varied in virulence; sometimes so mild as to be mistaken for chickenpox; sometimes of devastating severity with a mortality of over 50 per cent. When first introduced into a race or community the morbidity and mortality are very high. Formerly children led in incidence and death-rate, since adults had acquired immunity by an earlier attack. Of late years the tendency is for a rising number of adult cases as a result of neglected revaccination. Even in the unvaccinated, however, the disease of late years has assumed a mild form. Natural immunity is rare.

Smallpox is not extinct; few physicians realize that thousands of cases occur annually in the United States. There is every probability that the disease will assume epidemic proportions just as soon as a false sense of security results in a considerable unvaccinated population.

Age, sex, race and climate are factors less important than formerly believed. The disease has a higher mortality in infants and children; its incidence is greatest in mid-winter.

Etiology.—Smallpox justifies its inclusion among the virus diseases although its virus passes a porcelain filter with difficulty. The virus occurs particularly in the vesicles and crusts, but the disease has been transmitted to monkeys by a patient's blood. It is also contained in the exhalations, probably due to eruptive lesions of the mucous membranes. The specific inclusion bodies described in 1892 by Guarnieri are found in the cytoplasm of the epithelial cells of the skin in both smallpox and vaccinia as well as in cells of the rabbit cornea inoculated with the vaccine. It is not known today whether these bodies are forms of the virus itself or the reaction of the cell to the virus. The same is true of the intranuclear, Paschen, bodies. There are, however, good reasons to discard the earlier views that the bodies are protozoal in nature.

There is nothing to suggest that the virus of smallpox and that of vaccinia are not identical; the same may be said of smallpox and its milder forms, *varioloid* and *alastrim*.

Pathology.—The morbid anatomy of smallpox is best considered under three headings: (1) the exanthematous lesion of the skin and mucous membranes; (2) the hemorrhagic features which may appear in association with the specific changes, or elsewhere; and (3) the pathologic processes occurring usually late in the disease, or as complications in such organs as the lungs, liver, spleen, lymph nodes, ovaries, testes, kidneys, bone-marrow and adrenals.

Many have stressed that it is the reticulo-endothelial system or tissues which exhibit the most marked involvement, the changes being found in the spleen, bone-marrow and lymph nodes. In these areas there occurs a proliferation of the reticulo-endothelial tissues far more marked than that seen in any other infection.

1. In the skin the specific lesions commence as a degeneration of the cells of the lower layer of epidermis. In these early lesions the Guarnieri inclusion bodies occur in the cytoplasm of the epithelial cells. From this beginning, the lesion passes through the stages of papule, vesicle, pustule and crust. The content of the vesicle is clear; that of the pustule increasingly cloudy from cellular elements. On culture of the pustule, streptococci are usually found. A typical pustule on the skin is firm and umbilicated, perhaps from its multilocular structure, perhaps from the presence of a central hair follicle. The exanthem extends from the mouth into the trachea and esophagus; occasionally the lower portions of the digestive tract, the vagina and the bladder are involved. The mucous membrane lesions seldom reach the stage of vesicle and do not proceed to pustulation. The pulmonary complications may well find their beginnings in deep-seated exanthematous lesions.

2. Hemorrhagic phenomena are variable but not rare. One may speculate on their relation to degeneration of capillary endothelium as a part of a widespread involvement of the reticulo-endothelial system. Early purpura is of very bad prognostic import. Hemorrhage may also occur into single "pocks" or into the urinary passages; the sputum may contain blood, and extravasations may form in any part of the body.

3. The liver and spleen are usually enlarged, the latter more often in children up to the age of seven years (Cowie). Also the cervical lymph nodes are early enlarged. Streptococcic or pneumococcic pneumonia is unfortunately common. Occasional involvement of the adrenals, testes or ovaries occurs.

A most interesting feature is the affection of the bone-marrow. This may be very widespread in many bones. Although suppuration may occur, the usual cells of the granular marrow series are lacking. Again the possible relation of the process to the reticulo-endothelium comes to mind.

Symptoms.—*Incubation Period.*—The incubation period can frequently be measured with great accuracy and has been found to fall in most instances between ten and twelve days; occasionally, it may be as short as eight days, even more rarely as long as fourteen or sixteen days. Thanks to the long incubation period, it is possible, by prompt vaccination, to prevent the development of smallpox in the exposed individual.

Onset.—Characteristic of smallpox is the suddenness and severity of the onset. In general, the symptoms are those of the onset of other acute infections, but far more intense. Instead of a mere malaise the smallpox patient as a rule experiences agonizing headache, severe pains in the extremities and in the lumbar region. This latter has a diagnostic value, for it occurs more often and more painfully in smallpox than in other acute infections. At the onset, one or more chills with or without vomiting are common, and at this stage in children convulsions may develop. Following the chill, the temperature rises to 103° or 104° F. With this fever there tends to be such an unusual degree of mental confusion or delirium as to suggest drunkenness.

Initial Stage.—For two or three days following the onset the fever continues high, with but slight morning remissions. The headache persists, sometimes with stiffness of the neck muscles. In some instances the patient appears overwhelmed by the infection; in others, the condition is good. Occasionally the patient's chief complaint concerns the tonsils and pharynx.

Unfortunately for diagnostic reputations, very confusing rashes may appear on the second or third day of the initial stage. One form is scarlatiniform; another resembles measles. Either may be diffuse, but it is more usual for the rash to be limited to the lower half of the abdomen, to the genitals and to the inner aspects of the thighs. The diagnostic value of the roughly triangular shape of this area has been much emphasized, but there may be extension upward along the sides of the trunk to the axillæ. Petechiæ may occur with either of the above rashes or alone in the same distribution. While these may be omens of severe and hemorrhagic smallpox, this is by no means always the case.

Termination of the initial stage usually occurs on the third day with defervescence and an amazing disappearance of all symptoms. (See yellow fever, dengue and measles.) In severe cases the temperature may not fall to normal; in a mild case, on the contrary, the infection would seem to be at an end unless the true eruption is recognized.

Diagnosis.—Initial Stage.—It is of the greatest importance that the diagnosis be made during the initial stage; unfortunately it is difficult, and often perhaps impossible. During an epidemic the suddenness and severity of the onset with intense headache and lumbar pain will often suffice. Sometimes the initial rash will be typical. In a sporadic case, however, it requires great alertness to identify the infection so early. In the initial stage smallpox may be mistaken for meningococcic meningitis, influenza, fulminant scarlet fever, dengue, measles, streptococcic infection of throat or septicemia. It is most important to remember that previous successful vaccination, while it lessens the severity of the eruptive stage (varioloid) may have no such effect upon the symptoms of the initial stage. With the appearance of the true eruption on the third day the list of probable errors changes.

Stage of Eruption.—Characteristically the eruption appears on the third day, being first seen on the wrists, forehead and face. Small, dusky red macules, perhaps 1 to 3 mm. in diameter, appear in these areas. At first these will pale on pressure, but in less than twenty-four hours they have become papules and have invaded the trunk, extremities and, to a variable degree, the mucous membranes of the mouth and throat. The papules are set *deep* in the skin, which gives the "shot-like" hardness; this is of some value in identifying the rash of smallpox. Within two days (fifth or sixth day of disease) all of the papules have been transformed into tense, shiny, often umbilicated vesicles with a variable red areola. Each "pock" is multilocular and cannot be emptied by a single needle prick, a helpful difference from chickenpox. During the next two or three days the clear contents of the vesicle becomes purulent, and the pustule loses its umbilication. By the twelfth day of the disease, desiccation has usually begun, crusts form; desquamation sometimes of the scab, sometimes of larger casts often from the foot, continues for a week or more. The skin may be left markedly erythematous for months, or permanently stained with a brownish pigment, or after a confluent eruption permanently pitted. Pitting is greatly aggravated if the lesions are scratched as they are apt to be, owing to the intense itching of the desquamation period. The hair may be lost during convalescence, and in severe cases the nails may be shed.

Wide variation from the typical eruption occurs, in fact, cases without eruption are recorded. More often there may be very few lesions which crust early and leave no pitting in varioloid, or which stop at the vesicle stage in the so-called abortive form. Hemorrhage into the skin may occur early before the appearance of any true eruption; this is associated with mucous membrane hemorrhages and forms the invariably fatal "black" (purpuric) smallpox. Far less serious is hemorrhage into the pustules (hemorrhagic pustular smallpox). Also quantitative variations in the typical eruption occur; the lesions may be discrete or numerous enough to justify the term confluent. It is with this form that edema, especially noticeable on the face, is associated, and that pitting, also greatest on the face, results.

Symptoms during the period of eruption vary in nature and severity. The fever, which has fallen with the eruption, rises again with the appearance of pustule formation about the seventh or eighth day of the disease. Its degree and duration are proportionate to the extent of the suppuration; it may terminate in three days and not exceed 102° F., or it may rise to 105° F. and may persist for ten or twelve days. Also it may end by crisis or lysis. The fever is thought by many to be a non-specific manifestation of the suppuration. Schamberg has estimated that the pocks of a moderately severe case may contain a total of 5 quarts of pus.

Delirium is the rule, and the usual picture of any infectious toxemia is present. Pain in the areas of the eruption may be severe when the lesions are numerous and confluent. Edema adds to the discomfort and may close the eyes from swelling of the lids. In the mouth and throat the eruption causes pain; the voice may be husky. There may be a general lymphadenopathy, but it is the cervical nodes which are chiefly swollen and tender. The liver and spleen may be sufficiently enlarged to be readily palpable.

Diagnosis in Stage of Eruption.—While the diagnosis in the initial stage is extremely difficult, there is little excuse for failure once a typical eruption has appeared. Mild smallpox is apt to be mistaken for chickenpox with disastrous results. The differential diagnosis should, however, be possible. Chickenpox differs in that (1) onset symptoms are very mild, (2) constitutional disturbance is trifling, (3) eruption appears sooner (first day), comes in crops, lesions of differing age lie side by side (polymorphous), chiefly on covered surface, not on palms or soles, rapidly formed vesicles which are superficial, usually unilocular and soft, variable in size and shape, and lack umbilication. They dry up within three days, leaving a depressed blackish crust. Of course a vaccination scar, especially in children, argues against smallpox.

Other conditions with which the eruptive stage of smallpox may be confused include drug rashes, impetigo contagiosa, pustular syphilids and pustular glanders.

Laboratory Features.— *Urine.*—The urine is that of any febrile stage; scanty, high-colored and containing more or less albumin and a variable number of hyaline casts, according to the severity of the attack.

Blood.—The changes in the blood differ widely, according to the stage and the severity of the attack. Seldom, however, is there any anemia except in occasional severe pustular and markedly purpuric cases. In these, the anemia is of a secondary character and may rarely become severe.

In the usual pustular form of smallpox, there occurs at the onset a transitory slight neutrophil leukocytosis (10,000 to 15,000). If the attack is not to be very severe, the total white count falls during the maculo-papular stage, to rise again in the vesicular and still higher in the pustular stage (20,000 to 30,000). During desiccation the count declines: the lowering of the total count in the maculo-papular stage is the result of a diminution in the neutrophils which fall sharply in both actual numbers and in their percentage in the differential count, down to 40 per cent. This results in a relative lymphocytosis much emphasized in olden times and even in some recent texts.

In severer attacks the initial leukocytosis is higher and may continue high with a neutrophil increase throughout the entire course of the attack. Occasionally in severe cases this leukocytosis fails to appear and leukopenia evidences the severity of the infection in the manner analogous to that seen in other overwhelming infections.

In purpuric smallpox the neutrophils rapidly decrease in number, although the total count remains high from actual increase in the lymphocytes. Degenerative morphologic changes occur in the neutrophils, analogous to those seen in any intense sepsis or toxemia, but Ikeda believes those seen in purpuric smallpox to be specific. The bone-marrow is markedly affected; young neutrophils and myelocytes, normoblasts and polychromatophilic red cells, as well as atypical lymphocytes appear in the circulating blood.

The platelets are diminished in the first stage of all forms of smallpox. This reduction continues until death in fatal purpuric attacks; in the usual pustular form there occurs a rapid rise of platelets in the pustular stage. A prolonged bleeding time has been reported.

Blood culture is negative except in the later stages of very severe smallpox, when a streptococcic bacteriemia is usual.

Specific Diagnostic Tests.—1. *Cutaneous Tests.*—(*a*) A positive local reaction within forty-eight hours to the intradermal inoculation of vesicle material into a rabbit previously sensitized to cowpox vaccine, is strongly indicative.

(*b*) In the previously unvaccinated smallpox patient, after the third or fourth day of the disease, a local reaction will follow the intradermal introduction of diluted heated cowpox vaccine.

2. *Culture of Virus on Rabbit's Cornea.*—The inoculation of a slight scarification of the cornea with material from a smallpox vesicle will result in very tiny vesicles within thirty-six hours and distinct ulcers in three or four days.

3. The method of complement-fixation has been tried, using the fluid from the vesicles and a specific serum.

None of these tests has proved of great practical value.

Complications.—It is noteworthy how seldom the important organs of the body, heart, kidneys, liver, brain, for example, are damaged by smallpox. Such renal changes as occur are "febrile and transient." Almost all of the complications arise from the eruption and are of pyogenic character. The list includes laryngeal edema and ulceration, bronchitis, bronchopneumonia, furunculosis, corneal scarring, alopecia, purulent arthritis and osteomyelitis, otitis media and septicemia. These occur in the pustular stage and tend to prolong the fever and may determine a fatal outcome.

The complications affecting the nervous system belong in a separate category. They are not pyogenic, may occur early in the attack and are as common in mild as in severe cases. One cannot help but compare them with the involvements of the nervous system in other members of the virus disease group (encephalitis, poliomyelitis, herpes zoster). The list includes hemiplegia, aphasia, pharyngeal paralysis, peripheral neuritis and myelitis.

Miscarriage may occur, and the disease may attack the fetus *in utero*.

Prognosis.—No disease varies more in severity and deadliness. The prognosis is influenced by virulence of epidemic, type of attack, age and health of patient, but far more by the vaccinal state of the patient. Not only has vaccination protected innumerable individuals, but by lessening the frequency of the disease has lessened its virulence and spared many of the unvaccinated. In smallpox unmodified by vaccination the older figures show a mortality of over 60 per cent; this has gradually fallen to about 30 per cent. Purpuric smallpox, however, still takes its toll of unvaccinated children and pregnant women. A confluent eruption gives a bad prognosis; a discrete eruption a good. Even in the unvaccinated an occasional epidemic will have a very low mortality, sometimes with trifling eruption. So different from severe smallpox is the disease in these mild epidemics that it leads to great diagnostic difficulty, and some have attempted to identify a new disease **(alastrim).**

Smallpox modified by vaccination is named **varioloid,** and this is seldom, if ever, fatal.

Treatment.—Immediate indications include (1) isolation of patient; (2) notification of, and coöperation with, local health authorities; (3) segregation and vaccination of exposed persons, including doctors and nurses; (4) disinfection or destruction of contaminated clothing, bedding, and other fomites.

The patient should be in bed in an airy but screened room. The fluid intake should be high, the diet adequate but simple; often during the initial stage vomiting will prevent the ingestion of anything but ice, fruit juices or carbonated drinks, and during the eruptive stage swallowing may be so painful as to make impossible the taking of anything other than liquids. When ingestion is seriously limited, one must be prompt to avoid ketosis by administration of sugars, if not by mouth perhaps by vein. The vomiting itself may respond to intravenous injection of glucose. An initial purge is still strongly advised by some and, of course, the bowels must be kept open throughout the illness.

At the onset the lumbar pain and headache may demand relief by acetylsalicylic acid, 0.6 gram (10 grains), repeated in two hours if necessary, or by acetphenetidin, 0.3 gram (5 grains), or if these fail, by morphine.

Much of the nursing and treatment of smallpox have to do with the eruption. Not only are the measures common to all infections indicated, but special care of the eyes, mouth and throat is needed. In the hope of preventing scarring of the cornea, the eyes should frequently be cleansed (boric acid solution) and a mild antiseptic solution (mild silver-protein, 20 per cent), instilled several times a day. Similarly, cleanliness of mouth, nose and throat is important and comforting. An oily application after thorough cleansing will help to prevent crusting in the nose. Many treatments of the eruption on the skin have been tried and found wanting, both for relief of pain and for the avoidance of scarring. Once crusting and desquamation commences, phenol (2 to 3 per cent) in vaseline is useful and tends to relieve the itching which may be intense at this time.

Fever and delirium demand no special measures unless severe, when cold sponging is to be preferred to any drug. Toxemia is best combated by an abundance of fluid.

Prevention.—That inoculation with material from human smallpox was so long practised in many countries is the best evidence of the dread in which smallpox was justly held. Vaccination with lymph from the early lesions of cowpox has in the past one hundred and fifty years, wherever thoroughly applied, protected the individual, prevented the epidemic occurrence of the disease, and made smallpox such a rarity that the physician of today often encounters this test of his diagnostic skill only after years of general practice. That smallpox is not extinct, however, is shown by the 145 deaths from this cause in 1927, and 131 in 1928 in the registration area of the United States.

Cowpox.

The group of animals affected by pock diseases includes sheep, goats, swine, horses and cows. The causative viruses are either identical or related and similar not only to each other but to that of human smallpox. In each the virus causes lesions with cell inclusions; each virus is inoculable on each of the animals subject to pock diseases; each immunizes against all the others. In cowpox, the eruption is almost exclusively on the udder and teats of milch cows. Commercially, lymph for vaccination is obtained from inoculated calves; it is protected from bacterial contamination by preservation with glycerin.

Vaccination.

Vaccination with lymph from cowpox causes in man a local lesion accompanied by systemic reaction (vaccinia) and culminating in a profound but not permanent immunity to smallpox.

Method.—Custom indicates the outer aspect of the upper arm, but the outer aspect of the leg below the knee or the thigh may be selected; an area free of hair should be chosen. The skin should be carefully cleansed, preferably with a saturated solution of acetone; if any other antiseptic is employed it must be thoroughly washed off with sterile water. The area cleansed should be several inches square to permit both the vaccination and a control. Many methods have been employed; the following is the safest and most efficient. At the point chosen for vaccination a drop of lymph is placed on the skin; none is used for the control. First at the control site and then through the drop of lymph, a sterile needle is placed flat (parallel) to the skin surface stretched tight by the operator. The needle is gently pressed several times against the skin in such a manner that the point breaks the cuticle but does not bring blood. The skin should not be pricked nor scratched with the point of the needle. All excess lymph is wiped off. No dressing is applied. This latter point has been very much emphasized of late. Any type of dressing, whether shield or gauze, seems not only to be unnecessary, but greatly increases the danger of tetanus. Cleanliness should be maintained, but no dressing applied at any time. In the absence of a covering there is little maceration or weeping, and little tendency for the clothing to become adherent.

Course.—No reaction should at any time appear at the site of the control. In a primary vaccination or in a revaccination after immunity has disappeared, the site of inoculation should show nothing for three days. On the fourth day, one or more papules develop, becoming vesicular on the fifth day. At this time fever and slight enlargement of the spleen appear. Also at this time an erythematous areola forms about the rapidly growing vesicles. By the eighth day the fever has reached its height, perhaps reaching 103° F., local lymph nodes are distinctly swollen and painful; the erythematous areola rapidly widens, sometimes encircling the arm, which may be edematous and swollen. At this time a sling for the arm, or even rest in bed may seem desirable. The central vesicles and areola reach their acme by the eleventh to twelfth day; the erythema rapidly fades and the vesicles commence to dry with the formation of a brown or black crust which finally separates on about the twenty-first day. The typical pitted scar, at first dusky red, becomes pale and remains for years but may disappear.

Moderate neutrophilic leukocytosis appears with the papule but disappears with vesicle formation; actual leukopenia may be present at the height of the fever on the eighth or ninth days.

Such a description seems to overstate the severity of the process, even in the unvaccinated. Revaccination may theoretically not differ from primary vaccination if sufficient time has elapsed for immunity to have disappeared.

When immunity is present the result of vaccination is very different. Within twenty-four to forty-eight hours the site of inoculation exhibits an erythematous reaction, and if this is distinct without any corresponding reaction at the control site the patient may be safely declared immune and released from quarantine. The more marked the immunity the more promptly the local reaction develops, but the more transient and mild it is. The process may reach vesiculation, but drying comes by the sixth day with rapid loss of scab.

Indications for Vaccination.—Every healthy infant should be vaccinated in his first year, and revaccinated at about the age of seven years. In an epidemic, all save the very feeble should be vaccinated. Following exposure to smallpox, vaccination should be performed, even if several days have intervened.

Complications.—There are three main complications of vaccination: pyogenic infection, tetanus and encephalitis. Very rarely a generalized vaccinial eruption occurs. Local infection sometimes leading to cellulitis and sloughing occasionally develops, but is usually avoided by ordinary cleanliness. Tetanus has been greatly reduced by the use of glycerinized lymph and abandonment of all local dressings. When it does occur it appears unusually late, after the seventeenth day, but it has a very high mortality. Encephalitis follows vaccination very seldom and there is no satisfactory explanation for the complication. It is certainly more than a coincidence, but, on the other hand, there seems to be good evidence that no encephalitis virus is transmitted by the lymph. Possibly a latent virus is activated by the vaccinia. Encephalitis, when it occurs, appears about the tenth day after the vaccinial inoculation. (See Part IV, on Diseases of Nervous System.)

REFERENCES.

BLAXALL, F. R.: Animal Pock Diseases in a System of Bacteriology in Relation to Medicine, vol. **7**, p. 140, London, 1930, His Majesty's Stationery Office.
IKEDA, K.: Blood in Smallpox During Recent Epidemic, Arch. Int. Med., 1926, **37**, 660.
——— Blood in Purpuric Smallpox, Jour. Am. Med. Assn., 1925, **84**, 1807.
MOORE, J. W.: Textbook of Eruptive and Continued Fevers, New York, William Wood & Co., 1892.
WELCH, W. H., and SCHAMBERG, J. V.: Acute Contagious Diseases, Lea Brothers & Co., 1905.

RABIES.

Synonyms.—Rabies, from Latin *madness;* Lyssa, from Greek *madness;* Hydrophobia.

Definition.—An acute infectious disease of lower animals due to a neurotropic filterable virus occurring in the saliva, transmissible by a bite and causing, unless prevented by prompt inoculation, a disease characterized by a long incubation period, a short stage of excitement, a paralytic stage and death.

History.—Hippocrates and Aristotle, among the ancients, mention the disease, and Celsus described it. In 1804, the saliva was known to transmit the disease, but even after this date sufferers from this disease were sometimes put to death, by smothering for choice, from fear of contagion. Cauterization with a red-hot iron continued the only prophylactic until July 6, 1885, when

Louis Pasteur applied with complete success his experiments on dogs to humans in the case of the nine-year-old Joseph Meister. The Pasteur treatment has saved countless lives and has largely taken the horror from the cry "Mad dog!" In 1903 Adelchi Negri discovered the "inclusion bodies" which carry his name and which are so important in the recognition of canine rabies.

Etiology and Epidemiology.—Rabies is properly placed among the diseases due to filterable viruses for it can be transmitted by an ultramicroscopic filter-passing agent, which has not surely been cultured, but which exhibits strong cytotropism with the production of specific inclusion bodies. Also immunity can be developed.

Pasteur termed the virus as it occurs in the saliva and central nervous system of the rabid animal the "street" virus; while the virus passed through a series of rabbits he termed "fixed" virus. This latter exhibits reduced virulence for man, a shorter incubation period, and a failure to produce Negri bodies. The reduced virulence of the fixed virus opened the way for preventive inoculation.

The disease occurs in many mammals, but primarily in the canine family; it has been present throughout the world, but rigid quarantine and muzzling, wherever enforced, have largely eradicated it. Pre-infectional vaccination of animals will alone never control outbreaks of rabies.

Pathology.—The virus of rabies is strongly neurotropic, passing to the central nervous system from the site of inoculation along the nerve axis-cylinders. During the disease it is also present in the saliva, and occasionally elsewhere, as in the mammary gland and pancreas. At autopsy, the only gross findings of note are a general hyperemia of the central nervous system with minute hemorrhages. Microscopic lesions may be found scattered throughout the brain and cord, but tend to center in the medulla, the ganglia, the hippocampus major and the cerebellum. The changes consist of lymphoid collections about the vessels and nerve cells, degenerations of nerve cells, and the widespread appearance of the specific Negri inclusion bodies. These were at first assumed to be protozoal, but are now thought to be in some way related to the action of the still unidentified virus of the disease.

Symptoms.—The shorter the distance from the bite to the brain, other factors being equal, the shorter the incubation period. Wide variations occur, twelve days to twelve months, but in the great majority the onset follows the bite in from twenty to ninety days.

Toward the end of the incubation period there may occur slight fever, malaise, and a local irritation and tingling or pain at the site of the bite. Restlessness and apprehension at this time are common and, it is claimed, may occur even in those ignorant of their danger.

Stage of Excitement.—During the next two or three days, the horrible symptoms come and reach their acme. At first, there is only a slight huskiness of voice and sense of choking, but this rapidly increases until violent spasm of the muscles of deglutition and respiration occur. With these, there is great dysphagia and dyspnea. Any attempt to swallow brings on an attack, and the refusal to take even water led to the misleading name hydrophobia and a legion of absurd beliefs.

The spasmodic seizures become more distressing, more intense and more numerous, being excited by such trifling stimuli as a cold draught of air or a loud noise. Persistent priapism is reported. Generalized convulsions with opisthotonos may occur and death from asphyxia or exhaustion may end the suffering at this time.

The inability to swallow leads to the viscid saliva accumulating in and dripping from the mouth, and the dyspnea leads to harsh gaspings, but the patient with rabies does not foam at the mouth, bark nor bite unless there is a strong hysterical element present. Mental anxiety and terror are apt to be extreme unless delirium clouds the mind. Fever is absent or slight during this stage.

Unless death has come during these first three or four days, the patient passes into the second or paralytic stage.

Paralytic Stage.—Occasionally there may be no period of excitement, but, as a rule, it is severe and the patient only terminally sinks into paralysis and coma. The relief from the spasms may quiet the mental stress and the patient may seem better for a few hours—but the fever tends to rise, perhaps to 104° or 105° F., the pulse becomes more frequent, the paralysis more complete and death from exhaustion comes, as a rule, before the seventh day of the disease. Just before death the fever may be extremely high.

Laboratory Features.—The urine contains albumin. The blood count often reveals a high red cell figure due probably to dehydration or asphyxia. Moderate neutrophil leukocytosis, 10,000 to 20,000, is often observed and has been attributed to the convulsions. It has, however, been found in a case without convulsions.

Diagnosis.—Tetanus is seldom transmitted by a bite; it commences with trismus and the spasm is not intermittent. Hysterical mimicry of rabies may arise from fear of rabies after a dog bite; it can usually be recognized by its early onset and the too obvious barkings and snappings. Mania may sometimes be confusing. Occasionally an early case of botulism with marked difficulty in phonation and deglutition may suggest rabies, but ocular palsies do not occur in rabies and are quite constant in botulism. Acute bulbar palsy will scarcely be confused with rabies.

If an animal is merely suspected of being rabid it need not be killed, for if it is rabid it will die within a few days, and if alive and well at the end of two weeks its innocence is established. If it dies or is killed, the animal, or at least its head, should be taken to a reliable laboratory where, by a histologic examination, the diagnosis can be made from the presence of Negri bodies. Fortunately, these appear early and can be recognized even if the tissue is not promptly examined. Diagnosis by inoculation into rabbits is sure, but is too slow to serve as a criterion for treatment.

Treatment.—All wounds should be immediately and thoroughly cauterized with phenol or fuming nitric acid.

If there are bites on the face, or even on the hands, it is the course of wisdom to commence vaccine treatment promptly, because of the shorter incubation period with bites in these parts. Otherwise, it is safe to delay for the few days necessary to make sure that the animal was rabid. Never delay if the animal was surely rabid, nor more than a week under any circumstances. The vaccine contains virus which has been greatly diminished in virulence for man both by passage through many rabbits and by other measures, such as drying. The principles are unchanged from Pasteur's original method; an attenuated or "fixed" virus is used, daily injections of more and more active material being given. Active immunity is achieved before the disease develops. As a rule, an injection is given daily for from two to four weeks, according to the severity, extent and location of the wounds. Beckman advises intramuscular injection into the buttock. Local reactions may occur, rarely an urticaria. Today the vaccine is usually easily available in syringes ready for injection; it can be ordered by telegram and promptly delivered. It is well to keep the material in the refrigerator.

There are no contraindications to the vaccine treatment. Its success is almost invariable; failures are said to occur in less than 0.5 of 1 per cent of cases. No deaths occurred among 589 cases treated in 1930 at the Pasteur Institute in Paris. That as many as 107 deaths from rabies occurred in 1928 in the United States registration area is probably to be blamed on lack of treatment. Immunity probably does not persist for much over a year. Some even advise giving a second course of vaccine six months after the first.

Complications of Pasteur treatment are infrequent, but serious when they occur. Paralysis due to myelitis may follow the onset of treatment in one to three weeks and in a few instances proves fatal. This may be of the Landry type, a rapidly advancing flaccid paralysis without fever or sensory involvement, with a mortality of 30 per cent; or a milder subacute form with a mortality of 5 per cent. Polyneuritis also may occur. Remlinger found that paralysis had developed in 40 of 107,712 persons treated and that the mortality of postvaccinal paralysis was about 16 per cent. This cannot be considered a contraindication to the treatment; the method of attenuation of the virus does not affect this danger. Onset of paralytic symptoms does not necessarily indicate the abandonment of treatment (McCoy).

During and after the period of injections, it is most important to reassure the patient and quiet his apprehensions. Beckman, who himself underwent the treatment, comments on "a certain unwonted apprehension." In a neurotic this might easily go further, even to a mimicry of rabies.

Once rabies has developed, the only indication is to relieve the suffering; there is no excuse for withholding morphine unless other sedatives suffice. Cocaine in 5 per cent solution sprayed into the larynx is said to lessen the spasms, but general anesthesia may be the only method to give any relief.

REFERENCES.

BECKMAN, H.: Treatment in General Practice, Philadelphia, W. B. Saunders Company, 1930.
JONESCO, D., and VALTER, B.: Recherches hématologiques et cliniques dans la rage humaine, Hematologica, 1927, **8**, 213.
McCoy, G. W.: Antirabic Vaccine Paralysis, Jour. Med., 1931, **12**, 257.

MEYER, K. F.:   Rabies, Calif. and West. Med., 1931, **35**, 39.
REMLINGER, P.:   Les paralysies du traitement antirabique, Ann. de l'Inst. Pasteur, 1928, **42**, 71.
VALLERY-RADOT, R.:   The Life of Pasteur, New York, Doubleday, Page & Co., 1916.
VIOLA, J.:   Les vaccination antirabique à l'Institut Pasteur en 1930, Ann. de l'Institut Pasteur, 1931, **46**, 574.

YELLOW FEVER.

Definition.—An acute disease due to a filterable virus transmitted by the Aëdes ægypti mosquito, and characterized by an incubation period of two to six days, an acute febrile onset, a remission on the second day and a return of fever with jaundice, albuminuria, bleeding from mucous membranes, and the vomiting of blood.

History.—Yellow fever had its origin in West Africa and did not reach tropical America until shortly before its first recognition here in 1648. The early Mayan epidemics often attributed to yellow fever were probably typhus while that of 1520 was undoubtedly smallpox. In 1668 the disease appeared in NewYork, in Boston in 1691, and the great Philadelphia epidemic came in 1793. The disease was named yellow fever by Griffith Hughes in the Barbadoes in 1750. Carroll, writing in 1907, estimated that yellow fever had caused 100,000 deaths in the United States; of which 40,000 were in Louisiana, where in the final epidemic of 1905 there occurred 8000 cases and 900 deaths.

There is no more instructive chapter in medical history than the early observations and speculations concerning the cause of this disease whose erratic, non-contagious spread seemed to defy all logic. Many, including Benjamin Rush, noticed the coincidence of epidemics of yellow fever and increased numbers of mosquitoes. Nott, in 1848, is usually credited with advancing the hypothesis that the mosquito transmits the disease, but Wilson has recently pointed out that he did not actually reach this conclusion. The matter remained a mystery until 1900, when Walter Reed, James Carroll, Aristides Agramonte and J. W. Lazear of the United States Army proved in detail the part played by the mosquito. This was done at the cost of the life of Lazear, the exposure to the disease of a group of heroic volunteers, and the intentional production by inoculation of 22 cases of yellow fever, fortunately without a death.

Several mistaken claims of the discovery of the etiologic agent have been made, including Bacillus icteroides by Sanarelli and Leptospira icteroides by Noguchi, who lost his life from the disease while conscientiously disproving his own earlier claims. In 1901 it was demonstrated that the cause was a filterable virus.

In 1927 Stokes, Bauer and Hudson proved that certain species of monkeys are susceptible to yellow fever and are suitable as experimental animals. Stokes, in the same year, died of the disease. Further evidence favoring the classification of the agent responsible for yellow fever among the filterable viruses was supplied by the discovery of inclusion bodies in liver cells by Torres and their study by Cowdry and Kitchen.

Within the past few years, 29 cases of yellow fever with 5 fatalities have occurred among research workers in the field. Noguchi and Adrian Stokes have been mentioned; the others are William Alexander Young, Paul A. Lewis and Theodore B. Hayne. As Sawyer writes, "The knowledge that we have of yellow fever has been purchased most dearly."

Etiology and Epidemiology.—The agent responsible for yellow fever is still undiscovered. It is a filterable virus and the disease meets most of the criteria for classification in this group. Yellow fever differs, however, in that the virus is in the body fluids.

Recognition of the mosquito Aëdes ægypti as the vector of the virus of yellow fever explained not only the endemic continuance of tropical yellow fever, but also the epidemic occurrence of the disease by extension into new areas. Carter postulates for the existence of the disease (1) the causative agent, (2) functionally active Aëdes ægypti, (3) susceptible humans, the mosquitoes having access to both 1 and 3. Once the vector was known, quarantine and the destruction of the vector's breeding places promptly eliminated the disease wherever these measures were properly carried out. Endemic centers still exist in West Africa and Brazil; the United States has been free since 1905.

To transmit the disease the female mosquito must suck the blood of a yellow fever patient during the first three or four days of the disease. After about twelve days the mosquito's bite becomes infective and a non-immune individual bitten by an infective mosquito regularly develops the disease.

There is no racial immunity, the relative immunity of the negro probably being an immunity acquired from a mild attack in childhood. Adults appear less susceptible than children, perhaps for the same reason. Acquired immunity persists in most instances throughout life; blood taken from thirty to seventy-five years after an attack has successfully protected monkeys inoculated with yellow fever.

Pathology.—Yellow fever virus acts chiefly on the cells of the liver, causing widespread, scattered, non-inflammatory hyaline necrosis. The cells in the mid-zone of the lobules are the first affected, but the process may extend to implicate the cells about the central vein and at the periphery. In the nuclei of the damaged liver cells are found the acidophil "inclusion" granules which so closely resemble those found in certain other virus diseases. As a whole the organ is firm and smooth, yellow or brown in color, often mottled with areas of subcapsular hemorrhage. The skin is always jaundiced, the tissues usually so. Possibly the jaundice is related to the extensive damage of the Kupffer cells.

In the kidneys there is usually cloudy swelling of the convoluted tubules, occasionally progressing to necrosis. The heart muscle may be flabby; the lungs may exhibit hypostatic congestion. The spleen is congested but not constantly enlarged. From mouth to rectum the digestive tube is apt to contain blood and to be the seat of hemorrhages and oozings. Blood is usually found in the stomach, and may be red and fresh, or black from the action of the gastric juice. The duodenum is particularly the site of congestion and hemorrhages. Petechiæ are common not only along the gastro-intestinal tract, but on other mucous membranes, in other organs and the skin. The petechiæ and hemorrhages are due to degenerative changes in the capillary endothelium rather than to changes in the blood itself.

It is amazing how few organic sequelæ follow recovery from yellow fever; apparently "complete and scarless regeneration of the liver and kidney" occurs (Klotz and Belt). It denotes the non-inflammatory nature of the process.

Symptoms.—An *incubation period*, usually of three or four days, but varying in either direction, is followed without prodromal symptoms

12

by an acute onset. Invasion is featured by the symptoms common
to many acute infectious diseases; sometimes there is a chill, always
there is headache, malaise and fever. While not as agonizing as the
pains of this period in smallpox, the aching in the lumbar region, and
particularly in the calves, is severe.

Initial Period.—Few infections so rapidly progress to their full
symptomatic picture. The fever rises within a few hours to 102° F.,
occasionally as high as 106° F.; delirium may cloud the symptoms, but
epigastric pain, nausea and vomiting cause distress. An almost pathognomonic facies consists of a highly flushed face, marked injection of
the conjunctivæ, and in severe attacks already a hint of the coming
jaundice and hemorrhages.

Remission.—Except in very severe instances of the disease, the
fever falls on the second or third day. This may terminate a very
mild or abortive attack. In cases of average intensity the remission
lasts from a few to twenty-four hours during which period the patient
experiences symptomatic relief. The remission in yellow fever is by
no means as clear-cut or constant as that in smallpox. It is interesting
to note that somewhat analogous remissions occur in five of the so-
called "virus diseases:" smallpox, yellow fever, dengue, pappataci
fever and measles. (See Fig. 8, page 161.)

Final Stage.—After the brief remission the temperature returns to
103° or 104° F.; in spite of this fever the pulse-rate remains about
80 to the minute or even lower, a point of diagnostic importance. Jaundice becomes deeper, vomiting more pronounced and when there has
been sufficient mucous membrane oozing from mouth or stomach, the
vomitus contains varying degrees of altered blood; sometimes mere
specks, "fly wings," sometimes copious coffee-grounds material. Bleeding from nose or gums may be persistent. The fourth and fifth days
see all the symptoms at their height, often with anuria, an added and
alarming symptom. The patient is thirsty, nauseated and in pain, but
may be mentally lucid and alert. Death, if it is to occur, usually does
so by the sixth day of the disease. A return or improvement in the
urinary output heralds a turn for the better. In non-fatal but severe
cases the fever begins to fall by lysis about the sixth day.

Convalescence and Complications.—Jaundice and albuminuria may
persist for several weeks; but convalescence is usually uneventful, with
steady return to health. The swollen bleeding oral mucous membranes
favor extension of infection to the parotid; abscesses elsewhere may
occur. Relapses are infrequent; other complications very rare.

Laboratory Features.—It is generally accepted that albumin and
casts appear by the third day even when the disease is mild, but Berry
and Kitchen state that albuminuria was striking by its absence rather
than by its presence in their 7 cases of yellow fever accidentally contracted in the laboratory. In severe cases the urinary changes are
always very marked; heavy albuminuria, many granular and cellular
casts, bile pigment and often blood.

No change occurs in the hemoglobin or red cell figures, and the
majority of authorities state that the white cell count remains in the
normal range. It is interesting to note, however, that Berry and

Kitchen found a marked leukopenia commencing on the first day and sinking to its lowest level on the fifth day. Both neutrophils and lymphocytes are lowered in numbers. After the sixth day the count returns to normal within ten days. In fatal cases a distinct leukocytosis may be present before death. Vacuoles have been noted in the mature neutrophils during the leukopenic period.

The van den Bergh test gives a strong direct reaction and the icterus index is high. In experimental yellow fever in monkeys, Kerr found that an icterus index of over 10 units on the second day, or 15 on the third, indicates a fatal prognosis, while lower figures were associated with a mortality between 12 and 23 per cent. Kerr reports that the bromsulphthalein test of liver function gives analogous but less accurate results.

Differential Diagnosis.—Guiteras stresses the facies, the low pulserate in the presence of fever, and the urinary findings. Unfortunately, the facies is a treacherous basis for diagnosis, while the onset, fever curve and initial symptoms may closely simulate dengue, and the jaundice, bleedings and urinary findings are duplicated by Weil's spirochetosis icterohæmorrhagica. In dengue, the jaundice, hemorrhagic phenomena and urinary picture of yellow fever are extremely rare. Leukopenia is the rule in dengue and rare in yellow fever. Splenic enlargement is more often found in dengue.

Weil's disease presents a symptom picture so closely resembling yellow fever that it could readily be thought to be a mild form of the latter were it not for the demonstration of the spirochetes, either during the first few days of the disease in the patient's blood, or later in the urine, or by intraperitoneal injection of guinea-pigs with the suspected blood. Malaria, which may be coincident, should not cause much confusion.

Prognosis.—In young children the disease may be very mild and death seldom occurs. Unrecognized attacks in childhood probably explain the relative immunity of negroes. Epidemics vary in severity, the mortality in some being as low as 10 per cent, in others as high as 70 per cent. In general the severity of the symptoms is a good measure of the prognosis, but even apparently mild attacks may terminate in death.

Treatment.—The usual therapy of acute infections applies to yellow fever: rest in bed, limited diet, increased fluid intake, stimulation of bowel activity, and relief of malaise. In yellow fever, however, the routine is modified by the tendency to gastric irritability and the danger of kidney failure. Carter stresses the importance of (1) absolute rest, (2) the avoidance of all food for three days and a very limited dietary from then on, and (3) adequate fluid intake, by mouth if possible, or by rectum. He advises against hypodermoclysis, but says nothing about the intravenous route. It would seem that glucose solution by vein might quiet the vomiting and supply both fluid and nourishment.

Initial catharsis with calomel and a saline is popular, as in so many infections. The early malaise may be controlled by acetphenetidin, 0.3 gram (5 grains), but more severe headache and backache may require morphine. Carter advises cocaine, 0.03 gram (0.5 grains) for epigastric pain.

It is interesting to note that during the period that Leptospira icteroides was considered the cause of yellow fever, successful results were obtained with a curative serum and a preventive vaccine prepared with this now discredited organism.

Prevention.—The first indication is by careful screening to prevent mosquitoes from having access to the yellow fever patient; second, the protection of uninfected individuals from possibly infected mosquitoes and, third, the elimination of all Aëdes ægypti. Fortunately the vector shows little tendency to fly far from its breeding places, which are usually near human habitations. It prefers clear water, often finding it in artificial containers. Small collections of water should be drained, frequently emptied, or protected by screening or the addition of kerosene. Large pools may be stocked with larva-eating fish.

An efficient vaccine for immunization is obtained by mixing human convalescent serum with virus attenuated by repeated passage through mice by intracerebral inoculation.

REFERENCES.

BERRY, G. P., and KITCHEN, S. F.: Yellow Fever Accidentally Contracted in the Laboratory, Am. Jour. Trop. Med., 1931, **11**, 365.

CARROLL, JAMES: Yellow Fever, Osler's Modern Medicine, Chap. XXVII, vol. **2**, Philadelphia, Lea Brothers & Co., 1907.

CARTER, H. R.: The Early History of Yellow Fever (An Epidemiological and Historical Study of Its Place of Origin), Baltimore, Williams & Wilkins Company, 1931.

COWDRY, E. V., and KITCHEN, S. F.: Intranuclear Inclusions in Yellow Fever, Am. Jour. Hyg., 1930, **11**, 227.

KERR, J. A.: Use of Icterus Index and Bromsulphthalein Test in Experimental Yellow Fever, Am. Jour. Trop. Med., 1931, **11**, 139.

KLOTZ, OSKAR, and BELT, T. H.: The Pathology of the Liver in Yellow Fever, Am. Jour. Path., 1930, **6**, 663.

SAWYER, W. A.: Recent Progress in Yellow Fever Research, Medicine, 1931, **10**, 509.

STOKES, A., BAUER, J. H., and HUDSON, N. P.: Experimental Transmission of Yellow Fever to Laboratory Animals, Am. Jour. Trop. Med., 1928, **8**, 103.

WILSON, ROBERT: Dr. J. C. Nott and the Transmission of Yellow Fever, Ann. Med. History, 1931, **3**, 515.

DENGUE.

Definition.—An acute infectious disease due to a filterable virus transmitted by the Aëdes mosquito, and characterized by an incubation of three to nine days, an acute onset with severe malaise, a short variable diphasic febrile course, marked leukopenia, the absence of complications, and almost invariable recovery.

History.—Dengue cannot be surely identified in medical annals until toward the end of the eighteenth century. In Java, in 1779, David Bylon (often misspelled Brylon or Boylon), who was himself affected, saw 68 cases and left a description of the disease. Benjamin Rush accurately described it in 1780 in Philadelphia, terming it "bilious remittant fever." Throughout the nineteenth century frequent epidemics record the spread of the disease in many parts of the world. In 1873 it spread throughout the Gulf States and 40,000 cases occurred in New Orleans. Graham, in 1903, supplied the positive proof that the mosquito transmits the disease and measures taken to eradicate yellow fever have incidentally reduced the incidence of dengue. In the Philippine Islands the disease, owing to its high morbidity, has been troublesome to the United States Army, and much of our knowledge of the disease has been won from researches carried on by the Medical Department of the Army, including the proof by Ashburn and Craig in 1907 that the causative agent is a filterable virus. Bacteria, protozoa and spirochetes had each previously been described as the causative agent.

Throughout the history of dengue it has often been confused with yellow fever, especially as the two diseases often occur in the same districts. Today it is accepted as a distinct disease.

Etiology.—The filterable virus of dengue fever is presumably ultramicroscopic and has not been discovered. Nor has the virus been cultured satisfactorily as have others of this group. Perhaps, owing to the very limited opportunity for pathologic study no "inclusion bodies" have been described.

Epidemiology.—An amazing identity here exists between dengue and yellow fever (p. 179). In both, the virus is present in the patient's blood for the first three or four days; in both the Aëdes mosquito (in the case of dengue, Aëdes albopictus as well as Aëdes ægypti) is infected at the time of biting; in both an interval of eight to twelve days must elapse before the mosquito can transmit the virus and produce the disease in a susceptible individual.

The disease is endemic in tropical and subtropical regions and has never penetrated in the United States north of Virginia. There is no immunity other than that acquired following an attack and even this seems in many instances not to extend much beyond a year. In this fact lies the explanation of the rapidity of spread and high morbidity of the disease when it becomes epidemic.

Pathology.—Adequate data are lacking because of the small number of deaths due to the disease. The 1928 epidemic in Greece did, however, offer an opportunity for some postmortem studies. Catsaras reports on 10 necropsies, in only 3 of which, unfortunately, was death due to uncomplicated dengue. In these cases, there were moderate cloudy swelling of the heart, liver and kidneys, and petechial hemorrhages in various areas, but chiefly in the mucosa of the stomach and bowel. The spleen was not enlarged. Photakis also found the heart muscle soft, the liver more or less swollen, the spleen not enlarged, the liver cells had undergone cloudy swelling and fatty change. Some authorities mention pulmonary and cerebral inflammation.

Symptoms.—After an incubation of from three to thirteen days, usually five or six days, the onset is sudden, sometimes with a chill or chilliness. Fever promptly appears and great malaise with severe aching in the head, eyeballs, limbs and lumbar region. Within a few hours the temperature has reached 102° F., or even several degrees higher, the pulse-rate is 120 or more to the minute, the patient is prostrated by pain. At this stage the skin of the face and perhaps of the whole body is flushed, and the eyes and the mucous membranes of the mouth and pharynx are injected and reddened. Only occasionally does vomiting occur.

This picture may continue from one to four days, but the fever is apt to decline after one or two days. A stage of remission is mentioned by all observers, but is by no means as constant a feature of dengue as it is of smallpox or yellow fever. With remission, all symptoms vanish, only to return in most cases after twenty-four to forty-eight hours. The secondary fever comes, as a rule, on the sixth or seventh day of the disease; it is seldom as marked as the initial fever, either in height or duration. The pulse-rate tends to lag below the level appropriate to the fever. Pains return with the fever sometimes in greater severity, and may persist well into convalescence.

At this time appears the so-called "terminal" eruption, which varies greatly in character. It commences on the hands and is best seen on the back, chest, upper arms and thighs. It is described as resembling the rash of scarlet fever or of measles, or of being midway between the two. It is followed by a branny desquamation for several weeks.

Experimental dengue produced by human inoculation has been carefully observed in some 80 cases: incubation period averaged five and six-tenths days; a chill or chilliness occurred in 50 per cent; fever averaged four and eight-tenths days with records as short as one day and as long as nine days; it usually reached 102° or 104° F. The pains were chiefly in the head, eyes and back; 60 per cent had pains in the limbs, 45 per cent in the joints. The pains were not very severe.

A primary rash was seen in 38 per cent, the terminal eruption in 69 per cent. Enlargement of the cervical or inguinal nodes was common; 30 per cent complained of parotid tenderness, a few of testicular. Anorexia was common; 20 per cent vomited. The pulse-rate was only slightly accelerated during the fever. Complications were negligible; convalescence sometimes slow; there were no deaths.

Laboratory Findings.—Albuminuria is not uncommon but does not approach that of yellow fever, nor are casts and blood apt to be seen in the urine.

The blood count is of great importance. No change is found in the hemoglobin content nor in the number of red cells or platelets. As early as the second day the white cell count begins to fall, and progresses downward, until by the fifth or sixth day it is as low as 2000, or even 1200. Both granulocytes and lymphocytes are reduced in numbers. A relative lymphocytosis is revealed by the differential count, becoming more marked during recovery, for the lymphocytes increase ahead of the granular series. The granular cells which are present are chiefly young neutrophils and the Schilling index reveals a shift to the left. The few mature granulocytes which are present exhibit marked degenerative changes. This has led to the suggestion that the virus of dengue exhibits a cytotropism, localizing itself in the leukocytes. By the third or fourth day of convalescence the white cell picture has returned to normal.

Diagnosis.—No one can compare descriptions of dengue and of mild yellow fever without understanding the long-standing confusion between the two diseases. The etiology, vector, incubation period, onset, symptoms, and fever curve, remission and absence of sequelæ are all points of similarity. If the reported pathology of dengue is correct, both diseases display hepatic damage; but in dengue, jaundice, hemorrhagic phenomena and severe kidney changes are extremely rare.

Leukopenia occurs in dengue, but is usually stated not to occur in yellow fever.

Pappataci fever, another of the filterable virus diseases, has a different vector, but in every other way, including the leukopenia, simulates dengue very closely. Influenza, rheumatic fever and malaria may each, for a few days, be confused with dengue.

Prognosis.—Only in the debilitated, diseased or elderly does dengue ever cause death. It is worthy of note, however, that in 1928 there were recorded 20 deaths from dengue in the registration area in the United States (Georgia, 6; Florida, 4; Alabama, 3; Missouri, 3; Louisiana, 2; Texas and South Carolina, each 1).

Treatment.—Rest in bed, plenty of fluid, light diet and care of the bowels are indicated. Salicylates or acetphenetidin may relieve the pain, but morphine is often needed. The measures for prophylaxis are identical with those employed in yellow fever (*q. v.*).

REFERENCES.

ASHBURN, P. M., and CRAIG, C. F.: Experimental Investigations Regarding the Etiology of Dengue Fever, Jour. Infect. Dis., 1907, **4**, 440.

BYLON, DAVID: Korte Aantekening, Wegens eene Algemeene Ziekte, Doorgaans Genaamd de Knokkel-Koorts, Verhandlungen van het Bataviaasch Genootschop der Konsten in Wetenschappen, Batavia, 1823, 2 ed., pt 2, p. 1780.

CATSARAS, J.: Pathologisch-anatomische Beobachtungen zum Denguefieber, Arch. f. Schiffs- u. Tropen-Hyg., 1931, **35**, 278.

RUSH, BENJAMIN: Medical Observations and Inquiries, Philadelphia, 1789, **5**, 104.

SILER, J. F., HALL, M. W., and HITCHENS, A. P.: Dengue, Philippine Jour. Sci., 1926, **29**, 1.

SIMMONS, JAMES, S.: Dengue Fever, Am. Jour. Trop. Med., 1931, **11**, 77.

SIMMONS, J. S., ST. JOHN, J. H., and REYNOLDS, F. H. K.: Numerical and Morphological Alterations of Leukocytes During Dengue Fever, Philippine Jour. Sci., 1931, **44**, 128.

PAPPATACI FEVER.

Synonyms.—Sandfly fever; Phlebotomus fever.

Definition.—An acute infectious disease due to a filterable virus transmitted by the sandfly, and characterized by sudden onset, marked malaise, a brief fever sometimes with a secondary rise, distinct leukopenia and no sequelæ or mortality.

History.—Although probably often confused with dengue, the disease, under a variety of local names, has been recognized for many years, especially in the Mediterranean countries, Syria and India. It was not until 1908 that it was proved to belong in the filterable virus group by Doerr and Russ. The disease was prevalent during the World War among the troops in Gallipoli, Salonika and Mesopotamia.

Etiology and Epidemiology.—A filter-passing ultramicroscopic virus is the agent causing pappataci fever, and this virus is thought, perhaps, to be related to the viruses of yellow fever and of dengue. The sandfly, Phlebotomus, is the vector in this disease, which fact explains the names sandfly fever and phlebotomus fever, but as sandflies also transmit leishmaniasis it seems best to use the term pappataci fever, derived from the species of sandfly (Phlebotomus papatassii) which transmits the disease.

The genus Phlebotomus are minute hairy flies, widely distributed in the tropics and subtropics. A very little moisture, as for example on stone walls, is adequate for breeding. The adults have but a short flight, are attracted by light and, unfortunately, can pass through the mesh of the usual mosquito netting.

Only the females suck blood; their bite often causes local irritation. To transmit the disease, the sandfly must bite a patient during the first two days of the fever, and six days must elapse before the disease can be transmitted to a susceptible individual.

Symptoms.—The disease picture closely resembles that of dengue but is shorter and milder. An incubation of from four to ten days is followed by an acute onset. Usually a chill or chilliness marks the onset of the fever. Headache and pain deep in the eyes may dominate the picture, but generalized pains in the back, neck and legs are common. Flushing of the face and injection of the conjunctiva and mucous membranes promptly appear. No true eruption characterizes this disease. Mental depression may be profound.

Within twenty-four hours the fever reaches 103° F. or more and may stay at this level for two or three days. Sometimes after a remission there is a short secondary rise; in other instances the fever persists for twice its usual period. Bradycardia appears with defervescence. No serious complications occur; death does not result from the disease alone. Convalescence may be slow and a pulse-rate of below 50 to the minute may persist for two weeks. Immunity follows an attack, but this is not lasting and second attacks occur.

Leukopenia similar to that found in dengue is a constant finding. The low count results from a sharp reduction in the number of neutrophils.

Diagnosis.—Although pappataci fever may at first be confused with malaria, influenza or other fevers, it is with dengue that the greatest confusion arises. The pains of dengue are said to be more severe; its eruption more distinct. Dengue is said to be more prevalent in the late summer and fall; pappataci fever in the early summer.

Treatment.—The attack requires only symptomatic treatment. There is no specific; quinine is useless.

Prevention rests on protection of the infected and the susceptible individuals from the bite of the sandfly. The sandfly bites almost always at night. For safety a netting with openings not over 1.5 mm. in size, although oppressively hot, is necessary unless the sleeping quarters are more than 10 feet above the ground. Exposed parts of the body may be covered with a repellant substance (oil of citronella, for example). Many take few, if any, of these precautions. Measures to prevent breeding are difficult of success.

REFERENCES.

DOERR, R.: Ueber ein neues invisibles Virus, Berl. klin. Wchnschr., 1908, **45**, 1847.
MANSON-BAHR, PHILIP: Manson's Tropical Diseases, London, Cassell & Co., Ltd., 1929, p. 210.
RUGE, R., MÜHLENS, P., and ZUR VERTH, M.: Krankheiten und Hygiene der warmen Länder, Leipzig, Georg Thieme, 1930, **3**, 231.

INFECTIOUS COLD.

Synonyms.—Acute coryza; Common cold.

Definition.—An acute infection of the upper respiratory tract initiated by a filterable virus, but prolonged, as a rule, by increased activity of the local bacterial flora, often leading to sinusitis, bronchitis or pneumonia.

Etiology and Epidemiology.—Colds have been blamed on many of the pathogenic organisms, but studies by Dochez and his associates have demonstrated the presence of a filterable virus that will transmit the disease by intranasal inoculation to man and monkey.

Spread of the disease is by contact or droplet infection; the certainty of exposure to the virus and the high incidence of susceptibility readily permitting the disease to become epidemic. It is especially in the winter months that the disease and its sequelæ are common, but a typical cold follows inoculation with the virus even in midsummer.

Disease Picture.—Inoculation of human volunteers proves the incubation period to be about twenty-four hours. This agrees with clinical experience. The onset is moderately acute with chilliness, malaise and slight fever. Often this systemic reaction is negligible; in other cases severe, with anorexia, headache and depression. Transient diarrhea is not uncommon. Sneezing and local symptoms may be the first and almost the only manifestation. The mucous membrane of the nose and pharynx becomes swollen and an amazingly abundant watery discharge runs from the nose, irritating the nares and upper lip. Extension to the larynx, posterior pharynx, lacrimal ducts or Eustachian tube results in appropriate local symptoms. Herpes labialis is common. No change occurs in the blood count.

Sometimes the disease terminates within a few days without further symptoms, and at this time the true virus infection ends. In most instances, however, the discharge gradually becomes more purulent and less abundant. This marks the pyogenic stage of the disease, and it is in this period that sinusitis and otitis may occur. Even more serious troubles may develop, including pneumonia, either lobular or lobar.

In *diagnosis*, one must keep in mind allergic rhinitis and the coryza occurring at the onset of measles. Theoretically, at least, one should distinguish between the usual epidemic infectious cold and the nasopharyngitis initiated by chilling, wetting or irritant inhalations. In these latter, the infection depends upon the existing flora.

Treatment.—Avoidance of infection is almost an impossibility, although greater thoughtfulness on the part of those with "nothing but a cold" would accomplish something. Routine use of a mildly antiseptic nasal lavage and gargle during the winter months is firmly believed in by many, and a prompt recourse to these measures after exposure to infection is reasonable. Once the infection is established, treatment is directed to relief of symptoms on the one hand and the limiting of the pyogenic phase on the other. No specific for the virus infection is available. The onset symptoms are best treated by warmth, abundant fluid intake, best as water, and acetylsalicylic acid, 0.3 gram (5 grains), hourly for three doses. Sweating should not be induced unless the patient is in bed; a hot drink or full dose of Dover's powder may then be employed. Mild purgation may also be useful.

Local treatment at first consists of a cleansing nasal lavage followed by an oily spray. Ephedrin in 3 per cent solution dropped or sprayed into the nostrils will often relieve the local swelling, but only temporarily. Later, more distinctly antiseptic solutions may be used to lessen the secondary infection.

Vaccines to prevent colds probably have no influence on the primary virus infection, but may, especially if carefully prepared autogenous vaccines are used, be of some value in limiting the later phases and complications of the disease.

REFERENCES.

DOCHEZ, A. R., MILLS, K. C., and KNEELAND, YALE, JR.: Studies on the Mechanism of Upper Respiratory Infection, Trans. Assn. Am. Phys., 1931, 46, 200.

DOCHEZ, A. R., SHIBLEY, G. S., and MILLS, K. C.: Studies in Common Cold: Experimental Transmission of Common Cold to Anthropoid Apes and Human Beings by Means of a Filterable Agent, Jour. Exper. Med., 1930, 52, 701.

POWELL, H. M., and CLOWES, G. H. A.: Cultivation of the Virus of Common Cold and Its Inoculation in Human Subjects, Proc. Soc. Exp. Biol. and Med., 1931, 29, 332.

PSITTACOSIS.

Definition.—A disease of parrots due to a filterable virus, transmissible to man and characterized in man by an incubation period of from nine to fourteen days, a sudden onset, a febrile course of from two to four weeks with atypical signs and symptoms of lobular pneumonia, and a mortality of 10 to 30 per cent.

History.—Ritter, in 1879, is credited with being the first to describe the disease; 3 of his 7 cases died and were autopsied by Eberth. The syndrome was named by Morange in Paris, in 1894, from the Greek *psittacos*, a parrot. Nocard and others found bacilli which they believed were the cause, but recent investigators (Bedson, Krumwiede, and others) have demonstrated that the disease is caused by a filterable virus, still unidentified. In the United States the disease was first recognized by Vickery and Richardson in 1904. In the Wilkes-Barre epidemic of 1917 there were 140 cases with a mortality of 11 per cent.

Etiology and Epidemiology.—Little is known of the virus beyond the fact that it is ultramicroscopic and will pass a "bacteria tight" filter.

Psittacosis is a highly contagious disease of parrots, being readily transmitted to humans from the sick bird, but probably not from human to human. The exact method of transmission is not known, but some of the evidence suggests that only proximity is necessary. Not all those exposed acquire the disease, but the virus is highly infective as evidenced by McCoy's report, that of the 11 workers in the hygienic laboratory who developed the disease, 8 had been in no direct contact with the infected birds. The first case developed nine days after the research was started.

Parrots developing the disease come, as a rule, from an infected district (Amazon parrots, for example), but they may appear healthy when sold by the retailer. A carrier state may exist, the disease breaking out upon exposure to cold. Other birds than parrots may, perhaps, also transmit the disease. The United States Public Health Service has found psittacosis present in some of the breeding aviaries of California and human cases have been traced to parrots and parrakeets from this source.

Pathology.—There is close agreement between the older case reports and the recent pathologic studies in human cases and in experimental psittacosis in monkeys. The essential lesion is a primary diffuse bronchitis with patchy areas of pneumonia and of atelectasis. Microscopically, the hyperplasia of the lining epithelium of the alveoli and the exudate of phagocytic mononuclear cells are most characteristic. In the monkey the process commences near the hilum and spreads to the periphery. The spleen may be enlarged.

Disease Picture.—After an incubation period of nine to fourteen days an acute onset occurs with malaise and rapidly rising fever. There may be a chill. Gastro-intestinal symptoms are not marked, but the tongue is coated, the abdomen may be distended and vomiting occasionally occurs. The fever reaches 103° F. or more; the pulse lags behind. Because the lung involvement is central, it is often not recognized for several days, but the roentgenogram will constantly reveal it within the first forty-eight hours. Also respiratory symptoms are apt not to be severe; the respiratory rate is little accelerated, there is little or no sputum or pleuritic pain. Sometimes cough also is slight, but in other instances, severe.

From day to day the physical signs of the lung lesion change and shift—possibly more influenced by the areas of atelectasis than by those of pneumonic consolidation, with resulting confusion. The fever is irregular. Sometimes, especially in children, the disease terminates in ten days or two weeks, sometimes the fever and pneumonia drag on for a month. Deaths occur chiefly in the elderly; the mortality varies in epidemics from 10 to over 30 per cent. Many reports of a typhoid-like form without lung involvement and even with "spots" are in the literature; these seldom prove fatal.

Laboratory studies are of little diagnostic assistance; there is no change in the blood picture; the urine is that of any febrile state. Intraperitoneal inoculation of mice with sputum emulsions may bring about infection with characteristic changes in the liver and spleen.

Confusion in *diagnosis* is the rule. Influenzal pneumonia is the usual diagnosis; typhoid or paratyphoid may be suspected. Contact, direct or indirect, with a parrot, preferably one that is ill, is required to confirm the suspicion aroused perhaps by a pneumonia atypical in its distribution and symptoms, lacking the usual cyanosis, dyspnea, tachycardia and leukocytosis.

Treatment.—Prophylaxis demands quarantine of imported parrots; the problem is not unimportant, for as many as 500 cases have been reported throughout the world in one year (1928). Even an apparently healthy parrot should not be bought as a pet too soon after import; a sick one should be killed or isolated. At no time should the bird be kissed or fed from the lips.

In the attack the treatment is purely symptomatic. A trial of convalescent serum is perhaps justifiable.

REFERENCES.

BEDSON, S. P., WESTERN, G. T., and SIMPSON, L.: Observations on Etiology of Psittacosis, Lancet, 1930, i, 235, 345.

McCOY, G. W.: Accidental Psittacosis Infection Among Personnel of Hygienic Laboratory, U. S. Pub. Health Rep., 1930, 45, 843.

MORANGE: De la psittacose ou infection spéciale déterminée par des perruches, Thèse de Paris, 1895.

PETERSON, E., SPALDING, O. B., and WILDMAN, O.: Psittacosis: A Clinical and Roentgenological Study of Seven Cases with Postmortem Observations in One Case, Jour. Am. Med. Assn., 1930, 95, 171.

RIESMAN, D., and DAVIDSON, H. S.: Psittacosis with the Report of a Case, Med. Clin. North America, 1931, 14, 815.

RITTER, J.: Beitrag zur Frage des Pneumotyphus, Deutsch. Arch. f. klin. Med., 1897, 25, 53.

RIVERS, T. M., and BERRY, G. P.: Psittacosis Experimentally Induced Infections in Monkeys, Jour. Exp. Med., 1931, 54, 91.

FOOT–AND–MOUTH DISEASE.

Although Pasteur's researches on rabies strongly hinted at the existence of filterable viruses, it was in foot-and-mouth disease that a filterable virus was first shown to be a cause of disease in man or animal (Löffler and Frosch, 1898).

The cause of foot-and-mouth disease has not been identified, but it is an ultramicroscopic filter-passing virus, and the disease meets all the criteria for classification among the virus diseases. There is evidence that there are several variants of the virus of this disease. Practically all cloven-foot animals are susceptible to the virus, especially cattle, sheep and pigs; horses are resistant, and guinea-pigs are to be preferred for experimental infection. Man is relatively insusceptible, but undoubted infection has occurred, transmission being by means of infected milk or butter, or by direct contact in milking if the teats are affected. It does not spread from man to man, nor has it been transmitted in vaccination against smallpox.

Named from the distribution of the lesions, the disease is further described by the other terms applied to it: *epidemic stomatitis* and *aphthous fever*. The incubation period is variable—two days to two weeks; the onset fairly acute with moderate symptoms of commencing infection. Chilliness, malaise and perhaps vomiting occur with the rising temperature. A sense of heat in the mouth and pharynx precedes the appearance in these regions of many discrete vesicles. Swallowing may be difficult and painful; salivation occurs and swelling of the regional lymph nodes. Similar vesicles may appear on the lips, on the skin between the fingers and between the toes, rarely on the palms, soles or elsewhere. In cattle, vesicles appear near the hoof with great constancy.

With the appearance of the vesicles the fever drops, usually by the fourth day of the disease. The vesicles rupture and gradually heal without scarring. Complications do not occur; there is usually no mortality, but death has been reported. Immunity is transient.

No change occurs in the blood picture and laboratory diagnosis rests upon inoculation of a guinea-pig and the demonstration of the nature of the virus by cross-immunity tests.

Treatment is chiefly prophylactic through isolation of infected cattle. During an epizoötic, milk should be avoided or boiled. The local lesions in the mouth may be cleansed repeatedly with any mildly antiseptic wash, or an application of silver nitrate may be made to any accessible ulcers which are giving pain.

REFERENCES.

LOFFLER and FROSCH: Berichte der Kommission zur Erforschung der Maul- und Kleuenseuche bei dem Institut für Infektionskrankheiten in Berlin, Centralbl. f. Bakteriol., Abt. 1, 1898, **23**, 371.

MAITLAND, H. B.: Foot-and-mouth Disease, A System of Bacteriology, vol. **7,** Chapter V, London, His Majesty's Stationery Office, 1930.

OLITSKY, PETER K.: Virus Diseases of Mammals as Exemplified by Foot-and-mouth Disease and Vesicular Stomatitis, Filterable Viruses, edited by Thomas M. Rivers, Chapter VI, Baltimore, Williams & Wilkins Company, 1928 (extensive bibliography).

CHAPTER IV.

DISEASES DUE TO RICKETTSIÆ.

By ROBERT VAN VALZAH, M.D.

TYPHUS FEVER.	TRENCH FEVER.
ROCKY MOUNTAIN SPOTTED FEVER.	TSUTSUGAMUSHI DISEASE.

IN 1916, da Rocha-Lima suggested the term "Rickettsia"—in memory of Howard Taylor Ricketts—to designate certain small microorganisms occurring in lice. Extensive study has proved that several of these organisms are pathogenic for man and a number which are non-pathogenic have been described. Cowdry describes them as follows, "Gram-negative, bacterium-like organisms of small size, usually less than a micron in diameter, which are found intracellularly in arthropods, which may be more or less pleomorphic and stain rather lightly with anilin dyes." Cowdry also summarizes our present knowledge of the Rickettsiæ in relation to human disease by stating that there is strong evidence as to their causation of typhus fever and Rocky Mountain spotted fever; the evidence as to trench fever is highly probable, and that in relation to tsutsugamushi disease remains ill-defined.

He also points out that these diseases possess certain features in common, namely, that they are transmitted to man by blood-feeding insects, that they exhibit a fairly high fever, that one attack confers temporary or permanent immunity, that they show more or less nervous system involvement and develop a somewhat similar exanthematous eruption.

TYPHUS FEVER.

Synonyms.—Spotted fever; Jail fever; Ship fever; Camp fever; Typhus exanthematique; Fleck Fieber; Tabardillo; Brill's disease.

Definition.—Typhus fever is an acute specific infectious disease, occurring usually in epidemics, transmitted through the bite of an infected body louse or other insect vector; it is characterized by sudden onset, a high febrile course of about two weeks' duration, terminating by crisis or rapid lysis, and also by marked prostration, a characteristic eruption, and severe nervous symptoms.

History.—Although undoubtedly existing in epidemic form in ancient times, the earlier descriptions do not completely differentiate typhus fever from other pestilential scourges, notably the plague. From the beginning of the sixteenth century adequate descriptions of the symptomatology and epidemiology are available to differentiate it with reasonable certainty from other epidemic diseases, although the final differentiation of typhus and typhoid fever was only accomplished by Gerhard and Pennock in 1837.

Typhus fever has usually followed in the wake of war, famine, overcrowding and general unsanitary conditions. During the sixteenth century notable epidemics occurred in Italy, Hungary and England. During and following the Thirty Years' War (1618–1648) the disease ravaged central Europe and later, following the Napoleonic campaigns, it spread in the wake of the French Armies. Severe epidemics occurred in England and in Ireland in 1816–1818, 1826–1828 and 1846–1847. The French and the English armies, during the Crimean War (1853–1856) suffered heavy casualities from typhus fever. The Italian campaign of 1861 and the Turco-Russian War of 1878 were again accompanied by outbreaks of the disease.

In the Western Hemisphere typhus fever was introduced into Mexico soon after the Conquest and in modified endemic form, punctuated by several epidemics, has persisted in certain parts of Central America up to the present time. No widespread epidemics have ever occurred in the United States, although localized epidemics have been reported in New York and other Atlantic seaboard cities, as well as in California. Sporadic cases of mild typhus fever, known as Brill's disease, have occurred in New York and other American cities, notably those in the southeastern United States.

During and following the Balkan Wars and the World War, typhus fever appeared in epidemic form in all the countries of eastern and central Europe. Accurate statistics are not available, but it has been estimated that at least 1,000,000 persons died of typhus in these countries during and following the World War.

The high mortality among medical attendants of those suffering from typhus fever has been noted in all epidemics; among the names of those who have made the supreme sacrifice in the study of this disease may be mentioned Moczukowski, Ricketts, Husk, Cornet, Prowazek, Jochmann, MacGruder, Donnelly, Bacot, Conneff, Schussler and Weil.

Etiology.—*Exciting Cause and Transmission.*—The exciting cause of epidemic Old World typhus is the Rickettsia prowazeki, which is communicated to man usually by the bite of infected body lice, although there is some evidence that it can be transmitted by louse excreta, through abrasions of the skin. Attempts to cultivate the organism on artificial culture media have been unsuccessful. It, therefore, does not fulfill Koch's postulates; but, as Wolbach points out, there is evidence of equally conclusive character that Rickettsia prowazeki is the cause of typhus fever. The organism has been described as pleomorphic, occurring as minute, paired ovoid bodies, also as bipolar staining rods and in filamentous forms. It is best demonstrated by the use of Giemsa's stain. It has been demonstrated occurring intracellularly in the gut of lice, in endothelial cells from human lesions and in the lesions of susceptible laboratory animals. The recent work of Maxcy, Rumreich, Dyer, Badger, Ceder, Lillie, Workman, Mooser, Ruiz, Castaneda, Zinsser and others has stimulated new interest in endemic typhus. They have been able to infect insect vectors other than lice and transmit the disease through them to susceptible animals. It seems well established at present that the rat flea, Zenopsylla cheopis, is the usual vector of endemic typhus. It has also been suggested that the differences in pathologic findings, course and mortality between Old World typhus and endemic typhus may, in some way, be attributable to the passage of the virus through different arthopods.

Predisposing Causes.—(a) *Socal Condition.*—Even before the mode of the transmission of the disease was understood, it was noted by all writers that general unsanitary conditions such as prevail in times of war, famine and economic distress were likely to be followed by outbreaks of the disease. In civil life the presence of multiple cases in the same family is not uncommon. The lower classes of the population that tolerate the presence of lice, such as vagrants, emigrants, those living in labor camps, jails, workhouses and slums, are likely to develop the disease. Overcrowding, lack of facilities for, and lack of attention to, bodily cleanliness predispose to the spread of typhus fever.

(b) *Age, Sex and Race.*—Sex probably plays no rôle in the susceptibility of individuals, and the reason for greater prevalence in the male can be explained on the ground of other predisposing factors. Pregnancy, the puerperium and lactation have no influence on susceptibility to or immunity against typhus. The occurrence of the disease in infancy and childhood is less frequent than in adult life, probably due, not to any natural immunity, but solely to lessened exposure. Race and nationality play little part *per se* in susceptibility to or immunity against typhus fever. One attack usually confers a life-long immunity, although isolated cases to the contrary have been reported by several observers.

(c) *Occupation.*—Physicians, nurses, priests, and those employed in transporting the sick have always shown a high morbidity and mortality incidence—a fact easily explained by the known mode of transmission. In the case of endemic typhus, food handlers are especially predisposed.

(d) *Geographic, Climatic, Seasonal.*—Typhus fever has been epidemic in central Europe, Russia, northern Africa, Ireland, Manchuria and Mexico. It occurs most frequently in the temperate zone during the winter months. Wilder has pointed out that in Mexico it is prevalent in the highlands and rarely seen in the lowlands. Endemic typhus of the United States is more prevalent in the South Atlantic and Gulf States and occurs chiefly in the summer and fall months.

Pathology.—No gross pathognomonic changes are found at autopsy. The distinctive lesions are microscopic. The skin shows the petechial rash persisting after death and may show areas of skin necrosis and gangrene. The blood is of dark color and coagulates slowly. If death occurs during the first two weeks the spleen may be enlarged. Areas of bronchitis and bronchopneumonia are commonly found in cases terminating fatally. Thrombosis of the larger vessels has been reported. The brain and meninges may show no gross lesions, but congestion of the meninges with minute hemorrhages is not uncommon.

Microscopically, the distinctive lesions of the disease involve the smaller vessels, notably those of the skin and of the brain, thus accounting for the two most characteristic symptoms of the disease—the skin rash and the central nervous system manifestations. Proliferative changes of the endothelium of the small vessels, followed by degeneration and necrosis, are the earliest manifestation. This is succeeded by the formation of mural or obliterating thrombi in the capillaries, followed by loss of continuity of the wall and extravasations of blood. Perivascular infiltration with cells derived from the adventitia along with mononuclear and polymorphonuclear leukocytes, also occurs. In the vessels of the brain these minute lesions may simulate miliary tubercles.

Symptoms.—The period of incubation is usually about twelve days, although variations from eight to fourteen days are not uncommon.

During the later part of the incubation period, mild prodromal symptoms may be present that are in no way characteristic; weakness, malaise, headache and slight rise of temperature may occur. The actual onset is usually abrupt, with a chill and rapid rise of temperature. In some instances, more than one chill, and in milder cases simply a sense of chilliness ushers in the disease.

The temperature rises rapidly within twenty-four to forty-eight hours to a high febrile level (103° to 104° F.) and remains at this level with slight diurnal variations for a period of about two weeks, when it declines by rapid lysis or by crisis. In cases terminating favorably, wider diurnal temperature variations are noticed for several days preceding the actual crisis. During this period the general appearance of the patient is improved, and subjectively he feels better. Sweating, which is absent during the stage of invasion and the fastigium, occurs during this precritical period and at the time of defervescence of the fever. Prostration is usually marked from the onset. The pulse-rate and the respirations increase *pari passu* with the temperature. Severe headache, occipital, frontal or general, is present. Loss of appetite and a tendency to constipation are commonly met. Nausea and vomiting may occur early after the onset, but are comparatively rare symptoms. Muscular pains, although present, are usually not so severe as in influenza or smallpox. Restlessness and insomnia are seen early in the course of the disease followed by active delirium and later by stupor and coma. Cough, at first dry and harsh, later more productive, begins about the fourth day and may continue as a troublesome symptom well into convalescence.

Physical Signs.—In the early stages, the facies is indicative of anxiety in contrast to the dull, apathetic expression exhibited by patients with typhoid fever. The face is flushed. Mild conjunctivæ injection and dryness of the tongue may be present. Herpes labialis, although rarely seen, may appear. Wolbach, Todd and Palfrey report its occurrence twice in a series of 181 cases. Enlargement of the spleen occurs during the first week of the disease, but toward the end of the second week or later it is rarely palpable.

The Eruption.—The most diagnostic physical finding is the eruption; unfortunately for diagnostic purposes, it usually does not occur until the fourth or fifth day; its occurrence as early as the second and as late as the eleventh day has been reported. In contradistinction to the rash of typhoid fever, the rash of typhus comes out in a single crop. It is of a macular character, the spots varying in size from 1 to 5 mm. in diameter. At first they are pink in color, definitely defined from the surrounding skin and disappear on pressure; later the lesions tend to become larger, spreading peripherally, and the center of the lesion becoming darker red to purplish in color from extravasation of red blood cells. Still later the lesions become truly petechial in character. The eruption involves almost simultaneously the abdomen, shoulders and back, and at about the same time the front of the chest and the extremities. The face is rarely involved. The profuseness and the severity of the rash differ considerably in different epidemics and in different individuals in the same epidemic.

13

Factors that confuse the observation of the nature of the rash are dark pigmentation of the skin, the presence of bites, the secondary lesions of the skin due to scratching and, finally, the lack of cleanliness on the part of the patient. A blotchy erythema, appearing at about the same time, involving the same portions of the skin surface, lasting for several days and disappearing before the typical typhus lesions, is encountered not infrequently. The extent and hemorrhagic character of the eruption bear some relation to the severity of the disease, but probably not so much as the severity of the nervous symptoms.

With the onset of rash, the signs of toxemia and especially the cerebral symptoms become more marked; delirium of a low muttering type, but more frequently of active and violent nature, ensues. Subsultus tendinum, carphologia, loss of sphincter control and finally coma ensue. Crepitant, subcrepitant and sibilant râles may be met with early in the course of the disease, and in most cases appear or persist until convalescence is established.

Laboratory Findings.—Typhus fever is accompanied by a mild leukocytosis, averaging about 12,000 in uncomplicated cases. There is little change in the hemoglobin and red blood cell count.

The Weil-Felix agglutination reaction, performed by using standard cultures of Bacillus proteus X, is positive in almost all cases and either the macroscopic or the microscopic method may be employed. The urine shows nothing characteristic but, in common with other infectious diseases, albumin is frequently present in typhus fever. The blood pressure, both systolic and diastolic, remains low throughout the course of the disease. The cerebrospinal fluid is usually under slightly increased pressure; it may be clear or slightly turbid, and in cases with severe cerebral manifestations may show xanthochromia or the presence of red blood cells.

Complications.—Bronchitis is met with so frequently and at such an early stage of the disease that it should be considered as a part rather than a complication of the disease. Palfrey and Wolbach report bronchopneumonia as the chief cause of death in the epidemic in Poland, which they observed. The onset of bronchopneumonia may occur at the height of the disease or after an apparent crisis. It may be sudden and fulminant in onset and course, or it may be insidious in onset but accompanied by evidences of vasomotor collapse.

Suppuration of the salivary glands and otitis media have been observed. Skin lesions of sufficient severity to classify as complications are frequently noted as follows: boils, abscesses, bed sores and gangrene. Some of the skin complications are probably due to thrombosis of peripheral vessels and pressure; frost-bite may be a predisposing factor. Thrombosis of the larger vessels with gangrene has been noted by a number of writers.

Diagnosis.—Occurring sporadically, typhus in the early stage may be difficult to differentiate from other infectious fevers. Where the disease is epidemic, the onset of symptoms in the majority of cases is sufficiently similar to make the physician reasonably certain of its presence. Typhus fever must be differentiated from smallpox, typhoid fever, cerebrospinal meningitis, malaria, measles, scarlet fever and Rocky Mountain spotted fever.

At the onset of the disease backache is likely to be more severe in smallpox; the eruption likely to appear first on the face; the blood picture somewhat different and the pre-eruptive fall of temperature present. Typhoid fever differs in the insidiousness of onset, leukopenia, persistent enlargement of the spleen, the limited type of more localized skin eruption occurring in crops, and in the positive blood and stool cultures and Widal reaction.

Cerebrospinal meningitis may show the same sudden onset, but differs in the irregularity of the fever curve, the early rigidity of the neck, paralysis of cranial nerves, a positive Kernig's sign and the characteristic spinal fluid findings.

From malaria it is distinguished by the rapid decline and intermittent course of the fever, the leukopenia and the presence of the specific plasmodium in the blood. It is differentiated from measles by the early appearance of inflammatory mucous membrane lesions, the presence of Koplik's spots and leukopenia.

Scarlet fever usually begins with severe sore throat and the early appearance of a rash quite dissimilar to that of typhus. Rocky Mountain spotted fever occurs in a limited area. Should typhus fever be introduced into the same area, the diseases might be almost impossible to differentiate clinically. Splenic enlargement and jaundice are more common in Rocky Mountain spotted fever. Guinea-pig inoculation from cases of Rocky Mountain spotted fever usually gives characteristic lesions in the scrotum, which is not the case with typhus fever.

Prognosis.—The mortality varies greatly in different epidemics. The sporadic form, Brill's disease, has a mortality of less than 1 per cent. Among a civilian population with adequate provision for care, a mortality of 5 to 10 per cent has been reported. Murchison's statistics, based on 3506 cases admitted to the London Fever Hospital during a decade, indicate a 20 per cent mortality. In severe epidemics and under unfavorable surroundings a death-rate of over 50 per cent has been reported.

Age plays an important rôle in prognosis. During the first two decades of life the mortality is low; thereafter, with increasing years, the prognosis becomes more unfavorable. Undoubtedly the mortality can be cut down by early recognition of the disease and careful nursing. Sex *per se* has little influence on the course and prognosis. The mortality among the better classes of the population, when attacked, is supposed to be higher.

The presence, early in the course of the disease, of such symptoms as marked nervous and mental manifestations, early severe respiratory symptoms, diarrhea, profuseness of the rash with early and extensive skin hemorrhages, is of serious prognostic import.

Prophylaxis and Treatment.—The prophylaxis of typhus fever may be summed up in the control of lice. This may not be a simple procedure, particularly where numerous cases are being handled. Physicians, nurses and attendants should wear single-piece gowns with stocking-footed trousers; a head dress and rubber gloves are also employed. Gowns should be frequently deloused by dry heat, steam or chemicals. The use of naphthalene sprinkled upon clothing and placed in an air-tight container for about twelve hours has proved effective in killing lice. The patient should be removed to an isolation hospital and his surroundings and those in contact with him thoroughly deloused. Contacts should be quarantined and observed for a period of two weeks. On arrival at the hospital the patient should be stripped of his clothing, which, with bedding and stretcher, should be subjected to disinfection. The hairy portions of the body should be clipped, the patient bathed and dried and finally rubbed with a solution of kerosene before removal to his room or ward. The destruction of rats and their harborages is indicated in the prophylaxis against endemic typhus.

Treatment of the disease itself at present is purely symptomatic. In typhus, as in typhoid fever, the availability of good nursing should, and probably does, affect the mortality materially. Absolute bed rest is essential; precautions should be taken to prevent the patient, in his delirium, from doing himself harm. His diet should be liquid or soft in nature and fluids should be forced. The introduction of liquid food and fluids by means of a nasal catheter should be used, if necessary. Hydrotherapy similar to that used in typhoid should be practised. Especial routine care of the mouth is necessary. Constipation can be treated by enemata and the observation of retention and need for catheterization should be noted. Contrary to previously expressed opinion, Palfrey and Wolbach found morphine and codeine of distinct value in the treatment of their cases at Warsaw, and theoretically the indications in controlling cough, pain and restlessness seem obvious. Hyoscine may be useful in the more marked forms of delirium. In cases where the prostration is not too great the use of the coal tar drugs has some place. Stimulants such as digitalis, camphor and caffeine have been used. Bed sores should be guarded against by frequent change of position and by pressure pads. Parotitis in the earlier stages is treated by the use of ice-bags; later by heat and incision. Bed rest should be enforced for at least a week following the defervescence of fever and longer if the nervous, mental or other symptoms are severe.

REFERENCES.

Cowdry, E. V.: Rickettsiæ and Disease, Arch. Path., 1926, 2, 59.
Dyer, R. E., Badger, L. F., Ceder, E. T., and Workman, W. G.: Endemic Typhus Fever of the United States—History, Epidemiology and Mode of Transmission, Jour. Am. Med. Assn., 1932, 99, 795–800. *Note:* Complete bibliography of endemic typhus is included in this reference.
Fraenkel, E.: Zur Fleckfieberdiagnose, Münch. med. Wchnschr., 1915, 62, 805.
Palfrey, F. W., and Wolbach, S. B.: Typhus Fever, Oxford Med., vol. 5, pt I, p. 439.
Weil, E., and Felix, A.: Zur serologischen Diagnose des Fleckfiebers, Wien. klin. Wchnschr., 1916, 29, 33–35.
———— Merkblatt zur serologischen Fleckfieberdiagnose nach Weil-Felix: Münch. med. Wchnschr., 1918, 65, 17.
Wolbach, S. B., Todd, J., and Palfrey, F. W.: The Etiology and Pathology of Typhus Fever, Report of the Typhus Research Commission to the League of Red Cross Societies to Poland, Harvard Univ. Press, 1922.

ROCKY MOUNTAIN SPOTTED FEVER.

Definition.—Rocky Mountain spotted fever is an acute infectious disease, transmitted to man by the bite of infected ticks. It is characterized pathologically by an endangeitis of the peripheral vessels and clinically by sudden onset, with chill, headache, continued fever terminating by lysis, severe bone and muscle pains and a petechial eruption, appearing first on the wrists, ankles and back, later becoming generalized.

History.—Although apparently known to the Shoshone and Blackfoot Indians before the coming of the white man, the evidence of this is largely traditional. The disease was not differentiated from other febrile diseases by the early white settlers. E. E. Maxey, of Boise, Idaho, in 1899 first described it clinically and characterized it as a specific entity. Ricketts and his associates established the transmission of the disease by means of ticks. Further contributions to our knowledge of the disease have been made by Wilson and Chowning, Fricks, Wolbach and others. Rumreich, Dyer, Badger and others have recently established the facts that there is an Eastern type of the disease, occurring along the Atlantic seabord, and that the disease is transmitted to man by the bites of infected ticks, the most important of which is the common dog tick, Dermacentor variabilis.

Etiology.—The exciting cause of the disease is a minute microorganism belonging to the Rickettsia group. It is a minute, intracellular, pleomorphic, bacterium-like organism, demonstrated best by the use of Giemsa's stain. It can be recovered from human lesions, from infected laboratory animals and from ticks. In ticks there is probably a direct transmission of the organism from one generation to another.

Geographically, two forms of the disease are now recognized—a Western type and an Eastern type. Western type: Certain localities of Idaho and Montana furnish the majority of cases, although the disease has been reported from Wyoming, Utah, Oregon, Nevada, Washington, California, Colorado and South Dakota. The small wild life of this section acts as the host for the specific tick, Dermacentor andersoni. Squirrels, chipmunks, woodchucks and weasels are known to harbor infected ticks and are susceptible to the disease. In the laboratory the disease can also be transmitted to guinea-pigs, rabbits and monkeys. Larger animals of this region, both wild and domestic, also act as animal hosts of the tick, but whether susceptible to the disease or not has not yet been determined. The majority of human cases reported occur in the spring and early summer months—March to July. Both sexes are probably equally susceptible, and the preponderance in males is due to the greater liability to tick infestation. Eastern type: Cases have been reported along the Atlantic seaboard, east of the Appalachian Mountains from New York to Georgia. The most common vector is the dog tick, Dermacentor variabilis. It occurs slightly later in the season than the Western type; the majority of cases, however, occurring in late spring and summer. Cases in men predominate, although many cases in children have been reported.

Pathology.—Enlargement of the spleen is almost a constant finding; the organ is two or three times its normal size, firm, and dark red in color. Hemorrhages into the skin and subcutaneous tissues are a striking feature. This is due to the microscopic lesions in the smaller vessels. The arteries, veins and capillaries are all involved. Large hemorrhages and necrosis of the tissues of the scrotum are also common findings. Necrosis of the skin of the vulva, face, fingers and toes has been reported.

The distinctive lesions microscopically consist of localized proliferation of the endothelium of the smaller vessels, followed by thrombosis and necrosis, which may be either mural or obliterating. There is usually some perivascular infiltration with large mononuclear cells, but not to the extent of forming nodules, as in typhus fever. The lesions differ from typhus also in the predilection for the tissues of the genitalia and the lack of involvement of the central nervous system. Terminal bronchopneumonia may be present in cases coming to autopsy.

Symptoms.—The incubation period for most cases is four to eight days, although limits of two to twelve days have been reported. After a day or two of mild prodromal symptoms consisting of malaise, anorexia, chilliness and slight evening fever, the onset is usually abrupt with a frank chill, headache and severe muscular and joint pains. The patient complains most of the pain in the lumbar muscles and in the calves of the legs and in the larger joints. Injection of the conjunctivæ, photophobia, harsh dry cough and constipation occur. The fever rises rapidly following the chill, reaching a level of 102° F. to 104° F., on the second or third day. It continues high with slight morning remissions, attaining its maximum during the second week. In cases terminating favorably, at the end of the second week, the fever begins to fall by lysis, reaching normal by the end of the third week. In fatal cases death occurs usually between the sixth and twelfth day after the onset, and may be preceded by unusually high fever. The pulse, usually strong and bounding at first, soon weakens, becomes smaller in volume, and increases in rapidity, as do the respirations, out of proportion to the height of the fever. Nervous manifestations are marked throughout the disease; hyperesthesia of the skin, restlessness, insomnia, active delirium and, finally, coma may be present.

The two outstanding objective symptoms are the presence of a palpably enlarged spleen and the characteristic eruption. The eruption may occur as early as the second day or as late as the seventh day. Its usual time of appearance is the third day. Its order of occurrence, as agreed by all observers, is somewhat characteristic. The wrists, ankles and lumbar region are first involved; later on the neck, face, arms, legs and chest. The palms, soles and scalp are last involved. The skin of the abdomen may be practically uninvolved, or if the site of eruption, it is disproportionately sparse in comparison to the remainder of the skin surface. The rash may also appear on the visible mucous membranes. The character of the eruption in the early stages is that of small, discrete, rose-red macules which disappear upon pressure. These soon change to a darker red to purple color, persist on pressure and become petechial. The lesions may remain discrete, giving the so-called "turkey-egg mottling" to the skin surface, or they may coalesce, forming hemorrhagic areas of considerable size.

In cases terminating favorably the rash begins to fade with the defervescence of the fever, leaving brown pigmented areas which may persist for some time. In severe cases necroses of the skin, especially of the external genitalia, the tips of fingers and toes, the ears and soft palate, have been observed.

A mild form of jaundice may be present during the second week of the disease. The urine contains nothing that distinguishes it from other febrile conditions. The blood shows a mild leukocytosis, usually about 12,000, with an increase in the large mononuclear elements and a decrease of the eosinophils. A moderate to severe secondary anemia develops as the disease progresses.

Diagnosis.—In children, the rash of Rocky Mountain spotted fever may simulate that of measles. In measles, however, the more gradual onset, the prominence of inflammation of the mucous membranes, the presence of Koplik's spots and the absence of leukocytosis, together with the order of involvement of the skin surface by the rash, all serve in differentiating it. Typhoid fever differs from it in the more gradual onset, the relative slowness of the pulse in comparison to the fever, the leukopenia, the positive Widal and blood culture and in the character and distribution of the rash. Cerebrospinal meningitis and Rocky Mountain spotted fever may be somewhat similar in onset. The early rigidity of the neck and the presence of Kernig's sign, the mode of development and distribution of the rash, and finally the positive spinal fluid findings in the former should suffice to differentiate them.

Prognosis.—The mortality of the disease varies greatly with the geographic area of its occurrence. In Idaho the mortality is less than 5 per cent. In the Bitter Root Valley of Montana a much higher mortality prevails, reaching 90 per cent. Intermediate degrees of mortality are present in other localities. The theory has been advanced that the difference in intermediate animal hosts of the tick may play some rôle in this marked difference in mortality. The disease in children is comparatively mild, and the seriousness of the disease increases with age. Severity of the nervous symptoms, increasing pulse and respiratory rate and sudden increase in the leukocyte count are considered of grave significance. The severity of the rash is of little prognostic importance. The mortality for the Eastern type of the disease is 25 per cent.

Prophylaxis and Treatment.—Prophylactic measures may be classified as general and individual. General measures are largely concerned in tick eradication. A laboratory at Hamilton, Montana, under the control of various state agencies in collaboration with the United States Public Health Service, has made considerable progress in this direction. Fricks lists several methods that have been investigated, some with promising results: (1) clearing and cultivation of land; (2) proper grazing laws; (3) destruction of small wild life by poison, shooting and trapping; (4) dipping domestic animals; (5) sheep grazing; (6) burning over of waste land; (7) parasitization of ticks. Individual prophylaxis consists of the use of high boots with one-piece outer garments and a repellant oily protective cuff at the wrists and neck, together with frequent inspection of the skin surface for ticks. Spencer and Parker have perfected a vaccine from a phenolized emulsion of infected ticks which has been quite successful in preventing the disease in those exposed to tick bites.

The treatment of the disease is largely symptomatic. Bed rest and careful nursing are essential. A highly nutritious bland diet with plenty of fluids is indicated. The use of hydrotherapy to control fever and relieve nervous symptoms is of distinct value. Daily evacuation of the bowels can be obtained by the use of mild laxatives or enemata. Digitalis is of service and should be started before actual signs of circulatory weakness develop.

REFERENCES.

ANDERSON, J. F.: Spotted Fever of the Rocky Mountains, Bull. No. 14, U. S. Pub. Health and Mar. Hosp. Serv., 1903.
FRICKS, L. D.: Rocky Mountain Spotted Fever, Pub. Health Rep., 1913, 1914, 1915, 1916.
MAXEY, E. E.: Some Observations on the So-called Spotted Fever of Idaho. Med. Sentinel, 1899, 8, 433.
RICKETTS, H. T.: Contributions to Medical Science, Dedicated to H. T. Ricketts, Univ. of Chicago Press, 1911.
RUMREICH, A. S.: The Typhus and Rocky Mountain Spotted Fever Group, Jour. Am. Med. Assn., 1933, 100, 331.
SPENCER, R. R., and PARKER, R. R.: Rocky Mountain Spotted Fever, U. S. Pub. Health Rep., 1925, 40, 2159.
WOLBACH, S. B.: Jour. Med. Res., 1916, 34, 121; 35, 147; 1918, 37, 499; 1919, 41, 1.

TRENCH FEVER.

Definition.—Trench fever is a specific, febrile, infectious disease communicated from man to man by the bite of the body louse, Pediculus humanus. It is characterized clinically by sudden onset, with prostration, headache, pains in the back and in the legs, hyperesthesia of the skin, enlargement of the spleen, a skin eruption and a moderate febrile course with intermissions and relapses.

History.—The disease, heretofore unrecognized as a clinical entity, was very prevalent during the World War. It derives its name from the type of warfare in vogue, which was conducive to the spread of louse-borne disease. It was chiefly reported from the Western and Eastern fronts, the Italian front and from Salonica. The Allied Armies as well as the German and Austrian troops suffered heavy morbidity from this disease. It has been estimated that one-fifth to one-third of all illness in these areas might be attributed to it. It is worthy of note that in certain areas where the disease was very prevalent during the war, it has not since reappeared among the civilian population.

Etiology.—The exciting cause of the disease has not been definitely determined, although the evidence in favor of a specific Rickettsia body as the cause, is quite convincing. Such bodies have been found in the blood, but not in the tissues of patients during the active phase of the disease. Experimentally, the disease has been reproduced in man by the bites of infected lice, by the injection of blood, dried urinary sediment and saliva of known cases and by rubbing dried lice and their excreta into skin abrasions of healthy volunteers. The organism probably undergoes a developmental cycle in the insect vector occupying a period of seven to ten days, before it is capable of transmitting the disease to man by any of the above mentioned methods.

Pathology.—Little is known of the pathologic changes in the body tissues, as the disease is not a fatal one. Perivascular lymphocytic infiltration has been demonstrated in the excised skin lesions, but endothelial necrosis and vessel thrombosis common in the lesions of typhus fever and Rocky Mountain spotted fever do not occur.

Symptoms and Course.—After an incubation period of ten to thirty days the onset is usually sudden, with chilliness or a frank chill followed by moderate fever, accelerated pulse-rate, headache, prostration and muscular pain, especially involving the lumbar region and the calves of the legs. Tenderness of the muscles involved, as well as marked tenderness over the shin bones, is a common finding. The headache is usually frontal in situation or referred to the eyeballs or just behind them, and may be accompanied by photophobia, nystagmus, injection of the conjunctivæ and lacrimation. Mild gastrointestinal symptoms—anorexia, nausea, vomiting—may be present, but are not outstanding.

The febrile course is not constant, although three main types have been described: (1) a moderate, five- to seven-day febrile period followed by a few days' intermission and a short secondary rise; (2) a single prolonged continuous fever of six or seven weeks' duration with no appreciable intermissions; (3) periods of fever followed by a five- to seven-day intermission and then alternation of febrile and afebrile periods over a period of weeks. The most marked objective findings, enlargement of the spleen and the rash, may occur as early as the second day after onset. They may both recur with the onset of a relapse. The rash consists of pink erythematous macules, usually occurring on the chest, back or abdomen and varying in size from 2 to 5 mm. in diameter. The rash occurs in about 75 per cent of cases, is transient in character, lasting from a few hours to two days, and may reappear with a relapse.

The urinalysis shows nothing distinctive and the leukocyte count is variable. A moderate leukocytosis of about 12,000 is the rule, although a normal count or a distinct leukopenia may be present. According to various British observers, disordered action of the heart (neuro circulatory asthenia) was a common sequel of the disease.

Diagnosis.—Where the disease is epidemic the diagnosis is made on the symptomatology and clinical course. There is no specific laboratory test available. It may have to be differentiated from typhoid fever, paratyphoid fever and typhus fever by their specific agglutination reactions; from malaria by finding the specific causative organisms in the blood; and from influenza by the mildness or absence of respiratory symptoms and respiratory complications.

Prognosis.—The disease is a non-fatal one. Its importance in war results from the large numbers of men unfit for active service and the frequent prolongation of their disability. Return of convalescents too soon to active duty is frequently followed by relapses and convalescents returning to louse-infested areas may disseminate the disease, as their blood remains infective for long periods.

Prophylaxis and Treatment.—Prophylaxis consists of louse control. Patients with the disease should be treated in separate wards and attendants should be protected by louse-proof garments and gloves. The skin surface of the patient should be carefully cleansed with soap and water followed by alcohol. Particular care should be paid to the hairy spots of the body. Clothing and bed clothing should be sterilized by moist heat (70° C. or above). Disinfection of urine and sputum should be carried out during the active stages of the disease.

Active treatment is solely symptomatic. Bed rest, a bland nutritious diet and the use of acetylsalicylic acid, phenacetin or codeine for the relief of pain, will add materially to the comfort of the patient. Care should be exercised to keep the patient in bed until symptom-free, and until the usual time for a relapse has passed. Resumption of physical activities should be gradual and, if relapses occur, bed rest should be again instituted.

REFERENCES.

Byam, W., *et al.:* A Report of Clinical Observations and Research as to Etiology, Pathology, Prophylaxis and Treatment of Trench Fever among Troops, Jour. Am. Med. Assn., 1918, **71**, 21–26; 110–113 and 188–192.
Graham, J. H. P.: Note on Relapsing Febrile Illness of Unknown Origin, Lancet, 1915, **93**, ii, 703.
Trench Fever: Commission Report: Medical Research Commission, American Red Cross, Oxford, 1918.

TSUTSUGAMUSHI DISEASE.

Synonyms.—Japanese river fever; Akamushi disease.

Definition.—Tsutsugamushi disease is an acute specific infectious disease, transmitted to man by the bite of an infected mite, Trombicula akamushi. It is characterized by a small ulcer at the site of inoculation, enlargement of the regional lymph nodes, a macular eruption and a continuous fever of about two or three weeks' duration.

Etiology.—The specific causative agent has not been definitely determined, but the available evidence points to a specific Rickettsia. Sellards has been able to culture an organism which morphologically and in other respects is similar to the Rickettsia. The disease occurs chiefly in certain parts of Japan, although a milder form of the disease may be present in Formosa, Sumatra, and the Malay Peninsula. With the subsidence of the swollen streams, following spring and early summer rains, the akamushi mite appears. This mite, in the larval stage of its developmental cycle, attaches itself to some mammal, particularly the vole or water rat, and sucks its blood. The virus of tsutsugamushi is transmitted hereditarily in this mite. The disease can be transmitted to monkeys, either by the bites of infected mites or by the injection of infected blood, with the development of rather characteristic symptoms. It can also be passed through guinea-pigs without the production of any symptoms. Human beings exposed to the bite of an infected mite develop a small sharply defined ulcer at the site within a few days.

Symptoms and Course.—After an incubation period of about seven days, the onset is abrupt with headache, malaise and rapid rise of temperature. The regional lymph glands become enlarged and tender; toward the end of the first week generalized enlargement of the lymph glands occurs. The fever curve is a continuous, moderately high one (103° to 105° F.) of about two weeks' duration, declining by rapid lysis. Enlargement of the spleen is usually present. The eruption of a red maculo-papular variety—somewhat similar to that of typhus fever—appears at the end of the first week, reaches its maximum in a few days and fades before the decline in fever. Some of the spots may become petechial. Cough and active delirium may be present in the more severe cases. At the height of the disease there is a distinct leukopenia. One attack affords partial, but probably not complete immunity.

In Japan, the mortality varies in different places and in different epidemics, but as a rule is high (10 to 60 per cent). The seriousness of the disease increases with age. In Formosa the disease is milder and the mortality lower (5 to 10 per cent).

There is no specific treatment. Cauterization of the original bite should be employed.

REFERENCES.

KAWAMURA, R.: Studies on Tsutsugamushi Disease, Med. Bull., Coll. Med., Univ. of Cincinnati, 1926, **4**, 1.

SELLARDS, A. W.: The Cultivation of a Rickettsia-like Microörganism from Tsutsugamushi Disease, Am. Jour. Trop. Med., 1923, **3**, 529.

CHAPTER V.

DISEASES DUE TO SPIROCHETES.

By ALAN M. CHESNEY, M.D.

Syphilis.	Relapsing Fever.
Yaws.	Epidemic Jaundice.
Rat-bite Fever.	

General Considerations.—The term "spirochete" is rather loosely applied to a number of different organisms that have at least one thing in common, namely, that their shape is that of an elongated spiral. The nomenclature of this group of organisms is in an unsatisfactory state, and their precise position among minute living organisms is not yet definitely settled. Some regard them as bacteria, others as protozoa, while still others would place them in a special group midway between bacteria and protozoa.

Of the spirochetes pathogenic for man there are recognized, following the nomenclature of Noguchi, three varieties: (1) treponema, (2) spironema, (3) leptospira. Treponemes are the cause of syphilis, yaws, and Japanese rat-bite fever. Spironemes cause relapsing fever, and leptospiras cause epidemic jaundice (Weil's disease). For a while it was supposed that a particular leptospira, Leptospira icteroides, was the cause of yellow fever, but this disease is now believed to be due to a filterable virus.

Of the diseases mentioned above, syphilis is by all odds the most widespread and the most important. The others are quite uncommon in the continental portion of the United States. Yaws is common in tropical regions but extremely rare in the temperate zone. Rat-bite fever, relapsing fever and epidemic jaundice are more common in other countries of the temperate zone than in the United States.

SYPHILIS.

Synonym.—Lues.

Definition.—A chronic relapsing infection due to a particular species of spirochete, Treponema pallidum, characterized by widespread involvement of the tissues of the body and not infrequently leading to permanent anatomic damage or even death.

History.—The disease has been well known since the early part of the sixteenth century. Two schools of opinion as to its origin and antiquity have developed, the one believing that it occurred in Europe prior to the discovery of America, the other holding that it was unknown in Europe until after 1492, and that it was introduced into Europe from America by some of Columbus' returning sailors. Opinion upon this point is not yet settled. It is certain that syphilis spread rapidly through western Europe in the last years of the fifteenth and the early part of the sixteenth century. Hundreds of different names were applied to it, of which syphilis, lues venerea and pox are the principal ones which have come down to us. The frequent transmission of syphilis by sexual intercourse was not at first recognized; later the disease became confused with gonorrhea and soft chancre, but was finally separated from these infections as a result of accurate clinical observation, largely through the efforts of Bell in England, and Ricord and his pupils in France. The discovery of the causal agent by Schaudinn and Hoffman in 1905, the introduction of the complement-fixation test by Wassermann, Neisser and Bruck at about the same time, and the introduction, by Ehrlich and Hata, in 1909, of arsphenamine as a therapeutic agent in the treatment of the disease, represent important and more recent milestones in the history of this infection.

Incidence.—Reliable figures as to the exact incidence of syphilis in the general population are unfortunately rare or non-existent. It is an exceedingly widespread disease, more so than many physicians realize. Recent (1926 to 1930) one-day surveys of cities in the United States with populations over 700,000 revealed that from 4 to 10.9 cases per 1000 of population were under treatment for syphilis on a given date. The highest rates were encountered in the southern cities with large negro populations. In a large general hospital from 5 to 25 per cent of the patients may be shown to be affected. One-half or more of all prostitutes will have acquired the infection during their active professional careers. In negroes the infection is from four to five times as common as among whites. In general the disease is more common in males than in females, although the difference in incidence in the two sexes varies with different social groups.

Because of its tendency, if not properly treated, to result in grave anatomic damage to the cardiovascular or central nervous systems, syphilis is an economic factor of the first importance. Insurance statistics show that the normal expectancy of life is reduced in syphilitics by one-third. Stokes has estimated the cost of syphilis to the United States at $5,000,000,000 annually.

Etiology.—The causal agent of the disease is the Treponema pallidum, a delicate spiral organism 5 to 15 microns in length, with from 6 to 10 turns, all arranged in regular fashion. The organism rotates actively on its long axis and is extremely flexible. It does not survive drying or exposure to the common disinfectants. It is difficult to stain and is best examined by the aid of the indirect system of illumination afforded by the dark-field microscope. It cannot be grown on ordinary bacteriologic media; Noguchi claimed to have grown it, using special anaërobic methods, but this is now doubted by some. If virulent strains of Treponema pallidum have ever been successfully cultivated, the instances have been few in number as compared with the many unsuccessful attempts. Nothing definite is known concerning a complicated life-cycle of the organism, although more recently it has been urged by some workers that the organism assumes forms which are different from the typical spiral form and may constitute stages in a life-cycle. Some of the anthropoid apes can be infected with this organism. Rabbits are easily infected and show characteristic lesions; guinea-pigs and mice may be infected, but the latter do not develop lesions.

Transmission.—The disease is usually transmitted from human being to human being by direct and intimate contact, although it may be transmitted by indirect contact, as by handling infected utensils or linen, or by drinking from the same cup. The percentage of infections occurring in this manner is low, but the knowledge that infection may occur by some such means has been a matter of great comfort to many patients, and has often enough provided a satisfying explanation for the source of the infection and prevented the disruption of a family.

While in nearly all cases of syphilis in adults the infection is acquired through the act of sexual intercourse, still the total number of cases in which the disease is acquired through other means of direct contact, notably kissing, remains surprisingly high. This fact is perhaps not appreciated as it should be, even by physicians.

Syphilis may also be transmitted from the mother to the offspring *in utero*, in which case the result may be either a dead syphilitic fetus, or a living syphilitic infant. The term congenital syphilis is applied to this form of the disease. It is doubtful if direct infection of the ovum by spirochetes from the father occurs, although the possibility exists.

Clinical evidence has shown that syphilis may be transmitted from one person to another by sexual intercourse years after the infection was acquired, even without any superficial manifestations of the disease being present, and the semen of latent syphilitics has been shown by animal experimentation to contain virulent treponemes. It is evident, then, that the person with latent syphilis is a menace, and it is the writer's opinion that such a person plays a greater rôle in the transmission of the infection than is generally recognized.

General Course of the Infection.—There is no infectious disease which has as many different manifestations as syphilis, and there is scarcely any organ or tissue of the body which is not susceptible of involvement, although some bear the brunt more than others. It is this great diversity in the manifestations of the disease which makes it impossible to describe its natural history in a few brief paragraphs, and which led Osler to state his well-known aphorism, " Know syphilis in all its manifestations and relations and all things clinical will be added unto you."

The more common course of events in the acquired form of the disease is as follows. After an incubation period of from three to six weeks (four weeks on an average), a small papule appears at the portal of entry. This lesion increases in size, becomes eroded, the edges and base harden and a full-blown primary lesion or chancre is finally formed. The regional lymph nodes become enlarged and firm. The chancre does not heal promptly unless treated, but even without treatment it will heal after a period of several weeks.

After the initial lesion heals there follows a period, variable in length but lasting usually from four to eight weeks, during which there is an apparent quiescence of the disease. This quiescence is more apparent than real, however, for general invasion of the body by the parasite by way of lymphatics and the blood stream is taking place, and the groundwork is being laid for further disease manifestations. The general dissemination of the organism throughout the body is, as a rule, followed by the appearance of manifestations of the disease at the site of localization of the spirochetes. The most common manifestations at this stage are skin and mucous membrane lesions, joint pains, general glandular enlargement, iritis, and a positive Wassermann reaction. Involvement of the central nervous system may occur at this time, but rarely is there evidence of involvement of the thoracic and abdominal viscera. The lesions at this stage are not usually destructive or painful, and will heal spontaneously if given time. The constitutional symptoms are surprisingly mild when one considers that an intense spirochetemia must prevail at this period.

Following the disappearance of these secondary lesions, as they are called, there usually ensues a long interval, known as the latent period, during which, although the infection is still present and the serologic tests remain positive, there are no active clinical manifestations of the disease. Then, perhaps after a period of many years, there occurs a relapse, the disease for some unknown reason becomes active again, new lesions develop which differ from the earlier lesions in that now they are destructive and mutilating in character and have a tendency to involve important parts of the body, as for example the central nervous, cardiovascular and osseous systems. This, the so-called tertiary period, may be fraught with the gravest danger to the patient, and it is in this period that the tendency of the disease to show the utmost diversity is revealed. The skin, mucous membranes, bones, heart, aorta, brain, spinal cord, eye, liver and testis are the most common sites of late lesions of syphilis, but no tissue seems to be wholly exempt, and the resulting symptoms will depend upon the extent to which the various structures are involved.

Some writers like to divide the course of syphilis into precise periods, or stages, and recognize (1) the first incubation period, (2) the primary stage, (3) the second incubation period, (4) the secondary period, (5) the latent period, (6) the tertiary period and even (7) the quaternary period, this term being applied to that stage in which advanced lesions of the central nervous system such as paresis and tabes occur. To the writer, separation of the infection into so many periods seems unnecessary even for descriptive purposes, and a simpler division into three stages, (1) early, (2) latent and (3) late, is to be preferred.

While the foregoing account represents, in a general way, what transpires in most cases of acquired syphilis, it is important to remember that in a great many patients the course of the disease varies markedly from that which has been described. The primary lesions may be insignificant or absent altogether, the secondary lesions may be few in number or many, they may appear quite early or be delayed for months, they may relapse again and again, or they may never occur at all. The late lesions may be few or many, relatively benign or very malignant. Or again, some cases may run an entirely silent course, and the existence of syphilis never be suspected until one day a laboratory reports a positive Wassermann test or a baby is born with unmistakable signs of congenital syphilis, indicating that the mother is infected. It is this extreme degree of variation in the course of syphilis which makes one hesitate to say that there is any one clinical picture of the disease.

The congenital form is likewise apt to show great variation. In general, three things may happen when syphilis is transmitted from mother to offspring. The pregnancy may result in a still-birth, or in a baby with manifest signs of syphilis, or in a child apparently well at birth but who, later in life, will exhibit deformities or disorders associated with congenital syphilis. Sometimes the presence of a positive Wassermann test will be the only indication of the existence of the congenital form of the infection, and in such instances only a survey of other members of the family will establish the fact that it is parental in origin.

In congenital syphilis the tissues most commonly invaded are the skin, liver, bones, lungs, adrenals, eyes and internal ear. Of interest are the disturbances of the cornea (interstitial keratitis) and of the teeth (Hutchinsonian teeth) which are observed in later life and of which more will be said later.

Pathology.—Infection by the virus of syphilis may take place through minute abrasions of the skin or mucous membranes. Whether an abrasion of either of these structures is essential for human infection to occur is not definitely known, but animal experimentation has demonstrated that infection can take place through mucosal surfaces that are intact to the naked eye. Dissemination of the organisms from the portal of entry occurs early in the course of the infection, and takes place by way of the lymphatics. By the time the primary lesion appears at the site of inoculation the regional lymph nodes have already been invaded. Syphilis, therefore, should never be regarded as merely a local disease.

A better appreciation of the morbid anatomy and, indeed, of the symptomatology of the disease may be had if one remembers that for some unknown reason the Treponema pallidum, unlike the various cocci, is not a pus-producing organism. It does not call forth large numbers of polymorphonuclear leukocytes, relatively speaking, and does not lead to the formation of abscesses. The cells which predominate in syphilitic lesions are lymphocytes, plasma cells and large mononuclears. Moreover, the presence of Treponema pallidum seems to incite to the proliferation of fibroblasts, which, together with the dense round-cell accumulation, doubtless accounts, in part at least, for the hardness to touch that one so often encounters when feeling syphilitic lesions. Another characteristic is that the lesions of syphilis heal slowly in the absence of treatment. The body apparently cannot react to the treponema in such a way as to bring about a prompt disappearance of the organism and resolution of the inflammatory process. The reasons for this state of affairs are not clearly understood. The natural result, however, is a chronic process, and all the individual lesions of syphilis exhibit this chronicity.

The first manifestation of the disease, the *chancre*, begins as a papule, but soon shows necrosis of the epithelium so that a shallow ulcer is formed, the edges and base of which are firm to the touch. The lesion as a whole is elevated and does not dig deeply into the surrounding tissue unless there is secondary infection. Histologic examination of the lesion will show an accumulation of lymphocytes, plasma cells and mononuclear cells, proliferation of fibroblasts and the formation of new capillaries. The lymphocytes and plasma cells are distributed compactly about the smaller blood-vessels and lymphatics, so much so that this arrangement has been likened to a coat sleeve investing an arm. Thickening of the intima of the blood-vessels is observed and new blood-vessels are formed. The cellular infiltration does not subside promptly, but may persist for weeks if untreated. Ultimately it heals and usually leaves behind a tell-tale thickened scar which is frequently of great service in diagnosis.

The *lesions of the secondary stage* are in reality small focal inflammatory reactions arising at the spots where the treponemes come to rest. The reaction may be little more than a localized dilatation of blood-vessels with the presence of a few white cells, in which case it will appear to the eye as a pinkish spot (macule), fading on pressure. If the reaction is more marked and the cellular infiltration becomes greater, a circumscribed elevation of the skin ensues and a papule is formed which can be felt with the fingers. Such a papule may spread peripherally, healing in the center, thus forming a ring, and several such rings may combine to form bizarre patterns. Occasionally the reaction may be frankly pustular, although this is unusual. Except in the pustular form, the reaction is chiefly mononuclear in character. Papules located in warm moist areas, as the perineum and axillæ, tend to be large, broad, flat structures (*condylomata lata*). Early syphilitic lesions, the chancre excepted, almost always heal without scar formation, but not infrequently they leave pigmentary changes. These changes may be of the nature of deposition of pigment, on the one hand, or removal of pigment, on the other.

The *tertiary or late lesions* may for the sake of convenience be classified into two groups. One of these is the more circumscribed lesion that goes by the name of *gumma*, the other is the diffuse process which may be designated syphilitic granulation tissue.

The gumma, probably less frequently encountered now than formerly, derives its name from its rubber-like consistency. The central portion is composed of necrotic tissue, which is firm and somewhat elastic to the touch. Surrounding this area of necrosis is an accumulation of epithelioid cells, wandering cells and lymphocytes. Giant cells are found, but less frequently than in tuberculosis. Gummata vary in size from miliary lesions to nodules several centimeters in diameter. When they heal they leave scars.

The other type of late lesion results from a diffuse infiltration of the tissues with lymphocytes and wandering cells and a proliferation of the connective-tissue elements so that a species of granulation tissue is formed. The blood-vessels of the vicinity will show thickening of the endothelium and not infrequently thrombosis. This syphilitic granulation tissue heals even without treatment, and in doing so is apt to leave diffuse scarring and distortion of the parenchyma. It is this mutilation of important parenchymatous organs, either through direct involvement by the syphilitic process itself, or through changes secondary to syphilitic involvement of the arteries, which makes the late lesions of syphilis so dangerous to the individual. According to Warthin, this type of lesion occurs much more frequently than gum-

14

mata, and is therefore the more characteristic lesion of the late stage of syphilis. Unquestionably it is of the utmost importance because of its tendency to involve vital structures.

The late lesions of syphilis exhibit the greatest variety in their extent and locale and, therefore, in the resulting clinical manifestations. When they involve the skin they may range all the way from small purplish red, innocent-looking nodules, to extensive ulcers that cause great disfigurations. In the mouth they may give rise to perforation of the soft parts or even destruction of portions of the naso-palatal skeleton, so that the bridge of the nose gives way and that feature is flattened out against the face. The bones of the skull or of the extremities may become involved and show circumscribed areas where the bony substance is lost altogether. If the syphilitic process involves the central nervous system, lesions of the meninges, of the vessels, or of the parenchyma, or indeed of all three, may occur, resulting in the greatest diversity of clinical manifestations, of which hemiplegias, ataxias and mental deterioration are among the best known. The tendency of the late lesions of syphilis to attack the aorta and the leaflets of the aortic valve is well established, resulting in incompetency of the aortic valve or in aortitis and aortic aneurysm. The myocardium may be involved, leading to serious alterations in its function. Of the abdominal viscera the liver is by far the organ most commonly attacked. Here the lesions may take the form of gummata or of a diffuse cirrhotic process. Syphilitic lesions of the stomach and intestines are surprisingly uncommon, although syphilis is thought by many surgeons to be one of the principal causes of stricture of the rectum. The testes are often affected but the ovaries, according to Warthin, seem to escape the syphilitic process almost altogether.

The essentially destructive character of the late lesions of syphilis, as distinguished from the early lesions, which are not destructive, has been a matter for considerable speculation. Since the spirochetes have been difficult to demonstrate in late lesions, and therefore have been presumed to be few in number in them, the natural assumption to explain the destructiveness of these lesions has been that the tissue becomes more sensitive to the organism as time goes on, and finally reaches a stage where it is capable of reacting in a maximal fashion to a minimal stimulus. The name "Umstimmung" was given by Neisser to this change in the reacting capacity of the tissues; it is obviously another word for "allergy."

One encounters an occasional case in which the early lesions are destructive in character; in these cases the skin lesions consist of large ulcerations with heaped up, oyster shell-like crusts. Such cases are called malignant syphilis. They are not due to increased virulence of the infecting organisms, but in reality represent a precocious tendency on the part of the tissues of the host to react to the syphilitic virus in an exaggerated (allergic) fashion.

The lesions of congenital syphilis are not inherently different from those of the acquired form, although perhaps, if anything, more extensive. For some reason the fetus seems to be a particularly favorable medium for the growth of the treponemes, and may be invaded to such an extent that it is killed outright, or, if death does not occur *in utero,* such destruction of the parenchymatous organs (especially lungs and liver) may take place, followed by replacement with connective tissue, that the infant survives but a short while after birth. It is not uncommon to see at birth, or shortly thereafter, extensive involvement of the skin in the form of large blisters or ulcerations, involving especially the palms, soles and buttocks. The epiphyseal lines of the long bones are often involved, a syphilitic osteochondritis being produced. Lesions of the lips are frequent, producing fissures and later scars at the angles of the mouth. Hardly any tissue or organ is exempt from attack. In later life the patient may exhibit recurring attacks of interstitial keratitis or malformations of the teeth, of which the best known are those described by Hutchinson. Histologically, the lesions of congenital syphilis, as in the acquired form of the disease, are characterized by an infiltration of lymphocytes, plasma cells and wandering cells, together with the proliferation of fibroblasts and the formation of new connective tissue. Extensive scarring is the rule.

Symptoms and Diagnosis.—The diagnosis of syphilis is sometimes easy, but again may be very difficult, and may call for the exhibition of all the clinical skill that the physician possesses and for all the information that can be brought to bear. One must rely upon the history, the examination and the laboratory. The latter is an extremely important aid in diagnosis, although some feel that nowadays there is a tendency for too much reliance to be placed upon the outcome of the laboratory tests, particularly if they are negative. A critical evaluation of the history and a thorough examination of the patient should not be replaced by any known test, however helpful the latter may be. Most important is it that the examiner should know what syphilis can do, and that he should be on the lookout for it. It may be that at times, in order to make the diagnosis certain, the therapeutic test will have to be used. This consists in giving an antisyphilitic drug and observing its effect upon the lesions.

Much has been written of the value of the history in making a diagnosis of syphilis, but in the opinion of the writer its value has been over-estimated. Certainly, an absence of a history of the early manifestations of syphilis carries little weight. The Wassermann reaction has taught us that there are many individuals with syphilis from whom no history of early manifestations can be elicited, and this is not due, in the majority of cases, the writer is convinced, to an attempt on the part of the patient to deceive the physician, but is due to the fact that either there were no early manifestations of the disease, or else they were so insignificant that they escaped the attention of the patient and might easily have escaped that of more careful observers. This is notoriously the state of affairs in central nervous system syphilis, and it may be pointed out that the behavior of the experimental infection supports this contention.

Early Manifestations.—The initial lesion, the chancre, is usually a single, eroded, elevated area of the skin or mucous membrane, about 1 to 1.5 cm. in diameter, with distinctly indurated edges and base, the induration being sharply circumscribed so that the lesion feels like a button and can be easily picked up and moved about over the loose underlying tissue. If a crust is present, a clean raw surface will be exposed on removal of it, in contrast to the dirty, ragged, greenish-yellow necrotic base which a chancroid presents. The chancre is characteristically painless or only slightly so. Intraurethral chancres can be discovered by palpation of the urethra. Examination of the regional lymph nodes will reveal discrete, painless, indurated swollen nodes, the typical syphilitic *buboes*, and the lymphatics can frequently be palpated as firm cords extending from the chancre to the nodes.

While the typical Hunterian chancre is relatively easy to recognize, a positive diagnosis should not be made without demonstrating the presence of Treponema pallidum in serum from the lesion. Since so many chancres are not typical in appearance, particularly in the early stages, and their true nature often not suspected, search for the treponemes is all the more necessary in the case of doubtful or non-characteristic lesions appearing on the genitalia and elsewhere, particularly those that do not heal promptly. Any lesion on the genitalia and many on the lips should be suspected of being syphilitic until proved otherwise.

Demonstration of treponemes is not particularly difficult if the proper apparatus is available. The suspected lesion should be cleansed by simple washing until the crust and all contaminating material has been removed. By gentle pressure serum can be expressed from the deeper layers and will appear as little pools on the exposed surface of the lesion. It is a simple matter to convey this material to a slide and examine it with the aid of the dark-field microscope. Care should be taken to avoid excessive bleeding and the use of antiseptics. A physician not equipped to carry out the procedure should refer his patient to someone who can. He does not do his full duty by his patient if he relies upon clinical examination alone in the diagnosis of lesions suspected of being chancres. This point cannot be over-emphasized. Moreoever, a single negative test proves nothing. Repeated examinations should be made, especially if the patient has been using antiseptics, and patients with suspected lesions in which the Treponema pallidum cannot be found should be observed at regular and frequent intervals for weeks and even months for other possible manifestations of the disease, such as the outbreak of generalized lesions, or the occurrence of a positive Wassermann reaction.

The Wassermann test, or one of the newer precipitation tests (Meinicke, Sachs-Georgi, Kahn, Klein, Hinton, Eagle) may be of help, but all are frequently negative in the earlier weeks of the chancre. The history may be helpful in arousing the suspicions of the physician, but often enough it is confirmatory only and not decisive.

Cutaneous Reactions.—The early skin manifestations are extremely varied. They may be single or multiple (more often multiple) and may simulate those of a number of other diseases. They are usually general in their distribution and vary in their shape. As a rule they do not itch, at least to the extent that they cause the patient to scratch, and they are not painful. The most common forms are the macular and papular syphilides.

The *macular rash* is usually widespread, best seen on the trunk, especially the abdomen, and consists of pinkish or reddish spots which tend to become copper colored. At the outset they may require the closest scrutiny for their detection and may be overlooked if the patient is not examined by daylight. They may leave brownish areas of pigmentation on healing, or again may lead to the disappearance of the normal pigment, so that one may encounter dark spots on a light background or light spots on a dark background.

The *papular rash* is often widespread, frequently shows a tendency to grouping when profuse, and may exhibit marked lichenification and scaling. The papules are often closely associated with the hair follicles. The larger papules are apt to be oval in outline, arranged with their long axes parallel and following the lines of the ribs (the so-called "lines of cleavage" of the skin). It is not uncommon to find a few papules only on the face or genitalia, and sometimes these spread peripherally while healing in the center, giving rise to the ring-like (annular) variety of syphilide, so common in negroes. If several such rings occur close to one another they may coincide to form patterns with scalloped edges.

Papules developing in warm moist areas, where skin surfaces are in contact, as the axilla, perineum, female genitalia, are apt to be broad flat affairs with grayish surface due to the maceration of the superficial layers of the epithelium. Such papules are called *condylomata lata* and are to be distinguished from condylomata acuminata, which are not syphilitic in origin.

Pustular syphilides occur but they are less common than the macular and papular forms. Their differentiation from the lesions of smallpox is not always easy. They are more common in negroes than in whites.

Mucous Membrane Reactions.—The mucous patch is the characteristic early lesion of the mucous surfaces. It is an eroded inflamed area, frequently covered with a thin whitish or grayish membrane composed principally of macerated epithelium. Mucous patches do not form ulcers. They give rise to surprisingly little pain, and are commonly located on the tonsils, pillars, buccal mucous membranes and inner surfaces of the lips. Diffuse syphilitic inflammation of the pharynx and tonsils without membrane formation may occur.

Hair.—Patchy or general falling out of the hair is of fairly frequent occurrence.

Joint Reactions.—Symptoms referable to the joints are quite common in early syphilis. These take the form of joint pains, worse at night, or those of an actual arthritis, in which case the joints may be swollen, red and painful, with effusion of fluid into the joint cavity. The joints of early syphilitic arthritis, however, are never as angry as in cases of suppurative arthritis, and they heal without ankylosis.

Eye Reactions.—Involvement of the uveal tract is by no means uncommon in early syphilis. The presence of an exudate on the iris, a contracted pupil, and engorgement of the pericorneal vessels, should always lead one to suspect the presence of a syphilitic iritis. Lesions of the choroid and retina are much less common in early syphilis.

Lymph Nodes.—Enlargement of the lymph nodes is the rule. The nodes are hard, discrete and not usually painful. General glandular enlargement is the most common single manifestation of early syphilis.

Constitutional Symptoms.—The constitutional symptoms of early syphilis are surprisingly slight, in view of the overwhelming spirochetemia which must occur in so many instances. Cases with fever have been described, but the average case is afebrile, or at most shows only one or two degrees (Fahrenheit) elevation of temperature. Vague aches and pains, slight malaise, slight loss of appetite or a feeling of being generally below par, are about all that are complained of. Many patients with outspoken early syphilis will, upon questioning, insist that they feel entirely well.

Central Nervous System.—The central nervous system is invaded by the treponemes early in the course of the disease in a great many instances, but in most of these cases there are no clinical signs of nervous system involvement, and the brain and spinal cord seem to have escaped permanent injury. In a small number, however, invasion is followed by reaction so that a meningitis or a meningo-myelitis is set up, and in that case there will be observed the general signs and symptoms of meningitis (headache, drowsiness, stiff neck, positive Kernig sign) plus the special signs referable to those portions of the nervous system (cranial nerve palsies) which are involved in the process. This type of reaction is most often encountered in patients who have not carried out their treatment continuously during the early phases of the disease. To it the term "neurorecurrence" or "neurorecidive" is given. In general, the symptoms of syphilitic meningitis are less stormy than those of meningitis due to other microörganisms, and the signs of meningeal irritation are less marked. At times the meningeal symptoms may be absent altogether and only examination of the spinal fluid will reveal the presence of a syphilitic meningitis.

Viscera.—Although there is every reason to suppose that the viscera do not escape invasion by the treponemes during the period of early spirochetemia, definite clinical manifestation of such involvement is at most rare. It is true that jaundice does occur early in the course of the disease but it is a comparatively infrequent event at this period in untreated patients.

Serologic Reactions.—It is in the period of early generalized lesions that the serologic tests are of greatest value. Here they are almost 100 per cent positive. While the discovery of a positive Wassermann reaction in a patient with a generalized cutaneous eruption does not necessarily mean that the rash is syphilitic in nature, it is strong presumptive evidence that such is the case. On the other hand, the occurrence of a negative serologic test in a patient with a generalized skin rash is very strong evidence that the rash is *not* syphilitic. Negative serologic tests are of greatest diagnostic value, therefore, in the presence of generalized eruptions.

Latent Period.—The diagnosis of latent syphilis can only be made at the present time by the use of laboratory tests. If repeated examinations of the blood reveal a positive Wassermann reaction, a diagnosis of latent syphilis may be ventured. This statement applies, of course,

to the temperate zone. In the tropics the situation is different because
of the occurrence of diseases other than syphilis which give rise to a
positive Wassermann reaction. Of these, yaws is the most frequent.
The reliability of the newer precipitation tests in the diagnosis of
latent syphilis has not been finally established, although they will
probably be found to give substantially the same results as the Wassermann reaction. The growing practice of requiring routine Wassermann
tests on all patients has revealed how many syphilitic individuals
there are in whom one can find no evidence of the disease save, perhaps, moderate enlargement of the lymph nodes. A study by Turner
of 10,000 consecutive cases in an ambulatory syphilis clinic showed
that about one-third of them belonged in the category "latent,"
another third were cases of early syphilis, and the remaining third
were late cases with manifestations. More latent cases will be found
in women than in men. It is thought by some that pregnancy is an
important causal factor in this connection, tending to suppress syphilitic disease phenomena in the woman and to make the course of the
infection milder.

Late Manifestations.—*Cutaneous Reactions.*—The late cutaneous
lesions of syphilis are extremely varied and may be relatively insignificant in appearance, but very significant in diagnostic importance,
since they may point the way to a correct diagnosis in the face of a
negative serologic test. While many different types of late skin
lesions have been described, resulting in a very complicated nomenclature, the differences are really superficial and do not rest upon pathologic processes which are inherently different. One may recognize
the simple nodular form, the nodulo-ulcerative type, and the gumma.
The nodular type may, of course, develop into either the ulcero-
nodular form or the gumma.

In general the late skin lesions of syphilis are not numerous, as
compared with the early lesions. They are indolent, that is, they look
like discrete low-grade inflammatory processes, with a bluish-red discoloration of the skin, and are not painful, as a rule, in spite of the
destructive character which they frequently assume. The nodules
are infiltrated and when they coalesce they tend to form lesions with
borders composed of many arcs of a circle. This polycyclic or scalloped border is an important diagnostic point. On the upper extremities they are usually found symmetrically distributed on the extensor
surfaces, but asymmetrical distribution is certainly the rule elsewhere.
When ulceration takes place the margin is usually clean-cut and the
ulcer has what is often described as a "punched out" appearance.
When the lesions heal they leave scars, as a rule, which are often
covered with thin epithelium and may or may not be pigmented.

The differentiation of syphilitic ulcers occurring on the legs from
ulcers due to other conditions, such as varicose veins, is by no means
easy if one relies upon the appearance of the lesion alone. Frequently
one has to determine by roentgen-ray if there is an underlying syphilitic periostitis of the tibia, or make use of the therapeutic test, before
arriving at a definite diagnosis. In no domain of syphilis is the thera-

peutic test of greater help than in the recognition of the late cutaneous lesions.

Bone and Joint Reactions.—The late lesions involving the bones may take the form of diffuse or circumscribed areas of periostitis, gumma-like lesions involving the cortex or medulla, or both, either with new bone formation or with actual destruction of bone. Syphilitic periostitis in its early stages is accompanied by swelling, pain worse at night, tenderness and some local heat and redness. The tibiæ are the bones most frequently involved. Palpation will reveal a thickening and roughening of the bone, and roentgen-ray examination will reveal more minutely the extent and character of the change. Gummatous lesions involving the shaft of the bone usually present themselves as more or less sharply circumscribed areas of swelling which are usually moderately painful and tender. The overlying skin is commonly reddened and, if the process is allowed to go untreated, may break down to form an ulcer. The skull, clavicles, sternum and tibiæ are the bones most commonly affected in this type of lesion. Careful roentgenograms of the skeleton will usually reveal that more than one bone is involved.

Late syphilitic disease of the joints is more apt to be monarticular, or at most only a few joints are involved. While the swelling of the joint may be marked, pain and tenderness and local heat are not present to an equivalent extent, and the syphilitic joint may simulate even closely the tuberculous variety. Roentgen-ray examination of the neighboring bones, if it shows a periostitis, will indicate the true nature of the joint process. The knees are the joints most commonly involved.

Cardiac Reactions.—Under this term are included lesions of the myocardium, the valves and the aorta. Myocarditis due to syphilis is much less common than the rheumatic fever variety, but unquestionably does occur. There are no signs which may be said to stamp the condition as syphilitic in origin, but the relatively sudden occurrence of the classical signs of heart failure (dyspnea, enlargement of the heart, tachycardia, passive congestion of the viscera and edema) in an individual without hypertension, arteriosclerosis, kidney disease or a history of acute rheumatic fever, should lead one to suspect the presence of syphilis as the causal factor.

Of greater frequency, by far, is the occurrence of syphilitic disease of the aorta and the aortic valve. Symptoms of aortic involvement may occur as early as three years after the infection is acquired. It is about three times as prevalent in negroes as in whites. Important early symptoms of aortic involvement are shortness of breath and substernal pain, both paroxysmal in character and prone to occur at night, at times extremely distressing so that the pains resemble those of true angina pectoris. Examination at this time is apt to reveal some increase in the size of the heart, increased dulness beneath the manubrium on percussion, and an increase in the intensity of the aortic second sound which takes on a ringing, bell-like note. Roentgen-ray examination may or may not reveal dilatation of the aortic arch. Later, when the disease involves the leaflets of the aortic valve to such an extent that they become incompetent, massive hypertrophy of the heart ensues, and examination will reveal the classical physical signs of aortic insufficiency.

Abnormalities of rhythm of the graver sort, such as auricular fibrillation, are rare in syphilitic cardiac disease. This is of considerable diagnostic importance. Of course, gummata involving the conducting mechanism will give rise to abnormalities of rhythm, and cases of Stokes-Adams syndrome (paroxysms of unconsciousness associated with heart block) due to syphilis have been described, but in general, abnormalities of rhythm are much less common in syphilitic than in rheumatic heart disease.

When aneurysm of the aorta follows syphilitic aortitis the symptoms and signs are those resulting from the slow and steady growth of an expansile tumor within a restricted and already crowded space. The condition involves the thoracic portions of the aorta more frequently than the abdominal portion.[1]

Central Nervous System Reactions.—The late manifestations of syphilis of the central nervous system may be referred to involvement of either the meninges, the vessels, or the parenchyma, or any combination of these three divisions of that system. Pure meningeal involvement is probably rare at this stage. It is much more apt to be accompanied by lesions of the vessels or of the parenchyma, a meningomyelitis, either diffuse or circumscribed, being the most common combination. Isolated gummata are less common.

The symptoms of late syphilis of the central nervous system fall into two categories, (1) those which occur with such frequency and uniformity as to constitute definite clinical entities, easily recognizable as such, as for example paresis, tabes dorsalis, optic atrophy, and (2) those which are so indefinite or vary from one another to such an extent that it is difficult to separate them into definite clinical entities. The great variability of this latter group is due, of course, to the fact that the underlying lesions are most often multiple and diffuse, and also to the complexity of the anatomy and physiology of the central nervous system. The recognition that the symptoms belonging in this category are of syphilitic origin must often rest upon the results of an examination of the blood and spinal fluid, or their response to a therapeutic test, rather than upon the character of the symptoms themselves, or their association. For example, a gumma of the brain will give rise to the same symptoms of increased intracranial pressure as will a glioma located in the same area. Again, a cranial nerve palsy resulting from syphilis will give rise to local symptoms that are in no way different from those resulting if the same nerve is injured by other agencies. The important thing to realize is that the symptoms of syphilitic disease of the central nervous system may be extremely varied and are frequently so indefinite in the early stages that one must resort to the examination of the spinal fluid to establish their syphilitic etiology.

Although these symptoms are varied and often indefinite, they may, for the sake of convenience, be divided into two groups, (1) the general

---

[1] For a detailed discussion of the symptoms and physical signs the reader is referred to the chapter on Diseases of the Heart.

and (2) the local. The more common general symptoms are headache, "nervousness," fatigability and vague aches and pains. Drowsiness and even coma may be present in the more severe cases. The local symptoms, as already indicated, will be most varied, depending upon the location of the lesion. Paralyses of cranial nerves, monoplegias, hemiplegias and disturbances of sensation are the more prominent features encountered on examination. One of the earliest signs of syphilitic involvement of the nervous system is a slowing or a disappearance of the reaction of the pupil to light (Argyll-Robertson pupil). Not infrequently this is the only clue to the existence of syphilitic nervous disease that examination gives. Careful scrutiny of the pupils, therefore, constitutes a most important part of the physical examination of syphilitic patients.

While it is of the utmost importance to recognize cases of neurosyphilis as soon as there is any clinical manifestation of the disease, it is of even greater importance to recognize the existence of neurosyphilis before the occurrence of symptoms, for the ultimate outlook for arrest of the disease or complete recovery is greatly enhanced if treatment can be begun before clinical evidence of neuraxis involvement has appeared. It is possible to recognize many cases of neurosyphilis months or years before the onset of symptoms, through examination of the cerebrospinal fluid, for there is abundant evidence to indicate that involvement of the nervous system, if it is to take place at all in a given case of syphilis, will occur early in the course of the disease, and will often give rise to characteristic changes in the spinal fluid long before clinical symptoms become manifest. Such cases of asymptomatic neurosyphilis are by no means uncommon. They are frequently overlooked because of failure to examine the spinal fluid. Such an examination should be a routine procedure in the management of every patient with syphilis.

While many of the symptoms of neurosyphilis are so varied or so indefinite as not to permit of separation into distinct clinical entities, others occur with such frequency and constancy as to constitute definite clinical pictures. Pathologic examination shows that these clinical pictures rest upon characteristic anatomic changes. Of these disease entities, the most important are paresis, tabes and optic atrophy.

When syphilis involves the gray matter of the cerebral hemispheres it may bring about an extreme degree of change in the brain cells and lead to the gravest alterations of personality ending in complete mental deterioration. This condition, known as *paresis* or *general paralysis of the insane,* is uniformly accompanied by marked chemical and serologic changes in the spinal fluid, and is often progressive in spite of treatment. The earliest sign of mental change in these patients may be a slight slowing of the mental processes, slight disturbance of speech or writing, forgetfulness, or a change in disposition. Too often such cases are diagnosed "neurasthenia." The patient may become depressed or sad, more often apathetic and disoriented as to time and place. His memory fails, he may become euphoric and may develop ideas of grandeur, imagining that he is extremely clever or rich or powerful, and in some instances he may become even homicidal.

As the deterioration progresses, the tendency to apathy increases, the patient becomes more and more dull until finally he lives at a plane little above that of a vegetable, and ends his days a hopelessly bedridden paralytic, unless he is fortunate enough to have a convulsion carry him off earlier.

Involvement of the spinal cord by syphilis may bring about a degeneration of one or more of the tracts of the cord. The tracts most commonly affected are the posterior columns and when they are involved and undergo degeneration a condition called *tabes dorsalis*, or *locomotor ataxia*, develops. In this disorder there are commonly, at first, sharp shooting pains in the legs and disturbances of sensation. The sense of pain and of touch is diminished or lost, and there is loss of coördination, so that the patient does not know where his feet are, and when he walks, he steps with a wide base and flings his legs in an exaggerated fashion. He may lose control of his sphincters and dribble urine or pass feces involuntarily, and often he loses his desire and his ability to have sexual intercourse. The deep tendon reflexes disappear, the pupils no longer react to light. The most extraordinary changes in his joints (Charcot joints) may occur, these becoming swollen and very loose but without pain, and attended by comminution of the joint surfaces and underlying bone, so that the joint cavity is filled with bony fragments. Again, so-called "trophic" ulcers may develop; these may burrow deeply into the feet but all the time without pain.[1]

One of the gravest of late manifestations of syphilis of the nervous system is that of involvement of the optic nerve, leading as it may to ultimate blindness. This may take the form of an initial optic neuritis, and the disease process may be confined to the optic nerve, but often it is associated with disease of other parts of the central nervous system, notably tabes dorsalis. Ophthalmoscopic examination during the early stages will show swelling of the disk with blurring of the margins and engorgement of the retinal vessels. The process may go on to atrophy of the nerve, in which case blindness may ensue. Optic atrophy not secondary to a syphilitic optic neuritis is also recognized by ophthalmologists. The mechanism of the development of this condition is not fully understood, although it is of more frequent occurrence than secondary optic atrophy due to syphilis. Some ascribe it to the toxic products of the spirochetes, but nobody has ever succeeded in demonstrating that Treponema pallidum can produce a toxin. It is this type of atrophy which is apt to be associated with tabes dorsalis. Ophthalmoscopic examination in such cases shows marked pallor of the disk, with narrowing of the blood-vessels.

The serologic reactions of the blood are helpful in the recognition of syphilis of the central nervous system, but the examination of the spinal fluid is much more helpful. The interpretation of the findings in the spinal fluid is not always easy, but it can be stated that when the fluid gives a positive Wassermann reaction in the hands of a reliable

---

[1] For a complete description of the symptoms of tabes dorsalis the reader must consult the section on Diseases of the Nervous System. There is not space here to recite them all.

worker, the patient has syphilis of the nervous system. The reverse is not true, however. A negative Wassermann reaction in the spinal fluid does not mean that the patient has *not* neurosyphilis. Many cases of syphilis of the vessels of the brain give negative Wassermann reactions in the spinal fluid. The same finding is by no means a rarity in cases of tabes dorsalis. On the other hand, it is doubtful if there has ever occurred a case of paresis in which the spinal fluid before treatment gave a negative Wassermann reaction. He would be rash who ventured a diagnosis of paresis in such a condition.

Visceral Reactions.—Liver.—Of all the viscera, this is the most frequent site of late syphilitic lesions. If they take the form of gummata they may cause an enlarged liver with irregular surface which is readily palpable. If the syphilitic process is diffuse it may cause destruction of large areas of the parenchyma and the resultant scarring may produce an extreme degree of cirrhosis with portal obstruction, ascites, and esophageal and rectal varices. Jaundice is not always present in these cases, even though the pathologic process may be widespread. Acute yellow atrophy due to syphilis alone is said to occur, but is very rare in untreated cases. It is much more common in the cases treated with arsphenamine. The not uncommon association of fever with hepatic syphilis has been frequently pointed out.

Stomach.—Syphilis of the stomach is comparatively rare, although it does occur. Either a diffuse or a circumscribed process, it may cause pyloric obstruction or show constant filling defects in the roentgen-ray. There are no pathognomonic signs of the condition.

Intestines.—The small intestine is very rarely involved in late syphilis. The major portion of the large bowel also escapes involvement, but many of the strictures of the rectum are thought to be syphilitic in origin and to follow a syphilitic ulcerative process. They are much more common in women than in men.

Spleen.—Late syphilitic lesions of the spleen are quite rare. When present they bring about an increase in the size of that organ.

Pancreas.—Syphilis may involve the pancreas, although this is a rare event insofar as the acquired form is concerned. If the process affects the islands of Langerhans it is conceivable that diabetes mellitus may be established, but as a matter of fact the cases of diabetes mellitus that can be shown to be due to syphilis are extremely rare.

Lungs.—Late syphilitic lesions of the lungs usually take the form of gummatous processes which are sharply outlined and may be revealed by roentgen-ray examination. Their true nature is usually disclosed by their response to antisyphilitic treatment.

Kidneys.—Munk has described a type of nephritis which he considers to be frequently syphilitic in origin. It is characterized by edema, marked albuminuria, and the passage in the urine of casts containing doubly refractile lipoid bodies. The clinical picture is markedly similar to that now called nephrosis. Gummata of the kidney are certainly rare.

Testes.—The testis is a fairly frequent site of late syphilitic lesions, the process taking the form of circumscribed gummata or a diffuse syphilitic orchitis. It is entirely possible that such a condition may play a rôle in the transmission of syphilis years after the infection occurred.

Eye Reactions.—Late syphilitic lesions of the eye are more apt to involve the cornea, the choroid and retina or the optic nerve, while early lesions are more prone to affect the iris. Syphilitic chorioretinitis is apt to pass unnoticed unless it involves the macular region, in which case it will intefere with vision and cause the patient to seek the ophthalmologist.

Ear Reactions.—It is established that late lesions of syphilis can affect the inner ear and bring about partial or complete deafness. Involvement of the middle ear is extremely rare.

Serologic Reactions.—The blood Wassermann reaction is frequently positive in cases of syphilis with late manifestations of the disease, but there are many such in which it is negative. It is important to remember that the absence of a positive Wassermann reaction by no means excludes syphilis. This is particularly true in the late forms of the disease. There are cases of syphilis in which the Wassermann reaction may be negative at the time treatment is begun, but will show a positive Wassermann reaction after a single dose of arsphenamine. These are called provocative reactions and are sometimes used as aids in diagnosis. Not a few cases of syphilis with positive Wassermann reactions in the blood will continue to give positive Wassermann tests after the most intensive antisyphilitic treatment. Such cases are said to be "Wassermann-fast." They are usually encountered among the patients with syphilitic disease of the bones, aorta or central nervous system, or in patients with late congenital syphilis.

Congenital Syphilis.—Early Manifestations.—The principal early clinical manifestations of congenital syphilis are those of the skin, mucous membranes, naso-pharynx and bones. The more frequent *skin lesions* are the macular and papular varieties. As a rule, the lesions are multiple and large, and of the color of raw ham. Large blisters or bullæ may occur. Fissures may develop at the corners of the mouth, giving rise to radiating linear scars when they heal. Extensive areas of inflammation of the palms and soles are not infrequent, and broad condylomata about the ano-genital region are common.

Rhinitis and pharyngitis, with bloody purulent nasal discharge (snuffles) is a frequent early manifestation of congenital syphilis. If unchecked, the syphilitic process may involve the hard palate and the bones of the nose, causing the entire bridge of the latter to cave in and producing what is known as the "saddle-nose" deformity.

Other *bones* may also be involved, notably those of the skull. The frontal eminences may become unusually prominent, forming bosses, or actual destruction of portions of the skull may occur. When the long bones are involved there is usually distortion of the line of calcification, or perhaps an osteo-periostitis leading to marked thickening and irregularity of the shaft. Roentgen-ray examination is helpful in recognizing these changes.

Of the late lesions of congenital syphilis, the most frequent are the changes in *the teeth* and the ocular manifestations. Sir Jonathan Hutchinson described the changes in the teeth of the second dentition which are so characteristic of congenital syphilis. They consist in notching of the cutting edge of the upper incisors, which are usually spaced wide apart and taper from the base to the cutting edge.

The most common late *ocular lesion* of congenital syphilis is interstitial keratitis. This condition is apt to recur and is extremely difficult to treat. It is manifested by a clouding of the cornea and injection of the conjunctival blood-vessels. Some suppose it to be an allergic phenomenon.

Lesions of the *central nervous system* may occur in congenital syphilis, even paresis and tabes dorsalis. Deafness due to involvement of the eighth nerve is by no means rare. Amyloid disease of the liver, spleen and kidneys has been known to occur in long-standing, untreated, congenital syphilis.

The Wassermann reaction is of great help in the diagnosis of congenital syphilis, for it is nearly always positive. It is important to remember that a positive reaction may be the only manifestation of the congenital form of the disease, and that, in order to prove in such cases that the disease is parental in origin, a survey of all the other members of the family may be necessary. As a matter of fact, when a case of congenital syphilis is recognized the physician should insist upon examining all the other children as well as the parents. In families where syphilis has been transmitted to several children the manifestations of the disease are apt to be most marked in the child first infected, and to be less marked in each succeeding child.

Immunity and Second Infections.—Second attacks of syphilis are relatively rare; they almost never occur except in persons who have been well treated during the early stages of their first infection. A person in whom syphilis has been present for some time acquires an immunity to a second attack of the disease. For years it has been thought that this immunity was dependent upon the presence of living syphilitic virus. More recently evidence of an experimental nature has been brought forward which would indicate that the acquired immunity may persist after the infection has been eliminated.

Second infections, whether they occur on top of a preëxisting infection (superinfection), or whether they develop after the first infection has been eliminated (reinfection), follow in general the same course as the first infection. Relapsing lesions are frequently erroneously considered to be second infections.

It is not possible to produce immunity to syphilis by any artificial system of immunization. Only the infection itself can produce immunity. The serum of syphilitic individuals does not possess any preventive or curative power.

For years it has been observed that women who have given birth to syphilitic infants do not themselves often show manifestations of the disease. In the pre-Wassermann era this observation was interpreted to mean that these women were not syphilitic but were immune to the disease, and the proposition was stated in a law, called Colles' law. We now know that this law is not true. Such mothers are in reality syphilitic, having acquired the infection prior to the birth of the syphilitic infant, but for some unknown reason they do not show any signs of it. Some think that pregnancy is the factor that suppresses the syphilis in these women, but just how it might do so is not clear.

Prognosis.—The outlook for the complete cure of syphilis is good if the disease is recognized early in its course. By appropriate treatment at this time it can be completely eradicated or arrested in the majority of instances. If not recognized until it has reached the latent stage, the outlook is still favorable, provided no damage has been done to the important organs of the body. If, however, they have been damaged, then the outlook is serious and in direct relation to the particular structure involved. It is important that every patient with early syphilis should be regarded by his physician as a potential candidate for paresis, tabes, aneurysm, optic atrophy, indeed for any or all of the gravest disorders due to syphilis, and these possible end-results of the disease should always be kept in mind in advising the patient concerning treatment.

Prophylaxis.—There are two main lines of approach in seeking to prevent syphilis; one is that which seeks to eliminate illicit sexual intercourse; the other is that which seeks to treat the infected individual and to render him non-infectious as rapidly as possible so that he is no longer a menace to the community. The former can only be accomplished by educational methods, and the educational method has and will continue to have a limited value at best, unless the nature of human beings and their attitude toward sexual intercourse change greatly in the direction of abstinence. Of such a change there is now no indication. The great difficulty in this respect is that preaching self-restraint in the matter of sexual indulgence is likely to be least effective in those races or sections of the population in which syphilis is most frequent.

Much more hope may be looked for if the efforts to stamp out syphilis take the direction of attempting to recognize and cure the infected individual. This is a question, first, of improvement in the ability of physicians as a class to recognize and treat syphilis adequately; second, of providing a sufficient number of centers for the diagnosis and treatment of syphilis at a low cost, or none at all, to the patient. Provision for the latter is properly the business of the state, although private agencies may be very useful in an endeavor of that sort. The experience of Great Britain in respect to establishment of treatment centers has been very satisfactory and points the way.

Individual prophylaxis through the use, by the male, of cleansing measures, accompanied by inunction with 33 per cent calomel ointment, has proved effective in military establishments, but is not likely to be widely employed in civil life and cannot, therefore, be depended upon to accomplish much in the prevention of syphilis. The method is not applicable to females.

Treatment.—**General Principles.**—The essential object in the treatment of syphilis is the eradication of all the spirochetes from the body and the restoration of tissues to as near a normal state as possible. The human body cannot accomplish this result without aid; it must be supported by outside agencies. The ease with which the object may be attained will depend upon (1) the particular stage in which the disease happens to be at the time treatment is begun, and (2) the location and character of the lesions. While one may hope to eradicate all the spirochetes, one is not justified in supposing that all the damage resulting from their presence may be repaired. One cannot expect all scars to disappear, or dead nerve cells to come to life again. In the early stages of the disease one has to consider chiefly the problem of destruction of the spirochete, since damage to the tissues is not a prominent feature at this period. During the late stage of the infection attention must be directed to the question of restoration of structure and function, as well as to destruction of the spirochetes.

For the elimination of the spirochetes there are three general groups of drugs, namely, (1) compounds of mercury, (2) organic compounds of arsenic and (3) compounds of bismuth. The value of mercury in syphilis has been known for centuries; the others are of comparatively recent date. It is generally supposed that these three groups of substances owe their therapeutic action in syphilis to their ability to attack the spirochetes directly, but the precise mechanism of their antispirochetal action is not known.

For aid in the restoration of the tissue to normal we can resort to the use of potassium iodide. This drug has the property of hastening the resolution of late syphilitic lesions, but just how it does so is still somewhat of a mystery. It is of little or no value in early syphilis.

The ideal arrangement in the treatment of syphilis would be to have a drug which would kill all the spirochetes in the body at one stroke, and indeed, this is what Ehrlich hoped to accomplish when he introduced salvarsan (arsphenamine), but unfortunately his hopes were not fulfilled. Experience has shown that all of our spirocheticidal drugs are only partly effective at best, and must be employed again and again if we are to succeed in killing the last remaining spirochete.

The selection of the drug to be used and the method of its employment should vary with each individual patient. An intelligent selection must rest upon a knowledge of what a given drug will or will not do, and its potentialities for harm. While it is not possible to go into the details of the mode of action of the various antisyphilitic drugs, it may be said that in general the spirocheticidal action of the arsphenamine group is shorter but of greater intensity while it lasts, whereas the action of mercury and bismuth is slower and longer and less intense.

While it is necessary to adjust the treatment to fit the individual case, nevertheless it is best always to formulate a definite plan of treatment at the outset and to adhere to that plan as rigidly as possible under the circumstances, particularly as regards the duration of the treatment. It is easier to formulate a plan for the treatment of patients with early syphilis than in the case of patients with late manifestations, for the problem is much simpler in the early period of the disease. Indeed, the management of patients with late manifestations of syphilis frequently offers problems of great difficulty and demands therapeutic skill of a high order if successful results are to be achieved. It is always desirable to explain to the patient the nature of his disease and the great importance of continuing his treatment over a long period, even though he may feel entirely well. Every legitimate effort should be made to assure him that the outlook in most instances is favorable if he will but play his part, and he should not be allowed to become despondent and a victim of syphilophobia, a condition that is often worse than syphilis itself.

Early Cases.—For cases of early syphilis it is most desirable that the patient should be kept continuously under the influence of an anti-syphilitic agent. The best results are obtained when a combination of drugs is employed. The most widely used combination is that of one of the arsphenamines (arsphenamine, neoarsphenamine, silver arsphenamine or sulpharsphenamine) with one of the compounds of mercury or bismuth. Some prefer to alternate courses of the one with courses of the other; others prefer to give the drugs simultaneously. Courses may consist of six or eight injections at weekly intervals.

Arsphenamine (0.4 gram for men, 0.3 gram for women) and neo-arsphenamine (0.6 gram for men and 0.45 gram for women) should only be administered intravenously. Neoarsphenamine is used much more extensively than arsphenamine because of the greater ease of administration, although it is probably not quite so efficacious as the other.

Mercury may be given by mouth in the form of the bichloride (0.005 gram), by intramuscular injection in the form of the water soluble bichloride (0.01 gram), or succinimide (0.01 gram), or the insoluble salicylate in a vegetable oil (0.12 gram); or it may be given by inunction in the form of the blue ointment (4 to 6 grams). The oral route, while easiest so far as the patient is concerned, is least efficacious and some syphilologists take the ground that mercury should almost never be given in this way. The intramuscular method probably affords the greatest precision from the standpoint of administration, but the rapidity of absorption may vary considerably and nullify to some extent this very factor of precision. The inunction method is the safest method but has the disadvantage that it requires considerable coöperation on the part of the patient and is a messy affair as usually carried out.

Bismuth appears to be as efficacious as mercury, perhaps even more so, and may be administered intramuscularly in the form of a 10 per cent suspension of the salicylate in olive oil, 0.2 gram being the average dose. Some prefer the water-soluble bismuth compounds for intramuscular injection. While they are probably absorbed more rapidly they have a tendency to be more irritant. The writer prefers bismuth to mercury wherever the latter is indicated.

The patient should be cautioned against the dangers of allowing too great a time to elapse between treatments, especially during the first months, for all too frequently a lapse in treatment is followed by the onset of syphilitic meningitis of the neurorecurrence type, or other forms of relapse. The physician should be always on the lookout for this untoward event and should not hesitate to perform a spinal puncture if symptoms suggesting this condition develop.

It is difficult to set precise limits as to the duration of treatment of patients with early syphilis, for there is no single satisfactory criterion of cure of the disease. One must select a time period which must,

15

after all, be somewhat arbitrary. Some physicians set two years of
continuous treatment as the minimum for the uncomplicated early
case; others put it at one year after the blood Wassermann becomes
negative. The latter standard seems to be sufficient provided, of
course, that the spinal fluid is negative. It is important to remember
that the change of a Wassermann reaction from positive to negative
does not by any means indicate that the patient has been cured. No
patient should be discharged as cured until he has been under observation for at least two years following the discontinuance of treatment,
and unless both blood and spinal fluid are negative. If he can be
kept under observation for a longer period so much the better.

Late Cases.—Patients with late manifestations of syphilis call for
the greatest individualization in the matter of treatment. Here greater
caution is necessary because of the danger of sudden lighting up of the
syphilitic inflammatory process in vital organs, through the treatment
itself. For that reason many prefer to commence the treatment of
late cases with potassium iodide by mouth, or with bismuth or mercury, and only employ one of the arsphenamines later, lest too rapid
healing of the lesions result in damage to important structures. Certainly the treatment of the late cases in general need not be as intensive
as that of the early cases.

In cardiac syphilis the greatest caution is necessary in the employment of the arsphenamines, and some physicians decline to use them
at all in such cases, but they can be used with safety and will prove
beneficial if small doses, 0.1 gram, be employed and increased very
slowly. The same is true if other viscera are involved, although it is
probably better to initiate the treatment of such cases with potassium
iodide and either mercury or bismuth before changing to one of the
arsphenamines.

In the case of syphilis of the nervous system the problem is very
complex. Many cases will be improved by the usual method of alternate courses of one of the arsphenamines and either mercury or
bismuth. Others may show no improvement, either in the clinical
symptoms or in the serologic reactions. One may then resort to the
use of tryparsamide, a derivative of atoxyl, which is of great value in
this type of syphilis, but not without danger because of its tendency to
bring about atrophy of the optic nerve and thus result in blindness.
It can be given, however, if care is used, but it should not be employed
without a full realization of its dangers, and the vision of the patient
should be followed constantly during its exhibition, and the drug
stopped at once if the patient complains of dimness of vision or other
visual disturbances. It is of little value in other types of syphilis.

Patients with tabes dorsalis and optic atrophy are notoriously resistant to the ordinary antisyphilitic drugs. For these, the Swift-Ellis
method of treatment may be employed. This consists in the introduction into the spinal canal of serum obtained from a patient shortly
after he has received one of the arsphenamines intravenously. This
method has a definite but limited field of usefulness.

The treatment of refractory cases of central nervous system syphilis,
especially paresis, by giving the patient malaria, has been followed by

a considerable measure of success. Many cases of paresis treated in this way have been arrested, if not permanently cured. The method is not so effective in tabes, but it represents a distinct therapeutic advance in the treatment of paresis. Blood is taken from a patient with malaria of the tertian variety, citrated to prevent clotting, and injected subcutaneously or intravenously into the patient. Fever develops within a week or ten days and typical paroxysms of malaria occur. The patient is allowed to have from ten to fifteen typical chills, depending upon his general condition, and the malarial infection is eliminated by giving quinine. Some brilliant therapeutic results have been obtained with this method, but it is not without danger. It is contraindicated in the presence of heart disease, nephritis and severe malnutrition.

Pregnancy is no contraindication to active treatment for syphilis. Excellent results are obtained so far as both mother and offspring are concerned, the best results being secured when treatment is begun early in the course of pregnancy. In progressive obstetric clinics where treatment of syphilitic pregnant women is carried out routinely and actively, the incidence of syphilis as a cause of abortion or miscarriage has been enormously diminished, and to the same degree the number of syphilitic babies greatly reduced. This result represents one of the signal triumphs of modern medicine. It is wise to carry on the treatment of the mother after the birth of the child and also during succeeding pregnancies, if there are any.

The treatment of congenital syphilis is not, in its essentials, different from that of adult syphilis. In infants, because of the smallness of the veins, intravenous medication may have to be dispensed with, in which case sulpharsphenamine can be employed intramuscularly. The dosage of the drugs employed is of necessity lower. Early congenital syphilis needs more intensive treatment than the delayed form.

Treatment Reactions.—Arsphenamine therapy is not without its dangers. The occasional immediate reactions (nitritoid crises) in which the patient complains of a tightness of the chest, flushing of the face or pain in the back, are alarming to the patient, but not dangerous. The instances of exfoliative dermatitis, jaundice, or bone-marrow intoxication, occurring after arsphenamine, are more serious. Jaundice in such cases means destruction of liver tissue and the drug should not be repeated at once when it occurs. The occurrence of itching is a danger signal in these cases and should be watched for. Severe vomiting after the intravenous administration of arsphenamine often precedes an attack of arsphenamine jaundice and should put the physician on guard. Excessive use of mercury or bismuth may lead to the symptoms of heavy metal poisoning, but careful watch of the patient as regards the condition of his mouth (stomatitis), blood (anemia) and urine (casts and albuminuria) will enable the physician to recognize the onset of the intoxication and to discontinue the drug before serious harm is done.

Syphilis and Marriage.—The physician is often called upon to pass judgment upon the question of whether or not a syphilitic individual should marry. It is one of the most difficult questions he is likely to be called upon to face, and it is one that cannot be delegated to others. To lay down hard and fast rules is dangerous, but it is proper to say that an individual with active manifestations of the disease should not marry. If, however, he has been well and thoroughly treated, if physical examination and all the laboratory tests, both of the blood and spinal fluid are completely negative, then he may be permitted to marry, but he should be told, before he does so, of the possibility that he may transmit the infection to his wife and, through her, to his offspring. It goes without saying that the woman should also know the possibilities of the situation before the step is taken. The whole problem revolves around the question, how much treatment has the individual had and what is his physical status, insofar as syphilis is concerned, at the time he contemplates matrimony? Once these facts are obtained, the rest is a question of the good sense, judgment and experience of the physician who is to advise the patient.

YAWS.

Synonyms.—Framboesia; Pian; Bubas.

Definition.—A chronic relapsing infection due to a particular species of treponeme (Treponema pertenue), and characterized by a typical eruption.

Etiology.—The disease is due to Treponema pertenue, a delicate spiral organism first described by Castellani. The disease is widespread and common in the tropical regions of America, Asia and Africa.

Yaws is *transmitted* by direct contact, but it is not a venereal infection, since sexual intercourse plays almost no part in its dissemination. Many young children acquire it and transmit it to their parents. The disease is not believed to be transmitted to offspring *in utero*.

Pathology.—The histopathology of the early lesions is that of a granuloma of the skin in which there is marked thickening of the epithelium and a dense accumulation of plasma cells. The late lesions are destructive in character and produce extensive distortions.

Symptoms.—Three stages, primary, secondary and tertiary, are recognized.

The primary lesion (mother yaw) appears after an incubation period of from two to four weeks, and develops from a papule into a crusted lesion, the base of which on exposure is seen to be granulating. The lesion is not commonly indurated. The location of the primary lesion is usually extragenital, frequently on the breasts or hips in women, and on the extremities in men and children. The regional lymph nodes become enlarged and firm but do not suppurate. Treponemes can be demonstrated in the secretion from the lesion.

The secondary stage is characterized by the occurrence of a generalized eruption, consisting of lesions which begin as papules but which soon develop yellow crusts that are very characteristic. Removal of these crusts reveals a raw granulating surface. The lesions heal slowly and may leave pigmented areas or areas without pigment. Mild constitutional symptoms are not rare during this stage.

The tertiary lesions are nodular or ulcerative in character. They may involve the skin or the bones. Some observers consider that gangosa, an ulcerative process involving the nose, pharynx and palate, is in reality tertiary yaws. There is little evidence to show that the internal organs are affected.

The Wassermann reaction is positive and hence cannot be used to differentiate the disease from syphilis.

Prognosis.—The outlook is not grave so far as life is concerned, although death may result from secondary infection.

Treatment.—The best results are obtained with arsphenamine or neoarsphenamine. The latter has been widely used. Castellani recommends a course of three to six intravenous injections of neoarsphenamine at intervals of three to six days, the individual dose starting at 0.3 gram and increasing to 0.6 gram. Of late, spirocoid (stovarsol), a derivative of atoxyl, has been used with success. It is given by mouth in doses of 0.25 gram three to four times daily, depending upon the age. Mercury appears not to be very effective.

RAT-BITE FEVER.

Rat-bite fever, or *sodoku*, as it is known in Japan, is an infection caused by Treponema morsus muris, a short spirochete 2 to 5 microns in length, with two to six turns, and extremely actively motile. Man is infected by being bitten by a rat harboring the parasite. An inflammatory lesion develops at the location of the bite, the regional lymph node becomes enlarged and fever develops. The fever is irregular, the evening temperatures reaching as high as 104° F. The fever subsides in a few days or weeks but often relapses. There sometimes may be a moderate leukocytosis. The spirochete may be found in the blood, rendering the diagnosis certain. The prognosis is favorable. The disease can be cured by the use of arsphenamine or neoarsphenamine. Cases of rat-bite fever have been described in which a streptothrix was isolated from the lesion.

RELAPSING FEVER.

Synonyms.—Recurrent fever; Rückfallfieber.

Definition.—An infectious disease, due to several varieties of spirochetes known as spironemata, characterized by intermittent periods of fever during which the organism is present in the circulating blood. Different varieties of relapsing fever are recognized.

Etiology.—The spirochetes causing relapsing fever belong to the genus Spironema. The species causing European relapsing fever is called Spironema recurrentis and also Spironema obermeieri. It was first seen in 1868 by Obermeier. The East and West African varieties of relapsing fever are caused by Spironema duttoni and the American variety by Spironema novyi. These organisms differ from one another in serologic reactions and in some morphologic particulars. They are 7 to 10 microns in length, possess three to five coarse, irregular spirals and are actively motile, rotating very rapidly on their longitudinal axes.

Transmission.—The European, North African, Indian and Manchurian varieties of relapsing fever are transmitted to man by lice, not through the bites of these insects but as a result of cuts or abrasions of the skin being infected with the contents of the body of the louse. The tropical African and the American varieties of relapsing fever are transmitted by ticks, infection occurring through contamination of cuts or abrasions of the skin with the feces of the tick.

Symptoms.—After an incubation of about seven days, as a rule, there is sudden onset of fever, headache, pains in the back and limbs, chills, anorexia and sometimes abdominal pain and tenderness with constipation. The temperature rises abruptly to 103° to 105° F., remains elevated for about five days and then falls abruptly to normal or subnormal. During this febrile period there is usually nausea and vomiting, the liver and spleen enlarge, the pulse and respirations become rapid, and a moderate anemia with polymorphonuclear leukocytosis may develop. After an afebrile period of ten to fourteen days there may be a relapse during which the fever again mounts rapidly and the same symptoms occur again, the fever once more falling abruptly to normal at the end of three or four days. During the febrile period the spirochetes can be demonstrated in the blood without difficulty.

Prognosis.—The outlook is favorable, the mortality being low (5 per cent) and usually due to complications.

Treatment.—Arsphenamine or neoarsphenamine is curative, but should be given cautiously during the attack.

EPIDEMIC JAUNDICE.

Synonyms.—Weil's disease; Spirochætosis icterohæmorrhagica; Spirochetal jaundice.

Definition.—An acute infectious disease occurring in endemic and epidemic form, characterized by jaundice and due to a particular variety of spirochete, Leptospira icterohæmorrhagiæ.

Etiology.—The causal agent, Leptospira icterohæmorrhagiæ, was discovered by Inada and his coworkers in 1915. It is a small spirochete with very close spirals which are difficult to see while the organism is in motion. One or both ends may be bent around to resemble a hook. The organism is an inhabitant of wild rats and may be recovered from their urine.

Infection of human beings is thought to occur through the skin. It has been suggested that infection may also take place through the alimentary tract.

The disease is prevalent in Japan but exists in other countries as well. During the World War it appeared among the troops of the Allied Armies on the Western Front.

Symptoms.—After an incubation period of seven days, on the average, the disease begins suddenly with chills, fever, weakness and prostration. The liver and spleen become enlarged, and after an interval of two or three days jaundice sets in. Nausea and vomiting are not uncommon and there may be pain and tenderness over most of the body. The blood may show a moderate anemia with leukocytosis and the leptospiras may be found in the blood if careful search is made. In the severe cases there may be hemorrhages from the mucous membranes of the nose, pharynx or alimentary tract. The fever lasts from seven to ten days and ends by crisis or lysis. Relapses are not uncommon. The diagnosis is made certain by finding the leptospiras in the blood or urine, or through guinea-pig inoculation.

The outlook is grave, the mortality ranging around 30 per cent.

Treatment.—The arsphenamines have been found to be of no value. Horses have been immunized and a serum prepared.

REFERENCES.

CASTELLANI, A., and CHALMERS, A. I.: Manual of Tropical Medicine, 3d ed., New York, William Wood & Co., 1919.

Handbuch der Haut- und Geschlechtskrankheiten, Berlin, Springer, 1928.

Handbuch der Tropenkrankheiten, Leipzig, Barth, 1914.

HAZEN, HENRY H.: Syphilis, 2d ed., St. Louis, C. V. Mosby Company, 1928.

MOORE, J. E.: The Modern Treatment of Syphilis, Springfield, Charles C Thomas, 1933.

SOUTHARD, E. E., and SOLOMON, H. C.: Neurosyphilis, Boston, Leonard, 1917.

STOKES, JOHN H.: Modern Clinical Syphilology, Philadelphia, W. B. Saunders Company, 1926.

CHAPTER VI.

THE PROTOZOAL DISEASES.

By CHARLES F. CRAIG, M.D.

AMEBIASIS.
INTESTINAL FLAGELLATE INFESTA-
TIONS.
THE LEISHMANIASES.
Kala-azar.
Oriental Sore.
Espundia.

THE TRYPANOSOMIASES.
African Sleeping Sickness.
Chagas' Disease.
COCCIDIOSIS.
THE MALARIAL FEVERS.
SARCOSPORIDIOSIS.
BALANTIDIASIS.

AMEBIASIS.

Synonyms.—Amebic dysentery; Amebic colitis; Amebic enteritis; Intestinal amebiasis; Endamebiasis; Entamebiasis.

Definition.—By the name "amebiasis" is meant the infection of the intestine of man by the protozoan parasite, Endamœba histolytica, belonging to the Rhizopoda, and the cause of amebic dysentery. The infection may occur without observable symptoms or it may be characterized by attacks of diarrhea or dysentery, or by other symptoms connected with the nervous and digestive systems. Amebic dysentery is one stage only in the condition known as amebiasis, and dysentery occurs only in the most severe type of amebiasis.

History.—Endamœba histolytica was discovered by Losch, in 1875, in the feces of a Russian suffering from dysentery, but it was not until the classical work of Councilman and Lafleur appeared in 1891 that the parasite was shown to be the cause of a specific form of dysentery, often accompanied by abscess of the liver, to which the name "amebic dysentery" was given. In 1903, Schaudinn clearly differentiated the pathogenic ameba, Endamœba histolytica, from the harmless ameba found in the intestine of man, Endamœba coli, and gave them their present specific names. Walker and Sellards, in 1913, proved by actual experiment upon human volunteers that Endamœba histolytica is the cause of amebic dysentery and that Endamœba coli is a harmless commensal of man, although animal experiments by many other investigators had proven this to be true in experimental animals. In 1918, Cutler and in 1924, Boeck and Drbohlav succeeded in cultivating Endamœba histolytica.

Geographic Distribution.—Amebiasis is practically world-wide in distribution, for wherever it has been searched for it has been found in a certain proportion of individuals. While more commonly present in the tropics and subtropics, the infection is frequently observed in the temperate zones, and it has been conservatively estimated that from 5 to 10 per cent of the population of the United States are infected with Endamœba histolytica. The most severe symptoms of amebiasis occur in patients in the tropics, but acute amebic dysentery also occurs in the temperate zones, so that the term "tropical dysentery" as synonymous with amebic dysentery is not correct.

(232)

Etiology and Epidemiology.—While there are no less than five species of amebæ living in the intestine of man, three only are of importance, *i. e.*, Endamœba histolytica, Endamœba coli, and Endamœba (Endolimax) nana. Of the species of amebæ occurring in the intestine of man, Endamœba histolytica is the only species that is pathogenic, all of the others being harmless commensals, as proven by experiments upon man and the lower animals. The natural habitat of this ameba is in the tissues and lumen of the large intestine and there are three well-defined stages in its life-cycle in man: the motile, or trophozoite stage, the precystic stage, and the cystic stage. In the motile stage the organism moves actively in a progressive direction by means of extensions of the ectoplasm known as pseudopodia, while in the precystic and cystic stages there is no motility, the organisms being round or slightly oval in shape. The differential features of the various stages of this parasite as compared with Endamœba coli and Endamœba (Endolimax) nana are given in the section on Diagnosis.

Endamœba histolytica is capable of invading the coats of the intestine and normally is a tissue dweller. It produces its harmful effects by cytolyzing the tissues with which it is in contact, and cytolytic and hemolytic substances have been extracted from cultures of this organism. In the tissues of the intestine and, when conditions are favorable, in the lumen of the intestine, the active stage divides into two daughter amebæ and this division continues indefinitely until conditions become unfavorable, when the amebæ become round, lose their motility, and eventually form cysts which are covered with a resistant cyst wall and may contain from one to four nuclei. These cysts are excreted in the feces and are the infective agents, for it has been repeatedly proven that the active, or trophozoite stage, cannot pass through the stomach as the hydrochloric acid of the gastric juice kills it. When the cysts are ingested in food or drink they excyst in the lower portion of the ileum or the region of the ileocecal valve, each cyst liberating a single ameba containing four nuclei, when mature. These nuclei again divide, so that eight nuclei are produced and then the parent organism divides into eight small amebulæ which develop into motile trophozoites, and multiply as trophozoites as already described. Whether this species of ameba ever lives solely in the lumen of the bowel without invading the tissues has not been determined, but most authorities believe that in every infection with this parasite there is some invasion of the tissues, and that the extent of the invasion explains the great variety in the character and severity of the symptoms.

The *transmission* of amebiasis is through food or drink contaminated with the cysts of Endamœba histolytica. This contamination may occur through food handlers who are "carriers" of the parasite; through the use of sewage for fertilizing vegetables; through water contaminated with sewage; and through the agency of flies. The cysts are very resistant to various chemical agents, will live for weeks in water which is free from gross bacterial infection, or in fecal material which is kept moist and in the shade; and viable cysts have been demonstrated in the excrement of flies thirty-six hours after the insects have fed upon infected feces. Sunlight quickly kills the cysts, as does drying, so that infection of man through the contamination of food by dust is impossible. The usual method of infection in communities where there is a protected public water supply, a properly controlled disposal of sewage, and the food is guarded from fecal pollution, is through food handlers who are "carriers" of the parasite. "Carriers" may be either "convalescent carriers" or "contact carriers," the latter being most numerous and most active in the transmission of the parasite.

Pathology.—The pathologic lesions of amebiasis vary all the way from slight surface necrosis of the mucous membrane of the intestine to extensive abscess and ulcer formation destroying large areas of the mucous membrane, the submucosa, and even the muscular coats of the intestine. Amebic ulceration is practically confined to the large intestine, although the lower end of the ileum and the appendix may be involved. The first effect of the amebæ upon the intestine is a cytolysis of the surface of the mucous membrane resulting in areas of necrosis. Further invasion of the mucous membrane is followed by the development of minute pockets beneath the membrane containing numerous amebæ, necrotic and cytolyzed material and mucus, communicating with the surface through a minute opening. This lesion frequently breaks down and an ulcer is produced, having overhanging edges, the floor being formed either by the submucosa or the muscular coat of the intestine. Many of these ulcers communicate with one another beneath the mucous membrane and eventually may merge into one another and form ulcerations extending around the entire intestine. In such cases large sloughs of the mucous membrane may be present and necrotic shreds of tissue may cover the inner surface of the intestine, giving the "buffalo-coat" appearance described by the older writers upon this infection. The ulceration may extend to the peritoneal coat, and perforation may occur. The amebæ are found lying in the lumen of the glands, in the mucous membrane between and below the glands, in the submucosa and muscular coats and in the blood-vessels and lymphatics. In regions where secondary infection with bacteria has not occurred there is very little cellular infiltration of the tissues near the lesions or in contact with the amebæ. The lesions in symptomless "carriers" are unknown, but it is true that definite ulceration due to Endamœba histolytica may be present in the intestine in individuals who have never had symptoms of dysentery or diarrhea and who have died from some other infection.

Symptoms.—The symptoms of amebiasis vary from those of slight disturbances of the intestinal tract to those of severe dysentery. It is most unfortunate that the term "amebic dysentery" has become synonymous with amebiasis, for while dysenteric symptoms are quite characteristic of infection with Endamœba histolytica, the vast majority of such infections are not evidenced by dysenteric symptoms, but by much milder symptoms often unrecognized as being caused by this parasite. The belief, held by many, that this parasite is peculiar to the tropics because it is in such regions that amebic dysentery is most common, leads to failure in diagnosing and treating a very important parasitic infection of man present in all parts of the world.

(a) **Symptoms in "Carriers" of Endamœba Histolytica.**—While it is probably true that a majority of "carriers" of Endamœba histolytica present no definite symptoms of infection, it is also true that a very considerable proportion show symptoms, as shown by numerous investigators. These symptoms are not pathognomonic of the infection, but the fact that they disappear after treatment resulting in the disappearance of the amebæ is believed to be sufficient evidence of their causation. The symptoms in "carriers" are most frequently alternating constipation and slight diarrhea, lasting only a day or two; colic and gaseous distention of the abdomen; capricious appetite and anorexia; neuralgic pains in the lower right abdominal quadrant; chronic headache of dull character; sleepiness or disturbed slumber; neuralgic pains in the limbs with dull aching, especially in the early morning; and a general lack of ambition and energy. The physical signs are underweight; a sallow skin; moderate anemia; a weak and irritable pulse; flushing of the skin and excessive perspiration of the palms of the hands and the soles of the feet; tenderness on deep pressure in the right iliac region or over the ascending or descending colon; distention of the abdomen in the right iliac region or over the descending colon; and tenderness, in some instances, over the region of the liver. All, or some of these symptoms, are commonly present in "carriers" of Endamœba histolytica and should lead to an examination of the feces for the parasite.

Symptoms simulating those of acute or chronic appendicitis sometimes occur in carriers and such symptoms should always lead to an examination of the stools for Endamœba histolytica before operative procedures are undertaken.

(b) **Symptoms of Amebic Enteritis and Amebic Dysentery.**—The symptoms of *amebic enteritis* are those noted in "carriers" with the addition of attacks of enteritis lasting for several days, generally followed by constipation. The enteritis is usually chronic in type, but may be acute, and it may or may not be followed by the appearance of true dysenteric symptoms. The stools in amebic enteritis contain much mucus but not visible blood, and the motile trophozoites of Endamœba histolytica are usually numerous and easily demonstrated.

The symptoms of *acute amebic dysentery* are quite characteristic. The onset may be sudden or an enteritis may have preceded the dysenteric attack. The patient has severe pain in the abdomen followed by an intense desire to defecate. Vomiting may be present and nausea is common in very acute attacks. The first stools passed may be partly formed and contain mucus, but they soon become fluid, the amount of mucus is increased and blood appears. As the condition progresses, shreds of mucous membrane may appear in the stools, the latter consisting almost entirely of blood and mucus, while tenesmus is marked. The number of stools varies with the severity of the attack, the average being from 15 to 20 during twenty-four hours, but there may be as many as 30 to 35 or more. When the stools are numerous a little material only is passed with severe tenesmus, and in such cases the patient becomes very weak and greatly depressed. Generally there is no elevation of temperature, but slight fever is usual in the most severe cases. Death may occur during the primary attack of dysentery, preceded by severe vomiting and collapse. In the great majority of cases the acute symptoms subside after a variable period and another attack may never occur, or, more frequently, the chronic form of amebic dysentery supervenes. Fulminant cases very rarely occur, in which the symptoms resemble those of cholera and death occurs within a few days from toxemia. The so-called *gangrenous type*, characterized by the occurrence in the stools of large sloughs of necrotic tissue of the intestine, is sometimes observed.

The *physical signs* during an acute attack of amebic dysentery are not characteristic, as other intestinal conditions may simulate them. The abdomen is tender upon pressure, especially in the right iliac region, or the tenderness may be diffuse along the entire length of the colon, or localized over the ascending, transverse or descending colon; the tongue is coated and the breath foul; jaundice may be present and the skin has a sallow appearance; rapid emaciation may be present in severe cases and there is always a marked loss in weight during the attack.

Chronic amebic dysentery may follow an acute attack, or the infection may be chronic from the beginning. The history, in the latter class of cases, is of repeated attacks of colicky diarrhea with the appearance of small amounts of blood and mucus in the stools, accompanied by anorexia, indigestion, loss of weight, and the symptoms noted in "carriers." Between the attacks of diarrhea there may be a fair degree of health, but usually there is indigestion, lack of appetite, dull headache, disturbed sleep and general malaise. In the chronic form of amebic dysentery which follows an acute attack the symptoms are similar. This type of amebiasis may continue for years and the writer has observed scores of chronic amebic dysentery patients who have suffered from the condition for twenty or more years. In such instances a condition of invalidism invariably results. During the acute exacerbations of the infection the *physical signs* are similar to those observed during the acute attack, and between the attacks there is usually tenderness over localized areas of the colon and thickening of the colon can be felt, especially in the right iliac region and the transverse or descending colon.

Complications and Sequelæ.—Liver abscess is the most serious complication of amebiasis and occurs in approximately 15 to 20 per cent of cases who have suffered from attacks of amebic dysentery. (See Diseases of the Liver.) It should be remembered that "carriers" who have never had dysentery may develop amebic abscess of the liver. Amebic abscess of the brain, generally secondary to abscess of the liver, and of the lung, spleen and other viscera have been observed but are very rare. Perforation of an amebic ulcer into the bladder has been noted by several observers, and perforation of the intestine is not infrequently observed in fatal cases. Contractures of the intestine by adhesions and cicatrices of healed ulcers are common sequelæ and sometimes cause obstruction of the intestine. Some authorities have described forms of arthritis as being caused by Endamœba histolytica, but this is more than doubtful.

Appendicitis caused by the invasion of the appendix by Endamœba histolytica is a not infrequent complication.

Diagnosis.—The diagnosis of amebiasis rests upon the demonstration of Endamœba histolytica in the feces, as the clinical symptoms are often so atypical as to be of little or no service in diagnosis. While a typical attack of amebic dysentery may be diagnosed by symptoms alone by an experienced physician, the vast majority of cases of amebiasis present symptoms so often observed in other disease conditions that their causation can be ascertained only by finding the parasite in the feces. The methods available for this purpose are the microscopic examination of both fresh and stained preparations and the culture of the organism from the stools. The writer has devised a complement-fixation test which is useful in diagnosis, but owing to technical difficulties, is not yet widely used. The technic of examining the feces for Endamœba histolytica and of making cultures for diagnostic purposes is detailed in works upon clinical diagnosis which should be consulted.

In diagnosis it is necessary to differentiate Endamœba histolytica from Endamœba coli and Endamœba (Endolimax) nana, two common and harmless species of ameba found in the human intestine. Table 6 gives the chief differential features of these parasites:

The various phases of amebiasis are frequently mistaken for other infections or diseases, and *vice versa*. The most frequent disease conditions confused with amebiasis are bacillary dysentery; mucous colitis and colitis due to other causes; chronic enteritis; schistosome dysentery, and balantidial dysentery. Bacillary dysentery is differentiated by the constant occurrence of fever and the character of the stools, which contain more pus and cellular exudate than does the stool of amebic dysentery, while bacteriologic examination will demonstrate the presence of one of the dysentery bacilli. In the chronic form of bacillary dysentery the diagnosis is more difficult, and impossible without a bacteriologic examination of the feces. Dysentery or diarrheas caused by schistosomes or Balantidium coli cannot be differentiated without a microscopic examination of the feces. Mucous colitis and colitis due to other causes than Endamœba histolytica are frequently difficult to differentiate from the symptoms alone, but the absence of Endamœba histolytica from the feces definitely eliminates this organism as a cause of the colitis. The so-called flagellate diarrheas may be differentiated by stool examinations and the demonstration of the flagellates with the absence of Endamœba histolytica. It should be remembered that flagellates are frequently associated with Endamœba histolytica and the diarrhea present is actually due to the latter parasite.

The diagnosis of any of the phases of intestinal amebiasis should not be made unless Endamœba histolytica has been found in the feces, as a diagnosis based upon clinical symptoms and physical signs is usually worthless. It is also well to remember that combined infections, as with bacillary dysentery, are not uncommon, and that their recognition depends upon a thorough protozoölogic and bacteriologic study of the feces.

TABLE 6.—DIAGNOSTIC POINTS IN THE DIFFERENTIATION OF ENDAMŒBA HISTOLYTICA, ENDAMŒBA COLI AND ENDAMŒBA (ENDOLIMAX) NANA.

	Endamœba histolytica.	Endamœba coli.	Endamœba (Endolimax) nana.
	Vegetative or Trophozoite Stage. Unstained.		
Size	18 to 60 microns; average, 20 to 35 microns	15 to 50 microns; average, 20 to 30 microns	6 to 12 microns; average, 8 microns.
Motility	Actively progressive and directional	Sluggish; rarely progressive; not directional	Sluggishly progressive.
Pseudopodia	Finger-shaped, clear and glass-like	Shorter and more blunt; less glass-like in appearance	Broad and blunt; not glass-like.
Inclusions	Red blood corpuscles when feces contains blood; no bacteria in fresh specimens	Numerous bacteria, crystals, and other materials; no red blood corpuscles	Numerous bacteria; no red blood corpuscles.
Nucleus	Invisible	Visible	Visible.
	Vegetative or Trophozoite Stage. Stained.		
Nuclear membrane	Delicate; inner surface has single layer of minute chromatin dots	Thicker; inner surface lined with coarser chromatin dots	Intermediate in thickness; chromatin rarely seen on inner surface.
Karyosome	Very small; usually in center of nucleus	Twice as large, situated eccentrically	Large and may be divided into one large and one small mass, situated at one side or in center of nucleus.
Intranuclear chromatin	No chromatin between karyosome and membrane	Chromatin grains between karyosome and nuclear membrane	No chromatin between karyosome and membrane.
Inclusions	Red blood corpuscles; no bacteria in fresh specimens	No red blood corpuscles; many bacteria and other material	No red blood corpuscles; many bacteria.
	Cystic Stage of Development. Iodine Stain.		
Size	6 to 20 microns; average 7 to 15 microns	10 to 20 microns; average 12 to 18 microns	5 to 10 microns.
Shape	Generally spherical; may be oval and rarely irregular	Spherical; rarely oval or irregular	Spherical, oval or ellipsoidal.
Nucleus	One to four; minute karyosome in center	One to eight; eccentric karyosome	One to four; large karyosome central or to one side.
	Hematoxylin Stained Cysts.		
Size	As in iodine-stained specimens	As in iodine-stained specimens	As in iodine-stained specimens.
Nuclear structure	Delicate membrane, minute *central* karyosome, no chromatin between karyosome and membrane, minute grains on nuclear membrane	Thicker membrane, larger *eccentrically* located karyosome, chromatin grains between nuclear membrane and karyosome, and large granules of chromatin on nuclear membrane	Thick nuclear membrane, large central or divided karyosome.
Chromatoidal bodies	Bar, oval or thick rod-like masses; present in about 50 per cent of the cysts	Filamentous or spicular with square or pointed ends; present in less than 10 per cent of cysts	Small granular or bacilliform masses, not comparable with those seen in the other species.
Nuclei, number of	One to four	One to eight	One to four.

Proctoscopic examination should be reserved for those cases in which it is impossible otherwise to secure suitable fecal material for microscopic examination and, if employed, the diagnosis of amebiasis should not be made unless motile trophozoites of Endamœba histolytica can be demonstrated in the material obtained from the suspected lesions.

Prognosis.—With modern therapeutic methods, if patients are treated early, the prognosis is excellent. Unlike bacillary dysentery, death very rarely follows the first acute attack of amebic dysentery, but repeated attacks so weaken the patient that death may occur or a condition of chronic invalidism result. The occurrence of abscess of the liver renders the prognosis much more grave than it is in uncomplicated infections. In relapsing cases the treatment must be persistent, and it should be remembered that in old relapsing cases the prognosis as to a cure of the infection should be guarded, for the longer it has lasted the more unfavorable the prognosis.

Prophylaxis.—As this infection is derived from food and drink contaminated with the cysts of Endamœba histolytica, the usual methods of prophylaxis employed in preventing diseases in which the infection is so acquired, as cholera or typhoid, are equally efficient in the prophylaxis of amebiasis. The proper disposal of sewage, the protection and sterilization of water supplies, the avoidance of eating fresh vegetables, the protection of food from flies, and the prevention of the breeding of flies are all valuable prophylactic methods. Water must be boiled to render it safe, as the cysts are not killed by chlorine in any amount which can be used in water sterilization. The detection and proper treatment of "carriers" is most important and, while impractical upon a large scale owing to the number of people who harbor Endamœba histolytica, it is a method that should be applied to food handlers in the public services and, as far as possible, in public restaurants or hotels. The education of the public as regards the importance and methods of transmission of amebiasis is a valuable prophylactic measure. The usual rules of personal hygiene should be observed.

Treatment.—The treatment embraces the treatment of "carriers," those presenting mild symptoms of amebiasis, and those having acute and chronic amebic dysentery. The detection of "carriers" should be followed by treatment, whether or not symptoms be present, and for the treatment of carriers and patients presenting mild symptoms of amebiasis, chiniofon (anayodin or yatren) has been found most efficient in the author's experience. Chiniofon (iodoxyquinolinsulphonic acid) is a synthetic preparation containing about 28 per cent of iodine and is supplied in keratin-coated pills, each containing 0.25 gram (4 grains), the dose for an adult being 3 to 4 pills three times a day for a period of eight to ten days. If the stools still contain Endamœba histolytica upon the completion of this course of treatment, it should be repeated after an interval of one week.

Other drugs which are recommended in the treatment of carriers and patients presenting any of the symptoms of intestinal amebiasis are vioform (iodochlorhydroxyquinoline) and carbarsone (4-carbiminophenylarsonic acid). Vioform contains about 40 per cent of iodine and is administered in capsules containing 0.25 gram (4 grains), a course of treatment for an adult consisting in the administration of 1 capsule three times a day for ten days, a treatment-free interval of one week, and 1 pill three times a day for another ten days. Carbarsone contains 28.85 per cent of arsenic and is administered in capsules containing 0.25 gram (4 grains) of the drug. A course of treatment for an adult consists in the administration of 1 capsule twice a day for ten days, and it should not be given in amebic hepatitis or any condition in which arsenic is contraindicated. The author recommends vioform in preference to carbarsone, as he believes it is more efficient and less apt to cause toxic symptoms.

In the treatment of *acute amebic dysentery* emetin hydrochloride, emetin bismuth iodide and chiniofon are the drugs that have been found most efficient. *Emetin* is a specific so far as the relief of symptoms is concerned, the patient being well on the road to a symptomatic recovery within a few days after beginning treatment, but it is doubtful if it actually cures more than one-third of the cases treated, even if repeated courses are administered. This drug finds its greatest field of usefulness in the treatment of the acute symptoms which disappear rapidly under its administration. It is best given orally or subcutaneously, and never intramuscularly or intravenously. When given by mouth keratin-coated pills or capsules should be used, and not more than 0.1 gram (1.5 grains) should be given morning and evening in equally divided doses. The drug is seldom used alone by mouth, but the oral and subcutaneous methods are combined, 0.03 gram (0.5 grain) being given by mouth every evening, and 0.065 gram (1 grain) subcutaneously every morning, for ten or twelve consecutive days. The oral administration is often entirely omitted and 0.065 gram (1 grain) of emetin given daily until the dysenteric symptoms are controlled but never for more than twelve days, after which chiniofon should be administered. Emetin is a toxic drug and, when given in too large a dose or over too long a period, causes severe diarrhea, myocarditis, neuritis, nervous prostration and great muscular weakness, and death may occur suddenly from cardiac failure. Such symptoms should be carefully watched for, and if they appear, the drug should be discontinued at once. During the treatment the patient must be kept in bed.

Emetin bismuth iodide, the double iodide of emetin and bismuth, is a more efficient drug than emetin and is administered by mouth in keratin-coated pills and not more than 0.2 gram (3 grains) should be administered per day, preferably at night, for twelve consecutive nights. This drug usually causes nausea for the first three or four nights of administration and diarrhea is a common symptom during the latter period of administration, but these symptoms need cause no anxiety. The patient must remain in bed during the treatment, and overexertion should be guarded against during convalescence. Toxic symptoms similar to those produced by emetin alone may occur and indicate prompt cessation of the treatment.

Chiniofon is administered orally and by enema in the treatment of acute amebic dysentery. For an adult the course of treatment consists in the oral administration of 1 gram (15 grains) three times a day for eight to ten days, intermitted for a week to ten days, and the same dosage repeated. Severe diarrhea may be caused by the recommended dosage and, if so, the dose should be reduced one-half. To secure the best results with this drug, the use of enemas containing chiniofon should be combined with the oral treatment. If this is done, 0.5 gram (7.5 grains) of chiniofon should be administered three times a day by mouth and a daily enema should be given of 200 cc. of a 2 per cent warm water solution of chiniofon, which should be retained for several hours. The treatment should be continued for ten days. If the full dose of 1 gram of chiniofon three times a day be given, combined with the enemas, severe diarrhea is very apt to occur, and the results obtained with the smaller dosage are apparently as good. Throughout the treatment the patient must remain in bed. Chiniofon is a less toxic drug than either emetin or emetin bismuth iodide, and is apparently more efficient in curing amebic infections.

In *chronic amebic dysentery*, during the acute exacerbations, the treatment should be with emetin bismuth iodide or chiniofon, and if cysts still persist in the stools, a course of vioform should be given. It should be remembered that if the infection is of long standing, and many relapses have occurred, the prospect of cure with any known method of treatment is poor.

Among other drugs that have been found useful in the treatment of amebiasis may be mentioned the subnitrate or subcarbonate of bismuth, recommended in doses of 12 to 14 grams (180 to 210 grains) a day, combined with emetin in moderate doses; the arsphenamines; chaparro amargosa; simaruba; and kurchi bark. None of these is as efficient as the remedies discussed.

The treatment of amebic abscess of the liver is largely surgical, but if symptoms of amebic hepatitis develop, the administration of emetin subcutaneously, within the limits of dosage already noted in the discussion of the treatment of intestinal amebiasis, should be employed. Emetin will not only prevent the development of abscess of the liver but will actually cause absorption and healing of abscesses of considerable size, as reported by numerous authorities.

General Treatment.—Confinement to bed is necessary in patients suffering from acute dysentery or acute exacerbations of the chronic type. A proper diet is of great importance and the smaller the amount of food taken while there are acute symptoms, with due regard to conserving strength, the better. During acute symptoms the diet should consist of broths, barley water, egg albumin, and milk with lime water. Pure milk or malted milk may be used when the acute symptoms improve and eggs, soft puddings and a semi-fluid diet should be given after the subsidence of the acute symptoms. A full diet is gradually adopted during convalescence, care being taken to avoid foods that are known to irritate the intestine. Alcohol should be forbidden in all cases of amebiasis, especially in those presenting dysenteric symptoms, and even in "carriers" indulgence in alcoholic stimulants frequently results in the appearance of symptoms, while in the chronic amebic dysentery patient alcoholic indulgence is often followed by a relapse of the dysenteric condition. The use of tonics during convalescence is indicated.

The cure of amebiasis can be determined only by the permanent disappearance of the amebæ from the feces, and every treated case should have repeated examinations of the feces for a period of at least four months after the cessation of treatment. If trophozoites or cysts reappear treatment should be repeated.

REFERENCES.

BOECK, W. C., and DRBOHLAV, J. J.: The Cultivation of Endamœba Histolytica, Am. Jour. Hyg., 1925, 5, 371.
COUNCILMAN, W. T., and LAFLEUR, H. A.: Amœbic Dysentery, Johns Hopkins Hosp. Rep., 1891, 2, 393.
CRAIG, C. F.: A Manual of the Parasitic Protozoa of Man, Philadelphia, 1926.
WALKER, E. L., and SELLARDS, A. W.: Experimental Entamœbic Dysentery, Philippine Jour. Sci., 1918, 8, 253.

INTESTINAL FLAGELLATE INFESTATIONS.

TRICHOMONIASIS; GIARDIASIS; CHILOMASTIGIASIS.

Infestation of the intestine of man by protozoan parasites belonging to the Flagellata is common and there are three species of these flagellates which are frequently observed: Giardia lamblia, Trichomonas hominis and Chilomastix mesnili. Other species have been described, but occur so infrequently as to be of no practical importance. Of the three commonly observed species it is doubtful if any are of medical interest so far as the production of disease is concerned, although Giardia lamblia may be capable, under certain conditions, of producing pathologic lesions. As regards Trichomonas hominis and Chilomastix mesnili, while some clinicians believe that these organisms produce diarrhea and other intestinal symptoms, the claims for their pathogenic nature do not rest upon any scientific evidence and it is the consensus of opinion of those who have most carefully studied these parasites that they are harmless commensals living in the intestine of man. If present in very large numbers they may be instrumental in aggravating pathologic conditions in the intestine produced by other causes.

A condition known as "giardiasis" has been described as being caused by the presence in the intestine of Giardia lamblia, characterized by an intermittent diarrhea which may become dysenteric. The attacks are described as severe, simulating amebic dysentery or, more frequently, the symptoms are less severe, consisting of a mild diarrhea accompanied by colic. In the severe attacks blood and mucus are said to occur in the stools, there is marked tenesmus, and if the condition has been of long standing there may be anemia and general debility. The vast majority of patients presenting symptoms of this infestation have a chronic diarrhea, the stools being fluid or semi-fluid but free from blood or mucus. It should be remembered that all of the flagellates infesting the intestine of man occur in the active stage only when the stools are fluid or semi-fluid in consistence, the cysts being present in formed stools. This fact renders it difficult to be sure if the diarrheal condition present is really due to the flagellate, as any other cause producing diarrhea would result in the appearance of the flagellates in the feces. Some authorities have claimed that this parasite is the cause of cholecystitis, ulcer of the gall-bladder, and so on, because it has been found in duodenal drainage or in the gall-bladder at operation, but the causative relation is not proven as no examinations were made for possible bacterial infection in these cases.

The *geographic distribution* of these flagellates is world-wide but they are most commonly observed in the subtropics and tropics. Of the three parasites mentioned, Giardia lamblia is the most common, Chilomastix mesnili the next, and Trichomonas hominis the least common. From 1 to 7 per cent of the adult population of the world is estimated to harbor one or more of these parasites, and infestation in children is still greater, especially infestation with Giardia lamblia.

The *diagnosis* of infestation is possible only by the demonstration of the flagellates in the feces of the individual harboring them.

In fluid or semi-fluid stools all three of these flagellates are actively motile, swimming about in a jerky manner, propelled by their flagella. All are roughly pear-shaped and hyaline in appearance and Giardia lamblia and Chilomastix mesnili form cysts which are voided when the stools are formed. The vegetative or motile form of Giardia lamblia has eight flagella, two nuclei, and a prominent sucking disc by which it is able to attach itself to the mucous membrane of the intestine. The cysts are oval in shape and contain two to four nuclei. The vegetative stage of Chilomastix mesnili has three anterior flagella and a large mouth or cystostome in which there is a fourth flagellum, while the cysts are lemon-like in shape and contain a nucleus and suggestions of the mouth and its contained flagellum. Trichomonas hominis has from four to five anterior flagella, an undulating membrane extending the entire length of the body and ending in a free posterior flagellum, and an axostyle. Cysts of this flagellate are unknown.

Transmission of all three flagellates is through the contamination of food or drink by food handlers, poor personal hygiene, use of human excrement for fertilizing purposes, and through the agency of flies.

The *prophylaxis* consists in proper personal hygiene and the protection of food and drink from fecal contamination, as in amebiasis.

The *treatment* of these infestations is unsatisfactory and no specific drug has been found for infestation with any of these parasites. The treatments described for amebiasis have all been thoroughly tried, but neither emetin, emetin bismuth iodide, nor chiniofon has been found of much value. Acetarsone has been recommended by many, administered as in amebiasis, but it cures only a small percentage of the infestations with Giardia lamblia in the experience of the writer. This drug appears to be quite efficient in the treatment of infestations with Trichomonas hominis and Chilomastix mesnili. Methylene blue, thymol, gentian violet, the arsphenamines, salol, guaiacol, carbon tetrachloride, and numerous other drugs have been recommended in the treatment of these infestations, but their very number is proof of their inefficiency.

THE LEISHMANIASES.

The leishmaniases include infections caused by protozoan parasites belonging to the Flagellata, genus Leishmania. There are three such

244 *THE PROTOZOAL DISEASES*

infections occurring in man, one a general infection called kala-azar, and two limited to the skin and mucous membranes, called oriental sore and espundia.

Kala-azar.

Synonyms.—Dumdum fever; Non-malarial remittent fever; Black fever; Visceral leishmaniasis; Cachectic fever; Infantile splenic anemia; Infantile kala-azar; Infantile splenomegaly.

Definition.—Kala-azar, dumdum or black fever, is an infectious disease caused by Leishmania donovani and characterized by long-continued irregular fever, enlargement of the spleen, progressive emaciation, anemia and leukopenia.

History.—Clark, in 1882, was the first accurately to describe an epidemic of kala-azar, but it was not until the discovery of the parasite by Leishman, in 1900, in the spleen pulp of a soldier suffering from so-called "dumdum" fever contracted in India, and the finding by Donovan, in 1903, of the same parasite in material obtained by spleen puncture from patients suffering from this fever in India, that the disease was definitely differentiated from malaria, undulant fever and other infections occurring in the endemic centers of kala-azar. The name Leishmania donovani was given the parasite by Laveran and Mesnil in 1903. The method of transmission by sandflies was apparently demonstrated by the Indian Kala-azar Commission in 1931.

Geographic Distribution.—Kala-azar occurs endemically in all of the countries bordering upon the Mediterranean; in southern Russia; India, especially in Bengal, Bihar and Assam; in Mesopotamia; Russian Turkestan; North China; Sumatra; the Sudan; western Abyssinia, and the Blue Nile region near the Abyssinian border.

Etiology and Epidemiology.—Kala-azar is caused by the infection of man by a protozoan parasite belonging to the genus Leishmania, known as Leishmania donovani. The parasites are found in the peripheral blood, either free or enclosed in wandering endothelial cells, or in mono- and polymorphonuclear leukocytes, and also in the endothelial cells of the internal organs, especially the spleen, liver, bone-marrow and lymph glands.

Two stages in the life history of Leishmania donovani are known, one occurring in the body of man, called the aflagellar stage; the other occurring in insects, especially the sandfly and in cultures, known as the flagellate stage.

Leishmania donovani in man always occurs as an oval or round body measuring about 2 microns in diameter, consisting of cytoplasm which stains blue with the Wright or Giemsa stain, containing within it a large nucleus, the macro- or trophonucleus, and at right angles to this nucleus a minute rod-like body called the blepharoplast. Both the nucleus and the blepharoplast stain a bright ruby-red with the stains mentioned. These bodies may be found free in the peripheral blood but are usually engulfed in mono- and polymorphonuclear cells or in endothelial cells in the organs and those lining the blood-vessels throughout the body.

The flagellate forms of Leishmania donovani, occurring in cultures and in the transmitting insects, are fusiform bodies having the large nucleus and blepharoplast common to the aflagellar form but, in addition, a long slender flagellum arising from the blepharoplast or parabasal body. These forms measure from 15 to 30 microns in length, including the flagellum, and from 1 to 3 microns in breadth.

The aflagellate forms multiply within the endothelial cells, which eventually rupture, liberating the organisms which attack new cells, repeating the process of division. The aflagellate forms, when taken into the intestine of suitable insects, develop into the flagellate forms which in turn multiply by longitudinal fission and eventually become forms which are infective to man. The organism can be cultivated in various culture media, the most useful being the N. N. N. medium at 22° C.

Method of Infection in Man.—The Indian Kala-azar Commission has apparently demonstrated that in India the sandfly, Phlebotomus argentipes, is capable of transmitting Leishmania donovani to experimental animals through the bite of infected flies, and this is probably the usual method of transmission. However, experimental evidence that the infection may be transmitted to animals through the ingestion of infected material is on record and the parasite occurs in both the urine and feces of individuals suffering from kala-azar.

Kala-azar in India is practically found only in regions with alluvial soil, does not occur at altitudes above 2000 feet, and occurs in regions where the annual mean of daily humidity is at least 60 per cent. In other endemic centers these conditions are not essential. Kala-azar is sharply localized, except during widespread epidemics, and is a house and family infection.

White mice, hamsters, monkeys and dogs are susceptible to experimental infection, and in dogs the infection may be naturally acquired.

Pathology.—Patients dying of kala-azar are anemic and emaciated. The *spleen* is enormously enlarged, may be soft or hard, with a smooth capsule. The cut surface is congested, purple or brown in color, and the Malpighian corpuscles are not prominent. Microscopically there is a great increase in the reticular epithelium and the cells contain large numbers of Leishmania. The liver is enlarged, firm, friable and mottled. Fatty infiltration of the liver cells containing Leishmania is noted. Kupffer's cells and the endothelial cells of the vessels contain numerous Leishmania, are swollen, and may block the lumen of the capillaries. The *bone-marrow* is red and soft and contains enormous numbers of macrophages containing Leishmania, myelocytes and polymorphonuclear leukocytes, which may also contain Leishmania. The *heart*, usually dilated, appears pale and flabby, and may show microscopically some myocardial degeneration. The parasitized cells occur in the myocardium and there may be parasites in the endocardium. The *kidneys* show cloudy swelling, and macrophages containing Leishmania may occur in the interstitial tissue. The *lymph glands* are usually enlarged and parasitized cells may be found in the lymph spaces. Ulceration due to other causes may be present in the intestines and invasion of the submucosa by macrophages containing Leishmania occurs throughout the intestine, most marked around Peyer's patches and the solitary follicles.

Symptoms.—The *incubation period* is unknown. The mode of onset is usually insidious, the patient noticing slight attacks of fever at irregular intervals. Typhoid and malarial types of onset have been described in which the symptoms were similar to those of the onset of these infections. In some patients the enlargement of the spleen first attracts attention, other symptoms being absent or so slight as to have been overlooked.

In the beginning a double rise of temperature during the twenty-four hours is often noted, while in other cases the temperature may show great irregularity or there may be quotidian exacerbations. After the infection is fully established the important symptoms are irregular fever with often a double rise during the twenty-four hours, anemia with leukopenia, edema, emaciation, dysentery or diarrhea, and a gradually developing cachexia, with great enlargement of the spleen and enlargement of the liver. The duration of the disease varies and it may be acute, subacute or chronic in type. In the acute cases death may occur within a few weeks, in the subacute cases within a year, while in the chronic cases a fatal result usually occurs in from two to three years.

In the infantile type of kala-azar the symptoms are irregular fever, progressive anemia, mental dulness, constipation alternating with diarrhea, emaciation, abdominal distention, purpuric hemorrhages and cachexia, with progressive enlargement of the spleen. The duration in infants varies from one or two months to two or three years, and spontaneous recovery occurs in some cases.

Complications and Sequelæ.—Cancrum oris is a common complication and often the cause of death. Hemorrhages from the gums, purpuric hemorrhages, bacillary or amebic dysentery, bronchitis, bronchopneumonia, albuminuria, nephritis, septicemia, dilatation of the heart and cerebral hemorrhage are the most important complications in the adult form of kala-azar, while in the infantile form cancrum oris, noma, hemorrhages into the skin and from the gums, septic infections, otitis media, mastoid disease, lobar and bronchopneumonia, and diarrhea and dysentery are noted as complications. In both forms death is frequently due to one or more of these complications.

A sequela of kala-azar, especially in cases treated with antimony, is the condition known as post-kala-azar dermal leishmaniasis, first described by Brahmachari (1922). White patches are noted upon the skin about one year after antimony treatment, followed by the appearance of nodules, and successive crops of depigmented areas and nodules may occur for months. In the nodules Leishmania donovani may be demonstrated both microscopically and in cultures. In these cases the infection appears to be confined entirely to the skin, as the parasites do not occur in the peripheral blood or in the spleen.

Diagnosis.—The diagnosis of kala-azar is established by the demonstration of Leishmania donovani in smears from the peripheral blood, of splenic pulp, of glandular juice, or of liver pulp, or in cultures of these materials, and no diagnosis of this infection is accurate unless the parasite is demonstrated. The smears should be stained with the Wright or Giemsa stain. The aldehyde test of Napier, which consists in adding to 1 cc. of clear blood serum 1 drop of 30 per cent formaldehyde, has proven most useful in diagnosis. In cases of kala-azar which have lasted for four or more months the serum immediately becomes viscid, and in one or two minutes will have become solidified so that the tube can be inverted, and in from three to twenty minutes the entire serum will be solid and opaque, resembling the white of an egg.

Differential Diagnosis.—Kala-azar must be differentiated from typhoid and paratyphoid fevers, malaria, relapsing fevers, undulant fever and tuberculosis. The clinical picture of these conditions, together with the laboratory methods of diagnosis that are available in all, should enable a differential diagnosis to be made without real difficulty.

Prognosis.—In untreated adults from 90 to 95 per cent of cases are fatal, while in infants the mortality varies from 75 to 85 per cent. Severe anemia, marked leukopenia, and cachexia are unfavorable prognostic signs, and when severe complications arise, as cancrum oris, pneumonia or diarrhea, the prognosis is increasingly grave. Some cases are resistant to specific treatment with antimony and in these the prognosis is almost hopeless. It is probable that mild cases of kala-azar occur which are not recognized and the effect of such cases upon the rate of mortality is unknown.

Under proper treatment with antimony the prognosis is excellent, from 85 to 95 per cent of cases so treated being cured.

Prophylaxis.—The most efficient methods of prophylaxis have been segregation of the infected and contacts and treatment of the infected. Admitting that sandflies are the transmitting agents, measures directed toward the destruction of these insects, the prevention of breeding and protection from their bites, are logical prophylactic measures. Up to the present there is no experience available as to the best methods of destroying or controlling these insects.

Treatment.—In 1913, Vianna and Machado reported the successful use of tartar emetic in the treatment of American leishmaniasis, or espundia. Caronia and Di Cristina (1915), Rogers (1915) and Muir (1915) reported success with this drug in the treatment of kala-azar, and since that time antimony has been recognized as a specific for this infection. The form of antimony most used is sodium or potassium antimony tartrate given intravenously, a 2 per cent solution in distilled water being employed. The solution should be freshly prepared and the usual aseptic precautions exercised during injection. After adding the antimony the solution should be boiled for a moment or two. In adults the first dose should be 2 cc. of the 2 per cent solution, which would contain 0.04 gram of the salt, and increased 1 cc. at each administration, until 5 cc. are being injected, and this dose should be continued until the end of the treatment. The injections should be made on alternate days to secure the best results and should be continued until 4 grams of the drug have been administered. The fever does not disappear until after about four weeks' treatment, or twelve injections, but the general condition of the patient rapidly improves. A sharp rise in temperature frequently occurs after injections and coughing, headache and vomiting may be present. Pneumonia should be constantly watched for, as it not infrequently complicates antimony tartrate treatment. A papular eruption may occur following the injections.

For infants of three years, commence with 0.5 cc. of the 2 per cent solution and increase to 2 cc. as a maximum; for a child of twelve years, 1 cc., increased to a maximum of 3.5 cc.; and intermediate dosage for other ages. In weak individuals, commence with 1 cc. and increase to a maximum of 3.5 cc.

Certain pentavalent preparations of antimony have proven successful in the treatment of kala-azar, the most useful being stibosan and ureastibamine. These preparations are costly but are powerful, curing patients after a much smaller number of injections.

The general treatment consists in proper diet, the treatment of complications as they arise, and general tonic treatment after the completion of the course of injections.

Oriental Sore.

Synonyms.—Delhi boil; Aleppo boil; Biskra boil; Frontier sore; Tropical sore; Cutaneous leishmaniasis.

Definition.—A specific ulcerating granulomatous lesion of the skin caused by a species of Leishmania, Leishmania tropica. It is autoinoculable and produces immunity to subsequent infection.

History.—Although clinically oriental sore has been known for many generations, the cause of the condition was first described by J. H. Wright, of Boston, in 1903, and named Leishmania tropica. The rôle of the sandfly, Phlebotomus papatassii, in the transmission of the disease was elucidated between 1921 and 1929 by the Sergents, Parrot, Donatien and Beguet, and Adler and Theodor.

Geographic Distribution.—This form of leishmaniasis occurs in Crete, Cyprus, Sicily, Asia Minor, Morocco, the Sahara, the Sudan, Syria, Arabia, Persia, Nigeria, Mesopotamia, the Caucasus, India, Turkestan, and Palestine. Cases have been described in Central America and South America. While often occurring in the same country, kala-azar and oriental sore seldom occur in the same locality.

Etiology and Epidemiology.—Oriental sore is caused by a protozoan parasite belonging to the genus Leishmania called Leishmania tropica. It is identical in morphology with Leishmania donovani in both man and the transmitting insect, and is transmitted by a sandfly, Phlebotomus papatassii. Oriental sore is practically universal among the natives in the endemic areas, has a seasonal incidence, and infection with the causative organism occurs naturally in dogs in the endemic localities. Leishmania tropica can be cultivated from the lesion in cultures, and in the transmitting insect flagellate forms appear. Monkeys and dogs can be experimentally infected. Both sexes and all ages are susceptible to infection.

Symptoms.—The incubation period may be a few days or several months, cases having been observed in which the incubation period was over fifteen months.

The symptoms vary considerably and the sores may be single or multiple and generally occur on the exposed surfaces of the body.

Usually the lesion first appears as a reddish papule which gradually develops a covering of fine dry scales which later become moist, forming a crust, upon removal of which a shallow ulcer is seen. The ulcer gradually becomes larger and has sharp-cut, raised edges surrounded by an indurated area. Secondary ulcers may form which coalesce with the original one producing ulcerating areas of considerable extent. Secondary infections of the lesion are common and often markedly change the clinical picture. The sores are autoinoculable and inoculable. In many cases the papule does not break down into an ulcer but disappears after a period of weeks or months. In the usual case the ulcers granulate in a period of from two to twelve months, or longer, and heal, leaving a depigmented depressed scar. Several forms of the infection have been described, as the verrucose form, the keloid form and the lupoid form. General symptoms are usually absent unless secondary infections are present.

The *diagnosis* of oriental sore is easily made by the examination of smears of the material obtained by puncture of the indurated edge of the ulcer and staining with the Wright or Giemsa stain. The Leishmania are found in the cells of the granulating tissue and in endothelial cells and large mononuclear leukocytes. They are not found in the peripheral blood. If smears are negative, cultures of the same material should be made upon the N.N.N. medium. If these methods fail and the case is one of infection with Leishmania tropica, it will respond to the specific treatment with antimony.

As regards life the *prognosis* is excellent, as this form of leishmaniasis, of itself, is never fatal. Death may occur from secondary bacterial infections. If properly treated all uncomplicated cases may be promptly cured.

Treatment.—A protective covering should be worn over the lesion to prevent insect infection, and the treatment of infected individuals should be practised. Precautions should be taken to avoid auto-inoculation and the bite of the sandfly transmitting the disease. In this disease, as in kala-azar, antimony acts as a specific. The intravenous injection of a 2 per cent solution of tartar emetic in the same dosage as in kala-azar is recommended, but this infection is more easily cured than is kala-azar and it is seldom necessary to give more than a total amount of 1 gram to 1.5 grams of the drug. The local injection of 1 cc. of a 2 per cent solution into the indurated tissue around the lesion, repeated in from three to four days, is advocated by some authorities. The use of the pentavalent antimony compounds, as stibosan and urea-stibamine, is followed by just as satisfactory results in a shorter period of time. Other drugs, as acetarsone, phosphorated oil, permanganate of potassium, and berberine sulphate, have been used with success, but the specific treatment is to be preferred. Treatment by exposure to the roentgen-ray has been followed by marked success.

Espundia.

Synonyms.—Muco-cutaneous leishmaniasis; Forest yaws; American leishmaniasis; Brazilian leishmaniasis; Naso-pharyngeal leishmaniasis; Uta.

Definition.—Espundia is a disease characterized by ulcerative skin lesions and destructive ulcerative lesions of the mucous membrane of the mouth, nose, and pharynx, caused by a protozoan parasite, Leishmania braziliensis.

History.—This disease has been known in certain regions in South America for generations and was first proven to be due to a Leishmania by Lindenberg (1909) and Carini and Paranhos (1909). Vianna (1911), considering that the parasite was distinct from Leishmania tropica, gave it the name Leishmania braziliensis.

Geographic Distribution.—Apparently confined to the countries of Central and South America, the disease occurs in Brazil, the Argentine, Peru, Venezuela, Bolivia, Ecuador, Paraguay, the Guianas, Yucatan, Panama, Colombia, and Mexico. Imported cases have been observed in the United States. Similar lesions have been observed in patients in the Sudan and in India.

Etiology and Epidemiology.—The disease is caused by Leishmania braziliensis which some authorities believe to be identical with Leishmania tropica, and is probably transmitted by a sandfly, Phlebotomus lutzi. The disease occurs in both sexes and all ages and the parasite lives in the tissue cells, endothelial cells and large mononuclear leukocytes in the involved areas of the skin and mucous membranes, and has the morphology of a typical Leishmania. It can be cultivated upon the N. N. N. medium and in cultures, and in cultures it develops into flagellate forms like those of Leishmania donovani and Leishmania tropica.

Symptoms.—The incubation period is unknown. The primary lesion appears on some uncovered portion of the body as a papule which ulcerates, and after a duration of a few months to two years disappears. After the original sore has healed, and sometimes before healing has occurred, the characteristic lesions of the mucous membrane of the nose appear, consisting of thickening of the mucosa, with the formation of nodular masses which break down, forming ulcerations invading the mucous membrane of the mouth and extending to the hard and soft palates. The mucous membrane of the pharynx and larynx may be affected and the voice may be lost. The cartilage of the nose may be destroyed and necrosis of the tissues of the affected areas may occur, resulting in great deformity and total loss of the nose and mouth. The disease may last for years and death usually is due to some intercurrent condition, more commonly septicemia and broncho- or lobar pneumonia.

The *diagnosis* is established by the demonstration of Leishmania braziliensis in smears of material obtained from the lesions stained with Wright or Giemsa stain.

Before the discovery by Vianna of the specific action of tartar emetic in this infection the *prognosis* was very grave, but if this drug be given early in the disease the prognosis is excellent, and even advanced cases have a favorable prognosis so far as life is concerned.

As the exact method of transmission is unknown, *prophylaxis* is unsatisfactory. The treatment of insect bites and abrasions with iodine may prevent infection, and the isolation and treatment with antimony of those having the disease are logical prophylactic measures.

The *treatment* of this infection is like that of oriental sore by the intravenous injection of tartar emetic.

REFERENCES.

ARCHIBALD, R. G.:   The Practice of Medicine in the Tropics, Byam and Archibald, 1923, **2**, 1443.
BRAHMACHARI, U.:   A Treatise on Kala-azar, London, 1928.
CRAIG, C. F.:   A Manual of the Parasitic Protozoa of Man, Philadelphia, 1926.
LAVERAN, A.:   The Leishmaniases, Paris, 1917.
NAPIER, L. E.:   Kala-azar, London, 1927.

THE TRYPANOSOMIASES.

The trypanosomiases are infections caused by protozoan parasites belonging to the Flagellata, genera Trypanosoma and Schizotrypanum. In man there are three disease conditions caused by these organisms, *i.e.*, African sleeping sickness, caused by Trypanosoma gambiense and Trypanosoma rhodesiense, and South American trypanosomiasis or Chagas' disease, caused by Schizotrypanum cruzi.

African Sleeping Sickness.

Synonyms.—African trypanosomiasis; Negro lethargy.

Definition.—Chronic infections caused by trypanosomes and characterized by irregular fever, enlargement of the lymph glands, and cutaneous eruptions in the early stage, and later by gradually developing nervous symptoms, terminating in coma and death. Two types are recognized, both transmitted by flies of the genus Glossina, one caused by Trypanosoma gambiense, and the other by Trypanosoma rhodesiense.

History.—African sleeping sickness was first described by Winterbottom, in 1903. Trypanosoma gambiense was found in the blood of man by Forde, in 1901, and named by Dutton in 1902, and Castellani found it in the cerebrospinal fluid of cases of sleeping sickness in 1903. Trypanosoma rhodesiense was discovered by Stephens and Fantham, in 1910, in the type of sleeping sickness occurring in Rhodesia. Bruce and Nabarro (1903), and Kleine (1909) proved that Glossina palpalis is the transmitting agent of Trypanosoma gambiense, while Kinghorn and Yorke, in 1912, showed that Glossina morsitans is the transmitter of Trypanosoma rhodesiense.

Geographic Distribution.—Both types of African sleeping sickness are limited in distribution to tropical Africa. Infections with Trypanosoma gambiense occur along the west coast from Senegal to Angola; the regions around Lakes Victoria, Albert and Banguelo; French Equatorial Africa; the Belgian and Portuguese Congo; the Bahr-el-Ghazal region; western Mongolia; and the islands in the Gulf of Guinea. Infections with Trypanosoma rhodesiense occur in northeastern Rhodesia, the northern part of south Rhodesia, Nyassaland, and in German and Portuguese East Africa.

Etiology and Epidemiology.—The two trypanosomes are found in the blood and cerebrospinal fluid, are indistinguishable from one another morphologically, and in preparations stained with Wright or Giemsa stain consist of a spindle-shaped mass of blue stained cyto-

plasm containing a large, oval or round, red stained nucleus or trophonucleus, situated near the center of the body, and a minute red dot,
the blepharoplast, situated at the posterior end of the body, from which
arises a flagellum which forms the end of an undulating membrane
and becomes free at the anterior extremity. In well stained preparations a second red staining rodlet may be seen close to the blepharoplast which is called the parabasal body. The trypanosomes measure
from 16 to 30 microns in length by 1.3 to 2.5 microns in width, but
there are great variations, some forms being short and thick, while
others are long and thin. Multiplication is by binary longitudinal
division. They are actively motile in fresh blood preparations. In
the transmitting insects, Glossina palpalis and Glossina morsitans and
other species of Glossina, the trypanosomes undergo a cycle of development, the fly becoming infective to man in from twelve to twenty-five
days, but direct mechanical transmission is possible for about twenty-
four hours after the insect bites an infected individual. Under certain
conditions the infection with Trypanosoma gambiense occurs in virulent epidemics, but this is not true of infection with Trypanosoma
rhodesiense. Age, sex and race bear no relation to susceptibility, and
the infections are not hereditary in man.

Pathology.—The submaxillary, inguinal and femoral glands are
enlarged, as well as those of the bronchi and mesentery. The cerebrospinal fluid is turbid, increased in amount, and contains the trypanosomes, and a chronic leptomeningitis is noted. Microscopically the
characteristic changes are hyperplasia of the lymphatic system, and a
perivascular cell infiltration of the nervous system, especially marked
around the blood-vessels and lymphatics. The trypanosomes may
invade the connective tissue of all the organs as well as the tissues of
the nervous system.

Symptoms.—The incubation period in infections with Trypanosoma
rhodesiense is between ten and fourteen days, while in infections with
Trypanosoma gambiense it has been estimated as from fourteen days
to several weeks. In the acute stage the symptoms are irregular
febrile attacks, enlargement of the lymphatic glands, moderate enlargement of the spleen, asthenia, and skin eruptions, erythematous in
type, evanescent in character, and most common on the trunk. Localized edema may occur and headache may be a prominent symptom.
In the *chronic stage* the headache is pronounced, the patient gradually
develops mental dulness, asthenia becomes pronounced, and somnolence increases until it is difficult to arouse him even for food. This
condition is accompanied by localized paralyses, contractures, retraction of the head, incontinence of urine and feces, epileptiform convulsions, coma and death. Eye lesions are common in the chronic stage,
as iritis, cyclitis and chorioretinitis. The blood shows nothing characteristic, but anemia is marked toward the end. The symptomatology
of the two types of sleeping sickness is much the same, the only
difference being that in infections with Trypanosoma rhodesiense the
symptoms are usually more severe and the course of the disease much
more acute.

The duration of the disease caused by Trypanosoma gambiense

usually covers several years, while that caused by Trypanosoma rhodesiense covers only a few months. The acute stage in Trypanosoma gambiense infections may last for years, and some cases are so mild as to present no clinical symptoms characteristic of the infection.

Malaria and ankylostomiasis are frequent *complications*, and death often results from secondary infections or pneumonia.

Diagnosis.—An early diagnosis is essential, as treatment after the development of the chronic stage is usually inefficient. The diagnosis rests upon the demonstration of the trypanosomes in the blood, gland juice, or cerebrospinal fluid, or by animal inoculation. The parasites are most numerous in the blood during the febrile periods and can usually be demonstrated at this time in blood films stained with the Wright or Giemsa stain, or in the fresh blood where their active movement attracts attention. Preparations made from material obtained by gland puncture are very useful in diagnosis and, in the chronic stage, stained smears of the cerebrospinal fluid obtained by lumbar puncture usually show the parasite. Inoculation of blood, gland juice or cerebrospinal fluid into rats, mice or guinea-pigs is sometimes successful when other methods have failed. The occurrence of forms with the nucleus situated in the posterior portion of the body in subinoculated animals differentiates Trypanosoma rhodesiense from Trypanosoma gambiense.

Prognosis.—In early cases, properly treated, the prognosis is excellent, but after the development of the sleeping sickness stage, even with approved treatment, it is always grave. The prognosis is more grave in infections with Trypanosoma rhodesiense than with Trypanosoma gambiense. Untreated, most infections end fatally, although spontaneous recoveries have been reported.

Prophylaxis.—The following measures are most useful in prophylaxis: isolation and treatment of the infected; removal of the inhabitants from endemic areas; the protection of man from the bites of the flies transmitting the infections; the control of individuals coming from infected into uninfected districts; and the destruction of the breeding places of Glossina palpalis, Glossina morsitans, Glossina swinertoni, and other flies belonging to this genus.

Treatment.—Among the drugs that have been used with some success in the treatment of sleeping sickness may be mentioned atoxyl, antimony trioxide and tartar emetic, but these drugs are useful only in the acute stage of infection with Trypanosoma gambiense. More recently treatment has consisted in the administration of either tryparsamide or Bayer 205 (germanin). While both of these drugs are almost specific in their action in the early stages of infection with both Trypanosoma gambiense and Trypanosoma rhodesiense, Bayer 205 is said to be the most effective in infections with the latter parasite and tryparsamide more effective in the late stage of Trypanosoma gambiense infections.

Tryparsamide (N-phenylglycinamide-p-arsonate) is administered intravenously in doses of from 0.5 to 3 grams (7.5 to 45 grains), never exceeding 0.035 gram per kilogram of body weight. Four weekly injections are given, followed by a month's interval, when the injections are repeated. It is usually necessary to give the drug in this manner until from 70 to 80 injections are administered. Toxic complications are not troublesome with the dosage recommended, but amblyopia, jaundice and optic conditions should be watched for and the drug stopped if they occur.

Bayer 205, or germanin, is given intravenously, the average dose being 1 gram dissolved in 10 cc. of distilled water, once a week, and continued until 10 grams have been administered. Toxic conditions may follow the use of this drug as urticarial eruptions and nephritis.

Chagas' Disease.

Synonyms.—Brazilian trypanosomiasis; Schizotrypanosomiasis.

Definition.—Chagas' disease, or South American trypanosomiasis, is an acute and chronic disease caused by a trypanosome, Schizotrypanum cruzi, transmitted from man to man by biting bugs belonging to the genus Triatoma. It is characterized in the acute stage by fever, myxedema, enlargement of the lymph glands, spleen, liver and thyroid gland, and by keratitis; and in the chronic stage by myxedema, and symptoms referable to the heart, endocrine glands or nervous system.

History.—The cause of Chagas' disease, Schizotrypanum cruzi, was discovered in the intestine of a biting bug, Triatoma megista, by Chagas, in 1909, who later found the same trypanosome in the blood of children suffering from a disease prevalent in Brazil. The causative relation of the parasite to the disease was first proven by Chagas and has been confirmed by all who have studied the infection.

Geographic Distribution.—Until recently it was thought that Chagas' disease was confined to Brazil, Venezuela and Peru, but Miller and Clark (1931) have shown that it also occurs in Panama.

Etiology and Epidemiology.—Schizotrypanum cruzi is found in the peripheral blood of infected individuals as a typical trypanosome and in the tissue cells as a Leishmania-like organism. No multiplication occurs in the blood, but in the cells multiplication of the Leishmania forms occur with consequent destruction of the cells. In the blood the trypanosomes measure about 29 microns in length and have an unusually large blepharoplast, a nucleus, undulating membrane and free flagellum. In the tissues the Leishmania forms measure 1.5 to 5 microns in diameter and have a nucleus and blepharoplast. In the transmitting insects a definite cycle of development occurs, but the duration of the life-cycle either in man or insect is not known. Several species of Triatoma may transmit the infection but Triatoma megista appears to be the common transmitting agent. The armadillo is thought to furnish a reservoir of infection. The usual method of infection is contaminative, the dejecta of the insect, which contains the trypanosomes, being rubbed or scratched into the lesion produced by the bite, although Chagas and others believe that infection may occur from the salivary secretion introduced in the act of biting. The bug becomes infective in from eight to ten days after biting and retains its infectivity for life (from one to two years). The adult insect transmits the infection in nature but the larvæ and nymphs are experimentally infective.

The disease is very common in children and adults and is a principal cause of infant mortality in the endemic areas.

The recent discovery in California of triatomas naturally infested with Schizotrypanum cruzi renders it probable that unrecognized human infections with this parasite may occur in the southern portion of the United States.

Pathology.—The characteristic pathology consists in the invasion of the tissue cells by Schizotrypanum cruzi, where it develops Leishmania forms which multiply and destroy the invaded cell, afterward becoming trypanosome forms which appear in the blood. The cardiac and skeletal muscles, fat tissue, the lymphatic glands, adenoid tissue, spleen, bone-marrow and connective tissues are most frequently invaded, but the nervous system and practically every tissue of the body may be parasitized.

Symptoms.—Two forms are described, the acute and chronic. The *acute form* usually occurs in children and is characterized by a high fever, followed in about two weeks by a deposit of mucoid material in the tissues causing tumefaction of the entire body. The face is swollen, the eyes partially hidden by edema of the eyelids, and the whole appearance is characteristic of myxedema. The skin is dry and the tumefaction does not pit upon pressure. The thyroid, lymphatic glands, liver and spleen are enlarged and keratitis is a very characteristic lesion. The acute stage lasts from two to four weeks and, if death does not occur, gradually fades into the chronic stage. The trypanosomes may be found in the peripheral blood during the acute stage.

The *chronic stage* follows the acute stage in children, but may primarily occur in adults. The symptomatology varies greatly and depends upon the principal localization of the trypanosomes in the tissues and organs. Thus cardiac, nervous, myxedematous, ovarian and suprarenal types have been described, in each of which the principal symptoms are those of involvement of the heart, central nervous system, thyroid, ovary and suprarenal gland. Acute febrile attacks may occur during the chronic stage, and at such times the trypanosomes may be found in the blood.

The *diagnosis* of Chagas' disease can be made only by the demonstration of the trypanosomes in the blood or by inoculation of a guinea-pig with the blood or cerebrospinal fluid. It is not possible to make a diagnosis from the clinical symptoms alone.

While children sometimes recover, the *prognosis* is very grave and in adults it is hopeless.

As the transmitting insects live in the walls of the native huts, *prophylaxis*, by reason of the construction of these dwellings, is most unsatisfactory. Where possible, the destruction or fumigation of infested habitations should be followed and measures taken to protect individuals from the bite of insects.

Treatment.—Although the various drugs employed in the treatment of African trypanosomiasis have been tried in the treatment of this infection, the results have been disappointing and no specific treatment is known at present. Thyroid extract may be useful in the acute stage and in the myxedematous type of the chronic stage of the infection.

REFERENCES.

BLACKLOCK, B., and YORKE, W.: In: Practice of Medicine in the Tropics, London, Byam and Archibald, 1922.
CHAGAS, C.: Mem. Inst. Oswaldo Cruz, 1909, 1, 159.
CRAIG, C. F.: Manual of the Parasitic Protozoa of Man, Philadelphia, 1926.
LAVERAN, A., MESNIL, F., and NABARRO, D.: Trypanosomes and Trypanosomiases, English translation, Chicago, 1907.

COCCIDIOSIS.

The Coccidia are protozoan parasites belonging to the Sporozoa, which occur rarely in the intestine of man but are common in some of the lower animals. There is a sexual and asexual cycle of development similar to those of the malaria plasmodia except that both cycles are completed within the mammalian host. Until recently several species of coccidia were supposed to be parasites of man, but at the present time one species only, Isospora hominis, is generally accepted as a true parasite of man, although Wenyon believes that another species, Isospora belli, also parasitizes man. The three species described by Dobell as parasites of man, Eimeria wenyoni, Eimeria oxyspora and Eimeria snijdersi, have been proven by Thomson and Robertson to be identical with Eimeria sardinæ and Eimeria clupearum, parasites of fish, described by Thelohan thirty years before Dobell's descriptions.

Isospora hominis is apparently a true parasite of man and some 200 cases of infection with this organism have been described. Infections have been encountered in France, Gallipoli, Salonika, Macedonia, Mesopotamia, Tripoli, Senegal, Egypt, the Philippine Islands, South Africa and the United States. Transmission is probably through food and drink contaminated with feces containing the oöcysts which are the infective agents. The diagnosis of the infection depends entirely upon the demonstration of the oöcysts in the feces. These bodies have a double outline, are oval in shape and measure from 25 to 33 microns in length by 12.5 to 16 microns in breadth. They are colorless and one end is lengthened, giving it a neck-like appearance. Within the oöcyst, when freshly passed, there is a spherical mass of brightly refractile granules. Rarely oöcysts are observed in the feces containing two masses, the sporoblasts.

The parasite lives in the small intestine of man and no other stage of development than the oöcyst is known. There is no scientific evidence available that establishes Isospora hominis as a pathogenic parasite, but in some instances of infection intestinal symptoms, as diarrhea, have been noted, but other causes for these symptoms were also present. Most infections with this parasite are transient. The prognosis is always excellent and prophylaxis depends upon personal hygiene and protection of food and drink from contamination with feces containing the oöcysts of the parasite. There is no specific treatment, and in view of the lack of evidence connecting this parasite with disease, treatment is not indicated.

THE MALARIAL FEVERS.

Types.—Tertian malaria; Quartan malaria; Estivo-autumnal malaria; Remittent malaria; Intermittent malaria; Pernicious malaria.

Definition.—The malarial fevers are specific infectious fevers caused by animal parasites belonging to the Protozoa, genus Plasmodium, which live upon and within the red blood corpuscles of man, finally destroying them. These fevers are usually characterized by marked periodicity, and occur endemically or epidemically in regions where the transmitting insects, mosquitoes belonging to the genus Anopheles, are present.

History.—The malarial fevers were known early in the medical history of mankind, and Hippocrates gave clear descriptions of quotidian, tertian, quartan and semi-tertian fevers. While this is true, it was impossible to distinguish these fevers from other febrile conditions until after the discovery of cinchona bark and its specific action upon fevers of malarial origin. From this time dates the modern history of malaria, which may be divided into three periods.

First Period.—The introduction into Europe of cinchona bark by the Viceroy del Cinchon, in 1640. As this drug acted as a specific curative agent, it thus became possible to differentiate the malarial fevers from other febrile conditions. It was not until 1820 that quinine was isolated from cinchona bark by Pelletier and Couventou, which still further aided in the differentiation of the malarial fevers.

Second Period.—The discovery of the plasmodia of malaria by the French Army surgeon, Alfonse Laveran, in 1880, and the differentiation of the tertian, quartan and estivo-autumnal, or subtertian species, by Grassi and Feletti, Marchiafava, and Celli and Golgi.

Third Period.—The discovery of the method of transmission of the malarial fevers by mosquitoes belonging to the genus Anopheles. Sir Ronald Ross (1895–1898) demonstrated that certain developmental changes occurred in the malarial plasmodia within mosquitoes belonging to this genus, and the Italian observers Bignami, Bastianelli and Grassi (1898–1899) demonstrated that anopheline mosquitoes transmitted malaria by actual experiments upon man and confirmed the developmental changes in the mosquito first observed by Ross.

In 1912 Bass and Johns first succeeded in cultivating the plasmodia of malaria *in vitro*, while within recent years the production of malaria as a curative measure in the treatment of paresis has added valuable data to our knowledge of these fevers.

Geographic Distribution.—The malarial fevers have a wide distribution but are most prevalent in tropical and subtropical regions, especially in low-lying coast regions or the alluvial valleys of rivers, mountainous regions usually being comparatively exempt. In the United States the malarial fevers were once very prevalent in the New England States but at the present time they have almost disappeared. These fevers occur in the Southern States, especially in those bordering upon the Gulf of Mexico; in the Mississippi Valley and the valleys of the larger tributaries of that river; in California, in the valley of the Sacramento River; in the coastal region of Mexico and the coast regions and low-lying interiors of the countries of Central America;

17

and in Cuba, Haiti, San Domingo, Puerto Rico and other islands of the West Indies.

In South America malarial fevers are common in the coastal regions of Colombia, Venezuela, the Guianas, Brazil, Argentine, Peru, Chili and Equador. Malaria is rarely encountered in England, France and Germany, but in Italy, Greece, Crete, Sicily and Turkey these fevers are common and very frequently fatal in character. In Russia, in the valleys of the rivers Dniester, Dnieper and Volga and along the shores of the Black and Caspian Seas, the malarial fevers are common.

In Asia the malarial fevers are common and often pernicious in type in India, Arabia, China, the Federated Malay States, Palestine, Persia, and Siam, Japan and Formosa. In the Philippine Islands, especially on the islands of Luzon, Samar, Mindoro and Mindanao, all types of malaria are endemic and pernicious forms are frequently observed.

In Africa pernicious types of malaria are frequently observed along the eastern and western coasts, while the valleys of the Congo, Niger and Senegal Rivers are heavily infested. The malarial fevers are common in the jungle country throughout tropical Africa and are frequently found in all the countries bordering upon the Mediterranean.

While the résumé given indicates the most important distribution of malaria, it should be remembered that in numerous localities sporadic cases occur at intervals but in which the three fevers may become endemic provided certain species of anopheline mosquitoes are present together with individuals harboring the malaria plasmodia.

Etiology and Epidemiology.—The malarial fevers are caused by animal organisms belonging to the Protozoa, class Sporozoa, genus Plasmodium. The species that are generally accepted are three in number: Plasmodium vivax, the cause of benign tertian malaria; Plasmodium malariæ, the cause of quartan malaria; and Plasmodium falciparum, the cause of estivo-autumnal or subtertian malarial fever. Other species have been described, as Plasmodium falciparum quotidianum, by Craig, 1909; Plasmodium vivax minutum, by Craig, 1900, and by Ahmed Emin, 1914; and Plasmodium tenue, by Stephens, 1914.

Each of the generally recognized species of malaria plasmodia produces characteristic types of fever, and all are transmitted from man to man by mosquitoes belonging to the genus Anopheles, the plasmodia undergoing a definite life-cycle within the insect. No other method of transmission of malaria in Nature is known. The life-cycle of the plasmodia in man is called the endogenous or asexual cycle, and man is the intermediate host, while the life-cycle in the mosquito is called the exogenous or sexual cycle, and the insect is the definitive host.

In man all three species of plasmodia undergo a definite life-cycle varying in time according to the species. Plasmodium vivax, the tertian malaria plasmodium, completes its life-cycle in man in approximately forty-eight hours, Plasmodium malariæ in approximately seventy-two hours and Plasmodium falciparum in approximately forty-eight hours. All of these species at first appear as minute hyaline discs or ring-like bodies, devoid of pigment, upon or within the red blood corpuscles and are known as *trophozoites*. Those that reproduce in man gradually enlarge, develop pigment and are known as *schizonts*.

The schizonts finally divide into a number of segments, which are called *merozoites*, which are liberated by the destruction of the cell containing them. These again invade the red blood corpuscles and the life-cycle is repeated. The reproductive cycle in man is known as *schizogony*.

Among the merozoites which are liberated at the time of segmentation there are some which do not undergo schizogony but develop into sexually differentiated forms called *gametocytes*. The male gametocyte is known as the *microgametocyte* and the female as the *macrogametocyte*. These forms develop within the red blood corpuscles, do not segment as do the schizonts, but when fully grown become free in the blood, where they undergo no further development unless ingested by certain species of mosquitoes belonging to the Anophelinæ. When the blood of an individual containing the micro- and macrogametocytes of the plasmodia is ingested by the mosquito the microgametocyte extrudes several flagellæ known as *microgametes*. These are finally liberated from the parent body and swim actively about until they come in contact with the macrogametocytes, which are now known as the *macrogametes*, certain changes having occurred within them preparing them for fertilization. The microgamete penetrates and fuses with the macrogamete, fertilizing it, and the product is known as the *zygote*. This elongates, becomes motile and is then called the *oökinete*. These changes normally occur in the dilated portion of the mid-gut of the mosquito, which is called the stomach.

After the oökinete becomes motile it penetrates the epithelial lining of the stomach and between this layer and the elastic membrane develops into a spherical cyst known as the *oöcyst*. Within this cyst there are developed innumerable forms known as *sporozoites* which are liberated by the rupture of the cyst. These sporozoites, which are minute, actively motile, thread-like bodies, make their way to the salivary glands of the mosquito where they may be found in the cells of the glands, in the ducts, and in the salivary secretion in immense numbers. When the infected mosquito bites man the sporozoites are injected into the wound made by the bite and thus reach the blood where they invade the red blood corpuscles, develop into schizonts, and initiate the human life-cycle of the plasmodium. The reproductive cycle in the mosquito is known as *sporogony*, and is completed in an average period of from ten to fourteen days.

Morphology of the Malaria Plasmodia.—While the morphology of the three common species of malaria plasmodia differs markedly it may be stated that they all appear at first upon or within the red blood corpuscles as minute hyaline bodies which gradually increase in size, develop pigment and finally fill more or less of the invaded corpuscles which undergo characteristic changes produced by the growth of plasmodia. After attaining full growth the plasmodia divide into minute oval or round bodies, varying in number for each species, which are liberated by the dissolving of the degenerated red blood corpuscle, and which attack new corpuscles, repeating the cycle of development. At all stages of development the plasmodia are colorless, consisting of a hyaline cytoplasm containing a vesicular nucleus and more or less pigment derived from the hemoglobin of the invaded erythrocyte. In infections with the tertian and quartan plasmodium, the gametocytes are round in shape but in infections with the estivo-autumnal plasmodium they are crescentic in shape, the so-called "crescents."

In preparations stained with Wright's stain the cytoplasm of all forms of the malaria plasmodia stains a robin's egg blue, the chromatin of the nucleus a pink or deep red color, and the vesicular portion of the nucleus remains unstained. The earliest forms of all of the plasmodia appear as blue stained rings within the pink stained red blood corpuscle, with one or two dots of bright red chromatin at some portion of the periphery of the ring, the trophozoites. The stages intermediate between the ring and segmented forms show a blue stained cytoplasm containing pigment and scattered grains or clumps of red stained chromatin, the schizonts. In the segmented schizonts each merozoite or segment consists of a mass of blue stained cytoplasm containing a small dot or minute mass of red stained chromatin. The male gametocytes, or microgametocytes, stain a lilac or greenish-blue, the red stained chromatin being distributed in a skein-like mass across the parasite, while the female gametocyte, or macrogametocyte, stains a dark blue and the chromatin is collected in a dense red mass usually near the periphery of the organism.

Mosquitoes Transmitting Malaria.—Only mosquitoes belonging to the genus Anopheles transmit malaria. Thirty-nine species of anopheline mosquitoes have been proven experimentally capable of transmitting Plasmodium vivax, 15 of transmitting Plasmodium malariæ and 42 of transmitting Plasmodium falciparum. However, less than one-quarter of these species act as natural transmitters. Thus in Europe Anopheles maculipennis is the principal transmitter of malaria, while in the eastern, central and southern portions of the United States Anopheles quadrimaculatus is the insect principally concerned in transmission. In the tropics a larger number of species act as efficient transmitters of these infections. The development of the plasmodia in the mosquito is governed by many factors, the most important being proper temperature and humidity, while the infection of the mosquito depends upon the species of anopheline present, the number, sex and age of the gametocytes in the blood of the infected individual and the number of times the mosquito bites the infective individual.

Pathology.—Patients dying of malaria have an anemic, sallow appearance unless the infection is of recent development, and the internal organs present characteristic changes except in the very acute fatal cases when the diagnosis must rest upon the microscopic examinations of the blood and viscera. The most characteristic pathologic changes are noted in long-continued infections.

The *brain* is markedly congested and small hemorrhages may be present in the parenchyma caused by blocking and subsequent rupture of the capillaries by parasite-laden erythrocytes, leukocytes and free pigment, and the cortex may present a gray or brownish appearance. Microscopically, the capillaries contain plasmodia, both free and within erythrocytes, phagocytes containing plasmodia, infected erythrocytes and pigment, while thrombi may be observed produced by the accumulation of these elements.

The *spleen* is usually enlarged, sometimes reaching nearly to the umbilicus and in old infections is dark blue or almost black in color. In chronic infections the cut surface is the color of tar due to intense pigmentation, but in the more acute cases it may be only slightly pigmented or dark red in color due to congestion. The capsule is smooth and thin and the splenic pulp is soft except in the more chronic cases, when it may be firmer than normal. Microscopically the capillaries of the organ are filled with infected erythrocytes, macrophages, pigmented leukocytes and free pigment, and hemorrhagic areas are numerous. Large macrophages filled with infected erythrocytes and enormous amounts of pigment are characteristic features of the pathology of this organ. Smears of the splenic pulp show all the elements mentioned, and the number of plasmodia present is enormous in fatal infections.

The *liver* may or may not be enlarged, is usually pigmented and congested. The capillaries contain infected erythrocytes, macrophages and free pigment, and the liver cells show cloudy swelling and fatty degeneration, with areas of necrosis. In the liver, as well as in the spleen, yellowish-brown free pigment is observed, in addition to the darker malarial pigment.

The *kidneys* sometimes exhibit the lesions usually observed in an acute or subacute nephritis associated with those peculiar to the malarial infection, consisting of engorgement of the capillaries, especially of those of the Malpighian tufts, with infected erythrocytes, pigmented leukocytes and free pigment, and pigmentation of the tubular epithelium.

The *lungs* show no characteristic lesions beyond the presence in the capillaries of infected erythrocytes, pigmented leukocytes and free pigment, with small areas of acute congestion. The *stomach* and intestines sometimes exhibit marked congestion of the mucous membrane, with slight pigmentation, while ulceration due to blocking of the capillaries by pigment, infected erythrocytes and macrophages, may more rarely be observed.

In long-continued malarial infections the bone-marrow is dark red to almost black in color, due to pigmentation, and the capillaries are crowded with infected erythrocytes, free pigment and macrophages.

The pathologic change produced by *chronic malarial infection* is characterized by anemia, marked enlargement of the spleen, enlargement of the liver and fibrosis of these organs. Pigmentation of the cortex of the brain and of the spleen, liver and kidneys is invariably observed. In latent malarial infections there may be some enlargement of the spleen and the capillaries of that organ as well as those of the liver may contain a few infected erythrocytes, pigmented leukocytes and free pigment.

Clinical Pathology.—*Blood.*—There is present some degree of anemia, most marked in the acute, pernicious types of these fevers. In pernicious infections the erythrocyte count may be as low as 1,000,000 per c.mm. and frequently the count averages 2,500,000 per c.mm. in infections in which several paroxysms have occurred. Most frequently the erythrocyte count falls to about 3,000,000 to 3,500,000 per c.mm. and tends to remain at this level if no treatment is given or treatment is inadequate. The leukocytes are reduced in number and the large mononuclear cells relatively increased. During the febrile paroxysm there may be a marked leukocytosis. The hemoglobin is reduced from 10 to 40 per cent within a few days but, in rapidly fatal cases or those in which treatment is promptly administered, there is little or no reduction in the hemoglobin.

Morphologically, poikilocytosis and an anemic appearance of the center of the erythrocyte is generally observed if the malarial infection is of some duration, and in severe infections nucleated erythrocytes may be present and the blood picture may resemble that of primary pernicious anemia. Leukocytes containing pigment and free pigment are present in the peripheral blood. The changes observed in the infected erythrocytes are described in the section treating of Diagnosis.

Urine.—In most infections with the tertian and quartan plasmodia no changes of importance are noted in the urine. In estivo-autumnal infections, especially in those presenting pernicious symptoms, the urea is increased in amount, the specific gravity is increased, albumin appears and hyaline and granular casts are observed. In severe tertian and quartan infections albumin and casts may appear in the urine, and in all three forms of malarial infection hemoglobinuria may occur in rare instances.

Symptoms.—Clinically, malarial fevers may be divided into intermittent, remittent, subcontinued or continued fevers, but this classification is not an exact one from the standpoint of etiology. If a single generation of plasmodium be present the fever is intermittent in all cases, but if several generations are present we may have a subcontinued or continued fever, while two generations of the tertian plasmodium may give rise to a quotidian intermittent fever. Therefore, it is better to classify the malarial fevers from an etiologic standpoint and, thus classified, there are three distinct types each caused by its own species of plasmodium, to which the names tertian, quartan and subtertian, or estivo-autumnal, have been given.

Symptoms of Tertian Malaria.—This form of malaria is caused by Plasmodium vivax, which segments in the blood of man approximately every forty-eight hours, giving rise at the time of segmentation to the typical symptoms of an attack of tertian malaria.

The *incubation period* varies from nine to twenty-four days, the average being fourteen to seventeen days. Prodromal symptoms, as loss of appetite, general malaise and dull headache may be noted a day or more before the attack. The latter begins suddenly with a shaking chill, the face appearing slightly cyanotic and the skin presenting the well-known "goose-flesh" appearance over the extremities and trunk. The pulse is rapid, of low tension and may be irregular, and the patient complains of cold even though he may be covered with blankets. The urine is increased in amount and the temperature gradually rises through the period of chill which usually lasts from one-half to as long as two hours in very severe infections.

The period of chill is succeeded by the hot stage in which the temperature reaches 104° or 105° F. in the average infection. The face is deeply flushed, the eyes brilliant, the conjunctivæ congested, the skin of the entire body reddened and hot to the touch. The respirations are increased in number as well as the pulse-rate, the latter being increased in tension and often dicrotic. There is intense headache and pains in the back and extremities. Epistaxis may occur and there may be a slight cough due to congestion of the lungs. Delirium may be present in very nervous individuals and in very severe cases a semi-comatose condition may develop. During this stage herpes is common, especially of the lips, and erythematous or urticarial eruptions may occur.

The hot stage may last from four to six hours and is succeeded by the sweating stage, lasting from two to three hours in the average case. As the temperature begins to decline, perspiration appears upon the forehead, face, arms, hands and legs and the severity of the other symptoms decreases. When the temperature reaches normal sweating has become very profuse, the entire body perspiring to such an extent that the water may be seen trickling from the face, arms, trunk and legs. In rare instances symptoms of collapse may occur at this stage, the respirations becoming rapid, the pulse weak and the extremities cold. At the end of this stage all symptoms disappear and the patient feels comfortable although weak. In the intervals between the paroxysms the patient feels comparatively well and often resumes his occupation. Polyuria is frequently present between the paroxysms.

The entire tertian paroxysm usually lasts from ten to fourteen hours but in severe cases may last twenty-four hours. It occurs approximately every forty-eight hours, and the symptoms are due to a poison or poisons liberated at the time of segmentation of the plasmodia. When two generations of Plasmodium vivax are present, segmenting upon successive days, a quotidian temperature results and such quotidian temperatures are frequently observed in induced malaria for the treatment of paresis.

Physical examination may reveal an enlarged spleen, with some tenderness, and in a small proportion of cases there may be a slight albuminuria with a few granular and hyaline casts.

Symptoms of Quartan Malaria.—The symptoms of quartan malaria, caused by Plasmodium malariæ, in which the paroxysms of chill, fever and sweating occur at approximate intervals of seventy-two hours, are much like those occurring in tertian infections but are perhaps more severe, the headache being more intense, while mild delirium is more frequently observed during the febrile stage. The paroxysms usually last from eight to ten hours but may last as long as twenty-four hours in severe infections. Quotidian and irregular temperatures may be caused by several generations of the plasmodium segmenting at different times, but such infections are less frequent than in tertian infections. The *period of incubation* is about twenty-one days, but there is great variation due to personal resistance.

Death may occur as a result of either tertian or quartan malarial infections, but is very rare and practically unknown in many localities where these forms of malaria occur.

Symptoms of Estivo-autumnal Malaria.—The symptomatology of estivo-autumnal malaria, caused by Plasmodium falciparum, is much more varied than that of tertian or quartan malaria, for it is this variety of malaria that causes most pernicious infections. The *period of incubation* varies from seven to fifteen days, average ten to twelve days, but may be prolonged to weeks or even months. It is to this type of malaria that the term "remittent malaria" is frequently applied because of the irregularity of the temperature curve, but in uncomplicated cases the temperature is as typically intermittent as in tertian or quartan fever, the paroxysms occurring approximately every forty to forty-eight hours, although owing to infection with more than one generation of plasmodium, remittent or irregular temperatures are more frequently observed.

In the average infection with Plasmodium falciparum the onset of the paroxysm is usually more gradual than in tertian or quartan infections, the chill less pronounced and the sweating stage shorter and perspiration less marked. A severe shaking chill seldom occurs, there being instead chilly sensations noted along the spine, trunk and legs. Headache is intense, the face cyanotic, the eyes brilliant, the respirations increased in number and the pulse fast and decreased in tension. The temperature gradually rises to 103° F. or over during the cold stage which usually lasts one-half to three-quarters of an hour.

The symptoms of the hot stage are similar to those in tertian and quartan infections, the fever reaching 104° F. or more, but there is more severe pain in the back and legs and the nervous symptoms are more pronounced, delirium or stupor being frequently noted. Vomiting may occur, as well as diarrhea, and the urine often shows some albumin and a few casts. This stage lasts from sixteen to twenty-four hours, or even longer, in severe infections.

As noted, the sweating stage is not as marked as in other malarial infections, the temperature rapidly falling but with comparatively little perspiration. With the fall in temperature the symptoms rapidly disappear and the patient feels well although weakened by the paroxysm. In this type of malaria the interval between the paroxysms is short, not over a few hours, and succeeding paroxysms usually present more severe symptoms until, in many instances, those characteristic of pernicious malaria occur.

The temperature in uncomplicated infections with Plasmodium falciparum is most characteristic. The fever rises rapidly during the first two hours of the paroxysm to 103° F. or higher, after which there is a period of two or more hours during which oscillations occur, at the end of which time there is a drop in the curve, called the pseudo-crisis. This drop may be of several degrees, but usually not more than two, when another rise occurs to a point as high or higher than the initial rise, after which the true crisis occurs, the temperature falling rapidly to normal or below normal. The entire febrile paroxysm usually covers thirty-six hours or more, and the temperature curve may be divided into the initial rise, the stage of oscillation, the pseudo-crisis, the precritical rise and the true crisis or fall.

As already stated marked deviations from this classical curve are frequently observed due to infection with several generations of plasmodia, insufficient treatment with quinine and the anticipation or retardation of segmentation.

Pernicious Malaria.—This name is applied to malarial infections in which the life of the patient is endangered. The cause of perniciousness is not definitely known, but the vast majority of pernicious cases are infected with Plasmodium falciparum, the estivo-autumnal plasmodium. For this reason estivo-autumnal malaria is always serious, for at any time pernicious symptoms may develop which may cause death. Blocking of the capillaries of the brain by parasite-laden erythrocytes, free pigment and pigmented leukocytes, the amount and character of the toxin produced by the plasmodia and the lack of resistance of the patient are probably the most important factors favoring the occurrence of pernicious symptoms. These forms of malaria are generally classified according to the character of the symptoms which accompany the attack. Thus we have algid, bilious, cardialgic, comatose, choleraic, delirious, dysenteric, eclamptic, hemiplegic, hemorrhagic and pneumonic types, but it should be remembered that these are not disease entities but indicate the most prominent symptoms observed. Of these various types the comatose and algid types are most frequently encountered.

In the comatose type coma may develop suddenly or may come on gradually during the usual malarial paroxysm. When it develops suddenly the patient loses consciousness and, if working, falls to the ground and does not regain consciousness in fatal infections. The face is congested, the breathing rapid and stertorous, the pulse rapid and of high tension, and the temperature high but often only slightly elevated. Death may occur in a few hours or one or two days. When coma develops gradually the first symptoms are an increase in the headache and nervous irritability followed by drowsiness gradually deepening into coma. The temperature is often irregular, usually between 102° and 105° F., but in some instances may be little elevated or even subnormal. In fatal cases the pulse becomes very rapid and weak, the respirations shallow and death occurs through collapse. Most comatose malarial patients die unless promptly treated, but consciousness may be regained and the paroxysm may be repeated, the patient dying during the second or even third paroxysm. In rare instances spontaneous recovery may occur.

The symptoms in the algid form of pernicious malaria are those of profound collapse almost from the beginning of the paroxysm. The chill may be severe, the skin is pale and bedewed with perspiration, the pulse thready, rapid, irregular and of low tension, and there is marked mental apathy or stupor. Death usually occurs in untreated cases within twenty-four to thirty-six hours although some patients die within six or eight hours after the onset of the algid symptoms. The algid type usually develops after the occurrence of several previous attacks of malaria.

Blackwater Fever.—The condition known as blackwater fever is now generally recognized as being invariably associated with malaria, if not actually caused by these infections. It is found wherever malaria occurs, but usually only where the estivo-autumnal infections are prevalent. It generally follows repeated malarial paroxysms, but may occur during the first paroxysm. The attack commences with a chill, the temperature rising rapidly to 104° to 106° F., the general symptoms being like those of a malarial paroxysm. Within a few hours the urine becomes a reddish or dark mahogany-red in color, due to the dissolved erythrocytes; jaundice appears shortly after the hemoglobinuria; and anemia develops rapidly. In mild cases the temperature may fall within thirty-six hours but it may become remittent or continuous. Anuria may develop and this is usually followed by death. In mild cases the attack may terminate within twenty-four hours but severe cases last for several days and death frequently occurs from anuria or cardiac failure.

The symptomatology of the other forms of pernicious malaria mentioned is indicated by the name of the type.

Latent Malaria and Masked Malarial Infection.—In endemic regions of malaria the inhabitants, especially the children, frequently show plasmodia in their blood, although definite symptoms of malaria may be absent. These "carriers" of the infection, for most of them have gametocytes in their blood, are of the greatest importance in the transmission of the disease, and in these individuals the infection is said to be "latent." A change of climate or unusual hardships, which decrease resistance, will frequently bring about definite paroxysms of fever in these individuals. In addition, malaria may be masked by some other disease process, or may simulate pulmonary tuberculosis, severe anemia, chronic amebic dysentery, insolation, acute appendicitis, facial neuralgia, undulant fever, acute bronchitis and yellow fever. The diagnosis of these latent and masked infections depends entirely upon the result of blood examinations.

Complications.—Combined infections with other diseases are frequent and the symptoms observed under such conditions have been incorrectly described as disease entities. Thus, combined malaria and typhoid fever have been described as typho-malaria, a disease entity.

In the *nervous* system the chief complications are nervous prostration, hysteria, delirium, acute mania, paraplegia, hemiplegia and meningitis; in the *respiratory* system, acute bronchitis, bronchopneumonia and lobar pneumonia and pulmonary tuberculosis; in the *circulatory* system, functional heart murmurs, bradycardia and any of the organic diseases of the heart; in the *gastro-intestinal system*, amebic or bacillary dysentery, acute and chronic gastritis, enteritis or colitis; and in the *genito-urinary* system, acute, subacute or chronic nephritis, cystitis and the venereal diseases.

Sequelæ of Malaria.—It is not always possible to differentiate between a condition which may have developed during an attack of malaria due to some other cause and a similar condition which may be a sequela of the infection, and in reaching a conclusion we must depend upon recorded experiences and the clinical history of the case.

In the *nervous* system sequelæ are largely due to the blocking of the capillaries with pigment, parasites and leukocytes. These sequelæ are often slight and quickly disappear. Psychic disturbances are sometimes noted, especially defective memory, and mania or melancholia may occur as sequelæ of estivo-autumnal infections. Aphasia, hemiplegia and paraplegia, multiple neuritis, neuralgias and insomnia have all been noted as sequelæ.

Acute or chronic gastritis, gastric ulcer, acute or chronic enteritis, and a form of chronic dysentery have been described as sequelæ of malaria, while albuminuria and acute or chronic parenchymatous or interstitial nephritis may occur in old relapsing infections. Transient polyuria is a frequent sequela. A form of hypertrophic hepatitis has been described as a sequela, but it is doubtful if atrophic cirrhosis of the liver ever occurs as noted by the older writers. Chronic enlargement of the spleen is a common sequela in long-standing malarial infection and rupture of this organ may occur during acute attacks due to intense engorgement and softness of the organ. In two such instances observed by the writer the rupture was caused by accidental blows over the spleen.

A chronic form of anemia may occur as a sequela of repeated malarial infection and rarely the blood picture is identical with that of primary pernicious anemia. Sequelæ affecting the eye are amaurosis, retinochoroiditis, keratitis, paralysis of accommodation, while intermittent otalgia and attacks of deafness, as well as labyrinthine vertigo, have been noted.

The condition known as *malarial cachexia* develops after long-continued infection and is characterized by a sallow complexion, underweight, attacks of fever and a marked anemia. The spleen is enlarged, the so-called "ague-cake" spleen, and is firm on pressure and not painful. With improved methods of diagnosis and treatment malarial cachexia is much less frequently observed now than formerly.

Relapses in Malaria.—Unless properly treated, from 80 to 90 per cent of malarial infections relapse. The cause of relapse is probably the continued existence of the human life-cycle forms of the plasmodia in small numbers between relapses, the number being insufficient to produce symptoms. The relapse is the result of a decreased resistance of the individual, allowing more rapid multiplication of the plasmodia which eventually results in the production of symptoms. The time of relapse varies greatly but the first relapse usually occurs between the twentieth and thirtieth days after the primary attack, while relapses occurring later vary between fifteen and sixty days between attacks. The longest relapse period observed by the writer was one hundred and fifty-six days after the primary attack, but relapses after longer periods have been described. It is possible that some resistant phase of the plasmodia, as yet unrecognized, is responsible for these long period relapses.

Diagnosis.—The only method of making an accurate and scientific diagnosis of malaria is by the demonstration of the malaria plasmodia in the blood. In uncomplicated tertian and quartan infections the symptomatology is very characteristic and may be sufficient upon which to base a diagnosis, but it should always be confirmed by a blood examination, while in estivo-autumnal and mixed infections the symptoms are notoriously unreliable from a diagnostic standpoint, and the blood examination is absolutely essential. An enlarged spleen in an endemic malarial region is usually indicative of malarial infection, and should lead to a careful microscopic examination of the blood.

The plasmodia are most numerous in the blood a few hours after the chill, but in tertian and quartan infections plasmodia are always present in average infections. In some infections repeated examinations will have to be made, and this is especially true in relapses and in estivo-autumnal malaria. In the latter only the small ring forms and the crescentic gametocytes usually occur in the peripheral blood, while in tertian and quartan infections all stages of the human life-cycle, as well as the gametocytes, are found in blood obtained from the finger or ear. Between the acute attacks of fever the plasmodia are mostly situated in the internal organs and repeated examinations of the peripheral blood may fail to reveal them, although in the experience of the writer, if enough blood smears be carefully examined the plasmodia can generally be demonstrated. The thick blood film is most useful in the examination of latent infections or in the intervals between attacks when the usual method of examination has proven unsuccessful in demonstrating the plasmodia.

The therapeutic test with quinine is useful where the microscopic examination of the blood has failed. All malarial fevers respond to quinine when properly administered and any fever which resists from 1.5 to 2 grams of quinine for over six days is not malarial in nature. If the fever disappears under quinine it does not prove that it was really malarial, but if it is not affected it is proof that it was not due to the malaria plasmodia. The test should never be depended upon when a blood examination is possible.

The differential features of the three species of malaria plasmodia which are depended upon in diagnosis are given in Table 7, page 269.

Differential Diagnosis.—The diseases in which it is most important to make a differential diagnosis are tuberculosis, typhoid fever, paratyphoid fever, undulant fever, yellow fever, dengue, relapsing fevers, cerebral apoplexy, influenza and septicemia. The use of the laboratory methods, available for the diagnosis of these conditions and malaria, and a careful study of the clinical picture should enable one to make a differential diagnosis with comparative ease. A microscopic examination of the blood should never be omitted in any febrile condition.

Prognosis.—The prognosis in tertian and quartan malarial fevers, even if untreated, is excellent, so far as danger to life is concerned, but in untreated estivo-autumnal infections the prognosis is always grave as in this type of malaria pernicious symptoms, resulting in death, may arise at any time. However, even in these patients the prompt intravenous injection of quinine is usually followed by recovery. In patients whose resistance has been lowered by such factors as famine or war conditions, the prognosis should always be guarded as fatal infections with Plasmodium falciparum frequently occur, and, much more rarely, infections with Plasmodium malariæ and Plasmodium vivax may result fatally.

In properly treated malarial infections the prognosis is excellent.

TABLE 7.—DIFFERENTIAL FEATURES OF PLASMODIUM VIVAX, PLASMODIUM MALARIÆ AND PLASMODIUM FALCIPARUM.

	Plasmodium vivax.	Plasmodium malariæ.	Plasmodium falciparum.
Size	Larger than erythrocyte	Same as erythrocyte	Smaller than erythrocyte.
Size of infected erythrocyte	Larger than normal	Normal in size	Normal or smaller.
Changes in cytoplasm of erythrocyte	Schuffner's dots (eosinophilic granules) present	Schuffner's dots absent	Maurer's dots (basophilic granules) present.
Number of merozoites	12 to 24	6 to 12	10 to 30.
Gametocytes	Spherical	Spherical	Crescentic (crescents).
Schizogony	Complete in approximately 48 hours	Complete in approximately 72 hours	Complete in approximately 48 hours.
Stages in schizogony present in peripheral blood	All stages	All stages	"Ring-forms" and rarely small pigmented forms.

Prophylaxis.—The prophylaxis of malaria consists in the destruction of the mosquitoes transmitting the infection, the protection of man from the bites of the transmitting mosquitoes, and the destruction of the plasmodia in man, thus preventing the infection of the mosquito. The destruction of mosquitoes is accomplished by destroying their breeding places by drainage, filling in and oiling of bodies of water which cannot be abolished. The use of various fish which devour the larvæ and the spraying of a mixture of Paris green and dust is efficient, while the catching of adult mosquitoes by traps is a useful method of destroying the adult insects.

The protection of man from the bites of mosquitoes is accomplished by the proper screening of habitations, the use of mosquito nets over the bed, the use of the head net and gloves, and the smearing of various odorous substances upon the exposed skin, the most generally useful being a mixture of 1 part of oil of citronella and 5 or 6 parts of liquid vaseline.

The destruction of the plasmodia in the blood of man, thus preventing the infection of the mosquito, is accomplished by proper treatment with quinine or a combination of quinine and plasmochin. Quinine, as a prophylactic, should be given in doses of 1 gram daily, the smaller doses, previously recommended, having proved unsuccessful in preventing symptoms. The administration of 0.02 gram of plasmochin three times a day, has been very successful in preventing infection and is now being used very widely in prophylaxis.

The method to be adopted in the prophylaxis of malaria is a local question, as a method or methods suitable in one locality, may be impossible in another. The most valuable of all methods, if it can be applied, is the prevention of breeding of mosquitoes by destruction of the breeding places, but usually it will be found necessary to combine this with protection from mosquito bites and the proper treatment of the "carrier" of the plasmodia and of the patient suffering from the infection.

Treatment.—Quinine is a specific in the treatment of malaria, and if the drug is properly administered, in sufficient dosage, and is absorbed by the patient, it will cure every malarial infection if the treatment is instituted before the patient is practically moribund. Unfortunately, many individuals absorb quinine with some difficulty; others, more rarely, have an idiosyncrasy to the drug; and, most frequently of all, the drug is not administered in sufficient dosage and for a long enough time, to cure the infection. It cannot be too urgently stressed that to insure the cure of malarial infection, quinine must be given over a period of several weeks and unless this is done relapses will occur.

Whether quinine cures by acting directly upon the plasmodia or whether it acts in some other way is not definitely known, but however it acts it will cure malarial infections when properly administered. So far as is known quinine-fast strains of the plasmodia do not develop after prolonged administration of the drug and such administration is perfectly compatible with normal health in most individuals.

The salts of quinine generally used are the sulphate, dihydrochloride and tannate, but in ordinary practice the sulphate for administration by mouth and the dihydrochloride for administration intravenously are the preparations of choice. The best method of administration, as regards time, is to give the sulphate in divided doses every three or four hours, and the dosage used depends upon the type of infection. Intramuscular injections of quinine, recommended by some authorities, should never be used if it can be avoided, owing to the necrosis of tissue following their use. In pernicious infections the drug should always be given intravenously, if possible. By mouth the sulphate may be given in the form of solutions, pills, capsules, tablets or cachets. Tablets are preferable, if easily soluble, and quinine in solution should be reserved for mass treatment in camps and institutions. For intravenous injection the dihydrochloride should be dissolved in normal salt solution and sterilized.

As a routine treatment for the average malarial infection, that recommended by the National Malaria Committee, in 1918, is as good as any yet devised. If carefully and conscientiously followed it will result in cure in the vast majority of infections. This treatment follows:

For the acute attack, 0.65 gram (10 grains) of quinine sulphate should be given by mouth, three times a day, for a period of at least three or four days, followed by the administration of 0.65 gram every night before retiring, for a period of eight weeks. For infected individuals without acute symptoms the latter part only of the treatment (0.65 gram nightly for eight weeks) is essential.

The doses for children are: age less than one year, 0.035 gram; one year, 0.065 gram; two years, 0.125 gram; three and four years, 0.2 gram; five, six and seven years, 0.25 gram; eight, nine and ten years,

0.35 gram; eleven, twelve, thirteen and fourteen years, 0.52 gram; fifteen years and over, 0.65 gram.

In some infections it will be necessary to continue the quinine in 0.65 gram doses daily for a period of twelve to fifteen weeks. Bass states that this amount of quinine daily for four weeks cures from 60 to 70 per cent of cases; for six weeks, 80 per cent; for eight weeks, 90 to 95 per cent; and from twelve to fifteen weeks, 100 per cent.

In pernicious malarial infections quinine should be given at once intravenously, the dihydrochloride or bimuriate being used. Not over 1.3 grams (20 grains) should be given at one time and in most cases 0.65 to 1 gram is sufficient. This amount of quinine should be diluted with at least 150 cc. of normal saline solution, boiled and allowed to cool to 38° C. before injection. Aseptic precautions should be observed. If the dangerous symptoms have not abated within five to six hours the quinine injection should be repeated.

The proper treatment of initial malarial infections is most important from a prophylactic standpoint and with the advent of plasmochin, a synthetic quinoline derivative, it is now possible not only to cure the infection in man by combining this drug with quinine but also promptly to destroy the gametocytes, thus preventing the infection of the mosquito. In every malaria infection, after the symptoms have been controlled by quinine, plasmochin in doses of 0.01 gram, three to four times a day, should be administered for a period of five or six days in order to kill the gametocytes that may have developed during the infection, the usual treatment with quinine being continued. If later examiations of the blood show the presence of gametocytes, the treatment with plasmochin should be repeated.

In the treatment of latent and recurrent malarial infections quinine should be administered in full dosage if symptoms are present and continued in the usual dose of 0.65 gram a day for at least eight weeks. If the blood contains gametocytes plasmochin should be administered as recommended above.

The treatment of "carriers" of malaria (those individuals having plasmodia in their blood without symptoms) is a most important prophylactic method, as a large proportion of such individuals have gametocytes in the peripheral blood and are thus infective to mosquitoes. It is possible by administering 2 grams of quinine daily, in divided doses, to cause the disappearance of gametocytes in from three to four weeks, but this practice is being replaced by the administration of a combination of quinine and plasmochin known as chinoplasmin.

This preparation is available in tablet form, each tablet containing 0.005 gram of plasmochin and 0.15 gram of quinine sulphate. To adults 2 tablets should be administered three or four times a day for eight to ten days, the results being controlled by a blood examination. Usually the gametocytes will have disappeared from the blood at the end of this period, but if not, the treatment should be continued until the blood is negative. Toxic symptoms, as abdominal colic, cyanosis, cardiac irregularity, epigastric tenderness, headache and nausea have been noted after the administration of plasmochin, but in the dosage here recommended toxic symptoms have never been recorded.

Plasmochin should not be relied upon for the cure of malaria, but it should be used in connection with quinine for its destructive action upon the gametocytes, and in tertian infections it has been found that its combination with quinine results in a very much smaller relapse rate than when quinine is used alone.

Atabrine has recently been introduced as a specific for malarial infections. It is an alkyl amino-acridine derivative and is furnished in tablets containing 0.1 gram ($1\frac{1}{2}$ grains) and the dosage recommended is 1 tablet three times a day (or 0.3 grams daily) for five consecutive days in the treatment of tertian and quartan malaria, while in the treatment of estivo-autumnal malaria it is recommended that to this dosage of atabrine there be added 0.01 gram ($\frac{1}{6}$ grain) of plasmochin three times daily. For children $\frac{1}{2}$ to 1 tablet of atabrine should be given once to thrice daily according to age and, if plasmochin is used with it, the dose of the latter should vary from 0.005 gram ($\frac{1}{12}$ grain) to 0.01 gram ($\frac{1}{6}$ grain) once to three times daily according to age. Atabrine acts upon both the schizonts and gametocytes of the tertian and quartan plasmodia, while it destroys the schizonts of the estivo-autumnal plasmodia only, so that if it is desired to destroy the gameto-cytes of the latter species it is necessary to combine plasmochin with it. All reports confirm the specificity of atabrine in the treatment of malarial infections and it is probable that in this drug we have the most powerful remedial agent now known for the treatment of malaria.

Some individuals are unable to take quinine, and other drugs have to be used as substitutes. Plasmochin is efficient in tertian and quartan infections but useless in estivo-autumnal malaria except for its specific action upon the gametocytes. Atabrine is curative in all malarial infections and should be used wherever quinine cannot be tolerated. Euchinin, methylene blue and acetarsone have all been used as sub-stitutes with reputed success, but none of these drugs is as efficient as atabrine.

In the treatment of blackwater fever quinine should not be given unless parasites are present in the blood. Excellent results in the treatment of blackwater fever with plasmochin or atabrine have been reported and it is probable that they are safer than quinine in the treatment of this condition. In severe cases and those presenting anuria, intravenous and subcutaneous injections of normal saline or of alkaline solutions should be practised and fluids should be freely given by mouth. Otherwise the treatment is symptomatic.

General Treatment.—The patient should remain in bed until the active symptoms have subsided, the diet should be light or liquid during the febrile period and nourishing and easily digested during convales-cence. At the beginning of the attack calomel should be administered in minute doses followed by a saline purgative. The symptoms should be treated as they arise in the usual manner.

It cannot be too strongly stressed that the administration of quinine should be continued for at least eight weeks if relapses are to be avoided and the malarial infection actually cured.

REFERENCES.

BASS, C. C., and JOHNS, F. M.: The Cultivation of Malarial Plasmodia, Jour. Exp. Med., 1921, **15**, 567.
BOYD, M. F.: An Introduction to Malariology, Boston, 1930.
CRAIG, C. F.: The Malarial Fevers, New York and London, 1909.
———— Manual of the Parasitic Protozoa of Man, Philadelphia, 1926.
DEADERICK, W. H.: A Practical Study of Malaria, Philadelphia, 1912.
MARCHIAFAVA, E., and BIGNAMI, A.: The Malarial Fevers, XXth Century Practice, New York, 1909, vol. **19**.
THAYER, W. S.: Lectures Upon the Malarial Fevers, New York, 1897.
THAYER, W. S., and HEWETSON, A.: Malarial Fevers of Baltimore, Rep., Johns Hopkins Hosp., 1895.

SARCOSPORIDIOSIS.

Infection with Sarcocystis lindemanni, a protozoan parasite of man belonging to the genus Sarcocystis, has been described by a few authorities, the parasite invading the muscles of the human host, especially the tongue, heart, larynx, diaphragm, abdomen and the biceps. The fully developed sarcocysts are cylindrical, elongated or fusiform bodies, with rounded ends, measuring as much as 25 mm. in length, enclosed in a distinct membrane, and containing multitudes of spores (Rainey's corpuscles) which lie within small compartments in the sarcocyst, and which are round, oval, elongated or sickle-shaped. The method of transmission of this parasite is unknown but is probably through the contamination of food. The symptoms of infection, if any occur, have not been studied and it is very doubtful if it is pathogenic except very rarely, as infections of the lower animals with similar parasites frequently occur without the appearance of symptoms. It is still undetermined whether Sarcocystis lindemanni is a valid species or whether it is identical with one of the species of Sarcocystis parasitic in domestic animals as cattle, pigs, sheep and poultry.

BALANTIDIASIS.

Synonym.—Balantidial dysentery.

Definition.—An infection of the intestine of man with a protozoan parasite of the pig belonging to the Ciliata, genus Balantidium, named Balantidium coli. In man the infection is sometimes characterized by diarrhea and dysentery and is known as ciliate or balantidial dysentery.

History.—Balantidium coli was discovered by Malmsten, in 1857, and named by Stein in 1862. Its relation to disease in man and the lesions produced have been described by Strong (1894), Brumpt (1909), and Walker (1913), and the exact morphology of the parasite by McDonald (1922).

Geographic Distribution.—Probably wherever the natural host, the pig, is domesticated. Cases have been described from Norway, Sweden, Russia, Finland, Germany, Austria, France, Holland, Serbia and Italy, in Europe; from Siberia, China and Ceylon, in Asia; from Egypt, the Sudan and Abyssinia, in Africa; from Brazil, Venezuela and Honduras, in South America; and from the United States in North America. The infection is quite prevalent in the Philippine Islands and cases have been reported from Cuba and Puerto Rico.

Etiology and Epidemiology.—Balantidium coli is the largest of the protozoa infesting man, the trophozoites measuring from 50 to 80 microns in length and from 40 to 60 microns in breadth.   It is oval in shape, contains a cytostome, a large kidney-shaped nucleus, a small nucleus, or micronucleus, in contact with it, and two contractile vacuoles.   The body is covered with rows of cilia, and reproduction occurs by transverse division.   The trophozoites are actively motile and live in the large intestine, encysting in the descending colon and the rectum.   The cysts are round or oval in shape and measure from 45 to 85 microns in greatest diameter.   It can be cultivated upon suitable media.

Balantidium coli is normally a parasite of the pig and infection of man occurs by the ingestion of food or drink contaminated with the feces of pigs containing the cysts.   Thus infection with this parasite is most common in those in contact with pigs, especially those who handle the feces or intestines of these animals, as butchers, employees of packing houses or swineherders.   Infection may occur through eating pork products insufficiently cooked.   The cysts live in moist feces for weeks and food may be contaminated through flies or through the use of pig feces for fertilizing purposes.   Infection with this parasite is not common in any locality.   It can be experimentally transmitted from pigs to monkeys and from man to cats, monkeys and pigs.

Pathology.—Balantidium coli may live in the intestine of man without producing obvious lesions or symptoms.   When it does invade the tissues of the intestine the lesions produced so closely resemble those of amebic infection that a differential diagnosis is usually impossible without the demonstration of the parasite in the lesions. There is the same picture of abscess formation, ulceration and necrosis of the tissues as produced by Endamœba histolytica already described, and the balantidia are found in groups or singly in the tissues at the base of the ulcers, in the mucous, submucous and muscular coat and in the blood-vessels and lymphatics of the invaded tissues.   Even when there is no evidence of penetration of the tissue the mucous membrane may be hyperemic and superficial necrosis and hemorrhagic areas may be present.

Symptoms.—Many infections with this parasite present no definite symptoms.   Diarrhea and dysentery are the characteristic symptoms, often accompanied by colic, nausea or vomiting, and tenesmus.   Loss of appetite, or a capricious appetite, slight anemia, dull headache, insomnia, muscular weakness and loss of weight are frequently observed. In uncomplicated cases the blood count is normal except for a slight anemia and fever does not occur.   Physical examination may be negative but usually there is tenderness over the colon and the thickened intestine may be felt through the abdominal wall.   The diarrhea is intermittent and in the intervals there may be constipation.   The diarrheal stools are semi-liquid or liquid and when dysentery is present contain much mucus and blood.   The general clinical picture is that of amebiasis.

Numerous *complications* may occur as the infection may last for years. The most common *sequelæ* are cicatricial contractions of the large intestine caused by the healing of the ulcerations.

The *diagnosis* rests upon the demonstration of Balantidium coli in the feces of the patient. When diarrhea or dysentery is present the motile trophozoites are found but when the feces are semi-formed or formed the cysts only occur in the stools. The differential diagnosis of balantidial dysentery from that due to Endamœba histolytica or other causes can be made only by the demonstration of Balantidium coli in the feces.

The *prognosis* is usually good in otherwise healthy individuals. Spontaneous recovery occurs and many cases recover after treatment. In debilitated patients the mortality has been stated to be as high as 20 to 30 per cent. In probably 50 to 60 per cent of infections with this parasite no symptoms are noted and in these "carriers" the prognosis is excellent, especially if treatment is instituted.

Prophylaxis.—The prophylaxis of this infection consists in precautions against the contamination of food and drink by the feces of pigs and in proper personal hygiene.

Treatment.—There is no specific treatment for this infection, and many drugs have been used with apparent success by different authorities. The organic silver compounds in enemata, as protargol, are said to be efficient and acetarsone (stovarsol) administered as in amebiasis has been used with favorable results. Methylene blue enemata (1 to 3000) and the administration of this drug by mouth is recommended as efficient, but emetin appears to be useless. The general treatment is that recommended for amebiasis.

REFERENCES.

BRUMPT, E.: Demonstration of the Pathogenic Rôle of Balantidium Coli, C. R. Soc. Biol., 1909, **67**, 103.
CRAIG, C. F.: A Manual of the Parasitic Protozoa of Man, Philadelphia, 1926.
McDONALD, J. D.: Univ. of Calif. Pub. Zoöl., 1922, **20**, 243.
WALKER, E. L.: Experimental Balantidiasis, Philippine Jour. Sci., 1913, **8**, 333.

CHAPTER VII.

THE METAZOAL DISEASES.

By ERNEST CARROLL FAUST, Ph.D.

INTRODUCTION.
GENERAL CLASSIFICATION OF HEL-
  MINTH DISEASES.
NEMATODE INFECTIONS.
  Ancylostomiasis.
  Trichocephaliasis (Trichuriasis).
  Ascariasis.
  Oxyuriasis.
  Strongyloidosis.
  Trichinosis.
  Filariasis.
CESTODE INFECTIONS.
  Teniasis.
  Echinococcosis.
  Hymenolepiasis.

CESTODE INFECTIONS—*Continued.*
  Dipylidiasis.
  Diphyllobothriasis.
  Sparganosis.
TREMATODE INFECTIONS.
  Distomiasis.
  Schistosomiasis.
GENERAL CLASSIFICATION OF ARTHRO-
  PODS INVOLVED IN DISEASE.
  Ticks, Mites, Spiders and Scorpions.
  Blood-sucking Insects.
  Filth and Myiasis-producing Insects.
  Nettling, Vesicating and Stinging
    Insects.

Introduction.—Metazoal diseases are those which are produced by animal parasites of the kingdom Metazoa; that is, many-celled organisms which at some stage in their life history are usually visible to the unaided eye, although some species are likely to be overlooked without the use of a microscope. More particularly, the diseases considered in this chapter are those caused (*A*) by worms (helminths) belonging to the class of flatworms (Platyhelminthes)—including (1) tapeworms (Cestodes) and (2) flukes (Trematodes)—and to the class of roundworms (Nematodes); and (*B*) by the arthropods, including (1) centipedes and millipedes (Myriapoda), (2) cyclops, crabs and crayfish (Crustacea), (3) ticks, mites, spiders and scorpions (Arachnida), and (4) flies, fleas, lice, bugs, bettles, bees, wasps and ants, moths and butterflies (Insecta or Hexapoda). The more important of these forms from a clinical viewpoint are the ones which are obligatory parasites during the greater portion of their existence or, in the case of some of the arthropods, are intermediate hosts and transmitters to man of such infections as plague, typhus, yellow fever, Rocky Mountain spotted fever and malaria.

Some of these worms live unattached in the intestinal lumen (Ascaris); others, like the hookworms, are attached to the intestinal mucosa, and still others, such as the blood-flukes (schistosomes) and Bancroft's filarial worm, are intimately housed in blood and lymph channels. The damage to host tissues and therefore the host's reactions to the parasite are due to one or more of several factors. In the first place the mechanical trauma and irritation produced by such parasites as the hookworm are frequently important. Likewise the mere bulk of the parasite, as an obstruction to the passage of food, blood or lymph, may produce acute symptoms, as, for example, a bolus of Ascaris worms in the intestine, a single schistosome in the portal blood stream or a filarial worm in an inguinal lymph node. In the second place, toxic secretions or excretions of the parasite absorbed by the system are commonly registered by the blood stream or hematopoietic organs (*e.g.*, hookworm, trichina and fish tapeworm in the causative rôle of eosinophilia and secondary anemia). Blood-flukes stimulate an excess production of euglobulin. Trichina worms frequently paralyze the motor centers. Hydatid fluid when released by rupture of the cyst produces anaphylactic shock. Furthermore, these worms and their products, such as eggs and larvæ deposited in the tissues or migrating through the body, commonly cause local reactions. Ascaris larvæ *en route* through the lungs, particularly of small children, are responsible for a pneumonitis clinically similar to a pneumococcic infection. The eggs of the Oriental blood-fluke, Schistosoma japonicum, when lodged in the wall of the intestine or in the liver tissues, stimulate a round-cell infiltration and giant-cell production which constitute the essential lesions of this disease. The fibromata formed around the adult Bancroft's filarial worms occlude the lymph flow from more distal areas and give rise to elephantiasis and varicocele.

With the probable exceptions of the pinworm (Enterobius vermicularis) and Strongyloides, multiplication of helminths does not take place in the human body. Propagation of the species depends on the production of vast quantities of eggs or larvæ which must pass outside the body before they can develop further. In some cases, as in pinworm and dwarf tapeworm infections, the egg is already fully embryonated when discharged in the feces, and merely requires introduction by mouth into the next host in order to produce a new infection. The whipworm (Trichocephalus) egg requires a period for maturing outside the body. Ascaris eggs not only need time for development in favorable soil but, after the mature egg has been swallowed and hatches in the duodenum, the emerging larva is obliged to undertake a circuitous migration through the lungs before it is able to develop into the adult worm. Hookworm eggs mature, hatch and undergo metamorphosis in the soil before they are capable of entering the human body *via* the skin route. Certain species like the beef and pork tapeworms require the ox and pig, respectively, as an intermediate host in which the embryo hatching from the egg develops into a cysticercus larva ("measle") in the voluntary muscles. Consumption of the infested flesh, raw or rare, produces infection again in man. Filarial worms all produce larvæ (microfilariæ) which migrate into the peripheral circulation, are taken up by blood-sucking flies, undergo development in these insects, and in turn are introduced into man when the fly next takes a human blood meal. All flukes have a complicated life-cycle, in which the larva hatched from the egg actively penetrates a species of snail to which it has become adapted. In the snail the larva metamorphoses and, after a twofold multiplication, myriads of tailed larvæ (cercariæ) emerge to swim about in the water. In the case of blood-flukes these cercariæ actively penetrate man's skin. In other cases, as in Fasciola and Fasciolopsis infections the cercaria encysts on water plants and gains entry to the intestine when the plant is ingested. In lung-fluke infection the cercarial stage, on erupting from the snail, invades and encysts in a crayfish or crab and reaches man in this wise; in Chinese liver-fluke infection fresh-water fishes replace the crayfish in the scheme of the life-cycle.

In a few infections, such as that of the dwarf tapeworm (Hymenolepis nana), children are more susceptible than adults. In this case a partial age immunity appears to have been developed. Ascariasis is more common in children than in adults, but this is probably accounted for by the greater exposure of children to contaminations in the house and around the dooryard. In all other helminthic diseases infection does not confer immunity. In fact the lowered threshold of resistance produced by some infections such as hookworm disease (ancylostomiasis) and severe strongyloidosis makes reinfection and hyperinfection easier.

In evaluating the symptoms and before treatment is begun it is essential that the physician visualize clearly the position of the parasite in the patient's body and the probable effects of the parasite, both local and indirect, on the system. This cannot be done without estimating the number of parasites in the infection. In order to obtain an accurate diagnosis of the species and a rough determination of the number of parasites involved a careful laboratory examination of the body exudates or fluids is required. Experienced laboratorians are needed for the diagnosis of all but the commoner helminthic diseases. In considering treatment, in addition to a knowledge of the specificity of drugs for certain parasites and a balanced judgment with respect to the age, weight, complications and possible individual idiosyncrasy of the patient to anthelmintics, the physician should also keep in mind the necessity for the drug reaching the parasite in a dosage lethal to the worm but well within the tolerance of the patient.

Arthropods are important as causative agents of disease in the following ways: (1) They may produce trauma by inserting their heads (ticks and blood-sucking flies) or stingers (bees and wasps) into or under the skin; they may live in burrows in the skin layers (sarcoptic mite and chigo), or they may deposit on the skin or in flesh wounds their eggs, which hatch, so that the larvæ (maggots) feed on and damage the tissues. (2) They may inject venoms into the body, resulting in local inflammation and motor paralysis (ticks and spiders) or destruction of the blood cells, cardiac spasm and neuromotor paralysis (scorpions). (3) They frequently open a way for the entrance of pyogenic organisms into the body. (4) Many species are intermediate hosts and transmitters of specific types of pathogenic bacteria, filterable viruses, spirochetes, protozoa and helminths. Frequently the same arthropod is responsible for the production of two or more of these disease entities at one and the same time.

General Classification of Helminthic Diseases.—The helminthic diseases to be considered in this chapter are divided as follows:

1. *Nematode or roundworm infections.*
    (a) Ancylostomiasis (hookworm infection).
    (b) Trichocephaliasis (whipworm infection).
    (c) Ascariasis.
    (d) Oxyuriasis (pinworm or seatworm infection).
    (e) Strongyloidosis.
    (f) Trichinosis.
    (g) Filariasis (infection with the filarial worms).

2. *Cestode or tapeworm infections.*
    (a) Teniasis (beef and pork tapeworm infections).
    (b) Echinococcosis (hydatid cyst).
    (c) Hymenolepiasis (dwarf and rat tapeworm infections).
    (d) Dipylidiiasis (dog tapeworm infection).
    (e) Diphyllobothriasis (fish tapeworm infection).
    (f) Sparganosis.
3. *Trematode or fluke infections.*
    (a) Distomiasis (produced by intestinal flukes, liver-flukes and lung-flukes).
    (b) Schistosomiasis (blood-fluke infection).

NEMATODE OR ROUNDWORM INFECTIONS.

Ancylostomiasis.—This disease, which is widespread in warm climates, is produced by three species of hookworms, Necator americanus, Ancylostoma duodenale and Ancylostoma braziliense. In a broad sense other closely related roundworms, such as Ternidens deminutus, species of Trichostrongylus, Hæmonchus contortus and Mecistocirrus digitatus, also fall into this group. Hookworms have been known since ancient times but it was not until Dubini, in 1843, reported the worms (Ancylostoma duodenale), obtained from the necropsy of a Milanese woman, that an accurate description was recorded. In general it may be said that Necator americanus is the common hookworm of the tropical belt of the Old World and the only common form in the New World; that Ancylostoma duodenale is found in the Old World north of 20° N. latitude, and that Ancylostoma braziliense is a minor human hookworm of man in warm climates, although it is the common hookworm of the dog and cat in these latitudes. Migration of people, particularly along the China Coast and in Malaya, has within recent times mixed these three infections so that in East Asia there is no clean-cut geographic distribution.

The worm lives in the middle levels of the small intestine with its head firmly attached to the mucosa by means of hooks or cutting plates. By an enzyme secreted from its esophageal glands it digests the tissue substance and produces hemorrhage from the associated capillaries. These worms are cylindrical in shape, reddish-white, creamy or a dirty gray in color, and have their heads somewhat arched. The smaller males measure from 7 to 11 mm. in length by 0.3 to 0.5 mm. in diameter and have an umbrella-like posterior expansion. The females measure 9 to 13 mm. in length by 0.4 to 0.6 mm. in diameter and have a tapering conoidal posterior end. On the average there is a sex ratio of 1 to 1 in any given infection. Insemination is accomplished by the male applying its posterior end to the vulva of the female and the introduction of spermatozoa. Each female lays several thousand eggs per day. These eggs are oval in shape, hyaline in color, have a thin shell and are layed in an early stage of cleavage. They measure 60 to 76 microns by 36 to 40 microns, those of Necator being somewhat longer and narrower than those of Ancylostoma. When passed in the stool the eggs are usually in the 4- to 16-cell stage and require deposition in favorable soil for further development. Sandy loam is the most satisfactory ground and hard packed clay the least satisfactory for development.   Warmth, moisture and shade are also essential; direct sunlight is detrimental.   In the course of from one to several days the embryo within the egg shell has matured into a motile larva, which breaks through the weakened shell and begins to feed ravenously.   This larva (the *rhabditiform stage*) is distinguished from the similar stage of Strongyloides by the rather deep invagination of its integument into the oral end, forming a long capillary mouth cavity which is easily seen in a quiescent specimen under the microscope.   Within the first three or four days the larva passes through a molting stage, feeds again, then forms a new sheath, within which it becomes elongated and transforms into the more graceful *filariform stage*.   This stage is unable to feed but may remain viable for weeks or even months in a favorable *milieu*.   Upon losing its sheath it is infective for man.   The usual portal of entry is through the skin, although it may penetrate through the mucous membranes.   It is also possible for it to be swallowed and survive passage through the stomach. In any event it reaches the venous blood stream and is carried through the right heart to the lungs, where it breaks out of the capillaries into the bronchioles, is carried up the air passages to the epiglottis and down the alimentary canal to the small intestine, where it becomes attached to the mucosa and develops into the adult worm.   From the time it enters the body until the adult female worm begins to lay eggs, a period of about five weeks elapses.   This is the prepatent or incubation period.

The usual site of entry of the worm into the body is the interdigital spaces between the toes.   Laborers in contaminated mines may be inoculated on almost any part of the body and plumbers working under raised porches may be inoculated on the back from contact with infected soil.   Not uncommonly in these infections lesions develop at the site of entry of the infective (filariform) larva.   These lesions are popularly termed "ground itch" and consist of an edematous swelling with erythema, developing into a papular eruption which vesiculates.   Secondary bacterial contamination of the lesion may complicate the picture.   Apparently no reaction is produced by the migration of the larvæ through the lungs, except in heavy inoculations, when an acute bronchopneumonia may develop.   The significant lesions of the disease are produced by the adult worms attached to the mucosa. At each point of attachment there is an open wound, with seepage of tissue juice and hemorrhage from damaged capillaries.   This continues long after the worm has loosed its hold and become attached at another point.   The life of the hookworm is from one to several years, so that each worm usually produces many such open wounds.   In light infections (10 to 25 worms) there is ordinarily complete compensation for the damage produced; in moderately heavy infections there is partial compensation; in severe cases there is frequently complete decompensation, due to loss of blood, both relative and absolute, and to toxic secretions of the worms, which affect the hematopoietic and endocrine organs and retard sexual maturity.

Physical retardation is produced by nutritional and endocrine insufficiency. Digestion is poor, with undigested food commonly passed in the feces. The hemoglobin is reduced so that the pallor of the skin is marked, edema of the face and extremities develops and "pot belly" becomes characteristic. In severe infections emaciation is pronounced and the skin becomes dry like parchment. Heartburn, flatulence, a feeling of fullness of the abdomen and epigastric pain which is relieved by a full meal are other signs of the disease. Geophagia is not uncommon. Lassitude results from physical weakness, the so-called "laziness" of the southern "poor white" and the negro. In prolonged infections, vasomotor disturbances with dyspnea and heart murmurs develop. These symptoms are most severe in children, where growth and puberty are greatly delayed. Women are more seriously affected than are grown men. Accompanying the physical symptomatology is mental sluggishness. Moreover, hookworm infection lowers the threshold of resistance to pneumonia, tuberculosis, measles and other infectious diseases. In heavy hookworm infections of long duration the conditions described become more and more exaggerated, terminating in complete exhaustion, cardiac failure and anasarca, unless relief is affected by expulsion of the worms and adequate diet. Diets rich in blood-building properties can temporarily check the decompensation produced by disease.

Diagnosis of hookworm disease is based on finding the characteristic eggs in the stools. Occasionally in constipated stools the embryos within the eggs may have matured to the motile larval stage. Stools in which hookworm eggs are few in the unconcentrated film usually indicate an infection of subclinical importance. The most satisfactory simple method for concentrating the stools consists in centrifuging about 2 grams of the feces in 20 cc. of water, comminuted and passed through several layers of ordinary gauze to screen out the gross débris. The centrifuge is spun at a slow speed for thirty seconds. The eggs are in the bottom-most fraction of the sediment. The blood picture is that of an aplastic anemia, with marked reduction in erythrocytes and in the hemoglobin index. In general this reduction is directly proportional to the amount of the hookworm burden. There may be an eosinophilia but this is not constant. The clinical picture may be confused with profound malnutrition.

Hookworm *therapy* has passed through several stages. Thymol and oil of chenopodium have been replaced by carbon tetrachloride as a more efficient drug. Tetrachlorethylene has more recently been introduced as an anthelmintic having the same efficiency as carbon tetrachloride without the contraindications. Carbon tetrachloride should not be administered in patients with hepatic, respiratory or cardiac disorders, nephritis, or pyrexia of undiagnosed origin. It should not be given alone where ascariasis complicates the infection. Preliminary administration of calcium chloride orally will partially protect the liver from toxic fatty degeneration. An eminently satisfactory course of treatment follows:

1. Thoroughly purge with sodium sulphate the night before treatment.

2. Administer three 1-cc. capsules of tetrachlorethylene medicinal in the morning on an empty stomach.

3. Thoroughly purge with sodium sulphate two hours after administration of drug.

4. A light meal, without fats or oils, may be allowed after a copious bowel movement.

A single course of treatment usually eliminates 90 to 95 per cent of the worms and at times the entire number. In case several worms remain, as determined by microscopic examination for eggs several days after treatment, a second course may be given safely within a week. For small children tetrachlorethylene may be given on a teaspoon, 2 minims for each year of age. Where ancylostomiasis is complicated with ascariasis, 0.2 cc. oil of chenopodium should be added to the usual prescription of tetrachlorethylene.

Recently crystalline hexylresorcinol has been found to be a mild anthelmintic in cases with hookworm, whipworm and Ascaris infection. It may be given on an empty stomach without preliminary purge, as follows: 4 to 5 0.2-gram enteric-coated tablets, requiring the patient to abstain from food for five hours following administration of the drug. Precautions should be taken to prevent the patient from chewing up the tablets before swallowing them. This is a particularly helpful prescription for infections in small children.

"Creeping eruption" or "larva migrans" is an intradermal infection with the filariform larvæ of Ancylostoma braziliense, which, for some unknown reason, after penetrating through the outer layers of the skin is frequently unable to reach the peripheral circulation, and therefore continues to wander through the Malpighian layer of the skin for days or weeks, producing a serpiginous tunnel. The larva is usually some short distance ahead of the raised portion of the tunnel. The migration produces an almost intolerable pruritus, with attendant insomnia, loss of appetite and loss of weight. Frequently bacterial infection complicates the picture. This type of hookworm infection is found along the sandy coastal stretches of the southeastern Atlantic Seaboard and around the coast of the Gulf of Mexico. It is particularly prevalent in Florida. The disease is satisfactorily treated by local application of ethyl chloride spray or carbon dioxide snow. Dakin's solution is indicated where secondary infection has developed.

Prophylaxis in hookworm disease consists in proper disposal or sterilization of human excreta. In cities with sanitary sewage systems the disease is known only from country cases coming into the hospitals. Sanitary privies in the country will care for the situation, provided all individuals make use of the privy. Inoculation usually takes place when bare feet are exposed to contaminations where the infective larvæ have developed at sites of previous defecation. Good leather shoes are important as a protection for children. In regions where "creeping eruption" is prevalent the adult worms (Ancylostoma braziliense) parasitize dogs and cats, which defecate promiscuously. Such unsanitary conditions require control before the disease can be stamped out. Finally, in heavily infected areas, where practically all of the population are hookworm carriers, adequate treatment of all infected individuals is recommended.

Trichocephaliasis (Trichuriasis).—This infection, which is cosmopolitan in its distribution, but has both a higher incidence and more clinical importance in the tropics, is due to the whipworm, Trichocephalus trichiura (Trichuris trichiura). These worms (males, 30 to 45 mm. long; females, 35 to 50 mm. long) live in the cecum and appendix, with their delicate capillary anterior end inserted into the tissues of the wall and their enlarged posterior ends projecting into the lumen of the bowel. The female has a bluntly rounded, club-shaped posterior end while the male's is coiled like a watch spring. When several of these worms are attached to the tissue close to one another, as in the appendix, they frequently form a matted, tangled mass which prevents the proper evacuation of fecal particles and may give rise to an inflammatory reaction. They have the ability to digest mucosa cells near the site of attachment. There is also the possibility of bacteria, such as streptococci and tetanus bacilli, entering the blood stream around the points of insertion of their heads. Toxic symptoms result from the absorption of by-products of the worms, giving rise to a low-grade anemia, slight eosinophilia, insomnia and reflex symptoms. In heavy infection these symptoms are aggravated: the toxic edema and anemia may simulate the picture of severe hookworm disease. Each female lays about 150 eggs per day. These characteristic eggs, narrowly barrel-shaped, lemon or golden-brown in color, with a mucoid plug at each end, are immature when passed in the stool; they require a period of several weeks or months for development outside the body, and are extremely resistant to desiccation, fermentation and other unfavorable conditions of the environment. When taken into the mouth as a contamination the mature eggs pass through to the duodenum where they hatch, and the emerging larvæ migrate to the large bowel, attach themselves to the cecal or appendiceal mucosa, and develop into the adult worms. The recovery of the immature eggs (size 50 to 54 microns by 22 to 23 microns) from the feces is the only certain method of diagnosis. The most efficient drug on the market for eradication of these worms is crystalline hexylresorcinol. *Treatment* with this drug is similar to that given for ancylostomiasis (*vide supra*). Oral treatment should be accompanied by high irrigation of the large bowel with a pint of hexylresorcinol solution, 1 to 1000 alkaline (S.T. 37). Rather high incidence of this infection but with a small worm burden may be found even in cities with a good sewage system. The incidence is highest in children of the pre-adolescent period. Personal hygiene is the most satisfactory method of controlling the infection.

Ascariasis.—This cosmopolitan infection is caused by the roundworm, Ascaris lumbricoides. These worms are large cylindrical forms which live free in the lumen of the small intestine. The females may attain a length of 45 cm. but are usually about 25 to 30 cm. long. The males are somewhat smaller. At the anterior end of each worm there are three large distinct lips, arranged approximately in tri-radiate fashion. Both females and males taper abruptly to a point at their posterior end, but the males are more or less curved along the ventral line. The females lay several tens of thousands of eggs per day. Usually these are fertilized and measure about 60 by 42 microns; they are broadly rounded, have a thick hyaline inner albuminoid wall and a heavy outer covering which is characteristically mammillated and bile-stained. Occasionally this outer layer is lacking. At times only females are present in the infection, in which case unfertilized eggs occur in the stools. Such eggs are longer and narrower, measuring 88 to 93 microns by 38 to 44 microns; they have an irregular deposition of the outer covering and are filled with highly refractive globules resembling droplets of oil. The fertilized egg is immature when passed in the feces. When deposited in the soil it develops rather slowly but in the course of a few weeks this egg will contain a wriggling larva. On account of the two protective coverings it is extremely resistant to desiccation and chemicals, also to cold. However, it is killed by moist heat over 70° C. The mature larva, when swallowed as a contamination of food or drink, hatches in the duodenum and the emerging larva penetrates through the intestinal wall into the portal blood stream or the lymphatics. It is carried through the right heart to the lungs, where it escapes into the bronchioles, occasioning an inflammatory reaction, at times accompanied by consolidation of the region. Eventually it is carried up the bronchial tree to the epiglottis and passes down the alimentary tract to the small intestine, where it grows into the adult worm.

One or two or even a half dozen ascarids frequently produce no serious *symptoms*, although parasitized patients will usually at one time or another experience digestive upsets which may either be caused by the worms or be the occasion for the worms to become disturbed and to wander promiscuously through the intestine. In so doing they may form a tangled mass which will completely obstruct the bowel and call for surgical intervention; or they may migrate into the stomach and be vomited or passed through the nares. Rarely they perforate the bowel wall. They have a predilection for obstructing drainage tubes following jejunotomy. In addition to their mechanical and physical effects on the intestine their toxic secretions and excretions when absorbed usually cause a more or less appreciable effect on the system, including, at times, a severe asthma. Eosinophilia and a mild anemia are not uncommon. Nervous symptoms such as insomnia, picking of the nose and gnashing of the teeth at night frequently result. In children a low-grade pyrexia is common.

Diagnosis consists in finding the eggs in the stool, except where there are only one or more males alone, in which event the symptoms alone must be depended on for diagnosis.

The *treatment* of many years' standing for ascariasis has consisted in administration of santonin, with the following directions:

1. Fasting the night before and taking an efficient cathartic.

2. Remaining in bed the morning of treatment and taking nothing but water or tea or black coffee.

3. At 8 A.M. taking 1 capsule containing santonin powder, 0.065 gram (1 grain) and an equal amount of calomel.

4. At 9 A.M. repeating anthelmintic treatment.

5. At 10 A.M. taking 60 cc. of sodium sulphate or senna-leaf infusion.

While the above prescription is relatively safe, this procedure is far from efficient in producing evacuation of the worms. Oil of chenopodium may be substituted for the santonin-calomel administration (1 cc. in capsule at 8 A.M. and 1 cc. at 9 A.M.). However, this latter anthelmintic has the following contraindications: gastro-enteritis, alcoholism and pregnancy. Even in the hands of experienced persons oil of chenopodium has at times produced serious complications and unnecessary loss of life. Crystalline hexylresorcinol, as indicated for ancylostomiasis (*vide supra*), is probably the most efficient and safest ascaricide on the market at the present time.

Ascariasis is essentially a disease of dirty homes and dirty dooryards, where the yard is seeded with eggs of the worms. Sanitary toilets or privies for adults do not reduce the infection, since it is essentially one of early childhood. In heavy endemic areas, such as the clay hill regions of the southern Appalachian Mountains and the Ozark region, children are continually becoming reinfected and frequently harbor at one time adult and immature worms in the intestine and migrating larvæ in the blood stream and lungs. With unclean habits of defecation they perpetuate a seedbed of intense infectivity which saps the vitality of a large per cent of the younger members of such communities. Supervision of the child's habits and inculcation of personal hygiene are essential for the reduction of the infection.

Oxyuriasis.—This cosmopolitan infection is caused by the pinworm or seatworm, Enterobius vermicularis (Oxyuris vermicularis). The milky white worms (male, 2 to 5 mm. long; female, 8 to 13 mm. long) live attached to the mucosa of the ileum and, at times, the cecum and appendix. The male is shaped like an inverted question-mark and the female has a rather long attenuated caudal extremity. When the uterus of the female becomes crowded with eggs, she relaxes her attachment to the mucosa and wanders into the large bowel. Frequently her excursions may take her into the appendix where at times an inflammatory reaction is induced. More commonly she descends to the rectum and at night, when the patient drops to sleep, she migrates out among the perianal and perineal hairs, where the crawling movement produces an intense pruritus. When her body begins to dry it bursts and the eggs are scattered like seed from a ripened pod. This materially increases the pruritus. In female patients the worm may migrate into and up the genital organs and finally reach the abdominal cavity where the worm may become walled off by an adventitious capsule formation.

The intolerable pruritus caused by the female worm in her excursions invariably induces scratching of the itching area, thus producing a raw area open to invasion from bacteria. This in turn causes insomnia and nervous symptoms. Several cases of epilepsy and other nervous disorders have been attributed to this infection. The eggs are found most commonly among the perianal hairs and only occasionally in the feces. They are elongated, oval in shape, with a moderately thick hyaline shell, are more or less flattened on one side and measure 50 to 60 microns by 20 to 30 microns. They are fully embryonated when set free by the mother worm. Reinfection is caused by introduction of the eggs on soiled fingers into the mouth. It is also probable that in certain cases the eggs may be returned up the bowel to the region of the duodenum, where they hatch and the larvæ grow into adult worms. Dirty bed linen and nightclothes are a common source of infection for other members of the family. Children are more commonly infected than adults. The incidence of the disease is highest in children's asylums.

Since the eggs are not common in the stools of infected individuals fecal examination is not a reliable method of diagnosis. The history of pruritus, particularly after going to bed, and the recovery of the migrating females are the most satisfactory means of differentiating the infection. The migrating worms in the large bowel may be washed out by periodic hexylresorcinol S. T. 37 enemas. The younger worms attached to the wall of the ileum can probably be removed by tetrachlorethylene or crystalline hexylresorcinol, administered as for hookworm disease (*vide supra*). Mercurial ointments are effective in reducing the lesions in and around the anus and perineum.

Strongyloidosis.—This disease is endemic throughout the hookworm belts of the world. It is caused by the minute worm Strongyloides stercoralis. The parasitic female lives imbedded in the mucosa of the intestine. In mild infections these worms are usually confined to the duodenum and upper jejunum, but in heavy infections they may extend upward into the pyloric wall of the stomach and downward to the ileocecal valve. Occasionally the cecum, colon and rectum are involved. The delicate thread-like female parasite lays eggs into the tissues. These eggs closely resemble hookworm eggs. However, the time required for them to break through into the lumen of the upper intestine and pass down the bowel is usually sufficient for the enclosed larvæ to mature and hatch, so that fecal examination of these patients almost always reveals the presence of motile rhabditiform larvæ. In the majority of cases these larvæ, on reaching favorable moist soil, feed, ensheath and become transformed into filariform larvæ. They are then infective for man: they enter the skin and wander through the tissues in the same way as does the comparable stage of the hookworm larvæ. This mode of development, which is most common, is known as the *direct type*. In the tropics and occasionally in more temperate regions the rhabditiform larvæ passed in the stool, instead of developing into filariform larvæ, after feeding become transformed into "free-living" adult females and males, which mate and produce a progeny of "free-living" second-generation rhabditiform larvæ. These latter, in turn, feed and become transformed into filariform larvæ which are infective for man. This mode of development is known as the *indirect type*. Another type, the *hyperinfective type*, has recently been proved to exist in severely infected individuals in the tropics. In such cases the rhabditiform larvæ become transformed into dwarf filariform larvæ while still in the bowel, so that the latter stage is infective through the rectal mucosa.

In lightly infected persons a slight injection of the parasitized mucosa is apparently the only lesion produced. In heavily infested individuals there is a marked inflammation of the entire region parasitized and frequently erosion of considerable areas. Severe cases with ulceration of the pyloric mucosa and rectal involvement in cases harboring the hyperinfective strain are not uncommon in the tropics. Damage produced by this latter type may be pictured when it is known that the worms parasitic in the mucosa may live for twenty years or more, continuously producing eggs. Lightly infected individuals may have no clinical symptoms, although alternating diarrhea and constipation are frequently recorded in such cases. In severe cases there is a history of chronic diarrhea, dehydration and wasting. The larvæ *en route* through the lungs also give rise to an acute tissue reaction similar to that in ascariasis. Aberrantly wandering larvæ have been found in the pleural and pericardial cavities and in many tissues of the body.

Diagnosis consists in recovering the rhabditiform (and occasionally the filariform) larvæ in the passed feces. These larvæ require differentiation from the comparable stages of hookworm infection. Rarely unhatched eggs are passed in a watery stool following a drastic purge. Recent clinical studies by the writer have shown that adult parasitic female worms, which have ceased to produce larvæ, may still be present in the bowel wall, with symptoms of loss of appetite, digestive disorders, nervousness and profound malaise, with a blood picture of leukopenia with or without eosinophilia. These cases usually improve after specific therapeusis. Specific *treatment* consists in administration by mouth of two 0.035-gram (0.5-grain) enteric-coated tablets of gentian violet (medicinal), before meals, for a period of ten days. One course of treatment is usually sufficient to eradicate the infection. There is no known contraindication to this method of treatment and no special preparation of the patient or dietary restriction required. Prophylactic measures are similar to those recommended for hookworm disease.

Trichinosis.—This disease is endemic wherever raw pork is consumed. It is produced by infection with a microscopic nematode, Trichinella spiralis, the so-called "trichina worm." The adult male and female worms (measuring 1.4 to 1.6 mm. and 3 to 4 mm., respectively, in length) live attached to or imbedded in the mucosa of the duodenum and jejunum. The females give birth to motile larvæ, some of which are shed into the intestinal lumen but many of which get into the lymphatics and the portal blood stream and migrate to the striated muscle, where from the ninth day on for a period of several weeks the larvæ settle down and become encysted. Each female worm in the intestine produces about 1500 larvæ. During the period of migration they can be detected in centrifuged peripheral blood.

The cyst capsule is an adventitious ellipsoidal object, within which the larva is tightly coiled up. Eventually most of these cysts undergo calcification. Human infection results from the ingestion of lean pork containing encysted viable larvæ, which are digested out of their capsules in the stomach, pass through to the duodenum and jejunum and, becoming attached to the mucosa, develop into adult worms.

The disease is divided into three periods: (1) invasion, (2) migration of the larvæ, and (3) encystment and tissue repair. During the first period the symptoms consist of nausea, vomiting, diarrhea or dysentery and colic, caused by acute catarrhal inflammation and hemorrhage of the upper levels of the small intestine. This lasts through the seventh day. The second stage is one of profound myositis, involving the diaphragm, muscles of the arms and legs, intercostals, larynx and mouth, with frequent difficulty in respiration, mastication and speech. Edema and dyspnea may occur at this time. Marked eosinophilia and leukocytosis are pathognomonic. Occasionally interstitial myocarditis, thrombophlebitis and thrombo-enteritis have been observed. In a few cases hyperplasia of the bone-marrow has been demonstrated. The third stage is the critical one, with edema and cachexia and in grave cases delirium, profound dyspnea and coma. During the second and third periods the temperature is usually elevated to 40° C. and at times to 41° C. Gradual subsidence of the symptoms during the third stage constitutes a good prognosis.

Diagnosis during the first period consists in differentiating the disease clinically from ptomaine poisoning, cholera and dysentery of bacterial or amebic origin. Later, typhoid must be excluded. The absence of albumin in the urine rules out nephritis. Microscopically the hypereosinophilia (15 to 50 per cent or more) and the finding of Trichinella larvæ in the stool or centrifuged blood is diagnostic. Biopsy of a small piece of biceps muscle and examination of the pressed muscle strip for larvæ is also helpful. There is no specific *therapeusis*, but symptomatic treatment is required during the entire course of the disease. *Prophylaxis* consists in thorough cooking of all pork meat (one-half hour for each pound) and thorough inspection of country slaughter houses for infected rats which serve as a reservoir of the infection. Within recent years epidemics of trichinosis have become common in the northern United States. Many of these cases have consumed "pork sandwiches" and essentially raw "wieners." Autopsy reports also reveal the presence of larvæ in high percentages of cases which have given no history of infection.

Filariasis.—The term "filariasis" is used to designate several specific disease entities caused by worms of the family Filariidæ. The worms are thread-like in general appearance and live in the lymphatics, blood stream, subcutaneous tissues and body cavities. They all have males distinguished by a delicate corkscrew-shaped caudal extremity. They all lay eggs which become greatly elongated as they mature. Some of these hatch (loose their "sheath"), while others remain "ensheathed" in the human body. These larvæ, the microfilariæ, either reach the peripheral blood stream or wander through the subcutaneous tissues, so that they are picked up by blood-sucking flies. Within the body of the fly these microfilariæ grow, undergo metamorphosis and eventually reach the fly's proboscis and are transferred again beneath the skin of man. They then migrate to the site of their choice and develop into the adult filarial worms. Among these forms are the loa worm of Africa (Loa loa), which lives in the subcutaneous tissues and is noted for its migrations in and around the temples and across the front of the eyeball, producing "fugitive swellings" *en route*.

The microfilariæ are sheathed. This species has an intermediate stage in the mango flies, Chrysops silacea and Chrysops dimidiata. Because of the presence of large numbers of the microfilariæ in the peripheral blood-vessels in the daytime this larva has been called Microfilaria diurna. Two closely related forms, Onchocerca volvulus of Africa and Onchocerca cæcutiens of Central America and Mexico, produce, respectively, subdermal swellings resembling juxta-articular nodules and tumefactions around the eyes and ears with an inflamed erysipelatoid appearance. Species of black flies of the genus Simulium transmit these two infections. Another species, Acanthocheilonema perstans, lives in the body cavities and may be "sewed" in and out of the mesentery or other tissues like a basting thread. The microfilaria of this species is sheathless and is constantly found in the peripheral circulation. Species of gnats of the genus Culicoides transmit this infection. Another worm distantly related to the filariæ is the meter-long Medina or Guinea-worm, Dracunculus medinensis, which has an intermediate stage in the small water crustacean, Cyclops, and is transmitted to man through raw drinking water containing the infected Cyclops. In man it is confined to Southern Asia, Africa and a few foci in Tropical America, but it has been found several times in reservoir hosts in the United States. The mature, gravid female migrates from the viscera to the subcutaneous tissues, finally producing a blister on the skin, which ruptures on contact with water to allow discharge of the motile larvæ. During the migration period the patient usually shows marked allergic manifestations, which are alleviated by the administration of adrenalin.

The most important of the filarial worms is Bancroft's filaria, technically known as Wuchereria bancrofti. This infection is common throughout the tropics. The worms, which are extremely delicate (males, 40 mm. long by 0.1 mm. in diameter; females, 80 to 100 mm. long by 0.24 to 0.3 mm. in diameter), live in tangled groups in nodular dilatations of the distal lymphatics, in lymph varices, in lymph glands or between the glands. They give birth to elongated larvæ, the ensheathed microfilariæ which are typically characterized by being in the peripheral circulation only at night (nocturnal periodicity). Many species of mosquitoes, but particularly the tropical house form, Culex quinquefasciatus (Culex fatigans) serve as intermediate host for this microfilaria, which is taken into the mosquito's stomach when she secures a blood meal at night from an infected person. These larvæ migrate to the thoracic muscles, where they undergo a twofold metamorphosis and eventually migrate into the proboscis to be returned to man when the mosquito obtains a later blood meal. About a year then probably elapses before the worm matures in the lymphatics.

A high percentage of persons having Bancroft's filarial infection are symptomless. Later, however, they may and usually do have premonitory *symptoms*, including frontal headache and depression. This is followed by lymphangitis and filarial fever. More advanced manifestations of the disease usually consist of elephantiasis, due primarily to blockage of lymph flow, with cellular infiltration, hypertrophy, fibrosis and calcification in and around the worm tangles. The elephan-

19

toid enlargement most usually involves one or both legs, but the upper extremities may be affected. In males the penis and scrotum and in females the vulva and mammary glands may be involved. Other complications include varicose groin glands, varix lymphaticus and chylocele with chyluria. In this last type microfilariæ may be found in the urine. The inflammatory process around the site of the worms (lymphangitis) may be responsible for a recurrent fever with tenderness of the involved part, rigor and terminal diaphoresis. Likewise, streptococcic infection probably plays a rôle in complicated cases.

Diagnosis of Bancroft's filariasis consists primarily in recovering the characteristic larvæ in peripheral blood at night (10 P.M. to 2 A.M.) or from the urine in cases of chyluria. However, a considerable number of cases cannot be diagnosed in this way, due to induration and calcification of the worm sites. In such types the roentgen-ray is frequently helpful in locating the sites. The disease requires differentiating from streptococcic and syphilitic elephantiasis, varicose veins and fevers of non-filarial origin. The microfilariæ, when obtained, need to be differentiated from those of other filarial worms. There is no specific chemotherapy. Surgical removal of elephantoid tissue is at times helpful.

CESTODE OR TAPEWORM INFECTIONS.

Teniasis.—This disease is produced by infection with the beef tapeworm (Tænia saginata) or the pork tapeworm (Tænia solium). In both cases the adult worms live attached by their "heads" to the wall of the jejunum or anterior ileum. Behind the head is the "neck" or region of growth. There follow in turn several hundred segments, or proglottids, each more successively mature, those at the distal end being crowded with eggs. The heads of both species are provided with four quadrilaterally arranged suckers; that of Tænia saginata is unarmed, and that of Tænia solium is provided with a rostral corona of hooks. The segments of Tænia saginata are much longer, due to the presence of a greater number of lateral arms of the uterus (15 to 20) as contrasted with that of Tænia solium, which has at most 11 to 12. The egg, which cannot be distinguished in the two species, measures 25 to 40 microns in diameter, is provided with a thick wall pierced with minute capillary openings and contains a six-hooked embryo, the onchosphere (hexacanth embryo). On reaching the outside world and being ingested respectively by the ox or pig the egg hatches in the animal's duodenum and the larva migrates through the intestinal wall into the blood stream, being filtered out in the striped muscles, where it grows into a little oval bladder worm (cysticercus). This is the stage infective for man, and on consumption of infested lean beef or pork the larva reaches the human intestine and develops into the adult worm. Tænia saginata usually attains a length of 4 to 6 m. and Tænia solium seldom more than 2 m. Usually only a single worm is harbored by the patient at one time. Unless removed by an anthelmintic it may live for many years. Segments drop off single or in groups and are passed motile in the stools.

The intestinal parasite ordinarily produces no grave clinical *symptoms*. It may, however, cause chronic indigestion, with alternating diarrhea and constipation. In neurasthenics it may produce anorexia, hyperesthesia and other nervous disorders, due, no doubt, to absorption of toxins from the worm. The graver danger in Tænia solium infection is the hatching of mature eggs *in situ* and the production of cysticercosis or bladder-worm infection in the somatic tissues, in the heart, brain or orbit. Epilepsy is a rather frequent accompaniment of pork cysticercosis in man. Thousands of such cases are on record, some from contamination with feces of infected associates, some from autoinfection. For this latter reason differential diagnosis of the two species of Tæniae is important, and in treatment of Tænia solium infection care should be exercised not to produce emesis.

Diagnosis can be readily made from recovering the eggs in the stool. Differential diagnosis requires examination of the passed segments, which may be pressed between two glass plates and held up to the light to determine the number of lateral arms of the uterus (*vide supra*). *Treatment* consists in a preparatory sodium sulphate purge the night before and in the morning on an empty stomach the administration of 3 to 6 capsules (0.6 cc.—10 minims) of oleoresin of aspidium filix-mas in three divided doses at thirty-minute intervals. Two hours later another purge is given and the patient allowed to get up only after a copious bowel movement has been obtained. The stools should be saved for forty-eight hours and search made for the head. Failure to secure the head usually means unsuccessful treatment, since the worm can regenerate itself from its head and neck in about three months. Prophylaxis consists in proper disposal or sterilization of all stools of infected patients; also thorough cooking of all beef and pork.

Echinococcosis (Hydatid Cyst).—This is a disease produced by the larval stage of a relative of the Tænia worms which lives in the intestines of dogs. The worm is technically known as Echinococcus granulosus. The disease is most prevalent among sheep, cattle and hog raisers, since these animals are reservoirs of the larval or hydatid stage. The eggs of this species are indistinguishable from those of the human Tæniæ. When passed by the dog and accidentally ingested by man they hatch out in the duodenum and make their way into the portal circulation, usually being filtered out by the liver. Or they may pass through the hepatic capillaries and become lodged in the lungs, heart, brain, kidneys, or shafts of the long bones. If space permits they develop into hollow cysts filled with a serous or gelatinous fluid called hydatid fluid (the so-called *unilocular hydatid cysts*). Under such circumstances there is an outer laminated layer and an inner germinal layer, the whole being surrounded by adventitious tissue and more or less effectively insulated from the body tissues and fluids. The germinal layer produces buds which develop into daughter cysts that become free and float in the hydatid fluid. Granddaughter cysts may develop in a similar manner from the daughter cysts; or the germinal buds may become detached as such and fall into the cavity as "hydatid sand." If the cyst bursts, each bud or head is capable of producing a new cyst at a new location.

Sometimes the developing larvæ originally lodged or implanted in the body are crowded and the germinal buds are forced through the laminated layer and develop multiple metastases. They are therefore uncircumscribed and are known as *multilocular* or *alveolar hydatid* cysts. Unilocular cysts are regarded as benign and multilocular cysts are malignant. It may require as many as twenty years for the unilocular cysts to become large enough to be noticed by the patient. On the other hand the multilocular ones develop much more rapidly.

Diagnosis may be made by experienced physicians in eliciting the so-called "hydatid thrill," particularly if the cyst is unilocular and lies in the abdominal cavity. If leakage of the cyst occurs there may be an eosinophilia, or complement fixation may be positive. Roentgen-ray may aid in the diagnosis. But in most cases all of these criteria are less satisfactory than the intradermal Casoni[1] reaction, which is both rapid and specific. Surgical intervention is possible if the cyst is unilocular and lies in a cavity where operation is possible. The cavity is opened and the fluid is aspirated out of the cyst, care being taken not to spill any of the fluid into the extracystic space lest anaphylactic shock result or fertile heads become implanted at new sites. The cyst wall is then completely enucleated, or, if that procedure is not feasible, the cystic cavity is marsupialized and sterilized with 10 per cent formaldehyde. Open drainage is then employed until it is advisable to close the operative wound. Prophylaxis consists in personal hygiene, particularly of the hands and cooking utensils, for persons in contact with sheep dogs and cattle dogs, and dogs herding hogs.

Hymenolepiasis.—This disease is caused by infection with the dwarf tapeworm, Hymenolepis nana, or the rat tapeworm, Hymenolepis diminuta. The former infection is the more prevalent and is particularly common in children in the southern United States and Italy. The minute Hymenolepis nana has a length of 25 to 40 mm. and a maximum breadth of 1 mm. The worms usually occur in groups of a few to many individuals, and are attached to the jejunal mucosa. As their distal segments disintegrate the characteristic eggs are set free and are passed in the feces. These are spheroidal hyaline objects, 30 to 47 microns in diameter, having a thin outer membrane and an inner membrane with two polar prominences from each of which two to four pairs of filaments are given off into the intermembrane space. Within the inner membrane is the onchosphere, which has three pairs of hooklets. These eggs when passed are immediately infective for man. When swallowed they are carried to the duodenum, where they hatch and the larvæ enter into the villi of the jejunum and undergo metamorphosis. Soon they reappear, become attached by their heads and develop into mature worms. Rats and mice serve as reservoirs of the infection in place of man, although man is not as susceptible to the murine as to the human strain.

Hymenolepis diminuta is somewhat larger than Hymenolepis nana, has a subspherical egg, measuring 60 to 80 microns in greater diameter,

---

[1] The intradermal injection of 0.2 cc. pooled filtered sterile hydatid fluid. Reaction: typical urticarial wheal which almost immediately develops.

a lemon-colored outer membrane, a pair of polar prominences without filaments on the inner membrane and six very distinct lanceolate hooklets inside the onchosphere. This infection is transmitted by several insects, including grain beetles, which are probably the most common transmitter to man on account of their presence in precooked breakfast foods. Rats and mice serve as the common reservoirs of this tapeworm. Numerous human cases have been recorded from Tennessee, Texas, India and the U. S. S. R.

Infection with species of Hymenolepis causes indigestion and systemic toxic symptoms. In small children convulsions, epilepsy, insomnia and dizziness are commonly recorded, and cachexia is not infrequent. Eosinophilia is quite a constant accompaniment. Diagnosis is based on finding the particular eggs in the stools, and treatment is similar to that for teniasis. Hymenolepis nana is frequently a familial or institutional infection and can be controlled only by carrying out rules of personal hygiene. Hymenolepis diminuta infection can be eliminated by campaigns against rats and mice around bins and pantries where human food is stored.

Dipylidiiasis.—This is a relatively rare disease in children, although it is the common tapeworm infection in dogs and cats. The worm, Dipylidium caninum, which lives attached to the wall of the jejunum and upper ileum, discharges its gravid distal segments, which are melon-seed shaped and frequently brick-red tinged. The eggs in groups or singly are ingested by human, dog and cat fleas and dog lice, where they undergo development. Accidental swallowing of infected fleas or lice produces infection in man. The symptoms and treatment are similar to those for hymenolepiasis (*vide supra*).

Diphyllobothriasis.—This disease is commonly known as broad fish tapeworm infection or bothriocephalus anemia. It is produced by infection with the worm Diphyllobothrium latum (the Bothriocephalus latus of older authors). The worm lives singly or in groups attached to the jejunal wall. The delicate head is an elliptical spatulate object, with a pair of lateral grooves which constitute the only suctorial apparatus. The length of the worm varies from 3 to 10 meters. Eggs are discharged from the terminal segments, which are characterized by having a uterus coiled into a rosette. These eggs are broadly ovoid in shape, with an opercular cap at one end, measure 70 by 45 microns, have a corn-colored shell and an immature embryo within. As many as 1,000,000 eggs may be passed into the feces by a single worm. The egg matures outside the body in an appropriate water medium. The mature onchosphere which hatches from the egg has a ciliated epithelium, which allows it to swim about in the water. Appropriate species of minute water crustaceans, Cyclops or Diaptomus, ingest the larva, which bores its way into the body cavity of these water animalcules. There the larva metamorphoses into a procercoid. When the Cyclops or Diaptomus is taken into the stomach of a top-feeding fish, such as pike, pickerel, trout, salmon, white fish, grayling, perch or burbot, the larva works its way into the muscles and develops into a ribbon-shaped sparganum. On consuming raw or rare infested fish or caviar, man becomes infected. This disease was originally introduced into the northern United States and southern Canada by immigrants from northern, eastern and central Europe, who practised the same unhygienic habits in their new abode as they did in Europe. The disease has within recent years become quite widely distributed by shipping of infested fish throughout the country.

The presence of Diphyllobothrium latum in man at times produces a more or less profound secondary anemia. There is frequently hemorrhage of the oral mucosa, and slight toxic edema of the face and joints. The infection may cause an erythropenia (1,400,000 to 2,000,000 red blood cells), with nucleated reds, anisocytosis and poikilocytosis, and a leukopenia with more or less pronounced eosinophilia. The hemoglobin percentage may be as low as 25 or 30. Frequently a slight irregular elevation of temperature is observed.

Diagnosis is made by finding the characteristic immature eggs in the stool. Treatment is identical with that for teniasis, but filix-mas is contraindicated in gastro-enteritis, nephritis, marked pyrexia and pregnancy. In these cases pelletierin hydrochloride (0.3 to 0.5 gm.) or pelletierin tannate (0.25 gm.) may be substituted. Removal of the worm results in rapid improvement of the patient. Prophylaxis consists in thorough cooking of all infested fresh-water fish and proper disposal of feces from infected individuals.

Sparganosis.—This disease is produced by several larval types of Diphyllobothrium (Sparganum) infesting the somatic tissues. The organs and tissues particularly involved are the muscles and subcutaneous regions, brain and orbit. The disease may be occasioned: (1) by accidentally swallowing infected Cyclops in raw drinking water, or (2) by application of infected fish or frog meat as a poultice to a festered or abscessed member, whereupon the sparganum crawls into the tissue and produces a suppurative pocket. It is capable of multiplication by budding. There is no known method of reducing the infection except in superficial lesions where the worm may be removed surgically.

TREMATODE OR FLUKE INFECTIONS.

Distomiasis.—All of the diseases in this group are caused by hermaphroditic flat-worms, consisting of a single unit instead of the chain of units of the tapeworm body. These organisms are characterized by having two suckers (hence the terms "distome" and "distomiasis"), one around the mouth and a second blind sucker somewhat behind the mouth in the mid-ventral line. The egg is passed in one or more of the body exudates, eventually hatches outside of the body and a ciliated larva (miracidium) emerges, to swim about in the water. In the event that an appropriate snail is present in the immediate vicinity, the miracidium swims toward and actively penetrates the soft tissues of the snail. Within the snail this miracidium becomes transformed into a simple sacculate body, called the sporocyst, which is a mature organism. Egg, miracidium and sporocyst constitute the first generation of the life-cycle. Within the sporocyst there are developed numerous daughter individuals called rediæ (named after the Italian physician Redi). These rediæ constitute the second generation. With-

in the redia there are developed numerous tailed larvæ called cercariæ. The cercariæ when mature erupt from the snail, swim about
in the water and encyst on aquatic plants or in the tissues of aquatic
animals. Consumption by man or animals of the uncooked vegetable
or animal tissues harboring the cysts completes the cycle with the
development of the adult hermaphroditic worms in the human tissues.
Cercaria, encysted larva (metacercaria or adolescaria) and the hermaphroditic adult worm constitute the third generation. Thus there
are required three generations for the completion of the life-cycle of all
distomate species. The diseases under this heading will be considered
according to the location of the parasite in the host tissues, *i.e.*,
intestinal, hepatic and pulmonary.

Intestinal Distomiasis.—The most important of these diseases is
produced by the large fluke, Fasciolopsis buski, which lives attached
to the mucosa of the small intestine, particularly the duodenum.
The infection is common in certain areas in the Orient. The worms
are fleshy objects of a pinkish hue, are elongate-oval in shape and
measure 2 to 7.5 cm. in length by 8 to 20 mm. in width. These worms
lay immature eggs similar in shape to a hen's egg, 130 to 140 microns
in length by 80 to 85 microns in transverse diameter. Upon falling
into water in rice fields or other irrigation plots they mature and an
active ciliated miracidium breaks out through a small opercular cap
at one end of the shell. The larva then penetrates the soft tissues of
the small watch-spring snail and gives eventual development to many
cercariæ, each with an active caudal appendage. These cercariæ
burst forth from the snail, crawl upon water weeds or the edible water
caltrap (Trapa natans and Trapa bicornis) or the water "chestnut"
(Eliocharis tuberosa), and encyst on the plant. Consumption of the
plant by man or pig produces infection.

These worms produce a localized inflammation at the point of
attachment, frequently involving the capillaries of the intestinal
wall, causing hemorrhage, or provoking abscess formation with an
infiltration of round cells and eosinophils. Clinical *symptoms* first
develop about three months after inoculation. In light infections,
diarrhea alternating with constipation and epigastric pain are the
conspicuous symptoms. The latter is relieved after a full meal. Large
numbers of worms may give rise to esthesia. As the disease develops,
diarrhea becomes more and more persistent, the stools assuming a
greenish-yellow color, with much undigested food, and having a fetid
odor. Edema of the face, abdominal wall and lower extremities occurs
at this stage. Toxic ascites is common and in children the abdomen is
frequently protuberant. During this period generalized abdominal
pain is noted. The appetite is fair but anorexia, nausea and vomiting
are usual in heavy infections. There is no true anemia in uncomplicated cases. In the terminal stage dehydration is marked, the skin
becomes harsh and dry, the diarrhea is continuous and prostration is
extreme. Death results from toxemia-following anasarca.

Diagnosis is based on finding the typical eggs in the feces. These
eggs cannot be distinguished from those of the sheep-liver fluke,
Fasciola hepatica. Treatment with beta-naphthol (two administra-

tions of 2 gm. each after purgation) or with carbon tetrachloride (one administration of 3 cc. CCl₄ C.P.) causes evacuation of the worms, but great care must be exercised in heavy infections where toxemia is extreme. Except in cases having advanced prostration the prognosis following specific medication is good. Prophylaxis consists in abstinence from eating raw water plants in infected areas.

Another group of intestinal flukes of minute size (measuring 1 to 3 mm. in length by 0.3 to 0.6 mm. in breadth) is common as a human infection throughout the Far East and in the Balkans and Egypt. These species (Heterophyes heterophyes, Metagonimus yokogawai, etc.) are rather loosely attached to the mucosa of the duodenum, jejunum and upper ileum and produce a mild catarrhal inflammation of the affected areas. They are not known to burrow deeply into the villi. These worms are acquired from consumption of raw fresh-water fish harboring the encysted stage.

Liver Distomiasis.—This group of diseases is caused by flukes parasitic in the bile passages of man. The principal forms are Clonorchis sinensis, Opisthorchis felineus and Fasciola hepatica. Clonorchis sinensis, the Chinese liver-fluke, has a distribution throughout the Far East. The organism is a delicate, almost transparent spatulate worm, measuring 10 to 25 mm. in length by 3 to 5 mm. in breadth. It lives for the most part in the distal bile ducts and passages. The minute lemon-colored, fully embryonated, operculate eggs (28 by 16 microns) pass out in the feces. They are ingested by certain operculate snails of the genera Parafossarulus and Bithynia, in which they hatch and multiply. The cercariæ which erupt from the snail attack fresh-water fishes, finally encysting in the flesh. Consumption of the raw fish flesh is the source of human infection. Opisthorchis felineus, with a geographic distribution in the Balkans, eastern Europe and Sibera, and structurally very similar to Clonorchis, has a life-cycle which almost exactly parallels that of Clonorchis. Fasciola hepatica, the cause of liver rot in sheep and cattle, has been observed from time to time as a human infection, there being more than 100 cases on record. These worms live in the proximal as well as in the distal bile tracts. They are relatively large, fleshy worms, measuring up to 30 by 13 mm. The thin-shelled hyaline oval eggs, with a small opercular cap and a measurement of 130 to 145 microns by 70 to 90 microns, cannot be differentiated from Fasciolopsis eggs. In marshy grasslands they mature and hatch and the miracidia infect snails of the genus Lymnæa, within which the usual twofold multiplicative cycle occurs. The cercariæ which emerge from the snail encyst on water grass and man becomes infected from consumption of such grass. The larvæ excyst in the duodenum and burrow through the intestinal wall, migrate through the abdominal cavity to the liver and penetrate from outside inward to the bile ducts, where they develop into adult worms.

In clonorchiasis and opisthorchiasis the primary lesion is a hypertrophy of the bile tract epithelium; in fascioliasis additional damage is produced by the migration of the young worms through the liver substance *en route* to the bile passages. This is followed by cellular infiltration and fibrosis around the passages. Pressure on the liver cells causes necrosis and in turn obliteration of both these cells and the portal vessels, with hepatic cirrhosis as the end-result. In the early stage of these infections there are no appreciable *symptoms;* in the secondary stage diarrhea, edema and other symptoms due to hypertrophy of the liver are recorded, and in severe cases, with involvement of the portal circulation, ascites, nephritis and emaciation are found. The most common complaints of patients harboring the worms are loss of appetite, fullness and pressure after meals, and diarrhea. There is no significant alteration of the blood picture. This disease requires differentiation from malignancies of the liver, hydatid cyst, beri-beri, and from the usual types of hepatic cirrhosis.

Diagnosis is based on finding in the feces the eggs of the particular species of distome involved. In clonorchiasis and opisthorchiasis in the earlier or milder cases, administration of gentian violet by mouth (enteric coated pills, 0.065 gram (1 grain), three times daily, for one or two months) is usually effective in killing most of the worms. In later or more severe cases oral administration at times causes emesis, so that the dye must be given intravenously (0.5 to 1 per cent solution, 40 cc. on alternate days, until not more than 6 grams have been introduced). No successful treatment of human fascioliasis has been recorded. The prognosis in early cases of clonorchiasis is fairly good; in fascioliasis it is poor. Prophylaxis in the case of clonorchiasis and opisthorchiasis consists in the thorough cooking of fresh-water fish consumed in endemic areas. In fascioliasis care should be exercised not to eat watercress and other raw water plants in sheep-raising areas.

Pulmonary Distomiasis.—This term is applied to infection with the lung-fluke, Paragonimus westermani. The disease is prevalent throughout the Far East. Domestic and wild mammals are parasitized by a related worm in the United States. The thick ovoid worms, which measure 7.5 to 12 mm. in length by 4 to 6 mm. in breadth and 3.5 to 5 mm. in thickness, usually reside in adventitious cysts in the alveolar tissues of the lungs. Their thick-shelled, broadly operculate, immature eggs have a characteristic golden-brown tinge (measurements, 80 to 118 microns by 48 to 60 microns). These are coughed up and voided in the sputum or are swallowed and passed in the feces. The eggs mature in water, the miracidia hatch and invade the appropriate snail (a species of Melania), undergo metamorphosis in the snail and give rise to a progeny of styletted cercariæ with a miniature pyriform tail. These cercariæ after a brief period of free-swimming existence penetrate into the gills and liver of crayfish and crabs, where they encyst and await transfer to the definitive host (man, dog, cat) when the soft parts of the crayfish or crab are eaten uncooked. These larvæ reach the duodenum, excyst and burrow through the intestinal wall, migrate through the abdominal cavity, penetrate through the diaphragm, then wander through the pleural cavity, after which they work their way into the lung tissues and develop into adults.

The presence of these flukes in the lungs provokes a host tissue reaction, consisting of a leukocytic infiltration around the parasite, followed by a deposition of fibrous tissue, thus providing a more or less effective insulation between the parasite and the host tissues. These cysts usually lie in the deeper lung tissues and are about the size of a filbert. Between the parasite and the cyst wall there accumulates a blood-tinged purulent fluid, with minute rusty-brown flecks, which are agglomerated masses of the parasite's eggs. On occasion these worms may be found in other tissues of the body, including the liver, intestinal wall, mesenteric lymph glands, groin, muscles, testes, brain or are attached to the peritoneum or pleura, where a characteristic slaty-blue color identifies the cyst. In the lungs the cysts are usually perforated by bronchioles, through which the eggs and excretions of the worms are discharged. The lesions as a whole are grouped into: (1) non-suppurative, (2) suppurative, (3) tubercle-like and (4) ulcerative. The infiltration of eggs into the tissues produces a peppered rusty-brown appearance, frequently visible to the naked eye. The lesions in the lungs result in diffuse cirrhosis, cystic dilatation of the bronchi, pneumonitis and pseudotubercle abscesses, and are usually accompanied by cough and hemoptysic discharge containing eggs. The physical signs resemble those of bronchopneumonia or pleural effusion. The abdominal type produces vaguer symptoms. In the intestinal variety diarrhea occurs, with eggs in the feces. In glandular involvement, inflammatory reaction with fever may be observed. The cerebral type resembles Jacksonian epilepsy, with hemiplegia, monoplegia, aphasia, ocular disturbance or paresis. Local or generalized eosinophilia may be present.

Diagnosis is based on finding the characteristic eggs in the sputum or feces, in the clinical history and admission on the part of the patient of residence in endemic areas and consumption of raw crustaceans. There is no known specific therapeusis. Prophylaxis consists in cooking well all crayfish or crabmeat intended for human consumption.

Schistosomiasis.—These diseases are caused by infection with the blood-flukes, of which there are three important species parasitizing man, Schistosoma hæmatobium, Schistosoma mansoni and Schistosoma japonicum. The first of these infections is distributed throughout Africa. It is also common in the Tigris-Euphrates Valley and is found in Palestine and parts of Arabia. Its heaviest endemic foci are in Egypt and the Sudan. Schistosoma mansoni is found in Africa and in the Western World (Brazil, Venezuela and the Guianas; the Lesser Antilles, and Puerto Rico). Schistosoma japonicum is confined to the Far East, including Central and South China, particularly the Yangtze Valley; Formosa, and at least one center (Leyte Id.) in the Philippines.

The worms which produce this disease are unisexual, the males being relatively robust and the females very delicate filiform objects. The two suckers on each worm are close together near the anterior end. The ventral aspect of the male is curved outward from the ventral sucker to the posterior extremity to form a longitudinal groove or trough, called the gynecophoral canal, in which the female lies almost constantly during her lifetime.

In the case of Schistosoma hæmatobium the worms live in the vesical blood plexuses, and the light yellowish eggs, which are elongate oval with a sharp wedge-shaped terminal spine and measure 120 to 160

microns in length by 40 to 60 microns in cross-section, are deposited
with embryonated miracidia in the capillaries of the bladder wall.
By mechanical pressure and lysis they escape into the bladder and are
discharged in the urine. In Schistosoma mansoni and Schistosoma
japonicum infections the worms live in the mesenteric radicles and
discharge their fully embryonated eggs into the intestinal capillaries.
The eggs of Schistosoma mansoni are yellowish-brown in color, elongate
oval in shape, have a distinct lateral spine and measure 140 to 165
microns by 60 to 70 microns; those of Schistosoma japonicum are
hyaline or straw-colored, broadly oval in shape with a minute inconspicuous lateral spine, are usually covered with leukocytic débris and
measure 70 to 100 microns by 50 to 65 microns. Upon reaching an
aqueous medium eggs of all these three schistosome species hatch, the
miracidium swimming about until it finds the appropriate snail.
Within these snails the miracidia of the respective species undergo
a twofold multiplicative development, so that for each larva penetrating the snail about 10,000 or more cercariæ may emerge at the
end of the developmental period. These cercariæ, which are characterized by the absence of a pharyngeal sphincter and by the presence of a conspicuous forking of their caudal extremity, actively
swim about through the water, coming to rest on the underside of
the surface film. When man exposes his skin to the water containing these cercariæ, those at the surface film become attached to and,
dropping their tails, penetrate through the skin, eventually reaching
the peripheral circulation, whereupon they are carried through the
right heart to the lungs and pass through the capillaries into the
systemic circulation. The majority are directed by the blood current
into the abdominal aorta, but only those which get into the mesenteric
artery and are carried through the capillaries into the portal system
are able to develop into adult worms. The others soon become foreign-
protein emboli and produce local petechiæ wherever they lodge. Once
within the intrahepatic portion of the portal stream the young schistosomes begin to grow and in the course of five to seven weeks after
exposure to infection the worms are mature, migrate out of the liver
against the portal current to the vesical plexuses (Schistosoma hæmatobium) or mesenteric radicles (Schistosoma mansoni, Schistosoma
japonicum), mate and the females begin to lay eggs.

Since the lesions in Schistosoma hæmatobium infection primarily
involve the bladder this disease is known as *vesical* or *urinary schistosomiasis*. In Egypt it is frequently referred to as *bilharzia* infection
(bilharziasis) or endemic hematuria. The disease may be divided
into three stages: (1) the incubation period, (2) the period of egg
deposition and extrusion and (3) the period of tissue proliferation and
repair. The first stage extends from inoculation to the maturing
of the parasite. At the time of penetration of the cercariæ an itching
sensation is frequently experienced, followed by development of small
petechiæ over areas of exposed skin. No further *symptoms* occur for
at least three weeks, when toxic manifestations are noted, including
anorexia, headache, malaise and generalized pains in the back and
extremities, with elevation of temperature late in the afternoon,

accompanied by rigor and sweating. Urticarial wheals frequently develop at this time. Blood examination shows a leukocytosis with high eosinophilia. The abdomen becomes distended, the liver and spleen are enlarged and tender, pericardial pains are common and respiration may become labored. The second stage may immediately follow or there may be an intervening period of weeks or months. Finally there is a painless passing of blood at the end of micturition. This may continue for years without subjective symptoms. During this time myriads of eggs may be voided in the urine. Eventually there is a burning sensation between periods of urination and the periods become shorter. Dull pains in the loin and suprapubic region and colic of the bladder now appear. Examination will reveal a papillomatous condition of the bladder wall and calculi in the bladder. Eggs now infiltrate in and around the prostate and tubules and the external genital organs become involved. Similarly in women the genitalia become infiltrated. As soon as egg extrusion into the tissues is well under way tissue reaction is initiated. Hyperplasia of the bladder wall gradually assumes the condition of a chronic cystitis. Phosphatic deposits are laid down in the wall, the urine becomes definitely alkaline, and mucus, blood and pus cells accumulate in the bladder. Calculi form around these elements of débris as well as around eggs. The urethra and the ureters become involved and at times the kidneys. Elephantiasis of the penis may develop and pyogenic organisms may cause abscess formation. This late stage is accompanied by extreme weakness, emaciation and intense pain at micturition. Finally the patient wastes away or dies of secondary infection. Secondarily the liver partakes of the infiltration process and hepatic cirrhosis is initiated. In a large percentage of late cases malignancies of the bladder develop.

Infections with Schistosoma mansoni and Schistosoma japonicum involve the intestinal wall and the liver, hence these diseases are commonly referred to as *intestinal schistosomiasis*. The two infections are similar, except that the much greater number of eggs deposited by Schistosoma japonicum causes greater damage. During the incubation period the pathologic and clinical pictures of intestinal schistosomiasis exactly parallel those of the vesical type. Egg deposition into the intestinal capillaries almost immediately follows maturity of the worms. There is first a prodromal diarrhea, then as the eggs infiltrate the intestinal wall they begin to be extruded with blood and mucus, which is usually passed at the end of the stooling period. Other eggs are carried back into the liver where they infiltrate into the tissues. Wherever an egg becomes deposited, whether in the liver or the intestinal wall, an intense tissue reaction is provoked, causing an invasion of white cells, commonly eosinophils, and production of giant cells around the egg. This is the typical schistosomiasis abscess or pseudotubercle. Around these fibrous tissue formation takes place. Moreover, hematin pigment, discharged from the parent worms, is engulfed by phagocytes in the portal spaces and in the tubercle. The spleen becomes engorged and the mesenteric lymph nodes enlarged. The third period is characterized by the development of scar tissue in the intestine and liver, thickening of the mesentery and omentum so as to bind down the colon, thus forming a protuberant mass in the upper abdomen and one below. Weakness and extreme pallor are common and dyspnea develops on slight exertion. Emaciation is extreme as the liver becomes more and more involved and ascites more and more common. The thoracic viscera are pushed upward, due to enlargement of the abdominal organs. Hepatic facies is pronounced. The peripheral abdominal veins become very prominent. The blood pressure is subnormal and the temperature inconstant. The patient gradually weakens, or may die of bronchopneumonia, appendicitis or malarial cachexia.

Blood examination shows a reduced number of erythrocytes, with low color index and hemoglobin percentage. Precipitation and complement-fixation tests are usually positive, due to increased euglobulin in the blood. Eosinophilia is less extreme than earlier in the infection. The feces frequently contain poorly digested food, with flecks of blood and mucus and eggs of Schistosoma mansoni or Schistosoma japonicum throughout the entire fecal mass. These eggs are at times so few that centrifugation of the stool is necessary in order to detect them.

Diagnosis is made on finding the characteristic egg in the urine or the feces. It is reinforced by the blood picture, precipitation reaction and clinical manifestations. *Treatment* is specific. Sodium antimony tartrate is the drug of choice and should be given intravenously as a 1 per cent solution in amounts of 60 to 100 mg. every other day or every third day until a total of 1.5 to 1.8 grams has been administered. Frequently tolerance for the drug must be built up. In advanced cases of the intestinal type administration of the drug may cause more harm than good because of the small amount of vital liver tissue left. Gradually with administration of the drug the blood picture and the general physical appearance of the patient begin to improve, eggs become less and less common in the urine or stools and finally disappear altogether. In thirty to forty-five days the patient is usually freed of the infection but the damage in moderately developed or late cases can never be repaired. Treatment is contraindicated in cardiac block, pneumonia, nephritis and profound hepatic cirrhosis. Recently fouadin, for intramuscular injection, has partially replaced tartar emetic.

Schistosome dermatitis has been reported from several localities in the northern United States, England and Germany. This is caused by cercariæ distantly related to the human blood-flukes attempting to invade or partially invading the skin of persons wading or bathing in water harboring these larvæ. None of these individuals have become infected viscerally with these worms.

Prophylaxis in schistosomiasis is a most complicated problem. The hundreds of millions of the world's population who are exposed to these infections know little or nothing of sanitation and personal hygiene. Sanitary disposal of feces is probably the one measure which would control the problem, but in the infected areas it is impracticable. Destruction of the snail hosts is equally out of the question. Since the worms live for ten years or more and individuals in endemic areas are constantly exposing themselves to reinfection, therapy is of little avail as a prophylactic measure. Possibly sterilization of night soil will be found to be the eventual solution to this difficult problem.

GENERAL CLASSIFICATION OF ARTHROPODS INVOLVED IN DISEASE.

Of the 13 recognized classes of arthropods the following 4 are medically important, either as causative agents *per se* or as intermediate hosts or transmitters of disease-producing organisms: (1) Myriapoda, including the millipedes and centipedes, the bites of which produce skin lesions and at times systemic shock, particularly in children; (2) Crustacea, including Cyclops, which serves as the intermediate host of the Medina worm (Dracunculus medinensis) and is one of the hosts of the broad tapeworm (Diphyllobothrium latum), and crabs and crayfish, which are the second intermediate hosts of the lung distome, Paragonimus westermani; (3) Arachnida, including ticks, mites, spiders and scorpions; and (4) Insecta, with several orders directly or indirectly involved in human disease.

Members of these groups are all typically characterized by having bilateral symmetry, an axial gradient, a true body cavity, true segmentation, an exoskeleton and articulated appendages. Their anterior paired appendages are usually highly modified into sensory, grasping and feeding organs.

TICKS, MITES, SPIDERS AND SCORPIONS.

Ticks and Mites.—These forms (technically known as Acarina) are medium to microscopic species, which have a fused cephalothorax and abdomen. They are usually broadly ovate and are compressed dorsoventrally. Their mouth parts are adapted for piercing, cutting or sucking blood or serum. They have four stages in development, namely, the egg, the larva (with three pairs of legs), the nymph (with four pairs of legs but sexually immature) and the sexually differentiated adults.

Ticks are larger than mites and have a leathery integument. Their abdomen is capable of enormous distention when they become engorged with blood. The eggs are layed in the soil or under leaves and humus, where the larvæ hatch. Sometime during its development each of the three motile stages (larva, nymph and adult) must have at least one blood meal; between feedings it drops off the host. Ticks are usually capable of securing their food from any land vertebrate, but a few species have predilections for certain hosts. Many ticks are transmitters of pathogenic microörganisms to domestic animals; a few species are important as transmitters of human diseases. The ear-tick of Africa, Ornithodorus moubata, and its close relatives, Ornithodorus venezuelensis in Tropical America and Ornithodorus turicata in Texas, are the intermediate hosts and transmitters to man of tick-borne relapsing fever. The Rocky Mountain wood tick, Dermacentor andersoni, and its eastern relative, Dermacentor variabilis, are responsible for the transmission to man of Rocky Mountain spotted fever, while Dermacentor andersoni also transmits tularemia from rodents to man.

Any species of tick which attacks man produces trauma by the insertion of its mouth parts into the skin layers. Frequently more damage results from attempting to pull out the tick from its temporary anchorage than by letting it drop off of its own accord. However, a few drops of chloroform placed on its head will cause it to relax so that it may be removed by easy traction. Paralysis may result from salivary secretions of the tick injected into any site in the body, but the symptoms are most acute when the toxin is introduced near the spinal column or at the base of the brain. Children are the most common sufferers. The syndrome is that of generalized toxemia, with elevation of temperature to 40° C., rapid ascending motor paralysis, difficulty in swallowing and respiration, and frequently death. This disease requires differentiation from poliomyelitis. Dermacentor andersoni is the tick involved in North America. In areas where it abounds, care should be taken, particularly during the late spring and summer, to prevent young children from wandering into under-brush or bushes where they are liable to attack, and after picnic excursions or walks through the woods they should be stripped of clothing and carefully examined each day for ticks.

Mites are smaller and more delicate than ticks. The common red mite, Trombicula irritans, is the cause of severe dermatitis and pruritus throughout most of the United States, but particularly in the South, during the late spring and early summer. Its relatives in the Orient are the transmitters to man of Japanese river fever and pseudo-typhus. The rat mite, Liponyssus bacoti, has been shown in Texas to transmit endemic typhus from rodents to man.

Two species of mites, Sarcoptes scabiei and Demodex folliculorum, invade the human skin. The former infection is common, producing sarcoptic mange; the latter, uncommon, causing at times an inflammatory reaction around the hair follicles and in the sebaceous glands. The human itch mite, Sarcoptes scabiei, has a cosmopolitan distribution but is most frequently found in the lower strata of society, particularly in jails and asylums. The adult mites live in skin burrows, where the females lay their eggs, which hatch and migrate into secondary tunnels or get onto clothing or bed linen and are thus transferred to different sites on the body or to other individuals. The infection produces an intolerable pruritus, which causes scratching, usually resulting in bacterial invasion of the lesion. Infected individuals should have green soap vigorously rubbed into the sites, after which they should lie in a warm bath to soften the skin and open the burrows. After drying, the lesions should be treated generously with 5 per cent sulphur in lanolin, leaving the ointment on overnight. In the morning fresh boiled clothing should be put on and all soiled clothing and bed linen thoroughly boiled. The treatment should be repeated once after five days and before ten days, in order to destroy the freshly hatched larvæ. The unhatched eggs are not affected by the treatment.

Spiders.—Common belief to the contrary, the American tarantula is not usually dangerous. The only North American spider which can inflict serious injury is the black widow, Latrodectus mactans, which is characterized by having an orange hour-glass pattern on the ventral side of its abdomen, in contrast to the sooty-black appearance of the remainder of the body. Following its bite the patient is frequently dizzy and experiences weakness of the legs, abdominal cramps, in addition to local pain and inflammation at the site of attack. Although the patient may be seriously ill, death is rare.

Scorpions.—These arthropods can be recognized by their large cheliceræ, like those of a crab, and by the recurved stinger which is found on the tip of the abdomen. All true scorpions are venomous but only a few are capable of injecting their venom under the outer layer of the skin. Five dangerous species are known for the Southern United States. They are most common in the dry Southwest. The durango scorpion, across the border in Mexico, is the most deadly. The venom of scorpions contains hemolysins, hemorrhagins, neurotoxins and other harmful substances. Death among children, who unwittingly step on this animal, is not uncommon. Treatment is symptomatic only. No antivenin has been developed.

INSECTS.

Insects comprise that class of arthropods which have a separate head, thorax and abdomen, typically with three pairs of legs, attached to the thorax. Some orders have complete metamorphosis, with egg, larva, pupa and adult; others have incomplete metamorphosis, omitting the pupal stage.

Blood-sucking Insects.—This physiologic group includes many of the flies, the fleas, the sucking lice and the hemophagous bugs. In all of these forms the mouth parts are modified into a proboscis for piercing the skin and sucking up blood from the host. The most numerous species are those of the flies.

Blood-sucking Flies.—All of these species have their mouth parts adapted so as to form an elongate tube through which they are able to obtain a blood meal from the host. Like all flies (Diptera) they possess only one pair of wings, the second pair being replaced by halteres or balancing organs. The female usually requires blood before she can oviposit. Eggs of most species are layed in or near the water, and the larvæ (several stages) ordinarily require moisture for development. After a period of feeding and growth the larva is transformed into a resting stage, the pupa. Eventually the pupal case opens to free the adult fly.

Blood-sucking flies, small or large, are annoying pests to man and domestic animals. Some persons manifest a distinct allergic reaction to the minute amounts of saliva which they inject into the skin. Among the numerous species which serve as transmitters of pathogenic organisms the following are particularly important: (1) species of the small gnat Culicoides ("punkie," "no-se-um"), which is the intermediate host of two human filarial worms, Acanthocheilonema perstans and Mansonella ozzardi; (2) species of sand-flies (Phlebotomus), which cause sand-fly fever, and are probable transmitters of kala-azar, cutaneous leishmaniasis and verruga peruviana; (3) black flies (Simulium species), which are intermediate hosts of the filarial worms, Onchocerca volvulus and Onchocerca cæcutiens; (4) species of tabanid flies (Chrysops), which are transmitters of tularemia and also transmit the filarial worm, Loa loa; (5) species of tsetse flies (Glossina) which transmit the two types of African sleeping sickness (trypanosomiasis), and (6) mosquitoes. This latter group requires special consideration.

Mosquitoes are delicate flies with long, narrow wings having a fringe of scales on the veins and along the posterior wing border. They have long, multisegmented antennæ, with whorls of long hairs at the joints. The species of medical importance belong to two tribes, (1) the Culicini and (2) the Anophelini. The former group have the following readily distinguishable characteristics: the eggs are layed in rafts (Culex) or singly (Aëdes), but without air floats; the larvæ are provided with a long breathing tube, which makes it possible for the organism to swing at an angle from the surface film of the water; the pupæ have a long tubular (Culex) or short conical (Aëdes) breathing tube; the adult is "hump-backed," that is, the proboscis is not in line with the abdomen. In contrast the Anophelini (principally species of Anopheles) have eggs, which are layed singly and are provided with air floats; their larvæ have very short breathing tubes, which require the larvæ to lie parallel to the surface of the water and feed in the surface film; their pupæ have a pair of short, broad, breathing trumpets; the adults come to rest with the proboscis in a straight line with the abdomen, at an oblique angle from the resting surface. Their wings are characteristically dappled. Species of Culex are the principal intermediate hosts of Bancroft's filarial worm (Wuchereria bancrofti); the "yellow jacket" (Aëdes ægypti) and its close relatives are the transmitters of yellow fever, dengue, Bancroft's filarial worm and tularemia (experimentally); Anopheles is the only generic group known to transmit malaria. In addition, these and other mosquitoes provide a frequent opportunity for streptococci, staphylococci and fungi to enter the skin. There is no good mosquito repellant. Remedial measures are of two types, larvicidal, aimed to control or reduce mosquito breeding, and human, aimed at preventing adult mosquitoes from biting man.

Fleas.—Fleas (Siphonaptera) are golden to dark brown, wingless insects which are compressed from side to side, with a specially long pair of hind legs, used for jumping. They have complete metamorphosis. One species, the chigo (Tunga penetrans) lives in burrows of the skin of man, the dog and the pig. The interdigital spaces between the toes and the plantar surface of the foot are most usually involved. This infection is common in warm climates. All of the other fleas of medical importance are ectoparasitic. The tropical rat flea (Xenopsylla cheopis) and its allies, the common rat flea (Ceratophyllus fasciatus), the flea of the California ground squirrel (Hoplopsyllus anomalus), the human flea (Pulex irritans) and other species are con-

20

cerned with the transmission of plague to man. Ceratophyllus fasciatus also transmits endemic typhus. The dog flea (Ctenocephalus
canis) and the human flea are responsible for transmitting the dog
tapeworm (Dipylidium caninum) to man. Public health measures
against rats and other rodents are required to prevent introduction
of plague into plague-free communities. Individual prevention to
prevent breeding of human fleas requires frequent kerosene-soapsuds
baths for dogs on which they commonly breed, and cleaning with
kerosene of old wooden floors and matting in which the larvæ develop.

Lice.—Blood-sucking lice are dirty gray, wingless insects, compressed dorsoventrally. They have incomplete metamorphosis. Eggs,
larvæ and adults are all found on the host's body. Human lice belong
to two groups, the crab or pubic louse (Phthirius pubis) and the body
louse (Pediculus humanus) with its two varieties, corporis and capitis.
The crab louse is relatively broad and has large cheliceræ; it is usually
confined to the inguinal and pubic region of the body and sticks
closely to the skin so that it is removed with difficulty. Ten per cent
thymol in olive oil rubbed into the affected area brings prompt relief.
While this species is alleged to transmit granuloma inguinale, adequate
proof is lacking. The body louse, particularly the variety corporis,
is responsible for transmission of epidemic and endemic typhus, trench
fever and louse-borne relapsing fever. Pediculosis is common among
beggars, prisoners and soldiers. Delousing requires the thorough
sterilization (preferably by steam) of all clothing of infested groups,
together with scrubbing of the body of individuals with a kerosene-
soapsuds mixture and frequently shaving off the hair of head and
trunk in order to destroy the attached louse eggs.

Hemophagous Bugs.—These insects have incomplete metamorphosis.
Only the adult stage attacks man. On provocation several species
will take human blood, but the cosmopolitan offender is the bedbug
(Cimex lectularius) and its tropical relative (Cimex rotundatus), which
live in human habitations, breeding in cracks and crevices of the bed,
floor and wall. While this bug has been shown experimentally to
transmit several pathogens, it is doubtful if it is a common source of
infection for any human microörganisms. It is, therefore, primarily
a nuisance, particularly in old hospital wards with cracks in the floor
boards, old linoleum and old plaster. Where an infestation has gotten
out of control mattresses should be dry cleaned, joints of iron beds and
springs should be torch-flamed, floors should be thoroughly scrubbed
with undiluted kerosene and then with soapsuds, and old plaster should
be torn off and the walls replastered. Another bug, Triatoma megista,
and its relatives are the intermediate host of Chagas disease (due to
Trypanosoma cruzi), which is prevalent in Tropical America and
extends north into the southern border of the United States.

Filth and Myiasis-producing Insects.—All of the common and
important members of this group are flies, most of which breed in
filth, such as manure of human and domestic animals, and garbage.
Others, by choice, breed in decaying flesh, or flesh wounds or mucus
exudates of debilitated persons or animals, while a few deposit their
eggs on uninjured human skin. Flies which feed and breed in filth

are capable of and frequently do transfer pathogenic organisms to human food and drink. Among the diseases which have resulted from such contamination are the following: bacillary dysentery, typhoid and paratyphoid, tuberculosis, anthrax, tularemia, plague, Malta fever, cholera, streptococcus and staphylococcus infections, amebic dysentery, ascariasis, trachoma and yaws. In parts of the Southern United States a small gnat, Hippelates pusio, has been incriminated in the spread of epidemic ophthalmia ("pink eye").

The eggs of several flies, deposited on food, are swallowed, hatch out in the small bowel and produce a temporary or chronic intestinal myiasis. Eggs of other flies—particularly the screw-worm (Cochliomyia), species of Wolfhartia (W. vigil in the Northern United States and Canada), the African floor-worm (Auchmeromyia luteola), Sarcophaga hæmorrhoidalis (in the Eastern and Western Hemispheres), the nasal bot (Œstrus ovis), the warble flies (Hypoderma bovis and H. lineata), Gastrophilus equi (which produces "larva migrans" in man) and the human warble fly (Dermatobia hominis)—are deposited on the skin, hatch in contact with the body's warmth and tunnel into the skin or the flesh, frequently producing permanent disfigurement, particularly on the face and neck of small children. Excision of the maggot is the only remedy for dermal myiasis. Recently certain investigators have advocated the placing of maggots of certain species into septic wounds such as exist in osteomyelitis and tuberculosis of the bone, in order to clean out the necrotic tissues. Cultures of sterile larvæ are now used to avoid the introduction of pathogens into the lesions, and attempts are being made to prepare maggot extracts to take the place of living larvæ. The value of the procedure is still *sub judice.*

Nettling, Vesicating and Stinging Insects.—Nettling insects are those species having specialized hairs, spines or scales which produce a dermatitis, and at times systemic disturbance, when they come in contact with the skin. Such hairs are found on the caterpillars of numerous moths and a few butterflies. The hairs are hollow and have a poison sac at their base. The commonest offenders in the United States are the brown-tail moth (Euproctis phæorrhea); the white-marked tussock moth (Hemerocampa leucostigma); the puss caterpillar (Megalopyge opercularis); the flannel moths (Megalopyge crispata and M. pyxidifera); the saddle-back caterpillar (Sibine stimulea), and the io moth (Automeris io). No satisfactory treatment for the urticaria is known. Vesicating insects are those whose body fluid contains a blistering substance (cantharidin). In the United States one family of beetles (Staphylinidæ) possess this property. When handled roughly or crushed on the skin they produce painful blisters. The blister should be opened and dressed with an antiseptic lotion. Stinging insects possess a sting which is connected with poison glands. The stinger, together with its poison, is usually left in the wound. Several families of hymenopterans, including the honey bees, the bumble bees, the wasps and hornets, the digger wasps, the velvet ants and the stinging ants, are capable of producing painful stings, with resulting inflammation at the site and, at times, a distinct allergic reaction. The stinger should be first removed by pressure rather than by attempting to pull it out, after which the wound should be bathed with ammonia or baking soda to neutralize the poison (formic acid).

REFERENCES.

Helminths.

ANDERSON, JOHN: Filariasis in British Guiana. London School Trop. Med. Research Memoir Ser., 1924, **5**, 122 pp.. 23 pl.

BARLOW, CLAUDE H.: The Life Cycle of the Human Intestinal Fluke Fasciolopsis buski (Lankester), Am. Jour. Hyg., 1923, Monogr. Ser. No. 4, 98 pp.

CAMERON, THOMAS W. M.: Some Modern Biologic Conceptions of Hydatid, Proc. Roy. Soc. Med. (Sec. Trop. Dis. and Parasitol.), 1927, **20**, 272–283.

CHANDLER, ASA C.: Hookworm Disease. Its Distribution, Biology, Epidemiology, Pathology, Diagnosis, Treatment and Control, New York, 1929, 494 pp.

CORT, WILLIAM WALTER.: Recent Investigations on the Epidemiology of Human Ascariasis, Jour. Parasitol., 1931, **17**, 121–144.

FAUST, ERNEST CARROLL: Human Helminthology: A Manual for Clinicians, Sanitarians and Medical Zoölogists, Philadelphia, 1929, 616 pp., 297 figs.

FAUST, ERNEST CARROLL, and MELENEY, HENRY EDMUND: Studies on Schistosomiasis Japonica, Am. Jour. Hyg., 1924, Monogr. Ser. No. 3, 339 pp., 36 pl., 25 figs.

FAUST, ERNEST CARROLL, and KHAW, OO-KEH: Studies on Clonorchis Sinensis (Cobbold), Am. Jour. Hyg., 1927, Monogr. Ser. No. 8, 284 pp., 14 pl., 33 figs.

HALL, MAURICE C., and AUGUSTINE, DONALD L.: Some Investigations of Anthelmintics by an Egg and Worm Count Method, Am. Jour. Hyg., 1929, **9**, 584–628.

LAMSON, PAUL D., and WARD, CHARLOTTE B.: The Chemotherapy of Helminth Infestations, Jour. of Parasitol., 1932, **18**, 173–199.

Arthropods.

BAERG, E.: Some Poisonous Arthropods of North and Central America, 4th Internat. Congr. Entomol., Trans., 1929, **2**, 418–435.

BEYER, G. E.: Urticating and Poisonous Caterpillars, Quart. Bull. La. State Board of Health, 1922, **13**, 161–168.

BENSON, R. L., and SEMENOV, H.: Allergy in Relation to Bee Sting, Jour. Allergy, 1930, **1**, 105–116.

BISHOPP, F. C.: Flies Which Cause Myiasis in Man and Animals, Jour. Econ. Entomol., 1923, **8**, 317–329.

BUXTON, P. A.: On the Sarcoptes of Man, Parasitol., 1921, **13**, 146–151.

GREENWOOD, A. M.: The Danish Treatment of Scabies, Jour. Am. Med. Assn., 1924, **82**, 466–467.

HINMAN, E. H.: Mosquitoes in Relation to Human Welfare, Ann. Entomol. Soc. Amer., 1932, **25**, 613–623.

HIRST, L. F.: On the Transmission of Plague by Fleas of the genus *Xenopsylla*, Ind. Jour. Med. Res., 1923, **10**, 789–920.

KUMM, H. W.: The Geographical Distribution of the Yellow Fever Vectors, Am. Jour. Hyg., Monogr. Ser. No. 12, 1931.

MATHESON, R.: Medical Entomology, 1932, Springfield, Ill. 489 pp.

NUTTALL, G. H. F.: The Part Played by *Pediculus humanus* in the Causation of Disease, Parasitol., 1917, **10**, 43–79.

YAO, H. Y., YUAN, I. C., and HUIE, D.: The Relation of Flies, Beverages and Well-water to Gastro-intestinal Diseases in Peiping, Nat. Med. Jour. China, 1929, **15**, 410–418.

CHAPTER VIII.

THE CONTAGIOUS DISEASES OF CHILDHOOD.

By A. GRAEME MITCHELL, M.D.

DIPHTHERIA.
SCARLET FEVER.
PERTUSSIS.
MEASLES.
VARICELLA.

MUMPS.
ROSEOLA INFANTUM.
FOURTH DISEASE AND FIFTH DISEASE.
RUBELLA.

DIPHTHERIA.

Definition.—Diphtheria is an acute, specific, contagious disease which is characterized by the production of a membrane usually localized on the throat, and a toxemia due to the absorption of the toxin produced by the causative microörganism.

History.—The disease is one of the oldest of the contagious group. Reports of epidemics of unquestioned diphtheria exist from ancient times. Before the discovery and recognition of its specific cause, the diphtheria bacillus, by Klebs and Loeffler, it was known under various names such as membranous croup and suffocative angina, and it was not clearly separated from other diseases until that time. The name diphtheria was given to it by Bretonneau in 1826.

Etiology.—The etiologic agent is the *diphtheria bacillus,* often called the Klebs-Loeffler bacillus because the first-named bacteriologist discovered the microörganism and the second proved that it was the actual and only cause of the disease. It is a straight, or slightly curved, bacillus which is rod-shaped and has rounded ends, its length being about 2 to 3 microns. When prepared with Neisser's stain it appears as a brown rod with granules at the poles. It can be confused with other microörganisms found in the throat, the so-called pseudo-diphtheria group or diphtheroids.

Age is an important predisposing factor, the majority of cases occurring in children from one to ten years of age. There is usually a natural immunity in the first six months of life, although even newborns may occasionally be attacked. *Epidemics* occur but the disease is endemic as well, being always present in large communities. The *individual susceptibility* is not great and many non-immune persons will escape unless the exposure has been direct and intimate. Fomites may, however, carry the infection and healthy *carriers* are a not uncommon means of spread and the cause of local epidemics. Contaminated milk has been shown to be the cause of some epidemics.

Pathology.—The characteristic feature is the production of a membrane (pseudomembrane) which, while usually located in the throat or larynx, may be upon any mucous surface or upon the broken or wounded skin. This pseudomembrane is of the nature of a fibrinous exudate containing masses of leukocytes and epithelial cells; beneath it the tissues undergo necrosis. Secondary pathologic changes come about through the action of the diphtheria toxin which may cause more or less severe degenerative changes in many body tissues and organs. Prominent among these, because of the serious consequences, are the heart, the peripheral nerves and the kidneys.

Symptoms.—There will first be described the ordinary *faucial* type. The incubation period is about one to four days. At the onset there may be fever, headache, malaise and other symptoms of infection. Sore throat will be complained of and there will be found redness of the throat and, in patients with tonsils, swelling and perhaps a follicular tonsillitis. Within twenty-four hours the membranous character of the exudate will be evident. The grayish exudate is removed with difficulty, the attempt to do this causing bleeding; it spreads slowly so that it involves the uvula, palate and later, within two to five days, may become quite extensive. There is a foul odor which is rather characteristic—so much so that experienced clinicians may attach diagnostic significance to it. As the membrane spreads the general symptoms of infection correspondingly increase. The pulse is usually rapid, out of proportion to the temperature—the latter not being high at the onset. There is a polymorphonuclear leukocytosis. Prostration is great. All of these symptoms are modified by treatment with antitoxin.

Laryngeal Diphtheria.—While this localization of diphtheria may be primary, it is more frequently secondary to faucial or nasal involvement, following the throat lesion after four or five days. Nasal diphtheria may be unrecognized until the laryngeal involvement begins. The symptoms of laryngeal diphtheria are those of cough, hoarseness, cyanosis, inspiratory and expiratory obstruction with retraction of the episternal notch and of the ribs along the attachment of the diaphragm and cyanosis. The membrane may extend into the trachea and bronchial tubes, making casts of them. Laryngoscopic examination may be necessary to see the membrane.

Nasal diphtheria may be only a part of a generalized naso-pharyngeal involvement but it may also be primary. In the latter case it may spread to the throat and trachea, or, especially in infants, remain for a long time only in the anterior nares as an isolated form of the disease. It causes a purulent and irritating discharge, frequently bloody, which excoriates the upper lip.

Atypical Forms and Locations.—Diphtheria may be mild, causing little local irritation, and when a typical membrane is not formed it may simulate follicular tonsillitis. In severe cases the membrane may not only be extensive but develop rapidly and toxic symptoms may be great and purpura develop. Marked local swelling of surrounding tissues takes place in these cases and it seems quite likely that microörganisms such as the streptococcus are operative in adding their local and general effect to the diphtheria bacillus. These cases are often designated septic or malignant, and in them diphtheria bacilli may be found in the blood stream.

The more common locations of diphtheria have been mentioned but, as previously stated, it may involve primarily or secondarily the mucous membranes or skin in such areas as the conjunctiva, wounds such as those of circumcision, or the umbilical stump in the new-born, or the stomach and intestinal tract. In all of these places it forms a pseudomembrane, causes local irritation and swelling and usually a bloody discharge, and it may or may not lead to general toxic symptoms, depending largely on the extent of the area involved.

Complications.—Among the most frequent and serious are those of paralysis, often correctly designated *postdiphtheritic paralysis*, since its manifestations are seen three or four weeks after the onset. Early, reflexes may be absent. Paralysis of the palate is a frequent form and causes nasal speech and regurgitation of fluid through the nose. The ocular nerves may be involved, causing strabismus, and other nerves also affected causing a multiple neuritis. Very serious is paralysis of the thoracic muscles and the diaphragm. *Cardiac failure* comes on usually in the third to fourth week but perhaps early in the course of the disease. It is probably caused by damage both to cardiac muscles and nerves. Pulmonary complications such as *bronchopneumonia* are not uncommon, especially in the laryngeal type of the disease. *Nephritis* of the tubular (nephrotic) type may occur.

Relapse and Recurrence.—Relapse is more common than in the other contagious diseases. The same may be said of recurrence, as one attack of diphtheria by no means guarantees permanent immunity.

Diagnosis.[1]—Tonsillitis and sore throat due to streptococci do not usually cause the pseudomembrane, the onset is more abrupt and the initial fever and toxemia greater. Vincent's angina causes a punched-out ulcer and there are not such marked general toxic symptoms; smear and culture may be necessary in the differential diagnosis. In young infants thrush may occasionally be mistaken for diphtheria, but the tendency of the former to localize on buccal mucous membrane and tongue and the whitish rather than grayish color and patchy character should make the diagnosis even before a culture has been examined. The thrush fungus can be seen in properly obtained and prepared scrapings.

An irritating bloody nasal discharge should lead to close inspection for a membrane and a culture of the secretion.

Acute laryngeal obstruction and croup should be proved to be non-diphtheritic by laryngoscopic examination, if possible, and by culture.

In any location the tendency to form pseudomembrane, the irritating and often bloody discharge may be the suspicious circumstances which indicate bacteriologic study.

A serious situation sometimes arises due to diphtheritic infection of post-tonsillectomy wounds where the usual postoperative exudate may confuse the clinical picture. A culture should be taken on all tonsillectomy cases as a preoperative measure and repeated thereafter if indication arises.

Skill must be acquired not only in the examination of cultures, but in the taking of them since it is essential that the swab be thoroughly applied to the proper area. In deciding the virulence of diphtheria bacilli and especially in determining whether a person is carrying

[1] See also page 319 for differential diagnosis.

virulent or non-virulent diphtheria bacilli it may be necessary to perform the so-called guinea-pig test. Injection into this animal of true virulent Klebs-Loeffler microörganisms causes characteristic pathologic changes.

Both clinical and bacteriologic diagnoses are important. Inasmuch as the latter is not always certain and, furthermore, that it takes usually twenty-four hours before the reading of a culture can be made, it often becomes necessary for the physician to act upon his clinical judgment and treat the patient accordingly.

Prognosis.—The mortality varies with the severity and the location of the lesions but primarily with the time of administration of antitoxin. Laryngeal diphtheria is more serious than faucial and when the membrane involves trachea and bronchial tubes the mortality is very high. The death-rate is declining and, from a study of statistics, diphtheria was apparently becoming a milder disease even before the introduction of antitoxin. Infants and children under five years of age have a greater mortality than older persons.

Paralysis is somewhat more likely to occur following severe cases than mild ones and especially in those tardily or insufficiently treated with antitoxin. Paralysis of the heart and of respiratory muscles are especially dangerous forms.

Treatment.—**Prophylaxis.**—Many infants are immune in the first six months of life. After that and during childhood a large percentage of persons are susceptible, but as adult life is reached an immunity is again established in many instances. Although there is some argument to the contrary, this comes about in all probability from submorbid (subclinical) exposures so that antitoxin is developed without the occurrence of a clinically demonstrable diphtheritic disease. *Schick* evolved a test in which a small amount of diphtheria toxin is injected intracutaneously; those persons who are immune or, that is to say, can develop antitoxin, will have a negative Schick test, whereas those who are susceptible will have a positive Schick test and show within twenty-four to forty-eight hours a local, slightly raised erythema at the site of injection of from 0.5 to 2 cm. in diameter. Reading of the reaction may be made on the third or fourth day. A negative Schick test, while a good indication of immunity, does not necessarily guarantee this if there is prolonged exposure to virulent diphtheria infection. This test shows that about 8 per cent of newly born and young infants are Schick-positive (susceptible); 30 to 40 per cent are positive at one year of age, 65 per cent at five years, 30 per cent at ten years and 18 per cent by fifteen years—all of these figures being roughly approximate.

The value of the Schick test in determining those who are susceptible and who need quarantine and isolation or protection during an epidemic is evident. Recovery from the disease usually takes a few weeks and is determined by two or preferably three negative cultures. In the case of chronic carriers the guinea-pig test for virulence should be employed and, if this prove positive, various local antiseptics may be used or the tonsils removed if these be present.

Active immunization which is more or less permanent may be secured in almost all cases by the injection of toxin-antitoxin or toxoid. Toxin-antitoxin injections, as evolved by von Behring, are given in three doses subcutaneously at intervals of one to two weeks. Immunity as indicated by a negative Schick test does not develop for about three to six months and, if the test is still positive, the injection should be repeated. In immunizing large groups of children a preliminary Schick test may be dispensed with; in more individual work it may first be performed to determine the necessity of toxin-antitoxin injections. Since it may be possible that the amount of horse serum present in toxin-antitoxin is liable to sensitize the patient to subsequent injection of it or to be dangerous in a patient sensitive to horse serum, it has become the custom of many clinicians to employ toxoid. This, as recommended by Ramon, is toxin "detoxified" by the addition of formaldehyde. It is used in a manner quite similar to that for toxin-antitoxin (except that two injections given three weeks apart are usually sufficient for children under five years of age) and it is as efficient, if not more so, than the latter and produces a quicker immunity (six weeks to two months). Other methods, such as percutaneous administration or the injection of alum toxoid, are not to be recommended at the present time.

Passive protection may be secured by the injection of 1000 units of antitoxin. This acts almost immediately and continues to be protective for about two weeks. It is not necessary to protect in this manner every non-immune (Schick-positive), exposed person; observation and repeated cultures are usually sufficient.

Antitoxin Treatment.—In the average mild case seen early in the course of the disease 5000 units of antitoxin should be injected intracutaneously or preferably intramuscularly. In severer cases and those seen late the dose should be doubled or quadrupled and often should be given intravenously so that its action may be more rapid. Laryngeal cases especially need this urgent treatment.

General Treatment.—This consists of the measures carried out in any infection. Supportive and stimulating treatment is also indicated. Local treatment should consist mainly in cleansing with alkaline sprays or gargles but strong antiseptic applications should not be used. Ice-bags to the neck are acceptable to some patients, annoying to others.

Treatment of Complications.—The urgency of antitoxin treatment in *laryngeal diphtheria* has been emphasized. A croup tent and oxygen inhalations are helpful. Mechanical suction, especially when performed by direct laryngoscopy, may dislodge the membrane. Intubation may be necessary but tracheotomy should seldom have to be performed. Tracheo-bronchial membrane has been successfully removed in some instances by bronchoscopy and aspiration. In *cardiac failure* complete and total rest and the administration of morphine should be tried, digitalis being contraindicated according to many authorities. In *respiratory paralysis* the use of a mechanical respiration chamber may be life-saving. Peripheral paralyses recover eventually and antitoxin administration has little, if any, effect in them; strychnine is said to be helpful.

Serum Reactions.—In case of sudden shock following antitoxin, adrenalin and atropin injections should be given. Serum sickness appearing in from five to eight days after the antitoxin injection is characterized by an erythematous or urticarial eruption, fever, articular pains and perhaps asthmatic symptoms. Adrenalin injections should be given in this condition. Bicarbonate of soda applications, baths and antipruritic ointments may be helpful in caring for the eruption.

If a patient is known to be sensitive to horse serum or is asthmatic or, to follow the custom of some clinicians, in all patients who are to receive antitoxin, a preliminary skin test for sensitivity to horse serum may be performed. Even if this be negative, precaution should be observed in a known case of horse serum or horse dander sensitivity. When antitoxin must be employed under these conditions a subcutaneous injection of 0.1 cc. or less is given; in one-half to one hour this dose is doubled and so on until a total of 1 cc. can be given at a time without reaction—upon which it is usually safe to inject the remainder of the required amount in one or two doses. Intravenous injection must here be avoided and the most concentrated serum obtainable used.

REFERENCES.

KLEBS, E.: Ueber Diphtherie, Verhandl. d. Kong. f. inn. Med., 1883, **2**, 139.
LOEFFLER, F.: Untersuchungen über die Bedeutung der Mikroorganismen für die Entstehung der Diphtherie beim Menschen, bei der Taube und beim Kalbe, Verhandl. d. Kong. f. inn. Med., 1884, **3**, 156.
RAMON, G.: L'anatoxine diphtherique. Ses propriétés. Ses applications, Ann. de l'Inst. Pasteur, 1928, **42**, 959.
SCHICK, B.: Kutanreaktion bei Impfung mit Diphtherietoxin, Münch. med. Wchnschr., 1908, **55**, 504.
———— Die Diphtherietoxin-Hautreaktion des Menschen als Vorprobe der prophylaktischen Diphtherieheilseruminjektion, Münch. med. Wchnschr., 1913, **60**, 2608.
VON BEHRING, E.: Ueber ein neues Diphtherieschutzmittel, Deutsch. med. Wchnschr, 1913, **39**, 873.

SCARLET FEVER (SCARLATINA).

Definition.—Scarlet fever is an acute contagious, febrile, eruptive disease which is probably caused by a specific strain of streptococcus. The rash is generalized and punctiform in nature and is followed by characteristic desquamation.

History.—The disease seems to be an ancient one but it was probably not clearly described and separated from other eruptive fevers until about the middle of the seventeenth century, although according to some historians a convincing description of it was given in the sixteenth century. At the present time it is widespread and appears in all civilized parts of the world.

Etiology.—For many years it has been known that the streptococcus was associated with scarlet fever, some authors considering it a cause of complications rather than the specific etiologic agent of the disease. Numerous studies supporting the view that a specific strain of hemolytic streptococcus causes scarlet fever have been reported, among the most recent as well as important of which are those of Dick and Dick and Dochez, Avery and Sherman. The evidence consists chiefly of: (a) the recovery of the microörganisms from the throats, lym-

phatic glands, blood and other tissues of patients; (*b*) the classification
of these into a specific biologic strain; (*c*) the production of the disease
experimentally in human beings; (*d*) the development of a specific
skin test for immunity; (*e*) the preparation of an immune serum by
injection into horses. The view is held by some investigators that
while the sore throat and the local symptoms connected with it may
be caused by streptococcic infection, the rash is in the nature of an
anaphylactic reaction.

Scarlet fever often appears in *epidemics* which usually, although
not consistently, have their height in the winter or fall. No predisposing cause seems to have any great influence with the exception of
age. Few cases are seen in the first year of life and the greatest incidence is between five and twelve years of age. Nursing infants usually
escape the disease when the mother contracts it. Race is somewhat
of a factor, negroes apparently being less susceptible than white-
skinned races, although this may be because the disease is unrecognized.
A high individual *susceptibility* is not a feature of scarlet fever and it is
much easier to control its spread than in the case of measles. Only
about 10 per cent of those exposed contract the disease unless the contact is close and continuous. The immunity of persons who have never
had frank scarlet fever may be due to the fact that they have developed
antitoxin by repeated submorbid doses of streptococci—that is to say,
they have not actually developed clinically recognizable symptoms.
That this is not the entire explanation is shown by the fact that
certain persons, who have apparently never been exposed or subject
to the disease, have scarlet fever antitoxin in their blood and also have
negative Dick tests, thus indicating natural hereditary immunity.

Transmission is usually by direct contact but may exceptionally be
by fomites. Epidemics have resulted from infected milk supplies.
It is a demonstrated fact that a specific scarlet fever sore throat may
occur without recognizable skin manifestations of the disease and it is
apparently true that the scarlet fever streptococcus may be carried
for many weeks in the throats of well persons. In this sense there are
carriers and it must be emphasized, too, that the convalescent frequently spreads the disease through the medium of persistent infectious discharges from the ears, nose or a complicating lesion such as
empyema. That the desquamating epidermal scales of a scarlet fever
patient are contagious agents is decidedly doubtful.

Pathology.—In the necropsy of a case of scarlet fever little that is
characteristic is found. The skin and mucous membranes involved in
the eruption are the seat of vascular congestion and cell infiltration,
both of which processes are exaggerated in those cases with severe rash,
and the changes differ according to the stage of the disease at which
the examination is made. There is a generalized hyperplasia of the
lymphatic system, including the spleen. Any other changes are those
consequent upon existing complications.

Symptoms.—The *incubation period* is usually two to four days,
although it may be as short as twenty-four hours and rarely longer
than a week.

The *onset* is sudden, occasionally with a chill and in young children not uncommonly with convulsions. Vomiting, which is almost a constant initial symptom in children, may be replaced by nausea in older persons. Soreness of the throat is complained of by patients old enough to describe it and the general symptoms of infection, such as rapid pulse, headache and rise in temperature, are present, the last being as high as 102° to 104° F. If the throat and mouth are examined at this time it is found that there is a rash on the tonsillar pillars and on the hard and soft palates and perhaps also on the buccal mucous membrane. This enanthem consists of small, bright-red, pin-point macules which later coalesce to give a more uniform scarlet-red appearance.

In the typical case the *rash* develops in about twenty-four hours after the prodromal symptoms, invading first the neck and upper part of the body and thence spreading rapidly downward over the remainder of the body and the extremities. Usually the face is little involved, but it is flushed, with the exception of the area surrounding the mouth, this giving the appearance of the so-called circumoral pallor. Although viewed at a distance the exanthem may appear to be a uniform scarlet-red erythema, closer observation shows it to be in reality very finely punctate. Within twenty-four hours it has reached its greatest extent and by two or three days its greatest intensity of color. Fading begins soon thereafter and the normal color of the skin, except perhaps for a yellowish tinge, is attained in a week. *Desquamation* takes place in practically every case of scarlet fever—in fact, its absence casts grave doubt upon the diagnosis. It is somewhat obscured by oiling or anointing the body, as is so frequently done. It begins at about ten days to two weeks from the onset, occasionally in one week. On the trunk and neck and proximal parts of the extremities there is branny scaling but the hands and feet usually exhibit extensive peeling with large areas of the epidermis, sometimes in the form of casts, being shed. Desquamation ceases on the average after five or six weeks, lasting longest on the hands and feet. The teeth, nails and hair are sometimes affected.

The *sore throat* continues throughout the first three or four days of the disease and longer in severe cases with tonsillar exudate. The *cervical lymph nodes* become swollen and tender and there is *generalized adenopathy* as well. The *temperature*, which reaches its height about the second to the third day, falls by lysis in the average case by the end of the first week; the *pulse* is characteristically more rapid than expected from the degree of fever. Among the most diagnostic symptoms is the appearance of the tongue. At the onset it is covered with a whitish coating but by the third day or shortly thereafter this is lost and the denuded bright red "strawberry" tongue with its swollen fungiform papillæ is present. By the end of the first week the tongue has often regained a sufficiently normal appearance to be no longer diagnostic. The *urine* at the onset may contain a few casts and a trace of albumin. There is almost always a *leukocytosis* in the febrile stage with a relative and actual increase in the polymorphonuclear cells, the latter being more characteristic than the former. During early convalescence the eosinophilic leukocytes are increased in number. It was formerly taught that the Wassermann reaction may become positive in scarlet fever; recent studies seem to show, however, that this is only the case with cholesterolized antigen and that it is transitory—a strongly positive reaction indicating that the patient has syphilis.

Atypical Forms.—Scarlet fever may be very *mild* in all its manifestations. It may occur with little or no fever, the sore throat may be minor in character and the rash very evanescent or, indeed, apparently absent. Other symptoms and signs, such as the appearance of the tongue or the polymorphonuclear leukocytosis, may fail to be diagnostic. On the other hand, in *severe* cases all symptoms are exaggerated and the patient is extremely ill, the rash profuse and the angina intense. In certain cases, the disease is so malignant that death takes place in a few days. In the *hemorrhagic* forms there is bleeding from skin, mucous membranes and from the genito-urinary and intestinal tracts.

Complications.—The frequency of complications varies with epidemics. Among the most common, as might be expected, is *otitis media* which may eventuate in mastoiditis. The infection of the throat and the associated *tonsillitis* may lead to purulent or even pseudomembranous laryngitis and to pharyngitis. Other respiratory complications such as bronchitis, pneumonia and empyema are not common. The *cervical adenitis* which is practically a constant accompaniment of the disease may proceed to suppuration. The initial adenitis may subside and return in the second or third week when, although the local condition appears mild, the fever and general reaction may be severe. *Arthritis* and synovitis are occasional complications, usually occurring in the first or second week. The involvement is multiple, often affecting the smaller joints and usually lasting only a few days. *Nephritis* of an acute hemorrhagic nature is one of the most common sequels. It follows mild as well as severe cases and seldom occurs before the third or fourth week. While it may be severe and rapidly lead to uremia, this is rarely the case, and after several weeks the symptoms usually disappear and the urine shows nothing abnormal, the kidneys recovering without residual damage. In a patient without previous kidney abnormality it is rare for the nephritis to become chronic. *Circulatory* complications such as endocarditis, pericarditis or phlebitis are very seldom encountered. There are no other characteristic complications although secondary infections of various organs such as the skin, meninges and the like may take place. Associated with scarlet fever may be other contagious diseases, such as measles or pertussis, due to contact and exposure rather than because of any lowering of specific immunity.

Relapse and Recurrence.—There is no doubt that, while rare, both relapse and recurrence may occur in scarlet fever.

Diagnosis.—While the diagnosis is simple in typical cases, the mild types present great difficulties. Clinicians of wide experience may then be puzzled and the wiser ones will err on the side of positive diagnosis rather than run the risk of spreading the disease by failing to pronounce a doubtful but possible case as scarlet fever. Streptococcic sore throat with toxic rash is a diagnosis which may well be dispensed with. When it is realized that the rash in scarlet fever may be scanty, atypical or even absent, that the throat and tongue may not be characteristic, that cases may be seen late in the course, the difficulties can be visualized. In very dark-skinned races the erythema may be obscured although the enlarged papillæ are present. Not infrequently cases are recognized only when desquamation or some such complication as nephritis has developed, the diagnosis having previously been missed.

The *Dick test*, which should be positive in the first few days of the disease, may become negative about the seventh day, but to this there are so many exceptions that it is not reliable. The *Schultz-Charlton* extinction phenomenon is an acceptable diagnostic aid, although even it cannot be stated as an absolute test. About 1 cc. of scarlet fever convalescent serum or 0.1 cc. of active scarlet fever antitoxin is injected intradermally and the eruption, if due to scarlet fever, is blanched in a few hours over an area of several centimeters and remains so. The so-called *Pastia's* sign is an intensification of the eruption in folds and creases of the skin such as at the elbow. The *Rumpel-Leeds* phenomenon consists of the occurrence of punctate hemorrhage in the elbow region after compression has been made on the upper arm for about fifteen minutes. It is not diagnostic. The discovery of undifferentiated streptococci in throat cultures means nothing, inasmuch as they are so frequently normal inhabitants.

The differential diagnosis from measles, rubella and diphtheria may be detailed by Table 8 which is subject to the usual criticism of dogmatism.

In this connection may well be mentioned *surgical scarlet fever*. Experience teaches that it is better to regard it in all matters relating to isolation and treatment as identical with true scarlet fever. The rash may be similar in distribution to the ordinary form of the disease or develop first in the region of a wound and spread from there. In this same category may be placed those cases which develop after tonsillectomy, extraction of abscessed teeth and other operations on the nose and throat and mouth in which there is presumably release or activation of the specific streptococcus which was present in the field of operation.

Certain drugs such as belladonna, the salicylates, quinine and some of the coal tars may produce a scarlatiniform rash. There is, however, no sore throat nor are other symptoms of scarlet fever present.

Prognosis.—The severity and mortality vary greatly with epidemics and locality. In some countries of Europe scarlet fever is a relatively virulent disease but in most sections of the United States at the present time it is a mild one, so that the mortality may be as low as 2 or 3 per cent or even less. Its severity seems to vary, too, in the individual epidemic and the more ill patients are usually seen at the height of the epidemic. Death may occur rarely because of the extreme toxemia, but usually from septicemia, or as a result of some of the complications.

Treatment.—In *prophylaxis* isolation and quarantine of the scarlet fever patient should be carried out. The usual legal requirement for

TABLE 8.

	Scarlet fever.	Diphtheria.	Measles.	Rubella.	Remarks.
Onset	Sudden, mild or no catarrhal symptoms, vomiting almost an invariable symptom	No catarrhal symptoms, may be nasal discharge with nasal diphtheria	Slow, with marked catarrhal symptoms; photophobia	Practically no prodromal symptoms	Posterior cervical lymphatics especially enlarged in rubella.
Fever	High, sudden rise at onset, falls by lysis	Low grade	High, characteristically falls before eruption and rises again with it	Mild.	
Eruption	Brght-red, punctate, face not involved, later marked desquamation	Infrequent, scarlatiniform, but more erythematous than punctate, usually on body only	Brownish-red, macular, crescentic distribution, face always involved, later branny desquamation	Pale-red, macular, discrete, face involved, may be scarlatiniform, may be slight desquamation	Schultz - Charlton extinction test positive only in scarlet fever.
Mouth and throat	Punctate enanthem, strawberry tongue, tonsillar exudate usually follicular	Membrane grayish, adherent, involves extratonsillar structures	Macular enanthem, Koplik spots	No sore throat, no Koplik spots, may be mild enanthem	Diphtheria may complicate other contagious diseases.
Blood	Polymorphonuclear leukocytosis, usually marked	Moderate polymorphonuclear leukocytosis	Leukopenia, diminution of mononuclear cells	Leukopenia, relative increase of mononuclear cells.	
Bacteriology	Hemolytic streptococcus	Klebs-Loeffler bacillus.			
Tests	Dick test positive early. Schultz-Charlton test positive	Schick test positive.			

the latter is six weeks. Longer is necessary if any purulent discharge from the ears or elsewhere is present. If hemolytic streptococci are found in these discharges in large numbers their contagious nature is more certain although it must be remembered that such microörganisms are frequently present in normal throats, and may also be found in the pus from otitis media, from an empyema and the like when these diseases are of a non-scarlatinal nature. On the other hand, the absence of streptococci from the discharges is only presumptive evidence that they are non-contagious. While it is doubtful that the desquamating scales convey the infectious agent, patients who are still shedding their epidermis are for some reason apt to be contagious. The possibility of the existence of apparently healthy carriers has previously been mentioned. In certain epidemics the milk supply may need study.

Passive protection, lasting two or three weeks, may often be secured by the injection of 10 cc. of convalescent serum (some clinicians employ as much as 30 cc.), 20 cc. or more of convalescent whole blood or 5 cc. of scarlet fever antitoxin. These procedures are helpful in epidemics, particularly in institutions.

Active immunization, with protection lasting at least for two or three years and possibly permanently, is brought about by injections of scarlet fever toxin as recommended by the Dicks and others. Only about 5 to 10 per cent of those once injected need reinjection as determined by the Dick test. Immunity is not developed for ten days and perhaps not for a month, and active immunization is, therefore, of no great value in combating epidemics. Subcutaneous injections are made every week, from three to four being given in all, and they may begin with as low as 500 skin-test-doses and increase up to as high as 80,000 or 100,000 by the last one. It is often customary to perform a Dick test about ten days after the third injection and to give the last two only if the reaction be positive. The Dick test may be performed before the first injection to determine the presence or absence of immunity, but in the administration of prophylactic inoculations to large groups of children this plan may well be dispensed with. General reactions not infrequently occur, particularly in older persons, and attempts have been made to detoxify the product, especially by formaldehyde.

To determine whether a person is immune the *Dick test* is performed. A negative test indicating that the injected toxin has been neutralized by the patient's antitoxin, while not an absolute guarantee of immunity, is usually so except in the presence of exposure which is overwhelming in quantity or virulence. The test is carried out as follows: 0.1 cc. of a 1 to 1000 dilution of toxin is injected intradermally. The Dicks caution that the syringes used must be boiled in distilled water and not in alkaline tap water or sterilized with alcohol. The reaction should be read in eighteen to twenty-four hours and the slightest flush or reddening, no matter how faint the color, should be considered positive if it measures as much as 10 mm. in any diameter. It is also probable that variation in the intensity of the local reaction indicates degrees of immunity—that is to say, a markedly positive reaction would signify lesser resistance than a slight one.

The *general treatment* consists of attention to and relief of symptoms and complications. In addition to this, every patient should remain in bed for at least three weeks. The diet should be liquid with plenty of fluid and later a soft diet may be allowed as the fever declines. Daily baths may be given and later, when desquamation begins, the skin oiled or a mild ointment applied. Exposure to cold should be avoided. Local topical applications, such as one of the silver preparations, may be made to the throat if not too disturbing to the patient, and gargles and sprays may be employed. Irrigations of the throat are only necessary when severe angina is present and should then be given by non-susceptible attendants because of the danger of contagion. It is wise, in any case, to employ only nurses who have negative Dick tests and to secure this, active immunization should be carried out if necessary on all attendants in scarlet fever wards. There are no specific preventive measures for nephritis, which, as stated, may develop in mild cases as well as in severe ones. No acceptable clinical evidence exists that restriction of protein in the first three weeks of scarlet fever decreases the incidence of nephritis; it is, however, a widespread custom to eliminate meats and even eggs from the diet during that period.

The toxic symptoms may be relieved by intramuscular injections of *convalescent's serum*[1] or whole blood—10 to 60 cc. of the former and twice that of the latter. *Scarlet fever antitoxin* obtained by the injection of horses with the specific streptococci or toxin or both is widely employed intramuscularly or intravenously in treatment. Much controversy exists as to its exact place and value. An active antitoxic serum undoubtedly relieves toxic symptoms if given in the first two or three days of the disease, but it may be stated that many clinicians believe that it has little effect on prevention of septic complications nor is it useful in their treatment. In the analysis of the figures obtained from a controlled study at the Cincinnati General Hospital it seemed quite evident that serum-treated patients had a low incidence of complications when compared to patients who had no serum treatment. The usual commercial preparation is given in doses of 10 to 20 cc. Serum reactions are quite frequent and it is the custom of many clinicians who employ antitoxin in treatment to do so only in the severe cases. In the study previously mentioned serum reactions were twice as frequent in those patients who had had previous injections of horse serum in some form. It is obvious that due precautions should be observed to determine the patient's sensitivity to horse serum. (See Diphtheria, page 309.)

REFERENCES.

DEGKWITZ, R.: Zum Scharlachproblem, Münch. med. Wchnschr., 1922, **69**, 955, DICK, G. F., and DICK, G. H.: Experimental Scarlet Fever, Jour. Am. Med. Assn. 1923, **81**, 1166.

---

[1] Blood is obtained from non-syphilitic patients, preferably between the second and fourth week of scarlet fever, but it is active for longer than that time, and the blood of those who have had the disease years before may be employed in larger doses. The serum may be effective for several months after withdrawal if it is sterile. Three-tenths per cent tricresol or other preservative is added and it is kept at low temperature in the ice-box. Pooled blood is obviously more likely to be uniformly active.

Dick, G. F., and Dick, G. H.:   A Skin Test for Susceptibility to Scarlet Fever,
    Jour. Am. Med. Assn.,1924, **82**, 265.
———— The Etiology of Scarlet Fever, Jour. Am. Med. Assn., 1924, **82**, 301.
———— A Scarlet Fever Antitoxin, Jour. Am. Med. Assn., 1924, **82**, 1246.
———— The Prevention of Scarlet Fever, Jour. Am. Med. Assn., 1924, **83**, 84.
Dick, G. H.:   Résumé of the Literature on Scarlet Fever; the Hemolytic Strepto-
    coccus as the Cause of Scarlet Fever, Am. Jour. Dis. Child., 1924, **28**, 484.
Dochez, A. R., and Sherman, L.:   The Significance of Streptococcus Hemolyticus
    in Scarlet Fever, and the Preparation of a Specific Antiscarlatinal Serum by
    Immunization of the Horse to Streptococcus Hemolyticus-Scarlatinæ, Jour.
    Am. Med. Assn., 1924, **82**, 542.
Schultz, W., and Charlton, W.:   Serologische Beobachtungen am Scharlach-
    exanthem, Ztschr. f. Kinderh., 1918, **17**, 328.
Stevenson, F. E., Veldee, M. V., and Mitchell, A. G.:   Scarlet Fever Strepto-
    coccus Antitoxin in the Treatment of Scarlet Fever, Pub. Health. Rep., 1931,
    46, 3023.

PERTUSSIS (WHOOPING COUGH).

Definition.—Pertussis is an acute, contagious disease involving primarily the respiratory tract and characterized by severe, spasmodic cough.

Etiology.—The disease is one of some antiquity, being first described at least four hundred years ago. The usually accepted bacteriologic cause is a small Gram-negative bacillus described by Bordet and Gengou. It is found especially during the early stage of the disease in the sputum. Exactly why the microörganism should produce the peculiar type of cough is not clear.

Sex is supposed to have some influence and more females are affected than males; this may only be due to a greater opportunity for exposure. The greater number of cases occur in early childhood. Adults, however, unless protected by previous attacks not infrequently contract the disease and there is no immunity in the early months of life. It has even been reported that pertussis may be congenital—a fact that is hard to explain upon the basis of the commonly accepted bacteriologic cause.

Epidemics occur and these are usually more frequent in the winter. There is high *individual susceptibility* and most non-immune children will contract the disease upon relatively slight exposure. *Transmission* is by means of discharges from the respiratory tract and it should be remembered that the explosive cough may cause droplet infection at a distance of 6 feet or more.

Pathology.—While during life there is congestion of the upper respiratory tract, particularly the larynx and trachea, little may be found at necropsy. Among the secondary pathologic changes are those of bronchitis or pneumonia or dilatation of the bronchial tubes, hemorrhages in the brain or other organs, and cardiac dilatation. In so-called pertussis encephalitis there may be degeneration of the brain with loss of nerve cells.

Symptoms.—The *incubation period* is about seven to fourteen days, but sometimes apparently is shorter. The *initial stage* consists of catarrhal symptoms with cough and some nasal discharge and perhaps mild symptoms of infection, including low-grade fever. The cough at first is paroxysmal but usually does not become characteristically so for one to two weeks. The so-called *paroxysmal stage* then begins. A typical paroxysm is difficult to describe. It begins with explosive expiratory coughs which are so rapidly repeated that there is little time between them for inspiration. Redness of the face and cyanosis develop, tenacious mucus hangs from the mouth and finally there is a long, crowing inspiration which constitutes the characteristic whoop. These attacks may occur several times a day or with extreme frequency. Vomiting often occurs at the end of the paroxysm. The attacks continue during the night, greatly disturbing the patient's rest. The severe paroxysmal stage usually lasts about two weeks and then the severity and frequency of the paroxysms decrease during the following two or three weeks—the whole course of the disease lasting six weeks or more.

A most interesting *blood* change begins early in the course and sometimes before any recognizable symptoms. This consists of a leukocytosis with a very great relative increase in the lymphocytes. By the time of the paroxysmal stage the total count is often 20,000 or 30,000, and sometimes much more than this, and the lymphocyte percentage is as great as 75 or 80 or more.

Atypical Forms.—Pertussis may be very mild or extremely severe and great differences in severity may occur at the same time in the same epidemic and even in members of the same family.

Complications.—Bronchitis is almost a part of the disease rather than a complication. Bronchopneumonia is naturally a common and serious accompaniment. The severity of the cough may lead to hemorrhages in various parts of the body such as into the eye, from the nose, into the gastro-intestinal tract, and into the brain. In addition to this effect on central nervous tissues a degenerative change sometimes takes place which is in the nature of an encephalitis and may cause convulsions, hemiplegia and other paralyses and, as sequels, blindness, deafness and mental deterioration. The heart may be affected and dilatation occur. Pulmonary tuberculosis may be activated.

Relapse and Recurrence.—Relapse is not common but it is rather characteristic that even as late as five or six months after the attack of pertussis is over some other type of respiratory tract infection may cause a return of a paroxysmal cough and whooping. True recurrence of pertussis in a contagious form is very rare.

Diagnosis.—It is characteristic of pertussis that there is a cough, gradually increasing in severity but with little or no fever and only minor evidences of respiratory tract infection. If, with these symptoms, there is a lymphocytosis, the diagnosis becomes quite clear. The changes in leukocytes mentioned may not be characteristic. The paroxysmal nature of the coughing attacks usually becomes evident early in the course. By having the patient cough on a Petri dish held about 4 inches from the mouth, and containing special media, there may be obtained in a high percentage of cases a positive culture of pertussis bacillus early in the course of the disease.

Prognosis.—Pertussis is a serious disease and, because of its complications, may have a relatively high mortality. This is especially the case in young infants, and in those under one year of age the death-rate may reach 25 per cent; after six years of age it is much lower and in older children it is seldom over 4 or 5 per cent. Adults, unless of an advanced age, have a very low mortality. Stated another way, over three-fourths of the deaths from this disease occur in patients under two years of age.

Treatment.—Prophylaxis.—Quarantine should be for about six weeks, although, practically, the contagiousness is almost entirely confined to the first three weeks after the onset. Patients with pertussis are contagious often before the diagnosis is made. The consensus of opinion concerning the value of vaccination with the Bordet-Gengou bacillus is that it is of no great value in prevention, although recently Sauer has had success with it, using a vaccine which causes the development of immunity only after three months. It has been claimed that 3 to 5 cc. of convalescent serum from a pertussis patient has prophylactic effect. This again seems to have little value.

General Treatment.—Unless the patient is suffering from a severe bronchitis or pneumonia, or has a definite degree of fever, he may be allowed to be up and around and in the fresh air, but he should not be exposed to air that is too cold. Every attempt should be made to keep the patient in good nutritional state and it is often found that when vomiting occurs shortly after a meal the patient is able and willing immediately to eat again and that he may then retain the food.

Many local applications to the throat have been recommended but seem to have no great effect. An abdominal binder is helpful in protection against hernia and gives the patient comfort during the severe cough.

Sedative treatments by means of medication may be indicated, but it should always be remembered that no form of treatment cures pertussis. The most that can be expected is a relief in severity and number of paroxysms of coughing and shortening of the course. A popular antispasmodic drug is belladonna or atropine. A young child may be started with 2 or 3 minims of tincture of belladonna, three times a day, and this increased by 1 minim a day up to 8 or 10 minims or more, three times a day, depending upon the appearance of such symptoms as flushing of the skin, dilatation of the pupils or rise in temperature. Among sedatives may be mentioned phenobarbital or some of its modifications, and also antipyrin, of which a young child may take about 2 grains, three times a day. It is not possible to mention all of the antispasmodic and sedative drugs which have been employed in pertussis. The mere fact of their number demonstrates that none of them has marked effect.

Subcutaneous and intramuscular injections of ether seem to have some effect in controlling paroxysms. These cause much local pain and not infrequently a slough. Ether in oil is also said to be beneficial when given in doses of about 10 cc. by rectum about every eight hours. Roentgen-ray treatment of the chest has been advocated but the general opinion is that it has little, if any, value.

Vaccine treatment, employing the Bordet-Gengou bacillus, is another form of treatment which is certainly not curative. There is some evidence that freshly prepared vaccines given in relatively large doses have a beneficial effect and their use is not to be discouraged. It may be that vaccines given in the incubation period have a tendency to render the subsequent course milder. Some clinicians employ mixed vaccines which contain, in addition to the pertussis bacillus, pneumococci, staphylococci, streptococci, Micrococcus catarrhalis and other micro-organisms.

Convalescent serum has also been used in treatment.

REFERENCES.

BORDET, J., and GENGOU, O.: Le microbe de la coqueluche, Ann. de l'Inst. Pasteur, 1906, **20**, 731.
SAUER, L. W.: Whooping Cough: Résumé of a Seven Years' Study, Jour. Pediat., 1933, **2**, 740.

MEASLES.

Synonyms.—Morbilli; Rubeola; Masern.

Definition.—Measles is an acute, contagious, febrile disease in which there is a characteristic enanthem and a macular exanthem and catarrhal symptoms.

History.—In the seventeenth century measles was recognized by Sydenham as a disease distinct from smallpox, but its separation as distinct from scarlet fever came later.

Etiology.—Of the several predisposing factors age is the most important. Few cases are seen in the first six months of life because all infants whose mothers have had the disease seem to have a temporary immunity. In instances in which the mother has contracted measles within one or two weeks before delivery the infant may be born with the eruption and other symptoms, or, if exposure of the mother is shortly before labor, the mother and infant may develop measles simultaneously. Throughout childhood the incidence is high, but adults may contract measles quite readily on exposure unless they have been protected by a previous attack. In *epidemics* the influence of season is shown by a greater incidence in winter, especially late winter or early spring. There is a very strong *individual susceptibility* and many unprotected persons of all ages will contract the disease even from short exposure; it is, in fact, the most contagious of all the exanthemata. A peculiar inexplicable temporary resistance to the infection is occasionally encountered in those who may contract the disease on subsequent exposure.

There can be no doubt that measles is an infectious disease but it cannot be stated positively that its cause has been discovered. The more interesting of the studies on etiology are those relating to a form of diplococcus described by Tunnicliff and a streptococcus described by Ferry and Fisher, and those relating to a filterable virus. The microörganisms mentioned are green-producing ones, and it is said by some workers that their toxins produce a positive skin test when injected intracutaneously into susceptible persons; that this toxin is neutralized by measles convalescent serum; that the microörganisms are agglutinated by measles convalescent serum; that an antitoxin produced by their injection into horses and goats has some protective

value. Much the same studies have been carried out on both the
diplococcus and the streptococcus. The former is described as Gram-
positive, anaërobic and filter-passing, and the latter as aërobic. The
transmission of measles by a filterable virus has not been accepted by
all investigators, some of whom are unable to secure the experimental
results to be quoted. Goldberger and Anderson, Blake and Trask,
and others have apparently produced a disease similar to measles in
monkeys and other animals by intravenous and intratracheal inoculation with both filtered and unfiltered material from the nasal secretions.
Inoculation of animals with blood from patients with active measles
has also given positive results. Degkwitz claims to have successfully
carried out human inoculation experiments with a filter-passing virus
which could be cultivated.

Whatever the infective agent, it is easily destroyed and does not
persist in secretions for much more than two weeks, if that long. That
is to say, there are no long-time *carriers* and, for example, discharges
from ears, nose and the like are not potential sources of contagion as in
the case of scarlet fever. During the incubation period and the acute
course of the disease, however, transmission occurs with great facility
and, although this is often denied, some instances can only be explained
by carrying of the disease by a third person or fomites, or by air-borne
passage.

Pathology.—With the exception of pathologic conditions dependent
upon complications there is only the slight change which occurs in
skin and mucous membrane, consisting of round-cell infiltration and
dilatation of vessels.

Symptoms.—The *incubation period* is about fourteen days until the
appearance of the rash. The *onset* is generally slow with fever and the
usual symptoms of infection and the catarrhal symptoms of coryza,
conjunctivitis, and often cough. In two to three days the enanthem
appears in practically all cases and consists of numerous, tiny, red
macules which are first seen particularly on the hard and soft palate
and are followed by the *Koplik spots* which typically are very small,
slightly white spots surrounded by a red areola situated on the mucous
membrane of the cheeks and lips.

The *rash* is usually present by the third or fourth day after the
onset of catarrhal symptoms, appearing first on the face and by
twenty-four to forty-eight hours spreading downward and entirely
involving the trunk and extremities. It is sometimes preceded by a
prodromal eruption which is generally of an erythematous nature
and which fades before the true measles eruption comes out. At first
the measles eruption consists of discrete, pin-point-sized, pale-red
macules which later become larger, redder, papular and more numerous.
Many of the spots become confluent and the resulting grouping is
arranged in the form of a rough crescent separated from similar masses
by relatively normal skin. The height of the rash in extent and color
is reached in two or three days after its onset, when fading begins and
the skin returns to normal in another two or four days except for a
mottled, brownish-yellow appearance. A fine, branny desquamation
begins in a few days after the fading of the rash, starting first on the

face and in degree usually varying with the intensity of the rash. Itching of the skin may be present at this time and often also at the height of the eruption.

The *catarrhal symptoms* which are so characteristic persist from the onset and increase in severity as the rash becomes more profuse. Photophobia becomes marked. The conjunctivitis and the nasal discharge give a miserable appearance which has justifiably led to the widespread employment of the adjective "measly" to connote any type of disagreeable situation. Laryngitis and bronchitis are almost constant accompaniments of this stage, but all catarrhal symptoms subside as the fever and eruption disappear. The cervical lymph nodes and other superficial lymphatic nodes are enlarged and the spleen is enlarged and palpable in about one-half of the cases. The *temperature* curve is often, but not invariably, characteristic, and if a record has been kept at frequent intervals from the onset it will be found to be quite different from that of other eruptive fevers. At the beginning of catarrhal symptoms the temperature rises sharply to about 103° F. but on the second or third day falls to normal or nearly so, rising again to its former level or even higher when the eruption develops and then falling by lysis as the eruption disappears. Even before the catarrhal symptoms and the skin manifestations develop, a definite *leukopenia* will be found and during the eruptive stage this becomes more marked and is accompanied by a relative increase in the lymphocytes.

Atypical Forms.—Considerable variation may exist in the symptoms and signs of measles. The temperature may not be characteristic; the rash may be scanty and poorly developed; the enanthem may not be discoverable; and it is claimed that infection with the measles virus may take place and yet eruption and catarrhal symptoms be absent. In *severe forms* all symptoms are exaggerated and in some cases the rash becomes hemorrhagic in nature. According to the laity the rash may "strike in," this being a dangerous symptom. In reality this is due to the poor condition of the patient, and especially to circulatory weakness with consequent paleness of the rash.

Complications.—Among the most frequent of the complications are respiratory disorders of both upper and lower tracts, such as exaggeration of the rhinitis, bronchitis and conjunctivitis (which in milder forms are part of the symptomatology of the disease), otitis media and bronchopneumonia. Stomatitis is not uncommon, and a fortunately rare complication is marked infection of the cheek proceeding to necrosis and gangrene (cancrum oris). The circulatory system is seldom affected although endocarditis and thrombosis of blood-vessels may rarely occur. Nephritis is very rare. Osteomyelitis and arthritis are possible complications. Serous meningitis and encephalitis occasionally develop. Tuberculosis, pulmonary or otherwise, previously quiescent, may become active and it has been shown, too, that the tuberculin test may become negative during the febrile stage of measles, this being taken to indicate a lowered resistance.

Relapse and Recurrence.—Both relapse and recurrence are possible but rare.

Diagnosis.—The differential diagnosis from other eruptive fevers is tabulated on page 319. The constancy of catarrhal symptoms, the character of the rash, the peculiar enanthem and the leukopenia make the average case a simple diagnostic problem. The relatively few cases with scanty rash may cause confusion. Smallpox in its early stage may present a rash somewhat similar to measles. Most clinicians, and I think correctly, hesitate to diagnose measles in the absence of catarrhal symptoms. The enanthem is almost always present, but the diagnosis cannot be excluded because of its absence. The leukopenia may be replaced by a leukocytosis if some other infection is complicating the picture. Certain drugs, such as quinine, antipyrin and copaiba, may cause a measles-like rash, but not the other symptoms of the disease.

Prognosis.—The case mortality of measles in an average epidemic is usually not much greater than 4 or 5 per cent. Certain epidemics are of greater severity than others and have a consequently greater mortality due largely to complications such as bronchopneumonia, or to the activation of tuberculosis as previously mentioned. Young infants have a much higher mortality than older children or adults. Statistics indicate that the severity of measles may be increasing in recent years.

Treatment.—In *prophylaxis* the extreme contagiousness of measles should be remembered. It is greatest at the height of the eruption and ceases as it fades, but also before this, during the catarrhal stage and before the eruption, contact is dangerous. Unfortunately, therefore, the disease spreads through the medium of early unrecognized cases. *Quarantine* may be removed by two weeks from the onset.

Convalescent serum prepared in the manner previously described (p. 321) and collected preferably within one to two weeks after recovery from measles is usually, but not invariably, protective. It should be injected intramuscularly in the first two or three days after exposure, about 5 cc. being employed and at least twice that much in older children, or if given later. After six days from the time of exposure it is no longer protective but may lead to a modified, mild attack with subsequent permanent immunity. This fact may be taken advantage of in strong, healthy children and the injection deliberately postponed to accomplish it. Serum or whole blood in doses of 30 to 75 cc. obtained from adults who have had measles many years previously has some protective value. McKhann and Chu have recently found that extracts of placenta have protective power against measles. It has been claimed, although this needs confirmation, that passive protection has been secured by injections of horse serum and goat serum when these animals have been inoculated with the green-producing diplococcus or streptococcus previously mentioned.

Herrman has suggested and performed *preventive inoculation* by applying the specially prepared nasal secretions from patients with measles to the nasal mucous membranes of infants of about five months of age. At this age a certain amount of natural immunity remains and a mild modified form of measles is said to result with subsequent immunity.

The *general treatment* is primarily that for any acute infection with appropriate attention to the possible complications. The photophobia requires protection to the eyes and can be secured by local means such as dark glasses. This is the only reason for darkening the room as is so often done. Fresh air is much needed in a disease with the respiratory complications of measles, although cold air may be irritating to the mucous membranes and the temperature of the sick room should be kept at about 70° F. Special attention to the mucous membranes of the nose and throat is indicated, but only mild non-irritating solutions should be used (neosilvol) and as little manipulation as possible employed. Itching of the skin is combated by bland ointments or bicarbonate of soda baths. Simple sedative cough mixtures may be employed to relieve the cough of the associated bronchitis. Convalescent serum or whole blood has been used to combat toxemia and certain complications such as encephalitis. It probably does not have marked beneficial effect and the same can be said of the injection of the horse serum and goat serum mentioned under prophylactic treatment, the specificity of which has yet to be demonstrated.

REFERENCES.

ANDERSON, J. F., and GOLDBERGER, J.: The Infectivity of the Secretions and the Desquamating Scales of Measles, Jour. Am. Med. Assn., 1911, **57**, 1612.
BLAKE, F. G., and TRASK, J. D.: Studies on Measles, Jour. Exper. Med., 1921, **33**, 385, 413, 621.
DEGKWITZ, R.: Spezifisches Masernschutzserum vom Tier, Münch. med. Wchnschr., 1926, **73**, 181, 248.
FERRY, N. S., and FISHER, L. W.: Measles Toxin; Its Preparation and Application as Skin Test, as Immunizing Agent and for the Production of Antitoxin, Jour. Am. Med. Assn., 1926, **86**, 932.
GOLDBERGER, J., and ANDERSON, J. F.: An Experimental Demonstration of the Presence of the Virus of Measles in the Mixed Buccal and Nasal Secretions, Jour. Am. Med. Assn., 1911, **57**, 476.
———— The Nature of the Virus of Measles, Jour. Am. Med. Assn., 1911, **57**, 971.
HEKTOEN, L.: Experimental Measles; a Review, Jour. Am. Med. Assn., 1919, **72**, 177.
HERRMAN, C.: Immunization against Measles, Arch. Pediat., 1922, **39**, 607.
KOPLIK, H.: The Diagnosis of the Invasion of Measles, from a Study of the Exanthem as It Appears on the Buccal Mucous Membrane, Arch. Pediat., 1896, **13**, 918.
McKHANN, C. F., and CHU, F. T.: Use of Placental Extract in Prevention and Modification of Measles, Am. Jour. Dis. Child., 1933, **45**, 475.
TUNNICLIFF, R.: Further Studies on a Diplococcus in Measles; a Measles Skin Reaction, Jour. Infect. Dis., 1925, **37**, 193.

VARICELLA.

Synonyms.—Chickenpox; Glasspock.

Definition.—Varicella is a specific, acute, contagious, eruptive fever characterized by a superficial vesicular eruption which appears in crops.

History.—There is no doubt that this disease has been recognized for many centuries, although it is only in the last hundred years that it has been clearly separated from smallpox and accepted as an entity.

Etiology.—Varicella is a childhood disease, but many infants will contract it on exposure even in the first six months of life and young non-immune adults not infrequently suffer from it. While it occurs in epidemics in large communities with a greater incidence in winter than in summer, it is usually endemic as well. *Individual susceptibility* is great, but not so much so as in certain other diseases, some few persons apparently having a natural immunity. Contagiousness exists for at least a day before the beginning of the eruption and lasts until the original crusts of the lesions have all disappeared. *Transmission* is by direct contact but also in certain instances by the means of a third person or by fomites and quite certainly it is carried by air. The *infective agent* has not yet been determined. An interesting controversy which merits brief mention is the relationship of varicella and herpes zoster. There is an extensive literature on this subject and there are many case reports of varicella developing from herpes zoster or the reverse of this. It has been both affirmed and denied that attacks of one of these protects against the other, and that convalescent serum from one protects against the other. In complement-fixation studies the identity of the conditions is also a matter of controversy. The author's experience shows that an attack of either herpes zoster or varicella does not protect against the other disease.

Pathology.—There is no characteristic pathologic anatomy with the exception of the slight changes caused by the eruption in the upper layers of the skin.

Symptoms.—The average *incubation period* is about fourteen days, but it may be shorter than this and also as long as three weeks.

The *onset*, as a rule, is abrupt with the appearance of the first skin lesions; the prodromal symptoms, such as fever, being so slight that they pass unnoticed. Occasionally a measles-like or scarlatiniform prodromal eruption occurs.

The *rash* begins as a small macule, rapidly becoming vesicular. Often this development into a vesicle is so rapid—taking only a few hours—that no papular stage is observed. Within about twenty-four hours the vesicle has reached the size of a split pea, is round or oval in shape, is slightly depressed (umbilicated) in the center, is superficially located and is surrounded by a red areola. It ruptures with slight trauma. It is characteristic that not all the macules develop into vesicles and that the eruption, beginning in the face, spreads rapidly downward over the trunk and extremities in successive crops. At the height of it macules, vesicles and pustules are all found. The individual lesions have passed to the crust stage and dropped off by six or seven days from their onset, after which secondary crusts may form on some of them. There may be only a few lesions, or these may be extremely numerous. All parts of the body surface may be attacked, especially the trunk and back and proximal parts of the extremities, including the palms and soles in non-calloused portions, and usually lesions can be seen on the mucous membranes of the mouth. Lesions cluster also around irritated parts of the skin.

The *general symptoms* are those of a mild infection with fever lasting for a few days. The *blood* shows no typical or constant changes. If leukocytosis is present, it is mild in degree. Lymphocytosis and eosinophilia have been described by some authors, but none of these changes, although occasionally present, is constant or diagnostic.

Atypical Forms.—In very mild cases there may be no general symptoms and fever is absent. The skin lesions may be very scanty, only a dozen or less of them developing to the characteristic vesicle stage. On the other hand, marked general symptoms such as vomiting and convulsions may attend the onset and course especially in the adult, and the lesions be large or extremely numerous or the site of secondary infection or gangrene or hemorrhage.

Complications.—While complications are numerically uncommon, they may occur and some of them are serious. To be mentioned are nephritis, from which recovery generally takes place; hemoglobinuria; secondary infections of the skin lesions as noted in the preceding paragraph and also complication with impetigo and erysipelas; encephalitis, polioencephalitis and meningitis which, as a rule, have a good prognosis for complete recovery. Severe laryngitis requiring intubation is another complication worthy of notation.

Relapse and Recurrence.—Relapse is very uncommon. In rare instances, recurrence can take place, although this has been denied by a number of authors.

Diagnosis.—Varicella has occasionally been confused with impetigo contagiosa. The greatest difficulty is likely to arise with smallpox. In smallpox the initial general symptoms are more severe, there is absence of the successive crops of skin lesions which in smallpox are found mostly in the same stage of development, the individual lesions are more deep-seated and do not have the superficial vesicular character so typical of varicella, the eruption is more profuse on the face and distal parts of the extremities rather than as in varicella on the trunk and proximal parts of the extremities. It must be admitted, however, that the differential diagnosis is often difficult. In a few instances the diseases have been seen in combination.

Prognosis.—The mortality is very low in varicella. If death occurs it is practically always a result of complications or association with some one of the other eruptive fevers. Almost invariably some of the lesions leave a permanent, small, white, pitted scar.

Treatment.—*Prophylaxis.*—Isolation and quarantine should be carried out until all the primary crusts have disappeared, which is about a week from the onset of the eruption. In institutions and hospitals it is very difficult to control the spread of varicella, some of the cross-infections being explicable only on the basis of carriage by a third person or by currents of air. Vaccination similar to that against smallpox has been carried out by inoculation with material from fresh varicella lesions and also by intravenous inoculation with varicellous material. The value of these methods of producing active immunity is questionable and the necessity for them seldom arises. Passive protection by convalescent serum can frequently be obtained and indications for it are encountered in the attempt to terminate institutional epidemics or in the avoidance of varicella in a child whose general condition is poor, or who is suffering from some other disease.[1]

The usual treatment for infection is obviously indicated. Rest in bed need not be carried beyond the period when the crusts of the lesions

[1] See page 321 for preparation and dosage of convalescent serum.

disappear. The itching, which is often marked as the vesicles develop, may lead to rubbing and scratching. This should be avoided insofar as possible, especially around the face, else secondary infections will exaggerate the subsequent scarring. Restraint may be necessary in young children and even in older patients, as scratching may occur during sleep. An antipruritic powder containing camphor or small amounts of phenol (the latter not too freely applied) may be helpful and perhaps is better than ointments, such as carbolated vaseline, which tend to macerate the lesions. Painting the individual lesions with tincture of iodine diluted one-half with alcohol is the best treatment of the eruption if it is not too extensive. Daily baths are permitted, bicarbonate of soda often being added to them.

Intraspinal and intravenous injections of convalescent serum may be tried in the treatment of a complicating polioencephalitis.

REFERENCES.

HESS, A. F., and UNGER, L. J.: A Protective Therapy for Varicella, and a Consideration of Its Pathogenesis, Am. Jour. Dis. Child., 1918, 16, 34.
KLING, C. A.: Technik der Schutzimpfung gegen Varicellen, Berl. klin. Wchnschr., 1915, 52, 13.
MITCHELL, A. G., and FLETCHER, E. G.: Studies on Varicella; Age and Seasonal Incidence, Recurrences, Complications and Leukocyte Counts, Jour. Am. Med. Assn., 1927, 89, 279.
MITCHELL, A. G., and RAVENEL, S. F.: The Value of Convalescents' Serum in Protection Against Varicella, Arch. Pediat., 1925, 42, 709.
RIVERS, T. M.: Viruses, Jour. Am. Med. Assn., 1929, 92, 1147.

MUMPS.

Synonyms.—Epidemic parotitis; Parotiditis.

Definition and History.—Mumps is a specific, acute, contagious disease characterized by inflammation of the parotid and other salivary glands. It is evidently an ancient disease which has been recognized as an entity for over one hundred and fifty years.

Etiology.—Mumps is primarily a disease of childhood, although it may occur in young infants and also in adults who have not been protected by a previous attack. Epidemics of it in young adults occur when they are congregated in schools or army camps. It is an impression that sex has an influence and that there is a predominance in males, but statistics do not bear this out. It occurs in *epidemics*, particularly in early and late winter. The *individual susceptibility* is not so great as in several of the other contagious diseases and *transmission* is usually by close contact with a sufferer from the disease.

While many different microörganisms have been described in association with mumps and studies have been carried out with a filterable virus, the infective agent has not yet been fully determined.

Pathology.—There has been little study of the pathologic anatomy of mumps but the changes in the salivary glands are known to be chiefly in the nature of an acute interstitial inflammation and those in a complicating orchitis both of a parenchymatous and interstitial nature.

Symptoms.—The *incubation period* is usually about two to three weeks but may be shorter or longer and in some epidemics may be a week or less. For a day or two there may be low-grade fever and its attendant symptoms but often pain and stiffness near the angle of the jaw or the cheek in front of the ear or earache itself is the first symptom and at this time there is almost invariably some fever which lasts for a few days. The swelling is in the region of the parotid and in front of the ear; if it is great there may be marked local tenderness and edema of the surrounding structures of the cheek and even of the orbital area. Gradually the parotitis subsides, disappearing by a week to ten days. Rarely both parotids are involved at the onset but usually the second becomes involved within two or three days after the first. In about one-third of the cases the submaxillary salivary glands become involved and, in much less than this number, the sublingual; very rarely these glands are the seat of the primary involvement and the parotid swelling follows. In parotitis the opening of Steno's duct is swollen and inflamed. The *blood* shows little change but at the height of the disease there is often a slight leukocytosis and quite regularly a relative lymphocytosis.

Complications.—One of the most common is epididymo-orchitis, which seldom complicates in childhood but may occur in from 20 to 50 per cent of adults. It begins a week or two or even three after the onset of the disease; is usually unilateral; and in a certain number of cases is followed by atrophy. If atrophy should be bilateral, sterility may result but not necessarily loss of libido. Involvement of the ovary may take place but not so commonly as the corresponding complication in males. Mastitis and thyroiditis are still less common. Arthritis and nephritis are quite rare. The virus attacks central nervous tissue in a certain percentage of cases, causing a meningismus or a serous meningitis with lymphocytic increase in the cerebrospinal fluid. The cranial and peripheral nerves may be involved, causing multiple neuritis, optic neuritis, or auditory nerve neuritis. Rarely suppuration of the salivary glands may take place.

Relapse and recurrence occasionally occur.

Diagnosis.—This seldom occasions difficulty. Cervical adenitis should be recognized by its different location, its more chronic course and its tendency to suppuration. The Steno duct sign may be helpful as it would occur only in mumps. It is very rare for the parotid or other salivary glands to become involved in any inflammatory process other than mumps. Sour or cold substances often excite or increase the pain in mumps. Orchitis not due to gonorrhea may be due to mumps and in rare instances constitutes the only or first involvement of the disease.

Prognosis.—The mortality is almost *nil*. Even when the central nervous system is involved recovery may be complete. Very rarely blindness or deafness may follow as a result of the cranial nerve involvement.

Treatment.—Quarantine should be for three weeks. Adult males especially should remain in bed for two or three weeks as this lessens the tendency to orchitis. Convalescent serum (p. 321) has distinct protective value, and it is said also that it lessens the tendency to orchitis. Particular attention to cleanliness of the mouth is advisable.

An ice-bag or, perhaps better, hot applications may relieve the local swelling of the parotid. A 5 to 10 per cent guaiacol ointment is often used for the same purpose. Somewhat similar treatment might be indicated for an orchitis. Meningitis should be treated by spinal puncture if there is increased pressure and by intraspinal and intravenous injections of convalescent's serum.

ROSEOLA INFANTUM (EXANTHEMA SUBITUM).

This specific eruptive fever should be given brief mention. It was first described by Zahorsky and since then by many others. It is in all probability an independent infection, having no relationship to any other contagious disease. Its cause is unknown. It is only slightly contagious and attacks infants and occasionally older children. The onset is sudden with high fever which continues for four days (three to five days) without any other symptom or discoverable cause. The temperature then drops rapidly to normal as the eruption appears, after which it does not rise nor do any other symptoms appear. Very characteristic is a distinct leukopenia during the preëruptive and eruptive stages. The rash, which is most profuse on the neck, trunk and proximal parts of the extremities and disappears in forty-eight hours, consists of small, pale, rose-red macules, usually discrete and irregular in outline. The patients always recover and there is no treatment except as the fever indicates.

REFERENCE.

ZAHORSKY, J.: Roseola Infantilis, Pediatrics, 1910, 22, 60.

FOURTH DISEASE AND FIFTH DISEASE.

These need only be mentioned in passing. There is no proof that the fourth disease (Filatow-Duke disease) exists as an independent affection and what has been described as this is, in all probability, that form of rubella in which the rash has a tendency to be confluent and scarlatiniform in character. The fifth disease (erythema infectiosum) is a mild eruptive disease that has been claimed by Escherich and others to be a specific infection, an attack of which does not protect from measles, rubella or scarlet fever. General symptoms are mild; there is no enlargement of lymphatics, and catarrhal symptoms are absent or very mild. The eruption, appearing first on the cheeks, is a pale, red, confluent erythema; this same type of rash involves the buttocks and proximal parts of the extremities. It may be macular in character on the trunk and on the face is scanty and macular or patchy in distribution. If such a disease exists, it is certainly either uncommon or unrecognized by most physicians.

RUBELLA.

Synonyms.—German measles; Rötheln.

Definition and History.—Rubella is a mild, acute, contagious, febrile disease characterized by a macular exanthem and often by mild catarrhal symptoms.

The disease was clearly described at least as early as the beginning of the eighteenth century, but before that time, and even since, rubella has been confused with other eruptive fevers such as scarlet fever and measles.

Etiology.—The *cause* is undetermined, although it is undoubtedly of a bacteriologic nature or belongs in the category of the filterable viruses. *Age* is a predisposing factor since relative immunity seems to exist in the first few months of life and in adults, the greatest incidence being in early and late childhood. It is an *epidemic* disease and the *individual susceptibility* in childhood at least is relatively high, although not to the same degree as in measles. *Transmission* is largely by upper respiratory tract secretions but possibly also in infrequent instances by fomites or carriage by air or a third person. Contagiousness is probably present only at the onset and at the beginning of the eruption.

The *pathology* consists only in the mild changes in the skin.

Symptoms.—The *incubation period* is seven to twenty-one days. At the *onset* only mild catarrhal symptoms and slight fever are usually manifest and even these may be absent. In one to two days the *rash* appears, shqwing first on the face and within twenty-four hours or less spreading over the body. It consists of pale, rose-colored macules which may be slightly papular and usually discrete without the tendency to confluence or the crescentic grouping of measles. It disappears in two or three days from its initiation, fading first in the parts first involved. Usually the *catarrhal symptoms* are mild. An *enanthem* has been described which may appear at the same time as the exanthem and consists of slightly red, minute macules on the mucous membrane of the palate, uvula and cheeks. This is certainly of rare occurrence in the experience of most clinicians. Enlargement of the superficial lymphatics occurs at the height of the disease and is characteristically marked in the *posterior cervical lymph nodes*. *Leukopenia* is present. *Desquamation* consists of slight branny scaling which may or may not take place, beginning a few days after the fading of the rash.

Atypical Forms.—The general symptoms of infection may be more severe than in the average case and considerable variation may exist in the severity and also in the type of the rash. In certain cases it rather closely resembles measles and in others it is scarlatiniform.

Complications are very rare, but pneumonia, nephritis and arthritis have been reported.

Both *relapse* and *recurrence* are extremely uncommon.

Diagnosis.—The differential diagnosis from other eruptive fevers will be found on page 319. Confusion may exist with mild forms of measles, especially when the latter does not exhibit the characteristic enanthem. Diagnostic errors may also occur with scarlet fever. Enlargement of the posterior cervical glands is a helpful but not pathognomonic sign of rubella.

The *prognosis* is almost invariably good.

Treatment.—Prophylaxis consists in isolation during the first five to seven days of the disease. *Convalescent serum* has protective value, but its use is seldom indicated except in institutional epidemics. The general treatment is that for a mild infection.

CHAPTER IX.

DISEASES OF DOUBTFUL ETIOLOGY.

By VIRGIL PRESTON SYDENSTRICKER, M.D.

RHEUMATIC FEVER.
INFECTIOUS MONONUCLEOSIS.
INFECTIOUS JAUNDICE.
EPHEMERAL FEVER.

MILIARY FEVER.
AINHUM.
GANGOSA.

RHEUMATIC FEVER.

Synonyms.—Acute rheumatic fever; Acute articular rheumatism; Polyarthritis rheumatica.

Definition.—An infectious disease of unknown etiology causing fever and marked intoxication, characterized by the presence of minute focal proliferative lesions in the heart and many other organs and tissues. In acute phases there is exudation in and around the joints and at times in various serous cavities.

Etiology.—Predisposing Factors.—Rheumatic fever is a disease of temperate and subtropical climates, occurring more frequently in the colder, damper areas. Atwater found the average hospital admission incidence for rheumatic fever in northern Europe to be 3.7 per cent, while the records of the United Fruit Company for fourteen years showed only 0.53 per cent of over 220,000 patients. There are notable exceptions to this generalization. Holland shows a strikingly low incidence, while the disease is frequent in Ceylon, Cameroon and the West Caroline Islands. Newsholme has shown that there is a definite cycle in the prevalence of rheumatic fever, with peaks occurring every four to six years which coincide with periods of deficient rainfall and excessive dryness of the soil. Atwater found that parallelism seemed to exist between the incidence of rheumatic fever and the streptococcal diseases, erysipelas, scarlet fever and septicemia. There is a marked seasonal variation. In America and continental Europe the greatest number of cases occurs in late winter and spring, with the peak in April, while in England there is an autumnal maximum. Many students of the disease have insisted upon its familial incidence, positive family histories being obtained in as many as 50 per cent of their cases. In this respect there is a suggestive analogy with the familial occurrence of tuberculosis. The frequently stressed relation of dampness, poverty and unhygienic surroundings is probably of importance insofar as unfavorable environment increases individual susceptibility to infection.

Age is an important factor, the disease being preëminently one of youth. The decade from five to fifteen years shows the highest incidence, though infants are occasionally attacked and the condition is relatively common up to thirty-five years of age; after this, first attacks

(336)

being progressively more infrequent with each decade. The manifestations, course and outcome of the disease depend to a considerable extent on the age at which infection is acquired. Chorea is largely concentrated in the five to fifteen years age group. This group also furnishes the greatest number of recurrences with resulting carditis in later life.

Sex plays a less important part than age. If all manifestations are considered, females are affected more often than males. In the first two decades girls predominate in the ratio of 3 to 2. Arthritis is more common in men, heart disease in women.

Rôle of Infection.—The frequent occurrence of pharyngitis, sinusitis and tonsillitis shortly preceding rheumatic fever has been emphasized. More than one-half of all cases follow such infections and many more have a history of recent acute respiratory disease. The causative organism has not definitely been identified nor has the disease been reproduced in experimental animals. Whether this is due to inability of the animals' tissues to react to the virus as do those of human beings or to failure to isolate the virus is unknown. No record exists of an attempt to transfer infection from man to man. It has been shown that rheumatic fever commonly follows hemolytic streptococcal infection of the upper respiratory passages and that relapses in rheumatic subjects are almost invariably subsequent to such infections. Coburn and his associates have stressed these facts and have demonstrated precipitins and antistreptolysins quite regularly in the blood of rheumatic patients. Numerous investigators have cultivated non-hemolytic streptococci from the blood and occasionally from the tissues. These organisms largely have belonged to the viridans group, though some observers have recovered indifferent streptococci only. No common biologic or immunologic relationships have been established between the various organisms and in some instances more than one strain has been cultivated from a single patient. It has been suggested that the rheumatic state is one of hypersensitiveness to a group or indefinite number of strains of streptococci. This hypothesis explains the manifestations of the disease on the basis of an initial lesion, possibly slight, with production of sensitization; then in the presence of continued infection in the original focus or of dissemination from it more serious disturbances develop elsewhere in the body as allergic phenomena. With reinfection or renewed activity in old foci recurrences of these phenomena occur. It is possible, too, after removal of the original focus that the secondary lesions in the tissues may harbor the infection and themselves become foci. Others are convinced on account of the constant and characteristic lesions found in the heart and other organs that the disease is caused by a specific infectious agent not demonstrable by present methods of investigation.

Pathology.—The gross lesions are largely exudative. Affected joints show edema of the periarticular tissues; the synovial cavities are distended with turbid yellowish fluid containing flecks of fibrin. The synovial membranes are thickened and injected and in rare instances the cartilages are slightly eroded. When pleurisy occurs it is serofibrinous, occasionally with adhesions. Pericarditis is serofibrinous,

22

often with massive fibrinous exudate. The pericardial endothelium may be destroyed and the pericardial cavity obliterated by organization of the exudate. Myocarditis is usually recognizable and there is frequently a localized thickening in the wall of the left auricle. Endocarditis or more properly valvulitis shows in early cases minute grayish-pink vegetations along the line of approximation of the cusps with thickening of the cusps. Older cases show varying degrees of thickening, distortion and vascularization. The mitral valve is most frequently involved, though aortic and tricuspid disease is common.

Histologically the characteristic lesion is a minute submiliary nodule occurring in proximity to small blood-vessels in the interstitial connective tissue. In early lesions there is a central strand or clump of necrotic collagen and coagulated serum. Around this is a group or zone of conspicuous large basophilic cells containing one or more bulky vesicular nuclei. These cells are thought to originate from the endothelium of small vessels and perivascular spaces. Small mononuclear wandering cells and polymorphonuclears form an outer zone of infiltration. In older lesions the central collagen and the small cell reaction disappear, leaving only the large cells. Eventually plasma cells and fibroblasts replace the typical large cells and the lesion is converted into a tiny scar. The type lesion is the Aschoff body in the myocardium. Analogous foci of reaction modified by the structure of the tissue in which they occur are widely distributed. They are plentiful in the periarticular tissues and synovial membranes, the subcutaneous nodules being conglomerations of them. Numerous lesions are found in the walls of the larger vessels and when the pericardium is involved they underlie the epicardium. In the heart valves foci of infiltration occur in the interstitial tissue of the cusps, the entire valve is edematous and the characteristic vegetations are thrombotic masses of fibrin deposited on areas where the swollen endothelium is damaged by impact. In older cases the cusps are thickened and often distorted by scar formation. In chorea the brain shows vascular and perivascular lesions analogous to Aschoff bodies. Vasculitis of the smaller vessels with a proliferate containing cells similar to those which characterize Aschoff bodies may occur in many localities, notably the coronary arteries, the tonsils, gastro-intestinal tract and kidneys. In the pleura, pericardium and trabeculæ of the lungs extensive infiltration with the characteristic cells may occur.

Symptoms.—Prodromal symptoms are present in a large majority of cases. In children persistent loss of weight may be an important early sign. Over one-half of the patients give a history of sore throat or tonsillitis preceding the acute attack and coryza and bronchitis occur in some. General malaise, undue fatigue, anorexia and fleeting pains in the limbs are frequent complaints. When no prodromata occur the disease may follow immediately on severe chilling or exhaustion. Often the onset is with slight chilliness and occasionally there is definite rigor. The temperature rises rapidly and with the fever one or more joints become painful. Within twenty-four hours the attack is fully developed, fever ranges from 102° to 104° F. and the pulse is rapid in proportion to the temperature early in the disease; later marked increase in the pulse-rate with or without irregularity indicates cardiac involvement. There is marked prostration, profuse sweating and arthritis. The affected joints are severely painful, tender and rapidly become swollen, hot and flushed. The large joints are chiefly involved, one or several at a time. Those most subject to strain are apt to be first affected, and as the process begins in a new joint those first attacked tend to subside. The vertebral, sternoclavicular and phalangeal articulations usually escape. Tenosynovitis is frequent, particularly with arthritis of the wrists and ankles. The degree of swelling is variable and depends to a considerable extent on the amount of exudation into the joint cavities. The synovial exudate is turbid with leukocytes, but actual suppuration does not occur without secondary infection. No permanent damage remains after the resolution of the arthritis. Sweats are profuse and frequent, sudaminal eruptions are common and the perspiration has a peculiar sour odor. Thirst is often a distressing symptom and anorexia and constipation are seldom absent.

In mild cases the fever persists for ten to fifteen days, running an irregularly remittent course varying between 100° and 104° F. The arthritis extends from one group of joints to another with exacerbations of fever accompanying each new involvement. Each joint is acutely inflamed for four to six days, then resolves and is not again affected. After varying numbers of joints have been affected the fever terminates by lysis, the remaining arthritis clears up and the patient recovers. The severer cases fall into two groups: the polycyclic in which the completion of one series of arthritic manifestations is followed immediately by another, or before one series is complete joints which have resolved relapse; and the continuous type in which there is persistent activity in one or several joints. It is in these two groups that cardiac involvement is exceedingly likely to occur.

Evidence of heart disease is frequent in proportion to the care with which it is sought. Electrocardiographic studies show abnormal curves in 90 per cent of cases of rheumatic fever. Clinical signs of endocarditis are present in 50 per cent and of myocarditis in a somewhat higher proportion. The evidences of myocardial involvement may appear early in the disease, precordial pain and hyperesthesia without signs of pericarditis are suggestive, the presence of a wavy diffuse apex impulse and a palpable gallop rhythm are confirmatory of this. Auscultation may disclose various disturbances of rhythm; usually the palpable gallop is found to be due to a markedly accentuated third heart sound; premature contractions are frequent, and dropped beats due to partial heart block may be detected. Gross evidences of cardiac embarrassment are commonly associated with auricular fibrillation and complete heart block. Significant increase in the size of the heart is rare and usually due to acute dilatation. Heart murmurs heard during the acute attack are seldom to be interpreted dogmatically. Systolic bruits at the mitral and tricuspid areas are usually attributed to stretching of the valve rings with resulting relative insufficiency. A similar explanation is assumed for the diastolic murmurs which may occur over the aortic area in the absence of other evidences of aortic regurgitation. It is to be remembered, however, that interstitial valvulitis with thickening of the cusps and deposition of minute vegetations may well cause minor degrees of anatomic valvular insufficiency without recognizable functional disturbances of the circulation. Murmurs tend to disappear with recovery from the acute attack, often to recur later. They may reappear also during a relapse. It frequently requires months or even years of observation to evaluate the significance of auscultatory findings. Undoubtedly the valves are damaged very often but the gravity of the lesion depends on the persistence or recurrence of infection. The eventual injury may be wholly myocardial so far as physical signs can be interpreted, or may be predominantly valvular with the picture of mitral or aortic disease.

Pericarditis is a frequent manifestation and is of special importance on account of its common association with the severer grades of myocardial disease. It occurs in a large proportion of fatal cases. The development of pericarditis in a patient with signs of valvular injury and myocardial disease justifies the use of the terms carditis and pancarditis. An increase in fever and the pulse-rate may herald pericardial involvement. A friction, with or without precordial pain, is diagnostic. Pericardial friction may be faint and very evanescent or may be associated with fremitus and persist for days. With the accumulation of fluid, fremitus and friction sounds tend to disappear but they may persist even with a large effusion when there are masses of fibrinous exudate. The development of an effusion is ordinarily heralded by tachycardia, increasing dyspnea and cough; the area of precordial dullness increases rapidly in size; there are signs of compression of the left lung, and the systolic blood pressure falls. Accessory signs of pericardial effusion are frequently found. After recovery extensive pericardial adhesions may form with resulting grave cardiac insufficiency.

Arteritis is seldom recognized clinically, but it may be suspected when there is tenderness on pressure over a superficial artery. Aortic aneurysm due to rheumatic arteritis has been observed.

Pleurisy is occasionally the first manifestation of rheumatic fever, but it may at times indicate a relapse or recrudescence. Pleural pain, with or without friction sounds, occurs in some 10 per cent of all cases and is more frequent on the left side, often in association with pericarditis. Effusion is frequent and may produce dangerous respiratory or cardiac embarrassment. Pneumonia or more properly pneumonitis may occur in very severe infections, usually in association with pleurisy and carditis. Exacerbation of fever, cough and blood-tinged sputum are suggestive of pulmonary involvement but physical signs are not definite and it is probably impossible to differentiate rheumatic pneumonitis from complicating bronchopneumonia. Upper respiratory manifestations are common, and redness and slight edema of the pharynx without exudate are usually found with the prodromal sore throat. Tonsillitis and laryngitis may occur during an attack or with a relapse and nodules may develop in the vocal cords. Chronic infections of the paranasal sinuses are not uncommon in rheumatic patients and have been thought to have direct relation to the disease.

Nervous phenomena are relatively frequent. In children chorea may be the first manifestation of rheumatic infection. There may be little or no fever but subcutaneous nodules may develop and recurrences of chorea are apt to be associated with arthritis or carditis. More commonly chorea occurs during the course of a typical attack with polyarthritis and cardiac symptoms. In adult patients delirium and coma may appear when there is hyperpyrexia; lasting psychoses may result. Cerebral rheumatism is a rare condition which may supervene either during an acute attack or after convalescence is established. Intense headache, restlessness, delirium and coma with or without pyrexia characterize this form of the disease. It occurs exclusively in adults and is almost uniformly fatal. Rheumatic meningitis has been described. Nerve pain is not an uncommon complaint in older patients but peripheral neuritis is rarely seen.

Acute nephritis is an unusual but serious accompaniment of polyarthritis; it may be the presenting feature of a relapse. Fahr considered rheumatic fever an important factor in the production of chronic nephritis. It is to be remembered that albuminuria and hematuria may follow the administration of salicylates.

Various skin eruptions of the erythema multiforme type may occur with rheumatic fever but none are specifically identified with it since they cannot be differentiated from similar exudative dermatoses occurring in other infections. Erythema nodosum occurs occasionally and has been thought to be a result of rheumatic infection. The relation of Schönlein's disease and Henoch's purpura to rheumatic fever has not been established

Subcutaneous nodules are a specific and important manifestation of the disease. They are believed to indicate an unusually virulent and widespread infection and to represent an extreme proliferative response to the virus in a tissue peculiarly adapted to such a reaction. The nodules are firm, usually painless, varying from pin-head to hazelnut size, occurring most frequently about the elbows, knees and malleoli, though they may be found over the skull, vertebral spines and the sheaths of superficial tendons. Nodules are often better seen than felt and should be looked for by oblique light; they appear suddenly, often in crops, grow rapidly and resolve slowly. The administration of salicylates is without influence in hastening resolution.

Other manifestations of rare occurrence are iritis, peritonitis, parotitis and involvement of the thyroid, breasts or testicles. Phlebitis has been described.

Rheumatic fever in children presents many variations from the adult type. Polyarthritis is infrequent and when present is less severe and more transient. The occurrence of subcutaneous nodules, tonsillitis, chorea, pleurisy or carditis may usher in the disease. Rare cases are fulminating and rapidly fatal. Prolonged periods of prodromal symptoms are the rule. Anorexia, loss of weight, lassitude, growing pains or fleeting joint pains may precede frank rheumatic phenomena by weeks or months. Chronic non-suppurative tonsillitis with anterior cervical adenitis is common and may constitute the only definite finding. Heart disease may be well established before the real nature of a seemingly trivial illness is recognized. Relapses are frequent and, as a rule, the heart damage is increased by each exacerbation.

The blood shows a rapidly progressive anemia of secondary type with leukocytosis of 10,000 to 25,000. Persistence of leukocytosis after the subsidence of acute symptoms suggests the likelihood of early relapse. The urine is small in quantity, of high concentration, strongly acid and may contain small amounts of albumin. Numerous red blood cells may be present and persist over long periods of time, the urinary chlorides being reduced.

Diagnosis.—In the absence of any method of bacteriologic or serologic diagnosis entire reliance must be placed on the recognition of clinical phenomena. An acute migratory polyarthritis affecting the larger joints and showing marked response to salicyl therapy offers little difficulty. Where arthritis is slight or absent the presence of subcutaneous nodules, of chorea, or of evidences of heart disease is of prime importance. Multiple acute secondary arthritis may be mistaken for rheumatic fever. The joint condition is more acute, the synovial fluid is actually purulent and organisms may frequently be demonstrated, and a history of recent purulent tonsillitis, of dysentery or cerebrospinal meningitis may be obtained. Gonococcal arthritis is associated with demonstrable genital infection; the arthritis is not fleeting and organisms can usually be demonstrated in the cloudy joint fluid. Following scarlet fever and puerperal sepsis, multiple serous arthritis is not particularly rare but the history is diagnostic. In children acute osteomyelitis and septic arthritis may cause confusion. Severe rheumatic polyarthritis is rare in children, and the septic fever, frequent chills, profound intoxication and marked leukocytosis should differentiate these conditions. Scurvy and hemophilia may produce acutely swollen, painful joints but the other features of these diseases are obvious. Serum sickness beginning with arthritis may strongly suggest rheumatic fever but the history of serum treatment within a period of three weeks and the rapid appearance of other evidences of hypersensitiveness make differentiation easy. Chronic infectious arthritis may have an acute onset; the persistent involvement of the small joints and of the vertebral articulations with absence of cardiac symptoms is of diagnostic importance. Acute gout has caused confusion. The history, the location of the affected joints, the frequent occurrence of tophi and the characteristic roentgen-ray findings are conclusive; a marked increase in uric acid in the blood is always demonstrable.

Prognosis.—Fewer than 5 per cent of patients die in the initial attack, so that the immediate outlook is good. Myocarditis with sudden heart failure, embolism and bronchopneumonia account for most early fatalities. Cerebral rheumatism is frequently fatal but fortunately rare. Recurrences increase the gravity of the outlook and chorea and subcutaneous nodules are of bad import. The seriousness of the disease lies in the permanent damage done to the heart valves or muscle. Puberty is a period of great danger to those acquiring the infection in childhood, the rapid growth at this time frequently precipitating heart failure. Occasional instances of complete clinical recovery from rheumatic endocarditis have been observed.

Treatment.—Inasmuch as the drugs which notably allay symptoms in this disease have no effect on the causative agent, it is essential to employ to the fullest such general measures as may help protect the heart and prevent the prolongation or recurrence of the illness. Rest is of first importance. With polyarthritis the patient is immobilized by pain but with milder manifestations rest in bed may have to be enforced. A safe rule is to maintain absolute rest for at least three weeks after the resolution of all arthritis and cessation of fever. When fever is not a marked symptom, leukocytosis is valid evidence of persistent infection and may be used as a guide. The patient must be protected against cold and particularly against chilling during or after sweats. Light flannel gowns opening down the back and along the seams of the sleeves add not only to the patient's safety but to comfort and ease of nursing, and a flannel shawl around the neck and shoulders is helpful. Linen or cotton sheets should be replaced by thin woolen blankets. When the knee or ankle joints are inflamed the bed covers should be supported by a frame.

Fluids must be given liberally, and often must be forced to prevent dehydration from excessive sweating as well as to facilitate elimination. The food should be easily assimilable and of high caloric value. Milk, eggs, cereals, cream soups and fruit drinks fortified with lactose serve all purposes during the febrile period though it may be necessary to cater to the patient's appetite. With cessation of fever a full diet should be instituted.

The skin requires special care. After sweats the patient should be sponged with warm 50 per cent alcohol, thoroughly dried and dusted liberally with powder. The affected joints should be wrapped loosely with cotton batting, and frequently immobilization on light, well-padded splints affords great relief. The local application of 25 per cent methyl salicylate in oil, of lead and opium lotion or of saturated solution of magnesium sulphate is comforting. When pain and tenderness are extreme light application of the Paquelin cautery surpasses other forms of counterirritation. If the joints are greatly distended with fluid it may be justifiable to aspirate them, when the strictest asepsis must be observed. The pain of pericarditis is often relieved by an ice-cap over the precordium. Pericardial or pleural effusions of sufficient size to cause cardiac or respiratory embarrassment must be aspirated.

Salicylates in adequate doses control the arthritis and to some extent the pyrexia of rheumatic fever though the proliferative lesions are not influenced. Sodium salicylate is the drug of choice and should be given in doses of 1 to 1.3 grams (15 to 20 grains), every two hours, until mild toxic symptoms develop. Tinnitus, deafness, vertigo and nausea indicate saturation, which usually occurs after 10 to 13.5 grams (150 to 200 grains) have been ingested. The dose should then be reduced by 25 per cent and continued at this amount until all pain and fever have been absent for a week; after this the drug may be gradually withdrawn over a period of ten days to two weeks. The salicylate

is best tolerated in milk and each dose should be accompanied or followed by an equal amount of sodium bicarbonate.   If sodium salicylate
cannot be administered by mouth it may be given by rectum, 3 to
4 grams (45 to 60 grains) in 200 cc. of starch water every six hours.
The intravenous injection of the drug offers no advantages.   Acetylsalicylic acid may be used instead of the sodium salt, the dose and
method of administration being identical.   It is to be remembered
that salicylates may produce delirium and maniacal states in certain
individuals.   Neocinchophen produces effects similar to sodium salicylate and is sometimes better tolerated; the dose is the same.   Late
toxic effects may occur.   Amidopyrine is as actively antirheumatic as
the salicylates and may be better tolerated.   It is given in doses of
0.3 to 0.5 gram (5 to $7\frac{1}{2}$ grains) at four- to six-hour intervals.   This
drug must be used with caution in view of the recent reports of
granulocytopenia developing in patients who had taken it alone or in
combination with the barbiturates.   Morphine or codeine may occasionally be necessary to control pain, especially that of pericarditis or
pleurisy.   Digitalis is indicated if signs of heart failure develop; the
dose must be carefully controlled as toxic effects are readily produced
in the presence of active myocarditis.   Non-specific protein therapy
and "desensitization" with vaccines or nucleoproteins prepared from
hemolytic streptococci have shown encouraging results in the hands of
some.   Biologic methods of treatment are in the experimental stage,
however.

With convalescence iron is indicated in full doses and stimulants to
appetite are often required.   After the discontinuance of salicylates
the patient should remain in bed for two weeks after all symptoms
have disappeared.   Tachycardia and leukocytosis are as important at
this time as fever or pain.   Getting up should be very gradual and
walking must not be permitted until sitting up for four or five hours
no longer causes fatigue or a significant increase in the pulse-rate.
Carefully graduated exercise controlled by the heart's response to it
is an essential part of treatment during convalescence.   Recurrence of
any symptoms at any time necessitates cessation of all activity.   After
recovery is complete and the weight and hemoglobin have returned to
normal it is wise to have any foci of infection in the nose, mouth and
throat removed in the hope that recurrence may be prevented.

REFERENCES.

ATWATER, R. M.: Studies in the Epidemiology of Rheumatic Fever and Related
    Diseases in the United States, Am. Jour. Hyg., 1927, **7**, 343.
CECIL, R. L., NICHOLLS, E. E., and STAINSBY, W. J.: Bacteriology of the Blood
    and Joints in Rheumatic Fever, Jour. Exper. Med., 1929, **1**, 617.
COBURN, A. F.: The Factor of Infection in the Rheumatic State, Baltimore,
    Williams & Wilkins Company, 1931.
COBURN, A. F., and PAULI, R. H.: Jour. Exper. Med., 1932, **56**, 609, 633, 651.
COOMBS, C. F.: Rheumatic Heart Disease, Bristol, 1924.
PAUL, J. R.: The Epidemiology of Rheumatic Fever: A Preliminary Report
    With Special Reference to Environmental Factors in Rheumatic Heart Dis-
    ease and Recommendations for Future Investigations, New York, American
    Heart Association, 1930.
PAUL, J. R., and SALINGER, R.: Jour. Clin. Invest., 1931, **10**, 33.
SWIFT, H. F.: Rheumatic Fever, Oxford Med., 1921, **5**, 2, 11.

INFECTIOUS MONONUCLEOSIS.

Synonyms.—Glandular fever; Benign lymphadenosis.

Definition.—An acute infectious and contagious disease observed chiefly in children and young adults, occurring often in epidemics. It is characterized by malaise, fever, a peculiar type of pharyngitis and sometimes conjunctivitis, marked enlargement of the lymph nodes and spleen and a striking alteration of the leukocyte formula, usually with leukocytosis.

History.—Pfeiffer in 1889 presented the first adequate clinical description of the disease under the title "Drüsenfieber." Many subsequent authors confirmed his observations. In 1920 Sprunt and Evans used the name "infectious mononucleosis" and emphasized the blood picture. The following year Tidy and Morley identified the glandular fever of earlier writers with infectious mononucleosis.

Etiology.—The causative organism has not been identified. Nyfeldt has reported the cultivation of a small bacillus or vibrio from the blood of patients with infectious mononucleosis and the production of monocytosis in animals by inoculation with this organism. This work requires confirmation. Occurring more frequently as a sporadic disease, outbreaks are not uncommon. Children are chiefly affected, although epidemics have been observed among adults. Infection occurs by way of the upper respiratory passages and is transmitted by direct contact, though Tidy observed an instance of apparent transfer by a healthy carrier. Where individuals are intimately associated, as in schools and barracks, a large proportion of those exposed contract the disease. A majority of epidemics have occurred in winter and spring.

Pathology.—Of the morbid anatomy nothing is known. Sections of excised glands have shown marked hyperplasia with disappearance of the follicles, large numbers of young lymphocytes and numerous mitotic cells. Tuberculosis and Hodgkin's disease can be ruled out by microscopic examination of sections. The picture so closely resembles that seen early in lymphatic leukemia that a diagnosis cannot be made with certainty by this means.

Symptoms.—The incubation period varies from five to twelve days; it is most often seven or eight days. There may be prodromal symptoms, sore throat, headache and malaise. Sometimes granular conjunctivitis may be present for two to five days. The onset is usually abrupt with mild rigors, headache, prostration, anorexia and pharyngitis. Fever is apt to be present and may rise to 103° F. or over. Pyrexia commonly persists for two to five days though some cases are practically afebrile and others have continued mild fever for ten days or more. Defervescence is commonly by lysis but may be abrupt. Drowsiness is a striking feature; on the second or third day the patient may fall into a sleep lasting for twenty-four hours, and wake up free from fever and feeling quite well.

The skin is flushed during the febrile period and sweating may be marked. The eyes are apt to be congested and there may be a peculiar dry granular conjunctivitis, often unilateral and involving both the palpebral and scleral conjunctivæ. The nose is often obstructed by swelling of the mucosa and epistaxis is frequent. The pharynx is congested and presents a coarsely granular or pebbled appearance from enlargement of the lymph follicles. The tonsils are not enlarged and typically there is no tonsillar or pharyngeal exudate. Soon after the fever reaches its height there is rapid enlargement of the lymph nodes, the posterior cervical and submaxillary glands are most strikingly affected and may attain the size of walnuts; the adenopathy is sometimes unilateral at first. The axillary, epitrochlear and inguinal nodes become swollen but to a less striking degree. There may be a troublesome non-productive cough suggesting pressure from enlarged mediastinal glands and the mesenteric nodes may be palpable. The enlarged glands are soft, discrete and moderately tender. The spleen is almost invariably palpable at some stage of the disease and the liver is not infrequently swollen.

The blood shows no significant change in the hemoglobin content or the number of red cells. Depending on the stage of the disease the leukocytes may vary from 3000 to 35,000 per cubic millimeter. There is at first a slight polymorphonuclear increase followed rapidly by a relative and actual neutropenia and a marked mononucleosis which may reach 99 per cent of the total count. The predominating cells are typical lymphocytes with a variable number of abnormal forms with deeply basophilic, often vacuolated cytoplasm and round, reniform or lobulated pachychromatic nuclei. Immature cells are absent. Plasma cells are common; they may be numerous and the monocytes are frequently increased. The urine may contain a small amount of albumin. Transient hematuria is very frequent.

Complications.—Secondary infection of the pharynx and tonsils occurs rather often. Suppurative adenitis is a rare but serious complication, as septicemia has ensued. Death has resulted in only 5 recorded instances, perhaps always from secondary infection.

Diagnosis.—The blood picture has frequently led to a suspicion of acute leukemia. The presence of heterophile agglutinins for sheep cells in the blood in infectious mononucleosis offers a valuable diagnostic test in doubtful cases. The absence of purpura, of anemia and of immature cell types in the blood and the rapid subsidence of acute symptoms suffice to differentiate the two conditions. Hodgkin's disease and acute tuberculous adenitis are ruled out by the blood picture and the prompt disappearance of fever. It is noteworthy that the glandular enlargement and marked relative lymphocytosis may persist for many months after symptomatic recovery.

Treatment.—This is entirely symptomatic and the usual measures taken for the relief of discomfort in mild febrile diseases serve all purposes. Secondary infection of the pharynx requires local treatment; suppuration of infected glands may necessitate incision. Precautions against contagion should be taken, particularly in schools and hospital wards.

REFERENCES.

GUTHRIE, C. G.: Glandular Fever (Infectious Mononucleosis), Oxford Med., New York, 1927, **5**, 498.

GUTHRIE, C. G., and PESSEL, J. F.: An Epidemic of Glandular Fever in a Preparatory School for Boys, Am. Jour. Dis. Child., 1925, **29**, 492.

NYFELDT, A.: Klinische und experimentelle Untersuchungen über d. Mononucleosis Infectiosa, Folia hematol., 1932, **47**, 1.

PAUL, J. R., and BUNNELL, W. W.: The Presence of Heterophile Antibodies in Infectious Mononucleosis, Am. Jour. Med. Sci., 1932, **183**, 90.

PFEIFFER, E.: Drüsenfieber, Jahrb. f. Kinderh., 1889, **29**, 257.

SPRUNT, T. P., and EVANS, F. A.: Mononuclear Leukocytosis in Reaction to Acute Infection (Infectious Mononucleosis), Bull. Johns Hopkins Hosp., 1920, **31**, 410.

TIDY, H. L., and DANIEL, E. C.: Glandular Fever and Infective Mononucleosis, with an Account of an Epidemic, Lancet, 1923, ii, 9.

INFECTIOUS JAUNDICE.

Synonyms.—Epidemic jaundice; Epidemic catarrhal jaundice.

Definition.—An acute infectious disease of undetermined etiology occurring often in epidemics, presenting at the onset marked constitutional symptoms with the early development of jaundice.

History.—Infectious jaundice was first recognized in the United States during the War of 1812. In the following seventy-five years eleven outbreaks were noted. Since 1886 there have been several hundred epidemics of varying proportions.

Etiology.—Of the specific cause nothing is known, but careful investigations in several countries seem to indicate that it is not a bacterial nor spirochetal disease. There is a marked seasonal incidence, 72 per cent of epidemics having occurred in the fall and winter and only 6 per cent in the spring. Outbreaks are more frequent in rural districts and small towns than in cities. Children and young adults are attacked much more frequently than older individuals. There is good evidence that personal contact is necessary for the transmission of the infection and it is strongly suspected that the infective agent passes out from and enters by way of the upper respiratory passages. At times the disease seems to have been transmitted by fomites. No proof has been brought that food, water, milk, animals or insects play a part in its dissemination. During epidemics as many as 50 per cent of the population have been attacked.

Pathology.—In the rare instances of death from infectious jaundice changes have been observed grossly resembling those seen in acute yellow atrophy. There is intense icterus, often with hemorrhages into the skin, the serous and mucous membranes, the lungs and various other viscera. There are cloudy swelling, fatty degeneration and focal icteric necrosis in the liver. In cases of long standing there is marked diminution in the size of this organ with widespread necrotic changes and hemorrhage simulating acute yellow atrophy. There is no demonstrable obstruction of the larger bile ducts. Scattered areas of coagulation necrosis, both superficial and deep, occur in the gastrointestinal mucosa. The kidneys show acute parenchymatous degeneration, sometimes with necrosis of the tubular epithelium and tubular or interstitial hemorrhages.

Symptoms.—The incubation period varies from two to twenty-eight days; usually it is from seven to ten days. There may be prodromal coryza or bronchitis. The onset is apt to be sudden, with nausea, vomiting and constipation; headache, backache and pain in the limbs are seldom absent; epigastric pain is very common. There may be practically no symptoms until the jaundice appears. Moderate fever is the rule, though some epidemics are practically afebrile and occasional cases have marked pyrexia. On the fourth or fifth day the severer gastro-intestinal symptoms subside and with them the fever. Jaundice appears with the amelioration of symptoms and varies from slight scleral discoloration to deep bronzing of the skin. Jaundice may be evanescent or may persist for as long as six or seven weeks. Occasionally there is an erythematous rash followed by desquamation; pruritus may be troublesome. Epistaxis and other hemorrhagic manifestations may occur. The tongue is heavily coated, the breath foul. Frequently there are the signs of mild bronchitis. The liver is large and tender and sometimes the spleen is palpable. The blood shows no marked variation of the hemoglobin and red cells. Leukopenia may be found and leukocytosis up to 20,000 has been recorded. In the majority of cases there is no marked change in the white cell count or in the differential formula. The serum shows varying amounts of bile pigments. The urine is concentrated, contains small amounts of albumin and quantities of bile. The stools are clay-colored and often inspissated. Quite rarely there are pronounced mental symptoms, somnolence, stupor or delirium. Hemorrhages into the skin and from the mucous membranes are of grave import. Nephritis occurs in a few of the severest cases. Convalescence is ordinarily rapid although prostration, anorexia and mental depression may persist for a number of weeks. Relapses seldom occur.

Complications.—Actual complications are very rare. Nephritis and a tendency to bleed may be regarded as severe manifestations of the disease rather than complications. Pregnant women sometimes abort and bronchopneumonia is not rare in elderly patients. Death is exceedingly infrequent.

Diagnosis.—The pre-icteric symptoms and epidemic prevalence of infectious jaundice, together with its preponderance during the first three decades of life, serve to separate it from obstructive icterus. Acute catarrhal jaundice probably represents the sporadic phase of the disease and cannot be differentiated. Weil's disease is more acute in its onset, constantly more severe in its manifestations, is frequently relapsing and is readily identified by the demonstration of the causative spirochete. Dengue may be confused with epidemic jaundice in the pre-icteric stage but the severe joint pains, erythema and absence of icterus soon permit differentiation. Yellow fever and blackwater fever have in the past offered difficulties for which there is no present occasion.

Treatment.—During the febrile period, rest in bed should be enforced. Fluids are to be given in large quantities. If nausea prevents an adequate intake by mouth, rectal administration should be instituted. The diet should be liquid or soft and contain a minimum of fats and sugars; milk is often not tolerated. Analgesics such as amidopyrine or acetylsalicylic acid alone or with small doses of codeine may be required for pain. Cool sponges are serviceable when there is marked pyrexia. Preliminary purgation may be helpful but repeated catharsis only increases the gastro-intestinal distress. Persistent nausea may yield to gastric lavage or to small doses (0.05–0.2 gm.) of chloretone repeated frequently. Chloroform water is often recommended. During convalescence bitter tonics are useful.

REFERENCES.

BLUMER, G.: Infectious Jaundice in the United States, Jour. Am. Med. Assn., 1923, **81**, 353.

ROSS, E. A.: Pathology of Epidemic Jaundice, Lancet, 1928, i, 599.

SYMMERS, D.: Epidemic Acute Hemorrhagic Jaundice of Toxic Origin, Jour. Am. Med. Assn., 1920, **74**, 1153.

WADSWORTH, A., *et al.*: Infectious Jaundice Occurring in New York State, Jour. Am. Med. Assn., 1922, **78**, 1120.

EPHEMERAL FEVER (FEBRICULA).

Definition.—A febrile reaction of acute onset persisting for twenty-four to thirty-six hours, presenting no local or localizing manifestations and disappearing without sequelæ. When such a fever persists for several days it is known as febricula.

Undoubtedly a group of unrelated conditions is included, of which the causes are indefinite or unrecognized. During epidemics a considerable number of ephemeral fevers occur which probably represent abortive forms of well-known diseases. Gastro-intestinal disturbances, toxic or infectious, form another group. Extreme heat, particularly with high humidity, produces fugitive pyrexia in some persons. Formerly exposure to foul odors, particularly sewer gas, was thought to be an important factor. Children and young people are more frequently affected and individual susceptibility is probably important.

Symptoms.—Onset is sudden, often with mild rigor and fever which may reach 103° to 105° F.; headache and pain in the back and limbs are usual; restlessness and irritability or drowsiness may occur. Anorexia, nausea and either diarrhea or constipation are seldom absent; oliguria is almost constant. Fleeting erythema has been observed and labial or nasal herpes is very frequent. The tongue is coated; there may be pharyngeal injection. In the febriculæ fever shows a wide daily variation and constitutional symptoms are less marked. Termination is usually by rapid lysis.

Diagnosis and Treatment.—Diagnosis is always by elimination and is arrived at only after the illness has terminated without unfavorable developments. Treatment is symptomatic; hydrotherapy and analgesics are useful. Mild purgation and liberal administration of fluids are always indicated.

MILIARY FEVER.

Synonym.—Sweating sickness.

Definition.—An acute infectious disease occurring usually in localized epidemics. It presents an acute onset with fever, prostration, marked sweating and on the fourth or fifth day a papular or papulovesicular eruption.

History.—Major epidemics with high mortality occurred in Europe and England during the fifteenth and sixteenth centuries. Since 1700 more than 200 outbreaks have been recorded chiefly in continental Europe. The last one of importance was in France in 1907. The disease has not been recognized in America.

Etiology.—The cause of the disease is unknown. Epidemics are usually well localized and occur almost exclusively in rural districts during spring and summer. Many individuals are affected in rapid succession, persons of all ages being attacked.

Symptoms.—The onset is sudden, profuse sweating with fever may initiate the illness or there may be preceding chilliness, headache, myalgia and gastro-intestinal disturbances. The temperature ranges from 101° to 104° F., sometimes higher, the pulse-rate is disproportionately accelerated, sweating is persistent, prostration is great, dyspnea and a sense of epigastric constriction are commonly present. On the third to the fifth day a diffuse erythematous rash appears, followed rapidly by an eruption of papules or vesicles. With the development of the eruption fever subsides and after a few days there is diffuse desquamation. Severe cases present delirium, convulsions and sometimes coma. The eruption may be purpuric and associated with hemorrhages from the mucous membranes. Fatal cases usually have a fulminating onset with hyperpyrexia, extreme tachycardia, dyspnea and convulsions or coma with death before the appearance of eruption. The disease produces severe loss of weight, anemia and prostration. Convalescence is slow. Fatalities are exceptional though some epidemics have had a mortality of 30 per cent.

Treatment.—Treatment is entirely symptomatic. All precautions against contagion should be exercised.

AINHUM.

Definition.—A chronic disease causing spontaneous amputation usually of the fifth toe though other toes and sometimes a finger may be affected.

Of the *etiology* nothing is known. Individuals of colored races only seem to be susceptible. The condition has been observed most frequently in the natives of the west coast of Africa, of Brazil and of India. It occurs in the West Indies and rarely in the United States. A familial tendency has been noted; males between the ages of twenty-five and thirty-five years are most frequently attacked. Ainhum has been variously described as a trophoneurosis, a parasitic disease, a form of leprosy, a result of repeated trauma and a sequel to the wearing of toe rings.

There is primary hypertrophy of the epidermis with the production of a sclerodermatous ring. As fibrosis and contraction ensue there is a secondary endarteritis and eventually a rarefying osteitis which destroys the proximal phalanx of the affected digit.

Symptoms.—The disease begins as a persistent or recurrent crack in the digitoplantar fold, this extends to encircle the toe, scar tissue develops and after the lapse of two years or more the normal structures of the proximal phalanx are replaced by a fibrous cord, the distal portion becomes edematous and often so large that it interferes with walking. Eventually the toe drops off. Pain and systemic manifestations are absent.

In fully developed cases amputation is necessary. During the period of scar formation cure has resulted from multiple longitudinal incisions through the constricting tissue followed by the application of salicylic acid ointments.

GANGOSA.

Synonym.—Rhinopharyngitis mutilans.

Definition.—A chronic disease of certain tropical regions presenting progressive ulceration of the pharynx, palate, larynx, nose and eyes, with destruction of bone and cartilage as well as soft tissues.

Many observers believe the condition to be a late manifestation of yaws. No specific causative agent has been demonstrated, although upward of 35 per cent of patients give a positive Wassermann reaction. Gangosa occurs frequently in Guam and is found in the Philippine, Fiji and Ladrone Islands and in the West Indies; natives only are attacked. The lesion is primarily granulomatous with superimposed secondary infection.

Symptoms.—The onset is with sore throat followed quickly by the appearance of a papule on the soft palate or posterior pharyngeal wall, a membrane forms and under it ulceration begins. The ulcerative process spreads rapidly involving soft parts and bones until palate, nose and often larynx and upper lip are destroyed. By way of the nasal ducts it may extend to the eyes. After about two years spontaneous remission occurs, usually only after horrible mutilation has been produced. Death may result from exhaustion or sepsis or from interference with the taking of food.

Gangosa must be separated from leprosy, lupus, cutaneous leishmaniasis and syphilis.

Treatment.—The administration of arsphenamine, bismuth and mercury as in yaws or syphilis has given encouraging results. Local antiseptic treatment is always necessary.

CHAPTER X.

THE FUNGUS DISEASES (NON–BACTERIAL).

By ISAAC IVAN LEMANN, M.D.

INTEGUMENT AND SKELETON.	GASTRO-INTESTINAL TRACT.
SPECIAL ORGANS.	CENTRAL NERVOUS SYSTEM.
INTERNAL ORGANS.	GENITO-URINARY SYSTEM.
RESPIRATORY TRACT.	

Introduction.—By fungi are meant the higher fungi, mycetes (eumycetes), as distinguished from bacteria or lower fungi (schizomycetes). They are unicellular or pluricellular filamentous plants of larger dimensions than bacteria which multiply by processes other than simple cell fission, usually by means of asexual or sexual spores. These higher fungi are divided into three classes:

1. Fungi imperfecti—hyphomycetes.
2. Ascomycetes.
3. Phycomycetes.

These divisions and further subdivisions are made on the basis of morphologic and cultural characteristics. Numerous members of all classes are pathogenic for man and lower animals. Much confusion exists in the terminology used in the literature. The chief species pathogenic for man are: actinomyces (nocardia, streptothrix), monilia, oidium, torula, mycetoma, sporothrix, saccharomyces, coccidioides, aspergillus, trichophyton.

Although mycology came into existence long before bacteriology, the latter's marvelous advances since the day of Pasteur have cast into the shade the relative importance of fungi in the production of human disease. Hooke, in 1677, saw with a magnifying lens filamentous fungi on a damask rose and has left drawings of them. Langenbeck, in 1839, discovered the thrush fungus, and Gruber the fungus of ringworm in 1844. It is only in the past twenty-five years that systemic fungus diseases have attracted any attention whatever. The number of case reports have greatly increased, and numerous comments have been made on the fact that these infections must be much more numerous and frequent than is usually thought. Castellani estimates that more than 20 per cent of tropical diseases in the strict sense of the word are caused by fungi. A very cursory review of the literature will show that diseases caused by fungi are by no means confined to the tropics and subtropics. The epidermophytoses (athlete's foot) are found universally throughout this country. Sanford gathered 678 cases of actinomycosis in the United States. Every one of the states except Utah and Wyoming was represented, the disease being especially prevalent in the upper Mississippi Valley and the north-western portion of the country. Systemic infections with other fungi (monilia, torula, coccidioides, aspergillus, sporothrix) have come from widely scattered parts of the United States. Many of the torula infections were reported from California. Ashford, commenting upon the universal and overwhelming prevalence of these microscopic saprophytes of plant life, comes to the conclusion that it is only because of a peculiar immunity of the animal phylum coupled with a lack of adaptation and low aggressivity for animals on the part of the fungus that the comparative infrequency of mycologic disease can be explained. Once, however, the adaptation is complete, few parasitic organisms can equal the pathogenic fungus in tenacity and seriousness of prognosis. Warfield remarks that there is no part of the civilized globe which has not had its case or cases of sporotrichosis. After 200 cases had been reported in the French literature, 1906 to 1910, no one reported his cases unless there was something unusual about them. The economic importance of mycoses is considerable, especially because of their similarity to tuberculosis and syphilis. Many cases may go through protracted periods of improper treatment because of false diagnosis. The preponderance of cases of actinomycosis among farmers and of sporotrichosis among manual workers gives some indication of their importance in matters of industrial health. In general a similarity exists in the clinical picture and in the problems of diagnosis and treatment; in order to avoid repetition, therefore, these will be described under the headings of the various parts of the body invaded rather than under those of the invading organism. Prognosis depends not only upon the part affected but also upon the type of invading organism. Not a single tissue of the body escapes infection by some kind of fungus.

Fungus Disease of the Integument and Skeleton.—Reference has already been made to the universal distribution of skin disease caused by tinea and other fungi. The diagnosis depends upon the characteristic skin picture, the location and upon the finding of the organisms in scrapings. The treatment consists in application of salicylic acid preparations (Whitfield's ointment and the like), iodine preparations and other fungicides, as well as the use of roentgen-ray. In addition to these more common conditions there are numerous other dermatomycoses and trichomycoses. For adequate descriptions and details of treatment the reader is referred to treatises on dermatology.

Of particular importance to the student of general medicine are those fungi affecting the skin, but extending also to the skeleton and to the viscera. Among these actinomycosis, sporotrichosis and blastomycosis deserve a more detailed description. In more than one-half the cases *actinomycosis* attacks the head and neck. In this form it finds its analogue in "lumpy jaw" of cattle. Most cases originate from the buccal cavity and spread to structures in relation to it and the pharynx. There is a brawny induration of the skin and underlying soft parts, suggestive of sarcoma. Suppuration occurs and fistulæ appear. Ulcerated lesions of the skin may resemble lupus or syphilis. There may be fever as in the cases with general systemic invasion.

Blastomycosis of the skin begins as a papule which later ulcerates

23

and forms abscesses. It resembles tuberculosis. If it remains confined to the skin the disease does not affect the general health, and runs a chronic course through years, with remissions and exacerbations. Metastases occur to bones and joints as well as to lungs, spleen, kidneys and other organs.

Sporotrichosis rivals disgusting phases of syphilis and tuberculosis. Characteristic of the disease are subcutaneous, more or less painless nodes which tend to suppurate. The impression is then given of a cold abscess. Ulceration or spontaneous opening occurs and when the abscess has been emptied the palpating finger finds thick, raised margins around the central depression. The abscess fluid is at first thick and viscous, later greenish-yellow and oily, sometimes tinged with blood. The nodes or gummata may involve the periosteum. In another form there is a single chancre-like lesion, usually on the extremities (hand); on the nose it presents a rhinoscleroma-like swelling. Some other lesions have been described as eczematoid, verrucose, vesicular, pustular, follicular, pityriasiform, impetiginous, ecthymatous, varioloid or even pemphigoid. These and other lesions resembling syphilides and tuberculides may occur without nodes. Adenopathies are rare and constitutional symptoms are usually missing. Widespread visceral involvement may occur (see below). The testicle is the ultimate site of election.

Mycetoma.—Infection of the foot (Madura foot) usually follows a penetrating, sometimes a crushing wound. The foot swells, a small vesicle appears which later breaks and discharges a thin, bloody fluid. Following this a sinus is found extending into the deeper structures. The opening of the sinus is usually on the top of a button-like projection. The discharge is a thick, foul, oily fluid, containing granules suggesting fish roe. Similar sinuses appear in other places in the foot indicating a growth and spread of the fungus in the underlying tissue. While Madura foot is chiefly a tropical disease, a few cases have been reported in the United States.

Special Organs.—Fungus disease of the eye and the ear also occur.

Internal Fungus Disease.—Thrush, characterized by the production of creamy white patches on the mucous membranes of the mouth, is caused by various species of monilia, oïdium, endomyces and saccharomyces. Castellani found another type of thrush (yellowish or brownish patches) occurring in the tropics. He also described larger patches of thin pellucid film resembling leukoplakia which he found to be due to a yeast-like fungus living in symbiosis with a bacillus. The buccal cavity may also be attacked by actinomyces and sporothrix. (See under Tongue, below.) In acute tonsillitis, monilia, saccharomyces, cryptococcus, oïdium, hemispora and aspergillus have been found. The tonsils are covered with creamy white patches, extending sometimes to the soft palate and pharynx and even to the larynx. Diphtheria is falsely diagnosed. Chronic infections of the tonsils due to nocardias (actinomyces, sporothrix) cause not only sore throat but often an unpleasant odor to the breath. Objective evidence is the appearance of small, whitish, yellowish spots which represent the surface of granules contained in the tonsillar crypts. Aspergillus infection causes small superficial ulcers on the posterior wall of the pharynx and yellowish spots of various sizes on the uvula and faucial pillars.

Respiratory Tract.—Fungus disease may occur by extension from the mouth and fauces or by metastasis from skin lesions. Cases have been reported where the lesions in the respiratory tract apparently have been primary. The invading fungi reported have been actinomyces, sporothrix, monilia, coccidioides and aspergillus. Fungus disease of the lungs should by no means be regarded as rare, and its presence should be suspected where the clinical picture is that of pulmonary tuberculosis, but where repeated examinations of the sputum have failed to reveal acid-fast bacilli. Cough, profuse expectoration, hemoptysis, fever, sweats, emaciation, may all be present. The writer is convinced that the routine examination of sputa exclusively by staining of dried smears for acid-fast bacilli is wrong. A fresh, moist specimen should be mounted and examined; also the routine treatment of the specimen with caustic soda solution to permit the demonstration of mycelia would be profitable. Other cases of fungus disease masquerade as chronic bronchitis, subacute pneumonia and bronchial asthma. In some instances neoplasms of the lung, syphilis of the lung and abscess of the lung have all been considered in differential diagnosis. The diagnosis is, of course, dependent chiefly upon the finding of the causal organism in the sputum, but it must be remembered that fungus disease, tuberculosis and neoplastic disease are not mutually exclusive. Fungus disease may be superimposed upon either of the other two and constitute merely a complication. Both tubercle bacilli and fungi may be found in the same specimen. A patient with metastatic lung neoplasm may exhibit fungi in the sputum. The context of the history is, therefore, important. The physical examination yields evidence of bronchitis, of consolidation or of cavitation. Roentgen-ray examination of the chest contributes valuable information. Fungus disease of the lung produces fluffy, "cotton puff" shadows, usually scattered throughout the pulmonary fields. These are so characteristic that the roentgenologist often feels justified in making a diagnosis without knowing the results of the sputum examination. Such a report, however, is not infallible, for the writer has seen beautiful "fungus shadows" (so interpreted by a most competent radiologist) in the lung fields of a patient with multiple lung metastases from a sarcoma of the leg. Repeated examination of the sputum showed no fungi and none were demonstrated in the lung postmortem, while the metastatic neoplasms were proven.

Fungus Disease of the Gastro-intestinal Tract.—Actinomycosis rarely occurs primarily in the tongue. It may occur there by metastasis or by direct extension. Grossly, the lesion must be differentiated from tertiary syphilis, tuberculosis, epithelioma, inflammatory cyst, fibroma. It rarely ulcerates, and the sinuses so often seen in fungus disease elsewhere are not present. "Aspiration of the contents of the suppurating nodule is usually unsatisfactory; it is best to excise the entire nodule for diagnosis. Only a few of the characteristic granules necessary for a positive diagnosis may be present within the nodule, and unless these granules are secured in the small specimen removed

for microscopic examination it is impossible to make a diagnosis."
Sporotrichosis causing ulceration of the tongue and wrongly diagnosed
cancer has been proven by cultures from the ulcerated surface and
promptly cured by appropriate medication.

The writer has found no report of fungus affection of the stomach.
Ashford attributes sprue to Monilia psilosis infection of the intestine
which he has found in the stools as well as in the blood stream of
patients with sprue. Ashford's contention, however, is not universally accepted. Actinomycosis of the small intestine occurs, but
apparently is rare. More frequent are reports of actinomycosis of
the cecum and appendix. Here it may be symptomless for a while,
giving finally the picture of acute appendicitis, or it may cause a slowly-
growing mass, suggesting the probable diagnosis of neoplasm. At
operation the process may be found to have extended to the abdominal
wall, thus increasing the impression of malignant disease. Only the
histologic examination of the removed mass will demonstrate its true
nature. Such affections may occur without the presence of actinomycosis elsewhere, or at least its recognition. Sporotrichal infection of
the large bowel, causing sudden diarrhea with blood and mucus in the
stools, has been reported in a woman with sporotricosis of the finger
nails. She was in the habit of biting the nails. Sporothrix was
demonstrated in the scrapings from the nails and cultures from the
stools. Involvement of the liver has followed or accompanied actinomycotic infection of the cecum and appendix. Blastocystis has been
found in the stools of patients suffering with vague indefinite symptoms
or without any. Apparently it may be implanted in the lower bowel.
Whether it is to be regarded as truly parasitic and a cause of disease
is at this time uncertain.

Central Nervous System.—Torula infections have a predisposition
for the central nervous system. In 11 authentic cases of torula gathered
by Sheppe from the literature, the central nervous system was the part
chiefly involved in 9. Hemiplegias and monoplegias associated with
cranial nerve involvements are frequent. All of the clinical signs of
brain tumor may be present. The diagnosis of senile dementia and
dementia paralytica was made in 2 cases which proved to be torula
infections. When the cord is involved, the pressure of the spinal fluid
is moderately raised. The yeast cells may be found in the spinal
fluid obtained by lumbar puncture, but may be mistaken for leukocytes which they superficially resemble. A diagnosis of tuberculous
meningitis is frequently falsely made. The central nervous system
has been invaded by actinomyces, blastomyces, coccidioides, usually
as a part of a widespread systemic infection, producing as indicated
above the clinical picture of brain abscess, brain tumor and meningitis.
These organisms, too, may be found in the spinal fluid. Blastomycosis
of the meninges without lesions elsewhere has also been reported. In
such cases it would seem probable that the original focus had healed.

Genito-urinary System.—In Israel's first case of primary actinomycosis of the kidney (1889) no other focus was found and the patient
remained well eleven years after the nephrectomy. In his second case
the disease began with fever, cough and pain in the region of the

twelfth rib. The cough subsided after five weeks but the fever persisted. Edema developed over the region of pain and a diagnosis of perirenal abscess was made. When nephrectomy was performed, actinomycosis of the kidney was found. Six more cases are in the literature where the actinomycosis was apparently primary in the kidney. Some of them, however, have other parts of the body involved, lungs, brain, vertebræ and peritoneum. One patient presented the clinical picture of pyelonephritis and cystitis. In another there was a mass in the groin which softened and was incised several times, but a sinus remained. Later there was a mass in the right lumbar region which broke down and discharged pus containing actinomyces. The urine showed blood and pus. The patient remained well eleven months after the operation. Besides this apparently primary actinomycotic involvement of the urinary tract, infections of this tract with other varieties of fungi (blastomyces) have been reported, but only in connection with wide dissemination throughout the body. Castellani has reported a few cases of mycotic urethritis which is apparently rare. He had seen several cases in the tropics and a few in the Balkans and southern Europe, one in New Orleans. The urethral discharges were whitish, yellowish, or reddish, according to the type of invading organism.

Reference should be made to the predilection of sporotrichal infection of the testicle. Thirty odd cases of actinomycosis of the tubes and ovaries have been reported.

Pathology and Pathogenesis.—The extent of the pathologic changes caused by the various mycoses has been indicated to a large extent by a description of the clinical picture. The histopathology is essentially that of an infectious granuloma. The mode of infection probably varies considerably. The sporotrichal and mycetoma infections apparently occur as a result of punctured wounds and other local injuries. Infection with actinomyces apparently occurs frequently through the mouth. Chewing of infected wisps of hay or blades of grass or the presence of a carious tooth in which the saprophyte exists and develops pathogenicity have all been blamed. It has been suggested, too, that the respiratory tract may be primarily infected by fungi through inhalation of infected dust. Whether the primary infection occurs in the integument, through the respiratory tract, the buccal mucous membranes, or the intestinal tract, there is considerable evidence that it is conveyed through the blood stream to distant parts. Reports of the finding of fungi in the blood stream are not uncommon.

Diagnosis.—Diagnosis depends upon the recognition of the causative organisms in discharges, secretions from the sinuses and abscesses, or in the sputum, urine, spinal fluid, blood and removed tissue. Highly important is the attitude of suspicion upon the part of the observer toward all chronic inflammatory diseases marked by ulceration and chronic sinus formation. This suspicion should be still further strengthened by observation of the so-called sulphur granules peculiar to actinomycosis.

Prognosis.—The fungus disease confined to the integument has, as has already been indicated, a not unfavorable outlook. Visceral mycoses, however, have a most serious prognosis. Pulmonary infections with actinomyces and blastomyces are practically invariably fatal. So also are the cases of involvement of the central nervous system with whatever form of fungus. Gastro-intestinal mycosis carries a mortality of 60 to 70 per cent. Infections of the kidney, when the nephrectomy is done early enough, are apparently not very unfavorable.

Treatment.—In general, the iodides and various iodine preparations are of prime importance in the treatment of all mycoses. The iodides should be given in massive doses to the point of toleration. The intravenous use of arsphenamine has found some advocates. Roentgenrays and radium have often proven valuable. Where infected tissues can be removed, as by nephrectomy or by appendectomy, or where localized abscesses and sinuses can be properly drained or even excised, surgery is indicated. Amputation seems to be the only adequate treatment of mycetoma.

REFERENCES.

CASTELLANI, ALDO: Fungi and Fungous Diseases, The Adolph Gehrmann Lectures of Illinois College of Medicine, 1926, Arch. Dermat. and Syphilol., October, November, December, 1927; January, February, March, 1928.
D'AUNOY, RIGNEY, and BEVEN, J. L.: Systemic Blastomycosis, Jour. Lab. and Clin. Med., 1930, 16, 124.
FOERSTER, HARRY R.: Sporotrichosis, Am. Jour. Med. Sci., 1924, 167, 54.
JOHNS, F. M.: Five Cases of Pneumonia in Which Monilia Pulmonalis Were Demonstrated in the Fresh Sputum, New Orleans Med. and Surg. Jour., 1924, 77, 8.
NEW, GORDON B., and FIGI, FRED A.: Actinomycosis of the Tongue, Am. Jour. Med. Sci., 1922, 163, 507.
PAGENSTECHER, G. A.: Third Case of Mycetoma, Jour. Am. Med. Assn., 1924, 82, 1692.
PRUETT, J. F., and WAYSON, N. E.: Granuloma Coccidioides, Jour. Am. Med Assn., 1923, 81, 1607.
SANFORD, A. H.: Distribution of Actinomycosis in the United States, Jour. Am. Med. Assn., 1923, 81, 655.
SCHENK, B. R.: On Refractory Subcutaneous Abscesses Caused by Fungus Possibly Related to the Sporotricha, Bull. Johns Hopkins Hosp., 1898, 9, 286.
SHEPPE, W. M.: Torula Infection in Man, Am. Jour. Med. Sci., 1924, 167, 91.
SNOKE, P. O.: Actinomycosis: A Report of Five Cases—With Four Autopsies— Two Showing Involvement of the Central Nervous System, Am. Jour. Med. Sci., 1928, 175, 69.
STEINFIELD, EDWARD: Bronchomycosis, Jour. Am. Med. Assn., 1924, 82, 83.
WADE, H. A., and BEL, G. S.: Critical Consideration of Systemic Blastomycosis, Arch. Int. Med., 1916, 18, 103.
WARFIELD, L. M.: Report of a Case of Disseminated Gummatous Sporotrichosis with Lung Metastasis, Am. Jour. Med Sci., 1922, 164, 82.
WEIDMAN, F. D., and FREEMAN, W.: Yeast Cells, Jour. Am. Med. Assn., 1924, 83, 1163.
WILHELM, C. M.: The Primary Meningeal Forms of Systemic Blastomycosis, Am. Jour. Med. Sci., 1925, 169, 696.
WRIGHT, J. H.: Biology of the Microörganism of Actinomycosis, Jour. Med. Res., 1905, 13, 349.

PART II.

SYSTEMIC DISEASES.

CHAPTER XI.

DISEASES OF THE HEART

By FRED M. SMITH, M.D.

GENERAL DISCUSSION OF DISEASES OF THE HEART.
  Etiology.
  Symptoms.
RHEUMATIC HEART DISEASE.
BACTERIAL ENDOCARDITIS.
  Acute Bacterial Endocarditis.
  Subacute Bacterial Endocarditis.
ARTERIOSCLEROTIC HEART DISEASE (Hypertensive Heart Disease).
  General Consideration.
  Angina Pectoris.
  Coronary Occlusion.
SYPHILITIC HEART DISEASE.
THYROTOXIC HEART DISEASE.
CONGENITAL HEART DISEASE.
DISEASES OF THE PERICARDIUM.
  Acute Fibrinous Pericarditis.
  Pericarditis with Effusion.
  Adherent Pericardium (Chronic Adhesive Pericarditis).
CHRONIC VALVULAR HEART DISEASE.
  Mitral Valve Disease.
  Aortic Valve Disease.

CHRONIC VALVULAR HEART DISEASE.
  Tricuspid Valve Disease.
  Pulmonary Valve Disease.
MYOCARDITIS.
FUNCTIONAL DISORDERS OF THE HEART.
  Cardiac Neuroses—Irritable Heart.
DISORDERS OF THE HEART BEAT.
  Normal Cardiac Mechanism.
  Sinus Arrhythmia.
  Disorders of Heart Beat Due to Heart Block.
    Sino-auricular Block.
    Auriculo-ventricular Block.
    Bundle Branch Block.
  Disorders of Heart Beat Due to Abnormal Impulse Formation.
    Premature Contraction.
    Simple Paroxysmal Tachycardia.
    Auricular Flutter.
    Auricular Fibrillation.
    Pulsus Alternans.
TREATMENT OF CONGESTIVE HEART FAILURE.

GENERAL DISCUSSION OF DISEASES OF THE HEART.

Etiologic Types.—Rheumatic Heart Disease.—This is one of the most important forms of heart disease and is largely responsible for cardiac disability during early life. During the past five years it comprised approximately 28 per cent of all the heart disease at the University of Iowa. In the study by Wyckoff and Lingg, 80 per cent of the cardiac disease between the ages of ten and nineteen years, 70 per cent between the ages of twenty and twenty-nine years and approximately 58 per cent between the ages of thirty and thirty-nine years, were attributed to rheumatic fever. Other and more recent statistics, including a series of cases from New England and Virginia, are in general accord with these findings. This leaves a fairly large group during the first and second decades in which the etiologic factor is not known. It is quite possible that there are many instances in which the cardiac involvement is the only expression of rheumatic infection, and further study may show that certain of those which have heretofore been placed in the unknown group should be classed as rheumatic heart disease. The incidence of rheumatic heart disease appears to be considerably lower in certain of the southern states.

Other Types of Cardiac Infection.—Certain other types of infection are occasionally responsible for cardiac damage. In serious and fatal cases of diphtheria the myocardium may be extensively injured by the toxin. Fortunately this type of myocarditis may be prevented by early diagnosis and the administration of adequate amounts of anti-toxin. Scarlet fever is at times complicated by an endocarditis or pericarditis. The cardiac involvement in some cases, particularly those with arthritis, has been attributed to an associated rheumatic infection. In rare instances endocarditis has followed measles and whooping cough. The exact etiologic relationship between these diseases and the ensuing cardiac disorder is not known. Tuberculosis, pneumonia, typhoid fever, gonorrhea, erysipelas and septic infections represent other possible causes of heart disease. In tuberculosis the cardiac impairment is mainly dependent on involvement of the pericardium with the subsequent development of adhesions. The other infections of the latter group are more frequently instrumental in producing an acute or subacute bacterial endocarditis.

Arteriosclerotic Heart Disease.—This form of cardiac disease dominates the later years of life in an even more striking fashion than the rheumatic type does the earlier. In the etiologic study by Wyckoff and Lingg, comprising all age groups, 25 per cent were designated as rheumatic, and 40 per cent arteriosclerotic heart disease. The incidence in our series of 1329 cases was approximately 28 per cent and 50 per cent, respectively. This type of cardiac disability begins to be manifested in a significant manner after forty years and is largely responsible for the high mortality-rate from heart disease after fifty years of age. In New York State, exclusive of New York City, 90 per cent of all deaths from heart disease occurred after the age of forty-five years, and 60 per cent of these were assigned to the arteriosclerotic form (Halsey).

Syphilitic Heart Disease.—This is one of the more serious forms of cardiovascular disease. The course, after the onset of the symptoms, is usually progressively downward. The incidence in the United States, as determined by the various statistical studies, ranged from 4 to 39 per cent of the total cardiac disability. The highest incidence is reported from the southern states, where it would seem that the prevalence of syphilis among the negroes and the relative infrequency of rheumatic fever are important factors. Cardiovascular disability due to syphilis is occasionally observed between the ages of twenty and thirty years, but is seen more often between the ages of forty and fifty-five years.

Thyrotoxic Heart Disease.—The cardiac disability associated with toxic adenoma and exophthalmic goiter constitutes an important form of heart disease in certain sections. The incidence is greatest in the Great Lakes region and the Pacific Northwest, and relatively low in certain of the eastern and southern states. In a large series of cases of organic heart disease reported from Oregon (Coffen), 11 per cent were attributed to a thyrotoxicosis. The incidence in New York is 1.1 per cent (Wyckoff and Lingg), in New England 3 per cent (White and Jones), in Texas 1.3 per cent (Stone and Van Zant) and at the University of Iowa 8.7 per cent. This form of cardiac disease is most common between the ages of thirty and forty-five years. Within recent years a form of cardiac disability has been ascribed to hypothyroidism.

Congenital Heart Disease.—The various congenital anomalies of the heart and great vessels comprise only a small percentage of the total incidence of cardiac disease. The major defects are not compatible with life, and many of the victims survive at most but a few months or years. Many of the minor forms are not recognized during life and are of importance only insofar as they may contribute to the development of a cardiac infection.

Conditions Contributing to a Cardiac Disability.—Chronic pulmonary disease, such as bronchitis, fibrosis and emphysema, promotes the disability of an already damaged heart, and upper respiratory infections not infrequently precipitate cardiac failure. Deformities of the chest and spine, particularly kyphoscoliosis, by producing a displacement and possibly a compression of the great vessels, as well as by seriously curtailing the peripheral vascular bed of the lungs, may impose a serious handicap on the heart. Obesity increases the work of the heart and perhaps favors the development of arteriosclerosis. High-grade anemia, especially of the pernicious type, occasionally unmasks a latent cardiac disability; the cardiac symptoms may, in fact, be the first to attract the attention of the patient. Excessive physical exertion very often promotes the onset of cardiac failure after sixty years of age. Pregnancy is another factor which may contribute to an existing impairment in the cardiac function, especially if mitral stenosis is the antecedent lesion.

Symptoms.—Dyspnea, substernal or precordial pain and palpitation are the most significant symptoms. Other symptoms of a varied nature from a secondary impairment in the function of the different organs frequently occurs.

Dyspnea.—Various explanations have been advanced for the dyspnea in heart disease. According to the more recent investigations, however, the mechanism has not been established. At present it would seem that a reduced vital capacity is the most important factor. Shortness of breath on exertion is one of the earliest and most frequent indications of impaired cardiac function. In 100 cases studied by Pratt, it appeared as the initial symptom in 60. This reaction, however, is significant only when compared to the normal response to a given exercise and with other factors excluded. Certain individuals normally have a limited tolerance to exertion. In the early stages of cardiac failure the patient begins to notice that he becomes winded on exertion that ordinarily has not caused discomfort. Later, he finds that less exercise is required to induce the shortness of breath. Frequently, at this time, edema begins to appear in the ankles and if the impairment in the cardiac function progresses the dyspnea becomes more evident and possibly present while at rest even in the upright position—orthopnea. Under these circumstances, the mere change to a recumbent position may produce intense shortness of breath. This change in posture further reduces the already limited vital capacity. Usually, by this time there is extensive edema with marked congestion of the lungs, engorgement of the liver and possibly fluid in the pleural and peritoneal cavities. This constitutes the advanced stage of congestive failure.

Paroxysmal Dyspnea.—*Cardiac Asthma.*—This form of dyspnea is invariably associated with an advanced impairment of cardiac function, and is observed most frequently in the arteriosclerotic and syphilitic forms of heart disease. In the beginning the patient is awakened from a sound sleep, usually during the early hours of the morning, by intense dyspnea, and is obliged to sit up in order to get his breath. The dyspnea is usually accompanied by a hacking cough, wheezing and a tight sensation in the chest. In the more advanced stage the subject raises frothy sputum which may be blood-tinged. After a time the dyspnea gradually subsides and the patient is able to resume his sleep. As the condition progresses, the individual may be awakened many times during the night and finally reach the stage when he is no longer able to sleep in the recumbent position because of being awakened suddenly by the respiratory distress.

Acute Pulmonary Edema.—This is closely related to paroxysmal dyspnea and occurs in the same type of cardiac disease. The patient who is subject to paroxysmal dyspnea may at any time have an attack of pulmonary edema. This is manifested by the sudden onset of intense air hunger. The cyanosis is extreme, the coughing violent, copious, frothy, blood-tinged sputum is raised, and numerous moist râles are heard throughout the lungs. The prognosis is grave and should recovery occur there is always the possibility of a recurrence.

Cheyne-Stokes Breathing.—This form of breathing is commonly observed in advanced cardiac failure of arteriosclerotic origin, particularly that associated with a hypertension and is of grave prognostic significance. It also occurs in uremia and diseases of the central nervous system, especially with acute increase of the intracranial pressure. There are various grades of this condition. The earliest stage consists of a periodic increase and diminution in the size of the respiration. Periodic breathing of this general type is often noted during sleep in infants and elderly subjects, may follow the administration of hypnotics, such as morphine and chloral, and is common in high altitudes. That referred to in the present discussion and as originally described is characterized by alternating periods of apnea and hyperpnea occurring in regular sequence. In the beginning it appears only during sleep but in advanced stages is continuous. During the period of apnea which may last from twenty to thirty seconds the patient becomes drowsy and often falls asleep. With the subsequent onset of breathing the respiration gradually becomes more labored and when fully established the subject is aroused or awakened with a start at the height of the hyperpnea. The hyperpnea then subsides in the same manner in which it appeared and sleep is again resumed with the return of the apnea. Various explanations have been advanced for this condition and there is still diversity of opinion concerning the mechanism.

Pain.—Substernal or precordial discomfort, ranging in degree from a feeling of fullness or heaviness to the agonizing and terrifying pain which occurs in certain instances of angina pectoris and coronary occlusion, is a common complaint in cardiac disease. The pain of angina pectoris and coronary occlusion is the most distinctive of all cardiac symptoms. In the former, the distress is invariably precipitated by anything which increases the work of the heart, more particularly exercise and excitement. It is generally first felt somewhere under the sternum, usually over the upper or lower regions, and frequently involves the precordium. It may later extend to the left shoulder and down the left arm, and in the more severe form may be felt in both arms. In certain instances the pain is transmitted to the neck and head. The distribution varies considerably in different individuals. In some the pain or paresthesia may appear first at a peripheral point, as in the wrist, arm, neck or head, and later be felt in the chest; in others the pain may be confined to the lower sternum and epigastrium, or even entirely to the upper abdomen. The distress in its mild form consists of a substernal feeling of fullness or heaviness or of constriction. It is often first noticed while climbing a hill or going up stairs or during excitement, and promptly disappears after the exercise is discontinued or the excitement subsides. Later the distress is more easily precipitated, of a more severe character, and possibly transmitted to the various regions mentioned. The pain of coronary occlusion is of a similar character, but often more severe, possibly has a wider range of distribution, and may persist in a minor form even after repeated injections of morphine. It is likely to occur while at rest, and very often awakens the patient from a sound sleep. This pain is frequently most intense over the lower sternal region and may likewise be confined almost entirely to the epigastrium.

Precordial distress often assumes other forms. It may be dull and more or less continuous, or transient, sharp and stabbing in character. It is frequently a prominent feature of acute rheumatic heart disease, particularly when there is involvement of the pericardium. It is occasionally observed in chronic valvular heart disease, especially mitral stenosis and aortic insufficiency, frequently occurs with abnormal cardiac mechanisms, such as premature contractions, paroxysmal tachycardia, auricular fibrillation and auricular flutter, may result from the toxic influence of tobacco and is one of the outstanding symptoms of the effort syndrome. In such cases a hypersensitive state of the nervous system is often an important factor. If there is doubt concerning implication of the heart, the possibility of intercostal neuralgia, nerve root involvement from a destructive lesion in the spine, hypertrophic osteoarthritis, or a mediastinal tumor should be considered.

Palpitation.—This symptom is usually not of great importance as an indication of a significant impairment of the cardiac function. It is, however, frequently the first to direct attention to the heart, and often causes great concern on the part of the patient. The occurrence after violent exertion or intense and sudden excitement represents a normal physiologic reaction. It is frequently associated with premature contractions, paroxysmal tachycardia, auricular fibrillation and auricular flutter. Consciousness of the heart is a common symptom in thyrotoxicosis, a prominent feature of the effort syndrome, and may be one of the early complaints in pulmonary tuberculosis. It is not infrequently observed during convalescence from various infections, during the menopause and in high-grade anemias. Other factors, as abdominal flatulence, fatigue, coffee, alcohol and tobacco, may induce or aggravate palpitation. Since this symptom may be associated with such a variety of extracardiac conditions, a careful history and a detailed examination are necessary in order to determine its significance.

Other Symptoms.—Many of the symptoms of heart disease are produced by secondary disturbances in the function of such organs as the lungs, gastro-intestinal tract and brain.

A *cough* usually indicates pulmonary congestion and may be a prominent feature in cases in which the cardiac failure develops during acute or chronic bronchitis, in cardiac asthma, acute pulmonary edema and aortic aneurysm. The sputum is ordinarily scanty except in chronic bronchitis or in pulmonary edema. In the latter, the expectoration of a large amount of frothy, blood-tinged sputum is one of the characteristic symptoms. Slight hemoptysis is seen not infrequently in mitral stenosis, and occasionally a frank hemorrhage occurs. *Abdominal discomfort* which is not referable to angina pectoris or coronary occlusion is often a conspicuous feature of early cardiac failure. A feeling of fullness or heaviness and the consciousness of gas after meals are usually the first of these symptoms to appear. They are followed by soreness in the right upper quadrant caused by engorgement of the liver, and in some instances by anorexia, and even nausea and vomiting. The digestive disturbance is due to deranged gastric function consequent upon passive congestion, but it is frequently mistaken for a sign of digitalis intoxication. When the hepatic congestion develops rapidly the distress caused by distention of the capsule may be severe enough to simulate an acute surgical condition. The pain in pericarditis may be referred to the upper abdomen by way of the phrenic nerves.

Cerebral manifestations, such as headaches, dizziness and faintness, are common in arteriosclerotic heart disease and are not infrequently observed in association with aortic stenosis or insufficiency, various types of abnormal cardiac mechanism and in the effort syndrome. The Adams-Stokes syndrome is occasionally encountered. This syndrome includes dizziness, faintness, syncope, possibly convulsions and a very slow heart-rate; it is frequently accompanied by, but is not synonymous with, auriculo-ventricular heart block. Psychosis sometimes develops during the course of cardiac failure and may be very disturbing. An occlusion of a cerebral vessel sometimes occurs from an embolus originating in the heart.

Fatigability may be one of the earliest and most prominent symptoms and often progresses to a feeling of exhaustion. A loss of 10 to 20 pounds in weight is not uncommon in more prolonged and advanced forms of congestive failure.

RHEUMATIC HEART DISEASE.

Rheumatic heart disease includes the cardiac involvement associated with or following the various manifestations of rheumatic fever, and that which is represented at a later stage by mitral stenosis, even though the history of an etiologic factor is lacking. The present discussion deals only with the acute manifestations of this disease.

Etiology.—The etiology of rheumatic fever has been discussed elsewhere and here only certain features will be considered. Rheumatic fever is an infectious disease and, from a clinical standpoint, appears to be closely related to streptococcus infection. While the causative organism has not been demonstrated, clinical experience has focused attention on the upper respiratory tract, particularly the tonsils and lymphoid tissue in the naso-pharynx, as the site of the origin of the infection. Swift states that in more than one-half of the patients the acute onset of rheumatic fever is preceded by sore throat or tonsillitis, and that in others there is often a history of acute infection of the upper respiratory passages or lungs. Coburn has recently emphasized the importance of upper respiratory infections and the close association of the hemolytic streptococcus with the onset and recrudescence of rheumatic fever. The greatest incidence of rheumatic heart disease falls between the ages of five and fifteen years. In a large series of cases studied in New York City (Wilson, Lingg and Croxford), 98.4 per cent had the initial infection before the age of fifteen years, and the average age at the time of onset was seven and three-tenths years. However, it may occur at any time during adult life, appearing occasionally in the third or fourth decade or even later.

The incidence seems to be slightly higher in the female sex. All races are apparently susceptible. Certain statistics point to a greater prevalence among the Italians and Irish, but it is possible that other factors may explain this apparent difference. In the United States, the incidence is high in the North and relatively low in the southern states. This form of heart disease is, in general, more prevalent in the north temperate zone throughout the world and relatively rare in the tropics and subtropical regions. It occurs more frequently during the wet and cold seasons of the year. The social and economic status of the individual is perhaps one of the important factors, for it is well established that rheumatic heart disease is more common among the poorer classes in which the resistance to infection is no doubt reduced through crowded living quarters and inadequate clothing and food.

Pathology.—Recent pathologic studies have emphasized the systemic nature of the rheumatic infection. This would indicate that the heart is probably always involved. The Aschoff bodies characterized by a collection of large cells with vesicular nuclei, frequently multiple, lymphocytes, plasma cells and occasionally polymorphonuclear leukocytes about a small area of central necrosis is the typical lesion in the myocardium. These lesions occur about or in the immediate vicinity of the small arteries or arterioles, frequently invade the adventitia and produce intimal proliferation which may result in the closure of the vessel. They may be widely distributed throughout the heart but are usually more numerous in the left ventricle, especially in the subendocardial tissue about the valve rings. Lesions in the right heart are more likely to be found in close proximity to the fibrinous ring of the tricuspid valve. While the entire heart is implicated to a varying degree, producing a true pancarditis, the involvement of the valves usually dominates the picture. These structures are swollen and thickened even in the early stages of the disease. In the past, attention was focused on the changes in the endocardium of the valves, particularly vegetations, but now these are regarded as being secondary to the interstitial valvulitis. The vegetations are tiny grayish-pink bodies arranged in a row along the line of the closure of the valve leaflets. They are firm and adherent to the underlying tissue and when rubbed off leave a rough and granular surface. The location with reference to the margin of the valve is apparently determined by the continuous trauma to which this portion of the leaflet is exposed. The endocardium of the left auricle may also be invaded. These lesions were first described by MacCollum and have since been observed by Thayer, von Glahn and others. They occur with considerable frequency and usually appear in the form of corrugated or puckered patches of thickened endocardium extending upward from the root of the posterior leaflet of the mitral valve. The area of involvement may be small but is often quite extensive, and in rare instances, as pointed out by Sacks, may affect the entire endocardial surface of the left auricle.

The mitral valve is the one that is most commonly invaded and is probably always damaged to some extent. The aortic valves come next in frequency, followed in order by the tricuspid, and in rare instances, the pulmonary valve. The tricuspid valve presents structural alterations more frequently than generally believed. Libman reported typical rheumatic vegetations of this valve in 66 per cent and Thayer in 44 per cent of their cases. The involvement of this valve, however, is often confined to a limited area and therefore rarely permits the development of a high-grade stenosis. Usually more than one valve is damaged, particularly in the more extensive form of the disease. Occasionally the aortic valve alone is involved but this is rather rare and when it occurs other etiologic possibilities should be considered. The damage to the valve structures ultimately results in a combined insufficiency and stenosis in which either effect may predominate. The production of a significant stenosis usually requires years, and the more advanced form commonly follows the chronic and recurrent type of rheumatic fever in which, not infrequently, the joint manifestations are lacking.

The pericardium is frequently affected and, according to Coombs, the incidence is very high in those dying from rheumatic heart disease during the first and second decades of life. In certain instances the pericarditis, either because of the effusion or later through the subsequent formation of adhesions, may impose an excessive burden on the heart.

Symptoms.—The symptoms vary in a remarkable manner, depending on the activity of the rheumatic infection and the extent of the cardiac involvement. A child may have mild rheumatic fever for weeks, months and possibly years, accompanied by slowly progressive damage of the heart which can scarcely be detected. Cardiac manifestations lacking, the symptoms continue to be those of a systemic reaction to a low-grade infection, as evidenced by fatigability, poor appetite, malnutrition and pallor, with intervals during which there is a slight elevation of temperature. Other cases show varying degrees of arthritis, while in some the focal expression is that of a chorea, or these two manifestations of the infection may occur at different periods in the same individual. In general, the arthritis is more apt to predominate in the older individual, and the cardiac damage is less likely to be a conspicuous feature. Recurrent upper respiratory infections, particularly tonsillitis, less often otitis media and mastoiditis, or certain infectious diseases such as scarlet fever, precipitate the cardiac involvement. In certain instances the cardiac involvement may be the only evidence of rheumatic infection.

Symptoms referable to the heart do not ordinarily appear until there is extensive cardiac damage. There is not infrequently, however, a feeling of heavinesss or fleeting twinges of pain in the precordium. Occasionally it is more severe and referred to the left shoulder, the left axilla, or even down the inner side of the left arm and may thus resemble that of angina pectoris. Swift and Hitchcock made a careful study of the subjective sensations over the precordium in rheumatic fever and found that a fairly large percentage of their cases experienced discomfort at some time during the course of the disease. This discomfort was generally associated with a demonstrable involvement of the heart, and the frequency with which it occurred was roughly proportional to the intensity of the rheumatic infection. In a few cases they observed a recurring pain in the left shoulder which was at first ascribed to a persistent inflammation of the joint but finally attributed to the diseased heart. At times the patients are conscious of the heart because of premature contractions or other forms of abnormal mechanism. In some the palpitation is a part of an effort syndrome that may follow any severe or prolonged infection.

In certain instances the picture is complicated or dominated by a pericarditis with possibly marked dyspnea or perhaps severe precordial or upper abdominal pain.

Objective Signs.—These depend on the stage and extent of cardiac damage. In the early stage they may be so indefinite that the cardiac involvement is overlooked. The systolic murmur at the apex is usually the first feature to direct attention to the heart. In the beginning, this is probably more dependent on dilatation of the auriculo-ventricular ring than on an alteration of the valve leaflets. The murmur is soft and blowing in character and generally confined to the apical region. Later, it changes in quality and is heard over a larger area, particularly to the left toward the axilla and perhaps posteriorly in the left interscapular region. The subsequent alteration in the character, and particularly the later harsher aspect is dependent on changes in the structure of the valve. The accelerated cardiac rate, and possibly an elevation of the temperature out of proportion to the arthritis or other causes, and a demonstrable increase in the area of cardiac dullness, are the most important findings. Occasionally a faint diastolic murmur of aortic insufficiency is heard over the aortic area or along the left border of the sternum. Disturbance in cardiac rhythm, more particularly premature contractions are not infrequently encountered and may be among the earliest manifestations of a cardiac involvement. The cardiac sounds often undergo a change in quality, and a canter rhythm is commonly noted. The latter may occur early in the disease, and with the accelerated rate possibly overshadows other findings. When the heart is more extensively damaged the murmurs are generally more evident and the cardiac enlargement is at once apparent. These findings are usually associated with or follow other acute manifestations of rheumatic fever. In certain instances the disease is so overwhelming that cardiac failure and death follow within a few weeks or months. The occurrence of a pericardial rub is rather common but often transient, and occasionally the findings are greatly altered by the development of a pericardial effusion.

Electrocardiographic Findings.—Changes frequently occur in the electrocardiogram. These consist of irregularities in the cardiac rhythm, particularly premature contractions, increase in the duration of the $P-R$ interval and alterations in the $Q-R-S-T$ complexes. Premature contractions are usually readily identified by routine methods of examination. A delayed conduction, however, is seldom diagnosed except by instrumental means. The incidence of this finding, according to various reports, ranges from 30 to 40 per cent. It is an indication of cardiac damage and, while it occasionally occurs during the course of various acute infections, is far more common in rheumatic fever. Alterations in the $Q-R-S$ group, the $R-T$ segment and the T deflection are likewise significant findings. These changes were first recorded in rheumatic fever by Cohn and Swift and have since been confirmed by various observers. They are generally transient and while less conspicuous, resemble those following coronary occlusion. It has been estimated that through the combined electrocardiographic evidence it is possible to demonstrate a myocardial involvement in more than 90 per cent of the cases of rheumatic fever.

Diagnosis.—The diagnosis is at once apparent in those in whom definite structural changes appear in the heart during or subsequent to other manifestations of rheumatic fever. In some, particularly those with indefinite cardiac findings, and in whom other possible manifestations of a rheumatic infection are either lacking or questionable, the diagnosis is extremely difficult and often not possible until after a period of observation. Attention may have been directed to the heart through the discovery of a murmur in examining a child because of general ill-health, or during or after an upper respiratory infection or some of the acute infectious diseases. The murmur alone, except when diastolic in time, is not of any particular significance unless accompanied by an increase in the size of the heart. Other signs, especially canter rhythm, are invariably indicative of a damaged myocardium. Prolongation of the *P-R* interval in the electrocardiogram may be one of the deciding factors in the diagnosis. In the more chronic and insidious forms of rheumatic fever, a detailed history and careful survey of all possible evidences of the disease are of utmost importance.

The recurrence or exacerbation of a cardiac infection is likewise often difficult to establish. This is particularly true in the chronic form of rheumatic fever. Here again the history and the general condition of the child are extremely important. There is not likely to be any appreciable change in an already existing murmur, and the slight increase in the size of the heart may not be demonstrable except possibly by means of a teleoroentgenogram. The appearance of a new murmur, particularly the diastolic murmur of aortic insufficiency, a pericardial friction rub, even though transient, or the demonstration of significant electrocardiographic changes, confirms the diagnosis. In the young adult it is occasionally necessary to differentiate between a recurring rheumatic attack and subacute bacterial endocarditis. The clinical appearance, from the standpoint of the evidence of an infection, and possibly joint manifestations, may, in certain instances, be quite similar. The embolic phenomena and the isolation of organisms from the blood stream decide the question.

Course and Prognosis.—The prognosis is determined by the extent and duration of the infection. It is possible that the heart may recover from a minor involvement without later presenting evidence of structural changes. The disappearance of the murmur in certain instances following acute infection may perhaps be explained on this basis. The initial cardiac damage is frequently not recognized, and the resulting structural alterations are not discovered until years later and then perhaps accidentally. Some of these patients sooner or later develop symptoms and finally die from cardiac failure. Others may perhaps attain the usual life expectancy and never suffer any particular inconvenience from the heart. In children in whom the heart is extensively damaged by the initial infection the prognosis is not only poor from the standpoint of the more remote future, but there may be grave concern regarding the immediate outcome. However, they generally recover at least temporarily from the first attack, but may die within a few years or during early adult life, either from subsequent cardiac damage or as a result of the handicap imposed by the valve lesion, but more often from a combination of these factors. Others with less extensive cardiac involvement recover from the first attack without any significant impairment of cardiac function and perhaps have no symptoms until after twenty or thirty years of age. The repeated insults to the heart from recurrence or exacerbation of the infection are one of the most important factors in the progression of the cardiac disability.

Treatment.—*Preventive Measures.*—Even though our knowledge is still limited concerning the various factors influencing the onset of rheumatic fever, yet it is believed that much may be accomplished

24

toward reducing the incidence of the disease and curtailing the extent of the cardiac damage. It is generally agreed that there is a close relation between rheumatic fever and upper respiratory infections. A child who has repeated attacks of sore throats or tonsillitis and the various associated or complicating conditions, such as sinusitis, otitis media and mastoiditis, is constantly in danger of contracting rheumatic fever. Fortunately, these conditions in a child are usually very amenable to surgical treatment, and it is believed that if care is taken to eliminate them before they are firmly established, the incidence of rheumatic heart disease will be diminished. It is important to protect the child against various infectious diseases, such as scarlet fever, diphtheria, measles, whooping cough, that involve particularly the upper respiratory tract. Adequate supervision of the diet, proper clothing, plenty of sleep, exercise in the fresh air, sunshine and the administration of cod-liver oil during the winter months, are vital factors from the standpoint of general health and help to diminish susceptibility to infection. Every upper respiratory infection in the child should be regarded as a potential cause of heart disease. If, in addition to the above precautions, the heart is carefully observed during and subsequent to upper respiratory infections, a possible cardiac involvement may be recognized at an early stage and the progress very likely curtailed by adequate rest.

During the Active Stage of Cardiac Infection.—Rest in bed, relaxation, sleep, a simple, well-balanced diet, and careful nursing are by far the most important parts of the treatment. The bed rest should be continued until all evidence of the rheumatic infection has subsided and the general health is restored, as indicated by the disappearance of joint manifestations, subcutaneous nodules, fever, leukocytosis and secondary anemia, and reduction in the pulse-rate and restoration of the body weight. The important part played by adequate rest in curtailing the cardiac damage cannot be overemphasized. In patients with acute joint symptoms the administration of salicylates in the form of sodium salicylate or acetyl-salicylic acid for control of the pain is indicated. They also help to combat the pain of pericarditis, although the latter may be severe enough to require codeine or morphine. The long-continued use of salicylates has been suggested in the treatment of cardiac infection, but it is rather doubtful that it influences the course of the condition to any significant extent. Iron preparations may be employed to advantage for the secondary anemia. Digitalis is not indicated unless there is cardiac failure.

The after-treatment is concerned with gradually getting the individual on his feet and protecting him against a recurrence of the infection. The exercise should be carefully supervised, particularly in patients with extensive involvement of the heart. This is followed by systematic and thorough removal of all foci of infection. Tonsillectomy can hardly be expected to have the desired result unless it is thoroughly and completely done. This operation should include removal of the adenoids and other possibly infected clumps of lymphoid tissue about the naso-pharynx. The subject should be protected thereafter against upper respiratory infections and carefully observed for possible recurrence of the rheumatic fever and further damage to the heart. Finally, the physician should encourage the child's parents to educate him so that he may be able to gain a livelihood and yet live within his physical limitations.

BACTERIAL ENDOCARDITIS.

When pathogenic bacteria enter the blood stream and are carried to all parts of the body they start localized inflammatory processes more readily in some places than others. One of the commonest of these sites is the endocardium of the valve leaflets, and the disease which is produced in this way is known as bacterial endocarditis. It may be initiated by many different kinds of bacteria. The disease manifests itself as an endovascular infection, characterized chiefly by embolic phenomena. Two forms, the acute and subacute, are ordinarily recognized. They differ not only in their clinical course but also from an etiologic standpoint, in that the acute form is generally secondary to some other disease, as pneumonia, puerperal sepsis, furunculosis, gonorrhea, whereas in the subacute form the bacterial portal of entry is usually unknown.

Acute Bacterial Endocarditis. — Etiology. — Previously acquired or congenital disease of the endocardium seems to predispose it to attack. Various organisms have been described, but the Streptococcus hemolyticus, the pneumococcus, Staphylococcus aureus and the gonococcus are the causative agents in the vast majority of cases.

Morbid Anatomy.—The infection of the endocardium leads to tissue destruction and the formation of vegetations. In some of the more severe forms there may be extensive destruction of the valve and even ulceration of the adjacent myocardium. The vegetations are grayish, cauliflower-like masses of varying size, made up of fibrin, platelets, leukocytes, red blood cells and bacteria. The infection may invade any part of the endocardium or even the intima of the aorta, but is most commonly observed on the valves, particularly those of the left heart and about congenital defects. The pathologic changes outside the heart, aside from those of the primary condition (*e. g.*, pneumonia, furunculosis) consist of various types of vascular lesions, many of which are embolic in origin. These lesions are essentially perivascular hemorrhages about the terminal vessels. They ordinarily occur on the skin and mucous membrane as petechiæ and are observed on the serous surface of the internal organs in sizes varying from that of a pin-head to large areas such as are produced by occlusion of splenic or renal arteries.

Symptoms.—The symptoms in the beginning may be overshadowed by those of the primary condition (pneumonia, puerperal sepsis) and the onset of the acute bacterial endocarditis not recognized, but in many cases it is clearly defined. The patient who has perhaps not appeared seriously ill is suddenly taken with chills and fever. The symptoms in general are those of sepsis, with chills and profuse sweating at irregular intervals, high fever, marked prostration and often delirium. The discovery of a murmur or the knowledge of preëxisting heart disease may focus attention on the heart. The spleen is perhaps enlarged and may be tender. The leukocyte count ranges from 10,000 to 30,000. Sooner or later, petechiæ are observed on the skin or conjunctivæ. The urine frequently shows a trace of albumin and often red blood cells. The causative organism may be isolated from the blood stream. The disease is not infrequently complicated by occlusion of large vessels in the spleen, kidneys, brain, extremities and possibly mesentery. It invariably pursues an unfavorable course and terminates in death within a few days or weeks.

Diagnosis.—The first physical sign to appear is an endocardial murmur, or perhaps a change in the character of a preëxisting murmur; when this occurs in the course of severe systemic infection it suggests endocarditis. Embolic phenomena and recovery of the bacteria from the blood complete the diagnosis.

Treatment.—The treatment is that of any severe infection. Various drugs, serums and vaccines have been employed without influencing the course of the disease. When recovery occurs, as it does in rare instances, it is to be ascribed to high individual resistance rather than to any particular form of treatment.

Subacute Bacterial Endocarditis.—Subacute bacterial endocarditis is a more common disease than the acute form but is nevertheless comparatively rare. In a large series of cases reported by White and Jones, its general incidence was 2 per cent, and its incidence in the rheumatic group 4 per cent.

Etiology.—The Streptococcus viridans is the etiologic agent in 90 to 95 per cent of all cases. Although various other organisms may cause the disease, the influenza bacillus and the gonococcus are the most important causative agents in the remaining 5 to 10 per cent. Involvement of the endocardium is apparently facilitated by previous valvular disease or by a congenital anomaly. Chronic valvular heart disease precedes subacute bacterial endocarditis in a large percentage of cases. The principal predisposing congenital defect is a bicuspid aortic valve. The highest incidence falls between the ages of twenty and thirty years, the disease is seldom encountered after fifty years. In the older patients atheromatous or syphilitic changes occasionally furnish the predisposing factors.

Morbid Anatomy.—Here again infection of the endocardium produces destructive lesions which may be very extensive. In the more chronic form, less destruction occurs and various stages of healing may be encountered. The vegetations vary greatly in extent, appearance and consistency. They may be confined to a small section of a valve leaflet but are usually more extensive, involving possibly the chordæ tendineæ, the walls of the ventricles or auricles or even the aorta. They are usually small, nodular, with perhaps short pedunculated clumps, but not infrequently occur in the form of large irregular masses, club-shaped or strap-like projections. The large pedunculated formations are usually quite firm in consistency, often present fibrous tissue formation and occasionally calcareous deposits showing the tendency of the disease to heal. Certain of the vegetations are so friable that they are easily broken off and carried out into the circulation. These lesions usually occur in the left heart, involving either the mitral or aortic valves, possibly more often the latter, but both may be affected. In rare instances the infection may begin on the tricuspid or pulmonary valves. When emboli appear in both the pulmonary and general circulation, it generally means that the vegetations are clustered about a defect in the interventricular septum. Minute perivascular hemorrhages occur in the skin, mucous membranes and the serous surfaces of the internal organs, and large infarcts in various organs, particularly the kidneys, spleen and brain. In the kidney, partial thrombosis of the glomeruli produces a characteristic type of nephritis.

Symptoms.—The onset is usually insidious and the symptoms in the beginning often very indefinite. The patient may note that he tires easily and possibly has aches and pains in various parts of his body. He may relate his illness to some recent infection, particularly of the upper respiratory tract. While the patient may be aware of an old cardiac lesion, yet he seldom connects his disability with the heart. In time a daily fever is discovered and perhaps chilly sensations experienced. The onset is occasionally more abrupt with chilly sensations or even a frank chill and fever. Fever is usually present to a variable extent throughout the course of the disease, although there may be afebrile periods for days or even weeks. In mild cases, the temperature rises from perhaps 99° F. in the morning to 100° or 101° F. in the evening, with an occasional ascent to 102° F. In severe cases, high fever of a remittent type is the rule. The general symptoms of systemic infection, fatigability, anorexia, loss in weight and possibly joint pains, continue as the only manifestations of the disease until the embolic phenomena make their appearance.

Symptoms from emboli vary with the organ involved and the size of the vessel occluded. Hemiplegia may occur from the occlusion of a cerebral vessel, pain in the upper left quadrant of the abdomen and lower left chest from a splenic infarct and intense pain in the leg, possibly followed by gangrene from the blocking of a femoral artery. Occasionally a mesenteric vessel is occluded, giving rise to very severe abdominal pain, shock, nausea and vomiting, constipation or diarrhea with perhaps bloody stools and possibly later the signs of intestinal obstruction. Either of the above major embolic accidents may occur early in the course of the disease.

Objective Signs.—Pallor is common, and with the yellow, faint-brown or muddy tint to the skin may be the first feature to attract the attention of the examiner. The signs from the heart are generally those of a chronic valvular lesion of the mitral, aortic, or both. In rare instances the history and signs suggest one of the congenital anomalies, such as a defect in the interventricular septum or persistent ductus arteriosus. The spleen is usually enlarged and palpable. Embolism gives rise to a variety of signs. Gross infarction of the spleen or kidney, occlusion of the femoral artery or hemiplegia from cerebral embolism, may be among the earliest manifestations of the disease. In other cases there is at first nothing to suggest subacute bacterial endocarditis except the symptoms of infection, a valvular lesion or the history of heart disease, and an enlarged spleen, but diligent search is rewarded sooner or later by the discovery of petechiæ. These tiny hemorrhagic spots appear periodically in the skin, retinal and mucous membranes, perhaps most characteristically in the conjunctivæ, and pass slowly through the usual color changes before they disappear. Occasionally the hemorrhages are so large that they may properly be called ecchymoses. The appearance of tender areas in the pulp of the fingers and toes is a closely allied phenomenon. These areas are bluish-red in color, quite tender and occasionally palpable. They usually disappear within a few hours or days. Clubbing of the fingers not infrequently develops during the course of the disease.

Secondary anemia develops as the disease progresses and in some cases becomes a prominent feature. A hemoglobin of 40 to 60 per cent and a red cell count of 2,500,000 or 3,500,000 are common. The hemoglobin may, however, recede to 30 or even 20 per cent and the red cells to 1,500,000. The leukocytes vary in number. They generally range between 12,000 and 18,000 and occasionally increase to 25,000. In many instances there is no significant leukocytosis. The blood cultures usually show Streptococcus viridans, but it may be necessary to make repeated cultures using large amounts of blood before a positive result is obtained.

The urine usually shows a trace of albumin, hyaline and granular casts, and frequently red blood cells. The kidneys may be damaged extensively either by occlusion of the large renal vessels or as a result of multiple thrombosis of the glomeruli. Occlusion of the capillary loops by small emboli produces a characteristic type of nephritis which occasionally progresses to renal insufficiency.

Diagnosis.—The clinical course of subacute bacterial endocarditis, aside from the embolic manifestations, is not unlike that of any protracted infection. In the pre-embolic stage, it may be confused with various other infectious diseases, such as pulmonary tuberculosis, typhoid fever, malaria and undulant fever. Typhoid and undulant fever are generally eliminated by the agglutination test. Subacute bacterial endocarditis should be considered, and blood cultures made in any patient with a heart lesion and an obscure fever. The conjunctivæ, mucous membrane of the mouth and pharynx, skin and eyegrounds should be examined daily for petechiæ. In all cases the blood culture is the most important diagnostic measure and should be repeated until the diagnosis is established. Subacute bacterial endocarditis may occasionally be confused with acute rheumatic heart disease, but the embolic phenomena and positive blood cultures complete the differentiation.

Course and Prognosis.—While there is considerable variation in the clinical course, the end result is almost invariably the same in all cases. Some patients linger for months, others die in a few weeks. Occasionally a patient recovers, but the incidence of recovery is very small. Death usually results either from exhaustion, intercurrent infection (*e. g.*, pneumonia), cardiac failure, or from the occlusion of a large vessel, particularly of the brain. In some cases, renal insufficiency is an important terminal factor.

Treatment.—The treatment is that of any severe systemic infection.

Various drugs, vaccines and serums have been tried without any apparent influence on the course of the disease. The end is no doubt often hastened by the employment of radical measures, chiefly those which are followed by a severe systemic reaction.

ARTERIOSCLEROTIC HEART DISEASE.

HYPERTENSIVE HEART DISEASE.

Arteriosclerotic heart disease is the prevailing form of cardiac disability during late life. It begins to be manifested at about forty years of age, contributes to the other forms of cardiac disability contracted during an early period and is largely responsible for the high death-rate from heart disease after fifty years of age. The impairment in the cardiac function is primarily dependent on either an excessive cardiac load from an associated hypertension or an insufficiency of the coronary circulation from a sclerosis of the coronary arteries, or the combination of these factors. The first factor predominates in the group in which the early clinical manifestations are essentially those of a hypertension, whereas the second is of primary importance in the cases with angina pectoris and coronary occlusion. These two factors, however, are generally present to a varying extent in the same patient. There is thus often a hypertension or a history of an elevated blood pressure, not infrequently an anginal syndrome, even though it may be overshadowed by shortness of breath and other signs of congestive failure, and ever the possibility of a coronary occlusion. The hypertension and the arteriosclerotic form of heart disease are combined in the present discussion because the factors which produce the cardiac disability are intimately related and often associated in the same individual. While it is generally recognized that there are certain instances in which the hypertension is the outstanding feature, yet it is frequently difficult and often impossible to eliminate the possibility of a coronary sclerosis.

Pathology.—A sclerosis of the coronary arteries is invariably associated with similar changes elsewhere and is frequently a part of a general involvement of the arterial system. The arterial changes are likely to be more advanced in certain organs, as the heart, kidney and brain. The aorta is usually involved but often not to the same extent as the coronary arteries. In syphilis, on the other hand, the damage to the aorta is the outstanding feature and the coronary arteries are often not concerned to any significant extent except by an encroachment on their orifices through an extension of the aortic lesion.

There is a great variation in the extent of the involvement of the coronary arteries. In certain instances in which a hypertension has been a prominent feature, the larger coronary vessels at least may not show significant changes. The impairment in the cardiac function under these circumstances is presumably dependent for the most part on the hypertension. There are cases, on the other hand, in which the sclerosis of the coronary arteries is out of proportion to the clinical manifestations. This is more likely to occur in individuals who have never had a hypertension and in whom an adequate coronary circulation has been maintained through the development of the extensive collateral circulation. During the development of the arteriosclerosis, a thickening of the intima is often observed about the orifice of the subdivisions of the coronary arteries, which, through a progression of the process, may later occlude certain of the smaller branches at their point of origin.

In the more extensive sclerosis, nodular thickenings of the intima project into the lumen of the coronary arteries and produce varying degrees of occlusion. A complete occlusion often results through a gradual extension of the process or from a thrombosis. The sclerosis is usually more advanced in the anterior descending branch of the left coronary artery which accounts for the frequent occlusion of this vessel. Barnes and Whitten have recently called attention to a similar involvement of the terminal posterior descending branches of the right and of the corresponding divisions of the circumflex branch of the left coronary artery, both from the standpoint of the extent of the sclerosis and the incidence of occlusion.

The heart is usually increased in size and may be very large. The cardiac weight at necropsy is frequently 450 to 500 grams and occasionally 800, or in rare instances even 1000 grams. There are varying degrees of dilatation and hypertrophy. The hypertrophy, however, generally predominates, especially in the left ventricle, and is more marked in those with a prolonged hypertension. There is, on the other hand, no definite relationship between the extent of the hypertrophy and the degree of coronary sclerosis. An advanced sclerosis of the coronary arteries is occasionally seen in a relatively normal-sized heart. The dilatation especially concerns the auricles but often involves the ventricles and not infrequently produces a relative insufficiency of the mitral and tricuspid valves.

The alterations in the myocardium, except for hypertrophy of the muscle fibers, may be relatively insignificant. In general, the changes range from the small area of fibrosis resulting from the closure of the smaller arterial twigs, which may be detected only through histologic examination, to the extensive necrosis and fibrosis following the occlusion of a larger artery. In the latter, the extent of the damage depends on the degree of anastomosis and whether the occlusion is sudden or gradual. If the vessel is gradually occluded and the neighboring artery which contributes to the blood supply of the involved section of the cardiac musculature is not sclerosed, conditions are most favorable to the further development of the collateral circulation. Under these circumstances, more and more of the arterial supply involved is taken over by the second vessel and the complete occlusion of the first, even though terminated abruptly, may be followed by a surprisingly satisfactory recovery and possibly not be suspected during life.

The changes in the cardiac musculature predominate in the left ventricle. In general, there are three types of lesions. The first is represented by the small area of fibrosis resulting from closure of the small arterial twigs, some of which are detected only by histologic examination. The second is manifested by a more extensively localized area of degeneration and replacement by fibrous tissue. The most characteristic lesion of this nature is produced by the occlusion of the anterior descending branch of the left coronary artery. It involves the anterior apical wall of the left ventricle, the lower anterior section of the interventricular septum and to a varying extent the adjoining anterior wall of the right ventricle. There is a striking variation in the extent of the lesion, depending on the degree of the collateral circulation. In some, where the destructive process is extensive as the result of an inadequate collateral circulation, the lesion may progress to an aneurysm of the left ventricle. The third type of lesion is that of a disseminated degeneration and fibrosis of the endocardial and subendocardial layers of the lateral and posterior walls of the left ventricle and frequently involves a portion of the posterior section of the interventricular septum. This lesion is seen in the most typical form following the occlusion of the circumflex branch of the left coronary artery and to a less extent following the closure of the terminal descending branches of this vessel or the corresponding branches of the right coronary artery.

The damage to the papillary muscles and the mitral valve structures is an important feature in the sclerosis of the coronary arteries. The papillary muscles are likely to be involved by the occlusion of either of the main branches of the left coronary artery. The changes in these structures contribute to the alteration in the first heart sound at the apex and to the production of the systolic murmur frequently heard in this location. Sclerotic changes also occur in the aortic valve and occasionally a high-grade stenosis is observed.

Symptoms.—There is a marked variation in the clinical manifestations. This, however, is not surprising in view of the anatomy and pathology of the coronary arteries and the systemic nature of the disease. The onset may thus be very insidious and perhaps overshadowed or entirely masked by symptoms directing attention to some other organ, or, on the other hand, be extremely abrupt as in coronary occlusion. In many there is a history of a hypertension. The appearance of premature contraction or the occurrence of paroxysms of auricular fibrillation, which may later become permanently established, may be the first indication of an impaired cardiac function. Usually, however, the first symptom is that of shortness of breath or the consciousness of a substernal discomfort on exertion. The association of the latter with an upper abdominal discomfort often convinces the patient that he has a gastric disturbance. In some the initial manifestation is that of a paroxysmal dyspnea. The onset may follow an upper respiratory infection or be preceded by recurring attacks of winter bronchitis. More frequently the onset is precipitated by overexertion. Various other factors, as emotional upsets, loss of sleep or indiscretion in diet, may contribute to the onset of the cardiac symptoms.

The most common clinical picture is that of the congestive type of cardiac failure as manifested by shortness of breath and the appearance of other signs such as pulmonary congestion, edema of the ankles, engorgement of the liver and finally the development of a generalized anasarca. In many there is at no time significant cardiac pain. In some a history of varying degrees of precordial distress or even an anginal syndrome may be obtained. These features, however, are usually overshadowed by the shortness of breath and possibly not elicited except by a direct question. There is another group in which pain of the anginal type is the predominating symptom. In the beginning there may be no appreciable shortness of breath. Later, however, during the height of the distress, it frequently becomes more prominent. In some the course is terminated by an attack of angina pectoris or coronary occlusion. Others pass into congestive failure either through a gradual progression of the cardiac disability or possibly because of a coronary occlusion. The advanced forms of congestive failure are not infrequently complicated by pulmonary infarcts through the detachment of emboli from the dilated right auricle. Pneumonia and intercurrent infections represent other possibilities. A cerebral accident resulting in hemiplegia may occur.

Physical Findings.—There is frequently a hypertension or the history of an elevated blood pressure. In those with a hypertension there is invariably a significant increase in the size of the heart. This is more likely to be a prominent feature in those with congestive failure. Various forms of cardiac irregularities, particularly premature contractions and auricular fibrillation, are common findings. While auricular fibrillation is rarely associated with angina pectoris, it is frequently responsible for the onset of the congestive failure. Auricular flutter and heart block are occasionally observed. Muffling of the first sound at the apex, gallop rhythm and perhaps a faint systolic apical murmur may be the outstanding auscultatory findings. The first sound is occasionally accentuated or slightly rough. At other times there is a well-developed systolic murmur at the apex which may be soft, blowing, harsh, or even musical in character. If an auricular fibrillation is present, the first sound at the apex varies in intensity and when the rate is particularly rapid, likely to be "choppy" in character. The associated systolic murmur likewise varies in intensity from cycle to cycle. The aortic second sound is usually accentuated and occasionally slightly amphoric. There is often a faint systolic murmur transmitted to the vessels of the neck. This murmur is seldom rough unless associated with an aortic stenosis which is occasionally encountered in this form of heart disease. In rare instances a faint diastolic murmur is heard. If, however, there is a significant aortic insufficiency it is usually either syphilitic or rheumatic in origin. In uncomplicated arteriosclerosis it is rarely possible to demonstrate much increase in the size of the aorta except as manifested by an extension upward. Under the latter circumstances an impulse may be transmitted to the palpating finger in the supersternal notch. During the early course of angina pectoris there are not infrequently no significant cardiac findings. The diagnosis may thus be solely dependent on the clinical history and the demonstration of an arteriosclerosis elsewhere.

The kidneys are rarely spared in the arteriosclerotic process. The urine frequently shows a trace of albumin, and on microscopic examination, hyaline and granular casts are seen. In some the renal damage may be more extensive and occasionally renal insufficiency occurs. In men a bladder retention from an enlarged prostate may promote the development of a renal insufficiency.

The examination of the fundi is essential to a careful survey of the vascular system. The findings in the retinal vessels indicate in general the extent of the cerebral arteriosclerosis and are representative of the changes in the smaller arteries elsewhere.

Electrocardiographic Findings.—The changes in the ventricular complexes constitute the most important electrocardiographic findings in arteriosclerotic heart disease. A left axis deviation curve is very common, particularly with a prolonged hypertension. The T deflection is not infrequently negative in Lead I and occasionally in Lead II in a left axis deviation curve, more especially with an increase in the duration of the $Q-R-S$ group. These findings are generally regarded as being indicative of a significant alteration of the myocardium. A sharp negative T deflection in Lead I with the opposite effect in Lead III or the reverse, *viz.*, T down in Lead III and correspondingly upright in Lead I possibly associated with alterations in the $R-T$ and $S-T$ segment in the absence of an increase in the duration of the $Q-R-S$ group is suggestive of coronary occlusion and warrants progress curves. If these alterations are associated with a healed infarct they are likely to remain fairly constant until there is further damage to the myocardium. If, on the other hand, the lesion is of recent origin, subsequent curves taken daily or possibly at weekly intervals generally show consecutive changes.

Bundle branch block is not infrequently encountered and is usually associated with an extensive impairment in the cardiac function; minor changes in the $Q-R-S$ group as manifested by a splintering or slurring, and perhaps some increase in the duration of these complexes are of less importance. If, however, they appear in all leads and the slurring occurs near the apex of the most prominent deflection, they are interpreted as indicating an interference with the spread of the excitation wave within the ventricle and ordinarily associated with a sclerosis of the coronary arteries.

Diagnosis.—The diagnosis is usually evident, particularly in the cases in which a hypertension has been the dominating factor in the production of the cardiac disability. The cardiac enlargement and a murmur or perhaps an auricular fibrillation at once direct the attention to the heart. An advanced sclerosis of the coronary arteries, however, may not be recognized because of the absence of clinical manifestations. The symptoms in others may be indefinite and difficult to connect with the heart. The clinical history is by all odds the most important means of determining the functional efficiency of the heart and may alone permit a diagnosis, as in angina pectoris, even in the absence of definite physical findings. The possibility of coronary disease should be kept in mind in every individual of the arteriosclerotic age. An upper abdominal discomfort or an indefinite chest pain may mean angina pectoris. A persistent bronchitis or asthmatic-like attack often represents a beginning failure of the left ventricle. The appearance of an auricular fibrillation may be the

first manifestation of an impaired cardiac function. The history or
the presence of a hypertension warrants a careful survey of the cardiovascular system, regardless of the apparent nature of the illness. In
some the cardiac findings may seem unimportant and even possibly be
overlooked unless the attention is focused on the heart by the history.
A muffling of the first sound at the apex and gallop rhythm are occasionally the only findings that particularly attract the attention of the
examiner. A combination of these findings, however, always means
a serious impairment in the cardiac function. Occasionally the electrocardiogram may be the deciding factor in the diagnosis.

Prognosis.—The prognosis is dependent, not only on the state of
the myocardium, but on the associated damage of the arteries elsewhere, especially those of the brain and kidneys, and whether there is
a hypertension. There is always the possibility that the condition
may be terminated by a cerebral accident or a renal insufficiency.
Diabetes may still further complicate the picture, particularly in those
with an extensive sclerosis of the vessels of the lower extremities.

The prognosis relative to the heart is determined by the functional
response and the extent of the structural changes. The recovery from
the cardiac failure, however, is more difficult with each successive recurrence and the extent to which the function may be restored is gradually
reduced. The prognosis is always in doubt in angina pectoris. Even
though the angina may appear mild there is ever the possibility of
sudden death or a coronary occlusion.

The treatment of the congestive form of cardiac failure is discussed
at the end of this chapter.

ANGINA PECTORIS.

Angina pectoris is one of the most characteristic manifestations of
coronary artery disease. This syndrome is identified by the paroxysmal nature, the location, character and distribution of the pain and
the association with factors which increase the demands on the heart.
The distress usually appears after exercise or excitement, generally
first felt in the upper middle or lower substernal region, frequently
transmitted to the left shoulder and arm, occasionally to the right
arm or perhaps to the neck and head and except in the more severe
form subsides within a few minutes after the exercise is discontinued
or the excitement disappears.

History.—The syndrome was first accurately described and designated as
angina pectoris by Heberden in 1768. Isolated instances had previously
been cited by Morgagni, Rougnon and others. Jenner was the first to connect
the disorder with a sclerosis of the coronary arteries. The same view was
held by John Hunter, who died in an attack in 1793. Some of the more recent
ideas relative to the mechanism of the pain were anticipated by Allan Burns
(1809) who proposed the theory of intermittent claudication. Wall (1772),
Corrigan (1837) and later Allbutt ascribed the syndrome to a disease of the
aorta. Parry (1799), Stokes (1854) and, more recently, MacKenzie regarded
the condition as a form of cardiac failure.

Etiology.—This disorder is quite common and frequently seen in
cardiovascular consulting practice, although rarely encountered in

the public wards of hospitals. Statistics seem to indicate that the incidence is increasing in recent years. It occurs particularly in the better classes, especially in the business and professional groups. The stress and strain of this type of life is presumed to predispose to the condition.

Angina pectoris occasionally occurs between the ages of thirty and forty years and rare instances are encountered at an earlier age. The incidence increases rapidly after forty-five, is greatest between fifty and sixty, but remains high between sixty and seventy years. It is four to six times more frequent in the male sex. In the cases under forty years of age a syphilitic aortitis is an important factor and should always be suspected.

Pathology.—A sclerosis of the coronary arteries, which is usually extensive and associated with a partial or even complete obstruction of certain vessels, is the most common pathologic finding. In those instances in which the sclerotic process is confined for the most part to the aorta, as in syphilis of the aorta, there is frequently an encroachment on or an occlusion of the mouth of one or both coronary arteries. Keefer and Resnik, in a recent review of the mechanism of angina pectoris, considered in detail the pathology associated with the condition. They collected a series of 386 cases from the literature which came to necropsy and added 13 of their own. A sclerosis of the coronary arteries was demonstrated in 381 of the total 399 cases. These authors pointed out that an aortic insufficiency was the predominating lesion in the instances of angina not associated with coronary artery disease, and in the vast majority of these the valve leakage was secondary to a syphilitic aortitis. Angina pectoris, however, is occasionally noted in the rheumatic type of aortic insufficiency and has been observed in other conditions as arteriovenous aneurysm, paroxysmal tachycardia, high-grade anemia, hyperthyroidism and hypothyroidism. In some of these it is possible that changes in the coronary arteries were the basic factor.

Mechanism.—The mechanism has been extensively discussed and many hypotheses advanced. An aortitis, coronary artery disease, fatigue of the myocardium and, more recently, an anoxemia of the cardiac musculature, are the more favored explanations. All except the aortic theory are closely related and fundamentally dependent on an impaired coronary circulation. It is coming to be fairly generally believed that an involvement of the coronary arteries, either at their point of origin from the aorta or during their subsequent course, is primarily responsible for all except the occasional instance of angina pectoris. The fact that coronary occlusion produces pain which strikingly resembles that of angina and that the basic pathology in the two conditions is identical, suggests that the mechanism is similar. The experiments of Sutton and Leuth, the electrocardiographic studies of Feil and Seegal, Wood and Wolferth and others, and the more recent observation of Lewis, support this conception.

Under normal conditions the blood supply to the various sections of the myocardium is undoubtedly ample to meet the specific needs of the various structures, even during periods of stress. If, for any reason, the blood supply to a certain area is diminished, the efficiency of that section is reduced. This area of the myocardium may thus be overtaxed by a load that is well within the functional capacity of the remaining cardiac musculature. While it is well known that the occlusion of a coronary artery may produce severe pain, it is conceivable that a less extensive disturbance of the blood supply to the same area of the myocardium may, during periods of exertion, cause distress with the same fundamental characteristics but less severe, and it disappears soon after the excess exertion is discontinued. It is, therefore, probable that angina pectoris and coronary occlusion differ only in the extent to which the function of the myocardium is disturbed.

In the various conditions in which angina pectoris is occasionally observed, as rheumatic aortic insufficiency, arteriovenous aneurysm, paroxysmal tachycardia, high-grade anemia, hyperthyroidism and hypothyroidism, it is very probable that in some instances a disease of the coronary arteries is primarily responsible for the pain. Each of these conditions, however, imposes an extra demand on the heart which might very well precipitate the anginal syndrome.

There are, no doubt, other possible causes for angina, as a dilatation of the aorta, a dissecting aneurysm, the rupture of an aortic valve and perhaps, in rare instances, a spasm of the coronary arteries. In general, however, when a syphilitic aortitis can be excluded, the clinician is justified in attributing the angina to a sclerosis of the coronary arteries.

Symptoms.—There is a remarkable variation in the extent and distribution of the pain. In the beginning there may be no more than a mild uneasiness or an indefinite sense of discomfort, or perhaps a burning sensation in the substernal region after excitement or on walking up a hill. Later it may be described as a heaviness, fullness, or constricting sensation which may become so severe that the individual is afraid to move because of the fear that it may become even more intense or that perhaps death might occur. The pain is usually first felt in the upper or middle and not infrequently in the lower substernal region. It occasionally involves the precordium, may extend to the epigastrium and in rare instances is confined entirely to the upper abdomen. Later there is a tendency for the pain to involve a large area or radiate to the arms, neck and head, and occasionally to the back. It is frequently transmitted to the left shoulder and often down the arm on the ulnar side to the elbow or even to the fingers. The distress in the latter location is manifested by a numbness or a feeling of constriction. In the more severe form, the pain may be transmitted to the right shoulder and arm. The pain in some patients is first felt in the arm and later, if the exciting factor is continued, appears in the usual location in the chest. The distress in others may radiate to the head and neck and be felt in the pharynx, jaw, mastoid region, or even the ear, without appearing in the arms, or may begin in the neck or head and later reach the chest.

Even though the distress may vary in character and have a wide range of distribution, the type of pain, except for the degree of intensity and the extent of radiation during different attacks in the same individual, is constant. Furthermore, the attack of pain, except perhaps in the very severe form where there is always a question of coronary occlusion, is usually excited by factors which increase the demands on the heart. The exciting factor may be the added effort of walking or climbing stairs or it may be the increase in the work of the heart imposed by the elevation of the blood pressure and the accelerated cardiac rate accompanying excitement; or, again, it may be the interference with the cardiac function from an overdistention of the stomach by a full meal or possibly an associated accumulation of gas. In some instances the patient is awakened from sleep. It is possible that in some the pain is induced by the increase in blood pressure resulting from nightmare or other forms of sleep disturbances. When the pain occurs under these circumstances the possibility of coronary occlusion should always be considered. The attacks usually disappear within a few minutes after the excitement or exercise is discontinued.

Physical Findings.—The cardiac signs are variable or may be entirely negative. In those with demonstrable structural changes in the heart, the findings are as previously outlined under the general discussion of coronary artery disease. A roentgenologic examination and a Wassermann test are indicated in every instance where the possibility of syphilis is suspected. In the doubtful case the electrocardiogram may be of considerable value in detecting a derangement of the myocardium.

Diagnosis.—The typical form of angina pectoris is readily recognized. In those with an unusual distribution of pain the diagnosis may be difficult. When the distress is confined to the epigastrium and lower chest and particularly when associated with the accumulation of gas, the condition is frequently mistaken for gastric disorder or gall-bladder disease. Not infrequently the early manifestations of angina may appear to be entirely gastric and their significance not appreciated until later development. It is always well to bear in mind the possibility of angina in every individual of the arteriosclerotic age with a vague epigastric distress. Ordinarily a detailed history and a careful survey of the cardiovascular system will enable the physician to come to a fairly definite conclusion regarding the possibility of angina.

Coronary occlusion has frequently been mistaken for the severe forms of angina pectoris. The character and distribution of the pain may be identical. Pain in coronary occlusion is usually more lasting and, instead of disappearing in a few minutes, may continue for hours or days and perhaps persist in a minor form even after repeated hypodermic injections of morphine. Changes in the cardiac findings may be sufficient to permit a definite diagnosis, even when the history is atypical. The distant and indistinct cardiac tones, gallop rhythm and premature contractions, at once direct attention to the heart. The later appearance of a systolic murmur and the occasional pericardial friction rub on the following day are conclusive evidences of cardiac damage. Significant alterations are usually evident in the electrocardiogram, and in the doubtful cases may establish the diagnosis.

The differentiation of angina pectoris from minor forms of coronary occlusion is extremely difficult, yet very important from the standpoint of treatment. When an attack of angina pectoris is more severe than usual and comes on while at rest, the possibility of coronary occlusion should be considered and if in doubt the patient given the benefit of a period of absolute rest. If, in questionable cases, the heart is carefully watched for possible changes in the findings, the physician will occasionally be rewarded by detecting a gallop rhythm or pericardial rub, the latter definitely establishing the diagnosis. The electrocardiogram renders the greater service in the atypical cases. The alterations may, however, at times be overlooked unless progress records are taken.

The precordial or upper chest pain from intercostal neuralgia or nerve root pressure from a mediastinal tumor, tuberculosis of the vertebræ or a hypertrophic osteoarthritis of the spine, not infrequently arouses suspicion or even closely resembles that of an angina pectoris. The history, however, is usually different and the physical examination will ordinarily point to other possibilities.

Prognosis.—The future of a patient with angina pectoris is always in doubt because of the possibility of sudden death. The wife or some responsible member of the family should therefore be informed concerning the nature of the disorder. It is well to bear in mind, however, as pointed out by Herrick, that recovery occurs, improvement is common, and some have been known to live twenty years. The outlook is determined to a certain extent by the condition of the cardiovascular system. It is always serious in those with frequent and severe attacks. When associated with luetic aortitis, after the development of an aortic insufficiency, the course is usually downward. If the patient is seen prior to the onset of the insufficiency, striking benefit may follow the administration of iodides and mercury. The prognosis in general is more favorable in those in whom it is not possible to demonstrate significant structural changes in the heart and the attacks are of a mild nature and occur at infrequent intervals. The angina associated with thyrotoxicosis and high-grade anemia may frequently be eliminated by the treatment of these conditions. The general temperament of the patient should be taken into consideration. In those with a hypersensitive nervous system, the basic pathology necessary to the production of the pain may be considerably less than in the placid individual. This is a recognized factor in women and possibly contributes to the production of the syndrome in thyrotoxicosis. Finally, the patients who are careful in complying with the recommendations of the physician may add years to their lives, whereas the disregard of factors which excite the pain may precipitate a sudden termination.

Treatment.—The objectives are the same as in the treatment of congestive heart failure. Rest is one of the most effective means of restoring the cardiac function and controlling the pain. In the milder form, curtailment in exercise alone may produce marked improvement. This is obviously the opportune time to promote the maximum restoration of the cardiac function and possibly cure the condition. A careful analysis of the various factors which contribute to the production of the pain is essential to this objective. A reduction in the exercise to the point where the pain is not induced is the first step in treatment. A period of rest, with complete relaxation and perhaps additional sleep, is often advisable. It is important that the diet be simple and overeating be avoided. If there are digestive disturbances a more careful supervision of the diet may be necessary. In the obese a gradual reduction in the weight is indicated. If the blood pressure in patients with hypertension is not sufficiently reduced by rest, relaxation, regulation of the diet and reduction in the weight of the obese, the administration of nitrites is justified in order temporarily to reduce the work of the heart. This medication will in addition have a favorable influence on the coronary circulation. Nitroglycerin, 0.01 grain (0.6 mg.), frequently gives prompt relief from an attack and should always be available when the patient is caught with pain. This drug may be conveniently carried in the pocket and employed often if necessary without harm.

There are instances in which such factors as infections, enlarged prostate, diabetes and anemia may contribute to the angina. The various possibilities should be weighed carefully and judicious treatment employed.

Theophyllin and theobromin preparations have their place in the treatment of angina pectoris. The possibilities are not as great as in the arteriosclerotic form of heart disease with the congestive type of failure, but they should nevertheless be given a chance and favorable results are frequently observed. Theophyllin in the form of metaphyllin is favored by the writer and usually prescribed in 1.5-grain doses, three or four times a day. This medication should be continued over a long period of time in order to maintain the maximum benefit. After the patient is permitted to assume more responsibilities he should guard against the production of pain.

In the more severe forms of angina pectoris, the treatment is much the same as in the advanced stage of congestive heart failure. Every available means should be employed to reduce the work of the heart and improve the efficiency of the myocardium. A prolonged period of rest, relaxation and sleep may be indicated. Mild sedatives may be advisable or even morphine necessary to promote relaxation and sleep, and obtain the maximum of mental and physical rest. The administration of digitalis, 10 to 15 minims (0.6 to 1 cc.) of the tincture or 0.06 to 0.1 gram (1 to 1.5 grains) of the powdered leaf, is frequently indicated. Nitroglycerin may be an extremely valuable remedy in this stage of the disease and should be given as often as necessary to control the pain. After the patient is allowed to leave his bed there is a greater necessity for more detailed supervision of exercise and other factors which induce the pain.

Surgical Treatment.—The section of the various portions of the sympathetic chain and more recently the paravertebral injection of alcohol have been recommended for the treatment of angina pectoris. In some instances favorable results have been reported. The paravertebral injection is by far the simplest procedure, but even this should not be attempted except by one who has expert anatomical knowledge and experience. While these methods of treatment are

25

still in the experimental stage, the results to date would seem to indicate that they are only applicable to a limited number of carefully selected cases, particularly those who are in great distress and not able to obtain relief by other measures.

CORONARY OCCLUSION.

The occlusion of one or more branches of the coronary arteries with varying degrees of myocardial degeneration and replacement by fibrous tissue is the most important complication of coronary artery disease. Whereas in rare instances it may be produced by an embolus from a subacute bacterial endocarditis or other sources, it is generally dependent on a sclerosis of the coronary arteries. This condition is occasionally seen soon after forty years of age and is not infrequently observed between the ages of forty and fifty years. About 90 per cent, however, occur after fifty and the incidence is highest between sixty and seventy years of age.

History.—Coronary occlusion is very intimately associated with the development of our knowledge of coronary artery disease. The writings of Jenner and Parry were perhaps the first to direct attention to the possible relation between the obstruction of a coronary vessel and sudden death. It was not until the latter part of the nineteenth century, however, that it was recognized that the occlusion of a larger coronary artery was compatible with life. This initiated a fairly active period of investigation, during which it was demonstrated that animals might survive the experimental ligation of one of the main branches of the coronary arteries, and it was further shown by the injection method that there is a fairly extensive anastomosis between the branches of these vessels. In the meantime the clinical manifestations of this condition as such were not recognized. Excellent descriptions of certain of the aspects of coronary occlusion were recorded by Leyden, Krehl, Huchard, Osler and others under the heading of coronary sclerosis or angina pectoris. Dock was one of the first to report a case in which the clinical diagnosis was verified by necropsy. While the syndrome was first definitely identified by Obrastzow and Straschesko in 1910, the report by Herrick in 1912 and his subsequent publication particularly stand out in the subsequent developments in this new field of medicine. This stimulated a widespread interest in the subject, which led to an extensive investigation of the anatomy, physiology and pathology of the coronary arteries, experimental and clinical electrocardiographic studies, and finally a careful clinical survey of the various features of coronary artery disease.

Pathology.—The essential features of the pathology have been discussed. The changes in coronary arteries are comparable to those ordinarily associated with angina pectoris. In this connection, the findings of Klotz and Lloyd are of particular interest. These investigators made a comparative study of the clinical and pathologic findings in a series of 26 cases of advanced coronary arteriosclerosis and a series of 18 cases of coronary occlusion. They concluded that there were no significant differences between these series, either in clinical manifestations or in the postmortem findings. The incidence of angina pectoris was practically the same in the two groups. In a series of 86 necropsies studied by Willius and Brown, 21 (24 per cent) had angina pectoris without other symptoms of cardiac failure. This group had extensive sclerosis of the coronary arteries, and in 14 (66 per cent) there was pronounced occlusion of the vessels. These results are in general accord with the observations of Nathanson on the autopsies of 115 fatal cases of coronary artery disease. In 80 per cent, attacks of angina pectoris, or less often acute respiratory distress, were the outstanding clinical manifestations, while in the remaining 20 per cent the symptoms were those of a progressive congestive failure without pain. The sclerotic changes were advanced in all instances, but the incidence of occlusion was highest in those who had angina pectoris.

Symptoms.—In a typical case, the distribution, character and duration of pain, the accompanying shock and fall in the blood pressure, the symptoms and signs of cardiac damage and a later development of fever and leukocytosis, produce a distinctive clinical picture. There is, however, wide variation in the clinical manifestations, depending in a large measure on the extent of the myocardial damage. The damage to the heart may thus be so overwhelming that the patient dies suddenly or within a few hours, or, on the other hand, it is so slight that few or no symptoms are produced and possibly the condition not recognized. Again, in those instances in which the pain and accompanying shock predominate in the clinical picture, the associated symptoms and signs of cardiac damage may vary to a remarkable extent. In some there may be no significant dyspnea and perhaps no definite structural changes in the heart except as demonstrated by the electrocardiograph. In other instances dyspnea is a more prominent feature and possibly there are obvious signs of myocardial damage. Finally, in a small group the onset is manifested by intense dyspnea with little or no pain.

The pain is the outstanding and most characteristic symptom of coronary occlusion. Many give a previous history of chest pain which is frequently typical of angina pectoris. In another group the occlusion is the first evidence of a coronary artery disease. The onset of the pain is usually abrupt but occasionally gradual, extending over a period of several hours or even two or three days before reaching the severe form. The patient is frequently awakened from sound sleep during the night and often during the early hours of the morning by the terrific distress. The site of the pain is similar to that of angina pectoris except perhaps a greater tendency to the lower sternum or the upper abdomen. In rare instances, as in angina, the distress may be entirely confined to the abdomen. Usually the pain has a greater area of distribution; whereas in those with a previous history of angina pectoris, the pain may have extended to the left arm, after occlusion it will frequently be felt in both arms. The pain may likewise be felt in the neck and various locations about the head, and in rare instances may be transmitted to the posterior chest. In a mild form or in those with a gradual onset, the distress is often described as a feeling of oppression or heaviness in the chest. On the other hand, it may be the most agonizing, tearing, boring or constricting pain. The duration in the more severe types varies from a few hours to days and may persist in a minor form even after repeated hypodermic injections of morphine. It is ordinarily not influenced to any significant extent by nitroglycerin. While the above type of pain often follows occlusion of a larger vessel, instances of even fairly large infarction are not infrequently encountered at necropsy which were not manifested by significant symptoms. The pain, if present, must have been of a very mild nature or in the cases with angina pectoris, perhaps no more than that experienced during an ordinary attack. There are some in which the clinical picture is so dominated by the dyspnea that the pain is overlooked.

The extent of the dyspnea represents a measure of the response of the myocardium. Pain and dyspnea are thus not necessarily present to the same degree. Even with a severe pain there may have been no appreciable shortness of breath, but if cardiac failure later develops, the respiratory distress gradually assumes a prominent aspect in the clinical picture. In other instances, the dyspnea is a striking feature at the onset, and is an indication of an extensive impairment in cardiac function.

The onset of the severe pain is ordinarily accompanied by profound shock in which the ashen-gray color, profuse perspiration, the feeble and imperceptible pulse, and the fall in the blood pressure are conspicuous features. The normal color often returns and the perspiration disappears after the severe pain subsides. The exhaustion and feeble pulse, however, may continue for days, depending on the extent of impairment in the function of the myocardium. The systolic blood pressure may recede to 90 or even lower. In those with an unrecognized hypertension, the extent of the reduction in the blood pressure is likely not to be appreciated. Following the occlusion of a smaller vessel there may be no change in the blood pressure or perhaps only slight, and transient in nature. After the closure of a large vessel the blood pressure rises slowly but often remains at a level considerably below the original.

Physical Findings.—There is a great variation in the physical findings. Some patients give a history of hypertension and have the customary changes in the cardiovascular system. Again, the findings prior to the accident may be surprisingly negative. During and even after severe attacks of pain there may be very little alteration in the heart. The cardiac rate is usually accelerated but is seldom above 100 per minute. Premature contractions are not infrequently noted and may be helpful in establishing the diagnosis. The distant and poorly differentiated cardiac tones and a gallop rhythm are possibly the most constant findings and may be the only demonstrable physical signs of cardiac damage. A systolic murmur may be heard at the apex or appear later. It is often very faint in the beginning, but later may become more conspicuous. There may be no appreciable increase in the size of the heart. In the cases with extensive myocardial damage, the cardiac signs are more prominent, with perhaps additional manifestations of pulmonary edema and engorgement of the liver.

A pericardial friction rub is occasionally demonstrated and is a most distinctive physical sign of cardiac infarction. It may be heard on the second to fourth day, frequently between the apex and sternum, occasionally at a higher level and ordinarily disappears after one or two days.

The temperature and leukocyte count are of considerable importance in that they are apparently solely dependent on the extent of the myocardial infarction. The fever ranging from 99° to 102° F. is usually not noted until the following day and ordinarily reaches the highest peak on the third day, after which it gradually subsides. In occasional instances, however, it may persist for a week or longer. An increase in the leukocyte count has been observed as early as one to two hours after the onset of the clinical manifestations of occlusion. It in general parallels the temperature and ranges from 12,000 to 20,000 per cubic millimeter. These two findings may be helpful in estimating the extent of the myocardial infarction and degree of the collateral circulation.

Electrocardiographic Findings.—The alterations in the electrocardiogram are frequently characteristic and may be the only evidence of structural change in the heart. During the acute stage of the infarction the electrocardiogram is continually changing to a varying degree. These alterations may not be apparent in a single curve, but are generally evident in serial records taken at one- to two-day intervals during the first week following the occlusion. The most conspicuous changes usually concern the T-deflection and the R and S-T segments. Along with these changes a Q wave often appears in Lead III. Soon after the cardiac infarction, the T wave or even the entire R-T segment may be elevated in Lead I, and perhaps the opposite effect noted in Lead III. This is followed by the gradual reduction in this portion of the ventricular complex and finally changes to a sharp negative T in Lead I and to an upright deflection in Lead III. Occasionally the reverse order is observed in which the T negativity is greatest in Lead III. There may be, in addition, a significant reduction in the amplitude of the Q-R-S group. Premature contractions, particularly of the ventricular type, are common and ventricular tachycardia has been observed.

Diagnosis.—The diagnosis is usually apparent from the history alone in the typical case. When, however, the pain is confined to the epigastrium or extends to this region, particularly when accompanied by tenderness, rigidity, nausea or vomiting, the diagnosis may be extremely difficult. Patients of this age may have a perforating peptic ulcer, gall-bladder disease or acute pancreatitis. The history is extremely important. It may point to peptic ulcer, gall-bladder disease, or on the other hand indicate a previous angina pectoris. A careful survey of the heart may in most instances prevent the physician from overlooking a coronary occlusion. In doubtful cases the diagnosis is dependent on the demonstration of the acute myocardial damage. Under these circumstances the heart should be carefully observed for possible evidence of structural changes, as indicated by an alteration in the cardiac tones, gallop rhythm, the occurrence of premature contractions and finally the appearance of a murmur or a pericardial rub. The electrocardiograph may, in this respect, render distinctive service and thus establish a diagnosis. It is extremely important that progress curves be taken, otherwise the significant alterations may be overlooked.

The differentiation of angina pectoris and coronary occlusion was discussed in connection with the former condition. Coronary occlusion not infrequently precipitates, and often complicates angina pectoris. The possibility of coronary occlusion should be considered whenever the pain differs from that of the usual attack and particularly if it is more severe and occurs while at rest. A detailed study of the physical findings, blood pressure, temperature, leukocyte count and electrocardiographic observations will ordinarily permit a diagnosis.

Prognosis.—The occlusion of a large artery is compatible with life and not infrequently an efficient myocardium. In a study of a series of 117 cases by Conner and Holt, 109 (93 per cent) were in good health three months following the first occlusion and 25 (21 per cent) were well after five years. They furthermore cite 4 instances of ten years' survival and 1 of seventeen years. In general, the course is more favorable in those in whom the heart withstands the accident without signs of cardiac failure, whereas the outlook is grave in the cases with an extensive impairment in cardiac function during the initial stages of occlusion. There are, however, numerous exceptions as indicated in the study of Conner and Holt. In their series of 102 cases in which they were able to study the relationship of the severity of the symptoms to the immediate prognosis, almost one-third of those who recovered were in the group with extreme initial manifestations. In spite of the apparent course, the future is indefinite. Recurrences are frequent and there is always the possibility of embolic manifestations from the detachment of a bit of the clot which forms on the endocardium at the site of the infarction. Finally, the course is dependent to a remarkable extent on the treatment immediately following occlusion. Even though damage to the heart may not seem great at the time of the accident, the chances for recovery may be eliminated by allowing the patient on his feet too soon.

Treatment.—The early stage is the critical period. The protection of the heart at this time may not only determine the immediate outcome, but often has a deciding influence on the subsequent course. The patient should, therefore, be confined to bed at as nearly absolute rest as possible. Morphine is the most valuable drug at this stage of the treatment and should be administered in sufficient amounts to control the pain and induce sleep. Digitalis is indicated if there are signs of cardiac failure. It is important that the diet be simple and the patient spared all unnecessary exercise. Bed rest should be continued for six weeks or perhaps two months when a large vessel is occluded. In some it may be advisable to extend this period.

The extent of the infarction is determined by the size of the vessel occluded and the degree of the collateral circulation. It is possible to improve the collateral circulation by the administration of drugs which have a dilating action on the coronary arteries, as theophyllin and theobromin preparations. These drugs should be continued long after the patient is permitted on his feet. The management of the patient after he is allowed out of bed is deserving of careful supervision. Graded exercises serve an important function in this stage of the treatment. These should be carefully regulated and not extended to the point of shortness of breath.

SYPHILITIC HEART DISEASE.

This discussion deals with the cardiac disability occasioned by syphilitic involvement of the first portion of the aorta, exclusive of aneurysm. There are two important factors in the production of the cardiac disability: (1) aortic insufficiency, and (2) narrowing of the orifices of the coronary arteries by intimal proliferation. The aortic insufficiency increases the work of the left ventricle and the lowered diastolic pressure and the narrowing of the orifices of the coronary arteries diminish the volume flow of blood through the coronary vessels. In certain instances the work of the heart may be further increased by an associated hypertension. The excessive handicap thus imposed on the heart accounts for the progressive downward course frequently observed in this form of heart disease.

Etiology.—The Treponema pallidum is the causative agent. The organisms are distributed generally throughout the body during the early stages of syphilis and, while obviously carried to the heart and aorta, rarely, if ever, produce significant damage to these structures at this time. Certain of the organisms may, however, survive the various defense mechanisms of the body and after a period of years produce clinical manifestations. In some cases the infection never reaches this stage and is not discovered until after death. The symptoms ordinarily appear fifteen to twenty-five years after the infection. The disease, therefore, usually occurs in a clinical form between the ages of thirty-five and forty-five years. It has been estimated that 75 per cent of the cases fall between the ages of thirty and fifty-five years. When the disease makes its appearance after the age of fifty-five years the pathologic and clinical findings are often modified by arteriosclerosis. Physical strain is an important factor in precipitating the clinical manifestations. The disease is five or six times more prevalent in the male than the female sex. There are reasons for believing that the incidence has been very significantly reduced during recent years, particularly in those sections of the country where systematic treatment is employed early in the course of the original syphilitic infection.

Pathology.—Syphilis shows a predilection for the root of the aorta, but it often involves the entire ascending portion, less frequently the arch, and occasionally the descending aorta. In rare instances the lesion may be confined to the abdominal aorta. If the aortic valve area and the orifices of the coronary arteries are spared by the syphilitic processes, the heart is not likely to be damaged. The present paragraphs therefore deal only with those particular aspects of syphilitic aortitis which produce an embarrassment of the heart. The early lesion consists of an endarteritis obliterans of the vasa vasorum and a perivascular infiltration of lymphocytes in the adventitia. This is associated with degenerative changes in the media which are believed to be of a nutritional nature resulting in the destruction of the elastic structures and a weakening of the vessel wall. The process finally extends to the intima and the aortic valve structures, producing in the typical case varying degrees of wrinkling and puckering of the former with intervening areas of depression and a thickening and shortening of the valve leaflets. In some instances the valve leaflets may be so extensively deformed that they are reduced to fibrous bands. A widening of the commissures is one of the earliest and most distinctive manifestations of an involvement of the aortic valve area. Scott and his associates have suggested that the syphilis spreads from the aorta to the margin of the valve leaflets through small vessels at the commissure and believe that the earliest lesion is found in this location. The widening of the commissures, together with a deformity of the valve structures, produces an aortic insufficiency which is later increased by a dilatation of the aortic ring. In the extension of the intimal proliferation there is often an encroachment on the orifices of the coronary arteries which may occasionally terminate in complete occlusion of the vessels at this point. The coronary arteries are ordinarily not involved by the specific infection except in the immediate vicinity of the orifices. The alterations encountered distal to this location are usually of an arteriosclerotic nature. The above findings are generally accompanied by a dilatation and hypertrophy of the heart, which in some may be very extensive. The dilatation is at first confined to the left ventricle and may later involve all chambers. While the myocardium occasionally shows changes which may be attributed directly to the syphilitic infection, the findings in general are not distinctive and conform, for the most part, with those usually encountered in arteriosclerotic heart disease.

Symptoms.—Dyspnea and pain are the outstanding symptoms of syphilitic aortitis and each generally indicates an extensive impairment of the cardiac function. The dyspnea is usually the first expression of congestive failure and in time is followed by congestion of the lungs, engorgement of the liver and edema of the extremities. In the beginning it is either manifested by shortness of breath on slight exertion or occurs in the form of paroxysmal dyspnea. Paroxysmal dyspnea is not infrequently the first symptom. It may occur at any time, possibly precipitated by exertion but often appears during the night. Pain may be a very prominent symptom and may or may not be associated with dyspnea. It varies in character from an ill-defined distress over the precordium or a sense of constriction or burning over the upper sternum to the typical pain of angina pectoris. The pain may be constant, often comes in attacks and may be initiated by exertion. It may be confined to a relatively small area or transmitted to the neck, shoulders or arms. In some cases the pain is presumably aortic in origin, whereas in others it is probably dependent on narrowing or occlusion of the orifices of the coronary arteries.

Objective Signs.—The physical signs of structural changes in the heart and aorta are usually very evident after the onset of symptoms. They are frequently those of aortic insufficiency, possibly with aneurysm and cardiac failure. The aortic insufficiency, when fully developed, is at once betrayed by the violent pulsation in the vessels of the neck, the evident cardiac enlargement, with a heaving apex impulse, and a conspicuous diastolic murmur. This murmur is frequently associated with a systolic murmur at the base which varies in intensity and often in the more advanced cases is transmitted to the vessels of the neck. A systolic murmur produced by relative insufficiency of the mitral valve may also be heard at the apex. In the early stage of aortic insufficiency the diastolic murmur may escape detection unless careful search is made. At this stage there are usually other signs, such as a faint systolic murmur and accentuation of the second aortic sound with perhaps a peculiar metallic bell-like or tympanitic quality which should direct attention to the possibility of an involvement of the aorta. Occasionally a tympanitic character of the aortic second sound is the first feature to suggest syphilitic aortitis. In the more advanced cases there is usually a demonstrable increase in aortic dullness both laterally and upward. The pulsation of the aorta may be visible or palpable in the suprasternal notch. Fluoroscopic examination of the patient in different positions may reveal the dilatation of the aorta. The Wassermann reaction is positive in 75 to 80 per cent of all cases. There is often a history of the original infection and not infrequently there are evidences of syphilis in other organs, such as the nervous system, bones or testicles.

Diagnosis.—The diagnosis is usually evident in a typical case. The onset of cardiac symptoms and the signs of aortic insufficiency in an individual between thirty-five and fifty years of age who has not previously been aware of a cardiac lesion generally mean syphilitic aortitis. This disease should always be considered when the aortic valve alone is involved,· even though there is a history of possible rheumatic infection, and in angina pectoris, particularly when it appears before fifty years of age. A latent syphilitic aortitis not infrequently promotes the cardiac disability from arteriosclerotic heart disease. The character of the aortic second sound or perhaps a faint diastolic murmur usually directs attention to this possibility. A history of syphilitic infection, or of miscarriages or sterility, evidence of syphilis elsewhere in the body, roentgenologic signs of enlargement of the aorta and a positive Wassermann reaction are the deciding points in the diagnosis.

Prognosis.—There is usually extensive damage and often cardiac failure by the time the disease is recognized. The course, therefore, is in general progressively downward, and the patient dies within a few months or a few years from cardiac failure, angina pectoris, coronary occlusion, intercurrent infection or perhaps rupture of an aneurysm. There are, however, exceptions, particularly those in whom the disease is discovered and systematic treatment instituted before significant aortic insufficiency develops or before there is much encroachment upon the orifices of the coronary arteries. In not a few instances the syphilitic involvement of the aorta is either not suspected during life or its effects are overshadowed by those of coëxisting arteriosclerotic heart disease.

Treatment.—If heart failure is present it should be relieved before specific antisyphilitic treatment is begun.

There is considerable difference of opinion concerning the use of arsphenamine in the treatment of syphilitic heart disease. It is fairly generally agreed that a conservative plan should be adopted and that arsphenamine should be preceded by systematic preparation of the patient with mercury or bismuth and iodides. This should be continued for ten or twelve weeks, after which it may be safe to proceed with the administration of arsphenamine provided that the cardiac function has been sufficiently restored. The initial dose should not exceed 0.1 gram and the response carefully noted. Thereafter the dose may be gradually increased, but not beyond 0.45 gram, and the drug given at weekly intervals until eight or ten injections have been administered. This is alternated with courses of mercury or bismuth and iodides, and perhaps continued for one or two years or even longer, depending on the general response of the cardiovascular system. The individualized and cautious administration of neoarsphenamine with alternating courses of mercury and iodides is rarely a dangerous procedure and will in certain instances be followed by decided improvement in the cardiac condition.

THYROTOXIC HEART DISEASE.

Thyrotoxicosis is a relatively common cause of cardiac disability in the regions with a high incidence of toxic adenoma and exophthalmic goiter. In a recent analysis of 1329 cardiac cases at the University of Iowa, the cardiac disability in 116 (8.7 per cent) was attributed to thyrotoxicosis. This group included only cases with a persistent auricular fibrillation, a distinct cardiac enlargement or cardiac failure that could not be explained on another etiologic basis. Reference has already been made to the incidence of this form of heart disease in certain other sections of the United States.

Etiology.—Various theories have been advanced to explain the cardiac disability in thyrotoxicosis. The increased demand on the heart from an elevated basal metabolic rate is no doubt an important factor. This factor is present even at rest, and certain observations would indicate that it is disproportionately increased with exercise. Recent clinical and experimental studies by Andrus, McEachern and others point to a serious disturbance in the metabolism of the heart. The heart appears to share in the general increased metabolic rate and this in turn permits the rapid utilization of the glycogen content of the myocardium with an excessive accumulation of lactic acid. This, with the increased demands placed on the heart from the general augmented basal metabolic rate would seem to provide a very plausible explanation for the cardiac disability in thyrotoxicosis. In general, cardiac disability is likely to be a more conspicuous feature in long-standing thyrotoxicosis and often supplements that from other forms of heart disease.

Pathology.—There are no distinct pathologic findings. Although the heart is frequently enlarged, there is seldom a marked increase in weight and then other causes must be excluded. It seems probable that the usual enlargement of the heart is due chiefly to dilatation. Various histologic changes have been described, but these seldom differ in any essential respect from those encountered in the controls of a given age group. Occasionally the myocardium presents extensive degeneration but it is rather doubtful that this is primarily dependent on the thyrotoxicosis. The structural alterations incident to other forms of heart disease, particularly rheumatic and arteriosclerotic are commonly present.

Symptoms.—The symptoms in the beginning are those of a thyrotoxicosis. The increase in the cardiac rate which persists during sleep is one of the earliest and most distinctive signs. This is frequently accompanied by palpitation of the heart or an uncomfortable sensation over the precordium. With a progression of the thyroid disorder, the cardiac rate is further increased, the patient is more conscious of the heart and shortness of breath is readily induced by exertion. Finally more characteristic manifestations of an impaired cardiac function may appear, as evidenced by the paroxysmal or continued auricular fibrillation, or the onset of congestive failure. In the elderly subjects angina pectoris occasionally occurs.

Physical Signs.—The increased cardiac activity is at once evident through the exaggerated pulsation of the peripheral vessels which is most apparent in the neck. The increase in the cardiac rate is more or less proportional to the elevation of the basal rate and usually ranges between 100 and 120 per minute. The pulse is full and quick and resembles, to a certain extent, that of an aortic insufficiency. Occasionally, a capillary pulse may be demonstrated. The blood pressure finding is one of the most distinctive signs. There is generally some increase in the systolic phase, whereas the diastolic may be normal, but often slightly reduced. The area of cardiac dullness is frequently increased. In our 116 cases there was a distinct enlargement in 67 (57.6 per cent), as evidenced by the physical findings, or verified by the teleoroentgenogram. Systolic murmurs are common at the apex and over the pulmonary area. In the beginning, these are usually functional. Later, if the thyrotoxicosis is permitted to continue, a relative mitral insufficiency generally occurs. In an occasional instance the vibration of the chest wall from the accelerated cardiac rate may suggest a presystolic thrill of a mitral stenosis. A persistent auricular fibrillation is a common finding and was encountered in 46 (39.5 per cent) of our series. In all except 3, the absolute irregularity was associated with a definite cardiac enlargement. The onset of the continued auricular fibrillation is often preceded by transient attacks, and within a few weeks generally followed by the signs of congestive failure. The changes in the electrocardiogram are not distinctive. Auricular fibrillation is common and, not infrequently, alterations in the *T* deflection occur.

Diagnosis.—It is always well to bear in mind the possibility of a thyrotoxicosis in every case in which there is a question regarding the cause of the cardiac disability, for this is one of the etiologic agents of heart disease that may be completely abolished. Moreover, the cardiac disability from a thyrotoxicosis commonly supplements that of some other forms of heart disease, producing symptoms long before they would otherwise appear. The diagnosis is based on the history of a thyrotoxicosis and usually there is a distinct enlargement, commonly nodular, of the thyroid gland. In the more chronic types of thyrotoxicosis, particularly that associated with an adenoma, a significant impairment in the cardiac function may develop or even congestive failure occur without much evidence of a disordered thyroid function. Under these circumstances the possibility may be suggested through the discovery of a nodular enlargement of the thyroid or perhaps suspected because of an unexplained auricular fibrillation. The basal metabolic rate is frequently the determining factor. This examination should be repeated in doubtful cases and deferred in the presence of congestive failure until the cardiac function is restored.

Prognosis.—The prognosis depends on the extent of the cardiac damage and the possibility of other contributing factors. Auricular fibrillation often disappears after subtotal thyroidectomy or is frequently abolished by quinidine. Striking results are not infrequently obtained by operation, even after congestive failure. If the cardiac disability is primarily dependent upon other forms of heart disease, the outlook is not so favorable. Even in advanced forms of the latter, however, considerable relief often follows the control of the thyrotoxicosis.

Treatment.—There are two objectives in treatment: the conservation of the cardiac function, and the control of the thyrotoxicosis. With a congestive failure, bed rest, relaxation and sleep are essential. Diet should be simple and meet the body requirements. It is important that the diet contain an abundance of carbohydrates because of the body requirements and in view of the disturbed metabolism of the myocardium. Digitalis is indicated, and in auricular fibrillation, should be given in sufficient amounts to control the cardiac rate if possible. In certain instances, however, it may be very difficult to reduce the rate by digitalis. It is important that the above measures be supplemented by the administration of Lugol's solution. Ordinarily, after a week or ten days, the general condition will permit an operation. If the auricular fibrillation persists following the recovery from the operation, it may be frequently abolished by quinidine.

CONGENITAL HEART DISEASE.

Congenital heart disease is a relatively unimportant form of cardiac disability. The incidence is less than 3 per cent, and in a fairly large proportion the structural defects are so extensive that they are either not compatible with life or the subject dies within a few months or years. The possible anomalies are numerous and various combinations may occur. In the present discussion only the more common malformations will be considered.

1. **Anomalies of Position.**—Dextrocardia.—Dextrocardia, the transposition of the heart to the right side of the chest, may occur alone or with a similar alteration of other viscera. In an occasional instance there is a complete *situs inversus*. The heart is frequently otherwise normal. An acquired dextrocardia occasionally occurs, especially in the adult, and invariably results from a pulmonary condition which either retracts or displaces the heart to the right side. The differentiation from the congenital form may be possible from the history and physical findings but is not infrequently dependent on the electro-

cardiogram. In the latter, Lead I is inverted and Leads II and III are reversed.

2. **Anomalies of Structure.**—Defects in the Cardiac Septa.—(*a*) *Interauricular Septum.*—Abnormalities of varying extent are frequently encountered in the interauricular septum. In the more advanced form there may be a total absence of the septum. A patent foramen ovale, however, is the most frequent congenital anomaly involving this structure. This may occur alone or be accompanied by other structural defects, especially involving the pulmonary area. With a free communication between the auricles, the membrane which ordinarily closes the foramen is lacking. The defect, however, is very commonly limited to the membrane—septum ovale, represented either by an incomplete attachment producing a valve-like slit, or by a small fenestration and thus has no clinical significance.

(*b*) *Interventricular Septum.*—The development of the interventricular septum may likewise be incomplete. This defect is usually situated at the base at the site of the membranous septum or undefended space. The opening varies in size in different individuals and may occur alone or in conjunction with other lesions. In the former there may be no increase in the size of the heart or no impairment whatever in the cardiac function.

Anomalies of the Pulmonary Orifice.—The lesions in this location constitute the most important group of congenital anomalies. *Pulmonary stenosis* is the most common form of congenital heart disease. The stenosis may result from a fusion of the semilunar valves or in certain instances be located in the infundibular region or even in the right ventricle. These obstructive lesions are generally associated with defects in the ventricular or auricular septum or a patent ductus arteriosus. The combination of pulmonary stenosis, interventricular septum defect, dextroposition of the aorta and hypertrophy of the right ventricle (tetralogy of Fallot) is commonly found in adults with cyanosis from congenital heart disease.

Patent Ductus Arteriosus.—This structure ordinarily contracts soon after birth and is usually completely closed after two or three weeks. If, however, the pressure in the right ventricle is increased because of a pulmonary condition as an atelectasis, or more particularly because of an obstruction at the pulmonary orifice, it may remain open. Occasionally this is the only lesion, but it is usually accompanied by defects, especially involving the pulmonary orifice.

Coarctation of the Aorta.—This refers to a narrowing or a complete atresia of the aorta between the left subclavian artery and the ductus arteriosus. The circulation, under these conditions, is promoted by anastomosis between the subclavian artery and the thoracic and abdominal aorta, especially by the way of the internal mammary and the intercostal arteries. In rare instances a congenital aortic stenosis occurs.

Abnormalities of the Valve Cusps.—The valve cusps of the aortic and pulmonary orifices are not infrequently increased or decreased in number. The supernumerary cusps are usually rudimentary and more often at the pulmonary opening. A reduction in the cusps or a bicuspid condition, on the other hand, is more frequently encountered at

the aortic orifice.   The recent observation of Lewis has directed attention to the importance of this lesion in subacute bacterial endocarditis.

Symptoms and Signs.—Symptoms rarely occur except with extensive
impairment in the cardiac function.   They usually consist of shortness
of breath on exertion or, in certain instances, of paroxysmal attacks of
dyspnea with possibly angina-like pain.   The attacks of dyspnea tend
to increase in intensity, generally accompanied by pain and may be
very distressing.   Hemoptysis and epistaxis are occasionally encountered and syncope and epileptiform convulsions have been observed.

Cyanosis is one of the most significant findings.   It occurs in 40
to 50 per cent of all cases and is ordinarily associated with an extensive
lesion.   The extent of the cyanosis varies in individual cases, but is
particularly conspicuous in the more advanced form.   When present,
it is usually noted at birth and generally persists to varying degrees
throughout life.   Various explanations have been given for this phenomenon.   There appear to be at least two important factors: the
admixture of venous and arterial blood from an abnormal opening
between the right and left heart, and the deficient oxygenation of the
blood in the lung because of an impaired pulmonary circulation.

The patient with a high-grade cyanosis generally has a marked polycythemia and often presents a clubbing of the fingers and toes.   The
red blood count may range between 6,000,000 to 12,000,000 with a
corresponding increase in the hemoglobin.   This is believed to represent a compensatory mechanism and no doubt contributes to the
cyanosis.   There is seldom a significant increase in the leukocytes.
The alteration in the fingers and toes affects chiefly the soft tissue
covering the terminal phalanges.   It is said that it may be present
at birth, but usually does not develop until later.

In the examination of the heart, the thrills and murmurs are the
most distinctive findings.   They are generally located at the base of
the heart, over the region of the right ventricle, and may cover a
considerable area.   The thrill is usually coarse and accompanied by
a harsh systolic murmur.   In rare instances, there may be a diastolic
or presystolic murmur.   The transmission of the murmur does not
correspond with that of the ordinary valve lesion.   In pulmonary
stenosis, the pulmonic second sound is often diminished in intensity
and may be absent.   There is seldom much increase in the area of
cardiac dullness which is contrary to that usually encountered with an
acquired lesion.   In certain instances, particularly with an obstruction
at the pulmonary orifice and patent foramen ovale, there may be a
very pronounced venous congestion of the retinal veins, with possibly
a marked distention of the arteries.   The roentgenologic examination
is often helpful in determining the enlargement of the right heart and
in a patent ductus arteriosus, may reveal prominence in the region of
the pulmonary artery.   The electrocardiogram frequently shows a
right axis deviation.   The extent of the right axis deviation is greatest
with a pulmonary obstruction and may exceed that produced by any
other type of cardiac lesion.

Diagnosis.—In infancy and early childhood, a cyanosis or the history
of a blue baby and the presence of a thrill and a harsh murmur at the

base of the heart establishes the diagnosis of congenital heart disease. Later in life, particularly in the absence of a cyanosis, the condition is more likely to be confused with an acquired lesion. The history with reference to a rheumatic infection, the size and the shape of the heart, the roentgenologic and electrocardiographic findings generally permit a differentiation. Functional systolic murmurs over the pulmonary area occasionally suggest a congenital defect. These murmurs, however, are rarely harsh and not accompanied by an increase in size of the heart or a cyanosis. It is often impossible to come to a definite conclusion concerning the nature of the defect because of the frequent multiplicity of the lesion. The findings in certain instances, however, may be sufficiently characteristic to permit a fairly confident diagnosis.

Pulmonary Stenosis.—This is one of the most common high-grade lesions compatible with life. A vast majority of those who reach early adult life are said to have this type of malformation. It is usually associated with either a patency of the interauricular or interventricular septum, perhaps both, and possibly an open ductus arteriosus. In a typical case there is a thrill and a harsh systolic murmur with maximum intensity over the second and third left interspace. The pulmonic second sound is often reduced in intensity or may not be heard. Cyanosis is generally present and it is usually possible to demonstrate an extension of the cardiac dullness to the right of the sternum. The electrocardiogram generally shows a distinctive right axis deviation.

Patent Ductus Arteriosus.—If this anomaly is not complicated by other lesions, the subject may not experience any particular impairment in the cardiac function, and there is usually no cyanosis. The murmur is heard best in the second interspace a short distance from the sternum, begins after the first sound and may extend beyond the second sound. It is accompanied by a thrill and an accentuated pulmonic second sound. Fluoroscopic examination of the chest or a teleoroentgenogram frequently shows a prominence in the region of the pulmonary artery.

Interventricular Septum Defect.—This lesion occasionally occurs alone and may not produce any cardiac disability. In a case observed by the writer the heart was normal in size, the cardiac response was excellent and there were no alterations in the electrocardiogram. The murmur is systolic in time, seldom accompanied by a thrill, moderately harsh in quality, and heard best over the third and fourth left interspace near the sternum.

Coarctation of the Aorta.—When encountered in the adult, there is often a history of hypertension and possibly headaches, epistaxis, dizziness or ringing in the ears. The heart is usually enlarged to the left. The blood-pressure reading from the arms is usually elevated, whereas the pulsation in the femoral arteries is greatly reduced or may even be barely perceptible. With a fairly high-grade obstruction, the collateral circulation on the chest is sooner or later evident. The increased tension and tortuosity of the intercostal arteries may produce an erosion of the ribs which is responsible for the distinctive roentgenologic findings.

Prognosis.—The prognosis varies with the degree of cyanosis and the extent of the cardiac impairment. In the more extensive malformations the condition is either not compatible with life or the majority die within a few weeks or months. A marked cyanosis is an unfavorable sign, but some survive for years. The growth and the development of a child and, above all, the cardiac response are the determining factors. Murmurs, regardless of their intensity, are to be evaluated on this basis. Minor anomalies are of no consequence except insofar as they may permit development of a subacute bacterial endocarditis.

Treatment.—The treatment in infancy is primarily concerned with the general care of the child. Later it may be necessary to curtail physical activities. Not a few, however, are capable of leading a normal life. Cardiac failure is treated in the usual manner.

PERICARDITIS.

Acute pericarditis may exist with or without effusion, depending on whether the exudate is chiefly serous or fibrinous. The terminal stage, characterized by adhesions between the pericardium and heart, and the pericardium and surrounding structures, is designated as adherent pericardium or chronic adhesive pericarditis.

Etiology.—The etiology of pericarditis is extremely varied. There are, however, five important causes: rheumatic fever, pneumonia, tuberculosis, chronic nephritis and coronary occlusion. Rheumatic fever is the most common etiologic factor. The pericarditis may develop at any stage of the disease, but occurs most frequently during acute exacerbations. The incidence, as determined by necropsy findings, is very high in those that succumb from rheumatic heart disease during the first and second decades of life. This would indicate that the pericardium is very commonly involved in the more acute and rapidly progressing forms of rheumatic heart disease. A pericarditis not infrequently occurs during the course of acute infections, particularly pneumonia. It occasionally complicates scarlet fever, and may result from invasion of the blood stream in puerperal infection, osteomyelitis, furunculosis, gonorrhea and other types of sepsis. Although the pericarditis which is associated with pneumonia may be of hematogenous origin, it is usually produced by direct extension of the infection from a pneumonic lower lobe, particularly the left, or from an empyema. In tuberculosis, also, the pericardium is invaded by direct extension from the pleura, lung or mediastinal lymph nodes. Any infection of the neighboring structures, including the ribs, sternum, vertebræ, or even of the abdominal viscera, may extend to the pericardium. The pericarditis of chronic nephritis is usually a terminal event, such as is seen occasionally in the terminal stages of various other chronic diseases. In rare instances, the pericardium is involved by malignant tumors, generally metastatic, but at times by direct extension from adjacent structures. The pericardial changes incident to coronary occlusion are very important because the associated pericardial rub is the most distinctive sign of cardiac infarction (but unimportant from the standpoint of pericarditis).

The varied nature of the etiologic factors permits pericarditis to occur at almost any age. Cases have been reported in new-born infants. The incidence is perhaps highest during childhood and early adult life because of rheumatic fever. The disease is more prevalent in the male sex.

Acute Fibrinous Pericarditis.—Pathology.—This is the most frequent and mildest form of pericarditis. The fibrinous exudate is the most prominent pathologic feature. In the earlier stages the exudate forms a thin film which may be confined to a relatively small area, or covers the entire pericardium. The process may subside at this point and the exudate be absorbed. However, if the inflammation continues the fibrinous exudate increases in thickness and is thrown into ridges or strands by the constant movement of the heart. In addition, varying amounts of serous exudate are usually present. Rheumatic pericarditis probably never exists without rheumatic myocarditis. The pericarditis which follows coronary occlusion is confined to the area of infarction.

Symptoms.—There are often no symptoms referable to the pericarditis itself, so that it is either overlooked, detected incidentally or perhaps not discovered until extensive effusion has appeared. Even if symptoms are present, they are likely to be confused with those of a pneumonia or overshadowed by a terminal infection.

Pain is the outstanding symptom, especially in the rheumatic type. It is often sharp or even stabbing in character and may be aggravated by coughing, deep breathing or change of position. It is usually confined to the precordium, but may radiate to the neck or the left shoulder and arm as in angina pectoris. In rare instances, because of the involvement of the diaphragm, the pain is referred to the abdomen, simulating acute abdominal disease. Cough and dyspnea occasionally occur. The general system reaction is determined to a large extent by the primary disease. Although fever is usually present, it may be difficult to determine how much of it is due to the pericarditis alone.

Physical Signs.—The pericardial friction rub is the most distinctive sign. It is occasionally detected by palpation and may be heard anywhere over the pericardium or even in the back, but more frequently along the sternum or at the base of the heart. The rub usually occurs both in systole and diastole, but in some cases it is limited to systole. It often overlaps the heart sounds in a way which varies from cycle to cycle, or is influenced by respiration, which helps to differentiate it from a murmur. There is great variation in the intensity of a pericardial rub. In some cases they are very rough, whereas in others they are soft and readily mistaken for murmurs. A rub often varies also in the same individual from day to day or from hour to hour. The intensity may be altered by position or increased by gentle pressure of the stethoscope. The rub appears to be superficial, is not transmitted as endocardial murmurs are, and lasts for a period which varies in duration from a few hours to days or weeks. Effusion into the pericardium may change its location or character or dispel it entirely. In rheumatic pericarditis there is invariably evidence of structural change in the heart in the form of enlargement and murmurs, and under these circumstances it is frequently difficult to estimate the

26

extent to which accumulation of fluid contributes to the increase in area of cardiac dulness.

Diagnosis.—The pericardial friction rub establishes the diagnosis. It is ordinarily identified without much difficulty. In some instances it may be confused with an endocardial murmur, particularly the double murmur of aortic disease, but the murmur is more constant and is transmitted in the direction of blood flow. In cases in which the pericardium is involved by direct extension of infection from the lungs or pleura, there may be a pleuro-pericardial rub. This is recognized by its relationship to the respiratory cycle and by the fact that it may be temporarily abolished by the cessation of breathing.

Prognosis.—The prognosis is largely dependent on the gravity of the disease primarily responsible for the pericarditis. In rheumatic fever the immediate outlook is favorable if the pericarditis does not progress beyond the fibrinous stage. However, to the inevitable rheumatic myocarditis, there is added the possibility of further embarrassment through the formation of pericardial adhesions. In certain instances the inflammation progresses, with the formation of a more extensive serous exudate, and the condition changes to that of pericarditis with effusion.

Treatment.—Treatment is directed chiefly toward relieving the primary condition, and is largely symptomatic from the standpoint of the pericarditis. The application of an ice-bag and the administration of salicylates are valuable measures in patients with precordial distress. When the pain is severe codeine or morphine may be required. In rheumatic fever it is important that the patient be confined to bed until all evidence of infection has disappeared.

Pericarditis with Effusion.—This form of pericarditis is characterized by an effusion into the pericardial sac which may either modify or dominate the clinical picture. It commonly develops as a sequel of fibrinous pericarditis. In the beginning the simple fibrinous exudate produces no symptoms except a pericardial rub and possibly pain, but when effusion appears the patient becomes short of breath, the area of cardiac dulness increases and signs of encroachment on the lungs appear. Various combinations may thus occur, depending on the extent and character of the exudate and the nature of the primary disease. Rheumatic fever, tuberculosis, pneumonia and septicemia are the most common causes of pericarditis with effusion.

Pathology.—The effusion varies in amount and rate of formation. It may be serofibrinous, hemorrhagic or purulent, depending on the type of the primary disease. A hemorrhagic effusion is generally associated with tuberculosis or malignancy, and a purulent exudate with pneumonia or a blood-stream infection caused by some pyogenic organism. The amount of fluid ranges from a few hundred cubic centimeters to 2 liters or more. The largest effusions are seen in tuberculosis and rheumatic fever, more particularly in the former. There is a varying amount of fibrinous exudate which forms ridges or presents an irregular shaggy appearance. The pericardial layers are congested and perhaps show hemorrhagic areas. In the cases with a purulent exudate there is often a granular appearance and sometimes distinct erosions. The parietal layer is frequently thickened and may be of a leathery consistency. In the more chronic forms the exudate may be separated into pockets by the formation of adhesions between the visceral and parietal layers of the pericardium. The outer layers of the myocardium are usually involved to a certain extent.

In the pericarditis which is associated with rheumatic fever there is invariably a general invasion of the myocardium, which may be extensive.

Symptoms.—The symptoms vary with the nature of the primary infection, the character of the onset of the pericardial involvement and the extent and rate of accumulation of the effusion. In rheumatic fever the arthritis may be the outstanding clinical manifestation in the beginning, and the pericarditis, particularly when painless, not suspected until the onset of dyspnea. The pericarditis may, on the other hand, be the first significant sign of a rheumatic fever and, because of the pain, be recognized early. In other instances the effusion into the pericardium is of short duration and never of sufficient extent to embarrass the heart or produce evident pressure signs in the lungs. Under these circumstances, the condition may readily escape detection unless attention is focused on the heart through the discovery of a friction rub. The pericarditis of pneumonia and other pyogenic infections is likely to be overshadowed by the primary disease. In tuberculosis the onset may be very insidious, and the patient may not consult his physician until he suffers from symptoms of cardiac embarrassment.

Pain and shortness of breath are the chief symptoms. The pain may precede the shortness of breath or they may be associated. In some cases there is no pain and the dyspnea is the outstanding complaint. The respiratory discomfort results from embarrassment of the cardiac function brought about by the fluid in the pericardial sac and from compression of the lungs. The effusion handicaps the cardiac contraction, and may become so large as to encroach upon the venæ cavæ and hinder the return of blood to the right auricle. At the same time the distended pericardial sac projects posteriorly on both sides, particularly on the left, and compresses the lungs, bronchi and trachea. Dyspnea may thus be a very prominent feature, and in the more advanced stages is associated with extensive engorgement of the liver and edema of the extremities or dependent parts of the body. The patient at this stage is obliged to sit up and is more comfortable when leaning forward. There is not infrequently an irritating cough, occasionally dysphagia from pressure on the esophagus and in rare instances aphonia through compression or irritation of the recurrent laryngeal nerve. The patient is restless and often unable to sleep except with the help of drugs. In the later stages delirium and even coma may occur. The fever varies with the primary disease. It is generally high in pneumonia and sepsis and occasionally a prominent feature in rheumatic fever.

Physical Signs.—In the beginning the pericardial rub is usually the only distinctive finding and generally responsible for the diagnosis. There may be some increase in the area of cardiac dulness, but differentiation of this increase from that produced by cardiac enlargement, particularly in the presence of endocardial murmurs, may be extremely difficult. Other significant signs appear as the fluid increases. The area of cardiac dulness increases both to the right and the left, and in an upward direction. The extension of the area of dulness at the base of the heart in the first and second interspaces to the right and left of the sternum, and the fact that it shifts with the change from the recumbent to the upright position, may be one of the early signs of pericardial effusion. There is likewise a shift in the area of dulness at the diaphragmatic level with a change in posture, but here the shift is the reverse of that encountered at the base of the heart. In changing to the upright position, the extent of the dulness is reduced at the base and increases at the diaphragmatic level. The shape of the cardiac dulness in the sitting posture has been likened to that of a pear, and becomes more globular on lying down. As the fluid increases the apex impulse becomes less evident on inspection and finally may not be detected even by palpation. In some instances, when the apex impulse is no longer palpated in a recumbent position, it may be felt by having the patient sit up and lean forward. In the meantime the pericardial rub has probably either disappeared or changed in character or become limited to a small area at the base. Occasionally it may persist in a pronounced form in spite of an extensive effusion. The cardiac tones are usually reduced in intensity and at times barely heard. The pulmonary second sound may be accentuated.

When the effusion is large, important pulmonary findings are generally encountered. There is usually a reduction in the expansion of the left side of the chest, with possibly a lagging, or even no movement, of the left costal margin. Projection of the pericardial sac posteriorly often produces a significant compression of the lung. This is manifested by an area of dulness of variable extent at the angle of the left scapula over which bronchial breathing is heard. These findings occasionally lead to a diagnosis of pneumonia. There may also be displacement or compression of the anterior lateral margin of the left lower lobe, producing a tympanitic percussion note and tubular breathing in the axillary region about the level of the nipple. These findings, and also those at the angle of the scapula, may be altered by having the patient lean forward.

Cyanosis is common, and the superficial veins of the neck, upper extremities and chest are often distended. The pulse, particularly with a large effusion, is frequently of low tension and may entirely disappear during inspiration, the paradoxical pulse. This is usually associated with a distinct reduction in the systolic blood pressure. The liver is often pushed down by the weight of the effusion and may produce a prominence in the epigastrium. In patients with extensive impairment of the cardiac function there are frequently engorgement of the liver and edema of the dependent parts of the body, and occasionally fluid in the peritoneal cavity.

Roentgenologic Signs.—There is a general enlargement of the cardiac shadow which in the early stages is difficult to differentiate from cardiac enlargement. A bulging in the dependent portion of the pericardial sac is the earliest sign. This is seen best on fluoroscopic examination in the lateral view. Later, as the fluid accumulates, the cardiac shadow fills out in the first and second interspaces, and the normal curve, particularly along the left border of the heart, is eliminated. At this time a definite alteration in the shape of the cardiac shadow is apparent with a change from the recumbent to the upright position. The width of the cardiac shadow immediately above the diaphragm is increased and that at the base in the first and second interspaces is reduced. The cardiac pulsations are diminished in amplitude and may be absent entirely in the more extensive effusion. This is one of the most important roentgenologic signs of pericardial effusion and at once eliminates the possibility of confusion with cardiac enlargement.

Diagnosis.—The mild degrees of pericardial effusion are often overlooked. In many instances attention is first directed to the possibility by the discovery of a pericardial rub. The differentiation between cardiac enlargement and fluid in the pericardial sac may be difficult, and the difficulty may be still further increased by the presence of endocardial murmurs and other factors which might explain a cardiac enlargement. The roentgenologic examination generally yields more decisive information than the physical signs. In those instances in which the fluid develops while under observation, the diagnosis is at once evident. The signs are generally quite distinctive if the effusion is large. In some instances the findings in the chest may suggest pneumonia or pleurisy with effusion, on the left side. The marked enlargement of the cardiac dulness, both to the right and left and in an upward direction, usually points to a pericardial involvement, and the roentgen-ray establishes the diagnosis.

Prognosis.—The prognosis varies with the nature of the primary condition and the character of the effusion. The immediate outlook is generally more favorable in the rheumatic type. In many instances the fluid is slight in amount and disappears in a few days. Even with extensive effusion it is seldom necessary to aspirate the pericardial sac, for the effusion is ordinarily of a serous character and rapidly absorbed. (The associated damage to the myocardium is the most important aspect.) In the tuberculous form the onset is more insidious and the course often prolonged. Repeated aspirations of the fluid may be necessary. Because of the chronicity, there is a greater tendency to the subsequent formation of extensive adhesions. In an occasional instance the exudate is purulent. The purulent effusions are always serious and when associated with a sepsis usually fatal. The prognosis is likewise grave in the pericarditis of chronic nephritis, and the terminal infection of various chronic diseases.

Treatment.—The treatment is directed primarily toward the underlying condition and conservation of the cardiac function. The patient is confined to bed and relaxation and sleep promoted. The diet should be simple and meet the body requirements. The application of an ice-bag to the precordium frequently gives relief from oppression and pain, reduces the cardiac rate and may possibly retard the progress of the effusion. Morphine is frequently required in severe cases for relief of pain. Paracentesis is indicated if there is embarrassment of the cardiac function and should be repeated when necessary. If there is reason to suspect that the exudate is purulent, an exploratory aspiration should be done at once, and if pus is obtained surgical drainage of the pericardial sac instituted.

Various sites have been suggested for the introduction of the needle, such as the fourth and fifth left intercostal spaces near the sternum, the chondro-xiphoid angle and the fifth and sixth left intercostal spaces just outside the apex. The apical location is generally believed to be the most satisfactory in that there is less danger of puncturing the heart, and the fluid is perhaps more accessible. It is important that the aspiration be performed with as little inconvenience to the patient as possible. In some it may be advisable to administer morphine. After a few minutes the patient is then arranged in the most comfortable position, the precordial area prepared in the usual manner by the application of tincture of iodine and alcohol and the skin and subcutaneous tissues at the site selected for the puncture carefully anesthesized by 0.5 per cent novocaine solution. The aspirating needle is slowly introduced in an upward direction. Some resistance is often encountered on entering the pericardial sac. If the operator proceeds cautiously, contact with the heart is usually evident through the impulse transmitted by the needle and thus any damage may ordinarily be avoided. The fluid may be aspirated either with a large syringe or a negative pressure apparatus, as employed in the removal of pleural effusion.

Adherent Pericardium (Chronic Adhesive Pericarditis).—The formation of adhesions between the heart and the pericardium, or the heart, pericardium and the surrounding structures, may result from an acute pericarditis. This commonly follows rheumatic, tuberculous or pneumococcus pericarditis. A localized adhesion between the pericardium and the heart usually develops after a cardiac infarction.

Pathology.—There is a marked variation in the extent of the adhesion. The simplest form is represented by one or more localized adhesions between the parietal and visceral layers of the pericardium. This may in no way interfere with the cardiac function, and is therefore of no clinical significance. In other instances the adhesions between the heart and the pericardium are more extensive and may entirely obliterate the pericardial cavity (concretio cordis). In such cases the pericardium is usually thickened, contracted and possibly presents areas of calcification. The adhesions are dense and not infrequently attached to the chest wall, diaphragm and the mediastinal structures. The superior vena cava, inferior vena cava and the hepatic veins may be caught in the adhesions. Obstruction of the hepatic veins produces an engorgement of the liver which may eventually terminate in a cirrhosis (Pick's disease). The more extensive the adhesions, the greater the handicap placed on the heart, leading ultimately to marked cardiac enlargement and failure. The heart is not infrequently hypertrophied and dilated to an extreme degree. In the rheumatic type there is invariably an associated involvement of the myocardium and endocardium during the acute stage of the pericarditis.

Symptoms.—The symptoms vary with the extent of the adhesions and the structures involved. Isolated adhesions between the parietal and visceral layers of the pericardium may be suspected because of the history of pericarditis or cardiac infarction, but no symptoms are produced and their presence is not established until necropsy. The symptoms of more widespread adhesions are in general those of a gradual impairment in cardiac function and finally congestive failure. Recurring ascites is the most prominent feature in some cases. Although there are generally extensive structural changes in the heart, the ascites is out of proportion to the degree of impairment of cardiac function and is to be explained by portal obstruction secondary to stenosis of the hepatic veins or inferior vena cava.

Physical Signs.—Structural changes in the heart are at once apparent in the cases with extensive pericardial adhesions, in which there are not infrequently obvious signs of congestive failure, such as dyspnea, cyanosis and perhaps edema. The apex impulse is broad, often heaving, and may lift the entire precordium with each systole. It may extend to or even beyond the anterior axillary line and down to the sixth interspace. There may be a systolic retraction of the interspaces and the ribs in the region of the apex. In some instances there is a prominent diastolic rebound which is generally accompanied by a shock. This is one of the important signs of pericardial adhesions and is attributed to diastolic release of tension on the adhesions. If the diaphragm is involved there may be a retraction of the eleventh and twelfth ribs posteriorly (Broadbent's sign). This sign, however, is not pathognomonic of pericardial adhesions, for it may occur with a large heart without adhesions. There is usually a general enlargement of the heart, as indicated by an increase in the cardiac dulness both to the right and left of the sternum. Endocardial lesions are generally present in the cases with a rheumatic history. Even though the valve may have escaped damage from the original infection, murmurs produced by relative insufficiency of the mitral and tricuspid valves are common in the later stages of concretio cordis. Diastolic collapse of the veins of the neck is occasionally observed, and a paradoxical pulse may occur. The additional signs are those of congestive failure.

Roentgenologic Signs.—Important information may be obtained by roentgenologic examination. This is one of the means of estimating fairly accurately the degree of fixation of the heart. The border of the cardiac shadow may be irregular, more particularly on the left side, and small projections are not infrequently noted. These small projections may be made more evident by forced breathing. In addition, the excursion of the diaphragm is perhaps curtailed, or the diaphragm may be forcibly pulled upward with each contraction of the heart. The identification of calcium deposits in the pericardium, while rarely possible, is a distinctive sign of obsolete pericarditis.

The *electrocardiographic* method affords another means of identifying a fixation of the heart. The curve should be taken first with the patient lying on his back, then on the right side, and finally on the left side. In the normal individual the ventricular deflections are altered by such a change in position. The absence of a significant alteration is a fairly reliable sign of cardiac fixation.

Diagnosis.—Adherent pericarditis should be suspected in every relatively young individual with marked cardiac enlargement, and particularly in those with an associated ascites. The history of a previous pericarditis, and of tuberculosis or other forms of pulmonary infection, is important. The diagnosis in certain instances is fairly readily established on the basis of a distinct fixation of the heart and the demonstration of adhesions by the roentgen-ray. The signs are often indefinite, however. · Systolic retraction, apparent fixation of the apex, and even Broadbent's sign may occur without pericardial adhesions.

Prognosis.—The prognosis is largely dependent on the state of the myocardium and the extent of the hepatic involvement. The patient may live for years with extensive adhesions, but is often an invalid. Death usually results from cardiac failure, recurring ascites or intercurrent infection.

Treatment.—The treatment is primarily concerned with the conservation or restoration of the cardiac function or with relief of the recurring ascites. The cardiac failure is treated in the usual way by rest, sleep and digitalis. Ammonium chloride, 1.5 to 2 grams (20 to 30 grains) after each meal, or salyrgan, 0.5 to 2 cc. intravenously, every second day, may help to relieve the ascites. Salyrgan should not be used if nephritis is present.

Within recent years there has been a renewed interest in the surgical treatment suggested by Brauer in 1902. The object of this operation is to free the heart from its mechanical encumbrances by removing parts of the fourth, fifth and sixth ribs on the left side with or without a part of the sternum, and to divide some of the bands which constrict the great vessels. This form of treatment is applicable to patients with a fairly satisfactory cardiac function without ascites. In certain carefully selected cases striking improvement has been reported.

CHRONIC VALVULAR HEART DISEASE.

In certain forms of heart disease, more especially in the rheumatic type, the mechanical handicap imposed by an insufficiency or a stenosis or, more often, a combination of these effects, from a deformity of the valve structures, is a prominent aspect or may even dominate the subsequent course. This, however, is not the only factor in the development of the cardiac disability. The valve lesions are frequently progressive, and in the more advanced stages, particularly following rheumatic fever, are generally dependent on repeated recurrences or exacerbations of the infection with an associated involvement of the myocardium. The damage to the myocardium may thus be a significant feature of the disease and, in those that die within a few years following the initial infection, usually overshadow the valve lesions.

In the arteriosclerotic heart disease, the structural alterations in the myocardium are usually far more significant than the associated valvular defect. The aortic insufficiency from a syphilitic involvement of the aorta is customarily mentioned in connection with aortic valve disease. This, however, is primarily dependent on a dilatation of the aorta and the deformity of the valves is relatively unimportant.

Statistics as to the relative frequency with which the different valves are concerned vary somewhat, depending on the incidence of syphilis and whether the diagnosis is established clinically or by a postmortem. In the figures cited by White, including more than 3000 cases, with two series totaling 508 cases in which the diagnosis was established at necropsy, the mitral valve was involved in 70 to 85 per cent, the aortic 42 to 45 per cent, tricuspid 10 to 15 per cent and the pulmonic valve in approximately 1 per cent. There was a surprisingly close agreement in the two series of necropsy cases. The mitral valve was diseased alone in 50 to 60 per cent, and the aortic in 10 to 20 per cent. A tricuspid lesion is usually associated with an involvement of the mitral valve and seldom diagnosed clinically, except when manifested by an insufficiency. Tricuspid insufficiency is relatively common, but usually results from a dilatation of the valve ring rather than from a deformity of the valve structures. It is thus designated as a relative insufficiency. The mitral valve ring is frequently concerned in the same manner. In many instances, particularly when the patient is first seen during a cardiac failure, it may be difficult or even impossible to determine the extent to which a mitral insufficiency is dependent on a disease of the valve structure or a dilatation of the heart. The distinction, however, is frequently not of any great importance at this stage of the cardiac disability, since it may have little or no bearing on the prognosis or treatment.

Mitral Valve Disease.

Etiology.—Mitral valve disease results from valvulitis in the vast majority of cases, and rheumatic fever is by far the most important etiologic factor. A mitral stenosis is generally regarded as being pathognomonic of a rheumatic infection. The history, however, is not infrequently negative for rheumatic fever, more particularly in the latent form, which occurs especially in women. There still remains a group in which the nature of the infectious agent is unknown. If, however, the cases with a varying degree of stenosis and those in which an arteriosclerosis is probably the responsible factor are excluded, the remaining group is relatively small.

A thickening and sclerosis of the valve structures occasionally result from an arteriosclerosis. In rare instances, an extensive calcification may involve the entire valve ring. Under these conditions, the possibility of a previous infection is difficult to exclude. In most instances, the mitral insufficiency associated with an arteriosclerosis is dependent upon myocardial changes and a subsequent dilatation of the auriculoventricular ring. A relative insufficiency of the mitral valve also occurs in various other forms of myocardial weakness, particularly that associated with high-grade anemia and thyrotoxicosis.

The incidence is highest between ten and thirty years because of the prevalence of rheumatic heart disease during this period, and rapidly recedes after forty years of age. This disease, however, persists to a limited extent in the upper age groups and is occasionally observed after sixty years. The arteriosclerotic type begins to appear at about fifty years and increases thereafter. The females predominate slightly in the rheumatic group, more particularly in cases with mitral stenosis.

Pathology.—Healing probably occurs in certain of the milder forms of acute endocarditis without any significant residual damage or perhaps no more than a slight thickening or contracture of the valve leaflets. When, however, the involvement is more extensive, or there are repeated invasions of the valve structures, from exacerbations or recurrence of the infection, the valvular deformity usually becomes a more prominent feature. The entire valve structure, and often the mitral ring may be involved. In the more chronic cases there is fusion of the valve leaflets, shortening of the chordæ tendineæ, and not infrequently an extensive calcification. The valves are held in a partially open position. This frequently produces a rigid irregular or funnel-shaped structure projecting into the cavity of the left ventricle with an opening varying in size and shape. There is thus produced a combined stenosis and insufficiency in which either effect may dominate. The higher grades of obstruction are designated as pure mitral stenosis. The opening may be represented by an irregular narrow slit or be oval in shape, possibly barely admitting the tip of the little finger. A pure mitral insufficiency is seen in the earlier stages of the disease before the valve structures become rigid and is therefore the prevailing mitral lesion in childhood. It is also observed at a later age when there is a limited deformity of the valves. The stenosis represents a more advanced stage in the development of the valve defect and may not appear for five or ten years, or even for a longer period after the original valvulitis.

The additional alterations in the heart vary with the extent and character of the mechanical handicap and the associated involvement of the myocardium. If the valvular lesion is primarily a stenosis, an extra load is placed on the left auricle and right ventricle. There is at first a dilatation and hypertrophy of the left auricle. The capacity of the left auricle is normally under 50 cc. In the more advanced forms of obstruction, it may be increased to 500 or even 700 cc. The projection of the dilated chamber, posteriorly and to the left, produces one of the most distinctive roentgenologic findings of mitral stenosis. The obstruction to the flow of the blood into the left ventricle leads to an increase in the pulmonary pressure which may finally result in pulmonary congestion, fibrosis and possibly a sclerosis of the pulmonary vessels. This in turn adds to the work of the right ventricle which is later manifested by a hypertrophy and dilatation. As the right ventricle increases in size, it occupies more and more of the anterior surface of the heart and in the more advanced stage may, for the most part, make up the apex which is normally produced by the left ventricle. The left ventricle, under these circumstances, is not increased in size to any significant extent, and may be actually smaller than normal. When, however, the mitral stenosis is associated with a distinct insufficiency, the left ventricle is involved along with the left auricle and the right ventricle. In general, the heart is larger with a double lesion. The most extensive cardiac enlargement is seen in cases with rheumatic heart disease that die within a few years after the initial cardiac infection. An insufficiency is generally the outstanding lesion. The associated involvement of the myocardium, however, is a prominent factor. The insufficiency is thus produced not only by the deformity of the valve leaflets, but by a dilatation of the mitral ring. While, under these conditions, the mitral insufficiency contributes to the cardiac disability, it is not as important as the damage to the myocardium.

Mitral Stenosis.—Symptoms.—The symptoms in general are not characteristic in mitral stenosis. They seldom appear until there is an extensive impairment in the cardiac function and usually represent a beginning failure of the myocardium. Certain complications may, however, occur before the onset of the more evident signs of cardiac failure. In some the pulmonary congestion and possibly an associated respiratory infection is productive of blood-tinged sputum or even a frank hemoptysis. A cerebral accident or splenic infarct is occasionally the first manifestation of a mitral stenosis. In other cases the attention is perhaps first directed to the heart because of premature contractions, possibly paroxysms of auricular fibrillation, or more often the onset of shortness of breath.

Physical Findings.—The findings prior to the onset of the cardiac failure, except for certain complications, as mentioned above, are confined to the heart. The information obtained by inspection is not infrequently surprisingly negative. In some, particularly in thin-chested individuals, the apex impulse may be rather prominent and of a diffuse character. It frequently does not extend beyond the midclavicular line. Occasionally, abnormal pulsations are noted in the third and fourth left intercostal spaces from an overactive pulmonary conus. The presystolic thrill is one of the most distinctive signs of mitral stenosis. It is often confined to a small area, usually well within the outer border of the apex impulse and corresponds with the location of the murmur. In the beginning the thrill is only felt with an accelerated heart-rate. It is crescendo in character and terminates abruptly with the first heart sound which is often manifested by a sudden shock. There is, likewise, a diastolic shock over the pulmonic area. Occasionally, particularly in the more advanced forms, the thrill may be divided into two stages, the de-crescendo and the crescendo, corresponding to the two phases of the murmur. On percussion there is often no significant increase in the size of the heart. An extension of the dulness to the right of the sternum may be demonstrated, but this is often difficult to elicit until the onset of cardiac failure and a more extensive dilatation of the right auricle. The heart is likely to be globular in shape, chiefly because of the filling out in the region of the left auricle and pulmonary artery.

The passing of the blood from the left auricle to the left ventricle through the constricted and irregular opening sets up a vibration which is not only responsible for the diastolic thrill, but also the diastolic murmur. The latter is another distinctive finding in mitral stenosis. The murmur and the thrill, as well, obviously correspond with the the particular period during the diastole in which the velocity of the blood passing from the left auricle to the left ventricle is greatest. It therefore first appears in late diastole during the period of the auricular contraction, and ends abruptly with a snappy first sound. Later, as the obstruction progresses, it advances toward the mid-diastolic period and finally an early diastolic murmur is heard. The murmur may occasionally extend throughout the diastolic period, with perhaps a reduction in the intensity in the mid-section. With the onset of an auricular fibrillation, the presystolic phase of the murmur usually disappears and only that occurring during the first half of the diastole is heard. If, however, the cardiac rate is accelerated, the murmur may again take on a presystolic aspect because of the shortening of the diastolic period. The snappy first sound is a prominent feature and in certain instances may not be preceded by a murmur. An accentuation of the pulmonic second sound is generally very evident, and not infrequently there is a reduplication. The amplitude of the radial pulse may be reduced, but the tension is fairly well maintained. There may be some reduction in the systolic blood pressure.

The findings from the roentgenologic examination are often helpful in the diagnosis of mitral stenosis. The globular shape of the heart from the filling out in the region of the left auricle and the pulmonary artery is suggestive. The dilated left auricle projects posteriorly and slightly to the left. It is therefore apparent in the oblique position and is one of the most distinctive roentgenologic signs of mitral stenosis.

There is not infrequently a right axis deviation in the electrocardiogram, which, in some instances, may be quite marked. The *P*-wave is often more prominent, the duration generally increased, and the summit frequently notched. The findings are generally considerably altered by a significant mitral insufficiency. There is invariably a more evident increase in the size of the heart. In the more advanced forms, the heart may be very large. The apex impulse, under these conditions, is usually diffuse and often extends well outside the mid-clavicular line. The displacement of the apex is more outward than downward. The diastolic murmur is frequently not so prominent or perhaps only evident after exercise or excitement.

Complications.—The tremendous strain placed on the left auricle, the increased tension in the pulmonary circulation, and the added load on the right ventricle may produce a characteristic train of complications. In the hypertrophy and dilatation of the left auricle, a stage is frequently reached in which the auricles fail to contract in a normal fashion and an auricular fibrillation is established. This may be preceded by a period of irregularity from premature contractions. Mitral stenosis is one of the most common causes of auricular fibrillation. The dilatation of the auricles also permits other possibilities. In the more advanced forms, and particularly after the onset of the auricular fibrillation, the rate of the blood flow within these dilated chambers is greatly reduced. This not infrequently permits the blood to coagulate, especially in the crevices in the auricular appendages. Occasionally, bits are dislodged, pass into the circulation and go to the brain, spleen, kidneys, mesentery vessels or perhaps to the extremities. In rare instances, a ball thrombus is formed in the left auricle which may, intermittently, further obstruct the mitral orifice and produce distressing attacks of dyspnea and precordial discomfort. The increased tension in the pulmonary circulation is prone to produce pulmonary congestion. This, along with the increased susceptibility to respiratory infections, may lead to blood-tinged sputum, occasionally a frank hemoptysis and, in certain instances, findings very suggestive of pulmonary tuberculosis. The failure of the right ventricle is evidenced by a relative tricuspid insufficiency and an engorgement of the liver. A prolonged engorgement of the liver may ultimately terminate in cirrhosis and portal obstruction. In certain instances, the hepatic complications may be an important feature in a later stage of the disease.

Diagnosis.—A mitral stenosis is ordinarily recognized by the thrill and characteristic murmur. In the early stages of the lesion, however, the murmur may be readily overlooked. It may not be present at rest, and perhaps brought out only by exercise or amyl nitrite. The murmur is usually heard best in the recumbent position, and frequently made more evident by turning the patient on the left side which brings the heart more in contact with the chest wall. It should be remembered that after the onset of the auricular fibrillation, the presystolic phase of the murmur generally disappears. A short early diastolic murmur with possibly a snappy first sound may be the only auscultatory findings. An apical diastolic murmur (the Austin Flint murmur) of the same general character may be associated with an aortic insufficiency. The aortic lesion is identified by the enlargement of the left ventricle and the peripheral vascular phenomena. When, however, there is a combined aortic and mitral lesion, particularly the rheumatic type, it is frequently difficult, or even impossible, to differentiate between the Flint murmur and that of a mitral stenosis. In the aortic insufficiency from a syphilitic aortitis, it is generally safe to assume that there is not a mitral stenosis. The faint diastolic murmur to the left of the sternum, from pulmonary insufficiency, may be mistaken for an aortic insufficiency. The absence of the other signs of an aortic lesion is generally sufficient to exclude the possibility.

An apical diastolic vibration is not infrequently observed in the overactive heart of hypersensitive individuals, occasionally heard in the cardiac enlargement involving the left ventricle, especially with an adherent pericardium. The history and associated findings usually permit a differentiation.

Prognosis.—Mitral stenosis represents one of the most serious forms of chronic valvular heart disease because of the progressive nature of the lesion and the possibility of grave complications. The prognosis in general is dependent on the extent of the stenosis, the age of the individual and associated damage to the myocardium. The outlook is usually poor in a relatively young individual, and the majority die before the age of forty years. Isolated instances of fairly high-grade stenosis are observed after fifty or even sixty years of age. Occasionally, there is a history of repeated pregnancies without any impairment in the cardiac function. The instance of intercurrent infection, possibly recurrent damage to the myocardium, and the social and economic status of the individual are very important factors.   If the individual carefully conserves the cardiac function and is fortunate in escaping complications, the onset of the cardiac failure may be postponed for years and death possibly result from some other condition.

Mitral Insufficiency.—Mitral insufficiency was at one time considered to be the most frequent form of valvular heart disease.   If, however, the term is restricted to the insufficiency that is dependent on the deformity of the valve structures, and the cases with recognizable stenosis are excluded, it is not a very common lesion.   Mitral insufficiency is the earliest manifestation of an acute valvulitis.   In the beginning, particularly in the rheumatic type, the dilatation of the mitral ring from the associated involvement of the myocardium is an important factor in the production of the murmur.   The lesion continues to be an insufficiency until, through the subsequent healing and perhaps recurring damage, the valves are further deformed and their movement greatly restricted.   This may require three to five or even ten years, and then the evidence of a stenosis appears.   In certain instances, however, especially when there is a limited damage to the valve, the lesion continues as an insufficiency.   Mitral insufficiency in later life may be produced by thickening or curling of the edges of the valve leaflets or a shortening of the chordæ tendineæ from an arteriosclerosis. It is, however, more often a relative insufficiency produced by a cardiac dilatation.

Physical Findings.—There is a remarkable variation in the size of the heart with this lesion, depending on the stage and the extent of the myocardial involvement.   The character and location of the apex impulse is one of the most reliable guides in estimating the extent of the cardiac enlargement.   If it is forceful and displaced to, or beyond, the mid-clavicular line, it is generally safe to conclude that the heart is enlarged.   In the more advanced stages, there is frequently an extensive cardiac dilatation and hypertrophy involving both the right and left chambers.   The precordium, under these circumstances, is usually prominent and there is frequently a widespread pulsation extending from the left border of the sternum to, or even well beyond, the anterior axillary line.   The more definite apex impulse is usually located in the fifth or sixth interspaces.   The contraction of the heart is forcible and possibly lifts the entire left lower anterior chest.   The second sound, especially over the pulmonic, may be readily felt.   In the early stages of the cardiac enlargement, the dulness is only increased to the left.   Later, as the dilatation and hypertrophy progress, there is an evident general enlargement of the heart, as indicated by an extension of the dulness, both to the right and to the left.   The murmur is systolic in time and soft blowing, harsh or even musical in character.   It replaces partly or entirely the first sound and may be heard over the entire precordium.   The transmission is to the left toward the axilla and possibly backward to the angle of the scapula.   There is usually an accentuation of the second pulmonic sound.

Diagnosis.—The diagnosis is usually evident, but may be very difficult.   It is at once apparent when there is a cardiac enlargement and a systolic apical murmur transmitted to the left. The recognition is by far the most important during the acute stage of the valvulitis. At this time the murmur is generally soft blowing in character and possibly not transmitted to any significant extent. The apical region is, furthermore, a very common site for systolic murmurs, not dependent on an organic basis. Some are definitely of the cardio-respiratory type. The explanation in certain instances, however, is not clearly understood. Systolic murmurs are likewise encountered over the pulmonic area and may be heard well toward the apex. These physiologic murmurs are not infrequently mistaken for a mitral insufficiency. The diagnosis may be extremely difficult when a child is seen for the first time, particularly during an acute infection. The character of the infection, past history and possibly evidence of rheumatic fever are important. The size of the heart, however, is a deciding factor. In questionable cases the appearance of even a faint presystolic rumble at a later period in the development of the valve lesion establishes the significance of the systolic murmur. Theoretically, the endocardial type of an insufficiency should be associated with a certain degree of stenosis. Generally, these lesions are combined to such an extent that both effects may be recognized. In the mitral insufficiency that appears in later life, it is often impossible to differentiate between that due to a deformity and that resulting from cardiac dilatation. The history and findings relative to the blood pressure, the condition of the arteries, the myocardium and the possibility of an anemia and thyrotoxicosis are helpful in the diagnosis.

Prognosis.—The prognosis is largely determined by the condition of the myocardium. The outlook in children is always in doubt because of the possible recurrence of rheumatic fever and the extension of myocardial damage. It is unfortunately poor in those with an extensive cardiac enlargement. If, on the other hand, the rheumatic infection is recognized early, the child given adequate treatment from the standpoint of rest, and protected against a recurrence of the infection, there may never be any significant impairment in the cardiac function. The prognosis in the arteriosclerotic variety is even more dependent on the state of the myocardium and other factors. In those with minor damage to the valve structures, there is always the remote possibility of a subacute bacterial endocarditis.

Aortic Valve Disease.

Etiology.—Rheumatic fever, syphilis and arteriosclerosis are the most important causes of aortic valve disease. In rare instances an insufficiency may result from a rupture of a valve segment. The valve is usually already damaged by sclerotic changes or possibly by erosion from a bacterial endocarditis, and with the former there is frequently a history of trauma or excessive strain. Bacterial endocarditis alone may be responsible for an aortic insufficiency. A congenital anomaly, particularly a fusion of two cusps, is fairly common in the aortic valves. This malformation apparently renders the valve more susceptible to sclerotic changes or may permit the development of a bacterial endocarditis.

The etiologic factors responsible for aortic valve disease allow it to occur any time between early childhood and advanced old age. The incidence, however, is highest in middle life because of the prevalence of syphilis and the fact that there are still instances of the rheumatic form. Lesions of the aortic valve are far more common in the male sex. The dominance in this sex holds for each of the three main etiologic agents but is more striking in the syphilitic and arteriosclerotic groups.

Pathology.—The early lesion in a rheumatic valvulitis is that of an insufficiency. It is quite likely that the involvement of the aorta by the rheumatic infection may, in certain instances, permit a dilatation of this structure and thus contribute to the production of the insufficiency. In the subsequent healing the valves are deformed to a varying extent, depending on the magnitude of the valvular damage. The cusps are thus not only thickened and retracted, but their movement curtailed, which produces a combined insufficiency and stenosis. The stenosis, as in the mitral valve, is a later development but less often the outstanding feature. It seldom occurs in an advanced form until after thirty years of age.

The syphilitic variety differs from the endocarditic in that it begins and continues as an insufficiency. In the early stages the widening of the commissures may be responsible. Later a dilatation of the aortic ring is the most important factor. The disease process in the aorta often involves the aortic cusps to a varying extent and frequently encroaches upon the orifices of the coronary arteries.

In the elderly subjects sclerotic changes may occur, resulting in a thickening and deformity of the cusps and possibly limitation in their movement. This is usually associated with degenerative changes in the aorta which occasionally permit a slight dilatation of the aortic ring. A combined stenosis and insufficiency may be produced. In certain instances the process progresses to a high-grade stenosis in which the valve cusps are fused and there is extensive calcification. These alterations are not infrequently engrafted on a previous valvular damage or a congenital anomaly, and are often associated with a sclerosis of the coronary arteries.

Aortic Insufficiency.—*Effects on the Heart.*—The amount of blood which regurgitates back into the left ventricle during diastole varies with the extent of the lesion. In certain instances, particularly in the syphilitic form, it is probably extensive. This allows overfilling of the left ventricle, and the fall in the diastolic blood pressure incident to the regurgitation necessitates a stronger ventricular contraction in order to maintain an adequate circulation. These two factors produce a dilatation and hypertrophy of the left ventricle and in time a relative insufficiency of the mitral valve. In the beginning the left ventricle alone is concerned, but in the later development of the lesion, particularly with a more extensive impairment in cardiac function, the left auricle and finally the right heart are involved. The left ventricle, in compensating for the regurgitation, is obliged to contract with a much greater force on a larger volume of blood, which generally results in an increase in systolic blood pressure. The sudden rises in the arterial tension with systole and the abrupt fall during diastole are responsible for the characteristic pulse and the other vascular phenomena.

Aortic insufficiency is perhaps the most serious form of valvular heart disease. More work is required of the left ventricle and, in addition, there is a reduction in the coronary circulation from the low diastolic pressure. In the arteriosclerotic and syphilitic forms the coronary circulation may be further impaired by an involvement of the coronary arteries or an encroachment on the coronary orifices. Changes in the myocardium incident to the valve damage is another important aspect. The combination of these various factors accounts for the extensive cardiac enlargement frequently observed in this type of lesion.

Symptoms.—The symptoms are relatively insignificant until the onset of cardiac failure. These patients are perhaps more prone to palpitation because of the forceful cardiac contractions and may at times be conscious of the pulsations of the vessels in the neck. Precordial or substernal discomfort is not infrequently observed and occasionally anginal pain occurs.

Physical Signs.—The apex impulse is usually evident and generally displaced downward and outward. In the early stages of the lesion it is often well localized, possibly in the fifth interspace and little, if any, outside the mid-clavicular line. With the progression of the lesion, it may extend to the sixth or seventh interspace and well beyond the anterior axillary line. The impulse is distinctly heaving in character and may lift the entire anterior chest. The location of the apex impulse accurately indicates the extent of the cardiac enlargement. The increase in the area of cardiac dulness is for the most part downward and to the left. In the more advanced form, however, it may extend to the right of the sternum.

The diastolic murmur is the most distinctive sign. It may be heard at the base and generally best along the left border of the sternum, at about the level of the third and fourth intercostal spaces. This murmur, however, is often transmitted to other locations and may thus be auscultated at a lower level along the left border of the sternum at the apex or even in the axilla. It is usually blowing in quality and characteristically prolonged, with a gradual reduction in intensity. Occasionally there is a whistling or musical quality. A pronounced change in the character should suggest the possibility of a destructive lesion, as in a subacute bacterial endocarditis or rupture of a valve segment. In the beginning the murmur is usually faint and readily overlooked. It may thus be necessary to auscultate very carefully at the base and more particularly at the left border of the sternum. The murmur at this stage is more easily elicited by direct auscultation and is often heard best by having the individual exhale completely and then hold his breath. Occasionally it is more evident in the sitting position. There is frequently a systolic murmur over the aortic area transmitted to the vessels of the neck and the suprasternal notch. In certain instances, especially in the arteriosclerotic and rheumatic groups, this murmur may be harsh and perhaps accompanied by a thrill. A systolic apical murmur transmitted to the

27

axilla, resulting from associated deformity of the mitral valve or relative mitral insufficiency, is common.

Flint Murmur.—The diastolic murmur described by Austin Flint is not uncommonly present in aortic insufficiency. This murmur is confined to the apical region, occurs in the middle or late diastole, and is low-pitched and crescendo in character. It differs from the presystolic murmur of mitral stenosis in that it is rarely, if ever, associated with accentuation of the first mitral sound or a distinct thrill. The murmur has been attributed to a relative mitral stenosis but the mechanism is not clear. In the explanation usually given it is assumed that the regurgitant blood stream from the aorta holds back the anterior cusp of the mitral valve, in the way of the blood passing from the left auricle into the left ventricle, and thus produces a relative mitral stenosis. A similar murmur, however, may occur in a large heart without aortic insufficiency. White has suggested that the dilatation of the left ventricle may be sufficient, with a relatively normal-sized mitral opening, to permit the formation of a murmur.

The sudden increase and the abrupt fall in the arterial tension produces characteristic *vascular phenomena*. These features vary with the extent of the regurgitation and may thus be difficult to elicit in the early stages of the insufficiency, or are made less conspicuous by an aortic or mitral stenosis. With a free aortic insufficiency there is generally extensive pulsation of all the peripheral arteries which is particularly noted in the neck and arms. In the advanced form, especially when there is an associated anemia, the head may nod and perhaps the bed shake with each cardiac contraction. A pulsation of the retinal arteries is revealed by the ophthalmoscope. The capillary pulse may be demonstrated by slight pressure on the tip of the finger nail, by means of a glass slide on the lower lip, or by a gentle stroke across the forehead. This is manifested by a flush projecting into the zone of pallor with each cardiac contraction. The pulse is characteristically collapsing ("water hammer"—Corrigan). There is a sudden increase in the tension and an abrupt fall which is accentuated by slightly elevating the arm. This is reflected in the blood pressure by the abrupt increase in the systolic and a significant reduction in the diastolic phase. In the advanced stage it may not be possible to obtain a true diastolic reading. This produces an unusually large pulse pressure, which, in the extreme form, is not observed in any other condition. Certain additional findings are encountered in the further examination of the peripheral arteries. If a brachial or a femoral artery is auscultated, it is noted that the abrupt distention of the vessel with each cardiac contraction is accompanied by a sound or even a sudden snap, the "pistol-shot" sound. On compressing the vessel by the bell of the stethoscope, a point is reached when a diastolic murmur is heard, which is generally designated as the Duroziez sign.

The roentgenologic examination gives important information relative to the size and configuration of the heart but more particularly the condition of the aorta. It is indicated in every case where there is any reason to suspect the possibility of a syphilitic etiology, and is not infrequently desirable in the arteriosclerotic form. The electro-cardiogram frequently shows a left axis deviation. Changes in the T deflection and alterations in the Q–R–S group, however, are more significant from the standpoint of the condition of the myocardium.

Diagnosis.—The diagnosis of an aortic insufficiency is ordinarily established without difficulty by the nature and location of the apex impulse, the general configuration of cardiac enlargement, the character and distribution of the diastolic murmur and the peripheral arterial phenomena. An aortic insufficiency is not infrequently overlooked because the diastolic murmur is not detected. The Flint murmur may be confused with the presystolic murmur of mitral stenosis. The absence of the usual accentuation of the first mitral sound and the association with an early diastolic murmur along the left border of the sternum and other manifestations of an aortic insufficiency, usually identify the condition. In rare instances a faint diastolic murmur (Graham Steell murmur) from a pulmonary insufficiency occurs. This, however, is invariably dependent on a high-grade mitral stenosis which is usually apparent. In doubtful cases the diagnosis is based on the absence of peripheral vascular phenomena and roentgenologic findings with reference to the left auricle and the prominence of the pulmonary artery. The electrocardiographic findings may be helpful. In mitral stenosis a right axis deviation curve is usually encountered, whereas in aortic insufficiency a left axis deviation is more likely to occur. The diagnosis of an aortic insufficiency should always include the determination of the etiologic factor, along with the estimation of the extent of the impairment in the cardiac function.

Prognosis.—The prognosis is determined by the extent of the insufficiency, the etiologic factor, the presence of other valve defects and the state of the myocardium. An aortic insufficiency of the rheumatic variety may be borne for years without much impairment in the cardiac function. Here again, there is ever the possibility of a recurrence of the rheumatic fever with a further increase in the valvular deformity, new insults to the myocardium and perhaps the involvement of other valves. The outlook in the syphilitic form is usually poor. The changes in the aorta are generally advanced by the time the insufficiency is discovered, and the course is frequently steadily downward. There is seldom an extensive regurgitation in the arteriosclerotic variety but there is likely to be a significant involvement of the coronary arteries. A moderate stenosis, both in the rheumatic and arteriosclerotic forms, limits the extent of the insufficiency and thereby leads to a more favorable prognosis. If, however, the lesion is associated with an involvement of the mitral valve, a greater handicap is placed on the heart.

Aortic Stenosis.—An advanced aortic stenosis is a rare lesion. It generally follows either a rheumatic valvulitis or results from an arteriosclerotic process. Instances of the former are rarely encountered before the age of thirty years and of the latter seldom observed until after sixty years of age. The rheumatic form is often associated with involvement of other valves, particularly the mitral valve. An aortic lesion, either on a rheumatic or arteriosclerotic basis, usually produces a combined insufficiency and stenosis. Even in the high-grade stenosis an insufficiency is not infrequently evident.

The left ventricle is obliged to work against an increased resistance. In the early stages the change in the left ventricle is manifested chiefly by hypertrophy. The wall of the left ventricle is therefore often greatly thickened without much increase in the size of the left ventricular chamber. The systolic phase of the heart is prolonged in order to compensate for the obstruction to the passage of the blood into the aorta. This accounts for the well-sustained pulse tension noted in aortic stenosis. With the gradual impairment in the function of the left ventricle, dilatation is more evident, and the left auricle and finally the right ventricle are involved.

Symptoms.—There are ordinarily no symptoms until shortly before the onset of cardiac failure. Dizziness or fainting attacks from a cerebral anemia are not infrequently the first manifestations. These symptoms usually occur with exertion and are often associated with some shortness of breath. Substernal pressure or true anginal pain may be experienced. The anginal symptoms, however, are not so frequent as in aortic insufficiency.

Physical Findings.—The cardiac enlargement is readily elicited in the younger subjects but may be masked in the elderly individuals by an emphysema. The apex impulse is usually not a conspicuous feature, or perhaps the location is determined only by careful palpation. The attention is usually attracted at once by the rough grating or musical murmur over the aortic area, communicated to the suprasternal notch and to the vessels of the neck. The aortic second sound is seldom heard. In rare instances, particularly in the advanced form after the onset of cardiac failure, the murmur may be barely audible or perhaps entirely absent. The intensity of the murmur under these circumstances increases with the improvement in cardiac function. There is often a faint diastolic murmur, and a musical systolic murmur is rather common at the apex. A thrill accompanies the harsh aortic murmur and is likewise transmitted to the upper sternum and vessels of the neck. This thrill varies with the intensity of the murmur and in certain instances may be barely palpable or possibly not elicited. It may be brought out by having the patient lie on his anterior chest over a firm surface.

The change in the pulse is one of the most distinctive features. It rises very slowly and is well sustained, producing in the sphygmographic tracing the characteristic broad plateau-like peak. The systolic blood pressure is frequently low and possibly not more than 90 to 100, with a diastolic pressure at about the normal level. This gives a small pulse pressure, ranging between 15 and 25 mm. Hg. The character of the pulse- and blood-pressure readings is altered by the extent of the insufficiency. The electrocardiogram usually shows a marked left axis deviation. An inversion of the T-wave and alteration in the Q–R–S group are common, particularly in the arteriosclerotic form.

Diagnosis.—The diagnosis is based on the murmur, thrill and character of the pulse. The pulse is by all means the most distinctive finding. The systolic murmurs are common over the aortic area in arteriosclerosis, aneurysm, or in a subacute bacterial endocarditis of the aortic valve, without a significant stenosis. A thrill is likewise not necessarily indicative of a stenosis. A diagnosis of aortic stenosis is therefore justified only when the murmur and the thrill are associated with a characteristic change in the pulse. In certain instances it is possible that the arteriosclerotic lesion may be confused with pulmonary stenosis. In the latter, however, the murmur and thrill are transmitted slightly to the left and not to the vessels of the neck, and the characteristic alteration in the pulse is lacking.

Prognosis.—An aortic stenosis may permit many years of active life. At the onset of failure, however, the course is usually downward. The arteriosclerotic form is not infrequently a latent development. It may not necessarily reduce the life expectancy. Some have been known to live to ripe old age.

Tricuspid Valve Disease.

The tricuspid valves are occasionally involved in a rheumatic infection. The necropsy findings reported by Coombs would seem to indicate that the incidence is fairly high in the more extensively damaged hearts. In 97 cases these valves were concerned in 35. In every instance there was an associated involvement of other valves, more particularly the mitral valve. These lesions, however, seldom result in a significant insufficiency and stenosis. While a tricuspid insufficiency is relatively common, it is generally due to a stretching of the auriculo-ventricular ring from a dilatation of the right ventricle. A stenosis is rarely encountered and not usually diagnosed during life.

Tricuspid Insufficiency.—This condition may occur from a valvular deformity but generally results from a dilatation of the right ventricle (relative insufficiency). The relative insufficiency therefore is usually associated with congestive failure.

Physical Signs.—The transmission of a systolic pulsation to the veins of the neck, the upper extremities and particularly to the liver through the regurgitation of the blood from the right ventricle to the right auricle is one of the most distinctive signs. The pulsation in the neck is usually more evident in the right supraclavicular triangle lateral to the sterno-cleido-mastoid muscle, where the external and internal jugulars enter the subclavian vein. It is synchronous with the carotid pulse, but may be distinguished from the latter by pushing the vein to one side, or, in doubtful cases, by a polygraphic tracing. In the more advanced form the pulsation may be detected by gently palpating the external jugular vein between the thumb and forefinger. This phenomenon is frequently observed in the most characteristic form in the arms. It is brought out by slowly raising the arm to a point just preceding the collapse of the vein. Occasionally the pulsation may be observed in the veins of the shoulders and chest. The regurgitation of the blood in the inferior vena cava and the hepatic vein produces a systolic pulsation of the liver. This is expansile in character and may be differentiated from those transmitted from the aorta or right ventricle by palpating the edge of the liver between the two hands, or, in thin subjects, between the thumb and forefinger.

The area of cardiac dulness is generally increased both to the right and to the left. There are frequently widespread precordial pulsations which may be particularly forceful over the lower sternum from the heaving contraction of the right ventricle. Various murmurs are heard, depending on the associated valvular involvement. A tricuspid insufficiency produces a systolic murmur with maximum intensity over the lower sternum. With a relative insufficiency the murmur is usually soft blowing in character and limited in its distribution. In those in which the insufficiency is of valvular origin and generally associated with some degree of stenosis the murmur is more harsh or even rough in quality, transmitted to the right, possibly in some instances as far as the anterior axillary line. Edema is usually present particularly with the relative insufficiency, and a generalized anasarca often develops. Occasionally the edema in the legs may disappear and the ascites persist. This is due to the development of a portal obstruction from prolonged engorgement of the liver.

Diagnosis.—The diagnosis in the early stages is generally not possible except by means of the polygraph. The location and the transmission of the murmur may suggest a tricuspid insufficiency but the diagnosis is finally dependent on the demonstration of a systolic pulsation of the veins. In a more advanced form this is very apparent in the veins of the neck or arms or is readily elicited by palpating the liver.

Tricuspid Stenosis.—Tricuspid stenosis is very rare and is usually associated with mitral stenosis. Cyanosis to a moderate degree may be present for years and rapidly progresses with the onset of cardiac failure. Shortness of breath is the most frequent complaint and generally easily induced.

The venous congestion with a cyanosis of the lips, nose, ears and hands, and the engorgement of the jugular veins is a conspicuous feature. The cardiac findings are often masked by the mitral lesion. If, however, the stethoscope is moved from the apex toward the sternum there are frequently two points of maximum intensity, one over the mitral valve area and the other over the tricuspid area. The cyanosis and venous congestion, a decided extension of the cardiac dulness to the right from a dilated right auricle, a harsh murmur over the lower sternal region and the early enlargement of the liver warrant a serious consideration of tricuspid stenosis. The diagnosis, however, is established only by the polygraph. A faint pulsation of the jugular veins is normally produced by the contraction of the right auricle. In tricuspid stenosis with a sinus rhythm this is markedly increased and constitutes the most distinctive sign.

Pulmonary Valve Disease.

Lesions of the pulmonary valves, aside from congenital anomalies, are exceedingly uncommon. These valves are rarely invaded by rheumatic infection. In a series of 97 cases reported by Coombs, the pulmonary valves were involved in only 2 instances. Rare instances are recorded in which damage has resulted from various types of infections. Sclerotic changes are occasionally encountered and an involvement by subacute bacterial infection has been reported. A stenosis or insufficiency may presumably result from these various causes but they are exceptional occurrences. When a pulmonary stenosis occurs it is almost invariably from a congenital anomaly. The signs of this lesion are considered under congenital heart disease.

Systolic murmurs are extremely common in the pulmonary region. They are usually soft-blowing in character, occasionally have a harsh quality and are seldom transmitted to any significant extent. These murmurs are more particularly seen in children and thin-chested individuals, occur with fever, and are commonly observed in anemic states. They are often altered by posture and frequently influenced by respiration. Occasionally a systolic murmur of a mitral insufficiency may be transmitted to the pulmonary region. These functional or physiologic murmurs are distinguished by their location and character, the influence of posture and respiration, and the fact that they are not associated with demonstrable structural changes in the heart.

An *insufficiency of the pulmonary valve* is generally functional and usually associated with a high-grade mitral stenosis. It is manifested by a soft diastolic murmur (Graham Steell murmur) along the left border of the sternum. This murmur is strikingly similar to the diastolic murmur of aortic insufficiency. It is distinguished from the latter only by the absence of the vascular phenomena and by the associated findings of a mitral stenosis. The differentiation in certain instances may be extremely difficult and perhaps not established until after a period of observation. In most instances in which a pulmonary insufficiency is suspected, the murmur is finally proven to be that of an aortic insufficiency.

Treatment of Chronic Valvular Heart Disease.—These patients should be under the general supervision of a physician. When first seen the infection and other factors which may promote the cardiac disability should as far as possible be removed. The treatment therefore is largely a matter of protecting the subject against further cardiac insults and overtaxing the heart by physical strain. This form of heart disease frequently progresses through the return or an exacerbation of the rheumatic infection. It is therefore important that more than the usual precaution be taken against infection, particularly of the upper respiratory tract, and the individual confined to bed during the active stage of the infection or until the physician is certain that' the heart is not damaged. Reinfections of the heart are altogether too often not recognized and thus protective measures are not instituted. Excessive physical strain, more especially with a mitral stenosis or an aortic insufficiency, often contributes to a reduction in the functional capacity of the heart. The physical activities under these circumstances demand careful consideration and adjustments are not infrequently necessary. With the more serious forms of valvular lesions, as a mitral stenosis or an aortic insufficiency, competitive athletics are prohibited. If the cardiac lesion is discovered in childhood, the child should be encouraged to continue in school in order that he may be able to gain a livelihood without resorting to physical labor. In women the advisability of pregnancy at times comes up for consideration. Many with a moderate degree of mitral stenosis go through pregnancies without any apparent ill effect. A woman, aged sixty years, with a very evident mitral stenosis was recently seen by the writer. This woman had been aware of her cardiac lesion for years and had gone through five pregnancies without any difficulty whatever on the score of the heart. With a marked aortic insufficiency or a high-grade mitral stenosis, there is a likelihood of trouble and with an evident reduction in the cardiac function, pregnancy should always be avoided, or, if it occurs, terminated at an early date. The individual's great desire for a child may, in certain instances, justify chances that would otherwise not be taken.

DISEASES OF THE MYOCARDIUM.

Myocarditis.

An inflammation of the myocardium, aside from that produced by rheumatic fever, is a relatively rare condition and, except in diphtheria, usually is not recognized clinically. It may be caused by any acute infection, but occurs most frequently with diphtheria, scarlet fever, pneumonia, septicemia, pyemia and perhaps in milder grades with influenza and typhoid fever. In the majority of cases that come to necropsy, death has resulted from the primary condition and not the myocarditis. The incidence of myocardial damage during the course of various infectious diseases is not known. Recent electrocardiographic studies would seem to indicate that minor changes probably occur with considerable frequency. These patients, however, generally recover without any apparent cardiac disability. It is not unlikely that infections may contribute at times to a very significant extent to an already existing myocardial damage. Except for rheumatic fever, diphtheria is probably the most important single factor in the production of the advanced forms of myocarditis.

Morbid Anatomy.—The gross appearance of the heart varies with the extent of myocardial damage. In the more extensive form, the muscle is soft and flabby and frequently presents a mottled appearance. Occasionally, minute epicardial hemorrhages are seen. There is generally a diffuse parenchymatous degeneration involving especially the ventricles. In the microscopic examination, varying stages of degeneration are encountered. In the beginning, muscle fibers stain light pink and the cross striations are indistinct. Adjoining sections of the myocardium may show areas with extensive degeneration with an albuminous exudate and infiltration of polymorphonuclear and mononuclear cells between the diseased muscle strands. An advanced form of degeneration with areas of necrosis is seen in diphtheria. In the myocarditis associated with septicemia, bacterial emboli may lodge in the smaller arterioles and produce an abscess. The more chronic varieties of myocarditis show various stages of healing with connective tissue proliferation.

Symptoms.—In many instances the myocarditis is a terminal affair and there are either no symptoms directing attention to the heart, or they are overshadowed by those of the primary condition. The myocarditis associated with diphtheria is the one that is most generally recognized. It is most likely to occur in the more toxic forms, particularly when the administration of antitoxin has been delayed or not given in sufficient amount. This complication is usually not evident until the beginning of the second week. In certain instances, it may not be apparent until the patient is up and about and perhaps first suggested by marked weakness or collapse after slight exertion. This is more apt to occur in patients in whom the convalescence has not been carefully supervised. The possibility of myocardial damage should always be considered when a tachycardia persists after the fifth or sixth day. An increased irritability is frequently one of the first manifestations. In certain instances upper abdominal discomfort, and possibly nausea and vomiting, from distention of the liver are early symptoms. Structural alteration in the heart, as evidenced by an accelerated rate, the extension of the apex impulse to the left, change in the quality of the cardiac tones, possibly a gallop rhythm and a faint systolic apical murmur are generally present. The accelerated rate invariably persists until the onset of heart-block, after which it may be reduced to approximately one-half that of the original level. The electrocardiograph affords a valuable means of following the course of the myocardial involvement. In the advanced stages the curves frequently show varying degrees of auriculo-ventricular heart block, alterations in the $Q-R-S$ group, and different types of premature contractions. As the disease progresses, the ashen-gray appearance, the low blood pressure and the weak or perhaps barely perceptible pulse from the failure of the vasomotor system are prominent features. The prognosis is always grave and the mortality is extremely high in the more severe forms. Death may occur at any time. Fortunately, in those who survive the recovery seems to be complete without later evidence of a cardiac disability. Rare instances of chronic heart block have been attributed to diphtheria.

A myocarditis from other etiologic agents is occasionally seen. It is likely to be mistaken for some other form of heart disease and is usually not diagnosed until necropsy. In certain instances, the onset of the cardiac disability follows an infection, and the subsequent course justifies the clinical diagnosis of myocarditis. The cases observed by the writer have shown a marked impairment in the cardiac function. In some, attacks of angina pectoris were outstanding features. Usually the course is that of a progressive congestive failure. The area of cardiac dulness is generally increased, murmurs are commonly heard and premature beats or auricular fibrillation are not infrequently noted. A persistent tachycardia may be a prominent aspect, and in some a pulsus alternans is present. Electrocardiographic records often reveal valuable information, and the findings may be very similar to those encountered in diphtheria.

Diagnosis.—The diphtheritic type of myocarditis, particularly in the more advanced forms, is usually diagnosed. Minor alterations in the myocardium, even with this possibility in mind, are often not recognized, except perhaps through the use of the electrocardiogram. The prolongation of the $P-R$ interval is sufficient to ind cate myocardial damage. The myocarditis from other infectious agents is frequently not suspected. The patient dies from an overwhelming infection, and the involvement of the myocardium is discovered at necropsy. In other instances, the connection between the cardiac disability and the responsible factor is not apparent. The diagnosis, under these circumstances, may be extremely difficult or even impossible. An extensive impairment in the cardiac function, as indicated by the faint and muffled heart sounds, a gallop rhythm, a rapid and feeble pulse and a low blood pressure, are often prominent features. Other causes, especially rheumatic fever in the younger, and coronary artery disease in the older subjects, must be excluded. A bundle branch block in a young individual is probably the most distinctive sign.

Prognosis.—The prognosis in the miscellaneous group is likewise grave. The course is generally downward and in the cases observed by the author death usually occurred in a few weeks or months. In the more chronic varieties there is a better opportunity for the myocardium to compensate for the damage and it may be possible to restore a fairly satisfactory cardiac reserve. A minor involvement of the myocardium may readily escape detection and perhaps heal without any appreciable impairment of cardiac function, or possibly render the heart more susceptible to future insults.

Treatment.—The development of a myocarditis from diphtheria is generally eliminated by the early diagnosis, the administration of adequate amounts of antitoxin, and a carefully supervised convalescence. There is always a chance that the heart may be involved during any severe and prolonged infection. Care should therefore be exercised during the convalescence and the patient not allowed on his feet too soon. It is extremely important that the cardiac damage be recognized early. Treatment is mainly that of absolute bed rest, relaxation and sleep, in which every effort should be made to conserve the cardiac function through the reduction in the cardiac load. It may be necessary to administer bromides or other simple sedatives in order to promote relaxation and extend the period of sleep. The diet should be simple, easily digested and fulfill the bodily requirements. Carbohydrates, particularly sugars, favor the restoration of the cardiac function. In the more severe forms of myocarditis the administration of glucose intravenously is a valuable remedy. It may be necessary to prescribe digitalis. The response, however, is often not very satisfactory and, under these circumstances, it is not advisable to push the drug. An ice-pack may add to the comfort of the patient and reduce, to a certain extent, the cardiac rate.

The rest in bed should be continued until after all evidence of the infection has subsided and the cardiac rate returns to normal level. The supervision of the convalescence is an extremely important aspect of the treatment. Great caution should be exercised in allowing the patient on his feet and in extending the exercise in order to derive the maximum restoration of the cardiac function. Irreparable damage may result if this aspect of treatment is not adequately controlled.

Other Forms of Myocardial Involvement.

Fatty Infiltration.—In obese subjects an extensive deposit of fat may develop about the heart and often penetrates the myocardium between the muscle fibers (fatty heart). It is said that this may produce a degeneration of the muscles. Arterial changes are likely to be present and may contribute to the cardiac disability. The fat alone curtails the activity of the heart. There is, in addition, an extra load imposed by the excess body weight. Shortness of breath on moderate exertion is frequently noted in obese individuals. This may progress to the point where it is a distressing feature without any discernible structural alteration in the heart. The possibility of a coronary artery sclerosis, however, should always be considered. Striking benefit is frequently derived by reduction in weight. The reduction in weight should be gradual and overexertion avoided until the heart has had ample opportunity to accommodate itself to the new condition.

Fatty Degeneration.—This condition is to a certain extent associated with all forms of myocardial degeneration, and may be produced by various chronic poisonings, notably arsenic, phosphorus and chloroform. It is a particular feature in prolonged high-grade anemia. The heart, in the more advanced form, is inclined to be flabby, often dilated, and frequently presents a mottled appearance. On closer examination, small yellow streaks are made out along the finer subdivisions of the smaller arteries as the result of the fatty degeneration from a deficient oxygen supply. These fatty streaks are also likely to be evident beneath the endocardium, especially in the papillary muscles. Palpitation and shortness of breath are common symptoms in high-grade anemia. In some instances the patient first consults his physician because of the cardiac symptoms. Occasionally attacks of angina pectoris are observed. The area of cardiac dulness is frequently increased, and murmurs over the apical and pulmonary areas are common. The symptoms generally promptly subside with the restoration of the blood picture and the murmurs may disappear. Instances of recovery from angina have also been recorded.

FUNCTIONAL DISORDERS OF THE HEART.
(CARDIAC NEUROSES.)

Symptoms referable to the heart are common in hypersensitive and neurotic individuals. They usually consist of palpitation or precordial distress, or both, and are frequently associated with various other manifestations, more particularly pertaining to the digestive system. It is important that these symptoms be carefully analyzed and, if possible, the exciting factors located. In many instances an increased excitability of the nervous system is an important factor and the cardiac disorder not infrequently precipitated by an emotional upset, overfatigue or lack of sleep. A consciousness of the heart or precordial discomfort may result from the toxic influence of tobacco, coffee, tea or alcohol, frequently associated with digestive disturbance and are common in women, especially at the menopause. Palpitation is often associated with a simple tachycardia, frequently accompanies premature contraction, is usually present in paroxysmal tachycardia, and is commonly experienced in auricular fibrillation and auricular flutter. It may appear as an early symptom in anemia, thyrotoxicosis or pulmonary tuberculosis. When a precordial distress is the outstanding complaint, particularly in an individual of the arteriosclerotic age, coronary artery disease should be considered. In certain instances the distress is dependent on intercostal neuralgia or the nerve root pain from an arthritis of the spine.

Irritable Heart (Effort Syndrome, Neuro-circulatory Asthenia).— The term irritable heart applies to a syndrome in which shortness of breath, palpitation, fatigue and vasomotor disturbances are the predominating manifestations. This syndrome was frequently encountered during the Civil War (DaCosta), and again came into prominence during the World War. It occurs in civil life, but is seldom seen in advanced stages.

Etiology.—The vast majority have a hypersensitive nervous system and many are constitutionally inferior, particularly from a physical standpoint. They not infrequently give a history of a reduced tolerance to exercise since childhood. While in school they usually avoid athletics and perhaps later drift into a sedentary occupation. The mental and physical strain of the first few days in an army camp was frequently sufficient to precipitate the symptoms. In another group the condition was associated with chronic infections, particularly pulmonary tuberculosis, or followed some severe acute infection, as influenzal pneumonia. The irritable heart in certain instances appeared to be related to foci of infection about the head and elsewhere. Finally, in a number, the disorders developed while engaged in active warfare from the high tension, exhaustion and the effects of irritating gases. In civil life it is most commonly induced by some emotional upset or financial reverses, family troubles or follows an infection.

Symptoms.—The reduced tolerance to exercise is one of the most characteristic features. There are ordinarily no symptoms while at rest. On slight or moderate exertion, however, the subject experiences shortness of breath, palpitation of the heart and fatigue comparable to that normally produced by the more strenuous and sustained forms of physical effort. Pain may be a prominent symptom, but it is usually a dull ache generally confined to the precordium and often accompanied by tenderness. A consciousness of the heart action frequently follows excitement or exertion. Dizziness is often induced by a change in position and more particularly by exercise. In certain instances syncope may occur.

Physical Signs.—This condition is not necessarily confined to any particular physical type. While it is frequently encountered in the thin and flat-chested individuals, yet it may occur in well-developed subjects. There is often an anxious expression and the neck and face may be flushed. The cardiac rate increases rapidly following slight exertion and may reach 160 to 180 per minute. It ordinarily subsides to the original level of 85 to 90 within two minutes. The cardiac impulse is frequently diffuse but does not extend beyond the normal limits. Occasionally a questionable thrill is felt over the precordium. This, along with the accentuation of the first sound, may suggest a mitral stenosis. Systolic murmurs, soft blowing in character and usually of the cardio-respiratory type, are common over the apical and pulmonary areas. The blood pressure is normal but frequently shows considerable fluctuation in change from the recumbent to the upright position. The vasomotor instability is a prominent feature. The hands become cyanotic in the dependent position and are invariably cold and clammy. These patients often perspire profusely from excitement or exercise and during the examination it is common to see drops of perspiration trickle from the arm pits. A coarse tremor of the hands is apparent at rest and accentuated by exercise. In certain instances the entire body may shake after more strenuous exertion.

Diagnosis.—This condition is more likely to be confused with an organic heart disease or a thyrotoxicosis. In certain instances, particularly following a severe infection, it may be difficult to exclude myocardial damage, and occasionally a period of observation is necessary to establish the diagnosis. The fact that the heart is not increased in size is the determining factor in the exclusion of an organic lesion. A careful history alone from the standpoint of heat tolerance, appetite and weight generally rules out a thyroid disorder. Moreover, the cardiac rate while relaxed, and particularly during sleep, is normal. In some the determination of the basal metabolism may be required. The first determination in this type of individual, however, is likely to be unreliable. When in doubt it should be repeated until the true rate is established. In every case a detailed search for an etiologic factor should be made. The history often gives important information. It may show that the disability has existed to a varying extent since childhood or dates back to some infection or emotional upset. An irritable heart is not infrequently associated with pulmonary tuberculosis. Various other forms of infection may, at times, be responsible. In a case recently observed by the writer, the cardiac symptoms followed undulant fever. This patient, prior to the undulant fever, was in excellent health and accustomed to hard physical work.

Treatment.—These patients usually have a fear of organic heart disease. It is therefore essential that the nature of the disorder be carefully explained. This aspect of the treatment may require considerable time and demand a sympathetic attitude on the part of the physician. Encouragement, relaxation and sleep alone may go a long way in restoring the confidence of the individual. Every effort should be made to eliminate exciting factors. The physical activity and general habits of living should be accommodated as far as possible to the disability. Graded exercise and fresh air often serve a very useful purpose in gradually increasing the tolerance. This feature, however, should be carefully supervised; otherwise the objective may be defeated. Digitalis is distinctly not indicated. Mild sedatives may be helpful in relaxing the patient, promoting sleep and in improving the general health. The patient should be told that the improvement may be slow and that he may always have a somewhat reduced tolerance to exercise. Complete recovery not infrequently occurs and even the constitutionally inferior type may be restored to a happy and useful life.

THE DISORDERS OF THE HEART BEAT.

Normal Cardiac Mechanism.—Under normal conditions the impulse which initiates the cardiac contraction originates in the sinus node. This highly specialized neuro-muscular structure is embodied in the upper end of the sulcus terminalis at the junction of the superior vena cava and the right auricle. It receives fibers from the vagus and sympathetic nerves which exert a regulating influence on the rate of

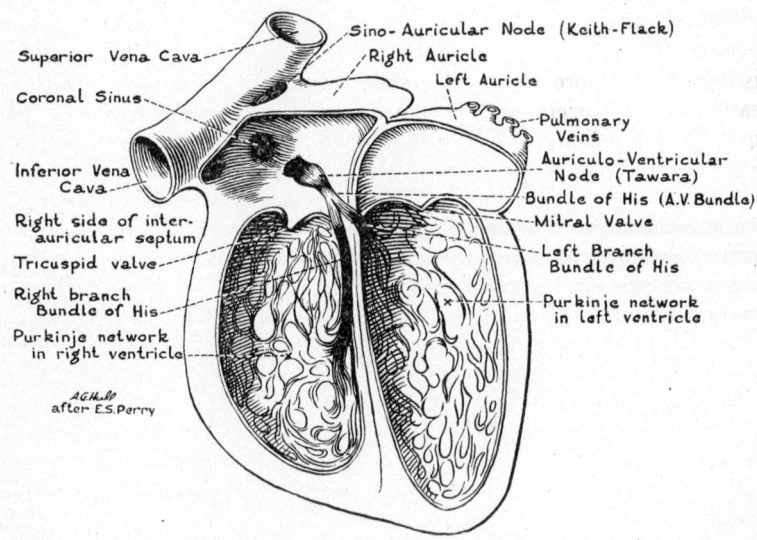

Fig. 9.—Specialized conduction system of the mammalian heart (diagrammatic). (After Frank N. Wilson, in Blumer's Bedside Diagnosis, Volume II, W. B. Saunders Company, Publishers.)

impulse formation. While any section of the heart is capable of initiating a contraction, the automatic rhythm of the sinus node, under normal circumstances, dominates that of any other section of the heart and therefore governs the cardiac rate and the mechanism of the heart beat. The impulses generated at the sinus node spread in a wave-like fashion over the auricles and are conveyed to the ventricle by the auriculo-ventricular bundle, which represents the only functional connection between the auricle and the ventricle. The auriculo-ventricular bundle begins with the auriculo-ventricular node, which is located in the base of the auricular septum slightly to the left of the coronary sinus. The bundle proceeds forward and to the left, to the anterior aspect of the membranous interventricular septum. At this point the bundle divides into two branches, the right and the left, going respectively to the right and left ventricles. The left branch passes through the membrane immediately below the junction of the right posterior and the anterior cusps of the aortic valves. This branch soon divides, and finally terminates in an extensive subendo-cardial network, the Purkinje system, which communicates directly with the muscle fibers. The right branch passes down the right side of the interventricular septum and follows the moderator band to the base of the papillary muscles before it begins to break up into its subendocardial ramifications. Passing through this highly specialized conduction pathway, the impulse which originates at the pacemaker activates all of the ventricular musculature. The contraction of the auricles is therefore followed in an orderly fashion by synchronous contraction of the two ventricles.

In the electrocardiogram (Fig. 10) the *P*-wave represents the spread of the excitation over the auricles. The conformation of the wave remains constant for a given individual so long as the excitation wave spreads in the normal fashion. It is necessarily altered if the impulse originates outside of the usual location. When the impulse arises in the base of the auricles, transmission over the auricle is, for the most part, in the opposite direction to that of the normal, and consequently the *P*-wave becomes inverted. The interval between the beginning

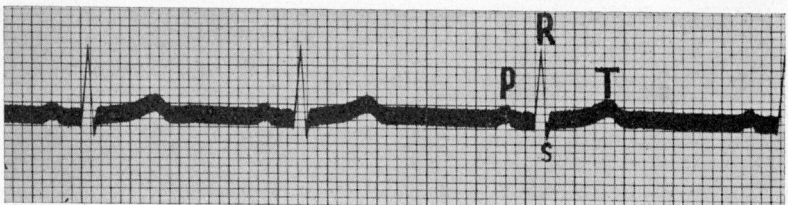

Fig. 10.—Normal electrocardiogram, Lead II.

of the *P*-wave and the beginning of the ventricular complex, the *P–R* interval, represents the time required for the impulse to travel from the auricle to the ventricle. Normally, this interval does not exceed two-tenth second. It might be added that the heavy perpendicular lines usually seen on the recording film or paper occur at intervals of two-tenth second. The *Q–R–S* group of the electrocardiogram is produced by the spread of the excitation wave through the ventricles. There may be still some doubt concerning the interpretation of the *T*-wave, but it is fairly generally believed that it represents a deactiva-tion of the ventricles. It is to be noted that the cardiac cycles as depicted by the electrocardiogram follow in an orderly sequence and are identical in every detail, indicating that the impulse in each instance arises from the same location and travels the same pathway.

Disturbance in Rate.

Normal Cardiac Rate.—The normal rate varies considerably in healthy adults, the average being between 70 and 75 per minute. It is, however, not infrequently 80 to 85, and in certain individuals may range between 50 and 60. The rate is rapid in infants, and at birth is usually between 130 and 140 per minute. It diminishes rapidly

during infancy and early childhood.   At six years the average is about
100, at ten years 90 and at fifteen years approximately 85 per minute.
The influence of the vagus becomes more apparent in later childhood
and is probably responsible for the gradual reduction in the cardiac
rate up to that time.

Sinus Tachycardia.—Various factors influence the rate at which the
impulses are generated in the sinus node.   Under normal conditions
the vagus nerve exerts a powerful inhibitory influence.   The subcutaneous administration of $\frac{1}{30}$ grain of atropine, a drug which releases
the vagus influence, is ordinarily followed in ten or fifteen minutes by
a sharp acceleration in the cardiac rate.   This response varies in
degree with different individuals and is more marked in the hypersensitive subject.   The increased cardiac rate that comes during the last
stage of meningitis is explained as the result of a reduction in the vagus
tone.   In a patient with a persistent tachycardia, recently observed,
the vagus nerves were almost completely destroyed by pressure from
a mediastinal tumor.

An increased cardiac rate develops normally with exercise and
excitement.   It occurs with fever, various infections and is a prominent
feature in tuberculosis, psychoneurosis and thyrotoxicosis.   In infections the influence of the elevated temperature on the sinus node is no
doubt a factor, for experimentally the application of heat and cold
to this structure is promptly followed by an acceleration or reduction
in the cardiac rate.   This, however, is by no means the only factor,
for in certain infections, notably typhoid fever, the heart-rate is not
elevated in proportion to the fever.   Simple tachycardia is associated
with nervousness and physical exhaustion, intoxication from nicotine
and low blood pressure.   Finally, in cardiac infections and myocardial
failure there is an increase in the rate.   The tachycardia of acute
cardiac infection is so constant a feature that it constitutes an important part of the diagnosis and serves as a guide in the treatment.   In
certain instances simple acceleration of the heart may be mistaken for
paroxysmal tachycardia.   The latter is characterized by a sudden
onset and abrupt termination.   This differentiation is ordinarily readily
established by the history.   The electrocardiogram in simple tachycardia shows that the impulses originate in the usual location and are
transmitted in a normal fashion.

The treatment should be directed toward the etiologic factor.   There
is no justification for the administration of digitalis unless the tachycardia is an expression of a cardiac failure.

Sinus Bradycardia.—Cardiac rates of 55 to 60 are occasionally encountered in normal individuals.   Lewis cites the case of a healthy
athlete whose heart-rate at rest ranged between 30 and 40 per minute.
The rate decreases somewhat with years, from fatigue, or during
exposure to cold.   It may be reduced by vagal stimulation from pressure on the carotid sheath or on the eyeball.   The slow rate associated
with brain tumors, cerebral hemorrhage and meningitis, is presumably
vagal in origin.   It occurs during convalescence from acute fevers,
more particularly in so-called vagotonic individuals.   A slow pulse is
frequently observed in certain cases of jaundice, and may result from

anoxemia or asphyxia. Digitalis, when administered to the point of intoxication in auricular fibrillation, may produce a striking reduction in the cardiac rate. An acute rise in the blood pressure is said to be accompanied by a reduction in the heart-rate from vagal stimulation through the direct effect on the medullary center. There is a fairly constant relationship between the pulse-rate and the metabolic-rate. The rate is thus accelerated in thyrotoxicosis and reduced in hypo-thyroidism or myxedema.

A significant reduction in the cardiac rate should always suggest the possibility of auriculo-ventricular heart block. When the rate is persistently 35 per minute, or below, there is usually complete heart block. Rates from 40 to 60 are compatible with partial heart block. In certain instances it may be necessary to resort to the electrocardio-graph to establish the diagnosis.

Sinus Arrhythmia.—The influence of the vagus on the sinus node is strongest in childhood and early adult life. Variation in the vagal tone may be sufficient to produce a distinct irregularity of the heart. This type of irregularity is often definitely related to respiration and

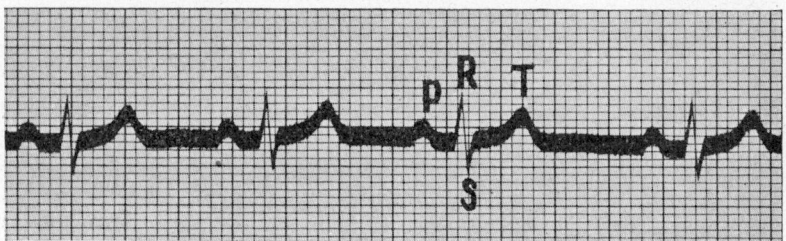

Fig. 11.—Sinus arrhythmia, Lead II from patient fourteen years of age.

is accentuated by deep and prolonged breathing. The rate is in-creased during inspiration and rather abruptly reduced shortly after the onset of expiration. This irregularity is distinctly dependent on changes in the vagal tone and may be promptly abolished by the administration of atropine. In the electrocardiogram (Fig. 11) it is to be noted that there is no alteration whatever in the character of the auricular and ventricular complexes. The condition is therefore entirely dependent on variation in the rate at which the impulses are discharged from the sinus node. Occasionally the inhibition becomes so pronounced that the pacemaker migrates to a lower level. There are rare instances in which the variation in cardiac rate is independent of respiration. Lewis cites cases of syncope from a cessation of cardiac contraction, and states that the condition is comparable to the cardiac standstill produced by stimulation of the vagus.

Sinus arrhythmia is frequently observed during convalescence from acute infection. In the adult it is far more common in the hyper-sensitive type of individual. It is occasionally associated with the slow pulse of meningitis or increased intracranial pressure, and may occur during the administration of digitalis. The diagnosis is at once evident when the relationship to respiration is noted. No treatment is required.

28

Disorders of the Heart Beat Due to Disturbance in Conduction—
Heart Block.

A blocking or interference with the transmission of the cardiac impulse may occur at various sites: (1) between the sinus node and the auricle—sino-auricular block; (2) in the auriculo-ventricular bundle—auriculo-ventricular block; (3) in the bundle branches—bundle branch block.

1. **Sino-auricular Block.**—This term has been applied to a condition in which a complete cardiac contraction drops out. In the electrocardiogram there is an absence of both auricular and ventricular complexes, producing a pause which is approximately double that of a

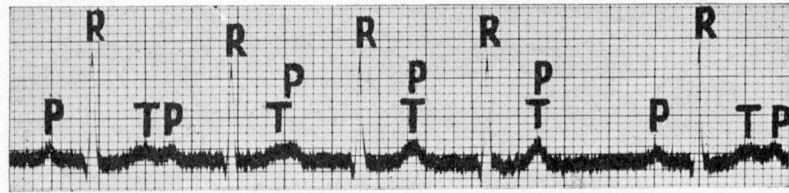

FIG. 12.—Partial auriculo-ventricular block with progressive lengthening of the *P–R* interval and "dropped beat."

normal cycle. This condition is occasionally observed in patients receiving digitalis. The fact that it may be increased by vagal pressure and abolished by atropine would indicate that in certain instances it is probably an expression of increased vagal tone.

2. **Auriculo-ventricular Block.**—In the past this was known as heart block because it was the first form recognized. The earliest stage is manifested by a slight increase in the time required for the

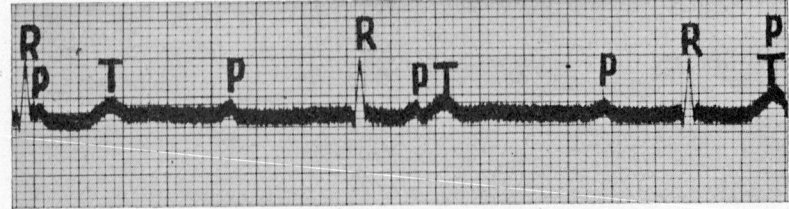

FIG. 13.—Complete auriculo-ventricular block, Lead I.

impulse to pass over the auriculo-ventricular bundle. In the electrocardiogram the conduction period is indicated by the *P–R* interval which is ordinarily well within two-tenth second. When this limit is exceeded it is designated as a prolonged *P–R* interval and represents the initial stage of auriculo-ventricular block. A slightly more advanced degree of block is characterized by the occasional dropping out of a ventricular contraction. Preceding the "dropped beat" there is a gradual increase in the duration of the *P–R* interval, and finally an impulse fails to pass (Fig. 12). With a further reduction in the conductivity of the bundle "dropped beats" occur with greater frequency, and a tendency toward the establishment of a simple ratio between the auricular and ventricular rate is observed. While various ratios are possible, 2 to 1 and 3 to 1 are by far the most common. The types of auriculo-ventricular conduction defects so far considered are included under the term "partial block." Finally, a state may be reached in which the bundle transmits none of the impulses to the ventricles. This condition is known as complete auriculo-ventricular block or auriculo-ventricular dissociation (Fig. 13). Under these conditions the auricles and ventricles maintain independent rhythms at rates of approximately 72 and 30, respectively.

Etiology.—This condition occurs at all ages. The earliest stage, namely, a prolonged $P-R$ interval, is common, but the more advanced forms are relatively rare. The former is frequently seen during various acute infections, more particularly in rheumatic fever, and often results from the administration of digitalis. Digitalis is likely to bring out a latent conduction defect, which probably accounts for the frequency with which it is encountered in the treatment of cardiac failure of arteriosclerotic origin. Higher grades of partial block, or even complete auriculo-ventricular dissociation are common in the more severe forms of diphtheria. Chronic heart block occasionally results from rheumatic fever. It may be associated with syphilis, but in the writer's experience is more commonly seen in arteriosclerotic heart disease. A few cases of congenital heart block have been reported.

Morbid Anatomy.—Minor alterations in conduction may occur with little or no significant anatomic change in the auriculo-ventricular bundle, but in cases of persistent high-grade block extensive pathologic alterations are generally present. The extent of the lesion, however, is not necessarily in keeping with the degree of functional impairment. In rare instances the pathologic changes have been negligible, or conversely, there has been considerable damage with normal conductivity. The lesion is commonly of the degenerative type, characterized by sclerosis and atrophy of the bundle or occlusion of the vessels which supply the bundle. In certain instances the inflammatory lesion of rheumatic fever, diphtheria, syphilis or subacute bacterial endocarditis is encountered. Gummatous changes, calcium deposits with fibrosis and even tumors have been described.

Symptoms.—The symptoms of auriculo-ventricular block are primarily dependent on the slowing of the ventricles. High-grade block may not produce symptoms if a ventricular rate of 30 or more per minute is maintained. In a 2 to 1, or 3 to 1 block, however, periods of ventricular slowing or even ventricular standstill are likely to occur, especially during a transition from partial to complete block. Various cerebral manifestations result, ranging from slight dizziness to syncope, and including even epileptiform seizures, depending on the degree of the cerebral anemia. When the condition progresses to the stage of syncope it is designated as the *Adams-Stokes syndrome*. While this syndrome is more commonly seen in auriculo-ventricular block, it also applies to the syncope associated with other types of ventricular slowing, such as that resulting from an increased vagal activity. In the milder attacks the patient may feel faint or temporarily lose consciousness. With a ventricular standstill of fifteen seconds or more, convulsive seizures may occur, involving first the face and upper extremities. There is always a possibility that these attacks may terminate in death. The writer observed a patient who on numerous occasions lost consciousness and often experienced convulsive seizures. When the patient was last seen, he had been free of these symptoms for more than a year. The cessation of these episodes was attributed to the establishment of a permanent complete block.

Diagnosis.—The diagnosis of delayed conduction is established only by means of a polygram or electrocardiogram. There are certain findings, however, which may be suggestive enough to make the clinical diagnosis reasonably certain. If delayed conduction occurs with a mitral stenosis, the characteristic presystolic murmur no longer merges with the first sound, and becomes distinctly separated from it, depending upon the duration of the $P-R$ interval. The auricular sound is normally not detected because of the short time interval between the auricular and ventricular contractions. However, when this interval (the $P-R$ interval) is prolonged, the auricular contraction may be audible and thus produce a reduplication of the first sound, or, if the conduction is still further delayed, possibly a reduplication of the second sound. It may also be possible to identify by physical examination the pauses occasioned by dropping of ventricular beats in partial heart block. During the pause there are no signs of ventricular activity. Partial heart block with "dropped beats" is likely to be mistaken for a sinus arrhythmia or premature contractions. There is, however, no relation to respiration, and the auscultatory findings of premature beat are lacking.

A ventricular rate of 40 to 50 per minute should always direct attention to the possibility of a 2 to 1 or 3 to 1 auriculo-ventricular block. Upon close investigation of the jugular pulse it is usually possible to determine that some of the auricular contractions are not followed by a ventricular response. If there is an associated mitral stenosis the murmur will occur either two or three times during the diastolic period, depending on whether the auriculo-ventricular ratio is 2 to 1 or 3 to 1. In complete dissociation the ventricular rate is usually under 40. Important information may be gained by a careful study of the jugular pulsation. Since the auricular and ventricular rhythms are independent of each other, the auricular contractions may occur at any time in the ventricular cycle. If an auricular contraction happens to coincide with the first or second sound, it may produce a noticeable increase in the intensity of the sound, or if it precedes the first, or follows the second, a reduplication is produced.

Prognosis.—In its early stage auriculo-ventricular block does not in itself interfere with the cardiac function, but the underlying myocardial change may be serious. In questionable cases of cardiac infection, as in rheumatic fever, the discovery of a delayed conduction definitely establishes the diagnosis. The more advanced forms of block increase the demands on the heart, and experimentally are associated with a reduction in coronary blood flow. Instances are occasionally seen, however, in which there is no apparent influence on the cardiac function. The damage to the myocardium in these cases is usually minimal. In general, the prognosis is based on the condition of the myocardium. Attacks of syncope are always serious and death may occur at any time.

Treatment.—The treatment varies with the cause, the condition of the myocardium and the extent of the conduction defect. If digitalis is responsible the drug should be discontinued. In the auriculo-ventricular block which is associated with acute infections, the treatment is directed toward the primary condition and the conservation of the cardiac function. In cardiac failure with a partial block the usual management is indicated, but caution should be exercised in the use of digitalis. Ordinarily, the conservative administration of this drug is not likely to produce ill effects, but on the contrary may increase the conductivity of the bundle through general improvement in the cardiac function. After complete block is established, it is then only necessary to avoid digitalis intoxication. Occasionally a partial block may be favorably influenced or possibly eliminated by atropine. In the Adams-Stokes syndrome thyroid extract, thyroxin, adrenalin, ephedrine and barium chloride have been employed to increase the ventricular rate. Ephedrine sulphate, 25 mg. ($\frac{3}{8}$ grain), three or four times a day, is probably the most effective remedy.

3. Bundle Branch Block.—The impulse may be delayed or blocked in its passage over either of the main branches of the auriculo-ventricular bundle. This condition is occasionally encountered in the more advanced form of myocarditis, particularly in diphtheria, but is seen most commonly in arteriosclerotic heart disease. With complete block there are usually extensive structural alterations and often a conspicuous functional impairment of the myocardium. The prognosis is generally poor. Relatively few patients survive longer than two years. The disorder may be suspected when the first or second heart sound is reduplicated, or when the apex impulse is bifid, but the diagnosis is established only by the electrocardiogram. The criteria are: (1) a prolongation of the Q-R-S interval; (2) a splintering or slurring of the Q-R-S complexes; and (3) a T-wave in the opposite direction to that of the chief ventricular deflection.

Disorders of Heart Beat Due to Abnormal Impulse Formation.

Premature Contractions.—The premature contraction is the most common form of cardiac irregularity. It is usually isolated and occurs at varying intervals, but occasionally appears at regular intervals, as every second, third or fourth beats.

Mechanism.—The impulses responsible for the normal cardiac contractions are released from the sinus node at regular intervals. Under certain conditions, impulses may originate outside the sinus node in the auricles, ventricles or junctional tissue. These impulses are capable of producing contractions if they are generated before the discharge of the normal impulse from the sinus node, while the ventricle is in a responsive state. They are therefore premature in the sense that they occur before the anticipated time, and replace the rhythmic beat since the heart is in a refractory state from the premature contraction by the time the normal impulse comes along. In the auscultation of the heart these abnormal contractions are usually identified by the early appearance and the subsequent pause.

The mechanism is at once apparent in the electrocardiogram. In the illustration (Fig. 14) the premature contraction is auricular in origin, as shown by the presence of an auricular wave (*P*-wave), and since the ventricles are activated in the usual fashion by transmission of the impulse over the auriculo-ventricular bundle and its ramifica-

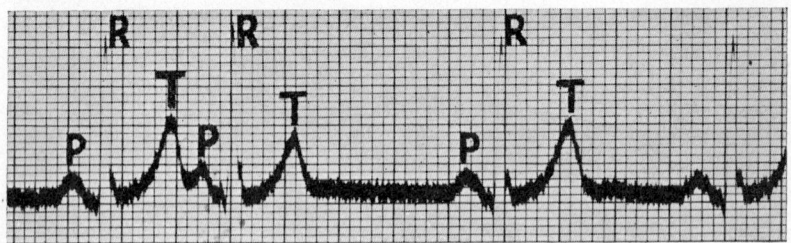

FIG. 14.—Auricular premature beat, Lead II.

tions, the ventricular complex is of normal configuration. The pause following the premature contraction is not fully compensatory because the distance between the two normal contractions separated by the premature beat is not quite equal to that between the first and third preceding rhythmic cycles. This is one of the characteristic features of a premature auricular contraction. Another electrocardiogram (Fig. 15) shows a ventricular type of premature beat. This abnormal contraction is not preceded by an auricular wave and furthermore the

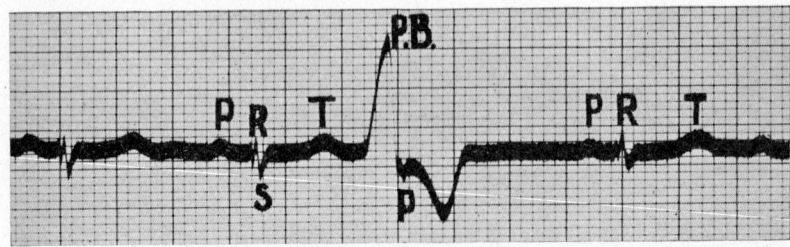

FIG. 15.—Ventricular premature beat, with retrograde stimulation of the auricles, Lead III.

ventricular complex is distinctly abnormal because of the aberrant course of the impulse in the ventricles. The pause which follows this type of premature contraction is compensatory, in contradistinction to that produced by a premature auricular beat. A third electrocardiogram (Fig. 16) shows the premature contraction occurring regularly after each normal cycle.

Etiology.—Premature contractions are seen at all ages and probably occur in most individuals some time during life, particularly those who live beyond the age of forty years. They are commonly associated with organic heart disease, but are frequently encountered in persons in whom there is no demonstrable evidence of cardiac disease. The incidence is highest after fifty years of age, no doubt because of the frequency of degenerative changes in the myocardium. Excessive smoking is occasionally an exciting factor and digitalis is commonly responsible. The appearance of premature beats during the administration of digitalis should at once suggest the possibility of intoxication from the drug. In hypersensitive individuals gastro-intestinal disturbances, particularly the accumulation of gas, are often associated with the occurrence of this irregularity. Premature contractions are not uncommon during the course of acute infections and may be the first indication of a cardiac involvement. They frequently follow coronary occlusion and at times may be helpful in establishing a diagnosis.

Symptoms.—There are frequently no symptoms, and the condition is discovered incidentally during routine examination. In those conscious of the irregularity the sensation is variously described. Palpitation is perhaps the most common complaint. This is usually attributed to the vigorous contraction following the pause. Others

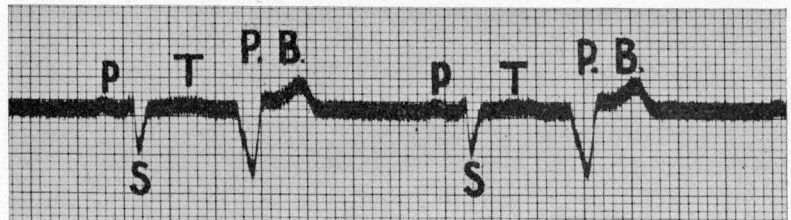

Fig. 16.—Regular recurring ventricular premature beats, Lead III.

have a feeling that the heart turns over with a premature beat, or experience a full sensation in the neck. Occasionally these symptoms cause grave concern on the part of the patient and perhaps lead to the development of an advanced psychoneurosis. In rare cases, particularly when the irregularity occurs at frequent intervals, there may be dizziness or faintness. The writer once saw a patient who was having so many premature beats, perhaps on account of an associated gastrointestinal upset, that he was not able to stand because of dizziness and and a fear that he might faint.

Diagnosis.—The premature contraction is usually recognized by the fact that it appears before the anticipated time, and by the subsequent pause. It produces two sounds if the aortic valves are raised; otherwise only the first sound. This, with the preceding normal contraction, produces a group of three or four sounds. If there is a systolic apical murmur, it is usually short and may be absent. Aortic murmurs are likewise reduced in intensity or are present only when the aortic valves are opened. Premature contractions are diminished in number by an increase in the cardiac rate. They are thus usually absent during fever and temporarily disappear with exercise or excitement. When they occur at frequent intervals the arrhythmia may be mistaken for auricular fibrillation. Under these circumstances, exercise is extremely helpful in making the differentiation. With an acceleration of the heart-rate the premature beats usually disappear, whereas in auricular fibrillation the irregularity is increased. It is rarely possible to determine the type of premature beat except by the electrocardiogram.

Prognosis.—The condition of the myocardium is the determining factor. If the premature beat is the only abnormality it is often of no significance, but all aspects of the case should be taken into consideration, particularly the possibility of infection. If there are no new developments after a few months, the patient may again be reassured.

Treatment.—Treatment is rarely necessary unless the premature beats are so numerous as to be primarily responsible for the symptoms. Occasionally it is possible to locate and remove the cause. The relatively innocuous nature of the disorder should be fully explained. Mild sedatives, such as bromides or luminal, may be indicated for relief of the subjective symptoms. In some the premature beat may be eliminated by quinidine, 0.2 gram (3 grains), two or three times a day. Careful inquiry should be made as to the time the irregularity is most likely to occur. It frequently appears after meals or is noticed only after retiring at night. Under these conditions the patient should be directed to take quinidine at least an hour before the irregularity is ordinarily expected. If there is evidence of a significant impairment in the cardiac function, the condition may be favorably influenced by digitalis.

Paroxysmal Tachycardia.—This disorder is characterized by its abrupt onset and sudden termination, absolute regularity and rapid rate, ranging from 120 to 200 per minute. The paroxysms vary in duration from a few seconds to a few hours but in exceptional instances may prevail for days. This condition is closely related to the premature beats and has been likened to a succession of these abnormal contractions. The impulses responsible for the abnormal mechanism originate outside the sinus node, in the auricles, the ventricles and in rare instances the junctional tissue. They are generated at regular intervals and at a rate far exceeding that of the normal rhythm. Consequently during the period of tachycardia the function of the sinus node is superseded by that of the ectopic focus.

Etiology.—Paroxysmal tachycardia is occasionally first noted in childhood. In the younger subjects it is usually auricular in origin and there is often no evidence of organic heart disease. The etiology is similar to that of premature contractions. Infection probably plays a rôle. The attacks are related to various factors as sudden exertion, excitement and digestive upsets. Excessive smoking, alcohol and digitalis intoxication may be responsible. The ventricular type is usually associated with coronary artery disease and is more frequently seen following a coronary occlusion.

Symptoms.—Short attacks lasting from a few seconds to a few minutes are not uncommon. The patient, while conscious of the sudden onset and the abrupt cessation of a fluttering sensation in the precordium and rapid pulsations in the neck, is rarely caused any inconvenience. Not a few who experience attacks lasting an hour or more may continue about their work without any particular discomfort. If the attack persists for a longer period a distinct precordial fullness, possibly pressure or pain frequently occurs, and shortness of breath may later appear. In the more prolonged attacks, cardiac failure finally develops with marked cyanosis, passive congestion of the lungs and engorgement of the liver. The rapid distention of the liver may give rise to abdominal tenderness and possibly nausea and vomiting. These manifestations of impaired cardiac function rapidly disappear after the restoration of normal cardiac mechanism. In the examination the marked pulsation in the veins of the neck, the rapid cardiac rate and the short and sharp cardiac sounds are the most prominent features. If the attack persists for an unusual duration, these findings are supplemented by signs of cardiac failure.

Diagnosis.—The history usually establishes the diagnosis. The patient is invariably conscious of a sudden onset but may be in doubt about the termination, particularly in the longer attacks. When seen during an attack the uniformity of the cardiac rate is a striking aspect. It remains constant in spite of a change in position or exercise, which is distinctly contrary to the findings in the sinus tachycardia frequently encountered in the hypersensitive individuals. The disorder may occasionally be mistaken for paroxysms of auricular fibrillation or flutter. There may be some difficulty in differentiating these conditions from the history, the onset and termination being similar in each instance. In fibrillation, however, the patient is generally conscious of the marked irregularity. This is usually not so evident in flutter but may be apparent to the patient, whereas in paroxysmal tachycardia there is no subjective sensation of an irregular mechanism. When seen during an attack the regular rhythm at once excludes fibrillation, but does not eliminate the possibility of flutter. The differentiation from the latter is frequently dependent on the electrocardiogram.

This condition may occur at varying intervals for years without any discernible structural alterations in the heart. A man, aged sixty years, who had been subject to this disorder since early adult life, was recently seen. This patient had never been inconvenienced to any great extent and the cardiac findings were essentially negative. The more prolonged attacks are always dangerous and may cause cardiac failure and death. The outlook is more serious in the ventricular form and grave if it occurs following coronary occlusion.

Treatment.—The treatment varies with the frequency and duration of the attacks and the condition of the myocardium. If the attacks are of brief duration and occur at infrequent intervals, treatment is rarely indicated. A careful survey should be made for possible exciting factors. In the more severe form, the treatment is concerned with a reduction in the number of attacks and the protection of the myocardium during the paroxysms. The regulation of the habits of living, the correction of digestive disorders, the removal of infection and, in some, the administration of sedatives may have a significant influence on the number of attacks. Quinidine sulphate, 0.2 gram (3 grains), two or three times a day, is the most valuable single remedy. This medication may be continued weeks or months and will frequently either abolish or curtail the number of attacks. Digitalis may be of value, particularly when the paroxysms first occur later in life and are associated with structural changes in the heart. The attacks are generally self-limited and in time the normal mechanism is restored. As a protective measure, the patient should lie down when possible if the paroxysms persist for more than a few minutes. In some, it may be advisable to attempt to stop the attack. This may be accomplished in some instances by firm pressure over a carotid sheath or on either eyeball. Quinindine sulphate, 0.2 to 0.3 gram (3 to 5 grains), every two to three hours, is often effective in reducing the duration of the attack. In the more prolonged paroxysms, it is important that the cardiac function be conserved. Relaxation and sleep are essential, even though it may be necessary to administer morphine. Digitalis is indicated if the heart begins to show signs of failure.

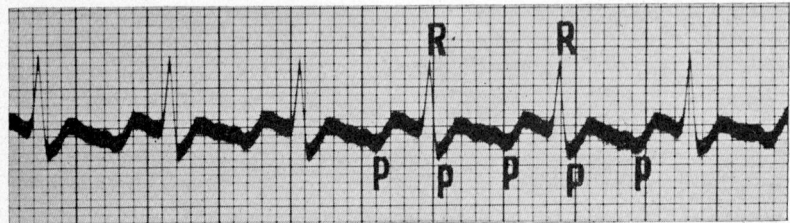

Fig. 17.—Auricular flutter, pure, with rhythmic ventricular response, 2 to 1 ratio, Lead II.

Auricular Flutter.—This disorder is characterized by an abnormally rapid and regular contraction of the auricles, ranging from 200 to 350 per minute, and associated with a partial auriculo-ventricular block. It is generally believed from the work of Garrey, Mines, and Lewis and his associates that the abnormal auricular activity is due to the development of a wave of contraction which circulates at a very rapid and constant rate in a ring of auricular musculature about the mouths of the great veins. The uniformity of the auricular complexes (*P*-wave) in the electrocardiogram (Fig. 17) indicates that the pathway of this circular contraction wave is for the most part constant. It is rarely possible for the auriculo-ventricular bundle to transmit all of the auricular impulses. Consequently a partial block is established in which the ventricle responds to every second, third or fourth auricular contraction. A 2 to 1 ratio is the most common, giving a ventricular rate of 100 to 175 per minute. The heart beat is perfectly regular so long as a constant ratio is maintained. The ratio, however, may change from time to time, producing varying degrees of irregularity. This is one of the features particularly noted following the administration of digitalis. In occasional instances the ventricles may for a short period respond to all the auricular impulses. Under these circumstances the subject often experiences distressing symptoms and syncope may occur. These episodes begin suddenly and terminate abruptly, and in this respect are quite comparable to the attacks of paroxysmal tachycardia.

Etiology.—Auricular flutter is a relatively rare form of cardiac irregularity. The incidence is highest after fifty years but it may be encountered in all ages. It is usually associated with an organic heart disease, either rheumatic or arteriosclerotic, but occasionally thyrotoxic in origin. In rare instances it may be difficult to demonstrate structural changes in the heart. The condition is closely allied to auricular fibrillation, both from the standpoint of mechanism and associated pathology. These two disorders are occasionally seen in the same individual and various gradations between the conditions are not infrequently encountered. Under the latter circumstances the irregularity is usually regarded as impure fibrillation or flutter, depending on the dominating mechanism.

Symptoms.—The symptoms are largely dependent on the condition of the myocardium. It is likely to be associated with manifestations of an impaired cardiac function, and frequently supersedes the onset of failure. The condition may occur in short paroxysms and the symptoms under these conditions are identical with those of simple paroxysmal tachycardia. Usually the disorder eventually becomes permanently established and in time promotes the development of more serious symptoms.

Diagnosis.—In certain instances the clinical findings are sufficiently distinctive to justify a probable diagnosis. A regular and persistent cardiac rate of 140 or more per minute in an elderly individual should at once suggest the possibility of flutter. This finding may be further supplemented by the occurrence of short paroxysms of a more excessive rate from the abrupt onset of a lower auriculo-ventricular ratio or in exceptional instances from the response of the ventricles to all auricular beats. Again the regular rhythm may be interrupted by the pauses from the transitory change to a higher ratio. This is fairly conclusive of an auricular flutter, but further evidence may be obtained from vagal stimulation through pressure on the carotid sheath or by the administration of digitalis. Because of the partial auriculo-ventricular block the stimulation of the vagus or the administration of digitalis reduces the ventricular rate and increases the irregularity. There are three forms in which the identification is entirely dependent on instrumental means: (1) the paroxysmal type with a constant auriculo-ventricular ratio; (2) a high auriculo-ventricular ratio, giving a regular ventricular rate of 70 to 90 per minute; (3) an ever changing auriculo-ventricular ratio, producing marked irregularity. The first simulates a simple paroxysmal tachycardia and the third an auricular fibrillation. The second type might be mistaken for a normal cardiac mechanism but flutter should be suspected from the very rapid movement in the jugular vein.

Prognosis.—A permanent auricular flutter is often a serious disorder. The outlook is largely determined by the condition of the myocardium, the ventricular rate and the response to digitalis. An occasional case may withstand an excessive cardiac rate for years; however, when seen in an individual past fifty years, there is generally evidence of an impaired cardiac function and, unless it is possible to control the ventricular rate, failure usually appears within a few weeks or months.

Treatment.—The paroxysmal form frequently may be abolished by quinidine sulphate, 0.2 gram (3 grains), two or three times a day. After the condition is more or less firmly established, the success of treatment is largely dependent on digitalis. Digitalis should be given in sufficient doses to reduce the ventricular response and, if possible, to convert the disorder into fibrillation. In an occasional instance the normal mechanisms may be restored upon withdrawing the digitalis after fibrillation is induced. The treatment is generally regarded as being highly successful if a fibrillation can be maintained by small doses of digitalis. In certain instances it may be possible to restore the normal mechanism by the combined use of digitalis and quinidine.

Auricular Fibrillation.—In this disorder the normal rhythmic contractions of the auricles are replaced by a fine fibrillary movement. The auricles, therefore, no longer serve as a contracting chamber but function from a mechanical standpoint merely as a reservoir for the inflowing blood. Lewis and his associates have demonstrated that the mechanism is dependent on a circus movement, as in flutter. It, however, differs from flutter in that the circular contracting wave travels at an irregular and more rapid rate in a pathway that varies somewhat from cycle to cycle. Impulses are thus transmitted over the auricles to the auriculo-ventricular bundle in an irregular fashion and at an extremely rapid rate. The ventricular beat is consequently grossly irregular and the rate will vary with the capacity of the bundle to transmit the impulse. There is thus always a partial block. In the untreated state the ventricular rate is usually over 100 and generally between 110 and 140 per minute. The conductivity of the auriculo-ventricular bundle may be diminished and the ventricular rate thereby reduced by vagal stimulation or the administration of digitalis.

Etiology.—This is one of the most common and important forms of cardiac irregularities. It may be transient and recurring but is usually persistent. Instances are occasionally encountered in childhood but auricular fibrillation is relatively infrequent before twenty years of age. The incidence thereafter rapidly increases and is possibly highest between thirty and forty and again after fifty years of age. The permanent form, with rare exception, is associated with demonstrable structural changes in the heart. Chronic valvular heart disease, particularly mitral stenosis, is responsible for the vast majority in early life, and accounts for more than 50 per cent of the total incidence. Many of the remaining are dependent on chronic degenerative changes in the myocardium from arteriosclerosis and hypertension. Thyrotoxicosis is a relatively important etiologic factor in certain sections of the country.

The paroxysmal form of auricular fibrillation has been attributed to various factors. It has been observed during the course of acute infectious disease, surgical anesthesia, in thyrotoxicosis and in intoxication from carbon monoxide, alcohol, digitalis or tobacco. In certain instances the abnormal mechanism has been associated with gastro-intestinal disorders. Occasionally emotional upsets have contributed to the production of the disorder. The occurrence of the irregularity in this form is not infrequently the only abnormal cardiac finding.

Symptoms.—During paroxysmal attacks the subject is generally conscious of the rapid heart action, frequently experiences an uncomfortable sensation in the precordium, occasionally feels dizzy or faint, and in the more prolonged paroxysms may become short of breath. In the persistent form the patient may possibly not be aware of the irregularity. Shortness of breath and other manifestations of cardiac failure are usually responsible for bringing the individual to the physician.

Physical Signs.—The irregularity in rhythm and in the force of the ventricular contraction is the most distinctive finding. This feature is increased by exercise, excitement or any factor which accelerates the cardiac rate. A gross irregularity with a rate of 100 to 120 per minute is generally dependent on auricular fibrillation. The heart sounds and associated murmurs vary in intensity from cycle to cycle, being more marked with the higher rates. During runs of rapid ventricular contractions, cardiac sounds are usually snappy and at times the second tone is lacking from the failure to raise the aortic valves.

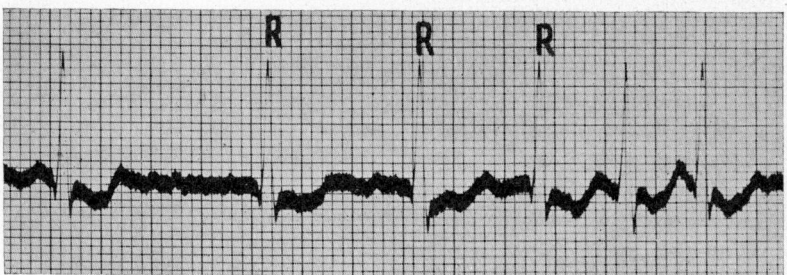

Fig. 18.—Auricular fibrillation, Lead II.

In a mitral stenosis the characteristic presystolic murmur produced by the rhythmic contractions of the auricles generally disappears after the onset of auricular fibrillation. The absolute irregularity is fully expressed in the pulse. With a rapid cardiac rate many of the beats are too weak to produce a pulse wave and are therefore not detected at the wrist, producing a difference between the ventricular and pulse-rate which is designated as the *pulse deficit*. The pulse deficit gradually becomes less and may finally disappear as the ventricular rate is reduced by digitalis. The electrocardiographic findings are characterized by the absence of a normal P-wave, the presence of fine fibrillary deflection from the disordered spread of the impulses over the auricles and the irregular spacing of the ventricular complexes. (Fig. 18.)

Diagnosis.—A grossly irregular and rapid heart action, particularly when associated with structural changes in the heart, is usually indicative of an auricular fibrillation. The diagnosis is generally established if the irregularity is increased by a further acceleration of the cardiac rate. The arrhythmia from premature contractions which is most likely to be confused with an auricular fibrillation is ordinarily reduced or completely abolished by the acceleration of the heart-rate. An auricular flutter with an irregular ventricular response may simulate fibrillation, but it is extremely rare and the differentiation is usually dependent on instrumental means. In certain instances sinus arrhythmia may resemble auricular fibrillation. However, in the former the irregularity is related to respiration or may be eliminated by atropine. Transient auricular fibrillation must be differentiated from paroxysms of flutter or from paroxysmal tachycardia. The diagnosis is usually evident when the patient is seen during an attack or may be apparent from the history. In the cases with complete auriculo-ventricular block the rhythm is regular, and consequently the diagnosis of auricular fibrillation is not possible except by the electrocardiogram or polygram.

Prognosis.—Paroxysmal fibrillation occurs under various circumstances and is not necessarily dependent on a significant damage of the myocardium. If it continues to occur there is always a possibility that it may become permanently established. The persistent form is ordinarily associated with a definite impairment in the cardiac function and the accelerated rate may impose a serious handicap on the heart. The prognosis, under these conditions, is largely dependent on the extent of the cardiac damage and the control of the rate. If the cardiac rate is not controlled, failure generally occurs within a few weeks or months. These patients often present varying degrees of failure when first seen. The prognosis is more favorable when it is possible to eliminate the exciting factor, as a thyrotoxicosis. Embolic manifestations may occur. The absence of the rhythmical contractions favors the stagnation of the blood in the auricles, particularly in the appendages with the formation of clots. Small pieces may be dislodged and pass into the general circulation.

Treatment.—The serious aspect of auricular fibrillation is largely dependent on the accelerated cardiac rate. The treatment, therefore, is primarily concerned with the control of this feature through the administration of adequate amounts of digitalis. When the disorder is associated with a cardiac failure, rest, sleep and other measures are essential. Digitalis normally has a depressing effect on the conductivity of the auriculo-ventricular bundle which is manifested to a marked extent in auricular fibrillation because of the partial auriculo-ventricular block. It is, therefore, generally possible to reduce the cardiac rate and maintain it at a reasonable level. The relief of the heart from the tremendous extra burden is largely responsible for the striking results so frequently observed in the treatment of the cardiac failure accompanied by an auricular fibrillation. The administration of 15 to 20 minims (1 to 1.3 cc.) of tincture of digitalis or 0.1 to 0.12 gram (1.5 to 2 grains) of the powdered leaf, three or four times a day, will usually reduce the ventricular rate to the desired level within a few days. Occasionally it may be necessary to prescribe larger doses. After the rate has been reduced to 70 or 80 per minute, the dosage then should be curtailed; otherwise toxic manifestations may appear. Thereafter it is important that the drug be given in sufficient amounts to control the rate. The amount of digitalis required to achieve this end varies, but often 10 minims of the tincture, twice a day, is sufficient. In some it may be advisable to continue the medication indefinitely.

The paroxysmal form is frequently abolished by quinidine sulphate, 0.12 to 0.2 gram (2 to 3 grains), three or four times a day. It is possible through this drug to restore the normal rhythm in at least 50 per cent of all cases of established auricular fibrillation. The sinus rhythm, however, is transient in the vast majority and seldom persists for more than a few days or weeks. This form of treatment is therefore not justified except in selected cases and then under careful hospital supervision. The extent of the functional impairment and the duration of the irregularity are the determining factors. Rarely is it possible to maintain a normal rhythm with quinidine after an attack of cardiac failure. The results are far more favorable in the fibrillation of relatively short duration and particularly in those instances where it is possible to eliminate an exciting factor, such as in thyrotoxicosis. The patient should be confined to bed during the active stage of the treatment and for several days after the normal rhythm is restored. In the beginning a test dose of 0.2 gram (3 grains) is given in order to make sure that the individual is not unduly sensitive to the drug. If

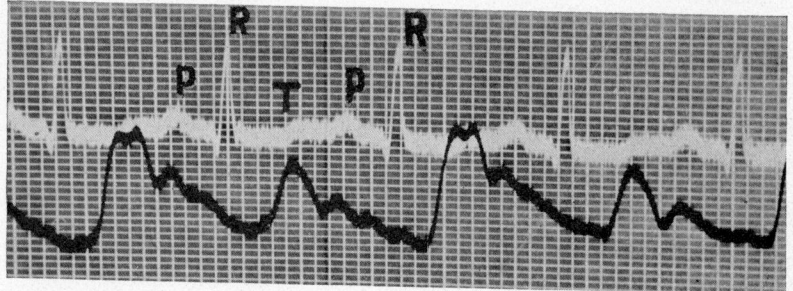

FIG. 19.—Top curve, electrocardiogram, Lead III. Lower curve, tracing from carotid artery showing pulsus alternans.

there are no untoward effects, the drug may then be prescribed in doses of 0.4 gram (6 grains) every three or four hours until normal rhythm is established or toxic symptoms occur. After the onset of the normal rhythm the dose may be reduced to 0.2 gram (3 grains) after meals. Occasionally it may be advisable to continue this dose for several weeks. In certain instances the quinidine is more effective after or with the administration of digitalis.

Pulsus Alternans.—This is a condition in which alternating strong and weak cardiac contractions occur in regular sequence with an even spacing of the ventricular systoles. It is expressed in the pulse by an alternating large and small beat and is at times manifested in the electrocardiogram by variations in the form or amplitude of alternate ventricular complexes. The disorder is usually recognized during the determination of the systolic blood pressure through the alternating occurrence of weak beats. If the pressure in the arm band is gradually increased, a point may be reached in which the small beats fail to come through. Occasionally, in the advanced stages, the condition is apparent on palpating the radial pulse. In many instances it is demonstrated only by an arterial tracing. The regular appearance of a premature beat after every normal cardiac contraction produces a condition simulating pulsus alternans. The pause following the ectopic beat usually identifies the latter disorder. However, with the premature contraction coming late in the diastolic period, a pause may not be apparent and graphic records are then necessary to establish the diagnosis. (Fig. 19.)

A transient alternans is common immediately following a premature contraction. A more persistent form is often encountered during the markedly accelerated cardiac rate of paroxysmal tachycardia and auricular flutter and has also been observed in infectious diseases and in patients receiving large doses of digitalis. Under these circumstances, however, the condition is usually not of any great importance. That resulting from a paroxysmal tachycardia and auricular flutter invariably disappears with the restoration of the normal cardiac mechanism. Likewise that dependent on toxic action of digitalis generally disappears following the discontinuation of the medication. The pulsus alternans associated with a relatively normal cardiac rate has a grave prognostic significance. It occurs particularly in arteriosclerotic heart disease and is generally accompanied by other manifestations of a serious impairment in the cardiac function.

TREATMENT OF CONGESTIVE HEART FAILURE.

Early Stages.—The restoration of the cardiac function in the early stages of failure is rarely difficult. This is usually accomplished within a few days by restriction of physical activities, relaxation, sleep and digitalis. When the patient is seen at this stage it is frequently possible to curtail the progression of the disease through a careful survey of the various factors which may be contributing to the cardiac disability. Infection should be removed when there is justifiable reason to believe that this is influencing the general health or promoting the progression of the cardiac damage, provided the risk and sacrifice to the patient are not too great. This is particularly important in infectious forms of heart disease. Striking improvement in the clinical course may follow the removal of the tonsils and other infections about the head. A young woman with a high-grade mitral stenosis was seen by the writer six years ago with cardiac failure which seemed to follow an attack of tonsillitis. Following the recovery from the cardiac failure, the tonsils were removed. There has been no recurrence of the cardiac failure and the heart is capable of considerable functional range. The elimination of the thyrotoxicosis by a subtotal thyroidectomy frequently produces a marked improvement or even may be followed by complete restoration of the cardiac function. Regulation of the diet in those who are inclined to overeat, and a gradual reduction in the weight of the obese, represent possible means of reducing the work of the heart, and perhaps favorably influencing the hypertension. The habits of living, in general, should be carefully studied and regulated, as far as possible, to fit the disability of the individual. Protection against upper respiratory infection, rest, relaxation and sleep have a decided influence on the course of the disease.

Occasionally, it may be necessary to administer a simple sedative to promote the proper relaxation and induce regular sleep. If there is auricular fibrillation, the continued or intermittent use of digitalis may be indicated to control the cardiac rate. The excessive rate of an auricular fibrillation is very often an important factor in promoting the return of the cardiac failure.

In the arteriosclerotic form of heart disease, an inadequate coronary circulation is frequently a significant aspect, or possibly primarily responsible for the cardiac disability. The theophyllin and theobromin preparations, because of their dilating action on the coronary arteries, are indicated. These drugs obviously have greater possibilities in the cases of less extensive coronary artery disease. The writer prefers theophyllin in the form of metaphyllin, 0.1 gram (1.5 grains), three or four times a day. This drug should be continued for weeks or months in order that the maximum benefit may be derived. Finally, the patient should be cautioned to avoid overfatigue or any exertion which induces shortness of breath. It is extremely important that the physical activities be gradually extended and maintained, as far as possible, well within the range of the functional capacity of the heart.

Advanced Stages.—The treatment of the advanced forms of cardiac failure is more difficult and generally demands detailed supervision. There are two primary objectives: (1) the reduction in the work of the heart; (2) the improvement of the cardiac function through the action of drugs. The importance of the former is often not fully appreciated and may explain the poor response to digitalis and other forms of medication. Here again, success is dependent on a clear conception of the condition and the factors influencing the cardiac disability.

Reduction in the Cardiac Load.—This is one of the most important aspects of treatment. Rest, relaxation and sleep are indispensable to this objective. The patient should therefore be confined to bed at as nearly absolute rest as possible. It is extremely important that the bed be comfortable and the head elevated. The patient should be spared all unnecessary effort in the taking of food, liquids and the use of the bedpan by careful nursing. Sleep represents the most satisfactory means of resting the heart and should be induced, if necessary, by morphine or codeine. Morphine is one of the most valuable drugs in the treatment of advanced cardiac failure and should be given in sufficient amounts to produce sound sleep. The writer usually prescribes 15 mg. (0.25 grain) hypodermically, at bed time, with directions to repeat if the patient does not sleep. Seldom is it necessary to continue the administration for more than two or three nights. In the meantime a simple sedative, as sodium bromide, 0.6 to 1 gram (10 to 15 grains), or luminal, 30 mg. (0.5 grain) after meals and at bedtime, is extremely helpful in promoting relaxation, and in a few days will permit the patient to sleep throughout the night and possibly part of the day. Sleep during the day should be encouraged provided it does not interfere with the rest at night.

Other Means of Reducing the Cardiac Load.—It may be possible to immediately curtail the cardiac load by other measures as a temporary reduction of the blood pressure in hypertension, by venesection, by

29

the removal of excess fluids from serous cavities and by the administration of oxygen. In patients with hypertension, nitroglycerin, 0.6 mg. (0.01 grain), under the tongue, every two hours or even more often, may produce a striking influence on the breathing and in turn promote relaxation and sleep. There is not only a reduction in the cardiac load, but the efficiency of the heart may be improved through the dilating action on the coronary arteries.

In certain of the plethoric cyanotic individuals, especially those with a hypertension, the rapid removal of 600 cc. of blood from a vein in the arm is often followed by immediate improvement in the condition. This procedure should not be employed when the hemoglobin and red blood cell count are below the normal standard. If the peritoneal cavity contains a large quantity of fluid, an abdominal paracentesis may be done following the venesection. Occasionally, it may be advisable to remove excess fluids from the pleural cavity. There is, however, a certain risk connected with this procedure which should be taken into consideration. The disturbance to the patient should be reduced to the minimum by the careful selection of needles, the use of novocaine and possibly a preliminary administration of morphine. Oxygen is a valuable adjunct and may be properly considered in this category. It reduces the dyspnea, lessens the cyanosis, and in general makes the subject much more comfortable. The administration by nasal catheter is quite satisfactory and ordinarily does not disturb the patient.

Diet.—The diet is an important factor and in the prolonged and more advanced forms of cardiac failure has a decided influence on the restoration of the cardiac function. In this type of patient the Karell diet is entirely inadequate in energy value and has not been necessary. During the past five years a diet has been employed which in the beginning consists of 45 to 50 grams of protein, 100 to 110 grams of fat and 200 to 220 grams of carbohydrates. This gives an energy value of approximately 2000 calories. It is served in the form of milk, cream, butter, eggs, puréed vegetables, cooked cereals, and fruit juices. The carbohydrates are further increased by the addition of sugars, such as dextromaltose, dextrose and lactose. Small and frequent feedings are given. When edema is present the liquid intake is limited to 1500 or 1800 cc., and the salt is reduced to the minimum. Usually on the third or fourth day other foods, as jellies, crackers (salt-free), toast and stick candy are added. After the first week, depending on the condition of the patient, puréed fruits and additional puréed vegetables are incorporated in the diet. The consistency of the food thereafter is gradually changed from that of the soft to the light diet. The diet is varied as far as possible to suit the needs and taste of the individual. If the patient with advanced failure is not able to take the usual amount of carbohydrates, it is supplemented by a daily intravenous administration of glucose. This, however, is rarely necessary.

The patient with cardiac failure should have a daily bowel movement. Should the bowels not move once during the twenty-four hours, a simple laxative is advised. The removal of excess fluid by the bowels, by means of cathartics, is not necessary. Furthermore, the violent purging incident to this form of treatment is liable to upset the function of the gastro-intestinal tract, and in addition impose an unnecessary amount of work upon the heart through the frequent use of the bedpan.

The Increase in Cardiac Efficiency through the Use of Drugs.— Digitalis is by far the most important drug in this group. The administration of 15 to 20 minims (1 to 1.5 cc.) of a reliable tincture, or 0.1 to 0.15 gram (1½ to 2 grains) of the powdered leaf, three or four times a day, is ordinarily sufficient to produce the desired results. Occasionally it may be necessary to prescribe larger doses. Eggleston and others have demonstrated that in general 1.5 cc. of tincture of digitalis for each 10 pounds of body weight, or 2 minims per pound, is required to produce complete digitalization. If the powdered leaf is employed, one-tenth of this amount is required. Rapid digitalization may be induced and the toxic action avoided by administering one-half to three-fourths of the total amount in the first three doses at six-hour intervals. Thereafter, the dose is reduced to 15 minims of the tincture or 1½ grains of the powdered leaf, three times a day. If there is nausea and vomiting from the extensive passive congestion, the initial dose may be given by rectum. It is well to clear out the lower bowel by warm water enemas at least one hour before the administration of digitalis. The digitalis is diluted up to 75 or 100 cc. by warm water or salt solution and injected slowly through a small catheter. The rapid administration of digitalis is not necessary, except possibly in the more extreme conditions. If the desired results are not obtained by the more conservative dosage, it has rarely been possible for the writer to promote recovery by increasing the dose. While there is no drug that will replace the digitalis group, yet in general too much reliance is placed on this aspect of the treatment and the first objective, namely, the reduction in the cardiac load, is neglected.

Even with the conservative method of administering digitalis, it is frequently necessary to reduce the dose after a few days or a week. This stage is reached in auricular fibrillation when the ventricular rate is reduced to 70 or 80 per minute. With a normal cardiac mechanism, the full therapeutic effect, or the onset of the toxic manifestations, may be indefinite. A feeling of exhaustion and loss of appetite are among the early indications of an intoxication. Coupling of beats is one of the most reliable signs and the drug should at once be discontinued for a few days. In auricular fibrillation it is extremely important that the cardiac rate be controlled. Ordinarily, after the cardiac function is once restored, 10 minims (0.6 cc.) of the tincture, or 0.06 gram (1 grain) of the powdered leaf, two or three times a day, is sufficient. The continued or periodic use of digitalis in small doses is often advisable in the arteriosclerotic form of heart disease with a normal rhythm after recovery from cardiac failure.

Oubain and amorphous strophanthin are the only other preparations that have an effective digitalis-like action. These preparations, however, are rarely employed except in an emergency. They are powerful in their action and thus dangerous if given in large doses, or if digitalis has already been used. The dose of oubain, intramuscularly or intravenously, should not exceed 0.5 mg. ($\frac{1}{125}$ grain), and that of the amorphous strophanthin, 1 mg. ($\frac{1}{65}$ grain). This may be followed by the usual oral administration of digitalis.

Theobromin and Theophyllin Preparations.—Until recent years these preparations were employed only as diuretics. Through their dilating action on the coronary arteries, however, they have another very important function, and are thus indicated in the treatment of the arteriosclerotic form of heart disease. They are most effective in congestive failure with extensive edema. Under these conditions, the heart profits from the combined action of the drug. The reduction in the cardiac load resulting from the diuresis adds to the benefit derived from the increased coronary circulation. Theophyllin preparations, metaphyllin and theocin, have the greatest effect on the coronary circulation. Metaphyllin, in doses of 0.1 to 0.3 gram ($1\frac{1}{2}$ to $4\frac{1}{2}$ grains), three times a day, is employed extensively in the treatment of arteriosclerotic heart disease. Theocin, which is more commonly used for its diuretic effects, may be used in doses of 2 to 3 grains for weeks without disturbing the gastro-intestinal tract. Theobromin, in the alkaloid form, or theocalcin may be employed.

In the more obstinate cases with extensive edema, the excess fluid may occasionally be eliminated after the above measures have failed by the mercurial diuretics novasurol or salyrgan. They are more or less toxic to the renal parenchyma, and the urine should be watched for granular casts and erythrocytes. Albumin alone is not a contraindication. Salyrgan is less toxic and has practically replaced novasurol. It is administered either intramuscularly or intravenously in 0.5 to 1 cc. doses at intervals of three to four days. A smaller dose is frequently effective. The diuretic effect is more certain and striking when combined with the administration of ammonium chloride, 1 to 4 grams (15 to 60 grains), three times a day.

The sudden cardiac failure manifested by acute pulmonary edema demands prompt and energetic treatment. When possible, the removal of 500 cc. of blood by venesection is one of the most valuable measures. Morphine sulphate (0.25 grain) and atropine sulphate (0.02 grain), hypodermatically, should be given at once. This is one condition in which the intravenous administration of digitalis is indicated. Oubain or strophanthin, because of their prompt and powerful action, should be given consideration. In the more extreme condition, the subcutaneous injection of adrenalin (1 to 1000 solution), 0.3 to 0.6 gram (5 to 10 minims), is indicated and may be repeated if necessary within a few minutes.

The treatment following the recovery from the cardiac failure should be carefully supervised. The restoration of the heart to the maximum efficiency is the ultimate aim. This may require a prolonged period of rest with a gradual rehabilitation of the cardiac muscle, and, finally, the removal or control of all possible factors which may be contributing to the cardiac disability. The exercise should be extended very gradually. If the patient avoids becoming "winded," he may be certain he is not placing an excess load on his heart.

REFERENCES.

Only a few of the more important references are listed and those in English are given preference.

General:
EDENS, E.: Die Krankheiten des Herzens und der Gefässe, Verlag von Julius Springer, Berlin, 1929.
LEWIS, T.: Diseases of the Heart, New York, Macmillan Company, 1933.
MACKENZIE, J.: Diseases of the Heart, Oxford University Press, 3d ed., 1913.
ROMBERG, E.: Lehrbuch der Krankheiten des Herzens und der Blutgefässe, 5th ed., Verlag von Ferdinand Enke, Stuttgart, 1925.
WHITE, PAUL D.: Heart Disease, The Macmillan Company, 1931.

Etiology of Heart Disease:
HALSEY, R. H.: Observations on the Mortality of Heart Disease in New York State, Am. Heart Jour., 1928, 4, 94.
WHITE, PAUL D., and JONES, T. D.: Heart Diseases and Disorders in New England, Am. Heart Jour., 1928, 3, 302.

Rheumatic Heart Disease:
ASCHOFF, L.: Zur Myocarditis Frage, Verhandl. d. deutsch. path. Gesellsch., 1904, 8, 46.
COOMBS, C. F.: Rheumatic Heart Disease, John Wright & Son, Ltd., London, 1924.
SACKS, BENJAMIN: The Pathology of Rheumatic Fever—A Critical Review, Am. Heart Jour., 1926, 1, 750.
ST. LAWRENCE, W.: Potential Cardiac Disease and Prevention of Organic Heart Disease in Children—A Study of Sixty-five Cases Under Continuous Observation for an Average Period of Four and One-half Years, Jour. Am. Med. Assn., 1922, 78, 947.
SWIFT, HOMER, F.: The Heart in Infection, Am. Heart Jour., 1928, 3, 629.

Bacterial Endocarditis:
BLUMER, G.: Subacute Bacterial Endocarditis, Medicine, 1923, 2, 105.
LEWIS, T., and GRANT, R. T.: Observations Relating to Subacute Infective Endocarditis, Heart, 1923, 10, 21.
LIBMAN, E.: A Consideration of the Prognosis in Subacute Bacterial Endocarditis, Am. Heart Jour., 1925, 1, 25.

Arteriosclerotic Heart Disease:
ALLBUTT, C.: Diseases of the Arteries Including Angina Pectoris, London, Macmillan & Co., 1915, vol. 2.
HERRICK, J. B.: Clinical Features of Sudden Obstruction of the Coronary Arteries, Jour. Am. Med. Assn., 1912, 59, 2015.
——— Thrombosis of the Coronary Arteries, Jour. Am. Med. Assn., 1919, 72, 387.
LEVINE, SAMUEL A.: Coronary Thrombosis—Various Clinical Features, Medicine, 1929, 8, 245.
LEWIS, T.: Ischemia of Muscle as Cause of Anginal Pain, Brit. Med. Jour., 1931, i, 941.
MORAWITZ, P., and HOCHREIN, M.: Zur Diagnose und Behandlung der Koronarsklerose, Münch. med. Wchnschr., 1928, 75, 17.
OBRASTZOW, W. P., and STRASCHESKO, N. D.: Zur Kenntnis der Thrombose der Koronararterien des Herzens, Ztschr. f. klin. Med., 1910, 71, 116.
OSLER, W.: The Lumleian Lectures on Angina Pectoris, Lancet, 1910, i, 697, 839, 973.
SMITH, F. M.: The Ligation of Coronary Arteries with Electrocardiographic Study, Arch. Int. Med., 1918, 22, 8.
——— The Electrocardiographic Changes Following Occlusion of the Left Coronary Artery, Arch. Int. Med., 1923, 32, 497.
WEARN, J. T.: The Rôle of the Thebesian Vessels in the Circulation of the Heart, Jour. Exper. Med., 1928, 47, 293.

Syphilitic Heart Disease:
  MARTLAND, H. S.: Syphilis of the Aorta and Heart, Am. Heart Jour., 1930, **6**, 1.
  MOORE, J. E., and DANGLADE, J. H.: The Treatment of Cardio-vascular Syph-
    ilis, a Study of the Duration of Life in 141 Treated and Untreated Patients
    with Aortic Regurgitation and Aortic Aneurysm, Am. Heart Jour., 1930,
    6, 148.
  SAPHIR, O., and SCOTT, R. W.: Observations on 107 Cases of Syphilitic Aortic
    Insufficiency, with Special Reference to the Aortic Valve Area, the Myo-
    cardium and the Branches of the Aorta, Am. Heart Jour., 1930, **6**, 56.
Thyrotoxic Heart Disease:
  ANDRUS, E. COWLES: The Heart in Hyperthyroidism: A Clinical and Experi-
    mental Study, Am. Heart Jour., 1932, **8**, 66.
  FAHR, G.: Myxedema Heart, Jour. Am. Med. Assn., 1925, **84**, 345; Am. Heart
    Jour., 1927, **3**, 14.
  RAKE, GEOFFREY, and McEACHERN, DONALD: A Study of the Heart in Hyper-
    thyroidism, Am. Heart Jour., 1932, **8**, 19.
  WELLER, CARL V., WANSTROM, R. C., GORDON, HAROLD, and BUGHER, JOHN C.:
    Cardiac Histopathology in Thyroid Disease. Preliminary report, Am. Heart
    Jour., 1932, **8**, 8.
  WILSON, FRANK N.: The Cardiac Disturbance Associated with Diseases of the
    Thyroid Gland, Jour. Am. Med. Assn., 1924, **82**, 1754.
Congenital Heart Disease:
  ABBOTT, M. E.: Congenital Cardiac Disease, Osler's Modern Medicine, 3d ed.,
    Philadelphia, Lea & Febiger, 1927, vol. **4**.
  ———— The Diagnosis of Congenital Heart Disease, Blumer's Bedside Diag-
    nosis, Philadelphia, W. B. Saunders Company, 1928, **2**, 430.
Pericardial Disease:
  CARTER, E. P., and DIEUAIDE, F. R.: The Electrocardiogram as an Aid in the
    Diagnosis of Adhesive Mediastinitis, Trans. Am. Soc. Clin. Invest., Jour.
    Am. Med. Assn., 1924, **72**, 2077.
  CONNER, L. A.: On the Diagnosis of Pericardial Effusion with Special Reference
    to Physical Signs on the Posterior Aspect of the Thorax, Am. Heart Jour.,
    1926, **1**, 421.
  MUSSER, J. H., and HERRMANN, G. R.: Chronic Pericarditis; the Clinical and
    Experimental Aspects, Jour. Am. Med. Assn., 1926, **87**, 459.
  ROLLESTON, H. D.: Pericarditis Pseudo-cirrhosis, Oxford Med., 1920, **3**, 342.
  WILLIAMSON, C. S.: Pericarditis with Effusion—A Clinical Study of 23 Cases,
    Jour. Am. Med. Assn., 1921, **77**, 2050.
Functional Disorders of the Heart—Irritable Heart:
  GRANT, R. T.: Observations on the After-histories of Men Suffering from the
    Effort Syndrome, Heart, 1925, **12**, 121.
  LEWIS, T.: The Soldier's Heart and the Effort Syndrome, New York, Paul B.
    Hoeber, 1919.
  WENCKEBACH, K. F., and WINTERBERG, H.: Die unregelmässige Herztätigkeit,
    Leipzig, W. Engelmann, 1927.
Treatment of Congestive Heart Failure:
  EGGLESTON, C., and WYCKOFF, J.: The Absorption of Digitalis in Man, Arch.
    Int. Med., 1922, **30**, 133.
  MARVIN, H. M.: The Value of the Xanthine Diuretics in Congestive Heart
    Failure, Jour. Am. Med. Assn., 1926, **87**, 2043.
  MUSSER, J. H.: Theophylline-Ethylenediamine in Heart Disease Associated
    with Pain, Jour. Am. Med. Assn., 1928, **91**, 1242.
  PARKINSON, J., and CAMPBELL, M.: The Quinidine Treatment of Auricular
    Fibrillation, Quart. Jour. Med., 1929, **22**, 281.
  SMITH, F. M., GIBSON, R. B., and ROSS, N. G.: The Diet in the Treatment
    of Cardiac Failure, Jour. Am. Med. Assn., 1927, **88**, 1943.
  WITHERING, W.: An Account of the Foxglove and Some of Its Medical Uses;
    with Practical Remarks on Dropsy and Other Diseases, M. Swinney, Bir-
    mingham, 1785.

CHAPTER XII.

DISEASES OF THE BLOOD-VESSELS.

By GEORGE E. BROWN, M.D.

DISEASES OF THE ARTERIES.
  Structures and Mechanisms of Disturbances in General.
  Functional, Localized, Vasoconstricting, Primary Disturbances.
  Raynaud's Disease.
  Functional, Localized, Vasoconstricting, Secondary Disturbances.
  Functional, Localized, Vasodilating, Primary Disturbances.
  Erythromelalgia.
  Functional, Localized, Vasodilating, Secondary Disturbances.
  Functional, Generalized, Vasoconstricting, Primary Disturbances.
  Essential Hypertension.
  Functional, Generalized, Vasodilating, Primary Disturbances.
  Hypotension.
  Organic Localized Forms.

DISEASES OF THE ARTERIES—Organic Localized Forms—Continued.
  Thrombo-arteriosclerosis Obliterans.
  Thrombo-angiitis Obliterans.
  Simple Thrombosis.
  Occlusion of Embolic Type.
  Aneurysm.
  Arteritis, Diverse Forms.
  Periarteritis Nodosa.
  Coarctation of the Aorta.
  Pulsating Carotid Arteries.
  Organic Generalized Forms and Forms Affecting Special Systems.
  Generalized Arteriosclerosis.
FORMS AFFECTING SPECIAL SYSTEMS.
ARTERIOVENOUS FISTULA.
DISEASES OF THE VEINS.
DISEASES OF THE LYMPHATICS OF THE EXTREMITIES.

Structures, and Mechanism of Disturbances in General.—According to their structure there are two types of arteries: those with strong development of elastic tissue, such as the aorta and its main branches, and those in which the muscular development is predominant, such as the peripheral arteries, especially the smaller arteries and arterioles. The arteries function not only as conveyors of blood, but they subserve the propulsive function of the heart by virtue of their rhythmic contractions and elastic properties. By virtue of control of tonus of the precapillary arterioles, the distribution of blood to the capillary circulation and maintenance of peripheral resistance is largely controlled. The caliber of arteries is regulated by vasomotor nerves, probably also by hormonal or chemical agents, and in addition they have an inherent tonus. Disturbances due to the peripheral arteries are found in the presence of the following: (1) imbalance of the vasomotor nerves, with intermittent disorder of temperature in the peripheral parts; (2) occlusion of the vessels by organic lesions such as thrombosis, or, in the smaller arteries, by excessive proliferation of the intima; (3) inflammatory disease of the arteries with local symptoms common to inflammation; and (4) structural defects such as obtain in aneurysm or arteriovenous fistula.

From the precapillary arterioles to the capillary there is progressive

(455)

diminution of the muscle fibers. The capillary is a continuation of the endothelial structure of the arterioles on which are contractile cells, Rouget cells, consisting of single muscle elements. These vessels have the property of independent contractility, mediated by vasoconstrictor fibers. The existence of vasodilator fibers is less certain. It is probable that hormonal and chemical, rather than neurogenic, agents produce vasodilatation. Substances are distributed to the tissue cells by the capillaries; their action is intermittent. They open and close according to the metabolic needs of the tissues. They are permeable to gases, water, salts, colloids and crystalloids, all of which are substances that enter into the metabolism of cells. The capillary pressure in the cutaneous vessels of man ranges from 9 to 15 mm. of mercury. The osmotic pressure maintains the balance between the blood and tissue fluids. Disease of the capillaries is manifested by disturbances in color, and in permeability, producing edema and ecchymosis. The release of tissue products (substances probably related to histamine), under certain conditions, affects the permeability of the capillaries and explains localized forms of edema, urticaria and angioneurotic edema. The size and number of the capillaries and venules, and of the contained blood, determine color of the tissue. A classification of arterial disease is given in Table 9.

TABLE 9.—TENTATIVE CLINICAL CLASSIFICATION OF ARTERIAL DISEASE.

Functional or vasomotor	Local in distribution	Vasoconstricting	Raynaud's disease
		Vasodilating	Erythromelalgia
	General in distribution	Vasoconstricting	Primary or essential hypertension, early stages
		Vasodilating	Primary or essential hypotension
Organic	Local in distribution	Thrombo-arteriosclerosis obliterans, including senile gangrene, and diabetic gangrene	
		Thrombo-angiitis obliterans	
		Simple thrombosis; thrombophilia; embolism	
		Arteriovenous communications, congenital or acquired	
		Aneurysm with or without thrombosis	
		Arteritis of diverse types, including periarteritis nodosa.	
		Coarctation aorta; certain forms of scleroderma	
	General in distribution	Arteriosclerosis, including atheromatosis and atherosclerosis	

The structure of the veins is similar to that of the arteries except that the muscular layer is less well developed. The column of blood is sustained by the tonus of the walls, by the valves and by the support and tonus of the surrounding muscles. The function of the veins is to return the venous blood to the heart. The "venopressure" function (Henderson), by which the amount of blood delivered to the right side of the heart is regulated, is of importance in maintaining circulatory efficiency. Failure of this mechanism is one factor in the production of shock or of cardiac insufficiency. Pressure of the veins is modified greatly by gravity. The gradient of pressure gradually diminishes, so that in the vena cava it is probably less than zero. Disturbances of the veins can be grouped as those due to: (1) disturbances of obstructive origin; (2) disturbances of non-obstructive origin.

THE ARTERIES.

FUNCTIONAL OR VASOMOTOR DISTURBANCES.

Circulatory disturbances of vasomotor origin have as their common attribute disturbances of color and of temperature of the skin. There are two forms: (1) those in which there is excessive constriction, and (2) those in which there is excessive vasodilatation. Normally, constriction and dilatation of the surface vessels is not accompanied by decided changes in color of the skin; there may be mild pallor, cyanosis or redness with exposure to cold or heat, although meanwhile there may be a wide range in the surface temperature of the hands and feet. The size and number of the capillaries and venules determine the color of the skin; the caliber of the arterioles determines its temperature. Decided changes in color, due to excessive vasomotor effects on the surface capillaries and venules, represent abnormality. If chronic, and associated with symptoms, this disturbance becomes a disease. Vasoconstrictor fibers are widely distributed in the skin, but the existence of vasodilator fibers is assumed. That there is independent neurogenic control of capillaries and venules is generally accepted (Krogh). There is also probably chemical or hormonal regulation of the vessels. Excessive constriction of the larger arteries does occur, but is rare.

Localized Forms.

Vasoconstricting Disturbances.—There are two groups of vasoconstricting disturbances: the primary type, which in its typical form is known as Raynaud's disease, and secondary forms.

1. **Primary Type, Illustrated by Raynaud's Disease.**—This is a vasomotor disturbance of the constrictor type, affecting the hands or feet, less frequently the nose, tips of the ears and acra. It is characterized by attacks or episodes of excessive constriction of the small vessels of the skin, with local coldness, ischemia, cyanosis and, if excessive recovery, rubor and increased local heat.

Raynaud's thesis, in 1862, described a new syndrome under the title of "De l'asphyxie locale et de la gangrène symétrique des extrémitées." He emphasized the presence of superficial gangrene of the digits without organic occlusion of the arteries. His second thesis, in 1874, included an additional group of cases. The type of gangrene was more clearly defined and its existence not considered essential to the diagnosis. Barlow, in his monograph, in 1899, made a complete report of the literature up to the time of his writing.

The criteria for diagnosis, postulated by Raynaud, were: (1) attacks of pallor, cyanosis initiated by cold or by nervous excitement, and relief with application of warmth; (2) bilateral distribution, frequently a symmetric nature of the disturbance; (3) gangrene, if present, superficial and confined to the skin; and (4) absence of occlusion of peripheral arteries. There is a further criterion: patients should be observed, or should have had the disease for at least two years to make certain of its primary nature.

Frequency.—One hundred and fifty examples of uncomplicated types of Raynaud's disease have been studied at The Mayo Clinic in ten years; this is an incidence of 1 to every 2800 new registrations. In a series of 1118 consecutive cases of circulatory disturbances of the extremities 20 per cent represented vasospastic disorders, of which 44 per cent were typical examples of Raynaud's disease.

Etiology.—The etiology is unknown. Analysis of our cases has shown that a large number of the subjects have a constitutional pattern similar to that of many subjects with psychoneurosis. Subjects are usually of asthenic build, with low blood pressure, small heart and other evidence of vascular inadequacy. Ninety per cent of our patients were women. It is a disease of adult life; it usually appears after puberty. A small number of patients exhibit the first signs of the disease at the menopause.

Pathology.—No pathologic changes have been found in the smaller arteries in uncomplicated cases. Intimal proliferation has been described, probably representing late changes secondary to ischemia. In the later stages of the disease occlusion of the digital arteries may occur; these are effects secondary to cutaneous infection and trophic lesions, a local fault as defined by Lewis. Pathologic studies of sympathetic ganglia have not disclosed characteristic changes. The large vessels are unaffected except as is compatible with age.

The disturbed physiology during the different stages of this disturbance is demonstrated by microscopic examination of the capillaries of the nailfold. In the stage of pallor, a diminished number of small or partially filled capillaries is visualized. The blood is stationary, and no blood is seen to enter the loops. The collecting venules are invisible. In the phase of cyanosis there is partial or intermittent relaxation of the arterioles and venules; blood slowly fills and distends the capillaries. Long periods of stasis of blood occur. A greater number of capillaries is opened. With prolonged stasis capillary blood becomes intensely cyanotic. The period of recovery is characterized by rapid opening of the arterioles, capillaries and venules, and resumption of flow, the blood rapidly changing from a cyanotic color to bright red. In this stage many more capillaries and small venules are open, and may dilate, thus giving the hyperemic color to the skin. During the ischemic and cyanotic stages the surface temperature is markedly reduced, the oxygen content of the venous blood is reduced to as low as 30 per cent of saturation. If recovery is complete, this rapidly increases to the normal or increased saturation for venous blood. Thrombosis of individual capillaries and death of the overlying skin produce minute, dry excavations.

Symptoms.—The symptoms of the disease are characteristic. The onset is usually in cold weather, in the form of attacks of pallor of one or more digits, and recovery is initiated by warmth and massage of the parts. The bilateral nature of the condition may not be evident for several months. Pain is absent or mild in the great majority of cases. This is modified by hypersensitivity of the patient. The disturbance gradually advances to other digits. The response to cold is more intense, and the attacks of pallor may be displaced by episodes of cyanosis. Recovery is less complete. The fingers may become more or less permanently cyanosed, and the skin, in place of its normal pink color, becomes excessively red or mildly cyanotic between attacks. Minute areas of gangrene (capillary thrombosis) which heal, leaving small excavated areas, are common. The subjective symptoms are numbness during the stages of pallor and cyanosis, and burning distress with the period of recovery. Oscillometric studies made during the period of ischemia may show some diminution in the amplitude, but not disappearance, of pulsations in the palpable arteries. Cases have been observed over a period of twenty years without gangrene or ulcers. The feet are usually involved to a less degree than the hands.

Diagnosis.—Diagnosis is not justified in the presence of any organic disorder which affects vasospastic disturbances, nor should the diagnosis be made in the presence of occlusion of the arteries in the extremities. In a survey of 25 unselected reports of cases of males with so-called Raynaud's disease, from German, English and American literature, in no instance were the criteria laid down by Raynaud fulfilled. Most cases represented the secondary ischemic changes in color which occur in organic disease of the arteries or nerves. Mild changes in color of the extremities, bilateral and without pain or trophic sequelæ in women are probably examples of mild Raynaud's disease. It is probably better to classify these mild cases merely as primary vasospastic disturbances.

Complications.—About 10 per cent of the patients who have had Raynaud's disease for a period of years eventually develops sclerodermal changes of the skin of the hands, arms, face and neck. In some cases the vasomotor and sclerodermal changes are consecutive, whereas in others the changes precede the vasomotor disturbance. In about 3 per cent of the cases observed at The Mayo Clinic, atrophic arthritis, with the usual destructive changes in the joint surfaces, muscular atrophy and deformity develop. In this group the symptoms of Raynaud's disease antedated the appearance of arthritic changes by a period of years. Epilepsy and amblyopia have been observed. Temporary attacks of aphasia and hemiplegia, with complete recovery, have been reported. Albuminuria and hemoglobinuria of the paroxysmal type have been reported by Hutchinson. One case of this type has been found in The Mayo Clinic series.

Prognosis.—The prognosis of the disease is subject to wide variations. There are two common groups: (1) There is a mild, slowly progressive type, eventually becoming stationary, without severe subjective symptoms or destruction of the skin. Probably this type is the most common. (2) A more progressive form has a rapid course. Secondary ulcers, of the felon type, may occur in the tips of the digits, with destruction of the terminal phalanges, and sequestration of particles of bone or deposition of calcified material. Rarely, this may give rise to a very distressing disabling condition. These suppurative lesions are extremely painful, but never, in the writer's experience, have progressed to the loss of more than the terminal phalanx. With the onset of scleroderma or arthritis, the disease becomes truly disabling.

Treatment.—In mild cases, measures to provide protection, if possible change to a warmer climate, contrast baths in which the hands are dipped alternately into hot and then into cold water, or so-called graduated baths, in which the extremity is immersed in water of decreasing temperature, can be tried. Frequently, reassurance is important in alleviating the nervous irritability which accompanies the presence of extreme changes in color in the skin, and fear of gangrene. This alone may be sufficient to give definite relief. In the more severe cases medical treatment is of no avail in modifying the disease.

The recent development of operations on the sympathetic nervous system has radically changed the therapeutic outlook. For diseases of the lower extremities, the second, third and fourth lumbar ganglia are removed through an abdominal route. Following this, there is permanent vasodilatation of the smaller arteries and absence of sweating of the feet, with complete cure of the disease. For diseases of the upper extremities the first cervical and the first and second thoracic sympathetic ganglia are removed through a posterior approach (Adson). If the operation is complete, as signified by complete absence of sweating of the skin of the upper extremities, head and upper part of the thorax, permanent vasodilatation results. Horner's syndrome follows this operation, which, when bilateral, is of no moment. Patients who have had this operation and have been observed for as long as six years were found to be completely relieved of attacks of vasoconstriction. In advanced cases, with involvement or thrombosis of digital arteries, vasodilatation is incomplete.

2. **Secondary Type.**—Changes in color accompanying vasoconstriction, such as pallor or cyanosis, are observed in many conditions; the most common are peripheral neuritis, atrophy from disuse, some cases of metallic intoxication, such as that from lead or arsenic, cervical rib, and organic diseases of the peripheral arteries such as thrombo-angiitis obliterans. Twenty per cent of the vasospastic disorders in our series were of the secondary type.

Vasodilating Disturbances.—The writer has observed that these disturbances are much more rare than vasoconstricting disorders. There are two main types: (1) the primary type, the best example of which is erythromelalgia (Weir Mitchell), and atypical forms which are usually unilateral, and (2) the secondary type.

1. **Primary Type, Illustrated by Erythromelalgia.**—This condition is a bilateral vasodilator disturbance of the extremities characterized by attacks of increased local heat, burning pain and local flushing. The name signifies a painful red extremity. The disease was first described by Mitchell, in 1872, and his second communication, in 1878, included additional cases.

Erythromelalgia represents an extremely rare disease. One case to every 40,000 persons registered represents the incidence at The Mayo Clinic; in the last ten years ten typical cases have been seen. The *etiology* is unknown. The disorder probably originates in the vasomotor centers of the spinal cord, affecting usually the feet, less frequently the hands. Sex is not of influence. There are no characteristic *pathologic manifestations*. The disturbance is functional, since in the interval between attacks abnormalities are not present.

The *symptoms*, as outlined by Mitchell, consist of the following: (1) there are bilateral attacks of burning pain of the extremities, which may be superficial or deep, usually confined to the soles of the feet, or, in the more severe attacks, extending to the lower part of the legs; (2) pain is accompanied by sharp increase in the surface temperature of the affected parts—the temperature parallels roughly the pain and it may rise to almost that of the mouth, and is associated with increased local sweating; (3) the superficial veins are distended and pulsate, and (4) relief is obtained by elevation of the parts or by placing them in cold water—the condition is usually worse in the summer and less severe or absent in the winter. Covering the feet frequently initiates an attack.

Mitchell emphasized the lack of amenability of this disease to treatment. The condition usually progresses or remains unchanged for an indefinite period of years.

There is a disturbance noted in older subjects of arteriosclerotic ages in which the complaint is a burning sensation in the extremities, usually the feet. This is differentiated from true erythromelalgia by the fact that the burning sensation exists with increased skin temperatures of the affected parts. (It is a subjective, not an objective complaint.) There is no dilatation of the veins or evidence of an increased volume flow of the blood during the episode of burning. This condition is designated as "burning paresthesia." It probably has a central origin on the basis of arteriosclerosis. The treatment is not satisfactory. Small doses of aspirin, salicylates, or barbituric compounds will give symptomatic relief. The condition usually disappears within one or two years.

2. **Secondary Type.**—Secondary vasodilating disturbances have been seen in a variety of conditions. Some cases of peripheral neuritis are initiated with clinical evidence of hot hands or hot feet, and there are symptoms of burning. The most common vasodilating disturbance is seen in cases of polycythemia vera. In about 20 per cent of cases of this disease an early symptom is a burning sensation of the hands or feet; in some cases there is paresthesia; other cases are examples of true vasodilator disturbances; the condition usually is localized, may be largely unilateral, may be excessively severe, and may be accompanied by local heat, flushing and a deep sensation of burning. The relative frequency of this condition should lead one to examine the blood carefully for evidence of polycythemia vera. Occasionally, arthritis is initiated by a period of vasodilatation. Recently vasodilating disturbances have been observed in cases of thallium poisoning. This represents, probably, a sympathetic neuritis. Thallium poisoning is not rare, and is due to the use of this drug in depilatory preparations. There is a form of so-called *infectious ganglionitis* in which burning vasodilator disturbance of the extremities is a prominent symptom. Seventy-five per cent of the dilator disorders in The Mayo Clinic series were examples of secondary forms.

From Cold or Heat.—Certain subjects exhibit abnormal grades of vasodilatation with cold. Edema of the angioneurotic type, of the exposed parts, usually the hands or feet, accompanied by marked vasodilatation, sharp rise in surface temperature, and occasionally subjective sensations of heat, is the course of events. The edema cycle usually endures for from eight to twenty-four hours. Repetition of exposures produces refractory periods. Similar examples have been noted with exposure to heat. These reactions have been designated as examples of physical allergy (Duke). Chilblain is a common example of this local vasodilating effect from cold.

A new syndrome has been described in which this reaction in the hands or feet is associated with a sharp systemic reaction, such as syncope, flushing of the face, tachycardia, a drop in blood pressure and a rise in concentration of gastric acids. The systemic reaction can be prevented temporarily by stopping the blood supply to the extremity. Biologic tests of the regional blood during the reaction show effects on nonstriped muscle suggesting that of histamine.

Generalized Forms.

This section, obviously, will include hypertension and hypotension. Consequently a few facts and opinions concerning normal blood pressure will be reviewed.

Normal Blood Pressure.—The normal blood pressure of the total population, for different ages and sexes, is unknown. Insurance statistics, or statistics based on large groups of selected types of persons, such as students in colleges, patients in dispensaries and inmates of prisons, although representing a close approximation of the normal values, are subject to selection and errors in sampling. A truer approximation of the mean values could be obtained by unselected sampling of large groups, representing the urban and rural inhabitants of all ages. At birth the systolic pressure varies from about 35 to 60 mm. of mercury, averaging 55 mm. (Rucker and Connell), increasing to about 82 mm. of mercury (Seitz and Becker) by the end of the first month. The average systolic blood pressure of subjects, fifteen years of age, has been found to be about 100 mm. for both sexes. Diastolic pressures do not change markedly from birth to puberty, and no differences between the pressure in the two sexes are noted in this period. There is a rise in pressure in adolescence, which falls in succeeding years (Alvarez). Between the ages of twenty and forty years the average systolic pressure for males is about 120 mm. of mercury, and for females, 113 mm. From then on, the pressures increase gradually, so that, at the age of sixty years, the systolic pressure is about 136 mm. for both sexes. In old age there is a tendency for the systolic pressure to rise without parallel increase in the diastolic pressure (Bower). The average systolic pressure for all age groups, based on insurance statistics (Fisher), is 123.2 mm., and the average diastolic pressure, 80 mm. of mercury (Bower). Among prisoners the modal, or most frequently observed, blood pressure does not increase from youth to old age (Alvarez and Stanley). This group of subjects is not comparable, however, with one composed of subjects living in non-restricted environments.

It may be stated that systolic pressure of more than 135 mm. and diastolic of 90 mm. or more in middle life, and that after middle life, pressures in excess of 150 mm. systolic and 100 mm. diastolic should be regarded as abnormal.

Blood pressure is not static. It is a variable, fluctuating physiologic response, held within certain limits, reacting to conscious and unconscious stimuli. If readings of the blood pressure of normal subjects, or of those with low blood pressure, are taken hourly over a period of at least twenty-four hours, under controlled conditions of rest and exercise, fluctuations of the systolic and diastolic pressures are within a relatively small range, from 15 to 20 mm. of mercury. (Fig. 21.) There is a daily rhythm, with an increase in pressure during the day, and a fall during sleep. In subjects with hypotension the fluctuations in pressure and in rhythm are less than in the so-called normal subjects. Among certain individuals in the "normal" group but with higher median pressures, the variations in the blood pressure and response to the same stimuli will be of greater magnitude. The normal rhythm and the hourly fluctuations are present, but exaggerated. In early cases of hypertension with blood pressure above the accepted normal levels, the rhythm and variations are of the same order but more exaggerated. If similar groups are examined, using a standard stimulus, such as placing a hand in ice-water (5° C.), there is a rapid rise in the blood pressure, occurring within thirty seconds, which usually returns to the pre-test level within one minute. Normal subjects and those with low blood pressures rarely show an increase in the systolic pressure of over 15 mm. of mercury, and in the diastolic of over 10 mm. of mercury (Hines and Brown).

There is a group of young normal subjects who reveal a hyperreaction to the cold test with increases in the blood pressure of two or three times that occurring in other normal subjects. Seventy-five per cent of these hyperreacting normal subjects give a history of hypertension in their immediate ancestors. There is evidence to believe that these hyperreacting normal subjects will eventually develop increased levels in their blood pressures, and what is recognized as essential hypertension. If the hypertension of subjects is established, the blood pressure response to cold stimulation is frequently as high as 60 to 100 mm. of mercury. In no other disease has this exaggerated vasomotor response been found. This difference in response of young subjects, in the author's opinion, is of great significance, since it reflects the order or pattern of the patient's vasopressor reactions.

Vasoconstricting Disturbances (Hypertension; Hyperpiesia; High Blood Pressure).

General Information.—Hypertension is the elevation of the intra-arterial pressure above the accepted range of normal for age, sex and body weight. Systolic pressure is the measure of the force of contraction of the left ventricle or the maximal pressure in the arteries immediately after ventricular closure. Diastolic pressure is the measure of the arterial pressure during the period of ventricular filling, an effect of the peripheral resistance in the arterioles. Pulse pressure is the difference between the systolic and diastolic pressures, and represents the force and volume of output of the left ventricle with each stroke.

Knowledge of hypertension is largely marked by five historic landmarks: (1) Richard Bright (1836), who noted the association of cardiac hypertrophy with a certain form of renal disease; (2) Sir George Johnson (1856), who demonstrated hypertrophy of the muscular layer of the arterioles as an expression of increased work; (3) v. Basch (1876), who adapted the sphygmomanometer to clinical use; (4) Allbutt (1895), who clearly separated the cases of primary high blood pressure from those of renal origin, which he termed "hyperpiesia;" and (5) Janeway (1912), who formulated the causes of death and laid down the facts on prognosis.

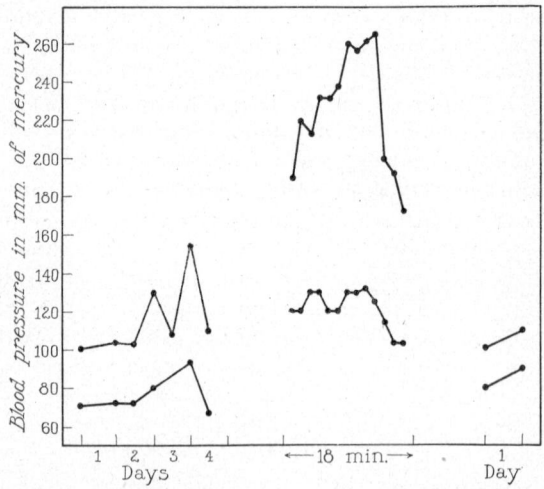

Fig. 20.—Blood pressures in a case of paroxysmal hypertension. (Mayo.)

Frequency.—Janeway showed that 11 per cent of patients in his private practice had blood pressures in excess of 165 mm. of mercury. Romberg's studies of his private patients indicated that 25 per cent of all organic cardiac disorders were due to hypertension. Statistics of The Mayo Clinic for 1930 showed an incidence of 7.9 per cent, or 3377 cases, of hypertension among new registrants for that year. Alvarez's statistics of healthy college students showed that in 20.7 per cent of males and 2.7 per cent of females systolic pressures were elevated above normal. Diehl and Sutherland found that 5.6 per cent of healthy male college students had transitory or permanent hypertension. Six and a half per cent of the applicants of a large life insurance company were rejected because of hypertension (Fisher). It is estimated that 140,000 deaths in 1924 were due to hypertension or its sequelæ. Twenty-three per cent of all deaths of persons who are more than fifty years of age can be attributed to hypertension. If accurate information were obtained, and all deaths due directly or secondarily to hypertension, with its consequent cardiac, renal and cerebral complications were recorded, including deaths from inter-current infections and pneumonia in cases of unrecognized hypertension, this figure would be increased.

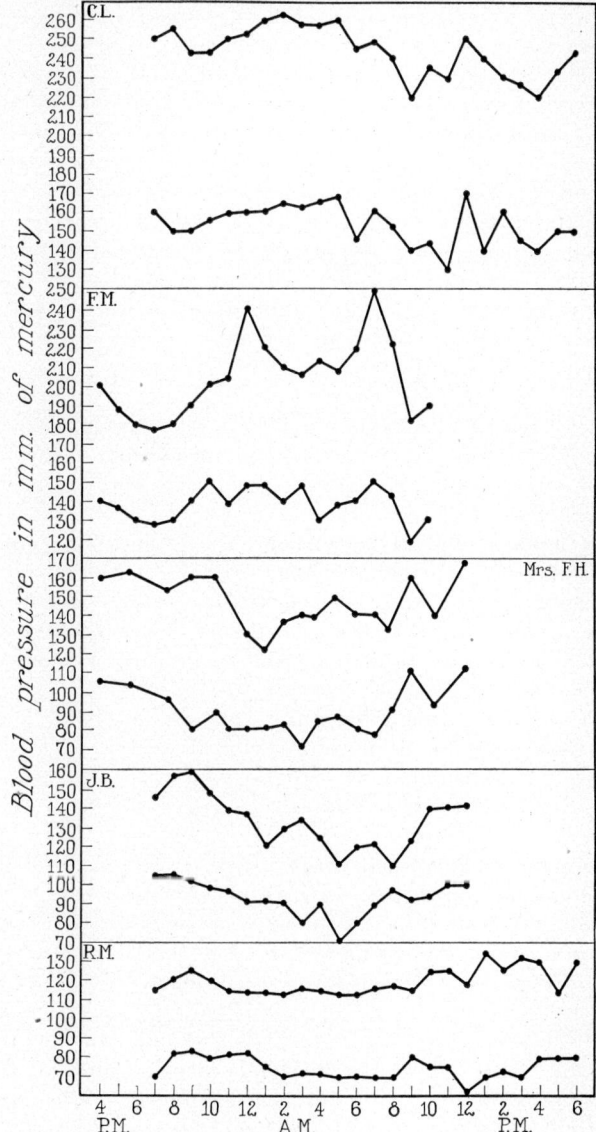

Fig. 21.—Hourly blood pressures of a normal subject and of subjects with hypertension.

Classification.—Cases of hypertension can be divided into two main groups: (1) Primary hypertension, of which the etiology is unknown, is the important type, and is the group usually known under the generic term "essential hypertension." There are two groupings of pri-

30

mary hypertension. One of these is known as (a) benign hypertension, which occurs in a mild and a severe form; the other is known as (b) malignant hypertension, and is fulminating in type (Volhard-Keith). (2) Secondary hypertension may be due to one or several causes: arteriosclerosis resulting in senile hypertension due to diminished elasticity of the arteries, with increase in systolic pressure but without parallel increase in diastolic pressure; glomerulonephritis; in advanced stages in cases of polycystic kidney and in the presence of obstructive lesions of the ureters; experimental hypertension has been produced by exposure of the kidney to roentgen-rays (Hartman); hyperthyroidism in which there is an increase in systolic pressure, due to cardiac overactivity and lowering of the diastolic pressure from vasodilatation; toxemia of pregnancy; aortic insufficiency and arteriovenous fistula with systolic hypertension; tumors of the suprarenal glands, of the form of paraganglioma, associated with paroxysmal forms of hypertension; intracranial lesions and trauma that causes increased intracranial pressure associated with an increase in blood pressure; coarctation of the aorta.

The distinction between primary and secondary hypertension is important. Measures to reduce blood pressure are valuable in the first, and of little importance, or perhaps deleterious, in the second. No further attention will be paid to secondary forms of hypertension in this chapter.

Primary or Essential Hypertension.—The following classification can be made based on organic changes in the arterioles, progression, and severity of the disease. The separation into exact groups is often impossible. Subjects followed over a period of years may exhibit all the various stages, with transition from a mild into a severe form of hypertension:

1. Pre-organic or functional stage;
2. Organic stage with following degrees of severity;
    (a) Benign or slowly progressive forms;
    (b) Intermediate forms;
    (c) Malignant or acute fulminating forms.

1. **Pre-organic or Functional Stage.**—The development of essential hypertension based on the excessive vasopressor responses to environmental and other stimuli permit of the following concept: the earliest manifestation of hypertension, so far as known, is the exaggerated vasopressor response to various forms of stimulation. It is not known whether this is present in the age before puberty, but there is some evidence to indicate that such is the case. During the younger adult ages this potentiality for hypertension is present in the individual, but without symptoms. No doubt many subjects in the pre-hypertension group are those in which the blood pressures are occasionally found higher than in the accepted range for young subjects. This has been brought out in the mass statistics on the blood pressure of college students.

2. **Organic Stages.**—(a) *Benign or Slowly Progressive Forms.*—This stage is believed to follow the functional stage. There is gradual thickening of the tunica media of the small arterioles, with a slow,

progressive increase in the levels of the diastolic pressures and a compensatory rise in the systolic pressures. This takes place slowly over a period of years, and organic changes are usually manifest in the arterioles of the retina in the fifth and sixth decades of life. Symptoms are not manifest until the arteries of the heart, brain, and kidneys reveal deterioration producing insufficiency of these organs. It is believed that the hyperreactions of the arterioles create overwork, eventuate in hypertrophy of the muscle layer analogous to that occurring in the left ventricle of the heart. There are certain variations in the course and behavior of the hypertensive disease.

There is an intermittent form which may be acute, subacute, or chronic. The blood pressure is normal until the patient reaches adult life and then hypertension develops. This may endure months or longer, and then subside. At intervals of years, with no clinical evidence of any renal involvement, or any other known primary cause, the episode may be repeated. In some cases the patients have indicated that the rise of blood pressure followed a severe mental strain. In others subclinical degrees of renal disease may be responsible for the hypertension. In women, toxemia of pregnancy may be the exciting agent. An attorney, while participating in a tense murder trial, developed hypertension. There was retinitis of severe hypertension and symptoms of cerebral origin. The blood pressure was taken daily by the patient for a period of years with no repetition of the hypertension except a very questionable residue of increased blood pressure. This form should not be confused with acute or paroxysmal type, secondary to or associated with tumor of the suprarenal gland. A small number of these cases has been reported, and several patients were cured by operation (Mayo-Pincoffs, Fig. 20). In others, exploration did not reveal a lesion of the suprarenal glands to explain the condition, and in such cases the condition progressed to a state of persistent hypertension.

There is the form of so-called remittent hypertension which has been observed in subjects who have mild grades of hypertension with exacerbations to higher levels for variable periods. Some, no doubt, represent the effects of bouts of intercurrent infections or unknown causes. Usually recrudescence is followed by residues of hypertension at higher levels, and other evidence of vascular injury.

During the menopause a mild form of hypertension is not infrequent, the so-called menopausal form. The systolic pressure is affected to a greater degree than the diastolic. Reisman noted that the patients tended to have robust bodies, were likely to be multiparas and that they exhibited excellent tolerance to the hypertension. There is no reason to believe that this is a distinct form of essential hypertension, but it is probable that it represents a phase of an essential hypertension accentuated by the endocrine disturbance of the climacteric.

(b) *Intermediate Forms.*—There is a group of cases in which the tempo of the progression of the hypertension is more rapid than in the preceding form of slowly progressive hypertension. Many of these occur among younger subjects, in the third, fourth and fifth decades of life. The mean diastolic pressures are high, in excess of 120 mm.

of mercury, and the fluctuations in the systolic and diastolic pressures are excessive. Symptoms are disturbances in vision, mental irritability, severe headache, vertigo, and other evidences of increased intracranial pressure. There may be objective and subjective evidence of cardiac or cerebral insufficiency. The prognosis in these cases is more severe than in the benign or slowly progressive form. Differentiation of this type from the malignant type is based largely on the absence of edema of the optic disk, and the presence of lesser grades of hypertrophy in the muscle arterioles, and absence of renal insufficiency. Otherwise the resemblance to the malignant form is frequently close. This type of hypertension may follow toxemia of pregnancy. In others no etiologic factor is evident except the familial.

(c) *Malignant or Acute Fulminating Forms.*—This is seen in two types: There is a pure type with pathognomonic changes in the eye, and another type in which these changes may be absent, but with the same fulminating course. In both forms diastolic pressures may be as high as 170 mm. of mercury; systolic pressures are often inordinately increased. Retinitis, disturbances in vision, changes of personality, mental irritability, vertigo, headache and evidences of increased intracranial pressure eventually occur. In many of these cases the diagnosis of brain tumor has been suspected. Cardiac hypertrophy and clinical myocardial insufficiency were usually demonstrable when the symptoms named were present. The age incidence in 81 cases ranged from nine to sixty-four years, averaging forty-two years. These ages were lower than those of cases of the benign form of hypertension. The prognosis of this disease is grave, the majority of the patients die within two to three years of the recognizable onset. Death usually is caused by cardiac failure or cerebral hemorrhage; more rarely, there is renal insufficiency, or all three may participate in the final breakdown. In the early stages of malignant hypertension, renal insufficiency may not be demonstrated by clinical tests (Keith, Wagener, and Kernohan). There is no impairment of concentrating or diluting function. Volhard and Fahr postulated that this syndrome is an expression of a toxic, irritative or inflammatory lesion superimposed on more slowly developing arteriosclerosis.

Etiology.—The cause of essential or primary hypertension is unknown, but various possible factors must be considered.

Sex.—There is no significant difference between the incidence of primary hypertension among males and that among females. In a series of 2154 cases of primary hypertension among patients of all ages, 48 per cent were men and 52 per cent women. Among patients who were forty years of age or less there was a rather marked predominance of women, the proportion of whom was 62 per cent, and of men, 38 per cent. There is a higher percentage among women than men in the fifth decade; in the seventh decade this is reversed (Gager).

Heredity.—The more carefully this factor is investigated, the more manifest the conclusion that constitutional predisposition is of great, perhaps major, importance. Patients with essential hypertension may inherit certain mental and emotional characteristics, as well as hypersensitive vasomotor reactions. There may be an inherited defect of arterial tissue, with a hypersensitive or overreactive affector mechanism. Similar familial trends have been observed in subjects with predisposition to premature, more localized arteriosclerosis, coronary sclerosis, coronary thrombosis, and renal and cerebral arteriosclerosis. The incidence of hypertension in families seems to follow the Mendelian laws of heredity (Weiss). The factor of heredity could be assumed to be present in 41 per cent of our series, in 47 per cent of cases reported by Steiglitz and in 60 per cent of cases reported by O'Hare. Vascular disease and its sequelæ determine longevity. Persons whose ancestors were long-lived have a tendency to low blood pressure.

Race.—Climate, geographic distribution and race are reflected on the systemic arterial blood pressure. The oriental races have lower systolic and diastolic blood pressures than similar economic groups of the occidental races. Among aboriginal negroes the incidence of hypertension is low (Donnison), whereas among American negroes the incidence is the same as among white people. Japanese residing in the larger industrial cities show the same incidence as the white races in comparable environment.

Diet.—The influence of diet on blood pressure in different races cannot be estimated. It is probably a factor in those undernourished, poverty-stricken groups of people, such as are present in China and India. A diet deficient in calories and low in vitamins has a depressing effect on energy, metabolism and vasomotor tonus. There is no proof that any specific food produces hypertension in man.

Body Weight.—Systolic blood pressures of obese subjects according to insurance statistics are higher than those of persons of normal weight. In compiling statistics of normal persons, correction should probably be made for increase in weight over the normal standard. Physique is probably a factor. Studies on constitutional pathology have shown that the tendency for vascular disease is increased among persons of sthenic or hypersthenic physique.

Obesity, like essential hypertension, is often an inherited characteristic; both tendencies can operate in the same individual.

Sleep and Rest.—The blood pressure, both systolic and diastolic, falls during sleep. Among subjects who have not hypertension the average fall in systolic pressure is as much as 20 to 30 mm. of mercury, and that in diastolic pressure somewhat less. The fall usually starts after onset of sleep. The average rise usually starts at 4 or 5 A.M. Among persons who sleep in the daytime and work during the night the rhythm is reversed. Disturbing dreams reflect sharp fluctuations in both systolic and diastolic pressures, and may explain cerebral accidents occurring during sleep.

Physical Work.—Addis has shown that in the normal subject, with moderate exertion, the rise in blood pressure is slower than the primary acceleration of the pulse. Under physical training, such as is obtained in the army, this reaction gradually becomes less. The vasomotor system becomes conditioned by repetition of stimulation. The person whose vasomotor system is hypersensitive may respond to exercise more than the person whose vasomotor system is hyposensitive, although this depends largely on the subject's mental attitude regarding the exercise. Competitive sports, such as golf, cause sharp responses, whereas leisurely forms of exertion, such as walking, may reduce the blood pressure.

Infections.—Differences of opinion exist as to the importance of infection in the etiology of hypertension. Since statistics on the point have not been properly controlled, positive deductions cannot be made. There is no convincing evidence that chronic foci of infection play any etiologic part in the development of hypertension. Removal of foci of infection has no effect on essential hypertension. The hypertension associated with glomerulonephritis is related to streptococcal infections, and the predisposing factor cannot be evaluated. This should in no wise be confused with the primary or essential forms of hypertension. Fulminating or malignant hypertension, following a streptococcal infection, with the development of characteristic changes in the arterioles, and without evidence of true glomerular nephritis, has been reported (Bannick). No doubt some toxic infectious agents affect the course of essential hypertension. These episodes are more likely incidental and not of primary etiologic significance.

Of 1287 patients forty years of age and younger, with hypertension, 208 (16 per cent) had histories of having had scarlet fever. Of these, 28 (13.4 per cent) had frank nephritis, whereas 178 (85.5 per cent) had primary hypertension; in 6 of the latter cases the condition was of the malignant type. This incidence of scarlet fever is the same as that in a control group with disease of the gall-bladder. This infection is probably of no importance in the etiology of primary hypertension.

Pregnancy.—Women with mild or early hypertension are more susceptible to the development of toxemia in pregnancy, which effects sudden, severe strain on the cardio-renal-vascular system. When of a fulminating form, this condition of toxemia and hypertension either is itself eclampsia or is indistinguishable from eclampsia. The nature of the intoxication is unknown. Renal and hepatic injury occur in the severe forms. Following delivery, hypertension may or may not persist as a residue. Successive pregnancies may or may not exert this toxic effect on the same person. It is a question of whether toxemia of pregnancy afflicts normal subjects who have no predisposition to hypertension. Of a series of 696 women, forty years of age or younger, with hypertension, approximately 11 per cent had histories of toxemia in previous pregnancies. This is probably a low figure.

Hypersensitivity of Sympathetic System.—The abnormal or excessive reactions of the vasomotor mechanism in many cases of early hypertension suggest that there is hypersensitivity of the (*a*) vasomotor center, or (*b*) of the sympathetic myoneural or vascular tissue, or (*c*) abnormal activity induced by pressor hormones. These may act alone or together. Evidence of localized forms of sympathetic hypersensitivity is seen in the extremities in Raynaud's disease. The systemic blood pressure is not disturbed, for only a small section of the total vascular bed is concerned. To explain the wide participation of the vascular system in hypertension, the stimulus must be assumed to act through the vasomotor center in the medulla. Inhalation of carbon dioxide in 10 per cent concentration produces an increase in the blood pressure comparable to that obtained with immersion of the hands in ice-water (Raab). In cases of essential hypertension the increase in blood pressure is exaggerated. Carbon dioxide acts on the cerebral centers; its chief peripheral action is to produce vasodilation. This is evidence of the increased sensitivity of the central mechanism in cases of essential hypertension. The thresholds of stimulation for the various vegetative functions differ greatly in different persons. Some subjects have abnormally labile heat-regulating mechanisms, with abnormal ranges of body temperature, reacting to environmental and psychic stimuli. Similar abnormalities are observed in the range of the pulse-rate and in the behavior of the sweat glands. Following severe psychic shocks or sudden states of anxiety, irritative phenomena affecting vegetative functions are observed. There are exaggerated reactions of the pulse and blood pressure, abnormal sweating and somatic symptoms. This constitutional predisposition to abnormal reactibility should be described as a hyperreactibility or hyperlability of the blood pressure. This abnormality precedes the stage of what we designate as essential hypertension. It may be the causal factor in producing increased levels of blood pressure. Hypertension is erroneously conceived as being a static stage; this conception at most should apply only to the advanced organic stages of the disease. A new term is necessary to describe the fundamental abnormality in hypertension, which would express the idea of abnormal lability and excessive vasopressor response.

Present, although incomplete, knowledge of the causes of essential hypertension could be summarized as follows: (1) there is a biologic or constitutional factor which is expressed by hyperirritability of the sympathetic vasomotor system, or by defective or inferior vascular tissue reacting abnormally; (2) there may be abnormal environmental conditions, affecting or producing excessive responses of the predisposed subject—the result may be failure of conditioning of the vasomotor reflexes; and (3) toxic or infectious insults may play a part. The second and third agents constitute "wear and tear."

Vascular tissues are perhaps capable of so much usage and so much replacement. The biologic life of this tissue in hypertension, with the rapid, excessive, intermittent strains of tension, is shorter than that of the tissue of the person with normal or low systemic blood pressures, whose vasomotor reactions are restricted. The life of the subject is complete, perhaps at sixty years, because the essential vascular tissues have been exhausted. This may be molecular fatigue, without demonstrable changes, such as apparently obtains in cardiac exhaustion. Finally, factors determining the distribution of blood are involved, with organic death.

Pathology.—There is a gradually diminishing gradient in the pressure of the blood from the left ventricle to the larger arteries, averaging 10 to 20 mm. of mercury. The sharpest decline is from the artery to the capillary, a drop of 70 to 80 mm. (Ellis-Weiss). In hypertension the arteriolar pressure averages 121 mm. of mercury (average normal arteriolar pressure is 55 mm. of mercury) (Weiss). The resistance offered by the hypertonic arterioles is then the crucial disturbance in the mechanism of hypertension. Increase in viscosity, and in volume, of blood, are not found in subjects with primary hypertension. Normally, the arteries have a reservoir capacity, depending on the elastic quality of the walls. At a point above the usual systolic pressure, the arteries receive the output of the heart without marked increase in tension. In healthy persons excessive strain is compensated for by reflexes set up through the aorta and carotid sinus, and transmitted to the medulla, with consequent vasorelaxation of the arterioles. The pressure in health ranges between moderately restricted limits. With tension increased above that limit, the vessels become more rigid. Relaxation of its intravascular pressure is compensated for either by back pressure on the heart, or by relaxation of peripheral resistance. In persistent hypertension, this adequate compensation is lacking. The elasticity of the large arteries becomes impaired. Ventricular hypertrophy is the inevitable result of persistent or maintained arterial hypertension. Only in this way can the need of the organism for blood be maintained. Hypertrophy, in this respect, is a compensatory, useful measure, and is compatible with health. It is of significance when the normal reserve of the heart is diminished. Until dilatation supervenes, the heart is adequate. Until this time, hypertension cannot be considered as seriously interfering with the integrity of the mechanics of circulation.

Pathologic studies of the vessels in early cases of essential hypertension disclose no characteristic changes; observation of patients who die accidentally, or from intercurrent disease, and examination of material obtained for biopsy have adequately demonstrated this. The conclusion is that there is a functional stage of primary hypertension, that comes before organic changes have taken place. At this phase hypertonus of the arterioles seems to be the primary disturbance. The earliest changes in tissue demonstrated in hypertension are hypertrophy of the tunica media of the smaller arterioles and lessening of the caliber of the lumen as compared to the thickness of the walls (Keith, Kernohan and Barker). This hypertrophy of the tunica media is independent of atherosclerosis, a process which has not been observed in arteries of this magnitude, except in those in the kidney. In larger arteries atherosclerosis may exist with this hypertrophy of the tunica media. It is necessary to remember that the arteriosclerotic process exists without hypertension, but that the process is accentuated or accelerated by the increased pressure. Many patients with hypertension die before the arteriosclerotic process is intense. In approximately 61 per cent of cases of hypertension in subjects who are less than forty-one years of age, when the patients are first seen, there are demonstrable organic changes in the arteries of the retina. The tenseness and thickening of the radial arteries that can be detected by palpation, in cases of severe essential hypertension, represent the hypertrophy of the medial coat and increased tonus; these qualities do not represent the changes of arteriosclerosis, which condition is so easily demonstrable in subjects of advanced age.

In malignant hypertension, material obtained for biopsy or at necropsy indicates widespread hypertrophy of the tunica media of the arterioles (Keith). A comparison of the material obtained for biopsy and that obtained at necropsy indicates that this process is widespread over the body. It may or may not be predominant in the kidneys. If present, there is quantitative diminution of the lumens of the arteries of the kidneys; this leads to ischemia of the glomerular tufts, with atrophy and tubular destruction, and the end stage of nephrosclerosis. Evidence seems to indicate that there is acute toxemia, which seriously injures or exerts major effect on the arterioles of 100 microns and less in diameter.

Ocular Manifestations.—Ophthalmoscopic examination of the smaller vessels gives direct information that cannot be obtained in any other vascular field. The value of use of the ophthalmoscope as a routine in cases of suspected or actual cardio-renal vascular disease cannot be overemphasized.

According to Wagener, the earliest changes observed in the retinal vessels are those of increased arterial tonus, in which the lumen of the arterioles is narrowed but uniform. There is a changed or altered relationship between the caliber of the arteriole and vein as compared with the caliber of these structures in normal subjects. These findings may be considered as representative of the stage of hypertension before organic change has taken place.

The second stage represents the beginning of recognizable organic change in the arterioles. There is hypertrophy of the tunica media, which causes narrowing of the lumen, and gives it an irregular appearance. There is greater reflection of light from the wall of the arteriole, giving it a coppery or steely appearance. Since the veins and arterioles are in the same sheath, the increase in thickness of the arteriolar wall and the increased intra-arterial pressure produce indentation in the more easily compressible veins, the sign designated as arteriovenous compression.

The third stage probably represents the beginning of the first recognizable phase of true arteriolosclerosis. There is more marked contraction and irregularity of the lumens of the arterioles, and exaggeration of the light reflex, associated with increased visiblity of the vascular wall, and at times with thickening of the vascular sheaths. In a more advanced stage, in the smallest visible arterioles, there is an appearance of obliteration, often with fine, punctate, white areas of hyaline or fatty degeneration and punctate hemorrhages (retinitis of arteriosclerosis).

Retinitis of hypertensive type is characterized by cotton-wool patches or edema of the nerve fibers distal to the points of arteriolar narrowing, occlusion or spasm. Mild edema of the retina and flame-shaped hemorrhages are usually present. This phase of retinitis may be superimposed on any of the preceding stages of organic change, and is the effect of some toxic agent, through spasm of the arterioles.

In the so-called malignant or fulminating forms of hypertension there are two ophthalmoscopic characteristics: (1) such marked constriction of the arterioles that they have the appearance of fine threads, and (2) edema of the disks, which may be measured, attaining at times a height of 4 diopters or more. These lesions are usually combined with the other features of retinitis, and may be superimposed on any degree of mesial thickening or of sclerosis in the walls of the arterioles. In young persons, especially, such lesions may precede the development of organic changes.

Symptoms.—There is a long period in the course of the benign forms of essential hypertension which is symptomless. Many of the subjects are extremely efficient. They possess great energy, high ambition and an inner spiritual drive necessary to fulfil their aims. Sixty-one per cent of the patients less than forty years of age seen in The Mayo Clinic were in this stage before organic change had taken place; the hypertension was found incidentally, in the course of general examination, either at the clinic or elsewhere. With the advent of arteriolar changes, impairment in local and general circulation is initiated, and symptoms of disease supervene.

Symptoms may be divided into two groups: general and local. The *general symptoms* are those of mental and physical fatigue, depression or abnormal stimulation, reduced endurance, insomnia and general slowing up of bodily energy. These symptoms are somewhat similar to those seen in cases of chronic nervous exhaustion; they are characteristic of a general stage of fatigue. Local symptoms arise by virtue of disturbance of circulation of special organs. In the malignant forms general irritability may be so pronounced as to simulate the irritability of hyperthyroidism. In about one-third of the cases the basal metabolic rate is definitely elevated. The general symptoms require no further comment, but several of the *local symptoms* must be considered, as follows:

Cerebral Symptoms.—Impairment of memory, failure of mental concentration and increased irritability may be the earliest symptoms. Headaches of the occipital type, usually appearing in the morning, are indicative of organic changes in the cerebral arteries. If migraine existed previously, this is aggravated by hypertension. With neuroretinitis, headache may be extremely severe.

Cerebral Hemorrhages.—Hemorrhages and apoplectic strokes vary greatly in degree. Some patients have slight, transient episodes of tingling and numbness in the extremities, mental confusion and aphasia; others suffer hemiplegia and death. Many of the milder episodes clear without residue. What part vascular spasm or hemorrhage plays in these minor cerebral crises is unknown. Spasm is observed in the retinal arteries (Wagener), and there is much basis to believe that similar episodes occur in those of the brain. Recovery from hemiplegia which has its origin in hypertension may be complete. Changes in mentality usually remain after recovery from the severer forms of hemorrhage. Cerebral thrombosis is more likely to occur in cases of arteriosclerosis without hypertension.

Cardiac Complications.—About 60 per cent of the patients with essential hypertension die from cardiac failure. The forms in which the failure appears are: (1) cardiac hypertrophy with myocardial fatigue, or (2) associated coronary sclerosis and myocardial infarction. In the hearts of subjects who die of myocardial fatigue no microscopic explanation of failure of cardiac function is found. Muscle fibers are hypertrophied, but have normal appearance. Thirty-three per cent of one series of patients who died of proved coronary disease had hypertension (Willius). The usual form of cardiac death of patients with hypertension is the congestive type of heart failure.

Renal Complications.—There is progressive thickening and probably associated spasm of the arterioles, with diminution of the amount of arterial blood which flows to the glomeruli and tubules. Ischemia is the basis of functional impairment and uremia. The changes terminate in the picture recognized as that of renal arteriosclerosis (nephrosclerosis) with atrophy of a focal nature. The earliest objective evidence of this is impairment of the capacity of the kidneys to concentrate urine, with polyuria and nocturia. There is increase in the number of formed elements in the urine. As impairment in function progresses, there is decreased elimination of colloidal dyes that are injected in tests of renal function, there is increase in the concentration of nitrogenous elements in the blood and the condition of the patient progresses into uremia. Passive congestion may precipitate acute renal failure. Anemia is rather constantly found at this stage. About 10 per cent of patients with essential hypertension die from uremia. The clinical picture is not typical of glomerular nephritis, and symptoms are related more closely to generalized arterial disease. Symptoms may be latent until uremia supervenes. Often this is well borne for long periods.

Intercurrent Infections.—During the compensated stage of hypertension, the incidence of intercurrent infections is low; that relatively high immunity to such infections exists is the clinical impression. With development of organic changes in the arteries, intercurrent infection is a potent factor in initiating general or local decompensation. There is, at this time, diminished immunity to infections, especially to those of the upper part of the respiratory tract. Bronchopneumonia is the cause of death of many of the patients. Complications of simple colds, grippe, respiratory infections and so-called influenza account for a still greater number. One reason why the vital statistics are not accurate in regard to this disease is that the high mortality in older subjects is ascribed to infection, which could be explained by the presence of underlying organic vascular disease.

Prognosis.—Among subjects who have systolic blood pressures in excess of 170 mm. of mercury, the actual mortality to be expected, according to insurance statistics, is as 100 to 219.6; among those whose systolic blood pressures are more than 200 mm. of mercury the actual mortality to be expected is as 100 to 827.5 (May). Among patients who are in the stage before organic change has taken place, and whose diastolic pressures definitely tend to remain over 100, but whose retinal arteries do not give evidence of definite organic change, the average length of life is approximately fifteen years after onset of the disease. No fixed rules or figures are valid in this connection, for too many exceptions occur. Every physician can recall embarrassing results of too rigid prognostication. Intercurrent disease may produce premature death, or hypertension remains stationary or regresses.

With diastolic pressures of more than 120 mm. of mercury, expectancy of life is less, probably averaging, for the group, five to eight years. In cases in which there is retinitis, renal insufficiency, significant electrocardiographic changes, or clinical evidence of cardiac insufficiency, or in which diastolic pressures are high and tend to be fixed, the expectancy of life would be less than five years. Again, many exceptions occur. Malignant hypertension carries with it a fixed prognosis; 90 per cent of the patients with characteristic changes in the fundi seen at The Mayo Clinic die within eighteen months.

Operative Risks.—In the preorganic and compensated stages of hypertension the risk of operative procedures is not increased. Infections and operative trauma are borne extremely well. With high grades of arteriosclerosis, or with insufficiency of vital organs, there is a definitely increased mortality. Renal or cardiac insufficiency, with terminal bronchopneumonia, thrombosis and embolism, accounts for a fairly high percentage of operative deaths.

Treatment.—There is no efficacious treatment for primary hypertension. If treatment is instituted, it should have its greatest effect in the functional stage, before organic changes have taken place. The word treatment has a broad inference as applied to this disease. The part played by heredity is paramount but uncontrollable. Treatment, then, must be directed toward modification of such factors as vasomotor hypersensitivity and environment. After organic change has taken place, treatment is limited largely to measures which will relieve the heart and kidneys of stress, or to supportive measures for renal or cardiac insufficiency.

General.—If possible, before instituting therapeutic measures, a sufficient number of observations of blood pressure should be made, under varying conditions, to allow the patient's vasomotor reactions to be determined. These observations can be carried out in a hospital by means of hourly readings of blood pressure, under conditions of rest and of exercise. Basal blood pressures can be determined after a period of rest, and increases from this level determine the magnitude of vasomotor response.

If marked fluctuations occur, and organic changes are not advanced, an attempt is made to lessen the sympathetic responses. Sharp changes in habits and methods of work, elimination of competitive forms of recreation and cultivation of the habit of taking periods of relaxation are vitally important. Analysis of a patient's habits, of the types of vacation and of rest he takes, and the type of work he does, reveals the necessity of readjustment. Vacations of Americans are far from ideal; the activities usually are of a competitive nature and consist in striving to increase the number of miles traveled each day or each hour, or the number of holes of golf played each day.

"Hypertension is not only a disease of the individual—it is a disease of American life. It extends to all our communal doings; it is reflected in the tension under which every individual in America lives.

"What are the causes of the American disease? They are, I believe, connected with our striving for wealth. We have created false standards, have deprived ourselves of peace and leisure and have lost the art of living wisely. We have had abundant material success, but have we not paid too dearly for it?" (Reisman.)

Unsuitable working conditions, excessive noise, interruptions and high pressure are distinctly deleterious. One sees definite eviden ce of diminished vasomotor irritability following careful readjustments along these lines. The entire problem requires great tact on the part of the physician, and willingness to coöperate on the part of the patient. A regimen can be initiated by a period of complete rest of a few days to a few months, demonstrating to the patient his ability to relax. When activity is resumed, it is broken up by rest at midday, for one-half hour to an hour, frequently in the office or place of work. Regular sleep of not less than nine hours should be had and part of week-end vacations may be spent in bed, eliminating largely the social features. The importance of this regimen, modified by the occupation and social status of the patient, is crucial to success in treatment of the stage before organic change has appeared.

Drugs.—The effects of treatment of hypertension by drugs are not impressive. Patients vary greatly in reaction to drugs, and a few days of trial of the effect of a drug should be had before prolonged administration is advised. Nitrites are useful to demonstrate lability of arteries; the effect is transient, but these substances may be given intermittently, one or two days a week, during the periods in which the levels of hypertension are highest. Potassium sulphocyanate, in doses of 0.1 gram (1.5 grain), three or four times a day, may exert some steadying effect on the blood pressure of some subjects who display marked fluctuations in blood pressures. Sedative drugs, for patients with excessive emotional reactions and "keyed-up" personalities, are frequently of great value. Drugs of the barbital group, in doses sufficient to produce definite slowing of the psychic reactions, reflect their effect on blood pressure, and are of definite value. These can be given for one or more days each week. The difficulty of evaluating treatment by drugs is due to the fact that wide variations in blood pressure occur without treatment. Control data are most important, but are difficult to obtain. The writer has patients who have taken their own blood pressures over a period of years. They have shown variations, some apparently related to seasonal changes and others spontaneous in nature, and these variations have been greater than the effects supposed to be due to drugs.

Physical Therapy.—Warm baths have a relaxing effect in many cases of hypertension. The effects on blood pressure should be determined. When favorable reactions are obtained, baths should be given at a temperature ranging upward to 105° F., for short periods, the length of the periods to be determined by the tolerance of the patient. Baths should be followed by periods of rest. Massage and diathermy are of some value when relaxation is difficult of attainment.

Diet.—Many forms of diet have been recommended for hypertension. The great diversity of opinion convinces one of their inefficacy. In the stage before organic change has taken place, the compensated stage, a diet reduced in calories, but well balanced from other standpoints, is advisable. If patients are obese, reduction of weight is indicated, although decisive effects on the levels of blood pressure are usually lacking. In the later stages, when there is interference with excretion of sodium chloride or urea, reduction of intake of these to minimal requirements is indicated. The basis of treatment for cardiac insufficiency is rest. When congestive cardiac failure is present, prolonged periods of rest, diets low in calories and digitalis in physiologic doses should be prescribed. Intravenous injections of salyrgan, 1 or 2 cc., preferably following a course of acid-producing salts, calcium chloride, ammonium chloride or ammonium nitrate given by mouth, in doses of 6 to 10 grams a day, until diuresis is evident or until untoward effects are noted (Keith) is most efficacious in refractory cases, in which there is marked edema and ascites. Frequently, withdrawal of 500 to 1000 cc. of blood is of help in cases in which there is cyanosis and marked dyspnea. With improvement of cardiac function, sharp restrictions in activity should be insisted on. These patients have low thresholds of safety, as regards infections and physical and nervous strain. Change of residence to a mild climate during the winter months may be most beneficial; by this measure prolongation of life is likely, because patients suffer less exposure to intercurrent infections, a most important factor in causing cardiac or renal "breaks." Usually two or more periods of decompensation may be experienced before death comes.

Surgical Measures.—The success obtained by removal of the sympathetic ganglia in the primary vasoconstrictive disturbance, Raynaud's disease, has opened up the question of whether control of hypertension by a similar type of operation is feasible. Unilateral or bilateral removal of the major and minor splanchnic nerves by the intradiaphragmatic approach has been carried out (Pierie-Craig). Moderate reduction in the levels and responses of the blood pressure has been noted in a few instances. More recently, section of the sixth thoracic to the second lumbar anterior roots by means of laminectomy has been carried out in a small group of subjects with severe advanced forms of essential hypertension (Adson). By this procedure the vasomotor nerves are removed below the diaphragm, including those to the suprarenal glands and the legs. There is denervation of the motor nerves of the abdominal wall with lowered intraäbdominal tension. After the operation there is a significant drop in the mean levels and responses of the blood pressure which has endured for months. Cerebral symptoms have been relieved. There is a relative hypotension of these subjects when in the standing position. Bilateral partial resection and denervation of the suprarenal glands has been reported to cause depressor effects on the blood pressure of subjects with essential hypertension (Crile-DeCourcy).

If apoplexy occurs, spinal drainage and bleeding can be carried out; if the blood pressure remains high, an ice-cap can be applied to the head and restlessness controlled by sedatives. Careful details of nursing are important; this includes attention to function of the bladder and bowels, avoidance of pressure sores and changing of position to lessen the incidence to pulmonary stasis. Profound, deepening coma is a grave symptom. Improvement, if it occurs, is obvious in from three to four days. A period of months may be necessary to determine the residue of paralysis. Physiotherapeutic methods, including passive and active forms of exercises, should be carried out for restoration of muscular function. Residual paresthesia in the affected extremities is most trying; symptomatic treatment with non-habit-forming sedatives offers some relief.

Vasodilating Disturbances (Hypotension; Low Blood Pressure).

General Information.—Hypotension exists when the systemic blood pressure, as measured in the brachial arteries of adults, is less than 100 mm. of mercury.

There are two types: (1) Primary or essential hypotension exists in the absence of any abnormality; it is not a disease, as it is present in about one-third of normal subjects; it is a constitutional attribute or state. (2) Secondary types may be acute, subacute or chronic; those that are acute are observed in shock, following hemorrhage; those that are subacute or chronic are associated with chronic infections, various forms of debility, malnutrition and Addison's disease.

Primary Types.—Primary hypotension is extremely common in adult life. Approximately 20 per cent of all adult patients observed at the Mayo Clinic have systolic blood pressures of less than 110 mm. of mercury. Fifty per cent of all postmortem examinations made by Symmer revealed small hearts and other evidence of hypoplasia and hypotension. It is more common among women than among men, and is more common in oriental than in occidental races.

Constitutional Characteristics.—More than one-half of the subjects with primary hypotension conform to a constitutional pattern. Usually they are of the thin, asthenic type, with small hearts and visceroptosis. They can be grouped as constitutionally inadequate types. Their resistance to infection is usually low, but from the vascular standpoint they are long-lived. Many have cold, moist extremities. Their vasomotor adjustment to cold and heat may be less effective than normal. Frequently there is inadequate adjustment of systemic blood pressure to changes in posture. In a few cases this inefficient postural accommodation produces serious symptoms known as postural hypotension with syncope.

Symptoms.—Usually there are no symptoms that can be ascribed directly to the lowered blood pressure. A large percentage of the patients have symptoms of chronic fatigue, nervous exhaustion and psychoasthenic disturbances. They are the antithesis of patients of the so-called hypertensive pattern. They are labeled neurotics. If the systolic blood pressure is persistently lowered to 60 or 70 mm., symptoms from hypotension are likely to be present. These are usually cerebral, and consist of vertigo, fainting, loss of memory, headaches and other symptoms suggesting cerebral anemia. That the symptom of fatigue is not produced by the hypotension itself can be demonstrated by the failure to produce symptomatic improvement by elevation of blood pressure. Hourly readings of blood pressures give evidence of diminished vasomotor response. Fluctuations in blood pressure are slight, only one-half or one-third as great as those seen in cases of hypertension before organic changes appear. The wear and tear on the vascular tree is minimal. This probably represents the major factor that contributes to longevity.

Postural Hypotension With Syncope.—Postural or orthostatic hypotension was first described in 1925 by Bradbury and Eggleston. As long as no primary cause of the condition is known, it seems logical to consider it as a primary type of hypotension.

The *symptoms* are characterized by the following common phenomena: (1) syncopal attacks and systolic blood pressure reduced to levels characteristic of shock on change of posture to the upright position; (2) slow and unchanging pulse-rate, with marked variation in blood pressure; (3) variable anhidrosis; (4) increased distress during the heat of the summer months; and (5) some decrease in the basal metabolic rate.

Other pertinent signs or symptoms which may be present are greater secretion of urine during the night than in the daytime; loss of sexual desire and potency; youthful appearance in relation to the true age; pallor of the skin and mucosa and secondary anemia. The fundamental disturbance in this interesting group of cases indicates an affection of the autonomic nervous system, both sympathetic and parasympathetic divisions. There is a diminished vasomotor response of the splanchnic vessels to shift in the blood mass. The blood sags into the abdominal regions when the patient is upright. Disturbance of the mechanism of sweating is further indication of sympathetic involvement. Diminished or absent response of the vagus mechanism to changes in blood pressure and to administration of atropine is evidence of involvement of the parasympathetic system. There is probably a disturbance of the myoneural structures. One of the patients observed at the Mayo Clinic was an elderly subject with arteriosclerosis. Other subjects were in the age before arteriosclerosis is generally seen. As has been indicated, no primary disease could be found to explain this circulatory disturbance.

Secondary Types.—Secondary forms of hypotension are the usual sequelæ of any debilitating or chronic disease, such as arthritis, tuberculosis, chronic anemia and many of the infectious diseases, such as typhoid fever, influenza and syphilis. In Addison's disease the lowered blood pressure is one of the most important diagnostic criteria. Persistent systolic pressures below 80 mm. should make one suspicious of the existence of this disease. Elevation of the blood pressure in Addison's disease does not alleviate the general symptoms of weakness and fatigue. Blood pressures taken hourly in cases of Addison's disease display slight, if any, variation.

Prognosis.—In primary forms of hypotension longevity is the rule, although resistance to intercurrent infections may be reduced. There is no information to justify the belief that chronic, low blood pressure in itself carries with it any untoward prognostic significance, either in primary or secondary types, with the exception of that found in Addison's disease. Increase in the blood pressure following debilitating illnesses is usually a sign of improvement and recovery.

Treatment.—There is no indication for treatment in the usual case of constitutional or primary hypotension. Elevation of the blood pressure by epinephrine or ephedrine does not produce alleviation of symptoms. In the presence of malnutrition and conditions of under-nourishment, increase in the amount of nourishment and periods of rest or graduated exercises may be indicated. There is some promise that the newer extracts of the cortex of the suprarenal glands may be of value in some of the exhaustive states associated with hypotension. Two cases of postural hypotension with syncope have been treated with ephedrine, 50 mg., every three or four hours, given by mouth, with satisfactory results. The use of a tight abdominal binder seems to give some temporary relief.

Treatment of secondary types is obviously directed against the underlying condition.

ORGANIC DISTURBANCES.

Localized[1] Forms.

Thrombo-arteriosclerosis Obliterans of the Peripheral Arteries (Arteriosclerosis With Thrombosis, Diabetic Gangrene, Senile Gangrene).—Arteriosclerosis is a generalized disease, but the condition may be more intense in some particular region and may dominate the clinical picture. The frequency of sclerosis of the arteries of the lower extremities is high in the later decades of life. Markings of calcification can be seen in the roentgenogram of many subjects who are more than sixty years of age. The condition can be designated as a disease when occlusion is produced by thrombosis. Diabetic gangrene is simply arteriosclerosis with thrombotic occlusion in which the sclerosis and the trophic lesions are intensified by the diabetes. (See Generalized Arteriosclerosis.)

Classification.—There are two types of sclerosis of the peripheral arteries: (1) Cases without thrombosis; pulsations are present but usually reduced in magnitude; the diagnosis is made by palpation of the characteristically nodular, arteriosclerotic vessels; frequently the condition is detected in the roentgenogram; the condition is usually symptomless, or the patients may complain of mild coldness of the extremities or of paresthetic symptoms. (2) Cases in which the arteriosclerosis is associated with thrombosis; arteriosclerosis obliterans, the disturbance of physiologic processes in this group, is similar to that in other types of arterial occlusion, modified by advanced age, with slower and less adequate development of the collateral circulation. Senile changes in the skin and diabetes predispose to infection.

Frequency.—Senile gangrene has been known from the time of Hippocrates. It is a relatively common condition. Forty-six per cent of the occlusive diseases of the peripheral arteries seen at the Mayo Clinic were of the arteriosclerotic forms; in 20 per cent diabetes was present.

---

[1] Pathologists do not admit that arteriosclerosis is ever exclusively a local process. From the clinical viewpoint, however, the process can be considered as localized in some cases.

31

Pathology.—The pathology of the arteriosclerotic process varies in some degree from that observed in the elastic aorta. (See Pathology under Generalized Arteriosclerosis.) The tendency to thrombosis in these cases is accentuated by the deposits of calcium which may project into the lumina, serving as a locus for the deposition of platelets and formation of the thrombus. There is marked predilection for thrombosis to occur in the arteries of the legs; three cases have been found in which the arteries of the upper extremities were involved. There is absence of the perivascular inflammation and fibrosis that is observed in thrombo-angiitis obliterans. Mixture of arteriosclerosis and thrombo-angiitis obliterans can be found in older subjects. Closure of the larger arteries probably never occurs from proliferation of the intima in itself; thrombosis is necessary for occlusion. In the smaller arteries, such as those seen in the skin, proliferation of the intima may progress to total closure; this is the true condition called endarteritis obliterans, which is a pathologic and not a clinical term. Sclerosis of the veins is observed in the arteriosclerotic process.

Ischemic changes are frequently demonstrable in the nerves of amputated limbs. These are due to occlusion of small vessels in the nerves; this process is more pronounced toward the periphery (Priestley and Kernohan). Diabetic neuritis has a similar ischemic origin on an arteriosclerotic basis (Woltman and Wilder).

Symptoms.—The symptoms of arteriosclerotic occlusion of the arteries of the extremities are those due to diminished supply of arterial blood to the distal tissues. There is lowered temperature of the affected foot. Claudication, or cramps of the muscles of the legs, with exercise, usually cause the patient to seek medical advice. Claudication most frequently occurs in the muscles of the calf, less frequently in the foot and rarely in the muscles of the thigh in the presence of closure of iliac arteries. Progression of the thrombus is accurately indicated by the patient's lessened tolerance to exercise. Trophic changes are recognized by diminished growth of nails, and tendency to infections of the skin bordering the nails. There is rubor when the part is in the dependent position and pallor with elevation. Ulcers, usually of the dry form, mark the onset of gangrene. When frank gangrene supervenes pain becomes continuous, although it is usually less severe than that observed in cases of thrombo-angiitis obliterans. Secondary types of infection are prone to develop, especially in cases of diabetic gangrene. Superficial phlebitis has not been observed at the Mayo Clinic and closure of the arteries of the arm is extremely rare in my experience. These constitute important points in the differential diagnosis of thrombo-angiitis obliterans. Arteriography of the peripheral arteries *in vivo* has shown a distinctive picture in arteriosclerosis obliterans. This method can be used in the differential diagnosis from other obliterative diseases of the peripheral blood-vessels (Santos, Allen).

Treatment.—If diagnosis of arterial occlusion is made before the development of trophic lesions, much can be done to prevent gangrene. Adequate care of the extremity, by avoidance of trauma, especially avoidance of instrumental injury, together with the care of the nails, instructions in care of the feet, frequent changing of shoes and protection from cold are important and should be reëmphasized. The most effective treatment for the pain of claudication has been obtained by the use of the newer tissue extracts. The "hormone" of Frey-Kraut (Padutin) obtained from the urine; the more effective pancreatic extracts of Gley (Kisthinios), and the extracts of the skeletal muscle (Schwartzman) when injected intramuscularly give significant increase in tolerance to exercise in more than 70 per cent of the patients with occlusive lesions of the arteries of the extremities. The basis of the therapeutic effect seems to depend on the supplying of some amine to muscle which is contracting in the presence of deficient supply of arterial blood. Vasodilatation is not uniformly produced by these extracts. Claudication is probably protective in nature, prevents overuse of the extremities and should be understood by the patient. Mild grades of radiant heat (110° to 120° F.) can be applied cautiously with ventilated bakers for increasing periods of time. Postural exercises and contrast baths can be carried out daily. Trophic lesions require careful handling. For moist lesions, with secondary infections, applications of saturated solution of boric acid or solution of normal sodium chloride or packs saturated in 50 per cent alcohol, or, if very painful, the frequent or alternate application of non-irritating anesthetic solutions are useful in controlling pain and promoting drainage. Immersion of the foot in physiologic solutions of sodium chloride may relieve the pain and secondary infection. In the dry forms of atrophic ulcer or gangrene the major consideration is control of pain. Intravenous injections of hypertonic salt solution (5 per cent) can be tried. Ethyl alcohol, given by mouth, 30 cc., every four or five hours, may be effective in producing vasodilatation and relieving pain. Theobromine given by mouth, in doses of from 10 to 30 grains (0.65 to 2 grams), three times a day, produces moderate degrees of vasodilatation. Anesthetic solutions of a non-irritating type applied directly to the ulcer may be effective in relieving pain. Section of sensory branches of the peripheral nerves supplying the affected digits has been used for control of pain (White). Methods to produce intermittent negative and positive pressures to the diseased extremities seem effective in increasing blood supply and in healing ulcers in arteriosclerosis obliterans (Herrman, and Landis and Gibbons).

Surgical attack on the sympathetic nervous system is not advisable. Excessive vasoconstriction, that might be relieved by sympathectomy, cannot be demonstrated in the majority of patients, and the operative risk is too high. If pain and progression of gangrene persist, amputation should be the operation of choice. This should be carried out above the knee.

Thrombo-angiitis Obliterans (Buerger's Disease; Presenile Gangrene).—Thrombo-angiitis obliterans is a clinical entity. Cases, probably representative of this condition, were described by Friedländer, in 1876, for which he introduced the term "arteritis obliterans." Von Winiwarter, in 1879, introduced the term "endarteritis obliterans,"

and described the pathologic changes in several cases which were
undoubtedly examples of what is now recognized as thrombo-angiitis
obliterans. Wedensky, in 1898, reported that arteritis obliterans was
prevalent in districts of Russia where the weather is severe. He
believed it occurred almost exclusively in males between the ages of
fifteen and sixty years. Buerger, in 1908, made the first complete
clinical and pathologic report of this disease. He introduced the
term thrombo-angiitis obliterans. This name has fulfilled the requirements and should be adopted. Since this time, the reporting of a
large number of additional cases has emphasized the importance and
relative frequency of this disease in the various races; it occurs in
practically all of them.

Frequency.—Statistics on the frequency of this disease are not
available. About 700 cases have been seen at the Mayo Clinic in the
last ten years, an incidence of 1 in 600 new registrants. This probably
does not represent the true incidence, for many mild cases are overlooked; that is, cases without symptoms and with closure of one or
two arteries. These 700 cases do not include those with superficial
phlebitis of a chronic relapsing type, many of which are examples of
thrombo-angiitis obliterans.

Etiology.—The etiology is unknown. It is believed to be due to
some infectious or toxic agent that acts mainly on the arteries and
veins of larger size in the extremities. The pathologic changes which
we tentatively accept as characteristic have been reproduced in man
by transplantation of infected veins to normal veins by Buerger, and
by Horton, who reproduced the pathologic picture in animals by a
similar procedure. There is much evidence to indicate that this
disease has a basis in infection, although the predilection for males
(98 per cent) arises to confuse this viewpoint. Tobacco has been
suggested as the etiologic factor (Meyers, Silbert). Barker showed
a higher incidence of thrombo-angiitis obliterans among excessive
users of tobacco than among control subjects of similar age and sex.
Recent work on the effects of tobacco has demonstrated that the
smoking of cigarettes has vasoconstricting effect on the peripheral
arterioles, as measured by the change in surface temperature of the
digits (Maddock-Coller). Testing the sensitivity of the skin of patients
with thrombo-angiitis obliterans to tobacco extract, in the hands
of some workers, has shown a higher sensitivity as compared with
normal subjects. Nicotine seems excluded as a factor (Harkavy,
Hebald, Selran and Silbert). However, the disease afflicts subjects
who have never used tobacco. Poisoning by ergot has also been
suggested as an etiologic factor.

Race.—This disease has been seen to afflict persons of practically
all races, except those of unmixed negro ancestry. There is a higher
frequency among Russian Jews, but this frequency varies greatly
according to the clientele.

Pathology.—The earliest pathologic lesion in the affected artery or
vein is active proliferation of the intima, with inflammatory reaction
in the media and adventitia. There is subsequent deposition of a
red thrombus, containing lymphocytes and leukocytes. This is fol-

lowed by organization of the thrombus by fibroblasts, and by gradual disappearance of hemoglobin pigment. Giant cells are seen. Grossly, the artery, vein and nerve are enmeshed in an inflammatory fibrous mass. The disease has a segmental distribution, involving small portions of the vessels, with closure, organization and canalization, and development of collateral circulation. After a variable period of time, a similar course of events takes place in other segments. The nerves frequently show trophic changes, producing ischemic neuritis.

Symptoms.—The symptoms of this disease are: (1) local pain, swelling and inflammatory reactions, due to local inflammation of the arteries or veins, and (2) symptoms which are due to occlusion of the larger arteries, with impairment of blood supply in the distal parts.

The earliest sign or symptom of the disease is frequently reduced temperature of either hand or foot. This is followed by decreased tolerance to exercise (claudication). This symptom may be present in the foot, arch, calf, thigh, digits or any part that is subjected to physical exercise, in which the blood supply is diminished. The foot develops reactionary rubor when hanging down and pallor when elevated (Buerger). Progression or regression in claudication represents accurately the progress of the disease. With the development of trophic lesions, usually on the nail margins, pain becomes constant. Small ulcers develop, either dry or moist. Gangrene may become progressive and pain becomes excruciating. This is modified by the sensitivity of the patient. If the condition is uncontrolled the patients become most pitiful objects. Loss of sleep, excessive use of tobacco and loss of appetite create a condition of complete mental and physical disability. Fortunately this picture is becoming increasingly rare.

Superficial phlebitis occurs in 40 per cent of cases and is an important visual evidence of the activity of the disease. It may precede the advent of any involvement of the arteries, or may remain confined to the veins. There are two forms: the linear, advancing form, in which the small veins of the skin become inflamed, visible as red, painful streaks, and the nodular forms, localized at the valves. The attacks of phlebitis usually last two to three weeks and then subside; after variable periods of time, similar episodes supervene.

In one or more of the palpable arteries of the lower extremities, including at times the femoral arteries, pulsations are absent. In 40 per cent of our cases one or more vessels of the hands were occluded, frequently without symptoms. In only 10 per cent were definite trophic changes present in the hands. Pathologic lesions, suggesting those of thrombo-angiitis obliterans in rare instances, have been found in arteries in other regions of the body, namely, the abdomen, the kidney, the brain and the coronary vessels. Coronary thrombosis, with sudden death, occurs in about 3 per cent of the cases of thrombo-angiitis obliterans.

Treatment.—Prognostic concepts have undergone radical changes in the last decade. This has been due largely to earlier diagnosis, and more effective forms of treatment. When diagnosis is made in the stage before trophic changes have taken place, and protective and educational measures instituted, and the patient is made cognizant of the dangers of maltreatment of the parts, the incidence of amputation is sharply reduced. Postural exercises and contrast baths are effective in some cases. Intravenous injection of solutions of sodium citrate, hypertonic salt solution and foreign protein, inducing non-specific responses in temperature of the blood, increases the surface temperature by inhibiting the vasomotor effects. The newer tissue extracts are effective in treatment of the pains of claudication. The treatment of trophic lesions is in general the same as that carried out in arteriosclerotic disease.

Surgical measures, such as sympathetic ganglionectomy, seem to have materially reduced the incidence of amputation. The basis of this procedure rests on demonstration of excessive amounts of vaso-constriction in the collateral circulation, by measures which produce relaxation of the vasoconstrictive element. Among patients who have high degrees of vasoconstriction, removal of the second, third and fourth sympathetic lumbar ganglia results in significant, maintained increases in the surface temperature of the feet. Increases of 200 to 400 per cent in circulation, by indirect measurement, can be demonstrated. Sympathetic ganglionectomy does not cure the disease, but allows maximal circulation by elimination of the vasoconstrictive factor, giving the extremity increased protection in the advent of subsequent trauma or further progression or relapse. Statistics of the Mayo Clinic disclose an incidence of less than 5 per cent of amputations in properly selected patients who have had this operation, and who have been traced for periods as long as six years.

If pain or gangrene cannot be controlled, amputation becomes necessary. The site of amputation is important, and preservation of the knee-joint is desirable. In approximately 75 per cent of cases coming to amputation, healing below the knee is successful. In the presence of occlusion of the femoral artery, amputation above the knee is probably best. Older subjects are less likely to have successful healing below the knee.

Simple Thrombosis—Thrombophilia.—Simple thrombosis represents a form of thrombosis without arteriosclerotic or demonstrable inflammatory changes in the arterial wall. The condition is usually due to changes in the factors which cause coagulation of the blood, or to injury to the walls of the vessels. Trauma, electric shock and burns cause the non-reactive or non-inflammatory type of arterial thrombosis. Symptoms of this group are similar to other forms of arterial obstruction. The thrombi frequently are of ascending type gradually closing off collateral circulation. Symptoms such as pain depend largely on the rate of formation and extent of the thrombus. Trophic changes in the distal parts, such as the hands, fingers or toes, are present if the thrombus occludes large segments of the artery. Treatment is similar to that of other forms of arterial insufficiency of the extremity.

Occlusion of Embolic Type.—Arterial occlusion of embolic type occurs in the following conditions: (1) endocarditis, with metastasis of vegetations; (2) separation and embolism of mural thrombi of coronary origin; and (3) thrombosis in fibrillating auricles or failing myocardium. The emboli are usually small and multiple. In cerebral localization there are signs of hemiplegia, aphasia or sensory disturbances. In the periphery with sudden closure of one of the main arteries there is sudden blanching of the distal parts and excessive pain. Recovery of the part depends on the development of collateral circulation. Renal, splenic or pulmonary infarction may give rise to local pain, hematuria or evidence of bronchopneumonia and pleuritis. Of the occlusive arterial diseases 3 per cent are of embolic form.

The *prognosis* in these cases is not good, since recurrence is the rule. *Treatment* of the peripheral forms is carried out by local measures: (1) preserving and accelerating the collateral circulation; (2) maintaining heat in the distal parts by insulating with cotton; (3) lowering of the parts; and (4) administration of opiates to control the pain. Embolectomy can be carried out if the diagnosis can be made early and if localization can be accurate. Unfortunately, recurrences in other arteries may take place.

Aneurysm.—The condition is due to localized dilatation of the coats of an artery. These dilatations may be small, discrete or diffuse. The true aneurysm involves one or more coats of the arteries; the false aneurysm is a perivascular extravasation of blood.

History.—Osler has reviewed the historic features of aneurysm. He mentioned Galen's familiarity with the traumatic forms. Vesalius was probably the first to recognize or diagnose thoracic aneurysm. The relation between syphilis and aneurysm was demonstrated by Lancisi and Paré. Morgagni, in 1761, described the symptoms and morbid anatomy. Knowledge of the primary changes in the media date from the studies of Helmstedter and Köster. Discovery of the Spirochæta pallida by Schaudinn, and demonstration by Warthin and others of spirochetes in the wall of the aorta completed the proof of etiology of syphilis in many of the aortic forms of aneurysm.

Frequency.—According to Osler, the proportion of aneurysms in the United States is higher than in Great Britain, Scandinavia, Germany or Austria. Lucke and Rea found an incidence of 1 in 117 at necropsy. In Vienna, an incidence of approximately 1.2 per cent was found at postmortem examination. In postmortem records of Guy's Hospital, the incidence was 1.7 per cent. For the Johns Hopkins Hospital, the ratio was 1 to 1.6 per cent. In the Mayo Clinic a total of 453 cases was seen over a period of ten years, approximately 1 to 1000 among new registrants. Of this number, 138 came to necropsy. This represents an incidence of 1.6 per cent in all postmortem examinations performed in this period. There were no negroes in this series.

Classification.—Aneurysms may be classified on an etiologic basis: (1) those caused by syphilis; (2) those incident to arteriosclerosis; (3) those that are congenital; and (4) those that are mycotic. In addition to these known types, there still remains a group in which etiology is not clear. According to distribution, aneurysms may be divided into: (1) those that are intracerebral; (2) those that are intrathoracic; (3) those that involve the abdominal aorta and its branches; and (4) those that involve peripheral arteries. Other so-called forms of aneurysm are: (1) arteriovenous fistulas, so-called aneurysms because of dilatation of the regional veins and arteries, and (2) false aneurysms, representing merely hematomas.

Etiology. — In the Mayo Clinic one-third of the patients were between fifty and fifty-nine years of age, whereas approximately 80 per cent were between the ages of forty and seventy years. Six patients were less than twenty years of age and 5 were more than eighty years of age.

Seventy-five per cent of the patients seen at the Mayo Clinic were men. In usual statistics the ratio is 5 men to 1 woman.

Congenital aneurysms are not infrequent. The studies of Forbus have demonstrated the pathologic basis. They are usually multiple; the miliary type is most frequently found in the cerebral arteries, less frequently in the abdomen. Seven proved examples of the congenital type were seen at the Mayo Clinic. The intracranial carotid system is the most frequent site of intracerebral, congenital forms.

Syphilis is the infection of greatest significance. There is involvement of the media, with rupture, usually localized, at a point of maximal intravascular strain. In 50 per cent of the cases seen at the Mayo Clinic, in which necropsy was performed, syphilis was proved pathologically. The point of predilection was the ascending aorta. Among the aneurysms involving the thoracic aorta syphilis was present in 77.8 per cent of cases. In bacterial endocarditis mycotic forms of aneurysm may occur.

Arteriosclerotic disease, with diffuse distention of the arteries, leads to destruction of the media, with bulging and frequent production of true aneurysms. This etiologic basis was present in 6.2 per cent of the cases in which the intrathoracic aorta was involved at the Mayo Clinic, or in 40 per cent of all cases which came to necropsy.

The factor of strain, both intrinsic and extrinsic, is undoubtedly important in initiating splitting of the intima and production of the aneurysmal sac. In cases seen at the Mayo Clinic a history of muscular effort was present in a small percentage of cases.

Obstructive lesions of the artery, such as thrombo-angiitis obliterans, rarely produce aneurysms in the peripheral arteries proximal to the obstruction. Infection of the walls of the arteries is probably the major factor. Two cases of this type were seen at the Mayo Clinic. Direct injury to the artery, as by a bullet wound, may cause a rupture, or a lacerating wound with partial penetration of the wall. An embolic form is seen in endocarditis, in which small, infected emboli produce inflammatory change in the walls of the arteries, with weakening of the media. These lesions are usually miliary and multiple. They have been observed in endocarditis caused by Streptococcus viridans. In our group of 7 cases subacute bacterial endocarditis was present in each case.

Pathology. — The aneurysm varies according to the etiologic agent. In syphilitic mesaortitis the earliest lesion is in the media. There is necrosis, with destruction of the elastic fibers, and round-cell infiltration about the vasa vasorum of both media and adventitia. Scarring of the intimal and medial structures is the terminal process. There is dilatation if the process is extensive, or true aneurysm if it is more limited. Clotting and spontaneous cure may take place in the sacculated forms, but not in the fusiform types. The changes in the arteriosclerotic group are those common to atherosclerosis. The primary factor is disease of the media, the supporting structure of the vessel. Repair and the replacement of muscle by fibrous tissue create a place of lessened resistance for the production of aneurysm.

Vessels Affected. — At the Mayo Clinic 72 instances of cerebral aneurysm were seen, in 45 of which the localization was proved by operation or necropsy; 6 involved a carotid artery, 20 a basilar or anterior communicating artery and 4 a vertebral artery. There were 257 cases in which the thoracic aorta was involved: the ascending and transverse portions of the arch were involved in 200 cases; the descending portion in 32. There was diffuse dilatation in 25 cases. There were 63 abdominal aneurysms: the aorta was involved in 31 cases, or approximately 50 per cent; the aortic branches, renal artery, celiac axis or cystic artery each in approximately 10 per cent of cases. Aneurysms of the iliac artery (common, internal and external) were found in 12 cases. There were 37 cases of aneurysm of the peripheral arteries, in 5 a femoral artery was involved, in 6 a popliteal artery, in 3 a brachial artery, in 3 a radial or ulnar artery and in 13 a subclavian artery. There were 7 cases of aneurysm of smaller arteries of the face or eyelid.

Signs and Symptoms.—The symptoms relating to aneurysm are predominantly from pressure on contiguous structures. With thoracic forms there may be compression of the vena cava, and consequent engorgement of the vessels of the head and arm, or of the subclavian vein with edema. There may be dislocation of the heart. The recurrent laryngeal nerve is frequently compressed, with paralysis of the vocal cord. This is more common in cases of aneurysm of the transverse and descending portions of the arch. The sternum may be eroded. Pressure on the trachea causes impairment of respiratory function, with paroxysmal coughing; or if the trachea is pressed on, dysphagia is present. The sac may grow into the lung and cause hemoptysis. Sudden rupture of a dissecting aneurysm is a frequent cause of death. Bronchiectasis or pulmonary abscess may result from pressure on a bronchus. Impingement on the carotid or subclavian arteries may reduce or obliterate the radial pulse. The most severe symptoms are observed in aneurysms of the descending portion of the arch, in which erosion of the vertebra, or compression of the spinal cord, produces intractable pain. Aneurysm of the abdominal aorta may be symptomless except for a pulsating mass; many were found on exploration. Smaller aneurysms in the aortic branches cause characteristic symptoms. In the presence of aneurysms of peripheral arteries, the common complaint is of a pulsating mass, with pressure on a nerve. Thrombosis may occur in the aneurysm, with occlusion of the vessel and symptoms of arterial insufficiency of the distal part as a sequela.

The symptoms of the cerebral group of aneurysms are most difficult of diagnosis. Among younger persons the onset of severe, intractable forms of intracranial pain or headache, the presence of blood in the spinal fluid and signs of increased vascular pressure suggest the diagnosis. The clinical signs, if present, will vary according to the underlying disease, the site of the aneurysm in the cranial cavity, the condition of the aneurysmal wall and whether rupture or leakage has taken place (Parker). In the presence of embolic aneurysms the general or local infections will dominate the picture, the most frequent of which is endocarditis. The patient may die with the aneurysm unruptured, and its presence unsuspected. If the aneurysm ruptures or produces leakage, a previously symptomless patient will have symptoms. There may be focal compression and neoplasm may be suspected. Usually aneurysms in the region of the circle of Willis leak or rupture before they reach a significant size. Basilar and vertebral aneurysms may become sufficiently large to produce signs of compression before rupture or leakage. The signs of rupture may be those suggesting epilepsy, without localizing signs. Spinal fluid is bloody, with intermittent leakage. There may be recurrent cerebral seizures, which eventually culminate in death. Signs of compression depend on the site of the aneurysm. Aneurysm of the middle cerebral arteries may cause pain in the region of distribution of the ophthalmic division of the trigeminus nerve, and paralysis in that of the third, fourth and sixth cranial nerves; exophthalmos; edema of the eyelid and severe supraorbital headaches. If there is intermittent leakage the focal signs may be suddenly intensified. The signs in cases in which the basilar or vertebral arteries are involved are usually those of sudden onset of hemiplegia, that disappears and reappears later on the opposite side, or alternates with paraplegia without loss of consciousness. When rupture occurs there are the same signs as in intracranial aneurysm generally, or the headache is more sharply localized in the occiput.

Diagnosis.—In regions susceptible to inspection or palpation, the diagnosis of aneurysm is usually made by detecting the presence of a pulsating tumor along the course of an artery. If, on the peripheral arteries, a mass is present without pulsation, and if pulsations in the distal branches of the involved artery are absent, the likelihood is that there is a thrombosed aneurysm. The diagnosis of the intrathoracic forms may be suspected when there is circulatory congestion of the neck and face or of one of the extremities, inequality of the pupils, or abnormal pulsations in the anterior thoracic wall. There may be a violent, diffuse, localized impulse, or a heaving, true aneurysmal pulsation. The impulse may be observed by inspection, or better by palpation. Tracheal tuggings, due to pressure on the trachea by the aneurysm, may be present. There may be areas of abnormal dullness to percussion, or widening of the ascending arch. There are no typical auscultatory findings, unless the aortic valves are involved. Roentgenographic study of the thorax has simplified the diagnosis of intrathoracic forms of aneurysm. Clinical diagnosis can be made now with an extraordinary degree of accuracy by this method. In all cases in which there is severe intrathoracic pain, or evidence of general or local intrathoracic pressure, or of syphilitic aortitis, fluoroscopic examination of the thorax should be made. If expansile shadows are seen, examination should be carried out in different positions. Difficulty arises in identifying non-expansile shadows of thrombosed aneurysms. Diagnosis has been made accidentally by broncho-scopy or esophagoscopy.

Prognosis.—In cases of intrathoracic aneurysm prognosis is grave, but it is less so if the aneurysm is of the small, sacculated type, which becomes organized. Fairly long life is compatible with intracerebral aneurysms of smaller size; leakage or rupture eventually occurs with death. In cases of peripheral aneurysm collateral circulation usually is adequate if the closure of the aneurysm proceeds at a slow rate.

Treatment.—There is no known medical treatment for aneurysm, except restriction of activity and prescription of diet low in calories, in an attempt to reduce arterial pressure. For intrathoracic, syphilitic aneurysms in which the aortic valves are involved, the usual measures for treatment of syphilis and cardiac disease are instituted. Control of severe pain may present a serious problem.

Attempts to produce thrombosis in the aneurysmal sac by intro-duction of foreign bodies such as wire and by electrolysis have been advocated. The risk is high, and results are not very encourag-ing. The more favorable results have been received with sacculated aneurysms. Excision of thrombosed aneurysms of peripheral arter-ies can be accomplished, and relief of symptoms of pain or pressure obtained.

Periarteritis Nodosa.—The first case of this condition was reported by Kussmaul and Maier in 1866; since then about 150 additional cases have been reported. Periarteritis nodosa is an inflammatory disease of the smaller arteries, and may be caused by a filtrable virus (Arkin). There is no basis for the belief that syphilis is the etiologic agent. Three stages are recognized pathologically: (1) a condition of peri-arteritis, involving perivascular lymphatic structures and vasa vaso-rum; (2) a subacute stage, or beginning of a stage of repair, with intimal proliferation and mesial necrosis; and (3) the chronic stage, with disappearance of the inflammatory elements, and closure of the lumens by proliferation or thrombosis (Watson). Aneurysm may form at any of these stages. The smaller arteries of the kidneys, the heart, the liver, the gastro-intestinal tract, the pancreas, the muscles and the peripheral nerves are affected. The nodules on the adventitia are composed of exudates of polymorphonuclear neutrophils and eosinophils. Subcutaneous nodules may be palpable.

Symptoms are usually those of sepsis, myositis, neuritis, general weakness, anemia and, when the abdominal vessels are involved, cramp-like pains in the abdomen. If renal lesions are present, hemor-rhagic nephritis is a part of the picture. The diagnosis is rarely made in life.

There are several forms of *arteritis* not well established, either clinically or pathologically. Arteritis has been described in cases of endocarditis in which there is an active proliferation and necrosis, with occlusion by disintegrating cells. Acute arteritis has been described in rheumatic fever, as well as in many infectious diseases, including the mycotic group. A relapsing form of arteritis of the temporal arteries associated with fever, weakness, anemia, and leukocytosis has been described.

Coarctation of the Aorta (Congenital Stenosis of the Isthmus).—
Coarctation of the aorta is a condition in which there is constriction
of the anatomic isthmus. According to Blackford, Paris, in 1791,
was the first to describe a case completely. In a survey of reports in
the literature, Blackford found that the condition occurs about once
in every 1550 cases in which necropsy is performed. About 200 cases
are reported in the literature; in 19 the diagnosis was made in life.
Eleven cases have been diagnosed at the Mayo Clinic.

The condition is a developmental anomaly. There are two main
types: (1) the infantile and (2) the adult. In the infantile forms
there is usually diffuse narrowing of the isthmus of the aorta, or this
segment may be represented by a fibrous cord, or it may be entirely
lacking. Usually there is no collateral circulation. In the adult
forms the degree of narrowing varies from mild constriction to almost
complete obliteration. Frequently the whole aorta is hypoplastic.
Atheromatous change and calcification may be found in the intimal
tissue lining the structure. The collateral circulation is carried on
through the anastomosis of the branches of the subclavian and intercostal vessels. The internal mammary arteries may be of accessory
importance. Hypertrophy of the heart is present in the majority of
cases.

Diagnosis of the infantile types is usually made after death. Death
may occur early in life, depending on the completeness of the constriction. There are no characteristic signs or symptoms. In older subjects the presence of marked collateral circulation, cardiac hypertrophy and elevation of the systolic blood pressure should lead one to
suspect this condition. Absence or diminution of pulsation in the
abdominal aorta or femoral artery usually confirms the diagnosis.
There may be signs and symptoms of arterial insufficiency of the lower
extremities, with claudication.

The majority of patients die of gradual cardiac failure and spontaneous rupture of the aorta; cerebral hemorrhage accounts for a small
percentage of deaths. In cases in which the diagnosis has been verified
at necropsy, death occurred in the first year of life in approximately
40 per cent of the cases (Bonnet). In the first decade of life an additional 44 per cent of patients died. Of the remaining 173 patients in
Bonnet's series two-thirds died between the ages of sixteen and forty years.

There is no known treatment. Sharp restrictions in activities of
life and avoidance of cardiac overstrain is important in delaying the
eventual cardiac failure.

Pulsating Carotid Arteries.—Pathologic pulsation in the carotid
arteries leads to erroneous diagnosis of aneurysm. There were 18
examples of this in the writer's series. This error arises from the fact
that the internal carotid artery may be kinked or buckled anteriorly,
thus simulating an aneurysm. This condition is usually found in
women, and all but one occurred in the right side of the neck, in the
supraclavicular region. The basis of this buckling is apparently the
elevation of the aorta and subclavian artery from hypertension. The
diagnosis usually can be made by careful palpation of the artery
(Brown and Rowntree).

Generalized Forms and Forms Affecting Special Systems (Arteriosclerosis; Atheromatosis or Atherosclerosis).

Generalized Arteriosclerosis.—Definition.—Arteriosclerosis is an inclusive term defining the pathologic changes occurring in the intima and mesial structures of the arteries during the span of life. These changes represent the response of the vascular structures to wear and tear (Virchow). Its inception in early life is initiated with the fatty subintimal deposits termed atheroma, and the process then is designated atheromatosis. In the older periods of life the lesion is more severe; there is chemical transformation of the fatty acids into calcium soap, there is necrosis, and destructive changes appear in the elastic laminæ; this stage is termed atherosclerosis (Marchand).

The entire process probably represents a specific disease of the supporting substance of elastic fibers. The calcium infarctions observed in other organs represent a similar reaction. The unitarian concept of the condition, implying progression from early to advanced age, is the most reasonable, and although the nature of these changes is not entirely clear, the concept serves as a logical basis for further work (Aschoff).

Classification.—There is no adequate classification of arteriosclerosis, nor is one necessary, if the appearance in the different periods of the disease is appreciated. Classification of arteriosclerosis into the "senile" or "low pressure" form, and that secondary to hypertension, is not valid. The process in the latter is the same, modified only by increased intravascular strain. There is the factor of time and intensity on the pathologic lesion with increased intra-arterial pressures. Nor is it advisable to designate the hypertrophy or thickening of the media that obtains in hypertension as arteriosclerosis. This is a normal physiologic response, comparable to that occurring in the heart as a result of increased work.

Frequency.—Arteriosclerosis is a universal disease. The intensity and distribution of the lesion increases with age, and conversely is milder in early life. Mönckeberg's statistics give the incidence of atheromatous lesions as 35.7 per cent among patients who are less than twenty years of age and 75 to 100 per cent among those who are between twenty and forty years of age. His material was derived from a selected group of generally healthy male adults who died while participating in the World War. If subjects are more than sixty years of age the lesion always exists, but again its intensity in different persons varies. Certain races and predisposed persons give early and intense expression to the process. Its incidence among males and females is approximately the same.

Etiology.—The most reasonable etiologic explanation of the pathologic changes in arteriosclerosis is that the process represents wearing or aging of tissue as a result of stress and strain (Virchow). This is borne out by the fact that it tends to localize in the aorta and in other structures that are subject to particular functional, intravascular strain, both constant and intermittent. Individual predisposition may be expressed through an abnormally reacting vasomotor system.

In the aorta there is strong development of the elastic lamellæ; it and its immediate branches are of the elastic type of vessel, and atheromatous changes appear strikingly in these arteries. In cases of atheromatous change in early life, localization appears in the posterior wall of the aorta, and in situations that bear the greatest mechanical burden, such as portions between the origins of intercostal arteries, the scar left by the ductus arteriosus, the bifurcation of the iliac arteries and in portions of the pulmonary circulation, in the presence of mitral disease. The accentuation of the arteriosclerotic lesions, such as those observed in diabetes, can be explained on the basis of changes in the lipoid content of the plasma (Aschoff). Experimentally, it has been shown that the cholesterol content of the diet plays a part in the production of atheromatous lesions. Similarly, the atheromatous changes in the rabbit, occurring after injection of bacteria, and after excessive intake of protein, can also be ascribed to increase in the cholesterol of the blood, or liberation of cholesterol by injury from infection. Of importance is the demonstration that the alimentary atheromatosis produced with feeding of lanolin appears more rapidly in castrated than in non-castrated animals (Murata and Kataoka). There are two factors involved in the atheromatous process: (1) that of the loosening of the subintimal elastic layers, which can be ascribed to internal stress and strain, and (2) the chemical factor of fat lipoid and cholesterol content of the plasma.

Pathology.—Assuming that the process of atheromatosis and atherosclerosis are one and the same, representing stages of the same lesion, the earliest change observed pathologically should be found in the small, intimal fatty plaques. There is separation of the elastic laminæ in the deeper layers of the intima by deposition of cholesterol esters in the intercellular cement substance. This is explicable, since the intima obtains nutrition by a process of imbibition from the plasma; the intima has no contact with the vasa vasorum. With advance of the process, there is increase in fat in the cement substance and deposition of fat droplets between the fibrils of the overlying intima and eventually fat droplets appear in the intimal cells. There is extension of the process to the surface endothelium, and the lesion becomes visible. This represents the atheromatous process of early life; whether retrogression of the lesion can occur is doubtful (Robertson).

The descending period of life starts at the age of forty-five years, and true sclerosis appears in the lesion; this is atherosclerosis (Aschoff). The process is more severe than atheromatosis, but varies greatly in different subjects, and is modified by individual predisposition; the process may be profound in some patients, at the age of fifty years, or relatively mild in others at the age of seventy years. The pathologic process is modified by vascular tissue that is older. There is deposition of fat in the cement or interfibrillar spaces; in addition, there is increase in the connective tissue of the intima. There is hyaline degeneration of the cells of the connective tissue in the deeper layers of the intima. The atheromatous areas are covered with newly formed connective tissue, probably an irritative reaction. This intimal proliferation undergoes hyaline change and represents the sclerotic intimal plaques. All degrees, sizes and ages of atheromatous plaques can be observed. Those in the early stage may simulate exactly those seen in youth, whereas in other stages the process may be much advanced. There is, in later stages, transformation of the deposits of lipoid, in which cholesterol is freed and calcium soaps are formed, with calcification of the atheromatous deposits.

In the muscular form of peripheral arteries the changes are more marked in the media. The forces of wear are exerted largely on the muscle fibers. There is separation of the muscle elements, with fatty changes and swelling of the cartilaginous matrix, brought about by mucoid softening. There is transformation of the fat to calcium soaps in the media, giving rise to mesial calcification, such as that described by Mönckeberg. The response in intimal proliferation is similar to that observed in the aorta.

With advanced arteriosclerotic changes in the arteries, there is atrophy of the capillary bed (Robertson). The disappearance of many of these vessels and atrophy of the parenchyma of the liver, kidneys and brain have been well shown by injection and corrosion methods for demonstrating the finer circulation. This atrophy of the capillary circulation explains parenchymatous atrophy and failing function of organs. The entire vascular tree participates in the process of ageing.

The characteristic picture produced in the arteries by increased arterial blood pressure is that of hypertrophy and thickening of the mesial or muscular layer. This is the same process as that which occurs in the heart, with hypertension. Arteriosclerosis proceeds in the arteries of the hypertensive subject as it proceeds in the subject who does not have hypertension. It is simply accelerated or accentuated in the latter, by the increased intravascular strain. Many subjects with hypertension die before advanced arteriosclerotic changes have appeared.

Physiologic Pathology.—Arteriosclerosis of marked grade may exist without clinical evidence of disease. Cardiac hypertrophy is absent in 35 per cent of all cases of marked arteriosclerosis (Ophüls). The omission of cases of persons who have had hypertension materially reduces this incidence of cardiac hypertrophy in arteriosclerosis (Bell).

Symptoms are initiated when there is interference or diminution in the flow of blood. This is produced in the smaller arteries by thickening or changes in the intima and quantitative reduction in the capillary circulation. These effects explain some of the earlier symptoms of general arteriosclerosis. In larger arteries intimal thickening probably does not progress to such a degree as seriously to interfere with adequate flow of blood. Thrombosis, with occlusion, is then a requisite, creating serious and rapid interference with the flow of blood, resulting in anoxemia of tissues, trophic changes and necrosis. A third factor is vasomotor effects on affected arteries, producing transient attacks of ischemia in digits and probably spasm of the coronary and cerebral arteries.

The importance of arteriosclerosis clinically depends largely on its localization. If the abdominal aorta is affected the presence of arteriosclerosis is compatible with health; if the coronary vessels are affected life is jeopardized; if the peripheral vessels are affected loss of a limb may ensue; if the renal or cerebral vessels are affected grave forms of disability or death occur.

The explanation of the rise in the systolic blood pressure in advanced grades of arteriosclerosis depends on loss of elasticity of the arterial tubes and impairment of vasomotor responses. With myocardial failure, the systolic blood pressure becomes lower.

Signs and Symptoms.—The general manifestations of arteriosclerosis of advanced grade are those which are generally grouped as senile changes. There are atrophic changes in the skin and muscles and general shrinking of the tissues. There is mental and physical impairment, loss of memory for recent events and increased irritability. There is increased intolerance to cold. In some cases this process is is extremely mild, in others greatly exaggerated. There is diminished resistance to infection. Bronchopneumonia is a frequent cause of death, as Osler has pointed out. Healing of wounds is slowed, and resistance to operations is diminished. Bones become more brittle; the serious fractures which occur in old age are frequently the cause of death.

Prognosis.—Prognostic factors in arteriosclerosis depend largely on the organ in which the process shows the greatest intensity. Coronary arteriosclerosis is one of the major causes of death. Attacks of angina pectoris, progressive dyspnea and significant changes in the electrocardiogram are of serious import. Death from renal arteriosclerosis is less frequent, and fairly long terms of life may be compatible with definite evidence of renal insufficiency. Intercurrent infections may precipitate uremia. Cerebral manifestations due to involvement of the larger arteries are of serious import, and death usually occurs from intercurrent infection or exhaustion. Diabetes may be mild or severe and may greatly aggravate the surface lesions due to arteriosclerosis. Thrombosis of the retinal veins has prognostic significance; the average life of the patients who have this condition is five years (Moore).

Treatment.—Arteriosclerosis in the descending period of life represents biologic old age. For old age there is no treatment, but regimens that will eliminate undue strain and allow avoidance of infections or toxic agents should be established. The most important single factor in prolongation of life of these patients is prevention of intercurrent infections, particularly those of the upper part of the respiratory tract. Subjects in the older decades of life do not stand cold, changeable climate well; their adaptive vasomotor adjustments are affected. Susceptibility of such patients to bronchopneumonia is well recognized. If conditions permit, residence where climate is mild and equable is highly desirable. In the presence of organic insufficiency the kidneys should be spared all avoidable stress, and the diet should be low in protein if there is abnormal retention of urea. If the patient is overweight, moderate reduction in weight is advisable. The treatment of heart disease is considered in the section on diseases of that organ. There is no treatment for cerebral arteriosclerosis. Adjustments (and frequently the physician can give useful service by assisting in making these adjustments) as regards work, relaxation and the more delicate matters of domestic relationships are advisable. There is no reason to believe that potassium iodide exerts any beneficial effect in this disease.

Forms Affecting Special Systems.—The localized clinical manifestations of arteriosclerosis are referable to the organ involved.

Cerebral Arteriosclerosis.—Cerebral arteriosclerosis may be manifested by the general signs of senility, or specifically by involvement of the more important arteries. With thrombosis of the cerebral arteries, hemiplegia, paresthesia or senile dementia occurs. Aneurysms may develop in the sclerotic plaque; these may be miliary or solitary and ischemia or pressure may develop. Degeneration and softening of the distal region supplied by the affected arteries are the ultimate results. If the terminal arteries are occluded, infarction of the hemorrhagic type or of the anemic type may result. The vessels most commonly involved are the middle cerebral arteries; such involvement usually produces permanent hemiplegia. If the smaller branches are occluded, hemiplegia may be symptomless or transient. If the lesion is on the left side it is associated with aphasia. There may be visual aphasia or there may be no symptoms except impairment of the intellect. Marked arteriosclerosis may occur in the arteries of the circle of Willis, without symptoms. In the retinal arteries the lumen is narrowed and the walls are thickened. There is loss of the normal light reflex. Thrombosis of the smaller arterioles is not observed but thrombosis of the veins with hemorrhage distally is common.

Renal Arteriosclerosis (Arteriosclerosis of the Kidneys; Senile, Atrophic Kidney).—The weight of the kidneys is decreased as compared to the normal weight. There is atrophy, contraction of areas on the surface and a mild, quantitative reduction in the circulation. The earliest symptoms are polyuria and nocturia, and lowered specific gravity of the urine. Unless death supervenes from other causes, there is progressive loss of ability of the kidney to excrete nitrogenous substances, and anemia and uremia develop. Edema is not present. This is the so-called senile form of renal disease.

Cardiac Arteriosclerosis.—Arteriosclerosis of the heart is concerned largely with the integrity of its own circulation through the coronary vessels. If the arteriosclerotic lesion is advanced, or thrombosis supervenes, the nutritional requirements of the cardiac muscle are imperiled. Angina pectoris occurs in 25 per cent of the cases of proved coronary sclerosis (Willius). Myocardial infarction occurs in about 25 per cent of cases in which there is proved coronary sclerosis. About one-fourth of the patients have progressive myocardial failure without painful attacks. Many cases are symptomless, the so-called occult coronary type of disease. Cardiac failure may be of the congestive or of the non-congestive type.

ARTERIOVENOUS FISTULA (ARTERIOVENOUS ANEURYSM; CIRSOID ANEURYSM; PULSATING VENOUS ANEURYSM).

History.—In 1757 William Hunter first recognized and described the signs and symptoms of arteriovenous fistula of the acquired type. Callander, in 1920, who made a review of the literature on the congenital type gave Bushe, in 1827, the credit for describing the first case. Lewis, in a recent review of the literature, credits Letenneur, in 1859, for the first description. According to Dandy, Steinheil, in 1895, was the first to describe arteriovenous fistula of the brain. Cushing and Dandy have both given classic descriptions of intra-

32

cranial arteriovenous fistula. Halstead's interest in the subject of arteriovenous fistula stimulated the researches of Callander, Reid, Holman and Rienhoff, Pemberton and Horton, who have contributed much to present knowledge of this subject.

Definition.—The term "arteriovenous fistula" is used to designate any abnormal communication or communications between arteries and veins. The different terms are confusing, and for the most part useless. The various descriptive terms, "cavernous," "racemose," "cirsoid" and "serpentine," whether applied to arteries or veins, are merely descriptive of a superficial expression of a lesion. The fundamental pathologic process is the same, regardless of whether the arteriovenous fistula is in the foot or in the cranial cavity.

Types and Etiology.—Arteriovenous fistulas are divided into two groups: (1) acquired and (2) congenital. Acquired arteriovenous fistulas follow penetrating injuries, such as bullet or stab wounds. The abnormal communication is usually single. In congenital arteriovenous fistulas the abnormal communications are usually multiple and have an embryologic basis.

Frequency.—Sixty-five examples of arteriovenous fistula have been seen at the Mayo Clinic in the last ten years; 49 were congenital, 11 of which were intracranial; 16 were acquired. Lewis reviewed the literature on congenital types; he found 24 reports, and added 6 of his own. Many cases of this type are unrecognized.

Pathologic Physiology.—Normally, blood from the heart flows through the arteries and capillaries into the veins and returns to the heart. With the establishment of arteriovenous fistula, the passage of blood is through arteries, communicating fistulas and veins, taking the path of least resistance. The capillary bed receives a lessened amount of arterial blood, and the resulting anoxemia is the basis of the trophic lesions. The amount of blood shunted through the fistula depends on the size of the fistula. The local, regional and systemic manifestations depend on the situation and size of the fistula, and on the length of time over which it has existed. The primary effects are those involving the veins, which become dilated and tortuous; the veins are "arterialized." These effects are due to the increased pressure of the arterial blood on the normally thin walls of the veins. The artery proximal to, and frequently distal to, the fistula shows similar changes. The larger the fistula, the more marked are these vascular changes. The regional effects are best illustrated by the congenital arteriovenous fistula which involves an extremity. The bone is lengthened as compared to the corresponding bone of the other normal extremity. The surface temperature in the region of the fistula is from 2° to 3° C. warmer than the same area on the normal extremity. The changes in bone are lacking in the traumatic form unless the defect is acquired in the period of growth. The systemic effects are important and concern the heart. With loss of blood from the arteries with each systolic contraction, the volume output increases to compensate for this. Cardiac hypertrophy and eventually myocardial insufficiency supervene. The cardiac dynamics are similar to those in insufficiency of the aortic valve (Holman).

Diagnosis.—The history of an injury, usually of a penetrating wound, associated with signs of vascular dilatation, makes diagnosis of the acquired type simple. A thrill usually can be felt over the lesion. If the fistula is closed by pressure there is a sharp drop in the pulse-rate (Branham's sign). In the congenital forms a thrill is absent in 80 per cent of cases. Attention is drawn to the diagnosis by over-growth of a hand or foot. There is increase in surface temperatures over limited areas. Branham's sign is usually absent. Arteriography *in vivo* by the intraärterial injection of an opaque substance has demonstrated arteriovenous communications in peripheral vessels (Yater, Horton). The most conclusive diagnostic sign is demonstra-tion of the arterial blood in a regional vein. This has been demon-strated, not only in the peripheral, but also in the arteriovenous fistulas of the head (Horton).

Treatment.—Surgical treatment has been successful in cases of single acquired arteriovenous communications. Closure of the fistula, or ligation of artery and vein may be necessary. Surgical excision of the multiple fistulous tracts, such as are usually seen in congenital forms of the disease, is impossible. Three cases of congenital type, with single communications, have been cured by surgical measures (Lewis). Treatment consists of application of heavy rubber bandages to the affected extremity in order to make the venous pressure greater than that of the arteries. Blood is then forced into the capillaries. Healing of ulcers can occasionally be affected by this means. Ampu-tation may be necessary if cardiac insufficiency is threatened.

DISEASES OF THE VEINS.

Classifications.—Diseases of the veins can be classified in two major groups: (1) obstructive and (2) non-obstructive. Symptoms and pathologic changes are diverse. The following is a tentative clinical classification (Barker):

Obstructive	Intrinsic	Inflammatory: thrombophlebitis Neoplastic: direct invasion
	Extrinsic (pressure)	Gravid uterus Neoplasms Arterial aneurysms Anomalies Trauma
Non-obstructive	Valvular	Primary varicose veins
	Traumatic	Arteriovenous fistula Rupture
	Congenital	Arteriovenous fistula Phlebectasia Hypoplasia
	Degenerative	Phlebosclerosis

The obstructive cases may be due to intrinsic occlusion such as occurs in thrombophlebitis, or direct invasion by neoplasms, which is rare, or from extrinsic pressure during pregnancy; from new growths and other gross lesions. The symptoms and signs of obstructive lesions of the veins vary according to the size of the vein involved. Clinical edema develops only with closure of the large veins. Homan believes that lymphatic involvement is also necessary. Suppurative phlebitis occasionally is observed in association with septic states. The thrombosis observed in association with certain diseases of the blood, and with cachectic states, stasis as in varicose veins and in thrombophiliac states is usually associated with some inflammatory change in the vessel wall, probably a secondary reaction. Secondary varicose veins may follow any of the obstructive lesions.

In the non-obstructive group, the most common variety is the primary varicose veins due to some constitutional defect in the valves, frequently plus occupational strain. Other less common conditions in this category are arteriovenous fistula and rupture of the veins. Degenerative phlebosclerosis has no clinical significance.

Etiology.—Thrombophlebitis is the most important group from the clinical standpoint. Three factors are recognized in its etiology: (1) A definite local injury of the vein due to gross trauma, chemicals, toxins or bacteria. (2) Stasis associated with bed rest or extrinsic pressure on the veins. (3) An increased tendency for the blood to clot—thrombophilia. In many cases such as the postoperative group and the types which complicate infectious diseases such as pneumonia and typhoid fever, all three factors may play a rôle. Thrombophlebitis is seen after chemical injury and as an extension of a local suppurative or infectious process, such as the sinus thrombosis associated with mastoiditis. It may occur spontaneously in varicose veins and in certain blood dyscrasias such as polycythemia vera. Primary idiopathic thrombophlebitis, frequently occurring in the superficial veins, and often relapsing in character, is seen in individuals where no causative agent can be recognized. It is probably due to local toxic or infectious injury to susceptible veins similar to the lesions of thromboangiitis obliterans.

Symptoms.—Symptoms of thrombophlebitis are due to local inflammation and venous obstruction. If superficial, there is often periphlebitis with local pain and heat. The thrombosed vein usually can be felt as a cord. Distal edema is rare except in the presence of extensive or multiple lesions. Thrombophlebitis of the deeper main venous trunks, such as the femoral vein, produces deep pain and tenderness along the course of the vein with varying degrees of distal congestion and edema. Rarely there may be severe pain in the entire limb due to the sudden production of intense congestion. The onset of these symptoms is usually rather sudden.

Non-inflammatory obstructive lesions may produce secondary varices, congestion, and edema, but the onset is slow and pain or tenderness is rare. Systemic reactions are absent.

Varicose veins, either primary or secondary, may be symptomless. If the varicosities are large or numerous there may be a feeling of distention, pressure, or definite aching after standing or walking which can be relieved only by elevation of the limb. Congenital phlebectasia and phlebosclerosis do not produce symptoms, as a rule.

Complications.—Local complications of venous insufficiency include chronic edema, lymphangitis, acute and chronic, local cellulitis, stasis ulcers, dermatitis and pigmentation. The most important complication of diseases of the veins, however, is the pulmonary embolism which is associated with thrombophlebitis. Thrombosis in the femoral or iliac veins may give rise to a fatal pulmonary embolism because of the large size of the clot; one of the principal causes of sudden death after operation. The embolus occurs soon after the clot forms and before there is much inflammatory reaction in the vein walls, hence local pain and tenderness is usually absent, and as a rule there are no clinical symptoms or signs referable to the extremities before embolus occurs. The greater the degree of local pain and tenderness of the affected vein, the less likelihood of fatal pulmonary embolism, for the thrombus closely adheres to the walls of the veins in the presence of inflammation. Twenty per cent of cases of pulmonary embolism occur in non-surgical cases. Of all surgical deaths, 6 to 10 per cent are due to fatal postoperative embolism and in 80 per cent of these cases the origin of the embolus is in the iliac, femoral or pelvic vein. Small and non-fatal emboli produce infarctions of the lungs with pleuritis, bronchial pneumonia, and sometimes abscess formation. The local suppurative types of thrombophlebitis may be the method of dissemination of pyemic processes.

Treatment.—The treatment of postoperative and postpuerperal phlebitis frequently applies to the leg. Measures consist of elevation of the leg and complete rest until the systemic temperature drops and local tenderness of the vein and the edema disappear. This usually requires from eight to fourteen days. Passive movements of the legs should then be instituted to assist in the maintenance of muscular tonus and prevention of residual edema. Walking is gradually resumed and daily measurements of the leg are made to determine the degree of edema and the need of bandages. Postural exercises to restore the normal supporting tonus of the wall of the vein and of the surrounding muscles should be carried out. Usually bandages are necessary for from three to six months following occlusion of the femoral or iliac veins. They are then omitted for short periods each day, and measurements of the legs to detect edema will indicate the necessity of their continuance. There are no known effective prophylactic measures for prevention of postoperative phlebitis. Movement of the body and limbs immediately after operation and breathing exercises may be beneficial. For the recurring, relapsing form of superficial phlebitis, foci of infection should be eliminated, or excision of the affected veins can be carried out. It is possible that these regions serve as foci for subsequent infection of other regions. Roentgen therapy applied over the inflamed regions frequently gives relief from pain. Rest and moist applications may be necessary in the rare cases in which pain is severe.

The treatment of varicose veins has been greatly facilitated by the injection methods. Sclerosing solutions are injected directly into the vein and the procedure is repeated until sufficient segments of the veins are obliterated. An inflammatory reaction of the vessels with thrombosis results. Embolic phenomena following this procedure are very rare.

DISEASES OF THE PERIPHERAL LYMPHATIC VESSELS (LYMPHEDEMA).

Lymph vessels possess an unbroken endothelial lining, are closed vessels and are well supplied with valves. Circulation of the lymph is carried on largely by action of the skeletal muscles and accessory action of the valves. Lymph contains fibrinogen and prothrombin; it coagulates when thromboplastic substances are added. Inflammation of the lymph vessels causes coagulation of the lymph and thrombosis. The clinical expression of lymphatic disease in the extremities is swelling of the tissues, lymphedema, and when inflammation is present, lymphangitis.

Classification of lymphedema (Allen):

A. Noninflammatory:
    1. Primary forms:
        Precox.
        Congenital.
        Simple.
        Familial, Milroy's disease.
    2. Secondary forms:
        Malignant occlusion.
        Surgical excision, lymph glands.
        Pressure.
        Roentgen and radium therapy.
B. Inflammatory:
    1. In primary forms.
    2. Secondary to:
        Venous stasis.
        Trichophytosis.
        Systemic disease.
        Local tissue injury.

Etiology.—The etiology of primary lymphedema is unknown. It occurs more commonly among women, 87 per cent in The Mayo Clinic series. The onset in the majority of cases was between the ages of ten and twenty-four years, inclusive. In 70 per cent of the cases the condition was unilateral. Evidence of the congenital form is present at birth or appears soon afterward. In the simple form the familial incidence is not present. In the familial form (Milroy's disease) the disease has a distinct familial incidence. In Milroy's original report, in six generations of a family of 97 persons, 22 had lymphedema. The secondary forms of non-inflammatory lymphedema occur as a result of interference to the flow of lymph by malignancy in lymph glands or removal of or pressure on them.

Symptoms and Signs.—Non-inflammatory forms of lymphedema may be symptomless, the limb gradually increases in size, the edema is pitting at first but later is firm and non-pitting. Reduction of swel- ling with elevation of the limb is slow and in later stages unusual.

The inflammatory form may be initiated by chills, fever, adenopathy of regional lymph nodes. The limb becomes hot, swollen and tender; with rest, this subsides in from four days to two weeks, leaving a resid- ual swelling in the leg. Recurrences are the rule. Foci of strepto- cocci in the tissues, resting infections, are believed responsible. Repe- tition of the cellulitis is followed by hard, brawny, persistent swelling, thrombosis of the lymph vessels, proliferation of connective tissue and lymphedema. In late stages the condition is truly disabling, the patient suffers with heavy, swollen legs, elephantiasis. Relapses of cellulitis with general systemic reactions are the rule.

Secondary forms of lymphedema result from lymphangitis of known causes; trichophytosis about the toes is a frequent etiologic agent. Systemic diseases, including filariasis and the puerperium may lead to lymphedema. Trauma, injury to tissue and infections may produce lymphangitis and lymphedema.

Treatment.—Lymphedema in the early stages may be controlled by drainage of the limb and application of heavy rubber bandages. These should be changed at least twice a day, and worn continually when the patient is up and about. The acute attacks of recurring lymph- angitis are treated with rest, moist dressings, and adequate bandaging to prevent lymph stasis after activity is resumed. Vaccines of mixed strains of streptococci are given in increasing doses to prevent, if possible, subsequent attacks. In the late stages with massive lymph- edema, the Kondoleon operation, or modification of it, is carried out with considerable success.

REFERENCES.

Vasoconstricting Disturbances Illustrated by Raynaud's Disease:
ALLEN, E. V., and BROWN, G. E.: Raynaud's Disease: A Critical Review of Minimal Requisites for Diagnosis, Am. Jour. Med. Sci., 1932, **183**, 187.
RAYNAUD, A. G. M.: De l'asphyxie locale et de la gangrène symétrique des extrémitées, Paris, Rignaux, 1862, p. 177.
———— Selected Monographs, London, New Sydenham Society, 1888, p. 199.

Vasodilating Disturbances:
HORTON, B. T., and BROWN, G. E.: Systemic Histamine-like Reactions in Allergy Due to Cold; a Report of Six Cases, Am. Jour. Med. Sci., 1929, **178**, 191.
MITCHELL, S. WEIR: On a Rare Vaso-motor Neurosis of the Extremities, and on the Maladies with Which It May Be Confounded, Am. Jour. Med. Sci., 1878, **76**, 17.

Hypertension:
ALLBUTT, T. C.: Diseases of the Arteries Including Angina Pectoris, London, Macmillan & Co., 1915, 2 vols.
FISHBERG, A. M.: Hypertension and Nephritis, 2d ed., Philadelphia, Lea & Febiger, 1931, 619 pp.
KEITH, N. M., WAGENER, H. P., and KERNOHAN, J. W.: The Syndrome of Malignant Hypertension, Arch. Int. Med., 1928, **41**, 141.
MAYO, C. H.: Paroxysmal Hypertension with Tumor of Retroperitoneal Nerve; Report of a Case, Jour. Am. Med. Assn., 1927, **89**, 1048.
PINCOFFS, M. C.: Paroxysmal Hypertension, Associated with Suprarenal Tumor, Jour. Am. Med. Assn., 1929, **93**, 63.

Hypotension:
  BRADBURY, SAMUEL, and EGGLESTON, CARY: Postural Hypotension: A Report
      of Three Cases, Am. Heart Jour., 1925, 1, 73.
  FRIEDLÄNDER, ALFRED: Hypotension, Medicine, 1927, 6, 147.
Thrombo-angiitis Obliterans:
  BROWN, G. E., ALLEN, E. V., and MAHORNER, H. R.:   Thrombo-angiitis Oblit-
      erans; Clinical, Physiologic and Pathologic Studies, Philadelphia, W. B.
      Saunders Company, 1928, 219 pp.
  BUERGER, LEO: The Circulatory Disturbances of the Extremities, Including
      Gangrene, Vasomotor and Trophic Disorders, Philadelphia, W. B. Saunders
      Company, 1924, 628 pp.
Aneurysms:
  MATAS, RUDOLPH: Surgery of the Vascular System, in Keen, W. W.:   Surgery,
      Its Principles and Practice, 1909, 5, 1.
  OSLER, WILLIAM, and McCRAE, THOMAS: The Principles and Practice of Medi-
      cine, 11ed., New York, D. Appleton & Co., 1930, 1237 pp.
  PARKER, H. L.:   Aneurysms of Cerebral Vessels; Clinical Manifestations and
      Pathology, Arch. Neurol. and Psychiat., 1926, 16, 728.
Periarteritis Nodosa:
  KUSSMAUL, A., and MAIER, R.:   Ueber eine bisher nicht beschriebene eigen-
      thümliche Arterienerkrankung (Periarteritis nodosa), mit die Morbus
      Brightii und rapid fortschreitender allegemeiner Muskellähmung einhergeht,
      Deutsch. Arch. f. klin. Med., 1865–1866, 1, 484.
  WATSON, C. J.:   Periarteritis Nodosa, Univ. of Minnesota Thesis, 1925.
Coarctation of Aorta:
  BLACKFORD, L. M.:   Coarctation of the Aorta, Arch. Int. Med., 1928, 41, 702.
Pulsating Carotid Arteries:
  BROWN, G. E., and ROWNTREE, L. G.:   Right-sided Carotid Pulsations in Cases
      of Severe Hypertension, Jour. Am. Med. Assn., 1925, 84, 1016.
Generalized Arteriosclerosis:
  ASCHOFF, LUDWIG: Lectures on Pathology (delivered in the United States, 1924),
      New York, Paul B. Hoeber, Inc., 1924, 365 pp.
Arteriovenous Fistula:
  HORTON, B. T.:   Hemihypertrophy of Extremities Associated with Congenital
      Arteriovenous Fistula, Jour. Am. Med. Assn., 1932, 98, 373.
  REID, M. R.:   Abnormal Arteriovenous Communications, Acquired and Con-
      genital. I. Report of a Series of Cases, Arch. Surg., 1925, 10, 601. II. The
      Origin and Nature of Arteriovenous Aneurysms, Cirsoid Aneurysms and
      Simple Angioma, Ibid., 1925, 10, 996. III. The Effects of Abnormal Arterio-
      venous Communications on the Heart, Blood Vessels and Other Structures,
      Ibid., 1925, 11, 25. IV. The Treatment of Abnormal Arteriovenous Com-
      munications, Ibid., 1925, 11, 237.
Lymphedema:
  ALLEN, E. V.:   Lymphedema of the Extremities, Proc. Staff Meet. Mayo Clinic,
      1934, 9, 112.
  DRINKER, C. K., and FIELDS, M. E.:   Lymphatics, Lymph and Tissue Fluid,
      Baltimore, Williams & Wilkins Company, 1933.
  MATAS, R.:   The Surgical Treatment of Elephantiasis and Elephantoid States
      Dependent on Chronic Obstruction of the Lymphatic and Venous Channels,
      Am. Jour. Trop. Dis. and Prev. Med., 1913, 7, 60.
  SISTRUNK, W. E.:   The Kondoleon Operation for Elephantiasis; a Report of
      the End Results, South. Med. Jour., 1921, 14, 619.

CHAPTER XIII.

DISEASES OF THE URINARY TRACT.

By WILLIAM SHARP McCANN, M.D.

GENERAL SYMPTOMATOLOGY IN RELA-
TION TO PATHOLOGIC PHYSIOLOGY.
NEPHRITIS.
HEMORRHAGIC BRIGHT'S DISEASE.
DEGENERATIVE BRIGHT'S DISEASE:
THE NEPHROSES.
ARTERIOSCLEROTIC BRIGHT'S DISEASE.
INFARCTS OF THE KIDNEY.
CHRONIC PASSIVE CONGESTION OF THE
KIDNEYS.
RENAL PAIN.

HYDRONEPHROSIS AND PYONEPHROSIS.
NEPHROLITHIASIS.
BACTERIAL INFECTIONS OF THE KID-
NEYS AND URINARY PASSAGES.
Non-tuberculous Infections.
Abscess of the Kidney.
Pyelitis and Pyelonephritis.
Tuberculosis.
TUMORS OF THE KIDNEYS.
POLYCYSTIC KIDNEYS.

GENERAL SYMPTOMATOLOGY IN RELATION TO PATHOLOGIC PHYSIOLOGY.

Since the principal function of the kidneys consists of excretion in the urine of various products of metabolism, it follows that disorders of kidney function, however they may be produced, result in some change, quantitative or qualitative, of the urine. It must be realized at the outset, however, that each normal individual begins life with vastly greater capacity for renal function than is needed for the ordinary demands of metabolic activity. In other words, the kidneys possess a large "factor of safety," to borrow an engineering term. Consequently, it must be apparent that a slowly destructive process may gradually reduce the number of functioning units within the kidney without seriously interfering with the function of units still intact, and that a high degree of anatomic change may occur within the kidneys before functional insufficiency results. Conversely, so dependent are the kidneys upon an adequate oxygen supply and upon an adequate supply of water, which is the principal constituent of urine, that extrarenal factors governing these supplies may determine a high degree of functional impairment of the kidneys with a minimum of anatomic change within them. Functional insufficiency of the kidneys, however produced, results in secondary changes in extrarenal structures and functions which are numerous and complex, such as the "altered quality of the blood," changes in the blood-vessels and heart, compensatory changes in the respiratory mechanism, or toxic effects upon the nervous system. In the stage of functional inadequacy the clinical picture is made up of a complex mixture of symptoms in extrarenal systems in which it is often difficult to separate those factors which are the cause from those which are the result of the functional failure of the kidneys. Such an analysis or sifting out of causes and effects

(505)

is usually made possible only by serial observations beginning before the onset of renal failure or continuing after it has been relieved. Lacking such serial observations one can frequently reconstruct the probable course of events in the pathogenesis of the disorder by a *careful, detailed, clinical history.* Only too frequently, however, progressive anatomic damage to the kidneys begins insidiously and advances so silently that severe functional impairment is encountered almost before the patient is aware that he is ill, and thus the history provides meager evidence as to pathogenesis.

It becomes of the utmost importance, therefore, to search among the multitude of symptoms and signs of renal disease for those which hold the important clues to the nature of the changes occurring *within the kidney,* as distinguished from those associated with disturbances in *extrarenal* structures and functions, and within this latter group to recognize the sequences of cause and effect.

The Urine.—The urine itself provides the most reliable clues to the nature of the changes occurring within the kidneys. It was with the urine that Richard Bright began his remarkable observations, and it is the urine to which Thomas Addis has brought us back after more than forty years of wandering in the wilderness of confused facts and theories. The nature of the proteins in the urine, the occurrence of casts, blood, leukocytes, epithelial cells and bacteria afford the most important indications of the qualitative nature of renal lesions.

Addis has given us valuable data regarding the amounts of protein, casts and cellular structures which may be found in the urine of normal individuals and a technic for their enumeration. Liquids are restricted for twenty-four hours. The twelve-hour night specimen is quantitatively collected and measured. If this specimen is sufficiently concentrated and acid in reaction a measured portion is centrifuged. The sediment is resuspended in a measured portion of salt solution and the formed elements are counted on a hemacytometer. In the twelve-hour night urine of normal men Addis found quantities of the various formed elements as shown in Table 10 of determinations made on 74 medical students.

TABLE 10.

	Range.	Average per twelve hours.
Red corpuscles	0–425,000	65,750
Casts	0–4,270	1,040
Leukocytes and epithelial cells	32,400–1,000,000	322,550
Protein	10–30 mg.	

If sediment counts are properly carried out the finding of an increase in the number of any or all of these formed elements indicates some lesion or abnormality of the kidneys or urinary tract. It must, however, always be borne in mind that the entire urinary tract must be considered, that extensive lesions may exist without abnormality of the urine specimen obtained, that casts may dissolve or disintegrate in dilute and alkaline urine and that red corpuscles may become practically invisible shadows under the same circumstances.

The study of other elements in the sediment is of no less importance. The finding of ova, fragments of tumor tissue, gravel, crystals and the demonstration of microörganisms by stain, culture, or animal inoculation, give the greatest aid in determining the nature of lesions in the kidneys and urinary tract.

Hematuria may be either occult or visible. Occult hematuria is said to exist when the red corpuscles exceed 500,000 per twelve hours in the night specimen. For the evaluation of hematuria it is of the utmost importance to determine whether the blood is uniformly distributed in all parts of the urine voided. Lesions of the urethra tend to give more blood in the first portions voided; lesions of the bladder give rise to more blood in the last portion voided. Those of the upper urinary tract give rise to a uniform suspension of the blood even though these lesions may be unilateral. Cystoscopic examination is sometimes necessary to determine the source of the blood, whether it be from stone, tumor, varices, parasitic or other inflammation of the lower urinary tract, and whether it comes from one or both ureters. The search for urinary tract purpura, calculus, tumor or tuberculosis must often be aided by pyelogram, and by the search for tubercle bacilli in stained specimens and by guinea-pig inoculations, combined with separate functional studies of the two kidneys. Calculi and tuberculosis may be bilateral. In both cases, however, the increase in urinary protein is proportional to the amount of blood introduced into the urine, and neither lesion causes cast formation. The suppurative lesions are accompanied by leukocytes in clumps.

The bilateral hematuria from the kidneys, which is accompanied by proteinuria, usually in excess of that contributed directly by the presence of blood, and by an increased number of casts, is characteristic of hemorrhagic Bright's disease. On histologic examination, as Volhard and Fahr and Addis and Oliver have shown, the kidneys in such cases exhibit various degrees of inflammatory changes of the glomeruli. In the presence of congestive heart failure, however, a slight increase in the urinary blood count may be attributed to passive congestion of the kidneys.

Cylindruria.—Casts consist of materials formed in the mold of the renal tubules. The materials originate either in an inflammatory exudate from the glomeruli or in the products of degeneration of the renal tubules. They vary from loosely packed débris, which rapidly disintegrates, to firmly coagulated structures. They are variously named according to their appearance or constituents as: *hyaline casts,* optically more or less homogeneous cylinders of a substance related to amyloid, giving a Gram-positive reaction; waxy casts; *granular casts,* containing a finely divided débris; hyaline or granular casts with fatty droplets adherent to or imbedded in them, the so-called *fatty casts; cellular casts,* in which leukocytes or epithelial cells are bound together in a hyaline or granular coagulum; *blood casts,* consisting of red corpuscles and their detritus; and certain broad casts to which Addis has given the name of "*renal failure*" casts, which are formed in the dilated terminal portions of the ducts of Bellini.

By the careful study of the casts Addis and Oliver have been able to draw surprisingly correct inference as to the morphologic processes occurring within the kidneys. The occurrence of blood casts in significant numbers was uniformly associated with exudative inflammatory lesions of the glomeruli. Renal failure casts were found only when great distortions of renal architecture existed, so that large numbers of renal units were functioning so poorly that the débris from them could accumulate in the terminal tubules of Bellini, either to remain there as broad loose plugs or occasionally to be flushed into the urine by the accumulating pressure of diuresis into the tubules above.

It should be remembered that failure to find casts may be due to their retention within the kidney, or to their disintegration in the urine. Particularly when the urine is dilute, of low acidity or actual alkalinity, will this disintegration occur. Blood casts are particularly liable to break up, though their fragments may frequently remain identifiable.

Proteinuria.—Proteinuria occurs in a wide variety of conditions, many of which are not associated with demonstrable lesions of the kidney or urinary passages. Addis found from 10 to 30 mg. of protein in the twelve-hour night urine of normal men. Occasionally a slight turbidity is produced when acetic acid is added to urines of normal men which contain chondroitin-sulphuric acid.

Proteins found in the urine include hemoglobin, fibrinogen, Bence-Jones albumose, unchanged food proteins (egg-white), parenterally injected foreign proteins (immune sera), as well as the ordinary serum proteins and other tissue proteins of the body.

Hemoglobinuria occurs in all conditions associated with hematuria. In conditions in which rapid blood destruction occurs unchanged hemoglobin may appear in the urine, *i. e.*, paroxysmal hemoglobinuria, malaria and black-water fever. In the latter condition obstruction of the renal tubules by massive deposits of pigment, resulting in oliguria or anuria, may occur. In malaria a true nephritis may be found, particularly in the estivo-autumnal variety.

Whipple and his co-workers have found that injected hemoglobin appears in the glomerular filtrate at a threshold level of 155 mg. per cent. Resorption of this hemoglobin occurs in the tubules until it is blocked by the filling of the cells with iron-containing pigment, after which hemoglobin appears in the bladder urine. Injury to the tubular cells by mercury interfered with this resorption of hemoglobin, and, conversely, previous blocking of the cells with iron-containing pigment exerted a protective influence against tubular injury by mercury.

Fibrinuria occurs when whole blood is extravasated into the urinary tract and is responsible for the formation of clots, which may at times become impregnated with salts to form fibrin calculi. In acute nephritis fibrinogen will at times pass through the kidney to produce a coagulum in the urine. Owing to the large size of the molecular complexes of fibrinogen it is rare for this protein to escape through the glomerulus. The fact of its escape is evidence of a serious increase in the permeability of the glomeruli.

The urinary proteins, which are commonly detected by testing with heat and acetic acid, occur in a wide variety of conditions, some of which are essentially benign in character, due chiefly to circulatory changes within the kidney, and others which are of graver portent. There is, however, no true parallelism between the amount of protein in the urine and the amount of anatomic change in the kidneys.

Orthostatic albuminuria is a benign condition in which protein appears in the urine only during standing in the erect posture. It disappears entirely during walking or sitting or recumbency, or during any posture which obliterates the lumbar lordosis with which it is associated. The amount of protein, which is usually small, may rise as high as 1 per cent, especially in the first voiding after recumbency and is usually associated with an increase in the number of hyaline casts. There is usually an orthostatic oliguria with a compensatory recumbent polyuria. The subjects are usually of asthenic habitus, with low pulse pressures. The condition is commonest in childhood and adolescence, but by no means confined to these age periods. The mechanism of its production probably depends upon venous stasis in the kidney.

A *"sport albuminuria"* is sometimes observed in athletes and others during muscular exertion. This is likewise believed to depend upon changes in the renal circulation. Likewise there is described an albuminuria during cold baths, due to reflex vasomotor changes in the renal circulation.

The albuminuria of chronic passive congestion of the kidney occurs in urines of high specific gravity, of high color, usually accompanied by an increased number of hyaline and finely granular casts and a slightly increased number of red corpuscles.

In nephritis the character of the proteins in the urine gives a clue to the nature of the pathologic process. This is particularly true of the ratio of albumin to globulin. Purely degenerative lesions usually give high ratios of albumin to globulin. In glomerulonephritis the intensity of the hemorrhagic or glomerular lesions is usually paralleled by the intensity of globulinuria, with corresponding variations of the albumin to globulin ratios. Low ratios are found when the hemorrhagic glomerular lesions are most intense. Diminution of globulinuria is a favorable indication either of healing or of transition into a stage in which tubular degeneration predominates.

The source of the urinary proteins in nephritis has been the subject of much investigation. There seems to be little doubt that serum proteins escape through the capillary walls of the glomeruli under conditions which increase their permeability, and no doubt that the cells of the tubules also contribute their quota by extruding semi-formed protein masses into their lumina. Andrews and his co-workers have found, in some cases, a highly dispersed and highly toxic protein fraction, which passes certain membranes more readily than ordinary serum proteins, and has suggested that these latter are excreted in combination with the toxic fraction. That the excretion by the kidney of abnormal proteins may result in renal injury is suggested by the observation by Thannhauser and Krause of a case of "nephrotic contracted kidney" in a patient with Bence-Jones albumosuria.

The loss of serum proteins in the urine may result in serious depletion of these substances, which are so important in the maintenance of a normal balance of fluid exchange through capillary walls. Low serum proteins contribute to the production of edema.

Edema.—Edema is an abnormal accumulation of fluid in tissue spaces, resulting in a swelling of the parts involved in which the application of pressure leaves an indentation.

Edema in renal disease may develop as the direct result of the pathologic processes which involve the kidneys, or as a result of heart failure consequent to hypertension and arteriosclerosis. At times it is probable that both factors may enter into its production. Still another form of edema occasionally encountered in renal disease is due to the inanition to which many patients are subjected in the course of treatment. In those edemas which are due to heart failure, the swelling is first visible in dependent portions of the body. In the early stages of some of the so-called "renal edemas" the first visible swelling may appear in the face and about the eyes, though in the later stages the effect of gravity upon the distribution of edema fluid usually becomes apparent. The edemas of inanition and of pure nephrosis are observed chiefly in dependent portions from the start, and in this respect resemble the edema of heart failure. Those edemas which are not confined to dependent portions are of the most vital importance, involving as they do important structures in the central nervous system, meninges, the eye and at times the lungs.

Our knowledge of the pathologic physiology of edema is in no case complete. In every case a multiplicity of factors are involved. To a rapidly increasing extent some of these factors are becoming known and appreciated. It has become apparent that an understanding of the physico-chemical mechanism of water-binding by the colloids of the body is fundamental in all forms of edema. In a broad, rough way certain features of this mechanism are known. Within cells, as well as within circulating fluids, a dispersed phase may exchange water with the dispersion medium. In general, the more finely a colloid is dispersed the greater are its affinities for water, the more it tends to swell at the expense of the dispersion medium. This tendency to swell may be measured as a pressure, *oncotic pressure*, analogous to the osmotic pressure of crystalloidal solutions.

Within the body the forces active at phase interfaces, capable of increasing or decreasing dispersion, or possibly of reversing the phase relationships, are just beginning to be guessed at, from the results of studies in general physiology.

Fluid exchanges across living membranes have received much study. The distribution of mineral salts and proteins on the two sides of such membranes obeys the same law which Donnan found for the equilibrium established with non-living membranes. Unlike collodion membranes those of the body are composed of living cells, within which changes may occur affecting their permeability.

In 1896 Starling made measurements of the swelling pressure of the plasma proteins, as a result of which we have come to an understanding of their importance in the exchange of water through the capillaries. The filtration pressure in a capillary is the difference between the hydrostatic pressure (capillary blood pressure) and the swelling or oncotic pressure of the plasma proteins. At the arterial end of the capillary the blood pressure normally is higher than the oncotic pressure, and at the venous end it is lower, while at some intermediate point the two balance exactly. Thus, a mechanism exists which provides for the filtration and resorption of fluid through the capillary wall.

Venous stasis, produced by a tourniquet or by congestive heart failure, by raising the capillary blood pressure, tends to increase the filtration pressure and to reduce capillary resorption. It may likewise, by dilatation of the capillary and possibly by injury to the endothelium resulting from anoxemia, cause an abnormal permeability of the capillary so that protein escapes. This extravascular protein, which is abundantly present in edema fluid in acute hemorrhagic nephritis, through its oncotic pressure, may further hinder the resorption of fluid by the capillary. In this way fluid may accumulate in the tissue spaces unless the increased filtration is balanced by an increased flow of lymph. This is the probable mechanism of the "hard" edemas of nephritis and inflammation. In the majority of instances the factors which produce venous stasis also produce lymphatic stasis, since the lymph-vascular system communicates with the veins.

When the plasma proteins are depleted by loss through the kidneys during albuminuria, or through an abnormal permeability of capillaries generally, or by reason of deficient formation in inanition, or experimentally by plasmaphoresis, the filtration pressure is increased and the factor favoring fluid resorption is diminished.

Von Farkas, Govaerts and others have found that serum albumin has a much larger oncotic pressure than has serum globulin. A loss of serum albumin is associated with greater tendency toward edema than occurs with corresponding loss of serum globulin. This is well illustrated in the nephroses in which low ratios of serum albumin to serum globulin are observed together with a marked tendency to edema.

No explanation of edema is complete which deals only with the exchange of fluid through the endothelial membranes of the capillaries. The mechanism of fluid resorption through the lymphatics must likewise be known, as well as the water-binding properties of connective tissue fibers and tissue cells. Concerning these latter factors our knowledge of clinical edema is meager. McClure and Aldrich and others have observed that physiologic salt solution, injected intradermally to form a wheal, disappears more rapidly in some edematous subjects than it does in normal individuals. The full significance of this phenomenon is not understood. The elastic resistance or turgor of tissues is doubtless of importance in determining the location of extravascular fluid accumulations.

Much has been learned by a study of the total fluid exchanges of dropsical individuals. Widal and Javal showed that the accumulation of fluid in the body in edema is accompanied by a retention of sodium chloride. By administering this salt, or by withdrawing it from the diet, the weight of dropsical subjects can be made to vary. Salt restriction has come to be fundamental in the treatment of all dropsies, however they may be produced. It is the sodium ion the restriction of which is important, not the chloride.

In many infectious diseases, as in pneumonia, ingested sodium chloride is retained within the body with an increase in body weight due to retention of water. During convalescence this retained water and salt are excreted, without edema having been observed. A similar phenomenon follows the parenteral injection of foreign serum, accompanied by urticarial or angioneurotic edema when serum sickness occurs.

Clinical observation has shown that the body weight of an individual with a tendency to edema will increase about 10 per cent before edema is detectable by the test of pitting on pressure. When a tourniquet is applied to an extremity the volume of the latter increases to this extent before edema can be observed.

Subjects of myxedema or hypothyroidism frequently exhibit a tendency to retention of salt and water with consequent fluctuations in the weight curve, without the occurrence of true edema. The administration of thyroid extract will frequently result in a reduction of edema, especially in those forms accompanied by degeneration of the renal tubules in which low values for serum proteins are observed. The writer has observed this to occur while the serum proteins were still below normal values.

In rare instances the administration of the parathyroid hormone has been followed by a reduction of such dropsies, possibly through its effect upon the calcium ion and the effect of this in turn upon capillary permeability. It is also possible that this hormone may relax angiospasm, thus relieving the glomerular ischemia which is sometimes responsible for oliguria.

The behavior of edematous subjects toward the administration of certain salts is interesting. Calcium salts, ammonium chloride, compounds of mercury and bismuth, and potassium citrate are all useful in combating dropsies of various types. Their administration is frequently followed by diuresis or watery stools with a loss from the body of water and sodium chlorides. The mechanism of their action is not entirely clear, yet it seems probable that they depend upon freeing sodium ions and water bound by colloids.

Hypertension.—**Symptoms Referable to the Heart and Vascular System.**—*Hypertension; cardiac hypertrophy; arteriosclerosis; so-called "albuminuric" retinitis.*—That disorders of the cardiovascular system are frequent concomitants of renal disease has been well known since the time of Bright, who observed the frequent enlargement of the heart, the hard, incompressible pulse in many cases, and speculated upon the relationship of these phenomena to "the altered quality of the blood." Since that time students of Bright's disease have continued to wrestle with the perplexing problems of these interrelationships, particularly those of cause and effect. The problems have grown somewhat clearer with the passage of the years, as pathologic physiologic correlations have improved, and as clinical knowledge of the life history of the various forms of Bright's disease has been increased by the early application of tests for renal function, chemical studies of the "altered quality of the blood," blood-pressure measurements and by the universal use of the ophthalmoscope.

Hypertension is now generally believed to be the cause of the hypertrophy of the left ventricle which occurs in the absence of valvular disease and adherent pericardium. Clinicians may watch its gradual development in persistent hypertension by the increasing cardiac dulness on percussion, by serial measurements on radiographs of the heart and by the progressive left axis deviation in the electrocardiogram.

Gradually there has developed a widespread realization that there are two great groups of individuals with persistent hypertension. In one group the hypertension is sometimes found to exist before any sign of renal disease is detectable, and usually before any serious functional disturbance of the kidneys is discovered. Death of these individuals from accident or intercurrent disease has permitted pathologic study which reveals entirely normal kidneys in many cases. Studies by Moschowitz, Fishberg, Branch and Linder, and many others indicate that the *arterioles* undergo degenerative changes as a *result* of hypertension, and that the renal lesions which may eventually appear in this first group of patients are the result of spasm, sclerosis, or endarteritis of the pre-glomerular arterioles. In the second great group the hypertension appears consequent to well-marked evidence of renal disease and disturbance of renal function.

Hypertension in the pre-nephritic group is found under a variety of conditions. In hyperthyroidism some degree of hypertension is usual. Certain adrenal tumors appear to be the cause in other cases. The association of vascular hypertension with erythremia is found in the Gaisboeck syndrome. In women an elevation of blood pressure frequently begins at the menopause. Among younger women Alvarez and Zimmerman found hypertension to be associated with evidences of subnormal sexual development. Finally there is a large group of individuals in which there appears to be an heredo-familial or constitutional predisposition to an "essential hypertension." Dawson and Ryle found that about two-thirds of their cases of hyperpiesis were of *pyknic* or *hypersthenic habitus*, with broad shoulders, thick neck, wide costal angle, ruddy and athletic, except when crippled by obesity from overindulgence. All observers of this group recognize the importance of psychic factors and the nervous tension of "high pressure" living in the production of hypertension in those constitutionally predisposed. Central vasomotor centers may be influenced by stimuli from all parts of the central, peripheral and vegetative nervous systems.

Numerous theories have been advanced to explain persistent hyperpiesis. The neurons of vasomotor centers appear to be stimulated in general asphyxial conditions, as well as by local partial asphyxia during increasing intracranial tension, so that it has been surmised that any local interference with their blood supply by vascular spasm or sclerosis would provide a mechanism. Search has been made for pressor substances. In particular Major has studied the effects of guanidine salts and their methyl derivatives. Hulse believes that hypercholesterinemia sensitizes the vascular system to pressor substances. Kylin finds abnormal ratios of potassium to calcium in the serum and believes that this ratio determines the character of the vascular response to adrenalin. Others have postulated a lack of depressor substances. Theories as to the mechanism of hypertension are legion; only a few of them may be mentioned here. The problem is still far from its final solution.

A rough but practical rule may be applied to the differentiation of "essential" hypertension from that which is secondary to nephritis. In the former the systolic blood pressure is usually over 200 mm. Hg before there is evidence of serious renal disease or functional impairment. In the latter the systolic blood pressure rarely goes above 180 mm. Hg without signs of profound renal disease and functional impairment.

The widespread use of the ophthalmoscope has done much to clarify the relationship of hyperpiesis to renal disease. By its aid one may directly observe the changes which occur in the retinal arterioles and the secondary changes in the retina. The old term "albuminuric retinitis" is now generally regarded as a misnomer, since it is clear that it is in no way due to albuminuria nor primarily to renal disease, but to hypertension. Volhard prefers the term *retinitis angiospastica*, indicating that the retinopathy is the result of arteriolar spasm.

The examination of the *retina in the early stages of essential hypertension* frequently reveals no lesion either of vessels or of retina, except perhaps a general narrowing of the arterioles. The longer hypertension has existed, the more likelihood there is of discovering evidences of arteriolar sclerosis, in which the vessels show some unevenness of caliber. The increased turgor of the arteries tends to displace the accompanying vein into the deeper layers of the retina at points where the vessels cross, giving the appearance of compression of the vein, which can usually be made out before sclerotic change is greatly advanced. The retinal veins in such cases often appear overfilled, in contrast to the narrow arteries, particularly when hypertension has reduced the myocardial reserve. A later change is the *hypertensive retinopathy*, characterized by the periodic occurrence of small flame-shaped hemorrhages and by the appearance of small glistening dots, so-called "exudates" in the macular region. These glistening dots are not true exudates, but owe their appearance to lipoidal accumulations in small areas of retinal degeneration. Both hemorrhages and "exudates" sometimes disappear without a trace. As the disease progresses the "exudates" become larger and appear flat and glistening, and frequently are arranged in some definite configuration about the macula. It is rare to find an entirely normal urine in the stage in which the retinopathy is seen. Albuminuria is the rule and casts are frequently found, though good renal function may exist. In many such cases the albuminuria is the result of passive congestion in hypertensive heart disease, since the renal units which are deprived of their blood supply by sclerotic closure of arterioles cease to elaborate any urine and hence contribute little to the albuminuria and casts. However, exquisite examples of hypertensive retinopathy have been observed in individuals suffering from adrenal tumors, in which both kidneys and urine were normal.

In the slowly progressing benign forms of "essential" hypertension the optic disks remain approximately normal, at least until the later stages when some blurring of the margins may be seen. In the *malignant forms of hypertension*, in which marked hyperpiesia rapidly progresses to widespread arteriolar necrosis and frequently to uremic death, the appearance of the retina is distinctive. In addition to arterial spasm, venous displacement and hemorrhages, there are seen *choked disk* and the "exudates," instead of being entirely flat and glistening, are more dull and less sharply marked, so that they are described as *cotton-wool exudates*. The changes in the disk are sometimes associated with increased intracranial pressure from cerebral edema, but this is not invariably true.

If one follows the course of retinal changes in glomerulonephritis one finds that the occurrence of pictures similar to those described above is dependent upon the presence of hypertension. In the acute stages of hemorrhagic or glomerulonephritis, hypertension is usually transient and not great. Cerebral edema may occur with various degrees of "choked disk," and occasional hemorrhages are noted. In chronic latent and nephrotic stages of glomerulonephritis both hypertension and retinopathy are usually absent. In chronic active cases, however, gradually rising blood pressure may result finally in the picture of "albuminuric retinitis." Many variations, of course, are observed in this disease, depending on the fluctuations of intensity and the duration of periods of activity and latency of the process.

Uremia.—The term uremia, originally introduced by Piorry, in 1848, to denote a state of intoxication due to resorption of urine, has now come to include all the toxic states which develop as the result of functional insufficiency of the kidneys in renal disease. The pictures of uremia in nearly every case are complicated by symptoms of disorders in extrarenal systems, so that it is very difficult to determine the exact symptomatology of pure uremia apart from the fundamental condition which causes the renal lesion or insufficiency. If the renal insufficiency is due to arteriosclerotic contraction of the kidney secondary to hypertension, the uremic picture is complicated by the widespread vascular disorder. If uremia develops in mercurial nephrosis it is complicated by symptoms due to extrarenal actions of mercury, or to water intoxication if diuresis fails to follow forced fluid ingestion. Some of the terminal symptoms of cholera are doubtless due to renal insufficiency. Even the simplest mechanism by which a dehydration could be produced would fail to give a purely uremic picture. Surgical removal of all kidney tissue gives a syndrome due to the retained products of normal metabolism resulting from complete absence of renal function, but this syndrome differs from the uremic states observed when renal insufficiency accompanies active disease of the kidneys, in which the possibility exists that toxic substances may be produced within the damaged kidneys, or as a result of a metabolic disturbance. This latter possibility is further suggested by the fact that experimental efforts to reproduce clinical uremia in animals by injecting normal urinary constituents have failed, even though symptoms of intoxication may occur.

Some writers (Volhard) would distinguish true from a false uremia. The *false uremic symptoms* are those which result from cardiovascular disorders and can arise in the course of hypertension without renal insufficiency. Volhard points out that lead encephalopathy without renal insufficiency may simulate in nearly every particular the acute eclamptic type of uremia. The term "hypertensive encephalopathy" (Fishberg) expresses Volhard's idea of an "eclamptic pseudo-uremia," which covers a wide range of symptoms due to generalized angiospastic crises (Pal) with increased intracranial tension due to edema of the brain, in those cases in which angiospastic ischemia and anoxemia injure the capillary walls and increase their permeability. Localized ischemias may also occur within the central nervous system, some of which may be due to localized angiospasm and edema and, at times, hemorrhage. These pseudo-uremic symptoms include "cardiac asthma" and Cheyne-Stokes respiration; symptoms of increased intracranial pressure such as headache, vomiting and slow pulse, and choked disk; focal neurologic symptoms such as amaurosis, hemiopia, aphasia and paralyses.

The term true uremia should be reserved for those toxic states resulting from renal insufficiency associated with some one of Bright's diseases. The commoner types of symptom complexes will be described without the attempt to separate entirely true uremic from pseudo-uremic mechanisms in the sense of Volhard. These composite pictures differ in actual experience according to the relative importance in each case of the variable factors of azotemia, edema, hypertension and vascular disease, and of renal acidosis.

Hypertensive encephalopathy, which is often called *acute eclamptic or epileptiform uremia* occurs frequently in the course of hemorrhagic Bright's disease and in the nephrosis of pregnancy. In hemorrhagic Bright's disease it frequently ushers in the first attack or occurs with an acute exacerbation of a chronic or latent process. The premonitory symptoms vary according to the preëxisting disease. With the onset of hemorrhagic Bright's disease there may have been a day or two of headache and hazy vision and slight edema when a *convulsive seizure* occurs with almost lightning-like suddenness. The convulsions are both clonic and tetanic, lasting for a minute or more, during which *cyanosis* and distention of veins in the neck are seen as a result of fixation of the respiratory muscles. This is often followed by clonic twitches with jerky, gasping respiration. As the cramps diminish the respirations become regular and deeper and often stertorous. In convulsions of this severity consciousness is usually lost and the patient may lie as if in a drunken stupor. Unfortunately, in rare instances, the kindly intervention of stupor or coma is lacking in the eclamptic seizures, and the tortured patient cries out to bystanders to hold him. The more frequent stupor or coma, from which the patient cannot at first be roused, gradually becomes more like normal sleep, from which the patient can be awakened.

Such attacks may be preceded by severe psychic disturbances of great variety, commonly mania or delirium, usually with some hyper-kinetic manifestations. Headache is often severe, usually occipital, and at times accompanied by stiff neck and Kernig's sign, slow pulse and vomiting. Amaurosis is usually marked, even with negative ophthalmoscopic findings. If lumbar puncture is done, the fluid is found to be under increased pressure in the majority of cases. The procedure frequently gives prompt relief from the acute seizures.

The convulsions often simulate epilepsy even to the aura. Repeated convulsions amounting to as many as 250 in twenty-four hours have been observed. The convulsions are sometimes unilateral or Jacksonian in type. Transient paralyses, monoplegias or hemiplegia may follow these convulsions. Other focal neurologic symptoms such as hemiopia, aphasia, ataxias and choreas are of frequent occurrence. In fatal cases it is difficult to find in the nervous system the anatomic basis of many of these focal symptoms, which are supposed to be due to local ischemia and edema.

Acute or eclamptic uremia is accompanied or preceded by marked oliguria or complete suppression. In favorable cases improvement sets in within two or three days, with gradual resumption of urinary secretion. There is always some elevation of blood pressure and usually some fever and leukocytosis.

The chemical alterations of the blood in acute eclamptic uremia depend somewhat upon the previous state of health of the patient. At the onset of an acute nephritis the acute false or eclamptic uremia may occur with no elevation of the non-protein nitrogen of the blood, and at times before renal function is impaired. In these cases the phenomena are purely those of acute hypertensive encephalopathy, such as may occur in eclampsia of pregnancy or in acute lead encephalopathy. Also at the onset of acute nephritis depletion of the alkaline reserve is not observed at once. Low values for plasma carbon dioxide combining power at the onset of acute uremia speak for a preëxisting chronic nephritis, as do low hemoglobin values. Renal acidosis and anemia frequently develop with considerable rapidity, however, in the course of a true acute nephritis, and if the acute uremia occurs in the later stages of the course of acute nephritis both anemia and low alkaline reserve may be noted.

Nellis Foster has isolated from the blood of patients with eclamptic uremia a toxic nitrogenous body in pure crystalline form, minute amounts of which are capable of producing convulsions in animals.

Traube's theory that edema of the brain is the basis of acute eclamptic uremia receives support from the postmortem appearance of the brain in some cases, but not in all. The dura is usually tense and, when a small opening is made in it, the brain tends to be extruded. The surface of the brain is pale and moist.   The convolutions are frequently so flattened that the sulci are scarcely recognizable.   On removal of the brain, the medulla and adjacent cerebellum may be seen to be molded conically within the ring-like impression of the foramen magnum.   When such a brain is cut the ventricles are often collapsed so that they appear as mere slits.

On lumbar puncture the spinal manometer usually records the increased pressure, often as much as 40 cm. of water pressure or more. The formation of a pressure cone may interfere with this measurement in some cases.   The frequent observation of edema of the optic disk is sometimes taken as an indication of increased intracranial pressure, though neuro-retinal edema may exist without cerebral edema.

Long ago Cohnheim pointed out that cerebral edema was not an invariable finding at autopsy in acute eclamptic uremia.   The phenomena are best explained by the theory that a vascular crisis occurs in the cerebral vessels with resultant ischemia and anoxemia, which is responsible for the nervous symptoms.   In the course of this angiospastic crisis a generalized or a focal cerebral edema may occur, depending upon the degree to which the permeability of the cerebral capillaries is increased by the ischemic-anoxic damage.

Chronic Uremia.—The *symptomatology* of chronic true uremia is that of a slowly developing chronic intoxication occurring when the last reserves of renal function are encroached upon.   At the beginning it expresses itself subjectively in a general depression and a sense of great weariness, and objectively in increasing asthenia and cachexia. Patients complain of dull headache, and of great fatigue.   They are drowsy and lethargic, frequently forgetful, apathetic, slow and uncertain in movement.   In the early stages the intensity of these symptoms abates with slight increases in urine volume, and grows worse when this declines.   The patient begins to look chronically ill, the skin takes on a muddy pallor, becomes dry and inelastic, the hair dry, dull and brittle, the eye loses its gleam of interest, and often there is a staring expression, approaching slight exophthalmos.   There is often weight loss, unless this is obscured by edema.   In non-edematous parts of the body the loss of panniculus adiposus may be noted; the myoedema may be elicited by mechanical stimulation of the pectoral or deltoid muscles.   Anorexia is usual and frequently amounts to loathing of food, and nausea and vomiting are frequent.   When this occurs dehydration is imminent, and a patient who is tormented by thirst may be unable to retain water given by mouth.

Drowsiness gradually increases into a stupor from which at first the patient can be aroused only by a loud noise to give rational responses to questions or commands.   Disorientation increases and mild delirium is observed in which the patient mutters to himself a queer jumble of ideas or repeats over and over again some word or phrase. Stupor changes to coma with deep (Kussmaul) breathing, which becomes stertorous with puffing out of the sagging cheeks.   This differs from the periodic breathing of Cheyne-Stokes, though like this it may be punctuated by apnea.   The breath has a urinous odor to which may be added a fetor due to neglect of cleanliness or to a stomatitis which is a frequent complication. The pupils are usually small, in contrast to the wide pupils of eclamptic uremia and of diabetic coma. Occasionally the skin becomes frosted with urea crystals unless the accumulation of these is prevented by frequent bathing. In the negro this "urea frost" gives a startling appearance. Tremor of the hands, small twitchings of the face may be succeeded by larger myoclonic movements, the tendon reflexes are hyperactive and death may be ushered in by clonic convulsions. Body temperature tends to be subnormal, though a pre-agonal rise is not uncommon.

The general picture given above varies from case to case, as different complications are encountered. The *stomatitis* may become pseudo-diphtheritic and spread through the pharynx to the trachea. *Parotitis* is a not infrequent sequel of neglected stomatitis. A diphtheritic *colitis* may occasion severe diarrhea. Terminal erysipelas, pneumonia, carbuncle, or sepsis may result from the generally *diminished resistance to infection*. The *uremic pericarditis*, however, occurs for the most part asymptomatically. Its presence is detected by the pericardial friction rub. Pain is absent. Occasionally large pericardial effusions may terminate life by the "tamponade" effect. In the majority of instances aspiration of the pericardium gives a sterile fluid. In slowly progressing chronic uremias signs of pericarditis may disappear during slight remissions in the intoxication, to recur with each exacerbation. The writer has observed several separate attacks of pericarditis in a patient with amyloid kidneys with glomerular lesions who was chronically uremic for a period of three years.

Pruritus is often an early symptom of uremia and one which may subject the patient to extreme torture, robbing him of sleep and rest. Various types of dermatitis are encountered. In some instances this is a *dermatitis medicamentosa* to which all patients with nephritis are unusually susceptible. A uremic peliosis may appear. Macules, papules, serous and hemorrhagic blebs may be observed. Extensive symptomatic purpura is sometimes seen, at times due to sepsis, at others to thrombocytopenia.

The blood in uremia gives evidence of three almost invariable concomitants, *azotemia, acidosis* and *anemia*.

Azotemia is expressed in the values observed for the various non-protein nitrogenous constituents of the blood. In 1821 Prevost and Dumas discovered that urea accumulated in the blood of a dog from which the kidneys had been removed. The increase of blood urea in nephritis was known to Bright in 1836. The level of total non-protein nitrogen at which uremic symptoms occur varies. In acute uremia severe intoxication may be manifest with values for "rest" nitrogen from 60 to 100 mg. per 100 cc., and in many cases with normal values. In more chronic processes in which there is a gradual accumulation of these bodies patients frequently exhibit only mild symptoms with values above 100 mg. per cent. In severe cases values up to 1000 mg. per cent may be observed. As the total rest nitrogen increases the fraction due to urea usually increases from the normal 50 per cent to

60 to 75 per cent of the total. In the beginning of azotemia uric acid is one of the substances to show a significant increase from its upper normal level of 4 mg. per cent. Slight increases (1.5 to 2.5 mg. per cent) of the so-called "creatinine" of the blood may occur early in the course of azotemia. "Creatinine" values of 5 mg. per cent have a serious prognostic significance as to the imminence of uremia, in which values of 5 to 60 mg. per cent may be observed. The writer has observed a return to normal of creatinine values after these had reached 12 mg. per cent.

The *acidosis* of renal insufficiency is reflected in the abnormally high values obtained for inorganic phosphate and sulphates, and in the low values for carbon dioxide combining power or alkaline reserve of the plasma. These chemical changes in the blood are brought about in two ways. The first of these is by retention of non-volatile acids, phosphoric and sulphuric, and by various toxic aromatic oxyacids, which are produced in the catabolism of protein. The retention of these acids reduces the amount of base in the plasma available for combination with carbon dioxide. This is influenced somewhat by the extent to which chloride is lost through vomiting.

The second mechanism by which renal acidosis is produced is the failure of the damaged kidney to form adequate amounts of ammonia for combination with the acids which are excreted. Benedict and Nash have proved conclusively that the ammonia of the urine is formed by the kidney itself. Normally the urinary ammonia increases in rough proportion to the amount of acid excreted, unless there is an excess of base available. By this means fixed base is spared to the body insofar as the kidney utilizes the volatile base ammonia for the neutralization of acids excreted. Due to functional insufficiency of ammonia formation plasma bases are depleted by the passage of fixed base into the urine in lieu of ammonia. Careful studies by Palmer and Henderson, in 1915, showed that in renal acidosis the pH of the urine was unusually low, and the ratio of ammonia to titratable acidity of the urine was low. The writer, in 1924, found that the same inadequate formation of ammonia occurs in diabetic coma as a result of functional insufficiency of the kidneys whether due to simple dehydration or renal disease, indicating that in the last analysis diabetic acidosis is renal acidosis. With normal renal function severe ketosis may exist without serious depletion of the alkaline reserve. The excessive loss of plasma base due to failure of the ammonia-forming function of the kidney may be compensated for by additional ingestion of bases in combination with organic acids which are capable of oxidation. The replenishing of the reserves of base is an important factor in treatment.

The *anemia of renal disease* depends upon a variety of factors. It is observed in the absence of uremia, but chronic uremia is rarely unaccompanied by anemia. In hemorrhagic nephritis the steady blood loss, continued often for weeks and months, represents a drain on the blood-forming organs of considerable magnitude. Whipple and co-workers have called attention to the importance of the kidney for the preservation and storage of materials necessary for blood regeneration. Next to liver, kidney tissue contains the greatest amount of those substances capable of stimulating blood regeneration in dogs which have been maintained at a constant level of anemia by bleeding. The writer has shown that kidney ingestion in pernicious anemia will produce remissions similar to those induced by liver or potent liver extracts. With these facts in mind, it is not surprising that anemia so frequently occurs in the end-stages of chronic nephritis. Added to this is the possibility that in some cases toxic substances may inhibit the normal regenerative activity of the bone-marrow, as the observations of Brown and Roth would indicate.

For the true chronic uremia the accumulation of toxic aromatic substances in the blood is of the greatest importance. Christison, in 1839, recognized the fetid odor of the serum from uremic patients. Obermeier and Popper associated this odor with the presence of increased quantities of indican in the blood. Becher has more recently developed a simple test for aromatic toxic substances, phenols and polyphenols and aromatic oxyacids which probably have their origin in the intestinal tract. This test is an extraordinarily reliable indication of the severity of intoxication in chronic uremia.

Estimation of Renal Function.—Until recently, theories of secretion of urine have had little relation to the tests applied for the estimation of renal function. The modern theory of Cushny finds ever increasing support. In an excellent recent review, Holten and Rehberg find that as yet few revisions are necessary. The theory starts with the postulate that an ultra-filtration through the glomerulus gives a protein-free fluid which is otherwise almost identical with the plasma and that this fluid is subsequently concentrated by resorption of water in the tubules. Since different substances occur in the urine in different concentrations, Cushny used the conception of "threshold substances" which were thought not to appear in the urine until their concentration in the blood had reached a certain "threshold value," that is, as long as the concentration in the blood was below this value they were completely reabsorbed by the cellular activity of the tubules.

Rehberg and Holten offer some modifications of the Cushny theory, particularly as it concerns the nature of the tubular resorptive process, which greatly reduces the number of so-called "threshold" substances. Beginning with the fact that, of all the common urinary constituents, creatinine is subjected to the greatest degree of concentration, *i.e.*, greatest difference between concentration in the blood and in the urine, it is calculated that 100 to 150 cc. of fluid must filter through the glomerulus per minute in order to accomplish the usual excretion of creatinine. The resorption of water from this filtrate by the tubules would concentrate all of its constituents, so that a difference in concentration of these substances between the fluid in the tubules and the blood would occur. This would tend to cause a backward diffusion of these substances through the walls of the tubules into the blood. Variable degrees of backward diffusion for different constituents would depend upon the relative degrees of permeability of the tubules for the substances in question. Thus the tubules would seem to be relatively impermeable to creatinine, and relatively less impermeable to urea, so that 20 to 50 per cent back diffusion of this substance occurs.

For substances like dextrose and sodium chloride, Rehberg is forced to assume an active and selective resorption, since both substances occur in the urine in concentrations less than that in the blood.

It must further be assumed that a true secretion may occur in the tubules in the case of ammonia at least, and possibly also of creatinine, if Benedict is correct in his belief that the so-called "creatinine" of the blood is not creatinine at all, but a nearly related precursor of urinary creatinine. If this were proved to be true it would seriously derange Rehberg's theory. Gaebler has confirmed the finding of Benedict that preformed creatinine does not exist in the blood.

Rehberg made calculations based upon the investigations of Vimtrup, that the human kidneys contain 2,000,000 glomeruli with a total surface for filtration of approximately 1.6 sq. m. The effective pressure for the filtration through the glomerular membrane is expressed by the following formula:

Filtration pressure, $P_f = P - P_o P_k$.

P = capillary blood pressure.

P_o = osmotic pressure of plasma proteins.

P_k = pressure of the filtrate in Bowman's capsule.

The pressure in Bowman's capsule must be sufficient to drive the fluid far enough into the tubules for resorption to begin. If tubular resorption is diminished P_k will rise and the amount of filtrate will be reduced.

If the number of glomeruli is reduced by disease, or if the capillary wall is thickened or rendered less permeable, or if the loops coalesce through inflammatory adhesions the amount of glomerular filtration will be reduced.

Similarly, fluctuations in the plasma proteins have a direct effect upon the degree of glomerular filtration, which is decreased if the protein content increases, other factors remaining constant.

In the study of glomerular filtration, Holten and Rehberg have devised the creatinine clearance determination. In this test 3 grams of creatinine dissolved in 50 cc. of water are given by mouth. The urine is collected in two one-hour periods. The blood samples are withdrawn at the end of the first and second hours. Enough liquid is ingested to ensure a suitable diuresis in the second hour. Creatinine is determined by analysis of the blood plasma and the urine and the creatinine clearance or glomerular filtration calculated by means of the following formula:

$$F = \frac{C V}{60}.$$

V = quantity of urine per hour.

$$C = \frac{\text{concentration of creatinine in urine}}{\text{mean concentration in two blood samples}}.$$

In normal individuals the filtration thus determined is rarely less than 100 cc. It varies when diuresis is less than maximal, probably due to inactive glomeruli. It varies with posture in normal individuals and with fluctuations in plasma proteins.

In patients with damaged kidneys the fluctuations were less. Blood non-protein nitrogen does not increase in patients with filtration rates above 50 cc. per minute. Uremic symptoms began to appear in patients with filtration rates below 30 cc. per minute.

In the writer's clinic the experience with this test is rapidly increasing its popularity. Many interesting data may be acquired by collateral determinations of the creatinine and urea clearance.

The *blood-urea clearance* is estimated by a formula devised by van Slyke, which expresses the relationship between blood-urea concentration, volume of urine and concentration of urea in the urine by means of which one may calculate the volume of blood which is completely cleared of its urea per minute. Van Slyke and his co-workers have applied this test of renal function to a considerable series of carefully studied patients with renal disease of various types, with the result that it has been established as one of the most valuable tests available. It has been found that a reduction of function to 40 per cent of normal, as measured by this test, may occur before functional insufficiency is detected by the phenolsulphonephthalein excretion, or by the blood urea or creatinine determinations. From the experience with the test it appears that two factors enter into the capacity of the kidneys to clear the blood of urea: (1) the actual amount of functionally efficient renal tissue, and (2) the amount of blood flow through the kidney. In the glomerulonephritis and in the nephroses it correlates well with the amount of structural change in the glomeruli which can be observed in the kidneys. In arteriosclerotic kidneys it is probable that the volume of blood flow through them, as effected by sclerosis or spasm of the arteries, is important, apart from the contraction of the kidney resulting from arterial closure.

For rates of diuresis below 2 cc. per minute the formula is as follows:

$$C_s = \frac{U}{B}\sqrt{V}.$$

C_s = standard urea clearance.
U = concentration of urea in urine.
B = concentration of urea in blood.
V = volume of urine in cubic centimeters per minute.

The average normal C_s for adults is 54 cc. per minute. For children or adults of unusual size a correction should be made, based upon the relative surface areas of the body, assuming average values to be based upon a surface area of 1.74 sq. meters.

For rates of diuresis above 2 cc. per minute the formula is:

$$C_m = \frac{U\,V}{B}.$$

C_m is the maximum urea clearance and has an average value of 75 cc. per minute for normal adults.

When both the standard and maximal urea clearance are determined in the same individual the same percentage of normal function is usually obtained with each.

The full significance and value of this test will not be known until it has been subjected to much more exhaustive clinical study than has yet been possible. As with all such tests its significance in any individual case will depend upon proper correlation with other data.

Among the simple tests of renal function which may be carried out by the practitioner without elaborate chemical laboratory equipment are the studies of variation in specific gravity of the urine and the response to water ingestion. A very valuable *concentration test* is described by Fishberg in which the patient receives his usual supper at 6 P.M., containing not more than 200 cc. of fluid. After this he neither eats nor drinks until after the test is completed on the following morning. The urine voided at bedtime or during the night is discarded. The urine is voided upon waking, and at the end of each of the next two hours. The specific gravity of each specimen is taken. With normal renal function the specific gravity of at least one specimen will exceed 1.022, often as high as 1.032. With severe impairment of function the maximum will not exceed 1.01. In patients with uremic symptoms the maximum is under 1.02 and usually approaches 1.01.

Low maximum specific gravity may be noted during diuresis in which edema fluid is being evacuated, in which case it is not a true measure of renal insufficiency. One must guard against being misled in cases in which the edema is larval or occult, as it often is in the early stages of hypertensive heart disease before outspoken congestive failure is recognized.

Dilution tests have been devised in which the patient, who remains in bed, ingests 1200 or 1500 cc. of water during one-half to three-quarters of an hour. The urine is collected in individual samples at regular intervals during four hours after water drinking. The entire amount should normally be eliminated within four hours, with the specific gravity falling to 1.002 in the largest specimen. Impairment of water excretion is shown by prolongation of the diuresis time. When this occurs in patients exhibiting normal concentrating power the disturbance in function is of extrarenal origin.

The older tests of Hedinger and Schlayer and of Mosenthal, in which the variations in specific gravity, nitrogen and chloride content of urine collected every two hours throughout the day, and during twelve hours at night, a standard diet being employed, have been abandoned in most clinics as too cumbersome in proportion to their value. The simple determination of specific gravity in two-hour day specimens, without control of the diet, reveals impairment of renal function in the "fixation" or constancy of specific gravity at subnormal levels. Normal individuals should show a variation of 9 to 10 points between the maximum and minimum.

The simple "two-hour test" will often reveal functional insufficiency of the kidneys in patients with severe pernicious anemia in whom other evidence of renal disease is lacking.

Of greater value is the determination of the volume and specific gravity of the twelve-hour night urine. Volumes above 600 cc. and specific gravities below 1.014 are unusual in normal individuals, unless these have taken unusual quantities of liquids with or after the evening meal.

The *phenolsulphonephthalein test* is the one most universally employed, because of its simplicity. It has many limitations, since the excretion rate of the dye may be influenced by extrarenal factors such as the amount of water ingested and the state of the circulation. A very considerable amount of damage to the kidneys may exist before insufficiency is revealed by this test.

To be of greatest value the conditions under which the test is performed should be more carefully controlled than is often the case. Each measurement of the amount of dye injected, care in selection of the site and manner of injection, standardized procedure with regard to amount of water ingested before the test are all factors of importance. If these details are carefully attended to it may be of some value to record the rate of excretion of the dye in fractions of the two-hour period, after allowing ten minutes for its appearance. Normally 60 to 85 per cent is excreted in two hours, about one-half the total appearing in the first half. When the total excretion decreases larger fractions appear in the later specimens.

The phenolsulphonephthalein test gives a rough estimate of the kidney function at the moment, as it is influenced by extrarenal factors as well as by renal disease. The excretion of this dye is greatly diminished in passive congestion of the kidneys, and also when diuresis is inhibited in states of dehydration. Abnormally high values may be obtained on the other hand if diuresis has been increased by excessive water intake, or during the subsidence of an edema.

NEPHRITIS, OR BRIGHT'S DISEASE.

Definition.—Bright's disease is not a single disease but a group of diseases which have in common bilateral non-suppurative lesions of the kidney, associated with albuminous urine and an abnormal number of casts. In every instance the renal disease appears to be but a part of a general systemic disorder. These diseases or disorders fall into three main groups, which may be classified according to the nature of the chief or characteristic renal lesion as: (*a*) glomerulonephritis, (*b*) parenchymatous or tubular nephritis, or nephrosis (Volhard and Fahr), or (*c*) arteriosclerotic nephritis or nephrosclerosis (Volhard and Fahr). Or they may be classified in the less consistent way of Addis as: (*a*) hemorrhagic, (*b*) degenerative and (*c*) arteriosclerotic. The terminology of Addis is translatable into that of Volhard and Fahr. Hemorrhagic Bright's disease corresponds to glomerulonephritis, degenerative Bright's disease to nephrosis, arteriosclerotic Bright's disease to nephrosclerosis.

History.—In 1827, Richard Bright, in his "Reports on Medical Cases," described postmortem findings in "diseases terminating in dropsical effusions," in which he said "I have never yet examined the body of patient dying with dropsy *attended with coagulable urine* in whom some obvious derangement was not discovered in the kidneys." In 1833, in a further report upon patients with albuminuria, to test for which he heated urine in a spoon over a candle or treated it with nitric acid, he said, "My conviction is complete as to the existence of some decided connection between three facts—anasarca, coagulable urine and *diseased function going on to diseased structure of the kidney.*" The final report of his work is in two papers in Guy's Hospital Reports for 1836.

The first, "Cases and Observations on Renal Disease Accompanied by the Secretion of Albuminous Urine," is followed by the second, the famous "Tabular View of the Morbid Appearances Occurring in 100 Cases, in Connection with Albuminous Urine." He began by commenting on the frequency of deaths with changes in the structure of the kidney, and on the want of success in treating it. This he believed to be due to the insidious nature of the disease, and to the fact that it is usually far advanced before it is detected. "There is great reason to suppose that the seeds of this disease are often sown at an early period; and that intervals of apparent health produce a false security in the patient, his friends, and his medical attendants, even when apprehension has been early excited."

In his tabular summary of morbid appearances he noted "the extraordinary manner in which the blood becomes impoverished." He was familiar with the increased content of urea, which had been discovered only a decade before by Prevost and Dumas, and with the reduced amount of albuminous substances in the blood of some cases.

Concerning the hypertrophy of the heart he remarks, "This naturally leads us to look for some less local cause for the unusual efforts to which the heart has been impelled; and the two most ready solutions appear to be, either that the *altered quality of the blood* affords irregular and unwonted stimulus to the organ immediately; or, that it is so affects the minute and capillary circulation as to render *greater action necessary to force the blood through the distant subdivisions of the vascular systems.*"

All the usually associated postmortem changes were known to him. The modes of death most frequently noted were apoplexy, coma or convulsions. Long before Riva-Rocci provided a convenient method of measuring it, he noted the hardness of pulse. In fact there is little to add to his nosographic treatment of the subject, except the results of a few modern functional tests, and the correlations with microscopic changes in the kidneys.

HEMORRHAGIC BRIGHT'S DISEASE.

Definition.—The use of this term in the sense that it is used by Thomas Addis applies to all those forms of Bright's disease in which an increased number of red blood corpuscles may be demonstrated in the urine, which may be correlated with diffuse or focal glomerular lesions in the kidney.

Since clinical and experimental investigations into etiology and pathogenesis have shown that there are wide differences between diffuse glomerulonephritis and focal glomerulonephritis, these two forms of hemorrhagic Bright's disease will be treated as far as possible as separate entities.

Diffuse glomerulonephritis may exist in acute, latent, chronic or active forms, which may heal completely, or may progress, usually with remissions and exacerbations to death from renal insufficiency. It should be differentiated as far as possible from focal glomerulonephritis, which occurs during the active course of infection and usually subsides when the causative infection subsides.

The latent form may become chronically active, the process very rarely may be reversed, or the latent form may have an acute exacerbation as may be seen in the diagram modified from Addis.

Etiology.—Diffuse glomerulonephritis has come to be associated most frequently with streptococcal infections of some form. It is the classical renal lesion of the convalescence from *scarlet fever*, as distinguished from that which may occur at the height of the disease.

When it follows *acute* tonsillitis a latent period of at least two to three weeks is usually observed between the onset of the infection and the appearance of the nephritis. The relationship of the renal disease to the preceding infection frequently cannot be determined, particularly in adults. The onset is often so insidious that all connection with the antecedent disease is lost, though the history may record one or more attacks of severe tonsillitis, otitis media, mastoiditis, sinusitis, rhinitis, bronchitis, or possibly some wound or skin infection with lymphadenitis. In war it is not infrequently associated with the "pyodermias" complicating scabies and pediculosis. It is extraordinarily rare in the course of erysipelas, the renal complications of which are usually focal and associated with bacteriemia.

In the long list of diseases associated with *hemorrhagic nephritis* the evidence is not always clear as to whether the renal lesion produced was of the diffuse or focal variety, or in fact whether intercurrent disease had merely produced an acute exacerbation of a previously existing chronic or latent diffuse glomerulonephritis. Aside from simple "cloudy swelling" and febrile albuminuria, the renal lesions occurring in the course of bacteriemias, such as typhoid fever, or malaria, are usually of the focal variety which disappear with the primary disease. This is true of the nephritis which occurs at the height of scarlet fever, and in relapsing fever and Weil's disease. Fishberg emphasizes the important difference between the two types of glomerulonephritis in endocarditis lenta. The diffuse form, which may progress with edema and hypertension to the uremic stage, is most commonly found in the "bacteria-free" phases of the disease. The focal embolic form, giving rise to the "flea-bitten kidney" so frequently found at autopsy in the bacteriemic forms of subacute bacterial endocarditis, gives few symptoms apart from hematuria.

Exposure to cold is a most important predisposing factor, though it is very doubtful whether it can cause nephritis apart from antecedent infection. Acute hemorrhagic nephritis occurred in outbreaks of epidemic proportions among troops during the World War, who were subjected to long exposures to cold in the mud of partly flooded trenches and shell holes, particularly in newly acquired terrain before more comfortable organization of defense was possible, with duckboards, well-dubbined boots and dry socks. Ancient clinical tradition has emphasized the importance of warmth and protection from chilling during the convalescence from scarlet fever as a means of preventing the occurrence of postscarlatinal nephritis.

Pregnancy also has a most unfavorable effect upon preexisting latent or chronic hemorrhagic nephritis. When an exacerbation of such a process occurs in the course of pregnancy it is rarely justifiable to permit the pregnancy to continue. A considerable number of women survive the first pregnancy under these conditions and few may survive two, or three, and, in rare instances, four pregnancies, before the renal reserves are entirely exhausted. Between the pregnancies the process may become latent or nearly so, though each succeeding pregnancy leaves the patient with a lower renal reserve.

Age.—Acute hemorrhagic nephritis is more common in childhood than in adult life. This is probably due to the higher incidence of streptococcal and other acute infections in childhood.

Sex.—In childhood the incidence is nearly equal in the two sexes. In adults there is a clear-cut predominance of acute hemorrhagic nephritis in males, possibly due to their greater exposure to wetness and cold.

Pathogenesis.—Evidence seems to be clear-cut that the phenomena of diffuse glomerulonephritis are not due to direct bacterial invasion of the kidneys. Blood and urine are usually sterile on culture. On the other hand, in those diseases characterized by bacteriemia in which bacteria are frequently found in the urine, diffuse glomerulonephritis occurs with extreme rarity. Such renal lesions as do accompany bacteriemia and sepsis are either acute focal embolic glomerulitis, acute interstitial nephritis or multiple abscesses or infarcts of the kidneys.

Trask and Blake demonstrated that the toxin of Streptococcus scarlatinæ was excreted in the urine of patients with scarlet fever at the height of the disease, but this does not explain the development of the postscarlatinal nephritis from two to six weeks later. Duval and Hibbard injected living streptococci and toxic filtrates from streptococci into animals. In animals which were non-immune no lesions were produced, unless sepsis resulted, in which case an acute interstitial nephritis might occur. However, if bacteriolysis were permitted to take place in the peritoneum of an immune animal, glomerular lesions were produced. This occurred also when the animals received filtrates from cultures treated with homologous immune serum.

Schick was the first to suggest that the postscarlatinal nephritis depended upon development of hypersensitiveness in the course of the process of immunity. Longcope studied the production of renal lesions by repeated injections of foreign proteins. With his co-workers Longcope studied the renal phenomena in serum sickness and observed the simultaneous occurrence of urticaria with glomerulonephritis. More recently he has studied the skin reactions to toxic filtrates from cultures of streptococci isolated from foci of infection in patients with glomerulonephritis, observing that these patients react more severely than do others without nephritis. In the majority of instances the streptococci were of the beta-hemolytic type.

Pathology.—**Acute Diffuse Glomerulonephritis.**—In the early acute stages the gross appearance of the kidney is very slightly altered from normal. In the majority of instances they are larger than normal and of softer consistency. The capsule can be readily separated and the underlying surface of the kidneys is smooth and grayish or reddish-brown in color. On section the cut surface may show little variation from normal, in other cases the dark medulla stands out sharply against a pale cortex, or in later stages the markings are indistinct, with a general cloudy appearance and evidence of fatty degeneration in grayish-yellow areas. These appearances are further modified by the presence or absence of venous stasis. The glomeruli can sometimes be made out as pale translucent points, in other cases they are dark hemorrhagic spots. Occasional red streaks of blood-containing tubules may be observed.

On *microscopic* examination the distinctive feature is the nearly universal change in the glomeruli, which show a variety of appearances depending on the intensity and duration of the process. Both intra- and extra-capillary lesions occur. The earliest changes are seen in the endothelial cells of the capillary loops, which enlarge and appar- ently increase in number. Later these cells appear to fuse. In still later stages hyalinization may be observed. The extra-capillary epithelium swells and proliferates. An increased number of leukocytes accumulates in the tuft. The result of these changes is that the glomerular tuft appears enlarged, the lobulation between capillary loops disappears by fusion or adhesion, the glomerulus appears poor in blood or is ischemic as a rule, and unusually rich in nuclei—endothe- lial, epithelial and leukocytic. Within Bowman's capsule blood, fibrin and desquamated cells, or an amorphous granular detritus may be found. *Nearly all glomeruli show changes*, a fact of importance in distinguishing the diffuse from the focal types of glomerulonephritis.

The tubules show various degrees of early degenerative change, cloudy swelling or early fatty changes. The lumina of the tubules contain the ingredients of the urinary casts, blood, leukocytes, granular detritus. Between the tubules there is little evidence of inflammatory reaction, such as may be seen in the focal type.

The arteries show few changes in the majority of instances. In some very severe cases a necrotizing arteriolitis, particularly involving the afferent arterioles, has been described.

Chronic Diffuse Glomerulonephritis.—This may present a wide range of anatomic pictures from large pale kidneys to small granular con- tracted kidneys. The time element is probably of the greatest impor- tance in determining the degree of contraction of the kidney. Cases which have run a relatively short course, in which non-cardiac edema has been prominent, usually show the larger pale kidneys. Those which have run a slower course, or have been more prominently charac- terized by hypertension, furnish the greater number of contracted kidneys.

When the kidneys are large and pale the capsule usually strips readily, revealing a grayish surface with a yellowish mottling and small hemorrhagic areas, or again a generalized yellow tinge due to lipids may be seen. This general appearance is further modified if chronic passive congestion occurs. The consistency is usually soft, and the weight is increased, sometimes greatly. On cut surface the dark medulla stands out against the wide, pale, grayish or yellowish cortex. The glomeruli vary in appearance, some pale and grayish, others seen as hemorrhagic dots. An irregular reddish streaking of the tubules may be noted.

At the other extreme stands the small hard granular contracted kidney, with thickened capsule which tears off with adherent cortex. Depressed scarred areas are dark brown against the paler grayish or

34

yellowish areas of partly degenerated cortical surface. On section the cortex is seen to be narrow and irregular, and in extreme sclerosis the fundamental architecture of both cortex and medulla is much obscured; irregular areas of scar tissue surround surviving but degenerated areas of fatty parenchyma.

Between the two extremes transition types are found. Histologically the gross appearance depends chiefly upon the relative proportions of surviving but degenerated parenchyma and the scars of replacement fibrosis.

On *microscopic examination* the essential diagnostic changes are those of the *glomeruli* in which all those remaining are involved. Some of these show changes such as were described in the acute stage with swelling, nuclear richness and ischemia. Others show that circulation has been reëstablished through them, though the tufts are distorted and often adherent to the capsule and various degrees of hyalinization are seen. In some glomeruli the capsular epithelium proliferates to form crescentic masses of cells. These processes of intra-capillary and extra-capillary change frequently progress side by side until a concentric thickening of the capsule encloses a homogeneous hyalinized glomerular tuft, both capillary and capsular space being obliterated. In the final stages no vestiges of glomeruli remain in the dense scars. The *tubules* show a great range of appearances from the earliest degeneration to more advanced fatty changes. Dilated tubules are seen here and there, lined by a low syncytial epithelium. Elsewhere nests of epithelial cells with pyknotic nuclei may remain as vestigial islets in the midst of extensive fibrosis and round-cell infiltration, which replaces the atrophied renal elements. The *arteries* in long-standing cases show changes in the majority of instances. These changes are of two main types, an endarteritis obliterans and arteriosclerosis. In the former the lesions consist of intimal proliferation and degeneration, which Fishberg believes to be due to the primary changes in the glomeruli, since they are confined to the renal arterioles. The arteriosclerotic changes consist in reduplication of the internal elastic membrane, hyaline deposits and other changes which are commonly seen in arterioles associated with continued hypertension.

Focal Glomerulonephritis.—Focal glomerulonephritis is the form of hemorrhagic nephritis encountered in the course of acute infections with bacteriemia. The gross appearance of the kidneys usually shows little change, though at times they may appear larger and darker with congestion. On section the architecture is nearly normal except for small hemorrhagic areas. In cases of subacute bacterial endocarditis the numerous small cortical hemorrhages may give the kidney a "flea-bitten" appearance.

On microscopic examination focal interstitial lesions are seen as accumulations of lymphocytes and monocytes. Only a part of the glomeruli show any lesions whatever. In some nothing may be detected except an escape of blood into the capsular space. In others intra-capillary proliferation is seen affecting one lobule only, or a portion of a lobule or a glomerulus, the remaining capillary loops appearing to be normal. The portion of the glomerulus involved often becomes homogeneous with necrosis. If this portion is adjacent to the capsule, either adhesions are formed or epithelial cells are desquamated. Here and there focal degeneration in the tubules is noted, consisting of cloudy swelling and early fatty change, with blood, leukocytes, and epithelial cells and detritus in the lumen. Many tubules are perfectly normal. In many cases bacteria can be demonstrated within the lesions by appropriate staining technic.

Symptoms.—The clinical pictures encountered are extremely varied. In the initial phase the onset may either be acute and fulminating or insidiously symptomless. The disease process may pursue a variety of courses. The initial phase can heal completely or it may pass through a subacute to a chronic active state, or again to a latent phase. The chronic active or latent phases can result in healing or

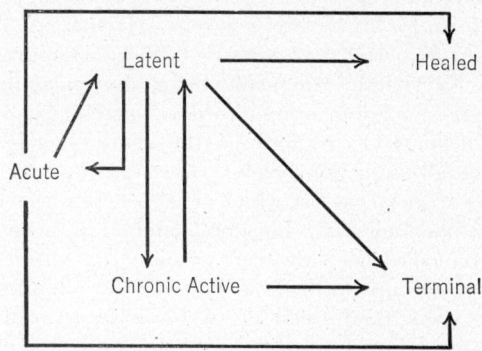

Fig. 22.—Possible courses of hemorrhagic nephritis (modified from Addis).

may progress to the terminal stage of renal insufficiency by a series of acute or subacute exacerbations of activity. A nephrotic form of hemorrhagic nephritis which is distinguished from true nephrosis with difficulty is often encountered in the subacute or chronic active stages.

Initial Stage.—The acute onset occurs typically in the third or fourth week after scarlet fever or an acute attack of tonsillitis. In the prodromal stage the patient feels tired and indisposed, pallor is noted, with slight puffiness of the face about the eyes, and occasionally of the hands and feet. In other cases edema almost escapes detection. A dull headache, usually occipital, may be complained of. High-colored, red or smoky urine is noted, and rarely a dull lumbar ache and slight burning on micturition may be felt. Slight fever and leukocytosis and moderate elevation of blood pressure are usually present. With rising blood pressure and diminishing urine volume the phenomena of acute "false" or eclamptic uremia may be ushered in by any of its varied forms—mania, eclampsia or coma, with meningismus, accompanied by various focal neurologic symptoms, previously described, such as amaurosis, hemiopia, hemiplegias, monoplegias, aphasias and choreiform disturbances. In favorable cases the hypertension diminishes, urine volume increases and in a few days the symptoms are entirely abated. Uninterrupted progress toward healing may be shown by the record of decreasing hematuria and albuminuria until the urine is entirely normal in two to four weeks. More commonly the disease is prolonged, passing from the acute initial stage into one of subacute activity which will be described below.

During the acute onset the blood shows almost no abnormal changes. There is often little or no increase of nitrogenous bodies, and during the initial edema the plasma proteins remain within normal limits. The phenolsulphonephthalein excretion is very temporarily decreased during the stage of oliguria, but promptly rises as good diuresis occurs. Even while the urine volumes are small, good concentration is observed. The blood-urea clearance remains subnormal even after phenolsulphonephthalein excretion has become normal.

It is more common for the acute sequela of the initial phase to persist in a subacute form for six to twelve weeks. Hematuria continues and frequently slight hypertension persists. The proteinuria increases, a large globulin fraction in the urine being not uncommon. Coincidentally a progressive fall in serum proteins, particularly of the albumin fraction, may occur. Occasionally in the acute sequela of the initial phase the serum albumin falls below 3.5 per cent and the total plasma proteins below 5.5 per cent, at which level a nephrotic edema usually appears. This phenomenon is far more common in the acute exacerbations of a chronic process, however. Unless the initial acute attack shows well-marked improvement in both urinary findings and blood-urea clearance tests by the end of twelve weeks, the disease almost invariably passes into the chronic active phase. Unfavorable signs, by which the development of chronic nephritis may be predicted, are progressive anemia, persistent elevation of blood pressure with gradual increase in heart size to the left, and decreasing blood-urea clearance and power of concentration. The transition to a hemorrhagic pseudonephrosis is an unfavorable development, though healing is still possible if this does not persist beyond six months from the onset. As an alternative to healing the process may come to a standstill in a symptomless *chronic latent stage* in which there is persistently lowered functional capacity as measured by urea clearance and concentration tests, even though the phenolsulphonephthalein tests and blood chemical findings may be normal. This latent phase may be prolonged for months, or even for years in rare instances, until some unfavorable influence, such as exposure, intercurrent infection or pregnancy, precipitates a renewed period of activity.

Acute exacerbations of a chronic hemorrhagic nephritis are symptomatically similar to the initial acute stage. The underlying chronicity of the disease may be recognized or suspected by the following signs, some of which are sure to be present. These are the cardiovascular or retinal sequelæ of hypertension, and anemia, acidosis and marked azotemia.

Cardiac hypertrophy and hypertensive retinal changes are rarely detected unless the process is of more than four months' duration. Severe anemia at the onset, marked elevation of blood urea and signs of renal acidosis are rare in the initial acute attack.

Chronic Active Stage.—This phase of diffuse glomerulonephritis is characterized at all times by *hematuria*, which may, however, be of such low grade that it is entirely overlooked in the casual microscopic examination of the urinary sediment. It is in this stage that the careful technic of the Addis sediment counts becomes most essential to a proper diagnosis, particularly when the clinical picture is dominated by edema with low plasma proteins, and when hypertension and increased blood urea are absent, as they frequently are.

Edema, a frequent symptom of this stage, may arise in three ways. The first has just been referred to, the nephrotic type. The second is the edema of heart failure resulting from hypertension and arteriosclerosis. The third is nephritic, which may occur in acute exacerbations. Combination forms may be encountered. Nephrotic edema is a feature of the earlier stages of chronic activity, which tends to disappear as the terminal stage is reached. The cardiac type of edema is more apt to occur as the terminal stage is approached.

Hypertension may characterize the chronic active phase throughout, though it is frequently absent in the presence of nephrotic edema. When this is true the clinical picture may exactly simulate that of true lipoid nephrosis, except for the evidence of hematuria contributed by the Addis counts. The total plasma proteins, the ratio of serum albumin to globulin, may be low. Blood lipids may be increased and albuminuria intense.

Hypertension tends to increase in progressing cases as the nephrotic phenomena subside. The writer has observed several instances of a remarkably rapid transformation from a nephrotic stage in which hypertension was absent to a non-edematous state in which elevation of blood pressure was marked. One patient lost 70 pounds of weight in twelve days, with disappearance of edema. The systolic blood pressure, which had been normal in the dropsical state, rose to 190, and retinal hemorrhages and exudates appeared, together with marked increase in the non-protein nitrogen of the blood.

The degree of cardiac hypertrophy and of vascular disease as seen in the retina depends upon the duration and intensity of the hypertension. In some cases this is practically absent until the terminal stage, except for transient elevations during acute exacerbations. In others some elevation of blood pressure persists throughout, progressively increasing as the terminal stage is reached, and in these cases the cardiovascular, cerebral and retinal phenomena may be pronounced. The degree of hypertension encountered is usually far below the levels seen in essential hypertension. In the nephritic hypertension of adults, before the terminal stage is reached, the systolic blood pressure is rarely over 170 to 180 and the diastolic pressure rarely over 110 mm. Hg. With children the degree of hypertension must be regarded in relation to the normal blood pressure for the age of the child. In some cases the phenomena of hypertensive encephalopathy or of hypertensive heart disease may become prominent in the picture. The more usual course is one of gradual progressive decrease in renal function until the terminal stage, characterized by true chronic uremia, anemia and renal acidosis is reached.

In the measurement of the progressive decrease of renal function in the chronic active phase, the urea clearance, phenolsulphonephthalein and concentration tests all give consistent results. Van Slyke separates the terminal from the chronic active stage by the fall in urea clearance below 20 per cent of the normal. The phenolsulphonephthalein test gives results which are misleadingly low when passive congestion of the kidneys supervenes, and perhaps misleadingly high results during the nephrotic stage. The progressive fall in concentrating power, as measured by the low maximum specific gravity on a "dry" day, or by the low specific gravity and large volume of the night urine, together with "fixation" of the densities of the day urine voided every two hours, all provide reliable evidence of the advance of diffuse glomerulo-nephritis to the terminal stage of contracted kidneys.

Terminal Stage.—This phase is separated, more or less arbitrarily by van Slyke, by the decrease in the blood-urea clearance to less than 20 per cent of its normal value. The symptomatology of the terminal stage has much in common with the final phases of arteriosclerotic Bright's disease, just as the final anatomic pictures in contracted kidneys are very similar. In the final shrinkage and scarring of the kidney in glomerulonephritis, arteriosclerosis often plays a large part. Just as the pathologist may separate primary from secondary con-traction by the observation of glomerulitis in the latter, so the clinician must depend upon the demonstration of *hematuria* by Addis counts in order to clinch his differentiation in those cases which have not been accurately observed in the earlier phases of their development. An exception to the rule, hematuria in "malignant" hypertension will be discussed later.

In the same way *hematuria* and *hypertension* serve to set this stage of hemorrhagic nephritis apart from the rare cases of nephrotic con-tracted kidneys, or amyloid kidneys with *degenerative* obliteration of glomeruli.

The transition to the terminal stage may occur directly from the initial acute stage, but more usually from the chronic active stage. It may in some cases occur suddenly, in a matter of two or three weeks, in others more slowly and gradually. The nephrotic phenomena dimin-ish, edema is less, plasma proteins increase, albuminuria diminishes as the transition occurs. *Hypertension* increases. The nitrogenous bodies of the blood increase. Gradually, or rapidly, the symptoms of true chronic uremia may appear, with its intoxication and cachexia, its anemia, its acidosis and its pericarditis, which have been previously described. The full development of chronic true uremia may be inter-rupted by the occurrence of apoplexy, hypertensive encephalopathy, intercurrent terminal pneumonia, or of heart failure, and edema when present is usually due to the latter.

As regards the tests for renal function, the loss of concentrating power shown in low constant specific gravities of the urine specimens, is extreme. The blood-urea clearances decrease from levels of 20 down to 5 per cent of normal. Patients may remain actively at work when urea clearance is between 10 to 20 per cent of normal. The writer has seen a case in which the patient, a young man, aged twenty-one years, worked actively in a factory up to ten days before the discovery that his urea clearance was only 10 per cent of normal, at which time the non-protein nitrogen of his blood was 100 mg. per cent. He was severely anemic. Moderate Kussmaul breathing was noted. The carbon dioxide combining power of the plasma was 25 volumes per cent. The blood pressure was 190 systolic and 110 diastolic. The heart showed evidence of both hypertrophy and dilatation. The exitus which occurred in a few days was due to a sudden edema of the lungs.

With extreme care and greatly limited activity patients may survive for months with a blood-urea clearance less than 10 per cent of normal, suffering at all times, but with varying intensity, from uremic symptoms.

Focal nephritis gives no symptoms apart from the disease in which it develops, except hematuria, albuminuria and casts. There may be lumbar pain or costo-vertebral tenderness at times. Edema and hypertension do not occur and renal insufficiency is extremely rare.

Differential Diagnosis.—The recognition of glomerulonephritis, diffuse or focal, depends upon the demonstration of bilateral renal hematuria. This demands careful standardization of conditions and quantitative estimation of the blood in the urine, as described by Addis. By this means only can one differentiate some cases of nephrotic hemorrhagic Bright's disease from the genuine nephrosis. Both conditions may exist without hypertension. The occurrence of nitrogen retention in some cases of true nephrosis with degenerative changes in the glomeruli makes it impossible to use this as a differential criterion.

In some cases, dangerously and erroneously called "essential hematuria," it may be necessary to exhaust all the resources of a urologic surgeon to rule out tuberculosis, tumors, stones or sources of blood other than the glomeruli of the kidneys. The diagnosis of "essential hematuria," arrived at by exclusion, should never be accepted as anything but some form of hemorrhagic Bright's disease.

The differentiation of hemorrhagic Bright's disease from hypertension with good renal function presents no difficulties. The presence of a quantitative increase of blood in the urine sediment is essential to the former. The degree of hypertension is also important. In hemorrhagic nephritis a blood pressure above 160 is nearly always accompanied by easily recognizable urinary abnormalities, and systolic pressures of 180 mm. or more are usually accompanied by severe symptoms. On the other hand, the primary hypertensive patients usually exhibit no urinary abnormalities and often no symptoms with systolic pressures over 200 mm. Hg. Edema occurs in this latter group only with heart failure, in which the systolic pressures may fall while at the same time passive congestion of the kidneys increases albumin, casts and even red cells in the urine. The Addis counts often reveal red cells to the number of 1,000,000 per twelve hours with chronic passive congestion of the kidneys. In such a case it is usually necessary to wait until passive congestion is relieved to get the true measure of renal function and the true pictures of the urinary sediment.

Patients with malignant hypertension present some difficulties, due to the fact that microscopic hematuria commonly occurs in this condition. Its recognition depends upon the peculiar appearance of the retinal lesions, and upon the appearance of marked hypertension and vascular phenomena before renal function has been seriously reduced.

Prognosis.—In acute diffuse glomerulonephritis the prognosis is greatly influenced by the age of the patient. Among children the great majority of cases heal completely. In adult life a far greater proportion become chronic. Of evil omen is the persistence of hematuria beyond four months. After six months one may be practically certain that a chronic process has become established. Also of bad prognostic significance is the persistence of hypertension and of high globulin fractions in the urine. If a latent stage is reached without too great reduction of renal function (urea clearance 50 per cent or better) it may be possible to arrest the disease by careful elimination of infectious foci, and careful avoidance of exposure, pregnancy and other factors predisposing to renewed activity of the disease. No rule can be formulated as to the rate of progress or duration of life. The rate of progress is best measured by serial determinations of urea and creatinine clearances.

The occurrence of hypertensive cerebral symptoms or of albuminuric retinitis in hemorrhagic nephritis is of serious significance. The duration of life is apt to be less than when these occur in non-nephritic cases. Anemia and renal acidosis are likewise evil omens portending rapid progress toward the end.

Prophylaxis.—Recognition of the possibility of renal complications in all streptococcal infections, in particular those affecting the upper air passages and pharyngeal lymphoid tissue, should lead to precautions particularly against chilling and exposure during the dangerous period of convalescence or subsiding infection. Surgical eradication of chronic active foci of infection is indicated when this is possible.

Treatment.—The therapy of hemorrhagic nephritis involves proper management in the acute stage of the oliguria or suppression of urine, the acute false uremia and the nephritic edema. After subsidence of the acute phenomena, eradication of infectious foci is in order. In the chronic stages dietary management is directed toward maintenance of good nutrition, the control of nephrotic edema and the regulation of protein catabolism to levels as nearly as possible within the range of the reduced functional capacity of the kidneys. For the rest the treatment is symptomatic.

Acute Stage.—The first efforts on putting the patient to bed should be to secure warmth. Flannel bed garments should be used. The patient may sleep between light blankets instead of sheets. Additional warmth may be provided by hot-water bottles or an electric pad over the lumbar regions, provided the patient is conscious. The room should be kept at a comfortable, even temperature, with indirect ventilation so as to avoid draughts.

The diet should be as nearly *salt-free* as possible. By use of salt-free bread and butter, avoiding milk and canned foods and salted meats, a diet may be prepared of common ingredients in any home with no more than 1.5 grams of salt. This restriction of salt is fundamental to the control of edemas of all types.

If the patient is not nauseated or vomiting, the protein should be restricted to 45 grams *per diem*, and carbohydrate and fat given as liberally as the patient can comfortably take them in order to lower the endogenous protein catabolism as much as possible. As the acute symptoms subside the protein should be raised gradually to 75 grams *per diem* to avoid excessive protein loss.

If the patient is nauseated or vomiting, glucose may be given parenterally by vein as 10 per cent glucose, or by proctoclysis or hypodermoclysis as 5 per cent glucose. Physiologic saline solution should not be used for this purpose, as it increases the edema. As soon as possible fruit juices with lactose should be given by mouth.

The total fluid intake needs careful consideration. Enough fluid must be given to balance the loss from the skin and lungs, which may amount to 1200 to 1500 cc. *per diem* in a warmed bed in a dry, steam-heated atmosphere. Beyond this point water should be given as a diuretic, being added in small increments (500 cc.) which may safely be increased if the urine volume increases with each addition. Water is a safe diuretic only when salt is excluded from the diet. With salt restriction its diuretic action should be sought.

No other diuretics should be used. Christian showed clearly how harmful their effects could be. This applies to purine diuretics such as caffeine or theocine, and those containing mercury, such as novasurol and salyrgan, should also be avoided.

If the bowels are sluggish milk of magnesia may be given in sufficient amount to produce loose stools without purging. It is well tolerated in the presence of nausea.

For the management of acute eclamptic uremia with the sudden onset of convulsions a wedge should be inserted between the teeth, if possible. Convulsions are usually well controlled by intramuscular injections of sodium amytal or similar preparations. In performing the lumbar puncture, which frequently gives prompt relief, care should be taken to permit fluid to escape slowly to avoid the formation of a pressure cone in the foramen magnum.

Magnesium sulphate is recommended by Blackfan for intravenous injection, 200 cc. of 1 per cent solution. Others recommend slow injection of 20 cc. of a 10 per cent solution. This may be repeated one or more times at two-hour intervals if necessary. The total magnesium sulphate injected should not exceed 0.1 gram per kg. body weight. The intramuscular administration of the soluble barbiturates is to be preferred, however.

In acute nephritis bed rest is essential until hematuria has subsided, not only because of rest but on account of the protection from exposure. Convalescence in a warm dry climate is desirable whenever feasible.

As a prophylactic measure against reactivation of the disease a careful eradication of genuinely infectious foci should be carried out. This should be done in any case when it is obvious that the acute process has become chronic. In spite of the fact that a tonsillectomy will frequently cause an exacerbation of the nephritis one frequently notes the first real improvement after this subsides. It should be said, however, that this eradication should be confined to definitely demonstrable foci of infection. Too often the program consists of a ruthless removal of foci which are merely suspected of activity. Needless to say the results in such cases are apt to be disappointing, aside from the mutilation of the patient.

In the chronic active stage with urea clearance above 20 per cent, every effort should be made to *maintain the nutrition* of the patient. It is not improbable that the great frequency of the nephrotic type of chronic hemorrhagic nephritis is due to the nearly universal habit of prescribing diets so low in protein that a "hunger edema" is superimposed upon the picture. This irrational procedure is due to the general ignorance of the fundamental principles of nutrition and of the importance of the plasma proteins. Patients with chronic nephritis should receive a diet high in carbohydrate and fat designed to lower the endogenous catabolism of protein, so that the lowest possible requirement of nitrogen excretion will be imposed upon the damaged kidneys. They should receive in the diet enough protein to balance this catabolism and enough more to replace the protein which is lost in the urine. If the plasma proteins are low, one may assume that the body has depleted its deposits of protein, and one usually finds food protein retained with avidity for regeneration of depleted tissue and plasma proteins, provided a high calorie diet is given, with care as to sources of vitamins. Foods with alkaline ash should be chosen to balance the acidity of the protein ash. Careful studies by Keutmann and the writer have shown that great improvement in nephrotic types of hemorrhagic nephritis may follow the procedure outlined above. Hematuria is not increased nor is the blood pressure elevated. With the higher protein intake a large water intake is necessary, and the *diet must be kept salt-free*. Albuminuria is increased somewhat but not enough to prevent the gain in deposit protein. It has been gratifying to observe improvement as regards disappearance of nephrotic edema and the anemia and in the increase of blood-urea clearance following such treatment. When the depleted body proteins are restored the protein intake should be adjusted to a normal balance level.

In the terminal stages it is often impossible to keep the rest nitrogen of the blood within normal limits by high calorie feeding even at a minimal level of nitrogen balance. Particularly does this become difficult when the nausea of uremia interferes. Vomiting and the reduction of fluid intake further increase the azotemia and uremic intoxication. Parenteral injection of fluid becomes imperative in such cases, and may be supplemented by proctoclysis if this is tolerated. By mouth, as far as possible, fluid is given in the form of fruit juices to which are added potassium citrate and lactose. (Potassium citrate up to 12 grams *per diem*.) Sodium citrate may be used in non-edematous cases. Such drinks help replace the depleted alkaline reserve of *renal acidosis*, and the lactose serves the double purpose of relieving ketosis and sparing protein. By this means the alkaline reserve of the plasma may be gradually built up.

The *anemia* of the terminal and chronic active stages presents a troublesome problem. Administration of liver is not feasible. The rest nitrogen of the blood is increased by it and hematuria is augmented. The problem is best met by transfusions in a series, which, together with a more liberal protein intake, where this is possible, often results in some improvement.

Congestive heart failure, manifested either by transient attacks of "cardiac asthma" with congestion and edema of the lungs or by more frank general congestive failure, is best treated by digitalization in full doses. Nitrites should be used in the asthmatic seizures. As an emergency measure in pulmonary edema venesection may give prompt relief if nitrites fail. It is well to collect the blood in a sterile flask with sodium citrate and re-infuse it later, if the patient is anemic.

DEGENERATIVE BRIGHT'S DISEASE: THE NEPHROSES.

Definition.—Degenerative Bright's disease includes those forms of degeneration of renal parenchyma which are not associated with inflammatory lesions of the glomeruli nor secondary to arteriosclerosis. Clinically they are characterized by albuminuria and an excessive number of casts and by the absence of hematuria. The tendency to edema is marked. In rare instances secondary contraction of the kidneys occurs, with nitrogen retention and uremia. Hypertension occurs only under special circumstances, as in some of the renal degenerations of pregnancy, and it is not characteristic of the group as a whole. The etiology of the group covers the widest range of causative agents or conditions and many are entirely unknown. For purposes of description the nephroses may be divided into the following types:

(a) Larval nephroses (febrile albuminurias, etc.).
(b) Necrotizing nephroses (mercurial poisoning).
(c) Chronic nephrosis, sometimes called "genuine" or "lipoidal."
(d) Amyloid disease of the kidneys.
(e) Nephroses of pregnancy.

Larval Nephroses.—These include a wide variety of conditions in which fever or mild intoxication produces albuminuria and casts without impairment of renal function. Pathologically the lesions are usually confined to cloudy swelling, the earliest changes of hyaline droplet, or fatty degeneration. The etiologic factors include infectious fevers, diabetes with glycosuria and ketosis, jaundice, severe anemias, mild intoxication with many drugs and chemical agents, notable among which are mercury, bismuth, arsenic, potassium chlorate, cantharides, phenols, chloroform and alcohol.

The symptomatology is entirely that of the infection or intoxication.

Necrotizing Nephroses.—**Etiology.**—The vast majority of cases are due to poisoning with bichloride of mercury, either taken by mouth or *per vaginam*. Occasionally large accumulations of insoluble mercury salicylate in the muscles have undergone a delayed but rapid absorption with fatal result. Mercurial nephrosis has also followed the internal use of "mercurochrome." With the increasing use of bismuth in the treatment of syphilis a bismuth nephrosis is sometimes encountered, particularly following the accidental entering of a vein during intramuscular injection of a soluble bismuth salt. Formerly it occasionally followed the injection of bismuth pastes into sinuses.

Necrotizing nephroses are reported among the anatomic findings in fatal cholera, in yellow fever and rarely in diphtheria.

Pathology.—The kidneys are usually enlarged, soft and pale, though they may at times show congestion. On microscopic examination the outstanding findings relate to degeneration in the tubules, which varies in degree from complete necrosis to simple cloudy swelling. Certain portions of the tubular system seem to be more vulnerable than others, particularly the proximal convoluted tubules. Here the swollen cells without nuclei fill the lumen of the tubule. Fatty degeneration is uncommon. More frequently vacuolar changes are seen. Calcium deposits in the necrotic tubules may be numerous. The beginning of regeneration is marked by the appearance of a low epithelium with deep-staining nuclei under the necrotic cells. Phagocytes of various types appear in the interstitium. The glomeruli appear congested, and degenerative changes in the capsular epithelium may occasionally be made out. The healing is often nearly complete in the kidney in those patients who do not die in the anuric stage but from subsequent complications.

Symptoms.—Apart from anuria, at first there are no symptoms due to renal lesions. The rapidity with which this develops depends upon the manner of poisoning. When bichloride of mercury is ingested with enough water to make a dilute solution the anuria may be complete in two or three hours, even when the stomach is emptied within ten minutes. With slower absorption oliguria may progress to anuria in two or three days, and sometimes complete anuria does not occur. The absence of symptoms is often striking. In other cases only the buccal, esophageal or vaginal lesions cause distress in the first days. Even in the asymptomatic stages leukocytosis may be marked, reaching levels of 20,000 to 40,000, apart from complicating infections.

With oliguria or anuria the non-protein nitrogen of the blood increases, the alkaline reserve is usually reduced and the blood chlorides fall to very low levels. As these changes occur the patient becomes apathetic and weak and shows various degrees of true chronic uremia without hypertension. Vomiting is persistent. When deep

Kussmaul breathing occurs it gives evidence of acidosis. The stomatitis is often very distressing. In the case of bismuth a black line forms in the necrotic margins of the gums. Colitis with bloody stools adds to the suffering. Stupor deepens into coma. If the anuria persists death occurs from uremia and circulatory collapse in from eight to twelve days. Even when diuresis is resumed death may occur from other causes than renal insufficiency. The urine passed after a period of anuria is usually of low specific gravity. Its volume quickly rises to high levels due to good glomerular filtration with poor tubular resorption. Hematuria and hypertension are not observed. Edema is rarely found and then only as the result of long-continued fluid administration in excess of the needs of an anuric patient.

Diagnosis depends chiefly upon the history and upon the chemical test for mercury or bismuth in the vomitus or stomach washings or in the stools or fluid returned from colonic irrigations.

Prognosis.—With prompt and appropriate treatment many patients will recover. Large doses of mercury in dilute solution are more apt to result fatally than when tablets are swallowed with little water. A high degree of leukocytosis is of bad prognostic significance. The longer the duration of anuria the less chance there is of recovery, though this has followed complete anuria for five days.

Treatment.—Milk and raw eggs should be given as soon as possible after the ingestion of bichloride and followed by gastric lavage. The eggs should be quickly beaten up in water or milk to prevent a dense coagulum from holding tablets in the stomach. After thorough washing, 30 grams of magnesium sulphate in solution may be administered through the tube.

Lambert and Patterson recommended giving every other hour potassium bitartrate, 2 grams in 250 cc. of lemonade with lactose. On alternate hours a glass of milk is given. The stomach is washed twice daily and colonic irrigations are given twice daily. Between irrigations a Murphy drip is given consisting of potassium acetate in 1 per cent solution. If the fluid absorption is small, due to poor retention of the rectal drip, it may be necessary to give hypertonic glucose solutions by vein in order to combat ketosis and to insure adequate fluid for diuresis.

If the stomatitis is severe it may not be possible to perform lavage. The mouth should be scrupulously cleaned four times a day. An alkaline mouth wash consisting of sodium bicarbonate and perborate is useful. Feeding may be made possible by the prior use of orthoform in 1 per cent solution.

Recently treatment with sodium formaldehyde sulphoxylate has been strongly recommended. Gastric lavage is performed with 1000 cc. of a 5 per cent solution, leaving 200 cc. in the stomach. Following this 200 cc. of a 5 per cent sulphoxylate solution is injected intravenously during twenty to thirty minutes. The injection of 100 cc. more may be given at the end of four to six hours in severe cases.

Chronic Nephrosis ("Genuine" or "Lipoidal").—The adjective "genuine" is proposed to distinguish chronic nephrosis from the nephrotic forms of glomerulonephritis, from which the differentiation is often made with difficulty. Genuine chronic nephrosis is an extremely rare disease, while nephrotic forms of diffuse glomerulonephritis are not uncommon.

Etiology.—Examples of true chronic nephrosis are encountered more frequently in pediatric practice than among adults. Among the latter some occur in the course of syphilis, usually though not invariably in the secondary stage. A distinction must be made between those cases due to the syphilis and those resulting from poisoning by antisyphilitic drugs. Among the non-syphilitic cases various infections may be associated with nephrosis, without certainty that they play a causative rôle in its production. Terminal pneumococcus infections are very frequent, but these are probably complications rather than causative factors. A few cases follow diphtheria or bacillary dysentery. Clausen and Marriott have shown the importance of chronic staphylococcus infections of the paranasal sinuses in children. The etiologic relationship of such sinus infections is suggested by improvement following treatment. The writer has seen one striking instance of this relationship in a young adult. True nephrosis, without amyloid, occasionally occurs in connection with tuberculosis and chronic suppuration of bone, though amyloid disease is more characteristic in these conditions.

In many cases the etiology remains obscure. For these, and possibly for the whole group, no better explanation remains than that of Epstein, who believes that the disease is due to a fundamental metabolic disturbance. Nephrosis discovered at autopsy in a case of multiple myeloma described by Thannhauser and Krause suggests injury to the kidney by the excretion of foreign proteins.

The *pathogenesis* of chronic genuine nephrosis remains obscure. The beneficial effects of thyroid administration led Epstein to suggest a fundamental metabolic disturbance in which thyroid abnormalities play a part. Clausen has demonstrated low surface tension of the urine and of the blood serum which suggests the possibility that the excretion of some capillary active substance has increased the permeability of the glomeruli to serum albumin.

Barker and Kirk found tubular degenerations in the kidneys of dogs subjected to plasmaphoresis, suggesting that these lesions were secondary to the low serum proteins or to the prolonged albuminuria. Leiter has vigorously protested against this view, holding that sufficient account was not taken of the spontaneous renal lesions of dogs, which are not uncommon.

There is no doubt that the edema is due to the lowered oncotic pressure of the blood plasma due to loss of serum albumin at a rate more rapid than its replacement by metabolic regeneration. That the capillaries generally throughout the body do not share the excessive permeability of those in the glomeruli is shown by the low protein content of the subcutaneous edema fluid and that of the transudates in serous cavities. This constitutes a major difference between nephrotic edema and the hard nephritic edema of the early stages of acute hemorrhagic nephritis.

The nature of the increase of fats and lipoids in the blood in nephrosis has not yet been satisfactorily explained.

Pathology.—The kidneys are usually enlarged, sometimes weighing 200 to 250 grams. The capsule is readily stripped. The consistency is soft. The surface, which is smooth, varies from a dirty yellow to a gray with yellowish blotches, which on cut sections may appear as radial yellow streaks, though the normal striations of the cortex are missing. The fatty change is often sufficient to impart a greasy feeling to the touch. The pale, wide, buttery cortex is sharply distinguished from the darker medulla.

On microscopic examination frozen sections stained with Sudan III show extensive fatty change, which may be missing when fat solvents are used in preparing sections. With a polarizing microscope doubly refractile lipoidal masses can usually be discovered. Not all the fat-like substances are anisotropic, however. The degenerative changes are most pronounced in the proximal convoluted tubules, less in the distal portions of the tubules, and least in the collecting systems. Epithelial cells are seen in all stages of degeneration, some large and swollen, nearly filling the tubules. Some tubules are dilated and lined by a low epithelium almost like a syncytium. Desquamation of epithelium and exudation of leukocytes into the lumen is seen, often in cast formation. The boundaries of tubules often disappear leaving islets of cells in various stages of disintegration. The interstitium often contains endothelial phagocytic cells which may be loaded with doubly refractile lipoid. Interstitial proliferative changes and cellular infiltration are sometimes of considerable extent. The glomeruli are usually intact. However, Fahr has described various degenerative changes which may affect the glomeruli. These consist of widening and swelling of the glomerular loops and of Bowman's capsule. Hyaline changes sometimes occur in the loops, and fatty changes may also occur in the cells of the capsule. Cellular proliferation affects the glomerular epithelium, and adhesions to the capsule may be found. These degenerative (not inflammatory) changes in glomeruli have been observed to go on to glomerular obliteration, according to Fahr.

A *nephrotic contracted kidney* is occasionally described, though the interpretation of the terminal anatomic picture is often debatable, particularly regarding the evidence of a pure degenerative change in the glomeruli. It is, therefore, difficult to be sure that such kidneys have not resulted from an original glomerulonephritis.

Symptoms.—The onset is often insidious. The patient usually feels tired and suffers from anorexia. Gradually increasing edema of the feet and ankles occurs, occasionally with facial or periocular swelling on first arising in the morning. The increasing dropsy usually leads to an examination of the urine which reveals the albuminuria. The anorexia is sometimes severe. Vomiting and watery diarrheas are extremely common. The edema reaches massive proportions in many cases. The skin assumes a pallor suggesting an anemia, but in such cases the blood counts are usually normal, or a mild secondary anemia is found which is far less than the pallor would suggest. The patient may come to a bed-ridden state with massive dropsy lasting for months, from which he suffers psychically as much as physically, from an attitude of hopelessness engendered by the obstinate persistence of the dropsy. Hypertension and cardiac hypertrophy are not encountered in such cases. Hematuria does not occur. The non-protein nitrogen of the blood increases only in those rare cases of true nephrotic contracted kidney with glomerular degeneration. The edema includes transudation into the serous cavities, particularly the peritoneum. These transudates are very poor in protein. The *urine* diminishes in volume during periods in which the edema increases. A steady state of dropsy may be reached in which fairly large urine volumes are attained, with normal or slightly reduced specific gravity. The concentrating power is somewhat reduced and the dilution tests usually show a delay in water excretion. The phenolsulphonephthalein excretion is often fairly good, particularly with the larger urine volumes, though it is reduced when oliguria is marked. The urine is usually very poor in chlorides and contains large amounts of protein, at least 90 per cent of which consists of serum albumin, amounting to from 15 to 25 grams *per diem*. Much larger amounts have been recorded. The Addis counts reveal a great increase of casts of the hyaline and fatty and waxy varieties and sometimes cellular casts. Doubly refractile lipoids may be demonstrated in the sediment. During periods of regression of edema a dilute alkaline urine is excreted in which casts readily dissolve and cast counts are of little value. Erythrocyte counts in the urine sediment show no increase above normal. Glycosurias are not uncommon. These are usually of the renal type with normal blood-sugar values.

The blood is frequently normal as to hemoglobin and red corpuscles, though in long-standing cases a moderate degree of secondary anemia is found. The most striking abnormality of the blood is its poverty of serum albumin. The serum globulin and fibrinogen percentage may even be slightly above normal. The normal ratio of albumin to globulin is reduced. Accompanying this change in serum proteins an increase in both fats and lipids of the plasma is usual, so that the plasma may have an opalescent appearance. The total non-protein nitrogen and urea are ordinarily not increased. The carbon dioxide combining power is usually normal or nearly so, owing to the fact that the ammonia-forming function of the kidney is not lost. The serum calcium is often below normal levels. Tetany, though rare, is occasionally encountered in chronic nephrosis. The whole blood and plasma chlorides vary considerably. Most frequently they are below normal. The plasma volume is normal, the blood volume is diminished only when the corpuscular volume is reduced by anemia.

The basal metabolism is low even after allowance is made for the increase of body surface due to the edema. It may not be increased appreciably by the administration of thyroid. Probably the severe wasting of the body due to prolonged protein loss is responsible for this low metabolism. The wasting is masked by the edema though it may readily be made out in non-edematous areas, such as the pectoral and deltoid regions.

The course of chronic nephrosis varies considerably. The onset of the edema may be marked by transudation into a serous cavity of an opalescent pseudochylous fluid. A previously dropsical patient may be observed to pass into an edema-free stage, going through a transition in which the only remaining sign of anasarca is an ascites. In the edema-free stage albuminuria and cylindruria remain as evidences of the activity of the disease. Edema is usually absent in the extremely rare cases of true nephrotic contracted kidneys and nitrogen retention sometimes occurs in these terminal cases.

Death from the nephrosis itself is of extreme rarity. When death occurs it is usually due to *complications*, of which pneumococcus peritonitis constitutes one of the most frequent. Pneumococcus sepsis and bronchitis or bronchopneumonias account for some deaths. Infections of the skin resembling erysipelas, which run a very chronic indolent course, are sometimes seen. In one instance of this sort in the writer's experience the skin lesions cleared up promptly following a blood transfusion, and in turn a sudden diuresis occurred with rapid and complete recovery of the patient.

Differential Diagnosis.—The chief differential points between lipoid nephrosis and amyloid disease are: (*a*) the greater frequency of azotemia and true uremia in the latter; (*b*) the recognition of splenic or hepatic enlargements due to amyloid; and (*c*) certain etiologic factors such as tuberculosis, late syphilis or chronic suppuration, which predispose to amyloid degenerations.

In many cases the differentiation between lipoidal and amyloid nephrosis is impossible. The rapid disappearance of injected Congo red from the blood stream, which was at first thought to be a specific test for amyloid disease, is now known to occur in genuine nephrosis as well. The differentiation from nephrotic forms of glomerulonephritis is based upon the persistent absence of hematuria, hypertension and cardiovascular changes.

Prognosis.—On the whole the outlook is favorable for the patient with chronic genuine nephrosis. Particularly is this true in the idiopathic cases in children and in the nephrosis of secondary syphilis, if proper therapeutic procedures are instituted. Even under the most skilful management the course may be greatly protracted, lasting for months. In such cases the process of recovery may commence suddenly and progress rapidly to healing without the introduction of any known new factor in the treatment of the patient.

In the few cases due to chronic suppuration of bone or tuberculosis, which are not amyloid nephroses, the prognosis is that of the underlying disease. When nephrosis follows diphtheria the prognosis depends upon the associated myocardial and nervous lesions more than upon the renal disease.

Treatment.—Guiding principles in the management of chronic nephrosis are as follows: (*a*) search for and attempt to eradicate underlying chronic infections if any are found; (*b*) limitation of edema by restriction of salt ingestion; (c) dietary regulation of the protein metabolism with a view to increasing the regeneration of serum proteins; (d) thyroid administration; (e) prophylaxis and treatment of intercurrent infections.

If previously untreated syphilis exists it should be cautiously treated in the secondary stage preferably with arsphenamine, or in later stages with preliminary preparation with mercury or bismuth. Even if no obvious sinus infection exists it should be carefully searched for clinically and by radiograph. The writer has seen rapid improvement follow diagnostic irrigation of an asymptomatic infection in the antrum of Highmore.

Dietary regulation consists of giving high protein, high calorie diets, which are minimal in salt content. The protein may be given in amounts varying from 150 to 200 grams *per diem* in some cases. It is well not to force this item to the extent of upsetting the patient, for the reason that fully as much can often be accomplished by giving large amounts of carbohydrate and fat for their protein-sparing qualities. The writer rarely uses more than 150 grams of protein *per diem*. Milk is avoided on account of its salt content. Fluids need rarely be restricted to less than 2000 cc. if the diet is salt-free. If watery diarrhea or vomiting is present the fluid loss should be replaced. In some cases with persistent vomiting it is necessary to resort to tube feeding.

Thyroid administration frequently produces excellent therapeutic results. Diuresis sometimes occurs before the serum albumin reaches the critical level at which edema usually disappears. Patients frequently tolerate doses of 0.2 to 0.4 gram *per diem* for a considerable period without any evidence of thyrotoxicosis.

Transfusion of blood aids greatly in the combating of complicating infections in nephrosis. It has a certain value in building up plasma proteins and is indicated even though the patient is not severely anemic. In nephritis and nephrosis the writer has never seen harm come from transfusion in which the cross-matching tests were perfect.

In the prophylaxis of terminal infections one must scrupulously guard against bed sores or any excoriation of the skin. Strict asepsis must be obtained in aspirations of ascitic or pleural fluid. Care of the mouth and nose should be thorough. Patients should be carefully protected from infection by contact with attendants or visitors with respiratory infections.

Amyloid Nephrosis.—Etiology.—Tuberculosis is responsible for the greatest number of cases. Chronic sinusitis with bone necrosis and chronic suppurative osteomyelitis are the other frequent factors. In some cases no causative factors can be found.

Both clinically and experimentally amyloid degeneration may occur with considerable rapidity. One of the writer's cases died in uremia within five months of the first symptom. Smetana produced amyloid deposits in mice in twenty-five days by daily injection of neutral sodium caseinate.

Pathology.—In gross appearance the amyloid kidney resembles somewhat that of chronic lipoidal nephrosis. The kidneys are usually large, though secondarily contracted amyloid kidneys are not extremely rare. In the large types the capsule strips readily. The surface appearance is smooth and pale ochre in color or it may be brownish. The consistency is usually more firm than that of lipoidal nephrosis. On cut section the same greasy appearance may be noted. The glomeruli stand out by reason of the translucent deposits of amyloid within them. When the cut surface is treated with dilute acetic acid followed by Lugol's solution, the amyloid deposits take on a brownish stain which turns greenish-blue when dilute sulphuric acid is applied. The presence of amyloid may be grossly demonstrated in this way, its chief locations being in the glomeruli and in the arteries. The iodine staining is often quite diffuse if there is amyloid deposited extensively in the tubules as well.

Microscopically the characteristic appearance of amyloid in the glomeruli, in the afferent arterioles and in the basement membrane of tubules, makes the diagnosis. The glomerular changes vary from those in which some circulation still persists to those in which there is complete glomerular closure and fibrosis. The tubular atrophy following glomerular obliteration results in extensive replacement fibrosis. If this process has reached a considerable extent a secondary contraction of the kidney may be produced, which grossly resembles the contracted kidney of arteriosclerosis or glomerulonephritis, except insofar as the presence of amyloid is recognized.

For the rest, tubular changes also occur which are precisely like those of chronic lipoidal nephrosis. The association with amyloid deposits in liver, spleen and other organs is usual.

Symptoms.—In many cases considerable deposits of amyloid are found at autopsy in which it was not suspected from the symptoms. In others, the symptomatology is entirely that of chronic lipoid nephrosis, without azotemia. In many cases the rest nitrogen of the blood is elevated, so that a nephrotic glomerulonephritis is suspected. Cardiac hypertrophy and hypertension are not found in these cases.

When secondary contraction of the amyloid kidneys takes place, mild hypertension with chronic true uremia may be observed. Such patients are usually not edematous. The writer observed one remarkable case of this sort with chronic uremia of more than three years' duration. During this whole period there was considerable azotemia, frequent periods of vomiting and oliguria, alternating with periods of hyposthenuric polyuria. Red blood corpuscles were never found in the urine. The systolic blood pressure rose as high as 170 mm. Hg, but cardiac hypertrophy was never demonstrated and retinal changes did not occur. The phenolsulphonephthalein excretion was less than 10 per cent in two hours when the patient was first seen. Uremic pericarditis recurred and disappeared on several occasions. At autopsy secondarily contracted amyloid kidneys were discovered.

Differential Diagnosis.—The differentiation from chronic true nephrosis has been discussed.

The secondarily contracted stage of amyloid may be differentiated from other conditions leading to contracted kidneys chiefly by the absence of hematuria, and the absence of hypertension sufficient to produce cardiac hypertrophy and angiospastic retinitis.

The *prognosis* is that of the underlying disease.

Treatment.—The management outlined for chronic true nephrosis applies equally to amyloidosis.

If the manifestations of chronic true uremia appear the main reliance must be put upon the induction of diuresis by forcing fluids with salt restriction. For parenteral fluid administration glucose solutions should be used.

Nephrosis of Pregnancy.—The inclusion of the "kidney of pregnancy" among the nephroses is chiefly due to the nature of the anatomic changes found in the kidneys at autopsy. These changes are tubular degenerations. However, the prominence of hypertension in the clinical picture sets this type of renal degeneration apart from all the other nephroses. The frequent association of the "kidney of pregnancy" with "eclampsia," which differs in no way from the encephalopathy of other hypertensive crises, would make it seem probable that the kidney of pregnancy is more closely allied to arteriosclerotic Bright's disease than to the true nephroses.

The literature of the subject is much confused by the frequent failure of the obstetrical observers to take account of preëxisting latent hemorrhagic Bright's disease or of hypertensive vascular disease, and the lack of data necessary to group the cases according to the newer orientation made possible by the studies of Volhard and Fahr and of Addis and Oliver.

Etiology.—The cause of this complication of pregnancy is unknown.

The renal lesions peculiar to it occur in the latter half of pregnancy, and are more frequent in primiparæ than in multiparæ. It is more common with twin pregnancies.

Pathology.—The most constant findings in the kidney of pregnancy are tubular degenerations, fatty and hyaline droplets. Vascular thromboses may occur with hemorrhagic infarcts. Volhard has called attention to pale anemic infarcts in support of his views that angiospastic ischemia is the cause of parenchymal degeneration of the kidney. Volhard further emphasizes the significance of the finding of glomerular ischemia in these cases. Fahr has described fatty changes in the glomeruli. The renal circulation is occasionally so impaired that complete cortical necrosis may occur.

In eclampsia the kidney of pregnancy is often found at autopsy. However, hepatic lesions are more uniformly present, and the kidneys may be practically normal in some cases. The changes in the nervous system in eclampsia are those described under acute eclamptic uremia or hypertensive encephalopathy.

Symptoms.—Cases with the kidney of pregnancy may be divided into three groups: (a) Those exhibiting only mild hypertension (blood pressure, systolic 150 mm. Hg and diastolic 90 mm. Hg) with albuminuria and casts, without edema. This group corresponds to the *low reserve kidney* in the terminology of Stander. The albuminuria rarely exceeds 1 gram per liter. (*b*) Those exhibiting *pre-eclamptic toxemia.* The blood pressure is higher than in the first group. Edema of the labia or of the lower extremities is common. The albuminuria often exceeds 1 per cent. In severe cases the hypertension reaches a high level. Dyspnea becomes marked and paroxysms of cardiac asthma may occur and a tendency to periodic breathing (Cheyne-Stokes) is noted. Visual disturbances are frequent, consisting of scotomata, spots or flashes. Spasmodic narrowing of the retinal arterioles can be seen in hypertensive crises. If the hypertension is prolonged large soft exudates sometimes appear and edema of the optic disk may be noted. Headache may be severe. The edema may increase rapidly as measured by daily weighing of the patient. (*c*) The third group exhibits *eclamptic convulsions.* These may follow upon the phenomena just described under pre-eclamptic toxemia, but in rare instances the eclampsia comes on with surprising suddenness, preceded by a marked and rapid rise in blood pressure and oliguria, usually with marked visual disturbances and all of the phenomena of hypertensive encephalopathy which have been described as acute eclamptic or false uremia. In a few cases albuminuria is lacking or minimal.

Eclampsia occurs in the latter part of pregnancy, in labor, or during the first four days of the puerperium. With delivery of the fetus the phenomena usually subside in a few days. The edema disappears with marked polyuria. Plass has called attention to the fact that azotemia may be observed during this period when it was absent before the eclampsia. The blood pressure usually falls promptly, though it occasionally remains elevated for some days, not exceeding ten.

Differential diagnosis during the pregnancy at times presents difficulties. The absence of hematuria differentiates the kidney of pregnancy from glomerulonephritis. Nephritic toxemia when it occurs is usually well marked in the earlier stages of pregnancy in which the true nephrosis gravidarum is not found. The finding of an elevation of blood pressure early in the course of pregnancy speaks for a preexisting hypertension or latent nephritis. The same may be said for cardiac hypertrophy and hypertensive retinal changes.

The phenomena associated with the true kidney of pregnancy disappear shortly after labor. Persistence of hypertension or urinary abnormalities after the puerperium is presumptive evidence of an underlying pathologic process which has been aggravated but not initiated by the pregnancy.

Prognosis.—The mortality among those who reach the eclamptic state varies from 10 to 20 per cent in different clinics. For those who survive the first four days of the puerperium the outlook is good. Eclampsia occasionally recurs in subsequent pregnancies, but frequently it does not recur. The same thing may be said for the milder forms of the kidney of pregnancy. Once the pregnancy is terminated the kidneys return to normal with unimpaired function.

Treatment.—From the standpoint of prophylaxis, the careful watching of the pregnant woman, frequent urine examinations, frequent observation for elevation of blood pressure and for edema, become of the utmost importance. If edema appears it should be handled upon the same general lines as outlined for the edema of glomerulonephritis, salt restriction being essential. If the hypertension reaches threatening heights the patient should be put to bed. As sedatives, chloral hydrate and morphine are used. Water is given by mouth freely. If this is impossible 10 per cent glucose is injected by vein. If the patient is at or near term she should be kept under the influence of sedatives until the cervix is fully dilated. If the eclampsia threatens earlier in the course of pregnancy it is often possible to treat the patient expectantly until the child is viable, when labor is induced. If severe hypertension exists or when the visual disturbances are marked, it is sometimes necessary to sacrifice the child, if it is not yet viable, to preserve the vision of the mother.

For the actual eclamptic seizures the treatment is that previously outlined for acute false or eclamptic uremia.

ARTERIOSCLEROTIC BRIGHT'S DISEASE.

Definition.—Arteriosclerotic Bright's disease is characterized by a nephrosclerosis resulting from the degenerative or inflammatory lesions of the renal arterioles occurring in the course of vascular hypertension. Clinically its symptomatology is dominated by that of the primary vascular disease, which usually produces death from the secondary lesions in the heart or brain before the nephrosclerosis has advanced to the point of renal insufficiency, though a small number of cases reach the uremic stage. The senile sclerosis of the medium-sized and larger arteries may give rise to renal infarcts with resulting scars, but not to true nephrosclerosis or primary contraction of the kidney.

Etiology.—The causes of essential hypertension have been discussed elsewhere. The etiology is still not clear, though the importance of certain factors have been recognized, such as constitution, certain nervous and emotional reactions, hormonal and metabolic disturbances and certain poisons.

Pathogenesis.—Arteriosclerosis has come to be regarded as the result of prolonged vascular hypertension, and is no longer regarded as its cause. Two main types of essential hypertension are recognized, benign and malignant. There is considerable difference of opinion as to whether these are two separate processes or whether they are merely different phases of a single pathologic process. As we shall see below, the anatomic lesions of the arterioles of benign hypertension are different from those of the malignant form. In both cases degeneration and eventual atrophy occur in the glomeruli and tubules from which the blood supply is reduced or cut off by the arteriolar disease. Those glomeruli and tubules of which the blood supply is intact may secrete an approximately normal urine, while those which are dying contribute only small amounts of abnormal urine. The functional capacity of the sclerotic kidney depends upon the relative patency of the renal blood supply and the degree to which the hypertrophied heart is able to maintain a circulation through them. Such urinary abnormalities as are found in nephrosclerosis are more often due to passive congestion of the kidneys than to the arteriosclerotic degeneration.

Pathology.—In cases of benign essential hypertension in patients who die from cardiac or cerebral lesions the kidneys may present a nearly normal gross appearance, or they may exhibit various degrees of granular contraction. The size may be increased and the color darker when passive congestion is present. The surface is marked by fine and coarse granulations, and the color is usually reddish-brown or gray. The consistency is firm. The capsule tears off with portions of adherent cortex. On section the cortex is narrow, the medulla less so, but medullary shrinkage enlarges the fat-filled space about the hilus.

On microscopic examination the glomeruli are seen in all stages, from those which are completely hyalinized and surrounded by fibrosis to those which are essentially intact. Intermediate glomerular changes consist of hyaline degeneration involving parts of the lobules with various degrees of patency of the tuft. The earliest arteriolar change is that of hyalinization of the vasa afferentia beginning at the glomerulus and extending directly under the endothelium. In the larger arterioles reduplication of the elastic lamellæ is seen. These processes eventually narrow the lumen and go on to obliteration. The glomerular and tubular atrophy are consequences of this obliteration. Atrophic elements are replaced by fibrous tissue in which round-cell infiltration is observed.

The *malignant types of essential hypertension* give rise to kidneys which sometimes present striking differences in gross appearance from those just described. The surface is characteristically marked by small hemorrhages, but the granular or pebbled appearance differentiates it from the "flea-bitten" kidney of bacterial endocarditis. Microscopically, in addition to the lesions described under benign nephrosclerosis a *necrotic endarteritis* is found in these malignant scleroses. This endarteritis consists of endothelial and subendothelial connective-tissue proliferation. These affected vessels frequently rupture. Sometimes this proliferative process extends into the glomerular tuft and causes some confusion of opinion as to the existence of a glomerulonephritis. Other glomeruli are frankly necrotic with hemorrhage into the capsule. Degenerative changes occur in the tubules.

The other pathologic changes of hypertensive vascular disease will be described elsewhere.

Symptoms.—Benign essential hypertension may exist for many years without symptoms in those who are unaware of its presence. In the vast majority of instances the symptoms are chiefly those of hypertensive heart disease or of hypertensive encephalopathy. The slow process of benign nephrosclerosis gives few symptoms and probably not more than 5 per cent of cases of benign hypertension die with renal insufficiency.

Nocturia is one of the earliest and commonest urinary symptoms. It usually antedates death by many years. It may depend upon nocturnal elimination of a larval cardiac edema which has accumulated during the day, or it may be caused by the hyposthenuric polyuria of the nephrosclerosis itself. In the former case the specific gravity of the urine is high, in the latter it is low.

Albuminuria may or may not be present and is usually slight in amount. When it is present it depends most frequently upon passive congestion of the kidneys. The number of *casts* varies considerably. They are more frequently preserved in the more concentrated urine of passive congestion than in the dilute pale urine of the nephrosclerotic polyuria. Red blood corpuscles of the urine are not increased in the absence of congestive heart failure. In this latter condition the increase is very moderate. True hematuria does not occur in benign nephrosclerosis.

The volume of the urine is reduced by congestive heart failure or by factors involving extra-renal water loss. As the contraction of the kidney progresses the specific gravity tends to become fixed, *isosthenuria*, and reduced, *hyposthenuria*. With the latter the volume of the night urine is increased. The dilution and concentration tests are of great value in the nephroscleroses. The phenolsulphonephthalein excretion is not impaired, in the absence of heart failure, until the urea clearance has diminished to about 50 per cent of normal. However, passive congestion of the kidneys occurs so frequently before nephrosclerosis is marked that the phenolsulphonephthalein test is not of great value in determining the extent of contraction.

The *urea clearance* test of van Slyke has proved to be of the greatest value in determining the extent of nephrosclerosis. Uremia does not appear until the urea clearance has reached levels below 20 per cent of normal.

The rest nitrogen of the blood may remain within normal limits until the urea clearance is less than 20 per cent of normal. Some degree of azotemia is usual at this point. Whenever congestive heart failure supervenes in the course of nephrosclerosis azotemia is usually increased.

The *uremia* which occurs in those patients in whom the urea clearance is greatly reduced is of a complex type. It consists of the phenomena described under chronic true uremia, modified by the coëxistence of the phenomena of "hypertensive encephalopathy," and frequently by the added factor of heart failure with cardiac edema.

The true uremic symptoms are those of the intoxication of azotemia, the renal acidosis and the anemia. Hypertensive encephalopathy accounts for convulsions and focal neurologic manifestations and Cheyne-Stokes breathing. Congestive heart failure is responsible for orthopnea and edema.

The symptoms of *malignant hypertension* are qualitatively the same as those of the benign with a few important exceptions. It occurs in a much younger group of patients, as a rule, and it may frequently run its entire course in less than a year. The majority of young patients with malignant hypertension survive cerebral and cardiac deaths until they have reached the uremic phase of nephrosclerosis.

The advance of malignant nephrosclerosis may be measured by the urea clearance, of which the rapid decrease is often surprising.

The urinary sediment may show considerable increases in the number of red corpuscles, probably accounted for by the arterial and glomerular ruptures seen in microscopic sections. These findings at first led some observers to the opinion that malignant hypertension was due to the superimposition of glomerulonephritis upon a benign nephrosclerosis. The hematuria is not as constant as in glomerulonephritis, however.

The *retinal lesions* in benign and malignant nephrosclerosis present characteristic differences. In the benign forms the lesions consist chiefly in narrowing and sclerosis of the arterioles and the formation of flat glistening exudates about the macula and elsewhere. The disks are generally normal. Small hemorrhages occur but rarely. On the other hand, the retina of malignant hypertension shows earlier and more extensive hemorrhages. The exudates which occur are larger and more dull and are frequently described as "cotton-wool exudates." Neuro-retinal edema is common and may progress to a considerable extent, resembling the choked disk seen with brain tumors.

Differential Diagnosis.—This rarely presents great difficulties. The occurrence of marked hypertension without significant abnormalities of the urine or serious impairment of renal function characterizes the earlier stages of arteriosclerotic Bright's disease. Even when renal function is decreased the vascular and cardiac lesions dominate the picture. When the uremic stage is reached the differentiation becomes more difficult, particularly when a good history does not supply the information which could have been obtained by prior observation. One point stands out as crucial to the diagnosis of nephrosclerosis, that is, the absence of significant hematuria, which betrays the presence of glomerulonephritis even in its terminal stages.

Congenital polycystic kidneys may occasionally cause some difficulty in differential diagnosis, especially if there is present some condition which makes it difficult to palpate the enlargement of such kidneys.

Uremia due to secondary contraction of amyloid kidneys lacks significant hypertension, and cardiac hypertrophy and hypertensive retinal changes are lacking in these cases.

Treatment.—The therapy of hypertension and of hypertensive heart disease has been discussed elsewhere in previous sections. The treatment of eclamptic phenomena of hypertensive encephalopathy or "false" uremia has likewise been discussed. The true chronic uremia of nephrosclerosis should be managed in the same way as that of the secondarily contracted kidneys of hemorrhagic Bright's disease.

INFARCTS OF THE KIDNEY.

Hemorrhagic infarcts of the kidney may arise by thrombosis, but more frequently by embolism. The basis of autochthonous thrombosis is *senile arteriosclerosis* of the larger arteries. Mechanical injury, and occasionally distortion of the pedicle of a mobile kidney may initiate thrombosis. Embolism results most frequently from endocarditis, or from mural thrombosis in the heart or aorta.

Pathology.—Fresh hemorrhagic infarcts are seen as wedge-shaped lesions with the apex in the medulla spreading toward the cortex. They may be uniformly red, or a gray necrotic center is seen with a hemorrhagic border. Healed infarcts are represented by deep scars. Occasionally an infarct may involve a whole kidney. *Differential diagnosis* can be made correctly only when sudden renal pain and hematuria occur in the course of some cardiac or valvular disease in which there is a tendency to embolism.

It may be suspected when transient asymptomatic hematuria occurs in connection with recognizable embolism in other organs.

The *symptoms* are obscure. Small infarcts frequently pass unnoticed. This may also be true of large unilateral infarcts. Larger infarcts may result in *renal pain* and in hematuria. Multiple large bilateral infarcts occasionally result in severe impairment of renal function with uremia.

CHRONIC PASSIVE CONGESTION OF THE KIDNEYS.

Stasis in the renal veins may result from several causes, the chief of which is congestive heart failure. Pressure upon the renal veins themselves and obstructions to the inferior vena cava are less frequent causes.

Pathology.—The kidney of stasis is enlarged, dark in color and rather firm in consistency (cyanotic induration). On cut section the vascular striæ are well marked. Microscopically tubular degenerations of moderate degree may be noted. The extent of degenerative change is proportional to the intensity and duration of the congestion. The *symptoms* consist entirely in alterations in the urine, which is scanty, dark in color and of high density. On cooling, a "brick dust" sediment composed of urates is usually observed. The degree of *albuminuria* depends upon the intensity of the congestion. In the sediment hyaline and granular casts are found in abnormal number. Enumeration of red corpuscles likewise reveals a moderate increase of 500,000 to 1,000,000 per twelve hours. The phenolsulphonephthalein excretion is temporarily decreased. A slight degree of *azotemia* may be observed as an expression of impaired excretion of nitrogen in severe cases.

The *diagnosis* of passive congestion must depend upon the recognition of the condition leading to stasis in the renal veins. When passive congestion is superimposed upon intrinsic renal lesions it is difficult to estimate the degree of functional impairment which is due to congestion. In the case of congestive heart failure one may observe improvement in phenolsulphonephthalein excretion after the exhibition of digitalis. In this way the congestive factor in functional impairment may be evaluated.

In *differential diagnosis* digitalis often plays an important rôle. For example, when a patient with contracted kidneys and hypertension is observed during congestive heart failure, the slight increase in red corpuscles in the urinary sediment due to passive congestion may lead one to suppose that the renal lesion is a glomerulonephritis. If relief of heart failure by the exhibition of digitalis reduces the red cell count to normal limits it is safe to assume that the renal lesion is a nephrosclerosis and not glomerulonephritis.

RENAL PAIN.

Sensations of pain originating in the kidney are of two main types: (a) The first type is a more or less continuous dull ache or burning sensation in the back. This may be rather vaguely localized in the lower dorsal or upper lumbar region, or it may be recognized as a rather sharply defined area of hyperalgesia, associated with tenderness on palpation in the costo-vertebral angle, or on bimanual palpation of the kidney. (b) The second type of pain is paroxysmal, the so-called *renal colic*, which is felt in all degrees of severity from barely perceptible discomfort to pain of sufficient intensity to cause loss of consciousness.

The distribution of pain in renal colic is unilateral and involves a zone from the eleventh dorsal to the second lumbar segments. Rarely it may be referred to the epigastrium or to the shoulder. The radiation of the pain is from the costo-vertebral angle around the flank into the testicle or labium majus. It also extends at times over the external and anterior thigh down to the knee. The paroxysms are usually accompanied by muscle spasm of the same segmental distribution, and frequently by nausea, vomiting, sweating and, in the most severe forms, by collapse. In the periods of relaxation between the paroxysms pain of the first type may persist.

Renal colic occurs in disease affecting the ureter or pelvis of the kidney. Many observers believe that it is only produced by acute obstructions to urinary flow. It may be produced by the distention of the renal pelvis by injection of fluid through a ureteral catheter. It is most commonly caused by the passage of a stone, less frequently by a blood clot, by a plug of fibrinopurulent exudate, or fragment of tumor growth, by ureteral instrumentation or any condition leading to sudden obstruction.

There is also colic due to ureteral tumors and to kinking of the renal pedicle due to abnormal mobility of the kidney, or compression by aberrant blood-vessels, in which there may be an intermittent hydronephrosis. Renal colic in such cases is probably not always due to hydronephroses. It is possible that it may be of vascular origin, or due to sudden swelling of the kidney with painful distention of the renal capsule. Renal colics associated with movable kidneys are known as Dietl's crises.

HYDRONEPHROSIS AND PYONEPHROSIS.

Definition.—Hydronephrosis is a distention of the renal pelvis and calyces by the accumulation of non-purulent urine produced by obstruction of a ureter or the lower urinary tract. Hydronephroses frequently become infected in which case pyonephrosis results.

Etiology.—Bilateral hydronephroses are caused by urethral strictures, hypertrophy or carcinoma of the prostate gland, carcinoma of the bladder, paralysis of the bladder in tabes dorsalis or other lesions of the spinal cord, in fact any obstruction of the lower urinary tract. Unilateral hydronephrosis is due to obstruction of one ureter by stricture of intrinsic or extrinsic cicatrices, by impaction of a calculus, by pressure upon it of intra-abdominal masses, by tuberculosis of the ureter and by congenital developmental anomalies of the ureter. Intermittent hydronephrosis is due to kinking of the ureter of an abnormally mobile kidney, by aberrant vessels or by a tumor at the ureteral orifice.

Pathology.—The kidney as a whole may be enlarged. On cut section the dilated pelvis and calyces are seen surrounded by a narrowed parenchyma, in which the microscope reveals varying degrees of degenerative change resulting from pressure atrophy.

Symptoms.—There are often no symptoms of chronic unilateral obstruction. A palpable enlargement of the kidney may be felt in thin individuals. At times there is dull pain in the region of the kidney. Bacterial infection usually results, in which case the symptoms are those of pyelitis.

With extensive bilateral hydronephrosis mild uremic manifestations gradually appear. These consist of anorexia, lassitude, nausea, headache, visual disturbances and frequently moderate elevation of blood pressure. The excretion of phenolsulphonephthalein is reduced. The rest nitrogen of the blood is elevated. These phenomena may occur in the course of chronic prostatic or urethral obstructions before retention of urine becomes complete, and their intensity increases in proportion to the volume of residual urine in the bladder. Their appearance is hastened when the urinary tract is infected. With paralyses of the bladder this organ is usually considerably distended and easily palpable, and this is also true in advanced cases of mechanical obstruction. Posture profoundly affects the renal function in such cases. It is usually impaired more in recumbency than when the patient is still ambulatory. Too rapid evacuation of the contents of the bladder frequently produces disastrous results, in that vesical and renal hemorrhage occurs and complete suppression of urine ensues. In such cases death often occurs in uremia, though renal function may be resumed.

Diagnosis.—The diagnosis of unilateral hydronephrosis or pyonephrosis can usually be made only by ureteral catheterization and the use of pyelograms, which reveal the shadow of dilated pelvis and calyces. (Intravenous pyelography without the aid of the cystoscope is increasingly successful.) Bilateral hydronephrosis should be suspected in every case of prostatic, urethral or paralytic obstruction in which there is incomplete evacuation of the bladder, also with extensive bladder tumors and perivesical masses, such as sarcoma. It becomes practically certain in such cases if the rest nitrogen of the blood is increased.

The differentiation from pyonephrosis depends upon the character of the urine obtained through ureteral catheters. The differentiation from ovarian cysts and other abdominal tumors, from renal tumors or congenital polycystic kidneys, depends chiefly upon the skilful use of the cystoscope, ureteral catheters and the interpretation of pyelograms.

Treatment.—It is highly important that the bladder be evacuated slowly by connecting a retention catheter to an elevated reservoir containing an antiseptic irrigating fluid, with an overflow adjusted to a suitable level to maintain the intravesical pressure. Depending upon the degree of obstruction and the azotemia the overflow is lowered a few centimeters at a time at intervals of several hours. In an average case the bladder may be "decompressed" in twenty-four to forty-eight hours. In such cases renal function gradually improves and an active diuresis may be maintained by forcing the fluid intake to a high level. Preliminary management along these lines is imperative if surgical relief is to be undertaken.

NEPHROLITHIASIS.

Definition.—Nephrolithiasis is the formation of calculi in the renal pelvis by deposition of substances which are normally dissolved in the urine.

Etiology and Pathogenesis.—The concretions vary in size from small particles like sand to large calculi which form molds of the pelvis branching into the calyces. Chemically they consist of phosphates, uric acid or urates, calcium oxalate or calcium carbonate, cystin or xanthin. Of these, stones with uric acid nuclei are the most common. Secondary incrustations on the original nucleus may occur, depending on the character of the secondary infection. The causes of nephrolithiasis are obscure. In children the passage of sand-like uratic deposits probably represents a sequel to the "uric acid infarcts" sometimes found in the kidneys of the new-born at autopsy. Knowledge of the solubilities of uric acid and urates indicates that high degrees of urinary acidity might rob urates of their basic ions and thus lead to deposition of the less soluble uric acid. Phosphatic calculi are more likely to be secondary to infections or other conditions producing alkaline urine. Excessive excretion of uric acid, as a result of excessive ingestion of nucleoproteins or as a result of excessive nuclear breakdown (following irradiation in leukemias) may influence the formation of calculi. The excretion of oxalic acid is increased by the ingestion of rhubarb, eggplant, spinach and certain foods. The excessive urinary excretion of calcium in hyperparathyroidism and osteitis fibrosa cystica is not infrequently associated with nephrolithiasis.

The movement of the stones with consequent trauma to the renal pelvis and ureter results in colic, hemorrhage and often secondary infection of the urinary tract. Persistent occlusion of the ureter or urethra results in hydronephrosis or pyonephrosis. Many fairly large calculi may pass without colic provided the ureter is not occluded.

Symptoms.—Nephrolithiasis may remain asymptomatic for long periods. Its presence may be indicated only by occasional attacks of dull pain in the flank or back. The disease may first become manifest in a severe attack of *renal colic* accompanied by sweating, nausea, vomiting and collapse. This is often accompanied by signs of infection, a *renal intermittent* fever, sometimes characterized by the occurrence of severe rigors and extreme intermittent hyperpyrexias, with *pyuria* and *hematuria*.

Diagnosis.—The diagnosis usually depends upon the demonstration of the calculus by roentgenogram and cystoscopy. Without these aids the *differential diagnosis* from intestinal colics, biliary colic, or Dietl's crises is frequently difficult.

Treatment.—A great many stones may be removed by ureteral instrumentation. If this fails, especially if renal function is being damaged, surgery should be resorted to. Palliative treatment and the frequent recourse to morphine for severe pain initiates far too many pathetic instances of morphine addiction. Following their surgical removal calculi are frequently formed again. Every effort should be made to correct dietary or metabolic faults underlying the excretion of the substances deposited in the calculus, and to avoid oliguria from dehydration. Adequate water intake must be insisted upon. Focal infection should be carefully sought for and eliminated as far as it is possible to do so.

BACTERIAL INFECTIONS OF THE KIDNEYS AND URINARY PASSAGES.

Non-tuberculous Infections.—The non-tuberculous infections of the kidneys and urinary tract produce a variety of clinical conditions the type of which depends in part upon the nature of the bacterial infection and partly upon local conditions in the urinary tract. In many bacteriemias organisms are excreted in the urine without exciting an inflammatory reaction. For instance, this occurs commonly in typhoid fever as a *bacilluria without pyuria*. In other instances typhoid bacteriemia is associated with a *focal nephritis*, in others a *pyelitis* or *pyelonephritis* may occur.

In hemolytic streptococcus sepsis the renal lesion is most commonly a focal *glomerulonephritis* or an *acute interstitial nephritis*. In the bacteriemic phases of subacute bacterial endocarditis one finds the characteristic focal embolic glomerulonephritis often described as the "flea-bitten kidney," which has been discussed under hemorrhagic Bright's disease.

In staphylococcal bacteriemia the renal lesions are commonly abscesses, single or unilateral, the so-called *renal carbuncle*, or multiple and bilateral abscesses.

The colon bacillus, which is responsible for at least 85 per cent of all bacterial infections of the urinary tract, produces most commonly a pyelitis or pyelonephritis.

Abscess of the Kidney.—Abscesses of the kidneys may occur in (*a*) an acute fulminating form, usually unilateral, known as *renal* *carbuncle,* or in (*b*) subacute or chronic forms; (*c*) multiple and bilateral abscesses may occur in the course of pyemic infections, in which (*d*) suppurative infarcts also occur.

The unilateral *renal carbuncle* usually occurs in the course of *furunculosis,* or a *whitlow,* or some *suppurative lesion* of bone, periosteum or joint.

Symptoms.—The onset is sudden, with a rigor. There is usually pain in the region of the kidney, accompanied by tenderness on palpation in the costo-vertebral angle. Tenderness on fist percussion is usually very marked. Sometimes an enlarged tender kidney may be felt on bimanual palpation.

The course depends upon the situation of the abscess. If this lies in the renal cortex perinephric inflammation aids in diagnostic localization. If rupture of a cortical abscess occurs a *perinephric abscess* develops. If, on the other hand, the abscess lies deep in the kidney it may give little or no localizing signs until its rupture into the renal pelvis results in pyuria. Prior to rupture the patient may suffer from a long-continued fever the cause of which remains obscure until pyuria occurs. The more chronic cases of this nature may present considerable diagnostic difficulty, being often confused with biliary disease when the right kidney is involved, or with splenic lesions when on the left. The puzzling nature of these cases is enhanced by the fact that the urine exhibits few abnormalities except for the presence of the infecting organism in urine cultures.

The course depends also upon the virulence of the infection. The outlook is grave in the fulminating cases unless a correct diagnosis is made and proper surgical treatment instituted. In the less acute cases rupture into the renal pelvis may result in spontaneous healing, though it is more commonly followed by a chronic pyuria. In such cases surgical intervention becomes necessary when improvement fails to follow upon expectant treatment.

Pyelitis and Pyelonephritis.—**Definition.**—Inflammations of the pelvis of the kidney are of two types, a descending or hematogenous infection and an ascending infection presumably due to lymphatic extension from the lower urogenital tract. In the descending type it is probable that the kidney is involved in a pyelonephritis in practically every case, though pathologic confirmation of this is difficult to obtain.

Etiology.—The descending infections usually appear spontaneously, and constitute a common ailment of women, frequently beginning in childhood. In such cases in little girls the right kidney is the one usually first involved. Bacillus coli is the infecting agent in nearly all cases. Attacks of pyelitis are frequently initiated by some intestinal disturbance, severe constipation or diarrhea. Attention has been called to the rich lymphatic connections between the cecum and ascending colon and the right kidney. Chronic infectious foci, about teeth, tonsils and gall-bladder, and furunculosis are important etiologic factors.

Ascending infections, secondary to some lesion of the lower urogenital tract, in which extension upward takes place along the lymph channels of the ureter, are also frequently due to Bacillus coli, though not by any means exclusively. Bacillus proteus and pyogenic cocci may be found in such cases. Ascending infections may follow urethritis, prostatitis, urethral or ureteral stricture. Instrumentation or the simple passage of a catheter may initiate the ascent. Urinary obstruction from any cause may result in it. It is not uncommon in pregnancy. Infection of the ruptured hymen sometimes results in a "defloration pyelitis." Occasionally it follows operation upon the female genitalia.

Contributory causes of pyelitis are important. Anemias and debilitating illnesses predispose to it, particularly in women. Neurologic conditions involving the control of micturition cause a great tendency to cystitis and pyelitis. Catheterization in such cases should be avoided except in special circumstances.

The possible influence of dietary deficiencies should not be overlooked. In experimental animals deficiency of vitamin A leads to metaplasia of cuboidal epithelium to a more squamous type. Such metaplasia in rats seems to predispose them to otitis media and pyelitis with great frequency.

Pathology.—The ureters and pelvis show various degrees of inflammatory change. The inflammation is sometimes pseudomembranous. At times small ulcers form. Cicatrization of the ureter or blockage by thick exudates sometimes leads to distention of the pelvis, flattening and distortion of the calyces. In severe cases the kidneys show streaks of suppuration in the pyramids of the medulla, which sometimes widen out through confluence. The cortex may be involved and small yellowish foci surrounded by a red areola may be seen on the surface. The papillæ may be destroyed. Such a process occasionally undergoes healing, leading to permanent distortion of the calyces and considerable scarring of the kidneys.

Symptoms.—The onset is usually acute, with rigor, and fever amounting to 104° F. The temperature is usually remittent and soon becomes intermittent. In many cases after four to six days it falls by lysis. Relapses at intervals of ten to fourteen days are frequent. In other severe cases remittent fevers of four to six weeks' duration are encountered. Afebrile cases are occasionally seen. Pulse and respiration are not much affected relative to the fever. Leukocytosis may not be marked unless there is pyonephrosis or severe pyelonephritis. Headache, nausea and vomiting are common.

At the onset, particularly in children, there are often no symptoms to draw attention to the urinary tract. The earliest and commonest is some degree of urgency and frequency, with burning or pain on micturition. Nycturia is frequent. Older children sometimes resume bed-wetting during a pyelitis.

Renal pain is often lacking, though at times it may be severe, particularly if a ureteral block occurs or if the kidney is severely involved. More commonly there is tenderness on pressure in the costo-vertebral angle or on attempts at bimanual palpation of the kidney.

Examination of the urine reveals pus and bacteria in it. The pus is frequently seen in threads. Bacteriuria may give an opalescent appearance. Casts are rarely present. Albuminuria varies from 0.5

to 2 per cent. The amount does not always correspond well with the amount of pus. Some degree of macroscopic hematuria is usual.

The reaction of the urine depends upon the nature of the infecting organism. Bacillus coli gives an acid urine, as do also Bacillus typhosus, paratyphosus and streptococci. In alkaline urine staphylococci and Bacillus proteus may be found. The organism should be identified by culture of a catheter specimen. During rigors a positive blood culture may frequently be obtained, particularly in the case of Bacillus coli.

Tests of renal function reveal some impairment in a considerable proportion of the cases. During the acute febrile stage the urine volume is usually reduced. The night specimen may be increased, however.

Chronic pyelitis may follow an acute attack, or may follow an asymptomatic period. During these asymptomatic periods persistent bacteriuria may be noted. Cystoscopic investigation in this stage reveals chronic inflammatory changes in the bladder in a considerable proportion of the cases. Differential studies of the urine from each kidney and pyelograms reveal a goodly number with damaged function and abnormalities of pelvis and calyces.

Prognosis.—In the spontaneously developing cases of Bacillus coli infection the prognosis *ad vitam* is good. The disease frequently becomes chronic and has a great tendency to relapse after apparent healing. In infants, however, the prognosis is grave.

In the case of ascending infections, particularly in association with urinary obstruction, the outlook is serious. Pyelonephritis in such cases not infrequently leads to uremic death. The nephrocirrhosis consequent to pyelonephritis results in some degree in permanent reduction in the reserves of renal function in many of the cases which heal.

Treatment.—In the acute stages of pyelitis every effort should be made to force fluids to insure active diuresis. The reaction of the urine should be changed if possible. In the case of infections by the colon bacillus, alkalinization of the urine by administration of sodium bicarbonate and citrates of sodium and potassium frequently gives prompt symptomatic relief. Neutral acriflavine also aids in the presence of an alkaline urine. If the infection fails to subside within seven to ten days the urine should be allowed to become acid again, and periods of administration of hexamethylenamine with acid urine should alternate with alkaline treatment. In those infections characterized by alkaline urine the order of procedure is reversed. In the alkaline infections due to staphylococcus the intravenous use of neoarsphenamine is frequently of great benefit. In all chronic cases of pyelitis cystoscopic investigation should be made to rule out the presence of obstructive lesions.

Collateral to the measures already mentioned, investigations should be directed toward the correction of chronic constipation, if such exists, toward the relief of chronic focal infection of teeth, tonsils, gall-bladder and so on. Anemia, if it exists, should be treated both symptomatically and from the standpoint of its cause. Careful investigation of

36

the diet is indicated, to ensure its adequacy in respect to vitamins, minerals and protein of good quality. Vitamin A should be specially added to the diet by means of a good cod-liver oil, especially during the winter and spring months.

TUBERCULOSIS OF KIDNEYS AND URINARY TRACT.

Tuberculosis of the kidneys and urinary tract may occur as part of a generalized miliary tuberculosis, in which both kidneys are simultaneously involved, or it may occur as a localized infection usually beginning in one kidney and spreading later to the lower urinary and genital tract and to the other kidney. The latter form is usually secondary to tuberculosis elsewhere in the body, especially of the lungs.

Pathology.—The initial lesions in the kidney may occur anywhere in the kidney, but most characteristically involve the pyramidal portion extending into the calyces, which may first show enlargement and subsequently destruction by ulceration. Caseation and fibrosis may gradually convert the involved kidney into a caseous mass. Very rarely the ureter may be sealed off by the extension of the process into it, a condition which is known as auto-nephrectomy.. More usually tuberculous products discharged from the kidney continue to pass to the lower urinary tract, first involving the ureter at its lower end and later causing a superficial catarrhal inflammation of the bladder, which may subsequently develop tubercules. Secondary involvement of the seminal vesicles, epididymis and prostate is not uncommon.

Symptoms.—The commonest symptom of onset is frequency of urination, which may later become painful. There may be mild renal pain, and occasional mild attacks of renal colic if the ureter becomes obstructed. The patient sometimes notes pyuria, and hematuria intermittently. The microscopic examination of the urine usually reveals a persistent hematuria and pyuria. In many cases vague indefinite constitutional symptoms may occur, loss of weight, anorexia, slight fever, fatigue and night sweats, such as one encounters in any tuberculous infection.

Investigation of the urine in the early stages usually reveals some pyuria *without the presence of non-tuberculous microörganisms*, though secondary infection may occur in later stages of renal tuberculosis. Tubercle bacilli may be demonstrated by appropriate staining technic, although this often requires frequent and persistently repeated examinations, in which one must use great care to exclude other acid-fast organisms. Inoculation of the urine into guinea-pigs is a more reliable method of demonstrating the organism than is staining. In diagnosis the careful examination of the seminal vesicles, prostate and epididymes is indicated, as the finding of hard nodular indurations may give a clue to the nature of the renal lesion, and of the extent to which the disease is advanced. Not infrequently draining sinuses in the scrotum are observed. Also the lower end of the vas deferens may be found to be beaded and indurated.

Tuberculosis of the kidney should be suspected in every case of frequency with pyuria occurring without demonstrable bacteria. A competent urologist should be consulted to carry out the diagnostic cystoscopy and pyelography upon which the early diagnosis depends. If such service is not available the internists may attempt to visualize the urinary tract by intravenous pyelography. This is of the greatest importance because of the necessity of doing a nephrectomy while the disease is still unilateral, if one expects to effect an arrest of the disease.

Prognosis.—If nephrectomy is done while the disease is unilateral and before involvement of the seminal tract occurs, a cure may be expected. Even when the seminal tract is involved a cure may be effected, or life greatly prolonged, especially when nephrectomy is combined with surgical treatment of the seminal tract.

It is not sufficient merely to treat the urogenital lesions, however. The patient himself must be treated in the same general way as with all other forms of tuberculosis, with proper attention to rest, nutrition, psychologic adjustments and the general hygiene of living.

TUMORS OF THE KIDNEY.

Ewing describes a variety of tumors of the kidneys: adenomas, adenocarcinomas, carcinomas and tumors due to adrenal rests within the kidneys, teratomas and sarcomas, as well as those of the renal pelvis, bladder and prostate. The student is referred to this excellent source for further information regarding their pathology and clinical peculiarities. They usually have in common the symptoms of hematuria, renal pain and frequently palpable renal masses. The details of their recognition by radiogram and cystoscopy are to be found in urologic texts.

POLYCYSTIC KIDNEYS.

This interesting condition, believed to be of congenital origin, is characterized by enlargement of the kidneys due to cystadenomas. It is often accompanied by similar cystic formations in the liver, and occasionally in the spleen and thyroid gland. Developmental anomalies of various sorts may coëxist, such as imperforate anus or congenital heart disease.

The condition is usually bilateral, but is not invariably so. When both kidneys are involved one may be larger than the other. The size may be enormous. Kidneys weighing more than 1000 grams are usual. The surface is studded with projecting cysts of 6 to 10 mm. in size. The cyst walls are thin and transparent. The contents may be fluid or jelly-like, pale yellow in color, though at times the fluid may be dark and turbid. Albumin, products of disintegrated blood, and crystals of cholesterin, and phosphates are often found in the fluid.

On microscopic examination there are found to be remnants of renal tissue in varying amount. It seems probable that the disease is progressive after birth, slowly displacing normal renal tissue. Not a few cases survive into middle life before renal insufficiency occurs, and in rare cases it does not occur.

The *symptoms* are of two main types, those due to the presence of large renal tumors and those of chronic hemorrhagic nephritis. The enlargement of the abdomen and the discovery of renal tumors may precede any evidence of disturbed renal function. In other cases recurring hematuria, progressive anemia, hypertension, cardiac hypertrophy, arteriosclerosis and diminishing renal function may lead to a mistaken diagnosis of chronic nephritis unless the presence of renal tumors is discovered. This error need only rarely be made, when renal enlargement is masked by some other factor such as ascites or obesity. The pyelogram of polycystic kidneys is very characteristic and a great aid in diagnosis.

The *treatment* is that of chronic nephritis. Some observers have noted improvement following aspiration of the cysts after surgical exposure.

REFERENCES.

Addis, T., and Oliver, J.: The Renal Lesion in Bright's Disease, New York, Paul B. Hoeber, Inc., 1931.
Bright, Richard: Cases and Observations on Renal Disease Accompanied by the Secretion of Albuminous Urine, Guy's Hosp. Repts., 1836, 1, 338; Tabular View of the Morbid Appearances Occurring in 100 Cases, in Connection with Albuminous Urine, ibid., 380.
Ewing, James: Neoplastic Diseases, 2d ed., Philadelphia, W. B. Saunders Company, 1922, p. 738.
Fishberg, A. M.: Hypertension and Nephritis, Philadelphia, Lea & Febiger, 1931.
Van Slyke, D. D., et al.: Observations on the Courses of Different Types of Bright's Disease, and on the Resultant Changes in Renal Anatomy, Medicine, 1930, 9, 257.
Volhard, F.: Nieren und ableitende Harnwege, in Handb. d. inn. Med., Bd. VI, Teil I u. II, Bergmann and Staehelin; II. Aufl., Berlin, Springer, 1931.
Volhard, F., and Fahr, Th.: Die Brightsche Nierenkrankheit, Berlin, 1914.

CHAPTER XIV.

DISEASES OF THE ALIMENTARY TRACT.

By ARTHUR L. BLOOMFIELD, M.D.

GENERAL CONSIDERATIONS.
DISEASES OF THE MOUTH, PHARYNX
    AND TONSILS.
    Medical Aspects of Dental Disease—
        Focal Infection.
    Vincent's Angina.
    Syphilis.
    Neoplasms.
DISEASES OF THE TONSILS.
    Acute Tonsillitis.
    Chronic Tonsillitis.
    Tuberculosis.
DISEASES OF THE ESOPHAGUS.
    Spasm.
    Cancer.
DISEASES OF THE STOMACH.
    Indigestion.
    Gastritis.
    Gastric and Duodenal Ulcer.
    Cancer.
    Other Tumors.
    Syphilis.
    Deformities, Displacements and
        Anomalies.
DISEASES OF THE INTESTINE.
    Intestinal Neuroses.
    Constipation.
    Diarrhea.
    Intestinal Obstruction.
    Appendicitis.
    Ulcerative Colitis.
    Tuberculosis.
    Tumors of the Bowel.
    Cancer of the Colon.
    Anomalies and Deformities of the
        Intestine.
DISEASES OF THE RECTUM.
    Infections.
    Tumors.
    Hemorrhoids.

DISEASES OF THE LIVER.
    Jaundice (Icterus).
    Hepatitis (Non-suppurative).
        Acute Hepatitis.
            Acute Yellow Atrophy.
            Infectious (Catarrhal) Jaundice.
        Subacute Hepatitis.
        Chronic Hepatitis.
    Hepatitis (Suppurative).
        Abscess.
    Syphilis of the Liver.
    Neoplasms of the Liver.
        Cancer (Secondary).
        Cancer (Primary).
    Anomalies of Form and Position.
DISEASES OF THE GALL-BLADDER AND
        BILE DUCT.
    Cholangitis.
    Cholecystitis.
        Acute.
        Chronic. .
    Cancer of the Gall-bladder and Bile
        Ducts.
    Cholelithiasis (Gall stones).
    Stenosis and Congenital Oblitera-
        tion of the Bile Passages.
DISEASES OF THE PANCREAS.
    Pancreatitis.
        Acute.
        Chronic.
    Cancer of the Pancreas.
    Cysts of the Pancreas.
    Pancreatic Calculi.
DISEASES OF THE PERITONEUM.
    Acute General Peritonitis.
    Localized Peritonitis (Abscess).
        Acute.
        Chronic.
    Chronic Adhesive Peritonitis.
    Tumors of the Peritoneum.

THE MOUTH, PHARYNX AND TONSILS.

General Considerations.—The mouth and pharynx include a number of anatomic structures which, in spite of their close proximity to one another, have little in common from the standpoint of the disorders which may affect them. Furthermore, while there are certain lesions

(565)

of these structures which are truly local, the pathologic changes in the main are part and parcel of, or incidental to, some widespread, constitutional or remote disease. Logical classification, therefore, immediately becomes difficult and in point of fact a complete consideration of the disorders of the mouth and pharynx would lead one into practically every by-path of medicine. Diphtheria, for example, exhibits its outstanding lesion in the pharyngeal region, but the disease certainly can be discussed more intelligently from the standpoint of infections in general than as a local disorder. Or, to illustrate further, in agranulocytic angina there may be picturesque mouth lesions but it is now known that they are usually secondary to more fundamental changes in the hematopoietic organs; and so on. Hence our discussion of the subject will consist first of a brief and diagrammatic synopsis of the implications of the various mouth and pharyngeal lesions to be followed by a more detailed discussion of those disorders which are in a strict sense local and proper to the structures under consideration.

Relations to Acute Infectious Disease.—In certain infectious diseases, especially diphtheria, scarlet fever and acute tonsillitis, the principal site of infection is in the pharyngeal and tonsillar region. With Vincent's angina the lesions may be more widespread through the buccal cavity or they may be confined to the tonsils. Most of the exanthemata, so-called, exhibit mouth lesions; one may mention the Koplik's spots and enanthem of measles, the curious erythema of the pharynx in influenza and the mouth lesions of varicella and variola. Anyone who has had a large experience with typhoid fever will recall the striking appearance of the tongue—tremulous, coated at the center and red at tip and edges—even if these findings are not characteristic. Many illustrations could be given.

Relations to Skin Diseases.—A variety of so-called skin diseases may exhibit mouth lesions. The student must consult the dermatologic texts, but erythema multiforme should be mentioned as an outstanding example, especially since, on occasion, the buccal lesions may overshadow the cutaneous phenomena. The swellings of angioneurotic edema, which so often affect lips, tongue or pharynx, are perhaps to be listed here.

Relations to Infectious Granulomata.—Interesting lesions may affect the mouth, tonsils and pharynx in syphilis, tuberculosis and leprosy. At certain stages of the infection these disturbances are to all intents and purposes local; they will be discussed more in detail below.

Relations to Diseases of the Blood.—A wide variety of unusual lesions occur in the mouth and pharynx in association with diseases of the blood. Of especial interest are the petechiæ and hemorrhages from the mucous membranes which are so prominent with the various types of hemorrhagic disease (thrombopenic purpura), the ulcerations of agranulocytic angina, the curious infiltrations of the tonsils in infectious mononucleosis, the atrophy of the tongue papillæ in pernicious anemia, and the nodular infiltrations of the gums and tonsils which sometimes occur with leukemia. Infiltrations of the tonsils with the specific lymphoblastomatous tissue are also seen occasionally in Hodgkin's disease and generalized lymphosarcomatosis.

Relations to Systemic Disease.—Here we have a wide and varied list. A few examples may be given, such as the buccal pigmentation of Addison's disease, the red, dry tongue of diabetic acidosis, the stomatitis of pellagra, the thickening of the tongue in myxedema and in acromegaly, the changes in the gums in scurvy and the stomatitis of mercurial poisoning.

The above list is obviously incomplete, but its purpose is mainly to impress upon the student the wide implications of different mouth lesions. Turning now to more strictly local disorders, one has to consider affections of the lips, teeth, gums, tongue, buccal cavity proper, tonsils and pharynx. We shall not, however, discuss the subject from a topographic standpoint but will merely describe some of the more important conditions.

The older physicians considered inspection of the mouth, and especially of the tongue, second in importance only to the study of the pulse. It is now known, of course, that most of their deductions were unsound, but none the less very important information can be gleaned by a careful examination of the buccal cavity. Under normal conditions the lips and buccal mucosa are clean and moist and the tongue presents a uniform pink appearance with prominent clean papillæ. The commonest and least significant deviation is the so-called "coated tongue." Often associated with constipation, indigestion and with an unpleasant odor of the breath, it must be admitted that many apparently perfectly healthy people habitually display this gray coating and seem none the worse for it. The condition is said to be due to an accumulation of desquamated epithelium and bacteria, but even an intensive scrubbing fails to correct it in those who are predisposed. More important are the changes which may occur with acute and chronic febrile disorders or with chronic debilitating disease. Here, unless special precautions are exercised, the lips become dry, cracked and fissured and covered with dark crusts which are spoken of as *sordes,* the buccal mucosa loses its normal gloss and the tongue is dry and shrunken. In extreme cases the tongue resembles a piece of horn, its tissues become fissured and they bleed on the slightest provocation. The pharynx is dry and secretions accumulate on its surface where they may form crusts which interfere painfully with swallowing. The above condition may be spoken of as "the mouth of neglect" since it can be largely avoided by proper local care and by the introduction of fluids in adequate amount. A tooth-brush should be used several times a day or the teeth, gums and tongue should at least be gently cleaned with gauze soaked in warm salt solution. In febrile cases it is especially important to clean the mouth after feedings. Bits of cotton on small applicators may be used to attack the crevices between the teeth. Secretions which accumulate in the pharynx should be removed by means of long swabs. If the patient can coöperate the mouth should be frequently rinsed with a mild alkaline lotion such as bicarbonate of soda and common salt, a teaspoonful of each to the pint of warm water, and a mixture of albolene 3 parts and glycerin 1 part should be freely applied to the lips and tongue to prevent fissuring. The importance of keeping the mouth clean during the course of prolonged fevers and chronic diseases of all sorts cannot be emphasized too strongly. First of all, there is the matter of comfort, and we do not wish our patients to have, like Kipling's Tommie "a mouth like a dried potato and a tongue like a button stick." Secondly, unless the mouth is in proper condition the patient cannot eat, and failure to take adequate nourishment is often disastrous. Finally, a dirty mouth sometimes promotes serious local infections, gangrene or parotitis, which may determine a fatal outcome for the case. In hospital work there is no better way of quickly judging the caliber of the nursing than to go through the wards and inspect the patients' mouths.

MEDICAL ASPECTS OF DENTAL DISEASE—FOCAL INFECTION.

The interesting dystrophies of the teeth which occur occasionally in congenital syphilis (Hutchinson's teeth), and in various nutritional disorders, as well as the rare hereditary anomalies of dentition cannot be discussed in detail here. Lack of proper denture always requires careful consideration; if the patient is unable to chew properly digestive and nutritional disturbances often result. It is hardly worth while, for example, to prescribe a liberal diet of meat and vegetables for a person who has only a few scattered snags. Certainly it is the duty of the physician to insist on proper attention to the teeth and to direct his patients to a competent dentist.

As to the actual causal relationship of dental disease to medical disorders, much has been claimed of recent years. It has been argued especially that local periapical tooth infections or alveolar abscesses act as foci of infection from which there may be either an absorption of toxic products or an actual distribution of bacteria which are responsible for remote lesions or for generalized disturbances of health. Hypertension, nephritis, arthritis, anemia, iritis, gastric ulcer and encephalitis are a few examples of the many conditions which have been alleged to result from such "focal infections."

The evidence upon which the focal infection theory has reposed is both experimental and clinical. On the experimental side the usual mode of procedure, elaborated especially by Rosenow, has been to make cultures from the infected area in some form of fluid medium which, after growth has taken place, is directly injected into rabbits in large amounts. It is claimed that specific lesions are produced in a high percentage of the experimental animals. If, for example, the dental abscess occurs in a patient with arthritis, then it is claimed that the cultures may produce arthritis in the rabbit. The organisms which have been isolated have, for the most part, been some variety of non-hemolytic streptococcus. However, most bacteriologists have been unable to confirm the doctrine of "elective localization" of Rosenow which has been outlined above; furthermore, it is very difficult to believe that such obviously unrelated conditions as chronic arthritis, gastric ulcer and acute poliomyelitis, to mention only a few, are all caused by non-hemolytic streptococci.

In spite of the uncertain state of the experimental basis for the focal infection theory it has won an astonishingly wide acceptance among clinicians, especially in America. Not only dental infections, but diseased tonsils, infected paranasal sinuses, localized infections in the genito-urinary tract, appendix, gall-bladder and elsewhere have been regarded as "foci" responsible for remote disease. Clinically, the usual mode of procedure is to eliminate the focus or foci, that is to say, to extract the suspected tooth, or extirpate the diseased tonsils, in the hope of curing or alleviating the condition such as arthritis, iritis, myocarditis, or what not, for which relief is sought. On the whole, the clinical results have been most disappointing and while every physician can recount individual miracles—which mean nothing, since chance, faith and uncontrolled variables, as well as possible foreign protein reaction, come into play—adequate statistics have failed to show that any consistent remote effects are obtained. The ardor of even the most enthusiastic has been dampened as years of experience have accumulated and while physicians still continue to advise elimination of "foci" the procedure is now hardly more than a gesture which lingers with us as the result of habit, and because it enables one to do something in chronic cases, in which there is so little to do. Let it not be understood that the writer is opposed to dealing with local infections if proper indications exist. Certainly abscesses at the roots of dead teeth deserve attention for their own sake, if for no other reason, and surely no one would advise the neglect of a severe chronic prostatitis. The most pernicious aspect of focal infection in practice has been the promises to patients rashly made but later not fulfilled. Over and over again these wretched creatures have been told "we shall remove your teeth and you will then be cured of your arthritis." This is, of course, inexcusable, and if the physician is disposed to have confidence in focal infection therapy he should at least represent his project to the patient as a purely experimental one.

REFERENCES.

For critical discussion of focal infection with extensive bibliography see:
   Holman, W. L.: Focal Infection and "Elective Localization," Arch. Path. and Lab. Med., 1928, **5**, 68.

VINCENT'S ANGINA.

Definition.—A disease featured by ulcerations of the mucous membranes of the gums, buccal cavity or tonsils, associated with the presence of spirillæ and fusiform bacilli. The primary causal agent is unknown.

Etiology.—In large aggregations of people such as military organizations the disease may occur in epidemic form (trench mouth). Most of the instances in civil life, however, are sporadic and cannot be traced to any other case. Age, sex and external conditions play no definite part and while dirty, ill-kept mouths are said to be specially susceptible, the disease may occur in spite of excellent oral hygiene.

Some of the cases are obviously secondary to some antecedent predisposing injury or disease, such as arsphenamine poisoning with granulopenia, agranulocytosis of obscure etiology (agranulocytic angina) and leukemia, but as a rule the trouble comes out of a clear sky. Bacteriologic study of the lesions usually yields an interesting combination of spirillæ and fusiform bacilli which were described by Plaut and by Vincent in 1894. The organisms are difficult to cultivate but are readily stained in smears made directly from the lesions. The Bacillus fusiformis is from 4 to 14 microns long and about 0.5 micron wide at its center from which it tapers to the ends. It is anaërobic, non-motile, non-sporeforming and Gram-negative. The spirillæ have from 5 to 8 wide convolutions, the ends are pointed, they are motile, Gram-negative and stain less readily than the fusiform bacilli.

It is doubtful, however, whether these organisms are the primary cause of the trouble, and both experimental studies as well as certain clinical observations indicate rather that they are secondary invaders which unfold their activities on soil damaged by some other undetermined agent.

Clinical Picture.—Ulcero-membranous lesions associated with the Vincent's organisms may occur in various situations such as rectum, vagina and lung (spirochetal pulmonary gangrene), but the present discussion will deal with the disorder as it affects the mouth. Two clinical types may be distinguished—diffuse ulcero-membranous stomatitis and the localized ulcerative form—although transition forms occur.

The diffuse form begins with a sore, raw feeling in the mouth and with tenderness and swelling of the gums. In the earliest stages only a reddening of the mucous membranes is visible, but there soon appear areas of thin adherent grayish membranous exudate. These are especially prominent on the gums near the dental margin but may occur diffusely through the buccal cavity. Attempts to remove the membrane reveal shallow ulcerations which bleed readily. There is marked fetor and salivation, and often great pain which makes it almost impossible to bite, chew and swallow. In extreme cases the teeth become loosened. The degree of constitutional reaction varies, but in many cases the patient is prostrated and there may be high fever. Moderate polymorphonuclear leukocytosis is the rule. The condition is a stubborn one and several weeks or even months elapse before complete healing takes place. The membranes gradually shrink and exfoliate, the ulcerations heal and the red sensitive mucous membranes slowly return to normal. Relapses are common, but the outlook is good, especially in the sporadic cases, which are rarely fatal. Local pyogenic abscesses may complicate the situation.

The localized form affects especially the tonsils. The lesions may predominate on, or be confined to, one side. With more or less violent constitutional reaction and fever, sore throat develops and on inspection the entire tonsil is red and swollen. An area of dense grayish membrane soon appears which covers a sluggish punched-out ulcer of variable size and shape. After persisting for a week or more the membrane resolves, the general tonsillar swelling subsides, the ulceration heals and the constitutional symptoms subside.

Diagnosis.—One should always take pains to exclude such conditions as agranulocytic angina and leukemia by examination of blood smear and by leukocyte count. Diphtheria and gumma must be distinguished from the local tonsillar form by means of cultures, smears and the Wassermann reaction. The diffuse form can hardly be mistaken for any other condition, although extensive syphilitic mucous patches may occasionally lead to confusion.

Treatment.—Even if the constitutional symptoms are mild the patient should be kept in bed or at least quietly at home. The same precautions against spread of the infection to others are in order as in acute tonsillitis (see below). Liquid and soft nourishment should be given freely, and even if the mouth is very painful the patient must be urged to eat. Mild general sedatives such as barbital, bromides, or codeine may be needed to secure rest at night. A vast variety of local applications and washes have been advised. In the writer's experience the following has been found useful: the mouth is thoroughly rinsed every hour or so with warm saline solution. Three or four times daily the teeth are cleaned and loose exudate is removed by means of pledgets of cotton (on an applicator) soaked in Fowler's solution. The procedure should be gentle but thorough and it is preferably carried out after a feeding. The excess of Fowler's solution is removed by a saline irrigation after each treatment is completed. In some cases painting the lesions with 2 per cent gentian violet has been useful. Arsphenamine intravenously (neo-arsphenamine, 0.3 grams) has been extensively advised and is said on occasion to be followed by prompt recovery. Our own experience with it has been disappointing. Above all, violent local manipulations with the use of strong antiseptics are contraindicated. They do not eliminate the infection and only serve to irritate.

REFERENCE.

Bloomfield, A. L.: Vincent's Angina, Oxford Loose Leaf Medicine, vol. **5**.

SYPHILIS OF THE MOUTH AND PHARYNX.

The mouth and pharynx may be affected in any of the stages of syphilis. Extragenital *chancres* occasionally occur on the lip; the tongue, buccal mucosa or even the tonsil may be involved. The lesion is modified by its situation but preserves the essential characteristics of an indurated mass with associated regional lymphadenitis. There may or may not be ulceration. Descriptions are of little value since one must be familiar with the appearances in order to have confidence in his diagnosis. The important point is that the physician keep the possibility in mind; he should not depend on the Wassermann test since it may not yet have become positive. In doubtful cases dark-field examination is often decisive.

The secondary manifestations, *mucous patches*, occur with the roseola and are analogous to it. Their appearance is usually characteristic— flat, grayish lesions with a tendency to superficial ulceration, especially abundant in the tonsillar and pharyngeal regions, although any part of the buccal cavity may be affected. The pharynx may be diffusely reddened in addition to the local lesions and the usual complaint is that of sore throat. The discovery of cutaneous lesions is especially helpful in confirming the diagnosis and the Wassermann test is uniformly positive.

Tertiary lesions, *gummata*, occur especially on the tongue and on the pillars, tonsils and pharyngeal wall. They may be painless and are discovered accidentally by the patient or there may be soreness and discomfort on swallowing. The lesions at first consist of nodular swellings which tend to ulcerate and finally leave scars which may grossly deform the affected regions. Complete erosion of the uvula, loss of part of the soft palate, perforation of the tonsillar pillars and adhesions of these structures to the pharyngeal wall are not uncommon end results. Gummata are to be differentiated from carcinoma, tuberculosis, and from rhinoscleroma. The Wassermann test and biopsy are valuable aids.

Treatment cannot be discussed in this section but general antiluetic measures are in order.

NEOPLASMS OF THE BUCCAL-PHARYNGEAL STRUCTURES.

The most important tumors of the buccal-pharyngeal structures are epitheliomata. The lip, tongue, buccal mucosa, tonsil and pharynx all may be involved. These conditions are essentially surgical and cannot be dealt with in detail here. However, every physician should be alive to the possibility and all lesions, even if they appear insignificant, should be seriously investigated, if necessary by biopsy, since early operation offers the only chance of cure and even at best the outlook is none too good. Malignant lesions present themselves either as indurated areas or as ulcerations, and the commonest errors are either to disregard them as being insignificant or to confuse them with gumma or tuberculosis. In the advanced hopeless stages with extensive sloughing and metastases the diagnosis is obvious.

ACUTE TONSILLITIS.

Definition.—Acute (follicular or lacunar) tonsillitis is an acute inflammation of the lymphadenoid tissue of the pharynx, especially the tonsils, caused by beta-hemolytic streptococci.

Etiology.—The specific bacterial agent is a hemolytic streptococcus (beta type of Brown). The evidence on which this fact is based is (1) the recovery of the streptococcus in practically pure culture from the tonsil in 100 per cent of the cases if poured blood agar plates are properly made, (2) the clinical and epidemiologic similarity to other known hemolytic streptococcus diseases such as scarlet fever, (3) the experimental production of the disease in volunteers by inoculation with hemolytic streptococci (Dick and Dick, Richey) and (4) the temporary immunity of carriers of the specific organisms (Bloomfield and Felty). While most writers recognize tonsillitis as a streptococcus disease they usually add that it may occasionally be due to staphylococci, pneumococci or other organisms. This is just as illogical as it would be to say that tuberculosis is usually due to the tubercle bacillus but sometimes to the colon bacillus or the plague bacillus. For a complete discussion of the subject and the detailed proof of the above statements the reader is referred to the articles of Bloomfield and Felty.

Most of the cases occur during the winter and spring months; the epidemiology is identical with that of scarlet fever. Young people are especially affected and those who are susceptible are liable to recurring attacks during successive seasons. The organisms are introduced by contact with other cases or carriers, or indirectly by ingestion of contaminated food, especially milk. After an acute attack the specific streptococci persist for a variable length of time in the tonsils; during this period the subject seems to be immune to further attacks.

Clinical Picture.—The disease begins with the constitutional reaction common to all acute infections—malaise, headache, anorexia and fever. There are often chills at the onset. Hand in hand with these symptoms the throat becomes sore, and within a day or two there is intense pain, especially on swallowing. It may be impossible to eat, and even sips of fluid are taken with difficulty. The glands at the angles of the jaw become swollen and painful.

During the first few hours the tonsils appear diffusely reddened and swollen. Subsequently they may assume immense proportions and they may practically meet in the mid-line. Exudate pours from the crypts as grayish patches (lacunar tonsillitis) or the swollen collections of lymphoid tissue may stand out as whitish nodules (follicular tonsillitis). The temperature rises to 102° to 105° F., the pulse is rapid and there is a variable degree of intoxication and prostration.

The disease runs its course, unless complications ensue, in from four to seven days. As a rule the temperature falls rapidly, the tonsillar swelling subsides, the glands in the neck resolve and there is an almost critical relief of symptoms. The mortality is negligible.

There is a polymorphonuclear leukocytosis (usually 12,000 to 20,000) and the urine shows the findings of an acute fever, high specific gravity with, perhaps, a little albumin and a few granular casts.

Complications and sequelæ are relatively infrequent. Local peritonsillar abscesses occasionally occur or streptococcus otitis media or erysipelas may supervene. Very rarely tonsillitis may be the starting point of a generalized streptococcus sepsis with multiple abscesses and bacteriemia. Acute hemorrhagic Bright's disease is known to follow tonsillitis, but it is less frequently encountered than after scarlet fever.

There is a much more severe variety of epidemic tonsillitis which has been described as *"septic sore throat."* A special streptococcus has been incriminated by Davis and the infection is acquired by the ingestion of milk contaminated with the organisms usually as a result of bovine mastitis. The disease runs a stormy course, with high fever, chills, great prostration and a tendency to suppuration of the local lesions and to widespread septic metastases. The mortality in some outbreaks has been as high as 25 to 40 per cent.

Diagnosis.—Diagnosis is made by inspection of the throat and usually presents no difficulty. Occasionally tonsillitis may be confused with diphtheria or with Vincent's angina. The membrane of diphtheria is, however, denser and more confluent and is likely to extend beyond the tonsil to the pillars or to the palate or pharynx. Vincent's infections of the tonsils usually lead to a solitary punched-out ulceration covered with dense adherent membrane. In doubtful cases cultures should be made, although any serious suspicion of diphtheria justifies the use of antitoxin even without a positive culture.

Prophylaxis and Treatment.—Tonsillectomy affords a high degree of protection and while the disease may still occur after the tonsils have been removed, in which case the seat of the streptococci is the bits of lymphadenoid tissue on the pharyngeal wall, the chances of infection are reduced about fourfold. Tonsillitis is not highly contagious and it is unusual to have more than one case in a family at the same time. None the less, the patient should be placed in a separate room, his dishes, untensils and linen should be isolated and the attendants should wear gowns while in close contact and should scrub the hands carefully on leaving the sick room.

The disease is essentially self-limited and treatment consists mainly of nursing and of attention to the patient's comfort. Complete bed rest should be enforced during the febrile period and for several days thereafter. Gradually increasing activity may then be allowed, but the patient should not go back to work until at least two weeks of convalescence have elapsed. The urine should be observed for a month or two to be sure that the kidneys have escaped. Any liquid or soft diet is allowable, but if there is great pain on swallowing, nourishment should not be forced. If necessary, fluids (salt solution) can be given by rectum—400 cc. every four to six hours. Small bits of cracked ice relieve the local discomfort, and if the cervical glands are much enlarged and tender a light ice-bag should be applied. For general discomfort and insomnia aspirin, barbital and codeine are useful. The local application of strong antiseptics to the tonsils is absolutely to be decried. It is futile to attempt to eliminate the infection by such measures and serious harm may be done by traumatizing the acutely inflamed areas. We have seen several cases of fatal streptococcus sepsis following ill-advised probing and swabbing. A gargle of warm saline solution should be used frequently. This is non-irritating and harmless and has a mild cleansing effect.

CHRONIC TONSILLITIS.

Many people possess tonsils which cannot be regarded as altogether normal. They may be very large, they may be scarred or adherent, they may have crypts plugged with caseous material or they may be subject to recurring attacks of acute inflammation. All of these changes have been loosely grouped under the heading of chronic tonsillitis. Tonsillar disease of this sort may be present in otherwise perfectly healthy and normal people; it occurs equally in those afflicted with every sort of ailment. The physician's concern, of course, is whether these changes have any bearing on the patient's general health, present or future, and whether they have a causal relationship to remote disorders such as arthritis or nephritis.

It must be admitted at the start that practically no one has tonsils which are histologically normal. Sooner or later the epithelial lining of the crypts is broken, bacteria penetrate into the substance of the tonsillar tissue and the evidences of chronic inflammation are present. So frequent is such a state of affairs that one must exercise the greatest caution in concluding that these changes have any important bearing on the general health, and when the laryngologist gazes wisely into the patient's throat and tells him that his tonsils are badly infected, the statement has just about as much meaning as if one told him that his colon was swarming with bacteria. The tonsils have been much incriminated as a "focus of infection" in the same sense as periapical tooth abscesses. The matter has already been discussed in the section on focal infection.

In practice the point at issue is the indications which justify *tonsillectomy*. Fortunately large series of statistics have gradually been accumulated so that fairly dogmatic statements can now be made. Tonsillectomy undoubtedly greatly lessens the likelihood of subsequent attacks of tonsillitis, scarlet fever and, to some extent, of diphtheria. There is no evidence that, by and large, "colds," influenza or otitis media are prevented. First attacks of rheumatic fever are said to occur somewhat less frequently in tonsillectomized children, but recurrences are certainly not materially reduced. Local mechanical difficulties with breathing or with the voice justify tonsillectomy. With regard to remote disorders such as arthritis or nephritis the evidence is not conclusive, but such statistics as are available bring no proof that tonsillectomy either prevents or has any special beneficial effect on remote or constitutional disease. In brief, the present practice of indiscriminate removal of tonsils on the slightest excuse or for no reason at all is certainly to be decried. The subject is an importance one, since the operation, while not usually difficult, has its hazards as well as its economic implications. Every physician should give the matter serious thought and one may fairly add "let your conscience be your guide." At any rate, one should become familiar with the published statistics, references to some of which are appended below.

TUBERCULOSIS OF THE TONSILS.

With the exception of the tonsils, the buccal and pharyngeal structures are rarely involved by tubercle. The tonsils are probably a primary portal of entry for the bacilli and careful histologic study of tissues removed, for various reasons, by tonsillectomy shows that tuberculous lesions are present in a considerable percentage (4.18 per cent, Crowe). As a rule the tonsils present no special appearances and there are no constitutional symptoms. Marked unilateral enlargement should, however, make one think of the possibility. With clinical tuberculosis of the cervical nodes the tonsils are very frequently involved (20 to 70 per cent) and they probably should be removed under these conditions.

Manifest tuberculosis of the lips, tongue and buccal mucosa is very rare. The palate, uvula and pillars are more frequently involved.

The lesions are primarily tubercles which break down to shallow sluggish ulcerations. The diagnosis may be suspected if there is outspoken tuberculosis elsewhere in the body; otherwise biopsy may be necessary. Local excision or cauterization can be done but, on the whole, one depends on the general regimen used in tuberculosis.

REFERENCES.

ALVAREZ, W. C.: Lessons to be Learned from the Results of Tonsillectomies in Adult Life, Jour. Am. Med. Assn., 1923, **80**, 1513.

BLOOMFIELD, A. L.: The Association of Susceptibility to Scarlet Fever and Acute Tonsillitis, Calif. and West. Med., 1928, **28**, 477.

BLOOMFIELD, A. L., and FELTY, A. R.: Bacteriologic Observations on Acute Tonsillitis with Reference to Epidemiology and Susceptibility, Arch. Int. Med., 1923, **32**, 483.

CUNNINGHAM, R. L.: Normal, Absent and Pathologic Tonsils in Young Women: A Comparison of Histories, Arch. Int. Med., 1931, **47**, 513.

FELTY, A. R., and HODGES, A. B.: A Clinical Study of Acute Tonsillitis, Bull. Johns Hopkins Hosp., 1923, **34**, 330.

KAISER, A. D.: Results of Tonsillectomy, Jour. Am. Med. Assn., 1930, **95**, 837.

MACCREADY, P. B., and CROWE, S. J.: Tuberculosis of Tonsils and Adenoids, Am. Jour. Dis. Child., 1924, **27**, 113.

RICHEY, D. G.: Experimental Streptococcic Tonsillitis, Jour. Infec. Dis., 1919, **25**, 299.

THE ESOPHAGUS.

Disorders of the esophagus usually manifest themselves by difficulty or pain on swallowing, with which may be associated an actual impediment to the passage of food. In the vast majority of cases the trouble is due to cancer, with spasm and stenosis next in order of frequency. Inasmuch as the esophagus is inaccessible to ordinary physical examination, diagnosis must be made from the story, together with certain instrumental methods of exploration and the roentgen-ray.

Congenital malformations (stenoses) are a rare group of special interest to the pediatrician and pathologist. The infants usually die shortly after birth of infection or inanition. *Diverticula* occur often enough to justify the physician's keeping the possibility in mind in cases of unexplained regurgitation of food or dysphagia. They may result from congenital weakness of the esophageal wall to which the effects of spasm, irritation or external adhesions are superadded. Many are situated at the upper end of the tube and are accessible to surgical extirpation. The diagnosis is confirmed by roentgen-ray, which usually reveals the size and position of the sac. Almost any unusual article may be accidentally swallowed and on occasion become impacted in the esophagus as a *foreign body*. The diagnosis is made from the history or by examination with the esophagoscope. Removal through the esophagoscope is necessary if the impaction persists. The most serious cases are those in which a sharp body such as a fish- or chicken-bone perforates the esophageal wall with resultant suppurative mediastinitis, since even prompt surgical drainage often fails to save the patient. *Benign tumors* are excessively rare, as are *tuberculosis* and *syphilis*. *Acute esophagitis* is said to occur occasionally with various infections, such as diphtheria and scarlet fever, but the most usual cause is the accidental or suicidal swallowing of acids (phenol) or caustics, such as lye. Pain, with dysphagia, are the outstanding symptoms, together with the constitutional effects of the poison or infection. There may be spasm with regurgitation of bloody, purulent or mucoid material. Instrumentation should be avoided during the acute phases for fear of perforating the esophageal wall. *Strictures* with partial or complete obstruction often remain as end results in those who recover, and offer difficult and complex therapeutic problems. In some cases instrumental dilatation may restore a passage, or gastrostomy for direct introduction of food into the stomach may have to be performed. Interesting cases of ulceration, especially of the lower part of the esophagus, have been described as *peptic ulcer of the esophagus* on the theory (not proven in all cases) that they arise in bits of misplaced gastric mucosa. The symptoms are not specific but epigastric or sternal pain, indigestion, regurgitation or bleeding usually occur in various combinations. Final diagnosis is made by esophagoscopy. Rest, small feedings of bland soft food and local applications (through the esophagoscope) of silver nitrate or bismuth subnitrate have been advised.

REFERENCES.

For systematic discussion of diseases of the esophagus, including malformations, injuries, foreign bodies, perforation, diverticula, tumors and infections, and for extensive references to the literature see article by FISCHER, in Henke and Lubarsch: Handbuch der speciellen pathologischen Anatomie und Histologie, 1926, **4**, Pt. I, 74.

JACKSON, C.: Peptic Ulcer of the Esophagus, Jour. Am. Med. Assn., 1929, **92**, 369.

JUDD, E. S.: Esophageal Diverticula, Arch. Surg., 1920, **1**, 38.

STURGEON, C. T.: Esophageal Diverticula, Jour. Am. Med. Assn., 1929, **92**, 379.

SPASM OF THE ESOPHAGUS.

Hollow viscera manifest ever-changing phases of tonus and motility and it is indeed remarkable that subjective sensations are ordinarily so completely absent. But if the series of reflexes which are responsible for the normal sequences of contraction and relaxation become even slightly deranged or "desynchronized," symptoms are likely to appear. Spasms of the pylorus (see article on indigestion) and of the lower end of the esophagus seem to occur in mild form quite frequently even in practically normal people; they may be associated with the symptoms of indigestion. But at times more persistent spasms of the esophagus arise, especially near the cardia and then quite outspoken and distressing consequences follow. In most of the cases, even if trouble persists for a long time, no structural changes occur except for hypertrophy of the esophageal muscle, and under proper therapy the spasm may be done away with and the patient is well, but occasionally there is associated a progressive dilatation of the tube above the constriction which eventually leads to serious results. Then the esophagus is greatly dilated like a loose bag, it may have a capacity of a liter or more, and the walls may sag down below the cardiac orifice

37

so that stagnation of food and secretions occurs with irritative esophagitis. The cause of esophageal spasms is not well understood. Developmental defects, disorders of the autonomic nerves (vagus) and psychic
influences have all been proposed and, while nervous influences obviously play a part, there is no explanation of why they should be
specially operative in a given individual so as to lead to persistent
spasm. The disorder can often, but not always, be correlated with
other nervous disturbances and it does not occur invariably in obviously neurotic or hysterical people. Women are affected much more
frequently than men and symptoms usually begin in young adult or
early middle life. Sometimes cardiospasm occurs as a reflex from
serious organic disease elsewhere in the gastro-intestinal tract, such
as cancer of the cardiac end of the stomach or gastric ulcer. This possibility must always be kept in mind to be excluded, if possible, during
the study of the case.

Symptoms.—The earliest symptom is usually a subjective feeling
that free passage of food down the esophagus is impeded. As a rule
there is more difficulty with solids than with liquids, but this is not
invariably so. Punctuated by periods of remission the general severity
of symptoms increases so that finally the patient has a definite feeling
that the food "sticks" in his esophagus, and there may be actual
regurgitation. Unpleasant sensations or pain, referred especially to
the episternal notch or epigastrium but at times to various regions
of the chest or back, accompany the bouts of spasm. On the whole
the symptoms are variable and at times the passage may seem to be
quite free. The patient soon learns that at certain hours of the day
or in certain situations it will "close up," and apprehension and
nervousness become superadded to the underlying difficulty. In the
severe cases with progressive dilatation of the esophagus nutrition may
be seriously impaired. Food, and its decomposition products, organic
acids and mucus accumulate in great quantity in the sac to be regurgi-
tated on occasion, usually without nausea or violent retching. But
on the whole the condition is essentially a chronic one and the patients
may go for years without serious impairment of health. They usually
die of some unrelated disease.

Physical Examination.—Physical examination shows nothing except,
perhaps, the evidences of impaired nutrition, which result in long-
standing cases. In extreme instances the patient is reduced to skin
and bones and the desiccated tissues give evidence of lack of proper
absorption of fluids. In one case of this sort, a woman who was
admitted as an emergency because of vomiting, an erroneous diagnosis
of pyloric obstruction and dilatation of the stomach led to a useless
laparotomy.

Further studies are necessary to determine the exact site and character of the disturbance and the roentgen-ray is indispensible. Following ingestion of a barium mixture (thick paste) a definite smooth
narrowing usually just above the cardia can often be clearly visualized.
There may be only slight dilatation above this or one may see a huge
irregular bag-like shadow. The smoothness of contour of the narrowing, as well as of the dilatated area, is suggestive of spasm in dis-

tinction to growth, but in doubtful cases direct inspection through the esophagoscope should be done and a bit of tissue taken, if necessary, for biopsy. It is inadvisable to pass sounds or bougies blindly for diagnostic purposes since, by ill-advised probing, one may rupture the esophageal wall with consequent suppurative mediastinitis, which is usually fatal.

Treatment.—One should try to discover and eliminate any mental hazards or adjustment difficulties, but most cases cannot be cured by psychotherapy. In mild grades of the disturbance regulation of diet by giving small meals of bland food to be eaten slowly and chewed well may give relief. To such a regimen may be added sedatives, sodium bromide, 1 gram after meals, and atropine or tincture bella-donnæ, 0.5 cc. or more one-half hour before eating. Drugs do not always help, however, and we have seen patients with the most marked symptoms even while under the full influence of atropine. By far the most satisfactory results are obtained by dilation, and Plummer's method seems to be the best. The patient first swallows a thread, and a day or so later when this has entered the stomach a bougie is threaded over it and passed until the obstructed area is engaged. The distance is measured and another bougie armed with a rubber bag is substituted. Dilation is effected by rapidly distending the bag with water under hydrostatic pressure. One forcible dilatation of this sort frequently effects a permanent cure, although there are some failures or relapses. The main disadvantage of this procedure is occasional rupture of the esophagus with its disastrous consequences, but in stubborn cases the risk seems worth while. The treatment is prefer-ably carried out by someone who has been trained in the method. In cases of advanced dilation of the esophagus with sac formation the problem is more complex. Dilation of the cardia may be tried. We know of one case in which cure followed gastrostomy, retrograde dila-tion of the cardia and resection of the redundant esophagus after it had been pulled through the cardia into the stomach.

ILLUSTRATIVE CASE—SPASM OF THE ESOPHAGUS (CARDIA).

H. C., American housewife, aged thirty-three years.

Complaint.—Tired and run down, loss of weight, and cough, indigestion and difficulty in swallowing.

Family History.—Negative.

Past History.—She has never been strong since birth of first child nine years ago. Six pregnancies in last nine years. She has worked very hard and has been under constant strain. For five to six years has had frequent attacks of indigestion with epigastric discomfort, sour stomach and vomiting with nausea.

Present Illness.—For the past year or so, in addition to her indigestion, she has had periodic spells of difficulty in swallowing. They seem to come without special provocation although they are likely to be worse when she is tired or nervous. There is a feeling that the food "sticks," and with this there is the indigestion described above and at times regurgitation of food. For the past three weeks has had a "heavy cold," with fever, general aching, cough and expectoration.

Physical Examination.—She was somewhat thin and she looked tired and worn. There was impairment of percussion note at both apices, and below right clavicle an area of definite dulness with bronchovesicular breathing and persistent moist râles was detected.   There were no other important physical findings. Blood pressure 110/75.

Laboratory.—Red blood cells, 4,600,000; hemoglobin, 78 per cent; white blood cells, 9000. Urine normal.

Sputum grayish, mucoid, *many tubercle* bacilli present.   Roentgen-ray of chest showed a sharply circumscribed triangular area of consolidation in the right upper lobe. There was also some fuzzy density in the left lung field. When the patient drank the contrast meal the esophagus was seen to be sharply and smoothly constricted at its cardiac end. Above, it was greatly dilated and tortuous (Fig. 23). Some barium entered the stomach and no abnormality was made out there or in the duodenum.

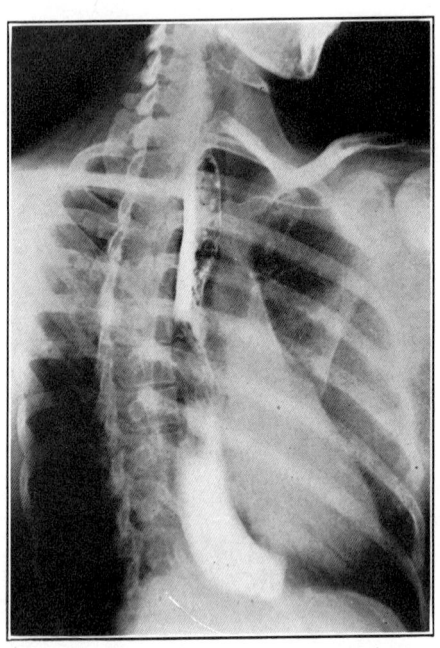

Fig. 23.—Cardiospasm. Note the constriction in the region of the cardia with marked dilatation above. Some barium may be seen entering the stomach.

Course.—The patient continued with moderate fever, cough and expectoration. After three weeks of rest in bed the cardia was dilated by means of a Plummer bag. All dysphagia immediately disappeared and a few days later roentgen-ray of the esophagus showed practically no arrest of barium at the cardia. The patient was sent to a tuberculosis sanitarium and six months later there had been no return of difficulty in swallowing or indigestion. However, roentgen-rays still showed some dilatation of the esophagus with a small amount of stasis just above the cardia. The pulmonary lesion seems to be arrested.

Comment.—The points to be noted are that in this case the cardiospasm led primarily to symptoms of indigestion. Difficulty in swallowing was a late and relatively inconspicuous symptom. All symptoms were relieved by dilatation of the cardia, although radiologically there was still some arrest of the barium six months later.

REFERENCES.

Hurst, A. F.: The Treatment of Achalasia of the Cardia, Lancet, 1927, i, 618.
Vinson, P. P.: The Diagnosis and Treatment of Cardiospasm, Jour. Am. Med. Assn., 1924, **82**, 859.

CANCER OF THE ESOPHAGUS.

The esophagus is one of the commoner sites for the development of cancer; in Ophüls' Stanford series, cancer of the esophagus occurred almost one-half as often as cancer of the stomach. The growth may begin in any part of the tube and often extends up or down for a considerable distance, sometimes burrowing under the mucosa to emerge here and there and give rise to a polypoid appearance; there are also localized ring-like forms. Ulceration and secondary infection are common. Histologically the tumors are squamous-cell epitheliomata with the exception of adenocarcinomata of the cardiac end of the stomach, which have extended up into the esophagus. Cancer of the esophagus rarely occurs in people under thirty-five to forty years of age, and men are much more commonly affected than women, in whom it is a relatively rare event. The explanation of this interesting discrepancy is not at hand. In 33 of our cases which came to autopsy the distribution of the metastases (or extensions) was as follows: liver, 7; larynx, 5; trachea, 4; stomach, 4; bronchus, 2; lung, 2; diaphragm, 1; thyroid, 1; neck muscle, 1; tongue, 1; lymph nodes, 20, including mediastinal, lesser curvature, cardiac, peribronchial, supraclavicular, retroperitoneal, liver hilum, cervical, iliac, submaxillary and mesenteric.

One should mention in passing the excessively rare cases of primary sarcoma of the esophagus.

Symptoms.—The earliest manifestations may be indistinguishable from those of spasm which have been described in the previous section, but as time goes by, constitutional symptoms—cachexia, fever and anemia—may be superadded. The latter are usually associated with ulceration and secondary infection of the growth. There may be regurgitation of foul, purulent or bloody material. A particularly interesting group of cases are those in which the local symptoms are insignificant and the picture is dominated by the effects of metastases or extensions. Perforation of a small carcinoma of the esophagus may, for example, lead to suppurative bronchopneumonia or mediastinal abscess. The primary growth may be entirely overlooked and the case masquerades as essentially one of lung abscess, empyema or pericarditis, or an enlargement of the liver may be the first clinical evidence of trouble. We have seen an instance which simulated a primary mediastinal mass with recurrent palsy. In another case there were numerous nodules in the lungs, obviously neoplastic, but the primary growth in the esophagus was obscure. Occasionally enlarged cancerous lymph nodes may be felt above the clavicle. The disease is usually fatal within a year or two from the onset of symptoms, in contrast to spasm, which may exist for decades without serious impairment of health. Death results from cachexia, secondary infection or the effects of metastases.

Diagnosis.—Persistent efforts must be made to rule out cancer in every case in which there is the complaint of difficulty in swallowing. Only too often slight symptoms are ignored by the physician, who tells the patient it is only nervousness and that it will go away by itself. Since operation offers the only hope of cure it is obvious that early diagnosis is paramount. Roentgen-rays are especially helpful; one often visualizes a ragged eccentrically placed narrowed area above which there may be a moderate degree of dilatation. Filling defects or irregularities occasionally extend over areas of esophagus several inches in extent. As a rule the findings are quite different from those of spasm, but especially in the early stages mistakes can be made and final diagnosis should be established by esophagoscopy and excision of a bit of the lesion for microscopic examination. Obvious metastases, of course, sway the diagnosis in an otherwise doubtful case, and in occasional instances the coughing up of food gives proof of esophageal-tracheal fistula.

Treatment.—Surgical excision is theoretically feasible, but in actual practice the operation has been successful in only a handful of cases. Technical difficulties, postoperative infection and ineradicable metastases contribute to the failures. The operation should not be considered unless the highest surgical skill is available. With advanced inoperable strictures gastrostomy may be done and food is introduced directly into the stomach. But such a surgical "tour de force" merely extends the patient's sufferings for a short time, and the wise and kind practitioner will rarely advise it. Careful dilatation may be tried in suitable cases but there is considerably more hazard of rupture than in cases of simple spasm.

Aside from surgical efforts the indications are to keep up nutrition as far as possible by small soft bland feedings and to take the edge off the patient's pain and distress by the free use of sedatives and analgesics, usually morphine in full doses. Fluids may have to be given by clysis. Radiation therapy is useless and some of the attempts have been followed by rapid sloughing and perforation of the growth.

ILLUSTRATIVE CASE—CANCER OF THE ESOPHAGUS.

M. S., housewife, aged forty-eight years.

Complaint.—Difficulty in swallowing for six weeks.

Past History.—Unimportant. No previous gastro-intestinal symptoms.

Present Illness.—Six weeks ago while eating some mashed potatoes she found she had difficulty in "getting it down." The food seemed to stick in her throat and part of it came up again. From this time on she had increasing difficulty in swallowing solids with a "sticking" sensation under sternum but no real pain. If repeated swallowing failed to dislodge the object she put her finger down her throat and relieved herself by regurgitation. At time of entry to hospital the trouble had progressed to a point where even liquids were swallowed with difficulty. She had lost 20 pounds.

Physical Examination.—Examination showed a very obese woman (weight, 230 pounds). The heart was slightly enlarged and the blood pressure was 170/110. Otherwise nothing remarkable was made out.

Laboratory.—Red blood cells, 4,700,000; hemoglobin, 80 per cent; white blood cells, 8000. Urine negative. Roentgen-rays: when the patient drank the barium meal it was arrested in the esophagus at the level of the third interspace and below this point there was a constriction of ragged and irregular outline. The barium gradually trickled into the stomach, which appeared normal (Fig. 24).

Esophagoscopy showed an irregular fungating tumor which bled easily on manipulation and had narrowed the lumen so that the smallest bougie was passed with difficulty. A small bit was removed, and on microscopic examination it was found to be a squamous-celled carcinoma.

A few days later the esophagus was explored surgically and the tumor was found to be about 8 cm. in length. The tumor and adjacent esophagus were resected and esophagostomy was performed. The patient failed rapidly and died in collapse on the third postoperative day.

Autopsy.—No metastases were found. The pleural cavities contained bloody fluid and the right lung was, for the most part, atelectatic.

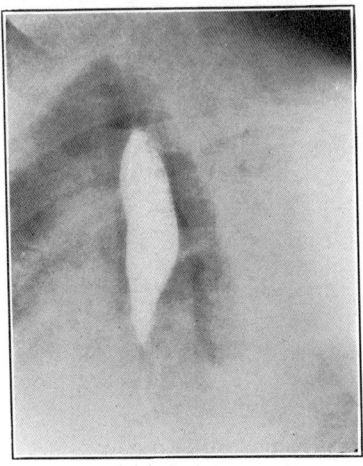

Fig. 24.—Cancer of the esophagus. Note the long, ragged, narrow area with dilation above it.

Comment.—There are several points of interest and importance. In the first place the patient was a woman. Second, the sudden onset of symptoms after the growth was well advanced suggests that spasm superimposed on the organic lesion played a part. Third, the good general nutrition and absence of anemia are noteworthy, and finally, the hazards of operation are well exemplified since this was, from a surgical standpoint, a favorable case for resection and no metastases were found at autopsy.

THE STOMACH.

THE CLASSIFICATION OF DISORDERS OF THE STOMACH.

In attempting to discuss systematically the disorders of the stomach one immediately encounters a serious difficulty, that of classification. This difficulty is not a new one, as a study of the tables of contents of modern text-books as well as of older treatises clearly testifies. Chapters on concrete anatomic disturbances such as ulcer and cancer are followed by discussions of less specific disorders such as gastric hemorrhage or pyloric obstruction; hyperacidity and anacidity may be presented as substantial clinical entities, while finally chapters on functional disorders, nervous indigestion or disturbances of motility make confusion worse confounded. Some writers have tried to beg the question by bringing everything under the heading of different types of "dyspepsia" or "indigestion," a procedure which offers no logical solution of the problem. Clearly the difficulty lies in the fact that such topics as the above are not mutually exclusive; they overlap. Ulcer and hyperacidity usually occur together and who can say to which, if either, the patient's symptoms, if he has any, are due. A separate discussion of pyloric obstruction and of dilatation of the stomach must obviously be a repetition of what has or should have been said in connection with certain types of cancer or ulcer. "Indigestion" may occur with ulcer and also in indistinguishable form in people who have a variety of other lesions or no anatomic disease at all. Obviously, then, some fundamental rearrangement of our concepts of stomach disorders, some workable definition of the "universe of discourse" must be effected before the subject can be approached in a constructive manner, and we shall not hesitate to clear the dead wood or, if necessary, to scrap existing structures and make a fresh start.

It may be conceded that a familiar group of symptoms—epigastric distress, fullness or burning with feelings of distention and eructations of gas or sour material—commonly designated as indigestion and often related by the subject to eating may fairly be referred to the stomach. The mechanism of their production will be discussed in detail later. These symptoms occur in people with gross anatomic disease of the stomach such as ulcer, they may occur in the presence of high or of low gastric acidity, and they may often be present in individuals without demonstrable organic disease of any sort. Conversely, patients with ulcer or cancer and patients with high acid or with anacidity may have no abdominal symptoms of any sort. In this brief paragraph lies, we believe, the explanation of the whole puzzle: lesions of the stomach are often essentially latent, although they may, on occasion, lead to reflex symptoms of "indigestion" which may, however, also be precipitated in identical form by extragastric lesions of great variety or by purely nervous influences. The details of the mechanism involved and the evidence on which the reasoning is based will be elaborated later.

Of course this is not the whole story. Other symptoms such as those associated with pyloric obstruction, perforation of the stomach, or bleeding into it will frequently be encountered. But their meaning is usually clear and their very grossness makes for simplicity.

With the above inherent difficulties in mind the following simple classification of stomach disorders may be proposed:

Indigestion (including "sensory and motor neuroses," hyperacidity and hypoacidity, pylorospasm, aërophagia, etc.).

Gastritis—acute and chronic.

Peptic ulcer (including pyloric obstruction, hematemesis and perforation of the stomach).

Cancer of the stomach.

Other tumors of the stomach.

Syphilis and other rare inflammations.

Deformities, anomalies and displacements.

A consideration of this classification leads to some pertinent conclusions as to the frequency and clinical importance of the various disorders. Of anatomic lesions gastritis in the sense of actual changes, inflammatory or degenerative, in the gastric mucosa is doubtless the most common. However, symptoms directly referable to gastritis are rare. Peptic ulcer and cancer, then, stand out as the two lesions frequently met with in the clinic, while other tumors, malformations and specific infections are only very occasionally encountered. The vast majority, however, of the patients who come to the physician with complaints referable to the stomach have no anatomic disease at all and their troubles will fall in the group which we have classified as indigestion.

DIAGNOSIS OF DISORDERS OF THE STOMACH.

Since certain general principles of procedure apply to the study of any case of digestive disturbance they may profitably be discussed in advance before dealing with special diseases. Diagnostic information may be derived from four sources: the history, the physical examination, gastric analysis and other laboratory examinations, and roentgenrays. Each will be discussed in turn.

History.—It may be assumed that the general anamnestic data have already been collected and that the physician's attention has been attracted to the possibility of stomach trouble. What particular line of inquiry may then be specially useful? First of all, one should inquire as to symptoms which suggest organic disease of the stomach, namely, vomiting of blood or passage of large amounts of blood in the stools, repeated vomiting of large quantities of material containing food which may be recognized as having been eaten on the previous day (obstruction at the pylorus), or intense epigastric pain and tenderness which might point to perforation with peritonitis, local or general. Aside from these symptoms the various digestive complaints dealing with appetite, nausea, fullness, gas, belching, epigastric discomfort or burning and sour eructations should be gone into, although, as will be pointed out below, they do not necessarily mean actual disease of the stomach, but may arise from extragastric or emotional reflexes. Duration of symptoms, their intensity, their persistence or periodicity, their relation to other troubles of which the patient complains, and the things which he has found give relief are also important, but while the experienced clinician may guess from such a questionnaire the nature of the trouble no actual diagnosis can be made without further data.

Physical Examination.—The stomach itself is peculiarly inaccessible to physical examination. Even large masses in the stomach wall usually escape detection by palpation unless perigastric inflammatory or neoplastic tissue has been superadded, although pyloric obstruction may sometimes be recognized by observing the characteristic large peristaltic waves which pass from left to right across the epigastrium. Even tenderness on pressure over the gastric region cannot be relied upon to indicate disease of the stomach except as corroborative evidence of other findings. However, useful points bearing on the diagnosis may be discovered during the general physical examination. Great prostration and emaciation, for example, usually speak for an organic rather than a functional disorder, or the discovery of metastatic nodules in the liver or in the rectal cul-de-sac may clinch a diagnosis of cancer then and there. But it is safe to conclude that an exact diagnosis of disease of the stomach cannot, as a rule, be made from the history and physical examination alone, and one must turn next to gastric analysis and the roentgen-ray.

Gastric Analysis.—There is no more obscure chapter in human physiology than that of the workings of the stomach. Certain crude facts are, to be sure, evident enough: the organ acts as a reservoir for recently ingested food, which is broken up and partly liquefied by the pepsin and hydrochloric acid of the gastric juice aided by mechanical trituration of the muscular stomach wall. Furthermore, milk is clotted by gastric rennin and fats may, to some extent, be dispersed or split. But the exact mechanism of these obvious performances is extremely complex, and the ultimate mode of formation of hydrochloric acid, the nature and mode of action of pepsin and the relative influence of autonomic nervous influences as against humoral agents in the control of gastric secretion and motility are as yet imperfectly understood. Of these matters the student must read in the special physiologic literature and it will be more profitable for the present purpose to approach the problem only in its clinical bearings.

For half a century physicians have attempted to correlate variations in the secretory activity of the stomach with different disorders as an aid to diagnosis. To this end some sort of "test-meal," consisting in its simplest form of a slice of bread and a glass of water, is eaten by the patient, and after an appropriate interval has elapsed, so that digestion is under way, the stomach contents are aspirated by means of a rubber tube and syringe and are analyzed for their content of acid and pepsin. At the same time abnormal elements, such as blood or pus may be detected, and information about the motility or emptying time of the stomach can also be obtained by determining how long the food remains in the stomach. As time has gone by, various modifications of the test-meal have been developed; that in most general use at present is the so-called fractional meal. The patient takes a special oatmeal gruel and, with the tube continuously in the stomach, samples are aspirated at fifteen-minute intervals in order to obtain a curve of "secretory activity." A consideration of these methods, however, shows that a great many errors are introduced which interfere with useful interpretation of the results. In the first place, the stimulus is not a standard one and variations will result from the patient's nervous reaction to the procedure, but above all the very introduction of the test-meal vitiates the findings, since one aspirates for analysis not pure gastric juice but mixtures of gastric juice diluted by unknown quantities of extraneous material. A simple example will make this clear. One gives bread and water and one hour later aspirates the stomach contents. If the pylorus has remained closed and the bread has remained in the stomach the gastric juice is diluted by the meal and the acidity will be relatively low. If, in the same subject, the stomach has emptied itself during the hour of the test, then there will be less bread and more gastric juice and the acid reading will be higher even if the actual secretion of the stomach has remained constant.

Attempts to introduce into practice tests for gastric secretion from which the element of a meal has been eliminated have met with objections from clinicians. It has been argued especially that the stomach must be given normal work to do, namely a meal, in order to test its function. This objection is obviously unsound as it might be argued with equal justice that the strength of a muscle could be tested only by digging ditches and not by a dynamometer. Furthermore, who can say what is the normal "test-meal" for any particular person. It might be a pound of roast beef or perhaps half a loaf of rye bread with some onions and red wine. The important point would rather seem to be that a standard stimulus be used which can be repeated in identical form on successive occasions, with the same or a different subject, and which is sufficiently powerful to bring out sharply differences in secretory capability. Histamine is a substance which on subcutaneous injection fulfils these specifications; by using it test-meals can be avoided and pure gastric juice is obtained for analysis. Normal standards of gastric secretion following histamine stimulation have now been worked out and with them the aberrations in disease may profitably be compared.

Technic of the Histamine Test.—The patient should be under "basal" conditions at rest in bed without having taken food or fluid for twelve hours. A small stomach tube is introduced. Any one of a great variety may be used, but we prefer the mercury-weighted type described by Wilkins. The fasting contents are then withdrawn by means of a Luer syringe; one of 50 cc. capacity is most convenient. They may vary from a few cubic centimeters to several hundred cc., although in normal people one rarely obtains over 60 to 75 cc. This material is best suited for study of abnormal constituents such as blood, pus and yeasts, and food particles, if present, indicate abnormal stasis since the preceding meal should have left the stomach within twelve hours. After the fasting contents have been removed, suction is kept up to discover if there is any continuous secretion, and the aspirated juice is measured over successive ten-minute periods. After two or three such periods histamine[1] is injected subcutaneously (upper arm) in doses of 0.1 cc. of a 1 to 1000 solution per 10 kilos of body weight. Aspiration is continued and, as a rule, it is evident within ten minutes after injection that the flow of juice is increasing and that it is becoming more watery and less viscid. The procedure is continued until the maximum flow is obtained, when the test may be discontinued. Within a few minutes after the injection of histamine a large wheal appears at the site of the puncture; this may be followed by flushing of the face, moderate increase in pulse-rate and fall of blood pressure. In some 2000 tests we have seen no alarming reaction. The patient must be urged not to swallow the saliva, and a convenient receptacle for expectoration is provided. Reflux of duodenal contents as indicated by the appearance of bile vitiates the test, which may be repeated on another occasion. The technic of adequate aspiration requires a good deal of practise and the quantitative results will be unrealiable unless done by someone proficient in the procedure.

[1] We have used the ergamine of Burroughs and Wellcome.

(1) **Interpretation of Results.**—The amount of juice obtained during each ten-minute period before and after histamine injection is measured and charted (Fig. 25). As a rule the greatest flow takes place during the third or fourth period and this value is suitable for comparing the rate of secretion in different people or in the same person on

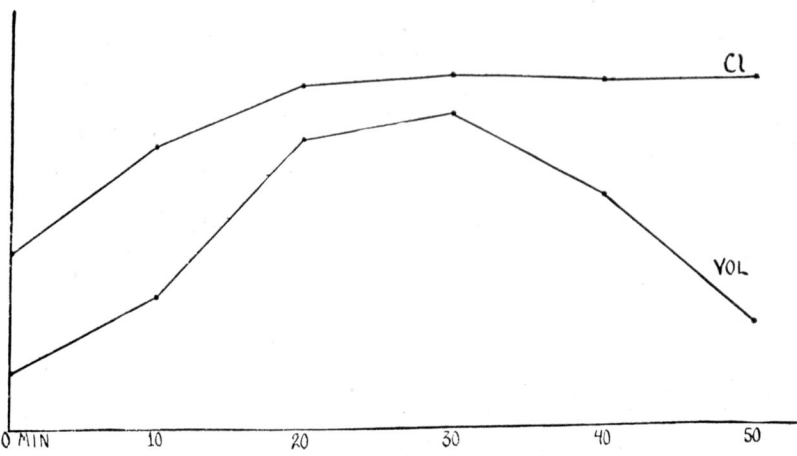

Fig. 25.—Form of curves of quantity of secretion (vol.) and of acidity (Cl) following injection of histamine.

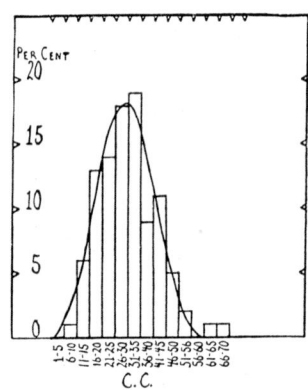

Fig. 26.—Distribution of curve of highest ten-minute secretory volume (cc.) after histamine in 100 normal people.

successive occasions. Fig. 26 shows a distribution curve of the highest ten-minute secretory volumes from 100 normal people. It is seen that while the majority of the values fall between 20 and 35 cc., some apparently normal people have a maximum ten-minute volume of as little as 10 cc. or as great as 60 cc. In certain diseases there is no increase after histamine and only a few cubic centimeters of mucoid material are obtained in each period.

Hypersecretion and Hyposecretion.—In the older literature a good deal of stress was placed on hyper- and hyposecretion as actual disease entities and it is true that with certain inflammations and atrophies of the mucosa the juice is diminished or absent, and that people subject to peptic ulcer usually secrete a large quantity. However, in view of what has been shown above, namely, that wide variations may occur in normal people, it may be safely asserted that large or small volumes of gastric juice do not in themselves constitute a pathologic entity, nor are these variations in themselves responsible for symptoms. It would seem wise to dismiss the terms hyper- and hyposecretion altogether because of the implication of disease which they convey and to speak simply of average, high or low secretory volumes.

(2) **Determination of Acidity.**—Samples of juice are titrated with $\frac{N}{10}$ NaOH in the usual way for free and total acid with dimethyl and phenolphthalein as indicators. In normal people the acidity rises following histamine and usually reaches a maximum within thirty to forty minutes (Fig. 25). The highest acidity attained during the course of the test represents a standard value which may be used in comparing different people or the same person on successive tests. Fig. 27 shows a distribution curve of the highest acid values (total

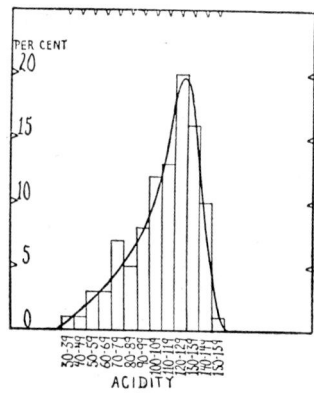

Fig. 27.—Distribution curve of highest acidity reached after histamine in 100 normal people.

acid) in 100 normal people. The majority are seen to lie between 90 and 140, although considerably lower figures are obtained from some apparently normal people. One hundred and sixty seems to be approximately the highest acidity which the human gastric juice can attain, no matter how powerful the stimulus.

Hyperacidity, Hypoacidity and Anacidity.—It has already been said that variations in volume of secretion cannot in themselves be regarded as diseases. The same is true of variations in acidity. While high or low acid values are, to be sure, often encountered in patients with stomach disorders, no symptoms can be attributed to the acidity itself, nor is there any evidence that extremely high or low acid is necessarily associated with disease or that it requires any special treatment. The syndrome of so-called "hyperacidity" of which physicians speak so glibly (to be discussed further under the heading of Indigestion) is usually spurious, and the alleged symptoms may occur in a person with average or low acid. Complete absence of acid after histamine rarely, if ever, occurs with a normal stomach. The significance of this finding will be discussed under "Gastritis."

There are many other interesting features of gastric secretion which cannot be gone into here, such as the decrease in volume and acidity with advancing years, but the most important point is that no narrow limits of normality can be set: the nearer to the average the values in the individual lie the more likely the stomach is to be normal, but wide variations occur in a minority of apparently healthy people. The significance of the findings in disease will be taken up later under the appropriate headings.

3. **Pepsin.**—The digestive power of the gastric juice depends, of course, primarily on the presence of pepsin, and the acid serves mainly to furnish a medium of suitable reaction for the ferment. Accurate quantitative determinations of peptic activity are extremely difficult and in clinical practice hardly seem to justify the effort involved. This is all the more true, since the presence of pepsin may be inferred from the acid values; unless there is a complete absence of acid, pepsin is almost always present in considerable amounts.[1]

4. **Gross Appearance.**—The fasting gastric juice varies greatly in its appearance, depending upon the presence of varying amounts of mucus, saliva and duodenal contents. After histamine the secretion usually becomes thin and clear and in many people is as limpid as distilled water. There are, however, variations which depend largely on the amount of mucus which is present. Within wide limits these variations cannot be correlated with disease and they have no clinical meaning. Under abnormal conditions, especially in gastritis, there may be no true secretion of gastric juice and the aspirated material consists of only a few drops of mucus.

5. **Other Examinations.**—The histamine juice is eminently suitable for various chemical examinations, since it is uncontaminated by admixtures of test-meal. Chloride, base and nitrogen may be measured, but in ordinary clinical work this serves no useful purpose.

In summary, then, for clinical purposes one needs to know the rate of secretion and the acidity of the gastric juice after a standard powerful stimulus. These values, as will be pointed out below, may be correlated with certain types of gastric disease. Determination of the presence of food stasis, pus and blood, or other gross abnormalities is also useful. Measurements of pepsin and other complicated chemical procedures are unnecessary in clinical work.

Roentgen-ray Examination.—Radiologic examination plays an indispensable part in the diagnosis of stomach disorders. Such questions, for example, as the exact size and position of ulcers, the presence of malformations, and the mode of emptying of the stomach often could be elucidated in no other way. It is a pity that this beautiful method is so much abused by physicians who demand of it more than it can give and expect the radiologist to furnish a complete diagnosis. Thus, it must be remembered that the roentgen-ray plate after all only reveals shadows and that at best one can but infer the nature of the lesion

---

[1] For fuller discussion the reader is referred to the papers of Polland and Bloomfield.

even though such inference is often quite correct. An irregular deformity at the pylorus, for example, may be produced either by ulcer or by cancer, and no matter how great the experience of the radiologist, differentiation is often impossible. A good deal of stress used to be placed on the character of the contraction waves and on the promptness and speed of emptying as well as on the shape and position of the stomach, but as thousands of observations have accumulated the variations in healthy people have turned out to be so wide that great caution must be used inferring the presence of disease from them. Pyloric obstruction with definite gastric retention is, however, one of the most useful findings of the roentgen-ray examination.

In brief, then, the roentgen-ray shows defects and deformities of the outline of the stomach and disturbances of motility. The former are much more reliable evidence of disease since the latter may occur without an actual lesion.

REFERENCES.

ALVAREZ, W. C.: The Mechanics of the Digestive Tract, 2d ed., New York, 1929.
BIDDER, F., and SCHMIDT, C.: Die Verdauungssäfte, Leipzig, 1852.
BLOOMFIELD, A. L., and KEEFER, C. S.: The Rate of Gastric Secretion in Man, Jour. Clin. Invest., 1927, 4, 485.
BLOOMFIELD, A. L., and POLLAND, W. S.: The Diagnostic Value of Studies of Gastric Secretion, Jour. Am. Med. Assn., 1929, 92, 1508.
CANNON, W. B.: The Mechanical Factors in Digestion, London, 1911.
CARLSON, A. J.: The Control of Hunger in Health and Disease, Chicago, 1916.
CARMAN, R. D.: The Roentgen Diagnosis of Disease of the Alimentary Canal, 2d ed., Philadelphia, 1920.
KEEFER, C. S., and BLOOMFIELD A. L.: The Significances of Gastric Anacidity, Bull. Johns Hopkins Hosp., 1926, 39, 304.
PAVLOW, I. P.: The Work of the Digestive Glands, 2d ed., London, 1911.
POLLAND, W. S., and BLOOMFIELD, A. L.: The Diagnostic Value of Determinations of Pepsin in Gastric Juice, Jour. Clin. Invest., 1930, 9, 107.
———— Normal Standard of Gastric Function, Jour. Clin. Invest., 1931, 9, 651.

INDIGESTION.

The vast majority of patients with disorders of the stomach complain of symptoms which may best be grouped under the heading of "indigestion." It has always been recognized that these symptoms may occur in people with a great variety of underlying disturbances and countless efforts have been made to classify and subdivide the complaints into groups or types which are sufficiently characteristic to have diagnostic significance. Thus we read of "primary dyspepsia," "nervous dyspepsia," "gastralgia," "sensory and motor neuroses," "ulcer indigestion," "gall-bladder indigestion" or "appendiceal indigestion." Careful study of this problem over a period of years has, however, convinced the writer of the complete futility of such classifications because they represent an attempt, as Sir James Mackenzie put it, to "differentiate what cannot be differentiated." In brief, the stomach, if trouble originates in it at all, can express itself only by certain symptoms (to be described below) and while the changes may be rung in various ways there is nothing inherently different in the indigestion experienced by a patient with peptic ulcer or by one with reflex disturbances brought on by worry or overstrain. The final diagnosis of the underlying condition depends on special phenomena other than those of "indigestion" itself. Hence it seems wise to adopt some such comprehensive and non-committal term as a basic designation which may, if possible, be further qualified in individual cases.

Symptoms.—Even the layman is familiar, in a general way, with the symptoms of indigestion. First and foremost, there is a curious disagreeable sensation in the epigastrium, often temporarilly related to the taking of food, and described as a burning, pressing or full feeling. We have never encountered a patient who could clearly describe the sensation, the reason being that unlike the accurately localizable and describable feelings of the body surface, one is dealing here with the crude elementary sensibility mediated by autonomic nerves. This distressful sensation may vary greatly in its intensity, duration and it may be more or less widespread. Sometimes it seems to flow upward over the front of the chest and there are burning or squeezing sensations in the throat with or without the actual regurgitation of sour fluid (*heartburn*). Next should be mentioned the belching of air which has been deliberately or unconsciously swallowed (*aërophagia*) and which, contrary to the opinion of the patient, is not generated in the stomach itself. *Nausea* may be present, although usually the appetite is good and vomiting rarely takes place unless provoked by the efforts or manipulations of the patient himself. When the layman says he has "sour stomach" or "indigestion" or "dyspepsia" or a "gas attack" or "biliousness," he is usually referring to what has been described above, and while the symphony of symptoms varies in its details in different sufferers—more elaborate in one, simpler in another—the same fundamental theme of epigastric distress and gas almost always can be recognized. Hand in hand with "indigestion" there often go a group of symptoms more properly referred to the bowel, namely, constipation, or irregularity of the bowel, perhaps with cramps and the passage of mucus (mucous colitis) and intestinal distention with passage of flatus.

The Frequency of the Symptoms of Indigestion.—Indigestion in some form or other is an almost universal experience and it is important for the physician to be aware of this fact in order that he may place proper emphasis on the patient's story. Does the nervous individual, for example, who complains to the doctor of gas have more real trouble than all of us are entitled to? Is he, perhaps, simply hypersensitive to the normal workings of the body which in most of us do not rise to the level of consciousness? To get light on this point we recently sent questionnaires to 200 college students who were at work and considered themselves to be normal healthy people. A surprisingly large number were found to be subject, in greater or lesser degree, to some of the symptoms of indigestion, although careful health examinations had revealed no evidence of any organic disease in them. This emphasizes the importance of the physician's acquiring a proper point of view. Certain symptoms are, perhaps, better ignored; on the other hand an indigestion which is a manifestation of serious organic disease of course requires careful consideration.

The Mechanism of Production of the Symptoms of Indigestion.— The symptoms of indigestion which have been described may conceivably be due either to actual sensitiveness of the stomach, just as a boil on one's hand is sore, or they represent reflex discomforts on the basis of the laws of referred pain. That the former explanation is untenable is admitted by all students of the subject, inasmuch as the stomach is not "sensible" to ordinary stimuli. In brief, heat and cold and mechanical stimuli of wide variety are not appreciated as such by the stomach as has been demonstrated over and over again since Beaumont's classical experiments with the gastric fistula of the temperamental St. Martin. Even actual ulcers of the stomach do not seem to be painful *in themselves;* we have frequently irrigated stomachs which were the seat of large peptic ulcers with $\frac{N}{10}$ HCl without the patient's being aware of the manipulations. It may be said that distention of the walls of the gastro-intestinal tube offers the only adequate stimulus whereby pain can regularly be produced, and many experiments are on record which describe the results of inflation of the stomach or bowel by means of balloons filled with air or in other ways. If, for example, a balloon is introduced into the first portion of the duodenum and inflated until symptoms appear, sensations of indigestion indistinguishable from those described above result. They are referred to an area between the xiphoid and the umbilicus extending to both sides of the mid-line, and they are described as burning or pressing pains or feelings of fullness or discomfort. On occasion, nausea and retching may also occur. Release of the distention leads to instantaneous disappearance of the pain.[1]

If it be admitted that "indigestion" represents reflex phenomena mediated through autonomic nerves rather than actual sensitiveness of the stomach, and if the immediate stimulus is abnormal tension or spasm of one or another portion of the gastro-duodenal tube, then the manifestations of indigestion as encountered in the clinic immediately become intelligible. Furthermore, if one considers for a moment the complex muscular mechanism of the stomach and its sphincters and the obvious possibilities for lack of proper synchronization it is readily understood how easily slight derangements may occur, even in normal people, which on occasion would produce indigestion.

The precipitating causes of indigestion will next be considered and they may be classed as follows:

1. *Lesions in the Stomach.*—Any lesion of the stomach itself may lead at times to abnormal spasm or tension, especially of the pylorus or of the cardia, which in turn sets up symptoms of indigestion. That an ulcer near the pylorus might be effective requires no stretch of the imagination. However, one must think of the ulcer as leading to spasm and hence indigestion only on occasion, perhaps during a certain phase of the digestive cycle, rather than as actually being the direct "*fons et origo*" of pain. Other lesions such as carcinoma also may cause indigestion indistinguishable from that precipitated by ulcer. The mechanism is the same and differential diagnosis must be based on evidence other than the purely "digestive" symptoms.

2. *Organic Abdominal Disease Outside the Stomach.*—When one con-

---

[1] For details of experiments and the newer evidence bearing on the matter, the reader is referred to the papers of Polland and Bloomfield.

38

siders the common sources of autonomic innervation of many abdominal viscera it seems evident that reflex spasms of the stomach and pylorus, with consequent indigestion, should result from extra-gastric lesions. The recent experiments of Smith, who showed by means of a recording balloon in the pylorus that inflation of the colon in dogs leads to pylorospasm, are supported by a host of clinical evidence. Every physician has had the happy experience of seeing his patient entirely relieved of indigestion by removal, for example, of a diseased appendix or gall-bladder, and in such cases the cure evidently is due to the elimination of reflex spasms of the stomach which were directly responsible for the symptoms. Indigestion may be a manifestation—sometimes an early one—of cardiac decompensation or of coronary disease.

3. *Abnormal Reflexes in the Absence of Any Organic Disease.*—Probably the vast majority of people with indigestion have no gross organic disease, and the abnormal spasms of the stomach which produce indigestion are set up by stimuli which are nervous or mental in origin. This is a matter of common experience so obvious as to be axiomatic: the gastro-intestinal tract acts as a sort of nervous safety-valve. Diarrhea is well known to occur under certain kinds of nervous stress; some unfortunate people are embarrassed at inconvenient times by audible rumbling of the bowels, the result of emotion, and we have all seen the vomiting of the intercollegiate half-miler at the end of the race or the nausea of the medical student at his first surgical operation. It is only a step further to grasp the idea that "indigestion" may result from purely nervous influences. These are too varied to enumerate, but in practice the subject is usually the high-strung type, and the actual symptoms are almost always directly related to worry, stress and tension or to poor habits of eating, especially rapid eating. One sees many patients who regularly have indigestion after rushing from the office to a lunch room but who in turn have no distress after a leisurely evening meal or when away on vacation. Lack of space forbids further elaboration of this most important point, and for a full discussion the reader is urged to study Alvarez' thorough treatise.

Physical Examination and Laboratory Tests.—The findings depend on the underlying condition and are too varied for systematic description. Physical abnormalities may be obvious, or the individual, as pointed out above, is normal on objective examination.

Gastric analysis shows nothing characteristic; every type of secretion is encountered and neither the degree of acidity of the gastric juice nor its amount can be related to the symptoms.

Treatment.—Successful treatment depends upon clear recognition of the cause of the patient's indigestion. If the symptoms are due to a diseased appendix or gall-bladder, psychotherapy or diet is not likely to work a permanent cure and conversely if the trouble depends upon nervous factors, removal of appendix or gall-bladder will turn out to be inadequate. In no department of medicine do physicians seem to be more at sea and to exercise less real judgment; there are those who incline to minimize all cases of indigestion and to prescribe a change of diet, perhaps with a bitter tonic, while others have only a little bag of tricks from which such diagnoses as gall-bladder trouble, duodenal ulcer or chronic appendix emerge more or less at random.

Clearly the physician's first duty is to determine, if possible, the presence or absence of actual disease of the stomach or abdominal viscera and to decide whether such disease, if present, is responsible for the symptoms of indigestion. This is no easy matter and often no absolute conclusion is reached, since one may, of course, have diseased viscera which are not the cause of the symptoms. If a definite causative lesion is discovered it should, of course, be eliminated by surgery or it should receive appropriate medical therapy. On the whole, it is unwise ever to attempt definite diagnosis of the factors underlying indigestion without careful and prolonged study. One must really come to know the patient intimately—his nervous make-up, his habits, his virtues, his vices, his social and professional problems, his reaction to stress—and sometimes the family must be studied as well. Not uncommonly it is not the patient but husband, wife or child that is at fault. At any rate, the greatest mistake one can make is to feel obliged to give a definite diagnosis on the first interview.

If it be concluded that the indigestion is dependent on nervous influences and not on some local abdominal lesion the following points must all be considered in planning the therapy:

1. *Relief from Strain.*—This is perhaps the most important consideration of all and involves in different cases adjustment of personal problems, regulation of daily activity so as to eliminate undue hurry and stress, arrangements for proper diversion, recreation and vacation, the securing of adequate restful sleep, and general provision for proper physical and mental hygiene. Under this heading should be mentioned the correction of any harassing minor physical defects such as, for example, eye strain.

2. *Diet.*—By weight of age-long tradition some form of dietary regimen has been the main feature of the treatment of indigestion. It must be admitted that some people do regularly have discomfort after eating certain special articles of food, but on the whole this fact is vastly overshadowed by a more important one, namely, that the stomach is marvelously indifferent to what is put into it. Certainly such discrimination as is expected by the physician who tells his patient that he may eat peas but not beans, and spaghetti but not macaroni can rest on no demonstrable physiologic basis. Indeed, we are convinced that nine times out of ten the dietary problem is not *what the patient eats but how he eats.* The most confirmed indigestion habitués not uncommonly relate that once away from hurry, worry and stress, tomales and zucchini may be taken with comfort, whereas even milk and crackers are followed by violent discomfort if consumed hastily in the middle of a strenuous day. Often the very act of prescribing a diet list with its ominous addendum of forbidden articles is enough to set up indigestion reflexes through fear or apprehension. We recall a patient who entered the hospital on a diet of brown bread and honey. She had been the rounds of physicians and each had eliminated one or another article. Finally, only brown bread and honey remained. No organic disease was found, she was reassured and on a

full and liberal diet promptly got well. One must remember, furthermore, that there is no phase of life about which people sentimentalize more than they do about food. Today we may crave a steak with a salad, tomorrow this may be quite unacceptable, and we desire fried chicken with corn on the cob. There is much physiologic and overwhelming clinical evidence to show that food which is distasteful leads to deranged digestive reflexes and indigestion. How unsound, then, to force on the patient an arbitrary diet which pleases no one's fancy except that of the physician. In brief, if one eats a varied and natural diet and one which is acceptable, the digestive processes go on unconsciously and they are not disturbed by psychic stimuli.

In any case the patient should be urged *to eat slowly and to chew well.* Liquids should be sipped and not gulped. Dental defects should be corrected so that mastication is effective. The meals should be of moderate size and any feeling of being "stuffed" should be avoided. Articles which the physician is convinced genuinely upset the patient should be eliminated; these will not be many. In general the food should be simple and plainly cooked and excessive quantities of coarse, highly seasoned and spiced dishes had better be avoided. However, the less the patient's attention is centered on his diet, "the less he lives around his stomach," the less likely is digestion to supervene.

An occasional exception to all that has been said is the patient who insists on having a diet list. There is a group of interesting mildly psychopathic individuals who thrive on restrictions. In mildest form this aberration expresses itself by undue attention to the inconsequential details of life in general; into this group fall those impelled to an excessive but fruitless orderliness in all their activities. To such patients one may be occasionally forced to give some sort of a diet list, but it should be carefully compounded on the above principles so as to eliminate fear and undue restrictions.

Coffee and tea in moderate amounts are allowable and an occasional alcoholic beverage, provided the patient experiences no discomfort in consequence, seems harmless. Some physicians feel that smoking promotes indigestion; we know of no real evidence to support this allegation. Rather it is that the nervous type of person who is subject to indigestion is also likely to be a heavy smoker; he does not get indigestion because he smokes, he smokes because he is plagued by indigestion. In those instances in which indigestion is said to have been cured by elimination of tobacco other factors have been operative at the same time. This is no brief for excessive use of tobacco; one should, of course, smoke in moderation. Different views have also been expressed as to the taking of water at meals, some advising a dry diet and others allowing fluids freely. We know of no physiologic evidence whereby the point may be settled and it would seem best for the patient to follow his natural inclination. The writer has observed a patient subject to indigestion who is never distressed, however, by hot flannel cakes, a favorite dish, which he washes down with copious draughts of ice-water.

3. *Care of the Bowels.*—The bowels should be carefully regulated (for details see article on Constipation).

4. *Drugs.*—In most cases the use of drugs can be avoided if the situation can be thoroughly explained to an intelligent patient. "Medicine" exercises, however, in all of us, a mysterious psychic effect, and especially at the beginning of the treatment its use may be advisable. We have had good results from mild antispasmodics such as a mixture of tincture of belladonna and sodium bromide taken after meals (Tr. belladonnæ, 0.3 to 0.6 cc.; Sodii bromidi, 1 to 1.5 grams) or a bitter tonic of tincture of gentian and tincture of nux vomica with a little soda may be given one-half hour before eating.

Treatment of Special Symptoms.—Patients with the indigestion syndrome frequently center their attention on some special feature of their symptomatology and they often rationalize about it in curious ways so as to make treatment very difficult. Most people who have "gas on the stomach" are convinced that the "gas" is generated in the stomach; they consequently devise means to rid themselves of it whether by violent eructations or by taking soda or other drugs "to bring the gas up." Often it is extremely difficult to convince the sufferer that he actually swallows the air which he belches forth; but he must be convinced before a cure can be effected. One particularly stubborn patient was taken to the roentgen-ray room and radiograms showing the stomach bubble were demonstrated to him. As soon as he was satisfied that everyone had some air in the stomach and that it did no harm there, his symptoms disappeared. The milder forms of belching usually improve as the indigestion is controlled. Another idea which harasses patients is that of biliousness. Convinced that their indigestion and constipation are due to accumulation of bile in the liver they plague themselves with fantastic and useless procedures and drugs to correct the supposed defect. Here again explanation of the actual meaning of the symptoms often at the price of shattering long cherished physiologic delusions is essential before relief can be obtained.

Finally it may be said that no one need expect to cure a stubborn case of indigestion in a few days. Persistent sympathetic effort on the part of the physician and coöperation by the patient are essential. Often one must explain to him over and over again the mechanism of his distress and emphasize the fact that, while things are not working properly, there is no organic disease. Do not tell the patient his trouble is imaginary; his discomfort is very real indeed. One must be prepared for exacerbations of symptoms at times when all seems to be going unusually well and one must support the patient against discouragement, remembering that he is usually dealing not with a disease but with a type of nervous make-up which cannot be fundamentally altered. During severe bouts of indigestion a day or two on a milk diet, bicarbonate of soda (0.5 to 1 gram) at times of distress, general sedatives such as phenobarbital in small doses, and in extreme cases rest in bed for a few days followed, if possible, by change of scene and diversion may be necessary. Where indigestion is one element in a widespread neurosis the services, or at least the methods of a trained psychiatrist should be invoked.

REFERENCES.

ALVAREZ, W. C.: Nervous Indigestion, New York, 1930.
BEAUMONT, W.: The Physiology of Digestion, 2d ed., Burlington, 1847.
HURST, A. F.: The Sensibility of the Alimentary Canal, Oxford, 1911.
———— Sphincters of Alimentary Canal, Brit. Med. Jour., 1925, i, 145.
POLLAND, W. S., and BLOOMFIELD A. L.: Experimental Referred Pain from the
    Gastro-intestinal Tract: Parts I and II, Jour. Clin. Invest., 1931, 10, 435, 453.
SMITH, F. M., PAUL, W. D., and FOWLER, W. M.: The Mechanism of the Epigas-
    tric Distress Associated with Irritable Colon and Chronic Appendicitis, Arch.
    Int. Med., 1931, 47, 316.

GASTRITIS.

General Considerations.—A considerable variety of somewhat unrelated disorders are usually included under the designation of gastritis: acute diffuse inflammations produced by poisons and irritants and rarely by infection, as well as a much vaguer group of chronic inflammatory and degenerative conditions. In the latter group "gastritis" takes on a significance analogous to that of chronic "nephritis," "hepatitis" or "iritis" and the evidences of actual inflammation are not always outspoken. There is great difficulty in clarifying the subject because of lack of adequate anatomic control of the clinical diagnoses. Clinicians speak glibly, for example, of gastritis in the case of people subject to indigestion who give a history of overindulgence in highly seasoned food, but whether any actual lesions exist is purely a matter of speculation.

Pathologists, on the other hand, are quite familiar with the anatomic appearances of gastritis. Alterations in the structure of the mucosa and of the glands, abnormal infiltrations of cells, increase of interstitial tissue and in extreme cases actual scarring of the mucous membrane or atrophy of its glandular cells are all described. The changes are complex and for details the student must consult the treatises on pathology. However, many of the people who at postmortem show the above-mentioned lesions gave no story of the alleged causes of gastritis during life, nor did they necessarily have any clinical symptoms.

With these reservations a clinical discussion may be attempted.

Acute Gastritis.—*Etiology.*—Acute inflammation of the stomach results from the ingestion of irritating substances. Extreme examples are phenol and bichloride of mercury, which produce actual necroses or eschars. Less violent are the effects of alcohol, whereas the milder grades of catarrhal inflammation may be supposed to result from spices, essential oils or perhaps mere overindulgence in coarse or rich food. Beaumont, with his fistula patient, observed the abnormal pouring out of mucus which followed irritation of the stomach. Acute bacterial inflammations (phlegmon) of the stomach are rarely encountered.

Symptoms.—Mild inflammations of the stomach undoubtedly often occur without any symptoms. Anorexia, indigestion, nausea and, in extreme cases, vomiting are, however, to be expected. Diarrhea is often associated with the gastritis of food indiscretion. Otherwise the symptoms are those due to other effects of the causal agent as, for example, the familiar picture of acute alcoholism. Fever of varying degree depending on the cause of the trouble may be present.

Physical Examination.—In extreme cases there may be epigastric tenderness but, as a rule, nothing is made out except the remote effects of the upset. If vomiting and diarrhea persist, the signs of desiccation—dry tongue, shrunken tissues, sunken eyeballs—develop. There may be collapse with rapid feeble pulse.

Laboratory Examinations.—After violent irritants or caustics, the vomitus shows evidences of the noxious agent. Blood may be present. Gastric analysis has not usually been done during the acute phases of a gastritis. It is said, however, that the normal thin acid secretion is diminished in favor of an outpouring of mucus, which perhaps serves a protective function.

Diagnosis.—The condition is suspected largely from the story, and the diagnosis is confirmed by the evidence obtained on gastric lavage.

Treatment.—In the ordinary instance of gastritis following dietary or alcoholic indiscretion the treatment is largely expectant. In the more extreme cases the stomach should be lavaged with warm water and the patient put to bed. A sedative such as barbital (0.5 gram) or a small dose of codeine or morphine hypodermically is advisable for restlessness or discomfort. As long as vomiting persists food should be withheld. It may be necessary to give fluid by rectum to avoid desiccation from loss of fluids. Four hundred cubic centimeters of water may be introduced every four to six hours. After starvation for from twelve to twenty-four hours, small amounts of milk which has been boiled and then cooled may be allowed. If well taken, toast is added, after which one progresses to a simple bland diet.

The severe cases following phenol, bichloride or other escharotics present special problems which cannot be gone into here.

Chronic Gastritis.—**Etiology.**—A great variety of causes are alleged to be responsible for chronic gastritis: overindulgence in highly seasoned or coarse food, rapid eating, chronic overindulgence in alcohol or focal infection. However, after examining the gastric secretions of many notable gourmets as well as those of chronic alcoholics and finding them perfectly normal, the writer confesses a complete skepticism as to the validity of such *a priori* reasoning. Some other and much more subtle cause usually lies at the bottom of these chronic gastric inflammations and the problem is as obscure as that of chronic nephritis. A somewhat different type of chronic irritation is associated with the stagnation of food and secretions in cases of pyloric obstruction; "gastritis" occurs with the congestion of chronic heart disease or cirrhosis of the liver and in stomachs bathed by the exudations of sloughing infected carcinomata.

Symptoms.—Aside from the evidences of associated conditions symptoms of gastritis, if they occur at all, are in no way different from those already discussed under indigestion. We know of no specific symptom-complex. Nor are there any special physical signs. Indeed, the only basis on which it would seem to be possible clinically to justify a diagnosis of chronic gastritis is by the demonstration of abnormalities of gastric secretion.

Gastric Analysis.—Very low acid or absence of acid, together with decrease in the quantity of the gastric juice and increase in mucus after histamine stimulation suggest strongly an actual anatomic defect of the gastric mucosa. Findings of this sort we have encountered in about 10 per cent of the general run of patients in whom we have made gastric analyses. The majority of these people have no digestive symptoms and may be to all intents and purposes well. Others may have minor digestive complaints which differ in no way from those encountered in people with normal stomach juice. To what extent anacidity (with gastritis?) of this sort is a precursor of later troubles, such as anemia or cancer of the stomach, is not clear. Certain it is that most of these people go for years without any evident trouble.

Treatment.—No treatment is indicated unless symptoms exist. Many of these people eat a liberal general diet without digestive complaints and they show no evidences of failing nutrition. If indigestion is present the methods of therapy outlined in the section on Indigestion should be followed. Hydrochloric acid may be given (HCl dil. 1 to 3 cc. in water with meals). Occasionally indigestion or diarrhea may improve on this therapy but the mechanism is not clear. Certainly the amount of acid which can be given in this way is too small to replace the natural secretion which amounts to perhaps the equivalent of 1.5 L $\frac{N}{10}$ daily. So-called "stomachics" such as nux vomica and gentian which are often prescribed with the idea of stimulating the flagging secretions are without avail if a complete anacidity exists. If benefit follows, it is because of stimulation of appetite or by psychic effect.

REFERENCES.

For complete discussion (with extensive literature) of inflammations of the stomach, see article by KONJETZNY, in Henke-Lubarsch: Handbuch, etc., 1928, 4, Pt. II, 768.

BLOOMFIELD, A. L., and POLLAND, W. S.: Gastric Anacidity, New York, The Macmillan Company, 1933. (For full discussion of anacidity and gastritis.)

GASTRIC AND DUODENAL ULCER.

"Peptic" ulcer, gastric and duodenal, is one of the commonest conditions encountered in medical practice. Clearly defined over one hundred years ago by the masterly descriptions of Abercrombie, Cruveilhier and Rokitansky, its cause and genesis still remain obscure, nor has any altogether satisfactory therapeutic approach been devised. Of recent years the amazing frequency of duodenal ulcer revealed largely by improvements in roentgen diagnosis has emphasized more than ever the importance of the ulcer problem.

No age period is exempt; the malady occurs literally from childhood to the grave. However, it is essentially a disease of young adult life and middle age. People of all classes and occupations are affected. Duodenal ulcer is more common in men than in women in the proportion of 3 or 4 to 1, whereas gastric ulcer is slightly more frequent in women. The pylorus is definitely the seat of war; the vast majority of ulcers develop near it either on the gastric or duodenal side, although involvement of the ring itself is rare. Chronic duodenal ulcers are limited to the first portion but acute forms may occur in the remoter reaches.

On the stomach side the lesser curvature is the site of predilection; ulcers of the greater curvature and body are distinctly rare. The ulcers may be single or multiple. There is usually only one, but two or three are not uncommon; as many as several dozen have been described, but in this case they are of the acute type (erosions). Elaborate statistical studies have been made of all of the above points and for details the reader is referred to Hurst and Stewart's recent monograph.

Etiology.—Virchow taught that the cause of chronic gastric ulcer is to be found in interference with the circulation to a localized area and in point of fact one sometimes discovers in the center of the lesion a sclerotic or occluded artery. The theory is not altogether satisfactory, however, since more often than not one is unable to demonstrate the vascular disturbance or it may be secondary and not primary. Furthermore, this theory does not explain the localization of ulcer on the lesser curvature or near the pylorus. Many other views have been proposed; one of the most popular and plausible is that highly acid gastric juice supplemented, perhaps, by pyloric spasm or the mechanical irritation of food leads to erosion of the mucosa and propagation of the ulcer. The experimental production of ulcers in animals has been adduced as evidence for this idea. Nervous and psychic influences, the presence of a superabundance of ferments, anemia, endocrine disturbances and chronic gastritis have all been blamed. Recently a good deal of stress has been placed on the influence of remote foci of infection such as diseased tonsils and periapical tooth abscesses. It is alleged that infected emboli pass from such foci to the stomach and initiate the lesion which may then be kept up by the action of acid gastric juice. The writer feels strongly that this theory is entirely gratuitous. The experimental evidence which has been brought forward in support bears only a remote analogy to human conditions and it remains to be proved that foci of infection are more prominent in ulcer patients than in other people. In a long series of cases carefully studied in our clinic in which foci of infection were as far as possible eliminated, the results after several years were no better than in a control series treated in other ways. Whatever may promote or propagate the ulcer once it is established, it is hard to escape the conviction that certain people have an inherent or constitutional predisposition to peptic ulcer. Often highstrung and nervous, they usually have a highly acid gastric juice and a tendency to indigestion. In some cases there is a definite familial tendency. Hurst especially has supported this view.

The association of acute duodenal ulcer with superficial burns is well established, but this interesting phenomenon has no evident relation to the problem of chronic ulcer.

Pathology.—Acute and chronic ulcers are to be distinguished, although transition forms occur. Acute ulcers, or rather erosions, are often multiple; they consist of shallow superficial losses of substance without great peripheral reaction or scarring; they rarely perforate but may be the source of large hemorrhages. To what extent they are early stages of chronic callous ulcer is not clear; at any rate the latter presents a somewhat different picture. The outstanding features are an actual loss of substance which may extend in a staircase-like manner through successive layers of the stomach wall, although more often the lesion looks as if a round bit of tissue had been neatly removed by a punch. The submucosa or muscularis usually forms the floor, but penetration to or even through the serosa not uncommonly occurs. There is a chronic inflammatory reaction in the base and at the edges of the ulcer where dense scar tissue may be heaped up in a projecting roll surrounding a central crater-like excavation. The ulcers vary greatly in size. In the stomach the diameter of the crater is usually not over 2 cm., although occasional instances of gigantic ulcerations are described. The writer has seen one ulcer as large as the palm of one's hand. Duodenal ulcers are usually smaller and rarely exceed 1 cm. in diameter. Ulcers may heal by scarring; the crater fills up and finally a fairly smooth surface devoid, however, of normal mucosa remains. The scar may contract and sometimes the pylorus is imbedded in a mass of inflammatory tissue, or the stomach may be distorted in various ways. As the ulcer penetrates, the stomach may become adherent to and perforate into surrounding structures such as the liver or pancreas, or large arteries such as the splenic or hepatic may be opened. In extreme cases a pathologic chaos of adherent and distorted tissues results which is disentangled with difficulty even at autopsy. Peptic ulcer is essentially a relapsing or recurring disease. Hence one may find signs of partial healing in one part of the lesion with extension in another direction, and scarred and active ulcers may coëxist in the same stomach.

Symptoms.—The ulcer may be latent for years and may heal without there ever having been any clinical manifestations. If symptoms are present they are those of indigestion or of hemorrhage, perforation or pyloric stenosis. So variable, however, are the complaints of ulcer patients that one can hardly paint a satisfactory composite picture. Illustrative cases will therefore be briefly presented.

1. **Ulcer with Indigestion.**—The indigestion of ulcer patients differs in no essential respect from that which has been described in the preceding article. Many writers stress the occurrence of symptoms at some regular interval after meals—one, two or three hours—and the fact that the taking of additional food or a dose of bicarbonate of soda when the indigestion is at its height may give temporary relief. It is pointed out that some of the patient's wake up in the night at a regular hour because of epigastric distress. All this is frequently true but the same events may occur in patients who have no ulcer, and many ulcer patients have no such characteristic sequence of symptoms. The writer is convinced there is nothing specific in the indigestion of ulcer and that indistinguishable symptoms may occur in people with other abdominal lesions or for that matter with no organic disease at all. During severe bouts of symptoms there may be vomiting and marked epigastric pains probably attributable to spasm of the pylorus but one cannot make a definite diagnosis unless the digestive symptoms are fortified by some more specific finding such as bleeding or positive roentgen-ray evidence. The symptoms persist for years or there may be interesting remissions during which the patient has no discomfort for long periods of time.

Physical examination in this type of ulcer case reveals no specific findings, and even when epigastric distress is present there is rarely any objective tenderness unless the ulcer has penetrated to the peritoneal surface.

Gastric analysis in the vast majority of cases shows a large volume of secretion of high acidity. After histamine, ten-minute volumes of 30 to 50 cc. or more are frequently found and the total acidity is usually above 110. While it is true that an occasional case of verified ulcer occurs in a person with low gastric acidity the high values are so constant that in a doubtful case low acid and volume weighs strongly against the diagnosis of ulcer. High values, on the other hand, while compatible with ulcer do not prove its presence since many normal people have similar findings. Blood may be present in the stomach contents or in the stools.

The roentgen-ray is indispensable in making a positive diagnosis and not infrequently an actual excavation is visualized in the wall of the stomach, especially on the lesser curvature. With duodenal ulcer definite filling defects are less evident but one encounters deformities in the shape of the duodenal cap which do not smooth out when the fluoroscopist presses barium through the pylorus. One must be cautious, however, in the interpretation of doubtful roentgen signs and our experience has been that if the roentgen-ray findings are equivocal the clinical features are also likely to be indefinite.

The above points are illustrated by the following cases:

ILLUSTRATIVE CASE—GASTRIC ULCER (LATENT).

E. O., seaman, aged seventy-five years.

Complaint.—Loss of weight, and blood in the urine.

Past History.—Appetite always good. Bowels regular. There has never been indigestion of any sort. No nausea, vomiting, gas, jaundice, hematemesis, colic, diarrhea, or bloody or tarry stools.

Present Illness.—One year ago noticed blood in the urine. This has continued to be present off and on and recently there has been pain on voiding. Moderate loss of weight and strength.

Examination.—There was marked emaciation and he looked sick and worn. There was generalized arteriosclerosis. The abdomen was negative.

Laboratory.—Red blood cells, 3,000,000; hemoglobin, 34 per cent; white blood cells, 5000. Stool, negative. No occult blood. Urine, grossly bloody. Cystoscopy showed a cauliflower-like bladder tumor which bled freely.

Course.—The patient refused operation and was followed for eighteen months until his death, which was the direct result of anemia and cachexia. *During this period there were never any digestive symptoms.*

Autopsy.—Aside from the cancer of the bladder there were found two typical benign gastric ulcers, 11 x 15 mm. and 5 x 5 mm. respectively, in size. They were situated 3.5 cm. and 0.5 cm. proximal to the pylorus.

Comment.—The case illustrates well the occasional complete symptomatic latency of gastric ulcer. The ulcers were evidently of considerable duration and were "active." They were not simply the scars of previous ulcers which had healed.

ILLUSTRATIVE CASE—DUODENAL ULCER.

R. P. W., laborer, aged thirty-six years.

Past History.—General health good until present illness. No previous digestive symptoms.

Present Illness.—Six years ago he began to have stomach trouble. The chief symptoms are a "gnawing pain" just under the xyphoid sometimes radiating a little to the right, belching, sour eructations and sometimes nausea. The discomfort comes two to three hours after meals and is relieved temporarily by food, olive oil and milk of magnesia. He says that soda makes it worse. At times lying down seems to relieve the pain, although it occasionally comes in the night and wakes him up. The symptoms have been intermittent; there are usually three or four bouts of indigestion a year lasting three to six weeks each. About a year ago he had a very severe attack which was not relieved by any of the ordinary measures. His physician then put him to bed for two weeks on a milk diet. He improved rapidly and went to work, but six weeks later the symptoms returned. Since then he has only been able to do light odd jobs.

Physical Examination.—Healthy looking, well nourished man. Physical examination entirely negative. He complains of discomfort on pressure in the epigastrium but there are no objective findings.

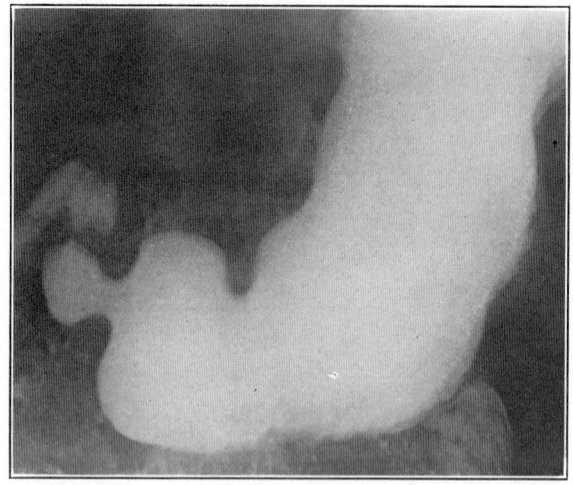

Fig. 28.—Duodenal ulcer. Note the normal stomach outlines, but the marked deformity of the duodenal cap.

Laboratory.—Red blood cells, 5,600,000; hemoglobin, 99 per cent; white blood cells, 5400. Urine, negative. Stool normal, no occult blood. After histamine the highest ten-minute volume of gastric secretion was 42 cc. with total acidity of 146. Roentgen-rays showed no irregularity in the outline of the stomach. The duodenal cap, however, was irregular and showed the typical "clover leaf deformity" which usually indicates duodenal ulcer (Fig. 28).

Course.—In view of the persistence of symptoms for six years and the patient's present disability, it was decided to operate and a pyloroplasty was done. The excised portion of duodenum showed three small areas of ulceration with induration of the adjacent tissues. The immediate postoperative course was uneventful. He was kept on a very much restricted diet (Sippy) but in spite of this all of the old symptoms returned within two months. Six months later, symptoms having persisted in the meanwhile, he committed suicide.

Comment.—This case illustrates very well the so-called typical story of duodenal ulcer. It will be found, however, that not all cases of ulcer give this story and also that similar symptoms frequently occur in people who have no ulcer. That the ulcer was not the direct cause of symptoms is further proven in this case by the fact that excision gave no relief (see below—treatment). This patient also illustrates the usual findings as regards gastric analysis and roentgen-ray.

2. Ulcer with Hemorrhage.—Bleeding into the stomach results most frequently from erosions or ulcer but there are various other causes such as the rupture of dilated veins in the stomach wall in connection with "splenic anemia" or cirrhosis of the liver (esophageal varices), polyps, ulcerating new growths, and certain blood diseases. Occasionally a large hemorrhage occurs without demonstrable lesion at operation or autopsy. The bleeding may be sudden and profuse and as much as a liter or more may be lost in a short time. In such cases the symptoms are those of any large hemorrhage—weakness or collapse with vertigo, dimness of vision, rapid feeble pulse and low blood pressure, or there is actual unconsciousness. Blood may be vomited, but sometimes it is undetected until a large "tarry" stool is passed; this is especially so with duodenal ulcer. On the other hand there may be slight continuous or repeated bleedings which reveal themselves by progressive weakness and anemia and by the finding of occult blood in the stools.

The majority of peptic ulcers probably bleed at some time or other during their life history; obvious clinical evidence is present in about one-fourth of the cases.

ILLUSTRATIVE CASE—GASTRIC ULCER (HEMORRHAGE).

V. H., housewife, aged thirty-nine years.

Past History.—General health good. From the age of fourteen to twenty years she had periodic attacks of lower abdominal pain which ceased after her appendix was removed. There were no digestive symptoms previous to the present illness.

Present Illness.—About four years ago she began to have indigestion, which came in periodic attacks followed by free intervals. The symptoms consisted of a feeling of gas and distention in the upper abdomen associated with a burning pain which radiated up under the sternum and spread fan-like to the back. The discomfort usually began about an hour after meals, and it was temporarily relieved by eating. It was often most severe at night. Three years ago following a severe and protracted attack she vomited a large quantity of blood. She went to bed for three weeks and then felt quite well. One night she felt warm and got up to open the window, when she suddenly became faint. She managed to get back to bed and then became unconscious. On waking she vomited "a quart of clotted blood" and also passed blood by rectum, whereupon she fainted again. She was brought to the hospital by ambulance.

Physical Examination.—No detailed examination was made on entry because of the recent bleeding. She was well nourished but looked very pale. The temperature, pulse and respiration were normal. She complained of discomfort in the epigastrium, where there was slight tenderness on pressure. Blood pressure 110/75.

Laboratory.—Blood: red blood cells, 2,500,000; hemoglobin, 35 per cent; white blood cells, 13,000; polymorphonuclears, 83 per cent. Urine normal. Stool black, liquid, almost pure blood.

Course.—She was kept in bed and no food was given by mouth. Fluids were introduced by rectum. She received a transfusion of 500 cc. of blood. After five days the stools no longer showed occult blood and small feedings of milk and cream were commenced. The blood count rose to red blood cells, 3,400,000 and hemoglobin, 54 per cent.

Roentgen-rays taken a few days later showed a deep niche in the lesser curvature, rather high up, probably above the middle of the stomach (Fig. 29). In view of the persistent symptoms and repeated large bleedings it was decided to operate. A large V-shaped piece of stomach wall bearing the ulcer was removed. No gastro-enterostomy was done. The specimen showed a chronic ulcer measuring 2.5 x 1 cm. in diameter which had penetrated into the submucosa. The base of the ulcer was covered with grayish necrotic tissue. No special vessel was demonstrated to be the source of the bleeding. Microscopically there were no evidences of cancer.

Following operation she did not do well and the old pain soon returned and persisted even with a very much restricted bland diet. There was occasional vomiting with traces of blood. Restudy of the patient in the hospital two months after the operation showed evidences of a new ulcer at the operative site. With rest and careful feeding she gradually recovered, however, and two years later considered herself practically well. She still had pain occasionally if she overate or ate too quickly.

Comment.—The case illustrates in a typical way the effect of sudden large bleedings from gastric ulcer. Some of the surgical difficulties are well exemplified. The complication of a recurrence of ulcer at the operative site is also of importance.

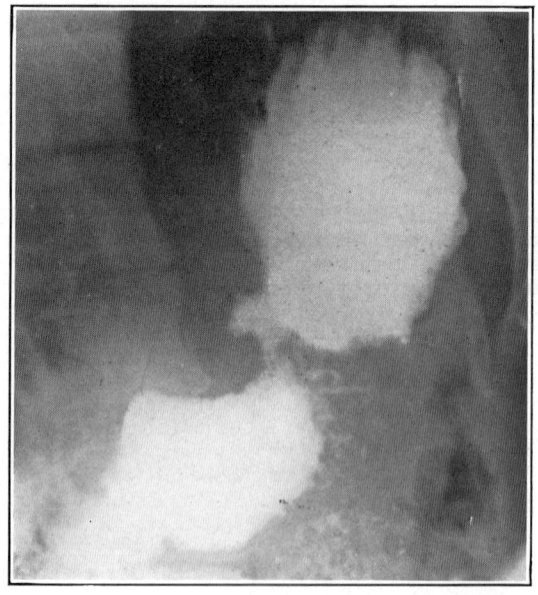

Fig. 29.—Gastric ulcer. Note the large crater on the lesser curvature with spasm opposite to it which gives an hour-glass appearance.

3. **Ulcer with Pyloric Obstruction.**—In some cases of chronic ulcer situated near the pylorus, scar tissue may be formed which gradually produces more or less constriction of the pyloric orifice or of the duodenum, or great inflammatory masses may develop distinguishable only with difficulty from a carcinomatous tumor. At times the actual organic narrowing is not so extreme but irritation and local edema, together with spasm, lead to an almost complete functional occlusion of the stomach outlet. When the process has extended so as to reach the peritoneal surface, adhesions with other organs develop and the pylorus may be almost inextricably bound up with adjacent structures. The incidence of this complication is estimated as not over 10 per cent.

Ulcer and cancer are by far the most common causes of pyloric obstruction, although it may result, on occasion, from extra-gastric adhesions, or from occlusion of the lumen by a polyp. We have seen no case in which the syndrome of greatly distended stomach with profuse vomiting occurred without an organic lesion at the pylorus, although cases of functional atony are described especially in the older literature. In children narrowing of the pylorus may result from developmental changes—the so-called *congenital hypertrophic pyloric stenosis.*

Symptoms.—It is astonishing to what an extent pyloric obstruction may progress before symptoms appear, and this, perhaps, is explained by the fact that as the narrowing develops, the muscular wall of the stomach hypertrophies and chyme is forced through the pylorus despite a partial occlusion. Finally, however, and often acutely as an immediate result of spasm or edema, the occlusion becomes so complete that there is a failure of compensation; contraction no longer serves to empty the stomach, food residues accumulate in large quantity and at last the organ may, as it were, give up so that its walls become distended and flabby, and peristalsis is weak and ineffective. Then quite a definite train of symptoms appears, featured by vomiting, often of huge amounts of material which consists of partly digested food remnants, accumulated gastric secretions and sometimes blood. The patient may recognize things he ate several days ago and he may himself be impressed by the great amount of the vomitus and speak, for example, of "throwing up a bucketful." As much as several liters of material have been ejected during a bout of vomiting. Once the stomach has been emptied there may be relief for a time until a further accumulation leads to a recurrence of the emesis. Aside from the vomiting there are various associated symptoms such as pain, indigestion, thirst and weakness.

Physical Examination.—On physical examination the most striking and pathognomonic finding is the presence of huge peristaltic waves which are seen to move slowly across the epigastrium from left to right. They are due to the forcible efforts of the stomach to push material through the narrow pylorus and hence are best demonstrated in relatively early cases. When the stomach has finally given out and become flabby and atonic the waves are no longer to be seen or at least they appear only occasionally. If vomiting goes on to a point where there is serious loss of food and fluid, emaciation and desiccation become evident. The tissues and skin are dry and loose, the tongue is dry and the thin, wasted extremities and sunken face stand out in contrast to the distended epigastrium.

The roentgen-ray is particularly helpful since the barium meal makes it possible to visualize the extent of pyloric occlusion, the degree of distention of the stomach, the character of the contractions and finally the emptying time. In extreme cases residues of barium remain in the stomach for days.

Laboratory Tests.—The urine is scanty and highly concentrated and the blood count may be abnormally high (5,000,000 to 6,500,000) as a result of desiccation. Of especial importance, however, are the changes in the ionic balance of the blood which are brought about by vomiting and the consequent loss of large amounts of gastric juice. The body becomes depleted of acid as can be demonstrated by actual measurement of blood chloride. Values as low as 250 mg. per cent instead of the normal of 550 to 650 have been observed. Hand in hand with this there develops an alkalosis and the blood carbon dioxide may rise to remarkable levels. There may be clinical evidence of tetany. Nitrogen retention also takes place; its mechanism is not clearly understood. The changes are obviously complex and the theoretical implications cannot be discussed here. The reader is referred to the studies of Haden and Orr and of Gamble and his associates. However, the practical importance of these perversions of blood chloride, nitrogen and bicarbonate is paramount, since we now know that operation is very dangerous (see below) unless the ionic balance has been restored and the loss of fluids corrected.

Illustrative Case—Gastric Ulcer (Pyloric Obstruction).

A. C., salesman, aged twenty-three years.

Complaint.—Stomach trouble for three years.

Past History.—Always well before present illness.

Present Illness.—Three years ago noticed that he was losing his appetite. Shortly after this he began having gnawing sensations in the stomach and a desire to vomit, especially in the afternoon. For the last two years vomiting spells have become more frequent and severe. He often vomits 2 quarts at a time and recognizes food remains from previous meals. There is no blood in the vomitus. His appetite has remained good and there has been no "indigestion," but he has lost 25 pounds in weight and feels weak. The vomiting spells are worse when he is worried.

Physical Examination.—Temperature, pulse and respiration normal. He looked tired and worn and was very thin. The upper abdomen was slightly distended and from time to time large peristaltic waves were seen to move slowly from the left costal margin transversely across the abdomen. No mass felt. No tenderness.

Laboratory Tests.—Red blood cells, 5,700,000; hemoglobin, 102 per cent; white blood cells, 9000. Urine dark, specific gravity 1024, trace of albumin. Stool negative, no occult blood. Blood chlorides (as NaCl), 449 mg. per cent; blood CO_2, 85 volumes per cent; blood urea, 45 mg. per cent. Gastric analysis: the fasting stomach twelve hours after lavage contained 800 cc. of clear, slightly bile-stained fluid. After histamine the highest ten-minute volume was 48 cc., with an acidity of 110.

Roentgen-rays.—The stomach is large and there is obvious obstruction at the pylorus. At six hours practically no barium has left the stomach; there is a small amount in the ileum. At twenty-four hours there is a two-thirds residue in the stomach (Fig. 30).

Course.—The stomach was lavaged twice daily with warm salt solution; no food was given by mouth. During the first twenty-four hours 500 cc. of 10 per cent glucose solution were given intravenously and 4000 cc. of salt solution subcutaneously. During the second twenty-four hours 3000 cc. of 5 per cent glucose in salt solution were given subcutaneously and 1200 cc. of salt solution by rectal drip. The blood chlorides rose to 540 mg. per cent and the blood CO_2 fell to 68 volumes per cent.

On the following day a laparotomy was done. The pylorus was found to be greatly thickened and scarred and no attempt was made to remove it. Gastroenterostomy was performed. For the first week there was persistent gastric distress with vomiting. This ceased following repeated lavage. He left the hospital ten days later on a limited semi-liquid diet. Six months later he reported that he felt perfectly well.

Comment.—It is to be noted that in this case there was no indigestion and that the symptoms were largely mechanical. The occlusion of the pylorus was of maximal degree; normally the stomach evacuates all the barium in about six hours. The alterations in the chemistry of the blood are of especial importance as well as the preoperative treatment (see below). The case is also of the type in which surgery is imperative and usually yields good results.

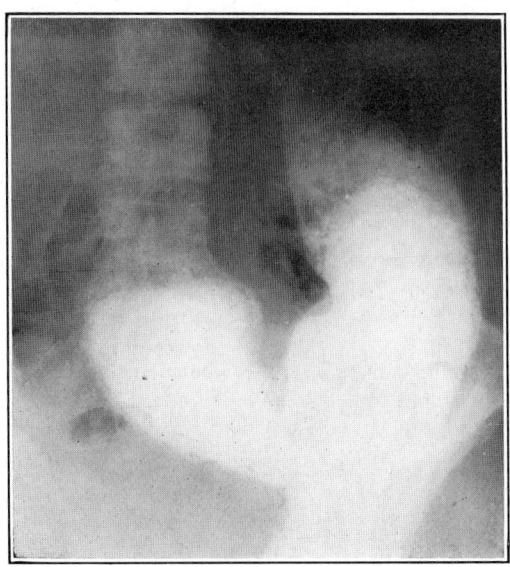

Fig. 30.—Gastric ulcer; pyloric obstruction. Note great dilation of stomach with obliteration of normal pyloric contour.

4. **Perforation.**—Perforation is the most dreaded complication of peptic ulcer. Even when the ulceration is deep, actual penetration of the serosa fortunately does not often take place, but occasionally there is a rupture into the free peritoneal cavity. As a rule, progressive ulceration is attended by local inflammation with adhesions which prevent free perforation. The ulcerated area becomes glued to the omentum or to some adjacent viscus whereby rupture is prevented, or at least is circumscribed. Perforation may come out of a clear sky in a person who is not even aware that he has an ulcer, or it may supervene at any time during the manifest clinical course of the disease. Perforation is infrequent, although autopsy series in which it is found in from 30 to 60 per cent of the cases testify to the gravity of this complication.

Symptoms.—With a varied pathologic picture of this sort, all sorts of symptoms may result. When ulceration has extended to the serous coat so that peritoneal reaction ensues there is often localized pain and tenderness in the upper abdomen such as one gets with any intra-abdominal inflammation. The symptoms are usually clearly distinguishable from those of the antecedent indigestion associated with the ulcer. Sudden rupture into the free peritoneal cavity results in the evidence of acute peritonitis—intense generalized abdominal pain with tenderness and rigidity of the abdominal wall, collapse, rapid feeble pulse and fever. Localized perforations into the lesser peritoneal

39

sac, liver and pancreas, produce variable symptoms; usually there are the evidences of a chronic septic infection—irregular fever with, perhaps, chills and sweats, abdominal pain and tenderness and sometimes special localizing signs. However, the findings may be slight or obscure and perforation of this sort is not uncommonly unrecognized until revealed at operation or autopsy.

Diagnosis.—This is to be made from the clinical features which have been described above. Chronic circumscribed perforations are occasionally suggested by the roentgen-ray appearances after the barium meal. In one of our cases free perforation occurred while the patient was under the fluoroscope and barium was seen to run out into the peritoneal cavity.

ILLUSTRATIVE CASE—GASTRIC ULCER (PERFORATION).

T. W., motorman, aged sixty-one years.

Complaint.—Indigestion and pain in stomach.

Past History.—Nothing remarkable before present illness.

Present Illness.—About six months before entry he began to lose weight and to have distaste for food. This was soon followed by "gas pains" in the upper abdomen and occasional vomiting without relation to meals. Four weeks ago he noted that the stools were black for several days. No vomiting of blood.

Physical Examination.—A poorly nourished elderly man. The general physical examination was not remarkable. There was definite tenderness over the upper mid-abdomen with a suggestion of muscle spasm on palpation.

Laboratory.—Red blood cells, 4,100,000; hemoglobin, 70 per cent; white blood cells, 8400. Urine, clear. Stool, occult blood present.

Roentgen-rays.—The outline of the stomach is very irregular in its lower third and the antrum is constricted about 5 cm. from the pylorus. At six hours there is a residue of 20 per cent.

Course.—On the day after entry at 1.35 P.M. he suddenly developed *intense pain* in the right upper quadrant. This soon became generalized. There was marked tenderness on pressure over the entire abdomen which was rigid and board-like. The pulse was rapid and small, he was slightly cyanotic and there was sweating. White blood cells at 4.45 P.M., 7800. On the following morning laparotomy was done (about eighteen hours after onset of pain). The peritoneal cavity contained a good deal of barium and gastric contents mixed with thin, yellowish turbid fluid. The peritoneum was intensely reddened. On the lesser curvature of the stomach there was a circular perforation about 0.5 cm. in diameter from which gastric contents were still exuding. The tear was repaired and the abdomen was closed. He failed rapidly and died thirty-six hours later.

Autopsy.—General peritonitis. At the pylorus there was a large crater-shaped ulcer about 4 cm. in diameter and 2 cm. deep, surrounded by an indurated mass of scar tissue. The perforation lay at the base of the ulcer. Microscopic study of the ulcer showed no signs of cancer.

Comment.—The recent onset of symptoms is of note, although the ulcer was evidently of long duration. Symptoms were apparently due in the first place to peritoneal irritation. Final rupture led to the picture of acute generalized peritonitis which was already well advanced in eighteen hours. If operation had been done sooner the patient might have been saved. The large size of the ulcer suggested cancer but the process was histologically benign.

Prognosis.—The course of peptic ulcer is too varied and the hazard of complications is too great to enable one to make exact statements as to the prognosis in the individual case. Ulcers undoubtedly often heal completely and permanently—witness the scars found in the stomach in a certain percentage of all autopsies. We have several times seen huge ulcer craters (roentgen-ray) disappear within a few weeks. However, peptic ulcer is essentially a chronic relapsing disorder and inasmuch as the tendency or "diathesis" is usually deepseated one does not usually expect a complete and permanent disappearance of the trouble, even with the most careful therapy. Small duodenal ulcers are, perhaps, most favorable; large deep ulcers, especially when pyloric obstruction exists, are more serious. Occurrence of complications of course alters the outlook at any moment. Ulcer of the duodenum rarely, if ever, becomes malignant, but the possibility of cancerous changes in a stomach ulcer is always to be considered. A lively dispute has gone on in the literature for the last fifty years as to the frequency of so-called ulcer-cancer and the matter is not yet settled. In brief it may be said that a certain percentage of gastric ulcers which clinically appear to be benign subsequently are shown to be carcinomatous by the fact that the patient dies of cancer of the stomach or, if the ulcer has been resected, of cancerous metastases. Whether the ulcer was actually cancerous from the start—a cancer with ulceration simulating that of peptic ulcer—or whether a benign ulcer underwent cancerous changes it is often difficult or impossible to say. Even the histologic interpretation of excised ulcers may vary in the hands of equally skilled pathologists. It is said that large ulcers, greater than 2 cm. in diameter, for example, are more likely to be cancerous than small ones, but certainly many huge ulcers are definitely benign. In summary, the writer's experience indicates that probably not over 5 per cent of gastric ulcers are malignant.

Illustrative Case—Gastric Ulcer (Carcinomatous).

C. V., housewife, aged twenty-six years.

Complaint.—Stomach trouble.

Past History.—Always well before present illness.

Present Illness.—Two years before entry (March, 1926) she began to have "indigestion." However, instead of the usual symptoms of fullness, gas and vague distress, she had severe pain localized in the mid-epigastrium which had no definite relation to the taking of food, although it was better when she was on a restricted diet. She was treated by her local physician, who put her through a standard ulcer treatment (rest in bed, Sippy diet) whereupon she improved and gained 30 pounds in weight. The symptoms returned, however, and in December, 1926, the abdomen was explored. The doctor reported that there was a large ulcer, apparently benign, high up on the lesser curvature. It was impossible to excise it and nothing was done. When she came to the hospital in March, 1928, the original symptoms were still present.

Physical Examination.—Her general appearance and nutrition were good. No abnormalities were found on physical examination. There was a well healed abdominal scar.

Laboratory.—Red blood cells, 4,800,000; hemoglobin, 85 per cent, white blood cells, 8500. Urine clear. Stool negative, no occult blood. Gastric analysis after histamine: highest ten-minute volume, 12 cc.; acid, 77.

Roentgen-rays.—There was a large niche (Fig. 31) just above the incisure. The pocket remained full throughout the examination. It was concluded that there was a large penetrating ulcer, and that the crater was about 3 to 4 cm. in diameter.

Course.—She was put to bed and placed on a simple bland diet, which was gradually increased. All symptoms disappeared and she left the hospital five weeks later. She continued to gain weight and was perfectly well for five months. She then developed severe abdominal pain with persistent vomiting and rapid loss of weight. She returned to the hospital very thin and desperately ill. The upper abdomen was full of hard masses and on exploration there was a general peritoneal carcinosis.

Comment.—It is impossible to say whether one was dealing with carcinoma from the start or whether a benign ulcer later became malignant. The youth of the patient is against primary carcinoma but does not exclude it. The large size of the ulcer crater and the small volume of gastric secretion with relatively low acidity should have roused one's suspicions of cancer. The case illustrates very well the difficulties of making a definite diagnosis. The relief of symptoms under treatment was especially confusing.

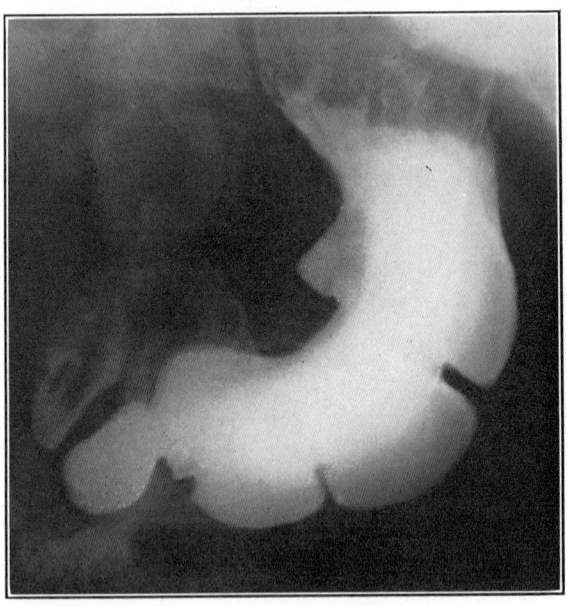

Fig. 31.—Cancerous ulcer of the stomach. Note the huge crater on the lesser curvature.

Treatment.—There are two main objectives in the treatment of gastric ulcer: first to relieve the patient's symptoms (indigestion) and secondly to eliminate the ulcer. Contrary to what one might expect these by no means go hand in hand. Symptoms may disappear entirely under treatment within a day or two when the ulcer is obviously not yet healed or, on the other hand, the ulcer may actually be removed by operation and the indigestion none the less persists. This apparent paradox is immediately clarified if one recalls that the ulcer itself is not painful but that it acts merely as a source of reflex irritation which sets up spasms which are in turn the direct cause of the symptoms. This mechanism has already been discussed in the section on indigestion. Furthermore, it seems likely that in many cases the ulcer, the abundant highly acid secretion and the symptoms all represent the results of a constitutional tendency and neither is the direct cause of the other. In brief:

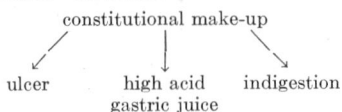

constitutional make-up

ulcer   high acid   indigestion
             gastric juice

may be the case rather than the conventional idea:

high acid gastric juice

↓

ulcer

↓

indigestion

That the former conception is probably correct is borne out by the very fact that high acidity and indigestion indistinguishable from that of ulcer patients are commonly encountered in people who have no ulcer at all. The ulcer which, to be sure, is probably promoted by the high acidity is really only an incident in the whole syndrome.

Treatment of ulcer may be medical or surgical.

Medical Treatment.—By weight of lengthy tradition the medical treatment of peptic ulcer centers on diet, and the name of nearly every prominent gastro-enterologist is associated with some scheme of ulcer feeding. These schemes have varied in accordance with the author's views as to the etiology of ulcer: some are based on the idea of keeping food (and alkali) constantly in the stomach so as to maintain neutrality or at least to avoid an excess of acid at all times; others emphasize protein and restrict carbohydrate, or *vice versa*, with the idea of either neutralizing or giving a minimal stimulus to secretion. Some advocate frequent small feedings; others prefer to give food at longer intervals. The end has not yet been reached, since no year goes by without the proposal of new dietary treatment schemes. Now when one studies the results obtained by various "ulcer diets" it is of interest that a certain percentage of the patients do well, whereas others continue to have symptoms or to relapse *regardless of just which treatment scheme is employed*. Indeed, the fact that no one diet is universally effective is witnessed by the constant proposals of new diets which are supposed to be better than the old ones. In brief, an approximately equal number of successes or failures is obtained with any one of the standard ulcer diets, even though they may be quite opposite in principle. It behooves one, therefore, to seek for the common factor and one then finds that they are all simple bland diets and that the patient is kept more or less at rest during the treatment. Long experience has convinced the writer that with a few reservations to be mentioned presently, it is not so much what the patient eats as how he eats it; that is to say, the general therapeutic regimen and dietary hygiene are all-important and the principles of treatment already discussed under indigestion must be invoked. We are convinced that except with the occasional neurasthenic patient who thrives on restrictions, detailed diet lists are unnecessary and do more harm than good. What can be more pathetic than the ulcer patient doomed at all costs to interrupt his work or play at two-hour intervals to consume an insipid mixture of milk and cream with the warning figure of the physician ever in the background as his evil genius! No wonder that most intelligent patients on this regimen sooner or later develop an inferiority complex which is almost worse than the disease itself.

In brief, it appears that drastic restrictions are usually unnecessary and in the ordinary case featured simply by indigestion the following points should be stressed.

1. *Rest.*—The term is used in the broadest sense and means not simply physical inertia but rest in the sense of *relief from strain.* *Hurry, worry* and *anger* must, if possible, be avoided or mitigated. A careful and sympathetic study of the patient's work, play, problems and background must be made; the mechanism of his symptoms (see article on Indigestion) must be explained to him and his full coöperation must be gained. Together with his physician the daily schedule must be revised. He must learn that the ulcer itself is only part of the picture and that despite the ulcer, comfort may be achieved if keyed-up nerves are let down, overstress mitigated, and undue hurry abated. A busy physician was promptly relieved of symptoms by making him get up one-half hour earlier so that he could linger over his breakfast and by spacing his appointments at longer intervals. In aggravated cases a change of scene or a preliminary period of complete rest in bed, preferably in the hospital, should initiate the treatment.

2. *Diet.*—As pointed out above it is more how the patient eats than what he eats that is of importance. He must be taught to eat slowly and chew well, and to sip liquids and not gulp them. This is paramount. Excitement, argument and tension must be avoided at meals. Most of us swallow our lunch hastily while talking shop with a group of associates, and at dinner, fatigued by a hard day's work, next winter's fuel supply and the children's schooling has to be discussed. All this must be avoided. It is better to omit the meal altogether than to eat in hasty excitement.

As to the actual content of the diet, one should never stuff. That pleasant feeling of being "full" must unfortunately be renounced by the ulcer patient. The food should be simple and plainly cooked, but it need not be insipid. The meals should be attractive so as to stimulate appetite and normal gastric reflexes. However, the following are to be avoided: (1) coarse foods such as corn, asparagus, cabbage, bran, tough meats, coarse fruits and berries, which may produce mechanical irritation; (2) highly spiced and seasoned dishes such as tomales, rich sauces, cheeses, and (3) fat, fried or greasy articles. All these are likely to set up discomfort and perhaps actually interfere with the healing of the ulcer. There remain, then, as a basis for the diet such things as fruit juices, strained cereals, eggs, toast, plainly cooked lean meat, fish and chicken, well cooked starchy vegetables, puréed green vegetables, jellies, junkets, custards, plain cake and ice cream. Milk may be taken freely and in our experience moderate quantities of tea and coffee are allowable if no indigestion follows. Alcohol is, on the whole, best avoided, certainly in excess, although some patients of the proper temper feel better for an occasional cocktail or glass of wine with dinner. No diet list is necessary after the above principles have been thoroughly explained to the patient.

In refractory or severe cases it may be well to initiate treatment by rest in bed and a few days of complete starvation except for small amounts of water. The idea is to put the whole organism completely at rest and despite the presence of acid in the stomach, symptoms often vanish as by magic within a day or two under such a rest cure. After from two to ten days of starvation milk and crackers may be given in increasing amounts, followed by a gradual transition to the diet outlined above.

There has been a good deal of futile discussion as to the relative merits of "ambulatory" or "bed treatment" of ulcer. Unless the patient is so nervous, worn out or depleted that bed is obviously necessary, ambulatory treatment should, of course, be tried as the simpler procedure. If the results are not satisfactory the rest cure may then be necessary.

3. *Drugs.*—The fewer drugs used the better. Small doses of tincture of belladonna (0.5 cc.) before meals to relax spasm, combined, perhaps, with sodium bromide (1 gram) are especially useful. Soda bicarbonate or burnt magnesia (0.5 to 1 gram) may be taken as necessary to relieve any particular bout of indigestion, but so-called alkalinization by continuous large doses is in our experience futile and inadvisable. The bowels should be regulated (see article on Constipation).

Preparations of gastric mucin have recently been advised with the idea of neutralizing acid and coating the ulcer with a protective covering, thus promoting healing. This form of therapy is still in an experimental stage.

4. *General Measures.*—Exercise, hours of rest, recreation and vacation should be carefully considered and regulated to suit the temper and needs of the individual case.

Under the above regimen the majority of patients with peptic ulcer improve rapidly and may indeed become symptom-free in a few days. Occasional days of discomfort or longer relapses are, however, not uncommon and the patient should be forewarned that this may occur so as not to be unduly disappointed. Whether or not the ulcer has really healed is, however, another matter, and this can only be judged by roentgen-ray appearances and by the cessation of bleeding. At any rate, it must be remembered that the ulcer tendency still exists and the usual story is that sooner or later definite symptoms are liable to recur—perhaps after years of comfort.

Treatment of Complications.—*Hemorrhage.*—Sudden hemorrhages, even if large, are rarely fatal but they demand absolute rest in bed. If the patient is in collapse a subcutaneous infusion of salt solution (1 to 2 liters) may be given, and the foot of the bed should be elevated. Warmth should be applied. Morphine (10 to 15 mg.) hypodermically is indicated for restlessness. As an emergency stimulant an injection of caffeine sodium benzoate (0.2 to 0.3 gram) is, perhaps, best. Some advise washing out the stomach with cold water if the bleeding persists, but we have not often found this necessary. After the initial shock has passed the patient should be kept quietly in bed for several weeks. Starvation is advisable during the first few days and fluids may be supplied by rectal or subcutaneous infusions. After the bleeding has stopped as evidenced by the disappearance of blood from the stools the usual treatment for ulcer may gradually be instituted, supplemented by measures to rehabilitate the blood such as feeding of liver or liver extract and iron. If the count is very low, transfusion of blood is in order. Surgical interference is to be avoided immediately after a large hemorrhage, since it is often difficult to find the bleeding point or to deal with it adequately at the time.

Persistent bleedings of lesser degree are usually controlled by general ulcer and anemia treatment. In occasional cases the bleeding persists intractably and chronic anemia and depletion result. Here one may be forced to operate with the idea of extirpating the ulcer. No positive rules can be given and experienced judgment is necessary.

Pyloric obstruction, if extreme, usually requires surgical relief by means of gastro-enterostomy or pyloroplasty. With lesser grades great improvement may result from rest, starvation with parenteral introduction of fluids, and daily lavage of the stomach with warm salt solution. Under such a regimen edema and spasm at the pylorus subside and small feedings of puréed bland food may then be adequately handled. Such efforts are useless, however, except with patients whose temper and material circumstances are such that they can coöperate in a tedious and trying treatment. If operation is to be done successfully proper preparation is all-important. This includes restoration of body fluids and salts by means of large infusions—rectal, subcutaneous or intravenous—of normal salt solution. Glucose solutions may also be given. The treatment must be pushed energetically until there is a free flow of urine and until the blood chloride and blood nitrogen have been restored to normal limits. This is usually accomplished in two or three days.

Acute perforation demands immediate surgical intervention. If operation is done within the first twelve hours many of the patients recover. Chances of successful treatment diminish rapidly as further time elapses and peritonitis spreads and the patient is more and more poisoned. Localized perforations may be unrecognized and they may in a sense heal themselves by encapsulation and scarring, but if abscesses or extensive perigastric adhesions form, operation is necessary. This should be done under the best possible conditions and preferably by skilled hands. Expert surgical judgment is necessary to get the best results.

Surgical Treatment.—Perforation of peptic ulcer affords an urgent indication for surgery. Pyloric obstruction also usually requires gastro-enterostomy or a plastic operation for its relief. Apart from these special conditions, however, the logic of surgical intervention has become less and less clear as time has gone by. Since the pioneer work of Billroth on surgical reconstruction of the pylorus fifty years ago, surgeons have continued with sublime and child-like faith in their art, but with inadequate understanding of the essential problem to devise new operations, always hoping to discover the happy combination of manipulations which will prove a cure-all for peptic ulcer. Now it is to make a gastro-enterostomy at some different point, now to cut and suture the pylorus in some new way, now to excise the so-called acid cell bearing area of the stomach or to divert a stream of alkaline duodenal contents into the stomach to neutralize the allegedly harmful acidity. The fact of the matter is that many patients have been improved or cured by any one of these procedures but the results are inconstant. There are always some brilliant successes, some partial improvements and occasionally the patient is worse. Here again, then, as with diet one is impelled to search for a common factor, and all that one can conclude is that frequently the operation, whatever it may be works so as to eliminate the pain-producing reflexes; but just what will happen in the individual case is quite unpredictable. Most surgeons have become aware of this uncertainty and realize that intervention is best restricted to those cases in which one is, so to speak, forced to do something. This will include, aside from perforation and pyloric obstruction, instances of ulcer in which symptoms have persisted over long periods of time despite intelligent medical treatment. It is wiser, in any case, not to promise the patient too much in the way of prompt or permanent relief and the availability of a surgeon skilled in stomach work should be taken into account in advising operation. An annoying sequel of operation may occur in the form of the so-called marginal or gastro-jejunal ulcer. A new ulcer, in brief, develops at the suture line of the gastro-enterostomy or beyond it in the jejunum. Such ulcers occasionally perforate into the colon with formation of gastro-colic fistula. These, and still other interesting complications, cannot be discussed here and the student is referred to the surgical literature.

Surgery of the autonomic nervous system may, in the future, have something to contribute to the ulcer problem if procedures can be devised to allay abnormal spasms of the gastric sphincters. Such efforts at present are still in the experimental stage.

REFERENCES.

GAMBLE, J. L., and McIVER, M. A.: A Study of the Effects of Pyloric Obstruction in Rabbits, Jour. Clin. Invest., 1924–1925, 1, 531.

GAMBLE, J. L., and Ross, S. G.: The Factors in Dehydration Following Pyloric Obstruction, Jour. Clin. Invest., 1924–1925, 1, 403.

HADEN, R. L., and ORR, T. G.: Chemical Changes in the Blood of the Dog after Pyloric Obstruction, Jour. Exper. Med., 1923, 37, 377.

HAUSER, in Henke-Lubarsch: Handbuch, 1926, 4, 361.

HURST, A. F., and STEWART, M. J.: Gastric and Duodenal Ulcer, London, 1929.

McVICAR, C. S.: Clinical and Laboratory Findings in Obstruction in the Upper Gastro-intestinal Tract, Am. Jour. Med. Sci., 1925, 169, 224.

MOYNIHAN, B. G.: Duodenal Ulcer, 2d ed., Philadelphia, 1912.

MURRAY, H. A., JR.: The Chemical Pathology of Pyloric Occlusion in Relation to Tetany, Arch. Surg., 1923, 7, 166.

SMITH, F. M.: Studies on the Mechanism of Pain of Peptic Ulcer, Ann. Int. Med., 1931, 5, 14.

CANCER OF THE STOMACH.

General Considerations.—Cancer of the stomach, one of the most dreaded and intractable of neoplastic diseases, is responsible for a large percentage, perhaps 30 to 40 per cent, of all cancer deaths. In gastric pathology it ranks next only to ulcer in importance and frequency. Males are more often affected than females in the proportion of about 3 to 1. Most of the victims are over forty years of age, but cases as early as the third decade are not extremely uncommon. There has been a great deal of discussion as to what factors predispose to and precipitate the development of cancer in the stomach; the weight of evidence points to chronic gastritis as the usual antecedent lesion and Konjetzny has actually demonstrated transitional changes.

Whether indiscreet eating, trauma and alcohol contribute is doubtful. The relation of cancer of the stomach to ulcer has already been discussed. The question of pathogenesis is most important in view of the possible development of preventive measures. For full discussion the reader is referred to the papers of Hurst and of Polland and Bloomfield.

Pathology.—The picture is varied. The majority of the growths are adenocarcinomata. There are infiltrating scirrhus types which on section look almost like cartilage. They may be of great extent but often are confined to the pyloric region. The pylorus is sometimes occluded or it may be held rigidly open as a result of infiltration of its wall. With other forms necrotic fungating masses are found. An interesting and unusual variety is the gelatinous or colloid cancer which invades great areas of the stomach wall. In rare cases the growth takes the form of a pedunculated polypoid mass which may attain the size of a lemon and sometimes becomes engaged in the pylorus. Ulceration can develop in any cancer of the stomach and perforation occasionally takes place. In about one-half of all the cases the growth is near the pylorus. In Ophüls' Stanford series of 97 cases, 54 were in the pyloric region, 17 at the lesser curvature, 5 in the fundus, 2 at the greater curvature and 1 in the anterior wall. The stomach was diffusely diseased in 12 cases, in 7 of which the growth was a scirrhus and in 5 of a more fungating character. In 77 cases the occurrence and distribution of metastases or extensions was as follows: liver, 31; peritoneum, 19; pancreas, 19; pleura, 8; adrenal, 7; diaphragm, 6; lung, 6; large bowel, 6; spleen, 5; kidney, 4; small intestine, 4; esophagus, 4; gall-bladder, 3; rectum, 3; bone, 2; duodenum, 2; ovary, 1; appendix, 1; lymph glands, 47, including regional, 21; retroperitoneal, 20; mesenteric, 12; mediastinal, 10; peribronchial, 7; liver hilum, 7; splenic, 5; cardiac, 5; supraclavicular, 2, and inguinal, iliac, cervical and aortic, 1 each. The distribution of metastases is especially important because of its clinical bearing on diagnosis and prognosis.

Symptoms.—It is useless to attempt any composite description of the symptoms of cancer of the stomach so variable are they in different cases. The disease may be entirely latent for long periods, perhaps years, and the first clinical manifestations appear when the roentgenray already reveals a tremendous growth. In other cases there are no local evidences of trouble but fatigue, anemia, wasting or fever bring the patient to the physician. Symptoms from metastases, especially to the liver, may entirely outweigh the local evidences of disease. As regards the gastric disturbances, loss of appetite, distress after eating, epigastric pain, nausea, vomiting, feelings of fullness, gas or "indigestion" occur in every possible combination. If the pylorus is narrowed by cancer the symptoms are those which have already been described in connection with obstruction from ulcer. If ulceration of the cancerous lesion or actual perforation with abscess formation takes place the case may present the evidences of septic infection or of intra-abdominal inflammation.

Physical Examination.—The primary growth is itself inaccessible to physical examination and the findings are those resulting from metastases and from the general intoxication of the disease. In advanced cases there are emaciation and pallor. If the growth extends through the stomach wall the omentum, seeded with cancer, becomes adherent over the lesion and one may feel the nodular, stony hard, transverse mass in the epigastrium so characteristic of cancer of the stomach. Nodules may be felt in the liver, which assumes great proportions as the cancerous lumps increase in size. Various abdominal masses usually due to infiltrations of the omentum are often felt and there may be ascitic accumulations in which cancer cells can occasionally be demonstrated. The fluid is usually clear but it may be bloody, or in the rare types of colloid cancer it has a curious gelatinous consistency. Metastases to the portal fissure can lead to jaundice and the enlargement of lymphatic nodes above the left clavicle due to seeding out of cancer cells *via* the thoracic duct is occasionally observed. Not infrequently nodules can be felt on rectal examination in the cul-de-sac between the rectum and bladder.

Laboratory Examinations.—Anemia is usually present. It is often extreme and the hemoglobin may fall to 20 per cent or less. This is especially so if the growth is ulcerated or if much blood is lost. Occasionally the blood picture may resemble that of pernicious anemia. The stools usually show occult blood if repeated examinations are made. Gastric analysis is especially helpful because of the frequent occurrence of anacidity. As a rule one recovers only a few cubic centimeters of mucoid material, sometimes mixed with blood or pus. In a minority of cases the juice may appear normal and some acid is present. The author has seen no instance, however, except those arising on a basis of ulcer, in which the volume of secretion and the acidity were both materially greater than the average normal values. Hence, in a doubtful case such findings are very much against the presence of cancer. On the other hand, low acid or absence of acid, while compatible with cancer, does not prove its presence, as these findings may occur in other conditions (gastritis, unexplained anacidity).

Roentgen-rays are of special value. Only very occasionally does a stomach, the seat of cancer, fail to show radiologic abnormalities, and in many cases the finding of annular lesions at the pylorus or irregular defects in the body of the stomach is practically diagnostic. However, roentgen-ray diagnosis is not absolute and mistakes may be made, especially in differentiating cancer from ulcer at the pylorus with scarring. The findings are always to be considered together with those of gastric analysis, as well as with the clinical features of the case.

Diagnosis.—Cancer of the stomach is to be considered *in every instance of digestive disorder in people over thirty-five years of age*. Occurrence of stomach symptoms in a person previously free of indigestion, especially if there is any general failure, weakness and pallor should strongly raise one's suspicions. If a mass can be felt or if metastases can be identified this suspicion is fortified, but gastric analysis and roentgen-ray are usually necessary to make the diagnosis final. The disease is especially to be differentiated from chronic peptic ulcer as well as from rare conditions such as lymphoblastoma and, perhaps, syphilis.

Treatment.—Medical treatment of cancer of the stomach is symptomatic and palliative. A simple diet must be worked out to best suit the symptoms of the particular case; aside from this, increasing restriction of activity and sedatives (barbital or, if necessary, morphine) for relief of pain as the disease advances are in order. Roentgen-ray therapy up to the present time has been ineffective. Surgery offers in theory the possibility of a cure by complete extirpation of the growth. In practice, however, even "early" operation is followed after a time by recurrences. What appears to be an "early" case from the standpoint of recent onset of symptoms, good general condition, absence of demonstrable metastases, and small local growth is none the less "late" in the sense that ineradicable metastases have already occurred. The writer has seen only one definite instance of surgical cure of cancer of the stomach. However, if the patient's condition allows and if the growth is not too large or too widely disseminated operation is distinctly indicated, since the patient often is rendered symptom-free for one or two years or occasionally longer before recurrence takes place. If the growth has occluded the pylorus such obstruction should, of course, be relieved by excision or gastro-enterostomy. Some writers advocate the surgical exploration and extirpation of all gastric ulcers because of the possibility of their being malignant and not benign. We are not prepared to favor an absolute rule of this sort, but it is the duty of the physician *to regard every ulcer with suspicion until prompt and intensive study followed, if necessary, by careful watching has convinced him of its innocence.*

ILLUSTRATIVE CASE—CANCER OF THE STOMACH.

Mrs. H. L. J., aged forty-four years.
Complaint.—"Can not eat anything solid."
Family History and Past History.—Unimportant.
Present Illness.—She never had any stomach trouble until six months ago. She then developed a feeling of a lump in the epigastrium on eating. This was followed by sensations of "gas" and finally by pain and tenderness in the pit of the stomach. At present she can eat practically nothing without having distress, and she thinks she would vomit if she ate more. No appetite. Slight nausea. She has lost 40 pounds and has become very weak.
Examination.—She looked thin, worn and very pale. The tongue was heavily coated. The heart was rapid, but otherwise normal. The abdomen was slightly distended and in the epigastrium one could feel a huge, transverse, stony-hard, irregular mass. The liver was not felt.
Laboratory Tests.—Red blood cells, 2,300,000; hemoglobin, 37 per cent; white blood cells, 11,000. Gastric analysis not done.
Roentgen-rays showed a huge irregular lesion which had reduced the upper two-thirds of the lumen of the stomach to a narrow channel.
Course.—She failed rapidly and died within a few days. Autopsy showed an extensive sloughing cancer involving the entire body of the stomach.
Comment.—This is the "classical" case of cancer of the stomach with emaciation, anemia, abdominal pain and epigastric mass. This picture is essentially that of the advanced, completely hopeless stages of the disease.

ILLUSTRATIVE CASE—CANCER OF THE STOMACH (PYLORIC OBSTRUCTION).

J. C., carpenter, aged thirty-seven years.
Complaint.—"Stomach trouble."
Family History and Past History.—Unimportant.

Present Illness.—Four months before entry he noticed a "gnawing feeling" about the umbilicus. The discomfort came on at any time without relation to meals. It was present for a few days at a time, with free intervals of from one to two weeks. Recently there had been occasional vomiting of moderate amounts of "sour" liquid containing food particles. He had lost 20 pounds in the past year.

Physical Examination.—He appeared well nourished and there were no evidences of cachexia. There were no striking physical abnormalities except a soft prominence in the epigastrium across which large peristaltic waves moved from left to right. There were no physical signs of metastases.

Laboratory Tests.—Red blood cells, 4,800,000; hemoglobin, 90 per cent; white blood cells, 9000. Urine, negative. Stool, negative. Vomitus: large amount of thin fluid (HCl, 0) with undigested food particles. Gastric analysis (histamine): free HCl, 0. Highest volume 10.5 cc. mucoid material.

Roentgen-rays showed a very large stomach with occasional vigorous peristaltic waves. After twenty-four hours most of the barium was still in the stomach (Fig. 32).

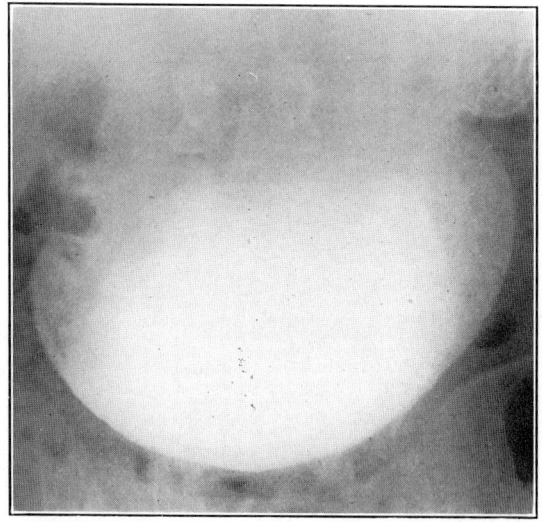

Fig. 32.—Cancer of the stomach—pyloric obstruction. Note huge dilated stomach with deformity of the pylorus.

Comment.—The brief duration of symptoms is of interest, as are the typical findings of pyloric obstruction, which are quite similar to those previously described with ulcer. The character of the gastric secretion, however, pointed strongly to cancer.

Operation.—At operation a small annular adenocarcinoma was found at the pylorus. The lesion and adjacent glands were excised.

Course.—He remained entirely well for two years. He then began to lose weight and developed cramp-like pain in the umbilical region with occasional vomiting. Physical examination was negative except for visible peristalsis in the epigastrium. No masses were felt on abdominal examination, there was no anemia and no occult blood in the stools. However, rectal examination revealed a definite nodular mass above the prostate (rectal shelf). On exploration a huge recurrent growth was found. The case illustrates the difficulty of curing cancer of the stomach even when the growth is small and circumscribed.

ILLUSTRATIVE CASE—CANCER OF THE STOMACH (PERFORATION, SEPSIS).

W. T., farmer, aged sixty-three years.
Complaint.—Soreness in stomach.

Family History.—Unimportant.

Past History.—There is nothing which bears on present trouble.

Present Illness.—For ten years has had attacks of "gas on the stomach." This usually comes on about one and a half hours after meals, without actual pain. Various medicines have given no relief. About four weeks ago an entirely different set of symptoms appeared featured by a dull boring pain in the epigastrium coming in attacks and sometimes relieved by food. He has lost weight and strength rapidly and has been confined to bed for two weeks. There has been no vomiting.

Physical Examination.—Very thin. Looks worn and ill. In the upper abdomen there is a slight fullness, and on palpation one feels a large, hard, irregular, transverse mass which descends on inspiration. The liver edge is palpable; it is firm and irregular. Rectal examination negative.

Laboratory Tests.—Red blood cells, 2,800,000; hemoglobin, 48 per cent; white blood cells, 6200. Stool, negative. Gastric analysis (histamine); only a few cubic centimeters of mucoid material; free HCl, 0.

Roentgen-rays.—There is a huge irregular filling defect involving practically the entire antral portion of the stomach. There is no evidence of pyloric obstruction (Fig. 33).

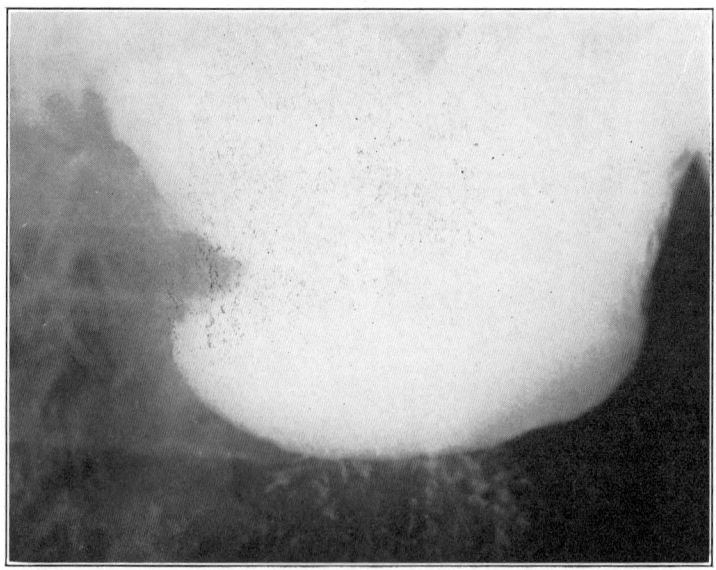

Fig. 33.—Cancer of the stomach. Note huge lesion of antrum without pyloric obstruction.

Course.—There was high irregular fever (up to 40.5° C.) with occasional chills. He failed rapidly and developed extreme tenderness in the epigastrium over the mass. A few hard nodules appeared in the skin near the umbilicus. Death occurred three weeks after entry with the picture of a septic infection.

Autopsy.—There were well marked adhesions between the pylorus and the liver and transverse colon. On separating these a large perforation into the stomach was found which communicated with an abscess cavity in the left lobe of the liver. The pyloric region of the stomach was extensively infiltrated with gelatinous tumor tissue. The inner surface was markedly ulcerated. Metastases were found in pancreas, liver and regional lymph nodes.

Comment.—The outstanding features are the perforation of the cancer with consequent abscess in the liver and the general picture of a septic infection. The story of the digestive symptoms illustrates well how non-specific they may be; certainly the history alone was not typical of any particular condition.

REFERENCES.

Ewing, James: Neoplastic Diseases, 3d ed., Philadelphia, 1928.
Hurst, A. F.: The Precursors of Cancer of the Stomach, Lancet, 1929, ii, 1023.
Osler, Wm., and McCrae, Thomas: Cancer of the Stomach, Modern Medicine, Philadelphia, 1900.
Polland, W. S., and Bloomfield, A. L.: Gastric Secretion in Cancer of the Stomach, Bull. Johns Hopkins Hosp., 1930, **46**, 307.
Smithies, Frank and Ochsner, A. J.: Cancer of the Stomach, Philadelphia, 1916.

OTHER TUMORS OF THE STOMACH.

Benign tumors are very rare. Fibroma, lipoma, myoma, lymphangioma, neurofibroma and others have been described. They are pathologic curiosities of little clinical importance, as are the rare myosarcomata, round cell, mixed and angiosarcomata. Under the heading of tumor one should probably mention *gastric polyposis*, although on occasion polypoid lesions may result from chronic gastritis. The polyps may be multiple (diffuse polyposis) or single; they usually cause no symptoms. Of clinical importance is the fact that they may bleed, that cancerous changes may supervene and that pedunculated polyps near the pylorus can prolapse into the canal and produce obstruction. The roentgen pictures may be characteristic and diagnosis is sometimes made before operation.

Lymphoblastoma (lymphosarcoma) is occasionally encountered. It may occur as the predominating lesion or it may be an incident in a generalized lymphosarcomatosis. The stomach itself is infiltrated to a variable extent; sometimes the lesion is very extensive and secondary ulcerations with hemorrhage may occur. The symptoms are not characteristic, but any of the types of referred discomfort from the stomach may be present. Diagnosis is suggested by the roentgenráy appearance which shows extensive and anomalous filling defects or by the discovery of other evidences of lymphoblastoma. In the 3 cases which we have seen the gastric acidity was within normal limits. Brilliant, if temporary, results may follow radiation.

REFERENCE.

For systematic discussion of tumors of the stomach other than cancer (with extensive bibliography) see article by Borrmann in Henke-Lubarsch: Handbuch, etc., 1926, **4**, Pt. I, 812.

SYPHILIS OF THE STOMACH.

In very rare cases syphilis seems to produce gastric lesions. The condition is certainly not nearly as frequent as one would be led to believe from the literature and in most of the reported series the criteria used for diagnosis are obviously inadequate. The writer has personally never seen a convincing case. There are a few instances on record in which spirochetes have been demonstrated in gummatous or cicatricial lesions. The diagnosis has usually been made on a basis of positive history or Wassermann test together with digestive symptoms and radiologic demonstration of filling defects or deformities. There is said to be an absence of gastric acid. Stress has been placed on the improvement of symptoms or the disappearance of roentgen-ray changes after antiluetic therapy. The writer feels that nothing short of the demonstration of spirochetes justifies the diagnosis.

REFERENCE.

For critical discussion of syphilis of stomach with extensive bibliography see Henke-Lubarsch: Handbuch, etc., 1928, **4**, Pt. II, 1015.

DEFORMITIES, DISPLACEMENTS AND ANOMALIES OF THE STOMACH.

Congenital malformations are rare. The most important, if it may correctly be classed with them, is the *congenital hypertrophic stenosis of the pylorus* of infants. Part or all of the stomach may enter the thorax through a *hernia* or an *eventration of the diaphragm*. There are usually no direct symptoms. *Diverticula* of the stomach are to be mentioned to contrast their rarity with the much greater frequency of such lesions in the intestine, especially the colon. *Foreign bodies* of every variety and description may be swallowed, including hair, nails and glass. They may become aggregated into large masses which eventually form a cast of the stomach; the subjects are usually mildly psychopathic. Symptoms, if present, are said to include fullness, pressure, pain and vomiting. Successful surgical removal has been practised in some cases.

Hour-glass stomach is not a definite entity. It is doubtful, according to Aschoff, whether a true congenital form exists, and the appearance is the result of scarring by inflammation or neoplasm. External adhesions to other viscera are usually associated. There is no specific symptomatology.

Ptosis, formerly much stressed in medical literature, is now known to be of little if any clinical importance. The demonstration, especially by roentgen studies, of the wide variations in shape and position of the stomach which occur in healthy people without symptoms have forced the conclusion that the symptoms which used to be blamed on "dropping of the stomach" were due to other things.

THE INTESTINE.

Introduction.—Disorders of the intestine, like those of the stomach, present a difficult problem from the standpoint of classification and discussion, and here again confusion arises through the fact that most of the conditions to be considered are not mutually exclusive. There are, on the one hand, definite anatomic lesions such as cancer and tuberculosis, and on the other, vaguer or more widespread disorders such as constipation, diarrhea or the intestinal neuroses. The two groups are usually combined, and while constipation or diarrhea may occur as isolated functional disturbances of a bowel which is anatomically intact, they are also to be expected with cancer or with dysenteries of various sorts, and intestinal obstruction, even though it is in a sense a definite entity, usually is incidental to, or the result of, some underlying anatomic disturbance such as a growth. In brief, as with the stomach, the variety of intestinal symptoms is limited and regardless of the underlying lesion, if such exists at all, constipation, diarrhea, pain or obstructive symptoms are the usual modes of expression. Final diagnosis, therefore, often depends on special studies of the stools (mucus, pus, blood, amebas, parasites, bacteriologic studies) or on the findings of the roentgen-ray, proctoscopy, or even exploratory operation.

The physician should follow a regular procedure: history and physical examination first; stool examination, only too often neglected, next; and proctoscopy and roentgen-ray study last. As a rule, attempts at hasty diagnosis are futile and the case must be carefully worked out. It is necessary, however, to keep in mind the important surgical emergencies: namely, acute appendicitis and acute intestinal obstruction. Here prompt action is essential in order that life may be saved and diagnosis must be made from the history and physical examination, together with such simple aids as the temperature and pulse curves and the leukocyte count.

In the following sections there will be discussed first what is by far the most common group of intestinal disorders, namely, the bowel neuroses. The symptoms include those which may also occur with serious organic disease and only after due consideration should the diagnosis be made. Next it seems advisable to take up the major "intestinal syndromes" of constipation, diarrhea and obstruction, recognizing that they are not specific diseases but only symptom-complexes resulting from a variety of fundamental disorders. Finally, the organic diseases—inflammations, tumors and anomalies, will be described and here again there will be some necessary overlapping with what has already been discussed.

Detailed consideration of the so-called "intestinal indigestions" and of "intestinal putrefaction" and "stasis" has been intentionally omitted. These alleged disorders are too indefinite both in their pathology and in their clinical manifestations to enable one to make any very sound representations for them; much of what has been said about them by others falls, we believe, more properly under the heading of the intestinal neuroses. The finer bacteriology of the intestine in relation to local or systemic disorders undoubtedly offers a field for important study. Up to the present, however, such conclusions as have been drawn about "intestinal intoxications" as well as the therapy which has been advised, including colonic irrigations, vaccines and attempts to alter the intestinal flora, fall, for the most part, in that shadowy borderland of practice which had better be avoided by conservative physicians.

INTESTINAL NEUROSES.

General Considerations.—Just as the majority of patients with indigestion have no organic disease of the stomach so there exists a large group of people with bowel symptoms which arise on a purely

40

functional basis. Very often gastric and intestinal symptoms coëxist in the same patient and their mechanism is essentially similar; indeed, the general considerations which were discussed in detail under indigestion apply with equal force to the intestinal neuroses and they need not be reiterated now.

Classification of the intestinal neuroses is difficult and there has been much confusion in the literature. However, under this general heading there fall the so-called "intestinal indigestion," unexplained capricious bowel irregularities and the syndrome of "mucous colitis" or "irritable bowel."

Symptoms.—The subjects of intestinal neuroses are likely to be of the high-strung, nervous introspective type and often there are neurotic symptoms referable not only to the bowel but to other domains as well. In some cases there is simply a vague abdominal discomfort with intestinal gas and mild bowel irregularity; these patients have been spoken of as "colon conscious." In other instances there are more severe discomforts often localized in some definite area such as the right upper or left lower quadrant or there may actually be attacks of colic. In classical cases of mucous colitis large lumps of mucus or casts of the bowel wall are passed in connection with attacks of pain (colic) but as a rule some mucus may be found in the movement at any time. Irregularity of the bowel is the rule, and while constipation predominates, there are sudden and violent attacks of diarrhea which may cease just as abruptly as they begin. It is not uncommon to have a fluid movement followed within a few hours by a constipated stool, with diarrhea again a few hours later. Obvious nervous influences may determine the character of the movement and any excitement is likely to be followed immediately by diarrhea. Sooner or later the patient begins to rationalize about his trouble and to blame it on one thing or another—certain articles of food, a past illness or injury, perhaps an operation or the finding of intestinal parasites. As the years go by he becomes more and more convinced that serious trouble exists and, as a rule, makes the rounds of the "colon cultists." Possibly a surgical operation or two has been done to relieve "dropping of the colon" or to mobilize his cecum. Despite all this his appetite and nutrition usually are preserved, and unhappy and worried as he may be about his interior workings he is likely to outlive his less harassed friends and relatives.

As with indigestion the immediate mechanism of symptoms is an abnormality of bowel motility, failure of proper coördination combined with spasm. This may be precipitated by local lesions or by irritation or inflammation of the bowel, or it may occur reflexly in association with various abdominal lesions. However, the vast majority of these patients have no demonstrable disease and their difficulties are of nervous origin.

Physical Examination.—The physical findings are not diagnostic, and it is obvious that all sorts of abnormalities may be found which have nothing to do with the chief symptoms. On abdominal examination localized areas of tenderness are frequently made out, especially in the lower quadrants or in the right upper quadrant. Sometimes there is general abdominal sensitiveness. But while the patient complains bitterly as the abdomen is manipulated there is no objective muscle spasm or resistance such as one gets with real inflammation. At times areas of spastic bowel may be rolled under the fingers; this finding usually varies from day to day. Fever is absent.

Roentgen-rays.—Roentgen examination usually shows a marked exaggeration of the colonic haustra—the so-called spastic colon of the radiologist. Occasionally a smoothing out of bowel outline is seen, although this is more characteristic of true colitis. Variations in length and position of the colon, in the size of the cecum and in the speed of emptying of bowel are described, but they occur no more strikingly than in people who have no symptoms and doubtless have little or no clinical meaning.

Laboratory Tests.—The most important findings are in the stools. A series of specimens should be examined to get the complete picture. Some of the movements are loose or even watery, others consist of small hard lumps of fecal material which have evidently been molded in the spastic bowel haustra, or there may be mixtures of hard lumps and fluid material. Mucus may be present in small particles or larger sheets or casts. The latter finding is rare. There are no special evidences of failure of digestion and *blood and pus are never present.*

Diagnosis.—No group of patients is more universally misdiagnosed and mistreated and most of the unfortunates who have been told they have "colitis" have a neurosis without any real organic disease. Every medical student should read in Axel Munthe's "Story of San Michele" the amusing but unfortunately true exposé of the colitis "racket." Others have their symptoms blamed on the shape or position of their colon, on cecal stasis, or mobile cecum, on the character of the intestinal flora, on a misplaced uterus or a chronic prostatitis, on a "chronic appendix" or a "gall-bladder" or on what they eat. It is true that things of this sort may, on occasion, disturb bowel function and lead to symptoms; there is an "honest trifle" there, but as a rule it "betrays us in deepest consequence" unless the whole picture is carefully surveyed. No attempt should be made to make a final diagnosis without prolonged study of the entire individual from the physical, mental and social standpoints. The problem is the same as with indigestion and the reader is referred again to that section. The main points which lead to a correct diagnosis, however, are (1) symptoms of long standing; (2) disproportion between severity of the patient's complaints and his general physical condition (good nutrition, absence of anemia, and fever); (3) characteristic type of bowel irregularity; (4) absence of blood and pus in the stools; (5) absence of evidence of organic disease of bowel, and (6) presence of other evidences of a neurotic make-up.

Treatment.—Successful treatment depends first and foremost on making certain whether the symptoms depend upon some definite organic disease or whether they are neurotic in origin. Great judgment must be exercised by the physician in reaching his final conclusion, since so often slight organic abnormalities may be found which are not necessarily responsible for the symptoms. No rules can be laid down. However, if one is convinced that a diseased appendix or a uterine malposition, for example, is the source of irritation this should be dealt with by proper methods, surgical or otherwise. On the other hand, if the case is to be treated along the lines of a neurosis it is essential not only to convince the patient of the absence of organic disease but the physician must be certain of this in his own mind in order to maintain his confidence. The situation must be explained over and over again to the patient and the most tactful medical "salesmanship" is often needed to convince a person who for years, perhaps, has cherished the idea of serious disease that there is really no organic lesion of his bowel. In brief, the ghost must be laid and nothing can be done unless complete understanding and coöperation exist. Never suggest that the symptoms are imaginary, they are only too real; emphasize the fact that things are deranged but not diseased.

In regard to general management of the case the reader is referred once more to the article on Indigestion. The principles are identical and include sensible regulation of activity, elimination of hurry and stress, and the solution of adjustment problems. With regard to diet, here again it is better, if possible, to get the patient's mind away from the workings of his intestinal tract. Once convinced that no real bowel disease is present a moderate general diet should be advised, from which it is necessary to eliminate only such articles as genuinely seem to upset the patient. We have time and again placed patients who, for years, had eaten only puréed or other forms of limited diet on full meals which to their surprise and pleasure go perfectly well, provided they are not afraid of them. An occasional patient insists on a diet list but this is to be avoided if possible. The meals should be light and they should be eaten slowly and chewed well. It should be pointed out that the bowel irregularity is of no serious significance and that it can to some extent be ignored. The regulation of constipation will be discussed in a subsequent article. Mild physical therapeutic measures such as warm baths before going to bed or general massage two or three times a week are helpful. Simple general sedatives may be given, such as a mixture of tincture of hyoscyamus and sodium bromide, or belladonna may be tried. On the whole, the less stress placed on medicine the better.

It should be recalled that the disorder is essentially the expression of a certain type of nervous organization; it is constitutional. Hence, improvement is usually gradual; complete cure is unlikely and relapses of symptoms are frequent. The physician must be prepared for "slumps" and the patient must be forewarned so as not to be disappointed. In really stubborn cases the treatment must be started along the lines of a formal rest cure, perhaps with isolation in a hospital, and the coöperation of a good psychiatrist, if one can be found, can be invoked to great advantage.

CONSTIPATION.

General Considerations.—Constipation is, perhaps, the most universal of all human complaints, and relatively few people, at least from middle life on, have an entirely unconscious and satisfactory bowel habit. Just where the borderline lies between the normal and the pathologic in this respect it is often difficult to say. Certainly if artificial methods of producing a bowel movement have to be resorted to and if the patient feels uncomfortable the condition demands clinical consideration.

Etiology.—Constipation may result from serious organic disease, such as adhesions or obstruction of the bowel from growth. In certain rare cases radical difficulties with the autonomic innervation of the intestine seem to lead to a form of paralysis with stasis, dilation of the colon and infrequent bowel movements (*Hirschsprung's disease*). As a rule, however, there is no serious anatomic lesion and the difficulty is the result of a combination of circumstances—irregular habits of going to stool, lack of exercise, obesity, inadequate diet or nervous disturbances. Attempts have been made to divide the cases into such groups as "spastic" and "atonic" constipation but in our experience this is not very feasible and serves no special purpose.

From the standpoint of pathologic physiology there seems to be an inhibition of, or an interference with, the normal defecation reflex which includes a rush of material from the lower colon into the rectum, together with coördinated relaxation of the rectal sphincters and contraction of the abdominal press.

Symptoms.—The most usual symptom is failure of the bowels to move spontaneously at normal intervals (once or twice daily) together with mild discomforts which are relieved when the bowels do move. These discomforts include fullness and pressure in the rectum or lower abdomen, lack of appetite, headache or general sensations of dullness, mental and physical. There is a very wide variation in the symptomatic reaction of the individual patient. Some people may regularly go several days without a movement and still feel perfectly well; others are miserable and unhappy all day if for any reason the morning evacuation is interfered with.

Just what the remote effects of constipation may be it is hard to say. Every manifestation of ill health has been blamed on the disorder and some go so far as to visualize the actual absorptions of toxic materials which have stagnated in the bowel, in which case such designations as intestinal auto-intoxication, or intestinal toxemia, have been applied. These syndromes are, however, too indefinite to allow any conclusive statements to be made and certainly one must be skeptical when he knows that many people are quite well despite a bowel movement only every few days or even longer. The immediate relief of symptoms which often follows an evacuation suggests rather a reflex basis for most of the discomforts of constipation. The stools may be constipated as to time, that is to say the movements are infrequent, or they may be constipated in quality—the individual movement is hard and is produced with difficulty.

Physical Examination.—As a rule this reveals nothing bearing directly on the symptoms. Attempts have been made to link constipation with certain body types, especially the feminine type with wide hips and narrow chest, flabby abdominal wall and dependent bowel and viscera in general. The correlation is not definite enough, however, to be diagnostic and it must be recalled that material passes through the bowel in any case by peristalsis and not by gravity. On the whole, well proportioned, physically fit people are less likely to be constipated, but this is by no means an invariable rule. Coils of spastic bowel may occasionally be felt; sometimes actual fecal masses are evident. In Hirschsprung's disease there may be obvious abdominal distention but it is remarkable how great an accumulation of material can collect in the bowel without external evidence. The examiner should always be on the lookout for signs of organic disease which may have a bearing on constipation, such as carcinomatous masses.

Laboratory Examinations.—The feces should be examined with care in order to rule out evidences of inflammation, blood and pus, and to make sure that the food has been properly digested. It is useful also to know if the fecal material is hard and inspissated or if its consistency is normal.

Roentgen-rays.—Roentgen-rays are especially helpful in revealing evidence of stricture, growth or dilatation. Minor deviations from the normal such as cecal stasis or ptosis must be carefully evaluated before concluding that they are of importance since they are found in so many people whose bowels are regular. It is remarkable that many constipated people pass the barium meal through to the rectum in normal time; their difficulty evidently lies with the mechanism of evacuation. Barium enemata are especially useful in ruling out tumors and strictures.

Treatment.—Assuming that organic narrowings and obstructions have been ruled out, treatment is directed toward promoting regular evacuations by cultivating proper bowel habits, by keeping the feces of normal consistency and by relaxing spasm. The patient's habits, diet and nervous and general make-up must be carefully considered. In order to habituate the bowel to regular defecation the patient must be urged to put aside fifteen to twenty minutes every morning, preferably after breakfast, when he will try to have a movement and to let nothing interfere with this routine. Hurry or excitement, as every one knows, is likely to inhibit the evacuation. The establishment of this regular routine is all-important and desire to defecate at other times should be suppressed because there will then be inadequate bowel content to stimulate the movement at the regular time. Habit formation should be supplemented by adding to the diet coarse breads and cereals, coarse vegetables such as spinach, cabbage, celery, turnips, carrots and corn, and plenty of fruit. Prunes, dates, figs and honey are mildly laxative. A glass of cold water on rising may stimulate the bowel. Exercise in general helps and gentle massage of the abdomen may promote the movement. With some people tobacco acts almost as a specific in stimulating peristalsis. If these simple measures do not suffice some mild laxative must be used. Mineral oil morning and evening in doses of a dessertspoonful to a tablespoonful is harmless for continuous use. If too much is taken the oil may irritate and run through the bowel without exerting its proper effect, namely, to keep the feces soft. Agar-agar may be combined with the oil; it acts by retaining water and making the feces soft and bulky. Some people obtain satisfactory results from bran or psyllium seed. Cathartics are to be avoided, if possible, but it must be admitted that many patients solve the problem by a mild laxative which they take day in and day out for years without apparent harm. Favorites are the various mineral waters or salines such as citrate of magnesia or effervescent phosphate of soda, to be taken early in the morning, or cascara (aromatic syrup of cascara, 2 to 8 cc.), aloes (compound laxative pill, 1 or 2) or phenolphthalein (0.03 to 0.2 gram) taken at night. Hundreds of other preparations are in use; we cannot attempt to catalogue them all. With cathartics "one man's food is another man's poison" and often several preparations must be tried before the one which suits the individual patient is found. Enemas are rarely necessary and once dependent upon them the habit is a hard one to break. However, in cases where only a slight stimulus is necessary to set the evacuation reflexes in motion an occasional small injection of water or soap suds or a glycerin suppository is harmless. Habitual "colonic irrigations" or "flushes" are to be decried. The unfortunates who get the idea that their comfort and health depend upon such unnatural manipulations reflect no credit on the physician who has initiated them into these mysteries, and in the end they are likely to require the services of a psychiatrist.

Fecal impactions may occur in people confined to bed for long periods of time or neglectful of their bowel habits. Rectal injections of olive oil (100 to 200 cc.) retained over night, enemata, oil by mouth and saline purges (Epsom salts 30 to 60 cc.) may be tried, but often manual removal of the impacted mass is necessary, perhaps under an anesthetic.

Hirschsprung's disease (idiopathic dilatation of the colon, megacolon) is a congenital disorder featured by obstinate constipation and great dilatation of the colon. The bowel may have a capacity of 3 to 4 or more liters and spontaneous movements if they occur at all are achieved at intervals of as much as several weeks. Sooner or later the general health suffers and most of the children are weak and retarded. Occasionally no symptoms occur until adult life. In outspoken cases the physical signs are striking: the belly is greatly distended, especially in its upper portion, which encroaches on the thoracic cage and the huge bowel may be visualized as it presses against the abdominal wall. The exact cause of the disorder is not clear and the student is referred to the special literature for discussion of the question. Irrigations and purges may be tried. Recently good results have been reported from lumbar sympathetic ganglionectomy, the operation being performed on the theory that the disorder is due to inhibition of colonic tone and motility as a result of sympathetic overstimulation. Excision of the colon has not been found satisfactory.

DIARRHEA.

Diarrhea is one of the commonest manifestations of intestinal disorders. It must be remembered, however, that it is only a *symptom* and not a disease in itself, and logically it should be discussed with the various conditions under which it occurs. But, for purposes of convenience, a general summary will be presented now so that repetition later will not be necessary. The term is used to describe any abnormal looseness of the bowel movement; as a rule the movements are frequent as well as of abnormal consistency.

Diarrhea occurs under a great variety of conditions. There may be local or diffuse lesions (inflammations, tumors, etc.) of any part of the intestinal tract, or without actual disease looseness of the bowels may result from nervous influences or from the indirect effects of remote disorders. The following outline gives some idea of the principal conditions with which diarrhea may be associated.

ACUTE DIARRHEA:

Infectious:
> Bacillary dysentery.
> Amebic dysentery.
> Typhoid fever.
> Cholera.
> Acute ulcerative colitis.
> Food poisoning diarrheas:
>> Paratyphoid.
>> Enteritidis.
> Intestinal parasites (trichinæ).

Non-infectious:
> Arsenic poisoning.
> Bichloride poisoning.
> Uremia.

CHRONIC DIARRHEA:

Infectious:
> Ulcerative colitis.
> Bacillary dysentery.
> Amebic dysentery.
> Tuberculous enteritis.
> Parasites.

Non-infectious:
> Amyloid disease.
> Pernicious anemia.
> Sprue.
> Leukemia.
> Addison's disease.
> Pancreatic disease.
> Cancer of the bowel.
> Hyperthyroidism.
> Chronic passive congestion of the bowel.
>> Heart disease.
>> Cirrhosis of the liver.
> Nervous diarrheas.

The list is not complete and some of the items may be incorrectly classified; however, the student will be impressed by the great variety of the mechanisms which may lead to looseness of the bowels.

Symptoms.—If the small bowel is especially affected the movements are likely to be less frequent than with a true colitis. Most of the serious chronic diarrheas are associated with trouble in the colon or sigmoid such as the various dysenteries. Abdominal discomfort of varying degrees of severity is the most frequent symptom; with an acute colitis there may be violent cramp-like pains referred for the most part to the mid- or lower abdomen, and when the rectum is involved tenesmus, a painful spasmodic or burning sensation in the anal region, occurs. In severe cases as many as twenty or more movements occur in twenty-four hours. The degree of weakness and prostration depends upon the severity and duration of the trouble, the amount of fluid which is lost (as in cholera), the patient's ability to keep up his nutrition and the toxic effects of the underlying disease or infection. The temperature is elevated in infectious cases.

One of the most frequent forms of diarrhea is that associated with a simple "intestinal upset." Usually out of a clear sky and without any obvious cause the patient is taken with loose bowels, mild cramps and perhaps nausea and vomiting. Some attempt is usually made to relate the trouble to a dietary indiscretion or to spoiled food but, as a rule, the effort is barren. The movements are watery but show no evidences of true inflammation (blood or pus). The condition clears up in a few days on rest and simple diet (see below).

Physical Examination.—Evidences of any associated or underlying disease such as pernicious anemia, hyperthyroidism or typhoid fever should be looked for. With mild diarrhea little is made out on physical examination. In severe or long-standing cases there is often abdominal tenderness and loops of spastic or thickened bowel can be felt. The general signs of wear and tear develop, and emaciation, desiccation of the tissues, prostration and pallor all may become evident. Proctoscopy, by means of which the rectum and part of the sigmoid can be inspected, discloses to the eye the character of ulcerations or inflammation and gives a clue to the appearance of the bowel higher up.

Laboratory Tests.—The character of the stool depends upon the underlying condition. Symptomatic diarrheas show no evidences of inflammation (blood or pus) and the movements are simply soft or liquid. Partly undigested food which has been hurried through the intestinal tract may be evident as in pancreatic disease. With true inflammations such as amebic dysentery or ulcerative colitis blood and pus are characteristic findings. In extreme cases little actual fecal material is present and the passages consist of small amounts of mucoid purulent material with more or less admixture of blood. Parasites (amebas) may be found. The blood count depends on the underlying infection or lesion. Eosinophilia may occur with parasitic disorders.

Roentgen-rays.—These studies are of especial value in large bowel lesions. Filling defects in connection with growths and ulcerations may be visualized or with colitis the characteristic smoothing out of the haustra may be seen.

Diagnosis.—A definite procedure should be followed and the first thing to be found out is whether a diarrhea is due to organic disease of the bowel or whether it is of functional origin. Study of the stools with special reference to presence of blood, pus and parasites, proctoscopy, roentgen-rays and stool cultures may be necessary. If no evidence of actual bowel disease is forthcoming some constitutional or nervous disorder should be sought for.

Treatment.—Specific treatment varies in different cases. If the diarrhea is due to Amœba hystolytica, emetine and other drugs are in order; if it is due to a carcinoma, excision is the ideal therapy. However, there are some general principles of treatment which may be emphasized now. First of all rest in bed is of great importance; just as exercise stimulates peristalsis, so rest in bed quiets it. Rest is usually also necessary because of the systemic symptoms of the underlying condition. The diet depends upon the type and duration of the diarrhea, but in acute cases until one gets his bearings it is never a mistake to restrict food for a few days. Milk which has been boiled and then cooled given in small amounts (100 to 200 cc.) every few hours is very satisfactory and to this, as the patient improves, may be added crackers or dry toast, soft eggs, scraped meat and tea or coffee. Water (uniced) can usually be taken in moderate amounts but if the patient is desiccated as a result of great loss of fluid, salt solution must be given by rectum or subcutaneously. In extreme cases (cholera) fluid may have to be introduced by vein in order to get in a sufficient quantity quickly. A hot-water bag or hot stupes give comfort if there is much abdominal distress. Of drugs paregoric (4 to 10 cc. every two to four hours) is perhaps the most useful because of its local and general analgesic and sedative effect. Bismuth subcarbonate (1 to 4 gm.) may be given at the same time. Other general sedatives or stimulants may be necessary.

In long-standing dysenteries anemia and cachexia usually develop and there may be the actual evidences of a deficiency disorder. Here general upbuilding measures with high vitamin diet, cod-liver oil, sunlight or ultra-violet light, liver and iron are in order. Bowel irrigations have been extensively used, but their value is somewhat questionable. It is obviously impossible to sterilize the colon, and we have the impression that some of the antiseptic flushes which are in common practice, such as silver nitrate, permanganate, mercurochrome and tannic acid, may irritate rather than soothe. At any rate it is wiser to begin gently with simple saline flushes and to be guided further by the patient's reaction to the manipulations and by the course of his disease. Surgical procedures designed to put the colon at rest are sometimes indicated with persistent colitis of various sorts (amebic, ulcerative). As a rule ileostomy is most useful. The large bowel remains then completely isolated and may be treated locally. If the condition heals continuity with the ileum can be restored by suture even after years.

INTESTINAL OBSTRUCTION.

General Considerations.—Obstruction is one of the most frequent and important bowel disorders. The occlusion may develop suddenly or slowly and any part of the intestine may be involved. Intestinal obstruction is always serious, partly because of the local lesion and partly because of the profound systemic effects. Diagnosis. is often difficult and in the acute types prompt surgical interference is usually necessary if life is to be saved.

Etiology and Pathology.—A great variety of causes underlie obstruction of the bowel, among which the most important are (1) twists, kinks, bands, adhesions and herniæ (through mesentery); these affect especially the small intestine and are often dependent on congenital abnormalities or disturbances following previous surgical operations; (2) tumors, especially of large bowel; (3) inflammatory strictures (tuberculosis). If the obstruction is due to a twist or a hernia the blood supply to the obstructed area is cut off with consequent hemorrhagic infarction and death of the bowel wall. If the block develops from within as a result of growth or stricture the effects are less drastic and one may simply have a distention of the bowel above the narrowed area. In gradually progressive occlusions the muscle of the intestinal wall above the lesion hypertrophies in its attempt to force material along the canal.

Pathologic Physiology.—One of the most interesting problems in medicine is the explanation of the profound poisoning ("shock," "toxemia") which is so characteristic of acute small bowel obstruction. A vast amount of experimental work has been done on this subject but no adequate conclusion has yet been reached. It does appear settled, however, that within closed loops of obstructed bowel secretions or exudate accumulate which are highly poisonous when injected into animals. Such material may be absorbed by the patient from his own bowel above the obstruction. Necrosis and autolysis of the bowel wall, decomposition of bowel contents by ferments or bacteria all may play a part in generating this poison. On the whole, the intoxication is more marked the higher up the bowel the obstruction lies; indeed, with large bowel obstructions this acute type of poisoning does not occur. It is because of this peculiar intoxication that intestinal obstruction is such a treacherous disease. Often the patient does not appear very ill and the diagnosis is in doubt for several days until sudden overwhelming poisoning and collapse occur and then treatment is no longer effective.

In addition to the action of the hypothetical poison described above dehydration and changes in the ionic balance of the blood somewhat similar to those which occur with pyloric obstruction take place, especially if there is much vomiting. Chloride and sodium are both lost, the blood chloride falls, blood nitrogen rises and there may be alkalosis. The exact explanation of why these changes sometimes occur even without much vomiting is not clear.

Symptoms.—The symptoms of small and large bowel obstruction differ and they must be considered separately. In the former case trouble usually comes on abruptly and any or all of the following may be present: severe pain, usually in upper abdomen, but sometimes diffuse and unlocalized; nausea; vomiting; weakness; prostration and collapse. The symptoms at first may differ in no way from those of any abdominal colic, but as time goes by the patient gets progressively worse instead of better. Evidences of collapse increase, vomiting may assume the characteristic so-called "fecal" character, the bowels no longer move and after a few days rapid failure with death usually occurs.

With large bowel obstructions, on the other hand, mechanical rather than toxic symptoms predominate. This is partly due to the fact that many large bowel obstructions develop gradually as a result of tumors and partly to differences in the pathologic physiologic results of small and large bowel obstruction. The onset of symptoms may be insidious and often the patient himself cannot tell just when the trouble began. Changes in bowel habit—irregularity as to time and character of the movements—and lower abdominal discomfort are usually the earliest complaints. As time goes by they increase in severity and finally there may be almost continuous cramps. If the obstruction persists and becomes more complete toxic symptoms appear, there is loss of weight and strength, general malaise, lack of appetite and nausea and vomiting. However, the picture in these cases is complicated by the underlying disorder, such as a cancer or tuberculosis of the bowel. Large bowel obstructions may also occur suddenly, as in the case of an annular carcinoma with narrowing of the bowel lumen which suddenly becomes plugged by fecal material. Colic is then the outstanding symptom.

Physical Examination.—Small Bowel Obstructions.—During the early stages little may be made out on physical examination. There are usually progressive evidences of shock, namely, weakness, prostration and rapid pulse. Fever may or may not be present and the temperature may even be subnormal. The abdomen may not be remarkable or there may be tenderness and distention. We have not observed the ladder patterns which have been described. The entire bowel often becomes inactive and there is absence of peristaltic gurgling on auscultation. As time goes by the picture is featured by progressive collapse, with dryness of the tissues from loss of fluid by vomiting, increased rapidity and weakness of the pulse and exaggeration of the local abdominal signs. Evidences of peritonitis frequently occur toward the end, reflex rigidity of the abdominal wall, signs of fluid in the flanks, and hiccough. Death occurs within a few days to a week in untreated cases. Stupor, delirium or coma may supervene or the sensorium may remain clear until shortly before the end.

Large Bowel Obstruction.—The positive findings, if any, are at first confined to the abdomen, which may show various degrees of distention. Tumor masses may be palpated. If the obstruction continues unrelieved a picture somewhat similar to that of small bowel obstruction develops and the patient gradually fails, with progressive weakness and wasting. Vomiting, toxic in origin, may then occur with its consequences (desiccation). After a variable but often lengthy interval (weeks to months) the patient dies of progressive failure if the underlying disease (tumor, tuberculosis) has not already carried him off.

Marked nutritional changes, which have recently been related by some to the dietary deficiencies, sometimes occur with chronic obstructions, and perhaps are bound up with improper digestion and absorption. An interesting group are those patients who develop pellagra-like lesions under these conditions.

Laboratory Tests.—The urine may be concentrated as a result of dehydration and in profoundly poisoned acute cases there is almost complete suppression. This has been related by some to toxic effects of the disorder on the kidneys.

There is often, although not always, a leukocytosis of moderate degree. With chronic large bowel obstructions anemia, often marked, may supervene.

Bowel movements cease shortly after an acute obstruction has taken place. The evacuated material may be modified by the lesion causing the obstruction; with cancers, for example, pus, mucus or blood may be present. Intestinal obstruction associated with strangulation or with hemorrhagic infarction of the bowel (mesenteric artery thrombosis) often is followed for a time by passage of blood in large quantities.

The vomitus varies. After the stomach has been emptied there is likely to be expulsion of a thin brownish fluid with a fetid odor. This is often spoken of as fecal vomiting but, of course, the material contains no feces in the usual sense.

Roentgen-rays are of especial value in the recognition and localization of large bowel obstructions. Barium should be given both by mouth and by enema. Acute small bowel obstructions can sometimes be visualized but the procedure is not of great use in actual practice.

Diagnosis.—Inasmuch as in acute small bowel obstruction the saving of the patient's life usually depends on prompt surgical intervention, early diagnosis is of the utmost importance—at the very time when it is most difficult. First and foremost is the keeping in mind of the possibility of obstruction in every case of acute abdominal upset. The demonstration of any possible predisposing factor such as past surgical operations which may have left adhesions is of great importance. If the symptoms become more marked after twenty-four hours and if there are any evidences of bowel paralysis (absence of stools, absence of peristalsis) the diagnosis should be seriously considered. Persistent diarrhea is a point against obstruction. Fever, rapid pulse, leukocytosis and vomiting are all important, but any or all of them may, on occasion, be absent, especially in the early stages. Later on when the bowel is necrotic and peritonitis has developed, the diagnosis is obvious but too late for useful action.

With large bowel obstruction immediate diagnosis is not so imperative and one may reserve an opinion until roentgen-ray and other studies have been made. In these cases the diagnosis is bound up with the recognition of the condition underlying the obstruction.

Treatment.—Prompt surgical interference is imperative with acute small bowel obstructions. Within the first few hours it is possible in many cases to cut adhesions and relieve twists before the intestine is seriously damaged. After twenty-four hours the bowel is likely to be necrotic and resection, which adds greatly to the hazard, is necessary. After several days when the gangrenous bowel has led to peritonitis, operation is only a gesture and the patient cannot be saved.

While it is possible that an obstruction may relieve itself spontaneously or by abdominal manipulation or by placing the patient in various positions, this is more luck than good management. Preoperative treatment is important. The stomach should be lavaged and salt solution and glucose should be given intravenously and subcutaneously in large amounts (see Pyloric Obstruction).

Slowly developing small bowel strictures are often multiple (tuberculosis) and they are not usually amenable to surgery. Here careful feeding of bland food and general therapy of the underlying disease must be practised; decision to operate requires skilled judgment and no rules can be laid down.

With partial large bowel obstructions palliative treatment may be employed if the underlying condition is inoperable. This includes washing out the bowel with enemas or irrigations, a diet from which coarse particles are eliminated and laxatives such as mineral oil or mild salines.

When these measures do not avail, surgical treatment is necessary and if the lesion cannot be excised a colostomy may prolong the patient's life.

Following abdominal operations of various sorts so-called paralytic ileus may occur. There is no actual obstruction but as a result of shock, infection or unexplained causes the bowel wall becomes paralyzed and the gut is distended and immobile. The outstanding symptom is persistent vomiting. As the patient's general condition improves the intestinal tone and motility are restored and normal bowel movements are resumed. Meanwhile repeated gastric lavage together with subcutaneous and intravenous introduction of salt solution and glucose are in order. Pituitrin, 1 cc. hypodermically, may be tried. Spinal anesthesia has given relief in some cases, presumably by paralyzing the sympathetic.

REFERENCES.

McIver, M. A., and Gamble, J. L.: Body Fluid Changes Due to Upper Intestinal Obstruction, Jour. Am. Med. Assn., 1928, 91, 1589.
Orr, T. G., and Haden, R. L.: The Treatment of Intestinal Obstruction, Ann. Surg., 1929, 89, 354.

APPENDICITIS.

General Considerations.—Acute inflammation of the appendix is a disease of definite symptoms and one of the most frequent and serious of abdominal disorders. Chronic appendicitis, on the other hand, is a much less clear-cut entity and while practically all appendices removed at operation show some pathologic changes such as fibrosis, thickening, kinking, adhesions, occlusion of the lumen with retention of fecal material or low-grade chronic inflammatory changes in the walls, it is often very difficult to be sure just how much clinical trouble the organ was actually giving. Undoubtedly reflexes from a diseased appendix may promote indigestion in some people or perhaps may be responsible for constipation or vague abdominal discomforts. But "the proof of the pudding is the eating," and only if the patient is relieved by appendectomy can one be fairly sure of the origin of the symptoms. Certainly the diagnosis is made much less often now than it was fifteen years ago and we see no way in which the syndrome can ever be put on a very firm foundation. If a person has had fairly definite attacks of acute appendicitis in the past a diagnosis of chronic appendicitis can, perhaps, be made later with more assurance.

The present discussion will concern itself, therefore, with acute appendicitis.

Etiology and Pathology.—Acute appendicitis is a bacterial infection. Streptococci and colon bacilli are commonly recovered on culture but other organisms including anaërobes may be implicated. Rarely fungi (actinomyces) are at fault. In the early stages there is an acute diffuse inflammation of the walls of the organ and if seen at this stage it presents a tense red swollen appearance. The lumen and to some extent the circulation become shut off by pressure so that necrosis soon results and infected material enters the peritoneal cavity where local abscesses are set up or general peritonitis may result.

The disease occurs predominantly in young people, although the aged are not always exempt.

Symptoms.—The early symptoms of appendicitis are reflex in origin and the diagnosis is often difficult. As a rule, out of a clear sky, the patient begins to feel "upset." There is distaste for food, nausea and perhaps vomiting. Hand in hand with this go epigastric discomfort or perhaps more widespread abdominal distress and cramps. Constipation is the rule and diarrhea is a point against the diagnosis. So far there is nothing very characteristic and often the condition cannot be distinguished from a simple stomach upset. The attack may subside and in point of fact many people probably get well without one ever being able to reach a diagnosis. But usually the symptoms progress during the second day, nausea and vomiting persist or recur and abdominal discomfort continues. There may be fever but it is rarely high and at times there are only slight elevations. After the first or second day symptoms of local peritoneal irritation develop and the patient may complain of soreness in the right lower quadrant. Various symptoms such as urinary frequency and discomfort may occur when the appendix extends into the pelvis or retroperitoneally. If the condition progresses to perforation the symptoms of peritonitis supervene.

Physical Examination.—In the early stages little is made out except that the patient "looks sick." Within twelve to twenty-four hours, however, some evidences of peritoneal irritation are usually evident in the form of slight tenderness or resistance in the right lower quadrant. Sometimes it is so slight that one is in doubt and then frequent examinations are important so that the slightest progression may be noted. By the time the appendix ruptures the signs are usually outspoken, and there is great tenderness or rigidity either locally or generally over the abdomen if diffuse peritonitis has set in. When the appendix is retrocecal or hangs into the pelvis there may be a confusing absence of local signs and rectal examination should always be done in order to elicit tenderness by this route.

The general signs of intoxication are important. Often the patient looks ill out of proportion to any objective findings and the pulse is usually but not always accelerated.

The leukocyte count is of special importance. While rarely elevated above 20,000 an increase, especially of the polymorphonuclears, is practically always found.

Complications.—Local abscesses and general peritonitis have already been mentioned. Abscesses may perforate into other viscera and fistulæ may result. In occasional cases there is thrombosis of veins at the base of the appendix and a progressive inflammation of the portal veins may result (*suppurative pylephlebitis*) with multiple liver abscesses. This condition is always fatal. Clinically it is featured by chills and sweats, prolonged fever of the septic type, swelling and tenderness of the liver and finally the picture of a general sepsis. Blood culture may be positive toward the end.

Diagnosis.—Diagnosis is based on the occurrence in a young person of malaise, nausea and perhaps vomiting with epigastric or diffuse abdominal distress in the absence of diarrhea, with fever, leukocytosis and rapid pulse and the subsequent development of signs of peritoneal irritation in the right lower quadrant. However, the picture is very variable and almost any one of the above manifestations may, on occasion, be absent. One may be badly misled, for example, by laying too much stress on the absence of marked fever. On the whole, the most common error is to misdiagnose a simple stomach upset and to temporize or perhaps make matters worse by purging, until perforation has occurred. Conversely appendicitis may be diagnosed when the actual condition is pelvic inflammatory disease, a urinary tract disturbance or other local abdominal inflammation. Typhoid fever has been mistaken in the early stages for appendicitis but the leukocyte count should make one escape this error. Acute pleurisy, with or without pneumonia, may be associated with referred pain to the lower abdomen which may lead to the diagnosis of appendicitis, but this is a gross mistake which no careful clinician should make.

As in so many other situations in medical practice the most important point in diagnosis is to have the possibility of the condition in mind. Appendicitis should be thought of in the case of every acute abdominal upset.

Treatment.—The more one sees of acute appendicitis the more one becomes convinced that early excision is the only safe treatment. If one waits until peritonitis has set in the results are poor and the mortality is high. Hence any *reasonable suspicion* of appendicitis justifies operation if adequate surgical talent is available. The old rule of waiting for the acute attack to subside and operating "in the interval" is obviously unsound, since one never knows in advance whether the attack *will* subside. Even if needless operation is occasionally done it is in the long run sounder practice to explore, and as a rule the physician will be rewarded by discovering an appendix which would soon rupture if not removed.

If, for some reason, operation cannot be done, the patient should be put absolutely to bed and attempts should be made to quiet the bowel so that if perforation occurs the infection will have a better chance to localize. This means starvation except for small amounts of fluid for a few days, mild sedatives or opiates such as barbital or codeine and a light ice-bag to the abdomen. Purgatives are absolutely contra-indicated.

REFERENCE.

KELLY, H. A.: Appendicitis and Other Diseases of the Vermiform Appendix, Philadelphia, 1909.

ULCERATIVE COLITIS.

General Considerations.—In addition to bacillary dysentery and amebic dysentery there have been known for a long time other types of acute and chronic colitis of less clearly defined etiology. They have been referred to in the literature under such designations as "simple colitis," "non-specific colitis" and "ulcerative colitis" and have been regarded for the most part as being caused by a variety of bacteria. But of recent years there has been a growing feeling that the disease is a more definite entity and, indeed, claims have been made for a specific bacterial etiology by Bargen. This investigator has been able to grow from material obtained directly from the ulcers (by means of the proctoscope and at operation) a non-hemolytic streptococcus which is said to be the specific cause of the disease. The evidence on which Bargen bases his views is the constancy of the finding of these organisms, the similarity of the strains from different cases, the experimental production of lesions in animals and the beneficial effects obtained in patients by use of vaccines and sera derived from them. However, Bargen's coccus has not been generally accepted; while streptococci have been isolated from the ulcers by others they have not always been of the same type and other bacteria such as colon bacilli may be found as well. It must be remembered that non-hemolytic streptococci normally abound in the bowel. The experimental lesions and the therapeutic results with vaccines and sera have also been questioned. The writer feels that the matter is not yet settled but that Bargen's work has been of great value in stimulating the study of this important disease.

Pathology.—The early lesions are best studied by means of the proctoscope. The mucosa shows an intense injection which gives it a reddish plush-like appearance and the surface bleeds easily on slight trauma. There is a diffuse exudate of muco-purulent material which is smeared over the bowel surface. Along with the injection tiny superficial erosions are seen; they vary in size from pin-point to several millimeters in diameter. Similar changes presumably exist throughout the colon. As time goes by, if the condition progresses the ulcerations become deeper and more extensive and there is an infiltration and induration of the bowel wall as a result of a diffuse chronic inflammation. Finally the bowel may become anchored and rigid like a piece of hose and the mucosa may be largely destroyed by confluent ulcerations leaving only islands of fairly normal tissue. A polypoid condition may develop in these islands and such areas occasionally undergo carcinomatous changes. Perforation rarely occurs.

41

Symptoms.—Most of the cases occur in young or middle-aged people. The onset may be stormy like that of an acute dysentery with abdominal cramps, frequent small stools with tenesmus and general prostration and fever. More often, however, the beginning is more insidious and aside from the fact that the bowel movements are increased in number and that they are loose the patient may be unaware of any departure from health. The course varies greatly in different people. Some, after a few weeks of diarrhea, are fortunate enough to recover and they may be permanently well, while others run a stormy course from the start with intractable dysentery, cramps, continued fever, rapid loss of weight and general failure. The majority, however, strike a middle course and with exacerbations and remissions go for years until the final stages are reached. Then, indeed, a pitiable state results. The patient is reduced to skin and bones and is bedfast from weakness, there is extreme anemia and the evidence of profound nutritional disturbances in the form of pellagra-like lesions or keratomalacia. Meanwhile he is plagued by perpetual cramps and diarrhea. The morale is affected and one may hardly recognize the plaintive querulous wreck of humanity which remains. Finally, an algid state with stupor and subnormal temperature terminates the picture.

Physical examination varies with the stages of the disease. There may be abdominal tenderness and in advanced cases thickened coils of bowel can be felt. Otherwise the findings depend on the patient's general condition and nutrition.

During the more active phases of the disease there is irregular fever, sometimes quite high, which may subside during a period of improvement or remission only to flare up later.

Laboratory Tests.—Leukocytosis of moderate degree is the rule during the active stages. There is practically always some anemia and in the advanced chronic types it may be extreme with hemoglobin of only 20 per cent or less. The stools vary, but the important findings are mucus, blood and pus. Amebas and the bacilli of dysentery are absent.

Roentgen-rays.—Roentgen-rays are useful in determining the extent and degree of the lesions. The smoothing out of the bowel haustrations so characteristic of colitis is usually demonstrable and in extreme cases actual suggestions of ulceration may be visualized.

Diagnosis.—Ulcerative colitis should be thought of in the case of any subacute or chronic dysentery if amebas and dysentery bacilli cannot be found. Proctoscopy is especially important since the process is usually within reach and the actual lesions can be seen. Local lesions such as cancer and tuberculosis must be ruled out.

Treatment.—It is generally conceded that treatment is unsatisfactory. Indeed, the multiplicity of therapeutic agents which have been advised make it clear that no real cure is as yet at hand. Rest in bed with fresh air and sunshine is of the utmost importance, especially at the start when progression into the chronic stage may, perhaps, be prevented. As to diet, it has been customary in the past to impose heavy restrictions, and patients have been carried for long periods of time on milk or on cereals, gruels and meat juices. We now know, however, that starvation of this sort merely superadds the results of dietary deficiency to the underlying disease and the pendulum has swung to the other extreme. A liberal general diet high in vitamins but low in roughage should be given. This will include plenty of butter, milk, eggs, fruit juices, tomato juice, puréed greens, tender red meat and liver. There is no evidence that such a diet produces local injury of the colon and prevents the healing of the ulcers as was formerly thought. Two thousand to 3000 calories should be taken in the twenty-four hours if possible. Cod-liver oil may be added. Most writers advise local irrigations of the colon and the number of medicaments which has been tried is legion. One may mention tannic acid, silver nitrate, permanganate, acriflavine, mercurochrome and gentian violet as a few of the long list. The writer is convinced from his experience that such measures are merely a futile gesture; obviously one cannot sterilize the colon and is likely to set up further irritation of the already acutely inflamed mucosa. In some cases irrigations make the patient feel better by removing fecal material and gas and perhaps by allaying spasm, and for this purpose one or two irrigations may be tried each day with warm salt solution. If discomfort is increased they should be abandoned. Aside from the above measures treatment is symptomatic and the suggestions made in the section on Diarrhea may be tried. Injections of foreign protein (peptone, killed typhoid bacilli) have been advised. Perhaps they deserve a trial in stubborn cases as do Bargen's vaccines and sera.

The question of surgical interference is always a difficult one and the indications for doing an appendicostomy or ileostomy are very hard to define. Ileostomy seems the procedure of choice since the colon is thereby at least put at rest, and if done at all it would seem wise to proceed before the bowel is hopelessly scarred. However, the inconvenience and the hazards connected with later restoring the continuity of the bowel make one hesitate, especially as the operation is frequently not followed by better results than may otherwise be obtained.

The writer has gradually reached the conviction that in the individual case the patient's course is somehow predetermined from the start regardless of therapy. This idea has come from the experience that some patients get well promptly under any form of therapy, whereas others seem totally refractory to all measures. Hence the essential points in treatment are rest and upbuilding with the high vitamin diet.

REFERENCES.

BARGEN, J. A.: Chronic Ulcerative Colitis: A Review, Arch. Int. Med., 1930, **45**, 559.

CROHN, B. B., and ROSENBERG, H.: Sigmoidoscopic Picture of Chronic Ulcerative Colitis, Am. Jour. Med. Sci., 1925, **170**, 220.

EUSTERMAN, G. B., and O'LEARY, P. A.: Pellagra Secondary to Benign and Carcinomatous Lesions and Dysfunction of the Gastro-intestinal Tract, Arch. Int. Med., 1931, **47**, 633.

HEWITT, J. H., and HOWARD, W. T.: Chronic Ulcerative Colitis with Polyps, Arch. Int. Med., 1915, **15**, 714.

LYNCH, J. M., and FELSEN, J.: Non-specific Ulcerative Colitis, Arch. Int. Med., 1925, **35**, 433.

PAULSON, M.: Chronic Ulcerative Colitis with Reference to a Bacterial Etiology: Experimental Studies, Arch. Int. Med., 1928, **41**, 75.

TUBERCULOSIS OF THE INTESTINE.

Involvement of the intestines occurs in most cases of generalized tuberculosis or of advanced tuberculosis of the lungs. As such it represents merely an incident in the course of a widespread disease. There are, however, more localized forms of intestinal tuberculosis which should be logically considered with other gastro-intestinal problems. The present discussion deals mainly with these.

Primary tuberculosis of the bowel is not uncommon in children and may be due to bovine strains of bacilli. In adults, even if it represents the outstanding lesion of the case, intestinal tuberculosis is usually secondary to tubercle elsewhere in the body. The pathologic picture is varied. The lesions commence in the lymphoid tissue of the bowel as tubercles which later coalesce and break down so that ulceration is a prominent feature. As with tubercle in general, fibrosis may be predominant and hence there may result localized hyperplastic infiltrations which present themselves as tumor masses especially in the cecal region. The lesions may be single or multiple. Sites of predilection are the cecum and appendix, ileum and colon with the sigmoid and rectum and the jejunum next in frequency. The duodenum and stomach are rarely affected. In extreme cases a large part of the bowel is riddled with ulcers of varying age and size. Healing may take place but scarring and stenosis as a result of annular lesions are likely to result. Multiple strictures are not uncommon. Other important complications or associations are tuberculous peritonitis which results from extension through the bowel wall, and tuberculosis of the mesenteric glands. Perforation is rare.

Symptoms.—Local or constitutional symptoms may predominate. The latter are those of tuberculosis in general—fever, malaise, weakness, anorexia, loss of weight. The local symptoms vary with the site and character of the lesions. Abdominal discomfort and diarrhea are especially prominent. In extreme cases the patient is reduced to skin and bones and tortured by perpetual cramps and diarrhea. Symptoms of chronic obstruction may develop, especially with the sclerotic fibrocaseous types.

Physical Examination.—This often reveals other evidences of tuberculosis, especially of the lungs. Abdominal tenderness, distention, and palpable masses of bowel may be made out, especially if the peritoneum is invoved.

Laboratory Examinations.—The blood count varies. There may be anemia, sometimes extreme, but this is not characteristic. The leukocytes are often reduced, but they may be normal or slightly elevated. Stool examination is of especial importance. If the process is active the movements are likely to be loose, and pus and blood are found. Large hemorrhages are unusual. Tubercle bacilli may be demonstrated by staining bits of bloody mucus or a concentrated sediment.

Roentgen-rays are very helpful in diagnosis but the specificity of certain appearances which was much stressed by tuberculosis specialists a few years ago has recently been questioned. Spasms, filling defects and stenoses are, however, often revealed and while single lesions especially in the colon may be indistinguishable from the picture of cancer the correct diagnosis can often be inferred if several filling defects or strictures are present.

Diagnosis.—Tuberculosis must be distinguished especially from chronic diarrheas of other origin and from cancer of the bowel. The discovery of tuberculosis elsewhere in the body together with the roentgen-ray findings are the most essential points, since the bowel lesions themselves produce no specific symptoms. Finding of bacilli in the stools is important but if active pulmonary tuberculosis is present the organisms may have originated in sputum which has been swallowed.

Treatment.—The general therapeutic regimen used in tuberculosis is, of course, in order—rest, fresh air and general upbuilding and, as with pulmonary lesions, better results are usually achieved in a sanatorium than at home. Some years ago a good deal of stress was placed on surgical resection of the major lesions but recent experience has shown that equally good or even better results follow medical treatment without the hazards of operation. The regimen includes systematic exposures to sunlight or to artificial ultra-violet rays and a liberal bland diet high in vitamins. Cod-liver oil and tomato juice are said to be especially helpful. For relief of symptoms the general measures and drugs discussed in the section on Diarrhea are in order; stupes to the abdomen may relieve pain and cramps and general sedatives, such as barbital, codeine or morphine may be necessary. Paregoric (8 to 12 cc.) is especially helpful with intractable diarrhea. Surgery still has a place, however, and may become obligatory in the case of tumor-like cecal masses or for the relief of obstructions.

REFERENCE.

Brown, L., and Sampson, H. L.: Intestinal Tuberculosis, 2d ed., Philadelphia, 1930.

TUMORS OF THE BOWEL.

General Considerations.—Malignant growths are among the commoner diseases of the bowel. The physician should be constantly on the watch for them since cure may be obtained by excision if the diagnosis is made in the early stages. The majority of bowel growths are primary carcinomata and they occur almost altogether in the large bowel. Carcinomas of the duodenum and small intestine are rare. Lymphoblastoma (lymphosarcoma), sarcomata, metastatic tumors of various kinds and benign tumors are occasionally encountered.

Cancer of the small intestine is rarely recognized clinically. When symptoms appear they include pain, indigestion, hemorrhage and the evidences of obstruction or metastases in various combinations. Jaundice which results from involvement of the ampulla of Vater is a frequent finding with cancer of the duodenum.

Polyps (adenomatous) occur in any part of the intestine. They may be large or small, single or multiple. Usually asymptomatic they come into clinical prominence on occasion because of bleeding or cancerous changes. Diffuse polyposis may be associated with dysenteric symptoms. Isolated polyps in the rectum may be removed through the proctoscope if they give trouble.

CANCER OF THE COLON.

Cancer of the colon is second in frequency and importance only to cancer of the stomach and rectum. Most of the cases occur in people between forty and sixty-five years of age, and men are affected more often than women. The sigmoid and cecum are most frequently involved, the flexures next and the transverse and descending portions least often. The growths are adenocarcinomata. They may be extensive, with necrosis and ulceration or, especially in the sigmoid, there is a tendency to formation of an annular sclerotic lesion above which fecal masses accumulate. Perforation leads to peritonitis or local abscess formation, and fistulas into adjacent viscera may develop. Metastases usually occur relatively late. In 27 of our cases which came to autopsy metastases were found as follows: liver, 10; peritoneum, 7; small intestines, 5; pancreas, 2; kidney, 2; diaphragm, 2; stomach, rectum, gall-bladder, duodenum, ovary, spleen, muscle, blood-vessels and brain, each 1. Lymph nodes were involved 19 times, for the most part intra-abdominally, but in 1 case each the peribronchial and supraclavicular glands were infiltrated.

Symptoms.—Carcinoma of the colon presents an interesting variety of clinical manifestations. The growth may be latent for a long time and symptoms begin suddenly with the evidences of intestinal obstruction when the lesion is already quite far advanced. As a rule, there will be some alteration in the patient's bowel habits, perhaps a failure to have the movements with the usual regularity, perhaps increasing constipation or alternating constipation and diarrhea. Large bleedings are rare. Pain, if present, is at first usually indefinite—mild cramp-like sensations or merely a vague abdominal discomfort in the mid- or lower abdomen. As the growth advances the local symptoms become more outspoken and the general health is affected. The appetite fails, there is loss of weight and strength, pallor and perhaps dyspnea on exertion. Constitutional symptoms or symptoms resulting from metastases, especially to the liver, may dominate the picture, even from the start, and the patient comes in complaining of upper abdominal pain or of distention or of actually feeling the hard lump (liver). Fever is the rule, especially with ulcerating growths or with extensive metastases; there may be perforations with secondary infection, local or general peritonitis or abscesses which are responsible for the symptoms of septic infection (chills, fever, sweats, pain and tenderness). Pellagra-like symptoms have been noted in occasional cases probably as a result of malnutrition.

Physical Examination.—Physical examination may reveal no signs of trouble of any sort; the patient appears to be in exuberant health. In other cases the evidences of intoxication and cachexia are present— loss of weight and pallor. The actual growth is rarely palpable except in the latest stages, and one must not depend on feeling a mass to make the diagnosis. Indeed, when one does feel a tumor it is usually largely impacted feces which have collected behind an annular narrowing. However, the abdomen should be palpated with the utmost care, especially in the cecal and sigmoid regions and at the colonic flexures and at times, even if the tumor is not palpable, thrill-like or squirting sensations are appreciated which arise from the forcible passage of bowel contents through a narrow lumen. This phenomenon may also give rise to squirting sounds on auscultation which must, of course, be distinguished from normal peristalsis. In doubtful cases the abdomen should be examined repeatedly, since the tumor mass varies in its accessibility to palpation from day to day because of different degrees of distention and bowel content. When obstruction is advanced, marked blowing up of the abdomen occurs. The liver may be large, hard or nodular. Peritoneal extensions are to be felt as lumps here and there in the abdomen and ascites may be detected. Proctoscopy may reveal growths in the lower sigmoid.

There is often an interesting difference between the effects of cancer of the right and left colon. The former are likely to be diffuse ulcerating growths which are associated with marked constitutional symptoms and frequently with a severe anemia. Left colon cancers are more often of the scirrhous annular type and signs of local obstruction without marked general poisoning predominate.

Laboratory Tests.—The blood may be normal. Anemia is common, however, especially with right colon growths. It may be extreme (hemoglobin, 20 per cent) and the blood picture may suggest pernicious anemia. The changes are not explainable by blood loss and are regarded as the results of intoxication. Leukocytosis (moderate) is often found, particularly with sloughing or secondarily infected growths. The stools may show no abnormality. Large amounts of blood are occasionally present, but bleeding on the whole is slight. Loose movements with pus and blood occur, especially with sigmoid and rectal growths. The alternating constipation and diarrhea with flat ribbon-like stools, which is stressed in the classical descriptions, has not been present as a rule in our experience; indeed, the ribbon stools are more likely to occur with mucous colitis and spasm.

Roentgen-rays.—Roentgen-rays, if properly used, are invaluable in diagnosis of bowel growths. A barium enema given after the bowel has been thoroughly cleaned out not uncommonly shows a definite filling defect or constriction. Two sources of error occur. The lesion may be overlooked because of looping of the bowel, or filling defects may turn out to be artefacts. The examination should be made by a conservative careful radiologist in coöperation with the physician and the roentgen-ray findings must be carefully correlated with the other features of the case.

Diagnosis.—So variable are the clinical manifestations of bowel growths that the possibility must be kept in mind in the presence of any obscure abdominal condition; indeed, *any alteration in bowel habits in a person over thirty or thirty-five years of age calls for a study to eliminate cancer of the colon.* Early recognition is of the utmost importance if successful surgical treatment is to be instituted, and exploration is often advisable in doubtful cases. Minor symptoms should not be ignored until it is obvious that advanced malignant disease exists. Common errors are to diagnose simple constipation or intestinal neurosis, chronic appendicitis or cholecystitis, or to have one's attention centered on metastases in the liver which may overshadow the primary lesion of the bowel. In the latter case the error is, of course, of academic importance only, as nothing can be done at this stage anyway.

The differentiation between tumor and abscess here as in other situations may be difficult. When there is irregular fever, perhaps with chills, anemia and leukocytosis one is often surprised to find on exploration that a cancer lies at the bottom of the trouble.

Treatment.—The only treatment of any value is surgical, and the importance of early diagnosis must again be stressed. In contrast to cancer of the stomach, bowel growths in a fair proportion of favorable cases are permanently cured by extirpation. Twenty-five per cent of those who survive resection are well for at least five years, even though recurrences may still take place. If the case is inoperable obstruction may have to be relieved by colostomy. Otherwise careful bowel regulation (see Intestinal Obstruction), rest, upbuilding and antianemic measures (iron, liver, transfusion) are all that can be done. In the terminal stages opiates should be used freely for pain.

ILLUSTRATIVE CASE—CANCER OF THE BOWEL (LATENT).

P. M., laborer, aged seventy-three years.

Complaint.—Dizziness.

Family History and Past History.—Unimportant.

Present Illness.—Three months ago patient began to feel weak and dizzy on walking. These symptoms have become worse. He has lost 25 pounds. There has been no abdominal pain, constipation or gastro-intestinal disturbance of any sort.

Physical Examination.—A thin, somewhat worn-looking old man. The head, heart and lungs showed nothing remarkable. The epigastrium was occupied by a visible fullness which, on palpation, was found to be the liver. This extended 4 cm. below the costal margin and the edge was hard and irregular. No other mass or abnormality was made out in the abdomen. Rectal examination negative.

Laboratory Tests.—Red blood cells, 4,000,000; hemoglobin, 75 per cent; white blood cells, 10,000. Urine negative. Stool normal. No mucus, blood or pus.

Roentgen-rays.—No obstruction or filling defects were visualized in the gastro-intestinal tract.

Course.—The liver increased rapidly in size, there was progressive failure and he died five weeks after entry to the hospital.

Autopsy.—Adenocarcinoma (annular) of the sigmoid; metastases to liver and to various other viscera.

Comment.—The case illustrates the complete latency of the primary growth which was quite overshadowed by the metastases to the liver. The failure of the roentgen-rays to reveal the lesion should also be noted.

ILLUSTRATIVE CASE—CANCER OF THE SIGMOID.

Miss L. S., clerk, aged twenty-seven years.

Complaint.—Abdominal pain, nausea and vomiting.

Family History and Past History.—Unimportant.

Present Illness.—The patient was perfectly well until seven months ago when she was suddenly taken with severe colicky abdominal pain, nausea, vomiting and obstipation. The attack lasted four days. Since that time she has had three similar attacks including the present one. This began four days ago with severe cramp-like diffuse abdominal pains coming at intervals of ten to fifteen minutes. She has vomited frequently since onset and there have been four to five very small bowel movements following oil enemas. There has been a great deal of gurgling and she has passed a small amount of gas.

Physical Examination.—She was a well nourished, well developed young woman. The general physical examination was negative. The abdomen was moderately distended. In the left lower quadrant there was a firm irregular mass about 5 cm. long and 2 to 3 cm. wide.

Laboratory Tests.—Red blood cells, 4,700,000; hemoglobin, 84 per cent; white blood cells, 12,800. Urine negative. Stool (enema) negative.

Roentgen-rays.—Barium enema showed marked obstruction in the descending colon at the point of the mass (Fig. 34).

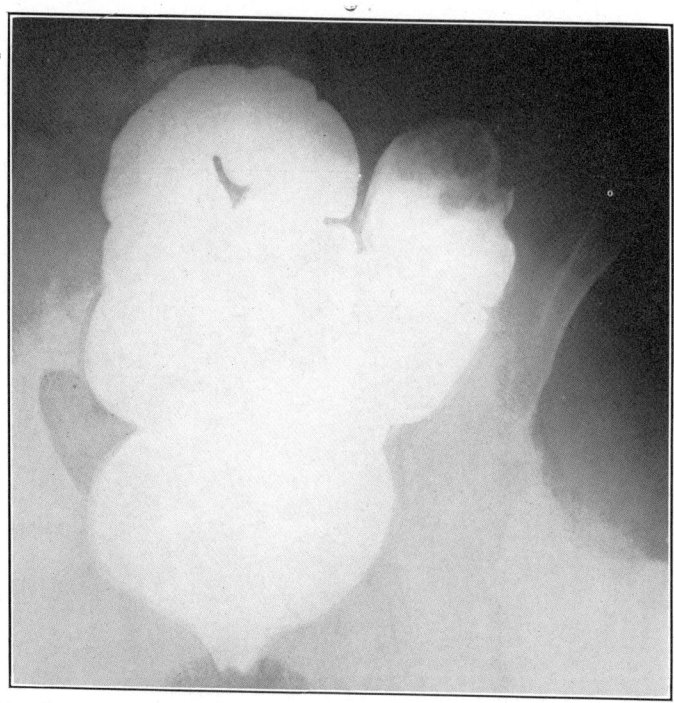

Fig. 34.—Carcinoma of the sigmoid—enema. Note sudden stoppage of barium in sigmoid region with filling defect.

Operation.—(Sept. 3, 1927). A huge tumor (adenocarcinoma) of the sigmoid was found. No metastases were seen and the mass was resected and a side-to-side anastomosis was done. Examination of the specimen showed that the growth had completely occluded the bowel, but that as a result of sloughing, a channel had become reëstablished. The patient was perfectly well four years later (September, 1931).

Comment.—The case illustrates very well the type of bowel growth with which obstructive symptoms are the outstanding feature. In this case there was no anemia, wasting or weakness. The youth of the patient is of interest and, above all, the fact that a four-year cure has been achieved despite the apparently advanced state of the growth.

ILLUSTRATIVE CASE—CANCER OF THE COLON (ASCENDING).

C. B., gardener, aged sixty-seven years.
Complaint.—Pain in right side and weakness.

Family History and Past History.—Unimportant.

Present Illness.—About five months ago he developed chills and fever and pain in the right upper quadrant of the abdomen. There was a dull heavy ache which has persisted up to the present time. There has been great loss of weight and increasing constipation, but no other bowel symptoms.

Examination.—The patient presented the picture of advanced cachexia. He was skin and bones and looked very pale and sallow. The abdomen was markedly distended in the right upper quadrant and toward the flank there was a bulge which looked like a segment of a large grapefruit. On palpation this was found to correspond to a hard irregular mass between the costal margin and the ileum about 14 x 10 cm. in diameter.

Laboratory Tests.—Urine, negative. Red blood cells, 2,700,000; hemoglobin 48 per cent; white blood cells, 24,000 (polymorphonuclears, 82 per cent). Stool, soft, homogeneous; no gross blood or pus; occult blood, *negative.*

Roentgen-rays.—Barium enema was introduced without obstruction as far as the hepatic flexure when the flow stopped abruptly. A large irregular filling defect was visualized in the region of the palpable mass. A small amount of barium trickled through to the ascending colon (Fig. 35).

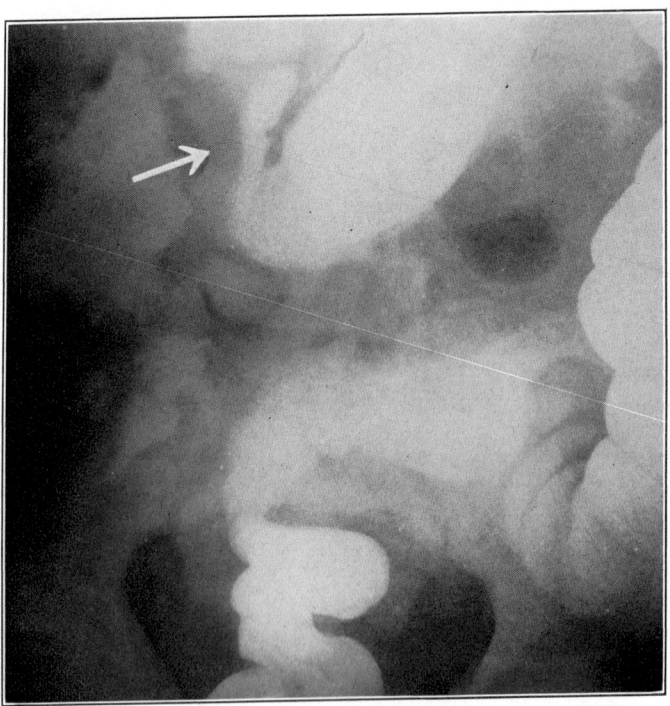

Fig. 35.—Carcinoma of the colon—hepatic flexure—enema. Note huge filling defect in region of hepatic flexure.

Course.—There was moderate irregular fever with chills. He failed rapidly and died within a few days.

Autopsy.—There was a huge carcinoma of the ascending colon with extensions to the surrounding organs (small intestine, peritoneum). The growth had perforated and there was a large subphrenic abscess. Metastases were present especially in the regional lymph nodes and in the liver.

Comment.—This case illustrates the extreme anemia which may develop with cancer of the ascending colon, even in the absence of bleeding. The complication of perforation and abscess is also important.

REFERENCE.

For systematic discussion of tumors, benign and malignant, with extensive bibliography, see article by OBERNDORFER, in Henke-Lubarsch: Handbuch, etc.,
1929, **4**, Pt. III, 717.

ANOMALIES AND DEFORMITIES OF THE INTESTINE.

Congenital Deformities.—Congenital deformities and imperfections
of the bowel, such as imperforate anus, occur occasionally; they concern especially the pediatrician. *Enteroptosis*, "dropping of the bowel,"
used to be regarded as a definite disease and all sorts of abdominal
symptoms have in the past been attributed to it. But since modern
roentgen-ray studies have demonstrated the frequency of dependent
viscera in clinically normal people little significance is attached to
such variations by most physicians. Just what the clinical significance
is of such minor anomalies as *mobile cecum*, *Lane's kinks* and *Jackson's
veil* which have been discovered by surgeons during abdominal operations it is hard to say. Unless actual obstruction results, one must
question their importance. The student, if interested, must pursue
this subject in the special surgical literature. Compression of the
duodenum by an anomalous mesentery or by a prominent spinal
column is said to produce on occasion a special syndrome featured by
bouts of headache relieved by vomiting or change in posture. *Chronic
duodenal stasis* and *dilated duodenum* are terms which have been used
to describe this disorder. *Congenital dilatation of the colon* (Hirschsprung's disease) has been discussed in the article on Constipation.

Diverticula are not uncommon. They may be congenital or acquired.
Incomplete obliteration of the fetal omphalo-mesenteric duct may
persist as a so-called *Meckel's diverticulum* in 1 to 2 per cent of all
people. The pouch varies from 3 to 10 cm. or more in length and
arises from the antimesenteric border of the bowel $\frac{1}{2}$ to 1 meter above
the ileocecal valve. It may be attached to the navel. Meckel's diverticula are sometimes the seat of inflammations or they may become
entangled with the bowel so as to lead to obstruction.

Multiple acquired diverticula occur frequently, especially in the
colon (diverticulosis). The mucosa herniates through defective areas
in the muscularis so that little pouch-like projections covered by serosa
stud the exterior of the bowel. They may vary in size up to 4 or 5 cm.
in diameter, although the majority are not over $\frac{1}{2}$ to 1 cm. in diameter.
The etiology is obscure, but congenital weakness of the bowel wall
probably plays a part. Diverticula are rare before middle age. As a
rule, the condition is asymptomatic and the lesions are discovered
accidentally on roentgen-ray examination. After evacuation of a
barium enema beautiful pictures may be obtained which show t he
barium retained in the sacs like clusters of grapes. Various symptoms
have been described, but they are probably coincidental rather than
due to the diverticula unless certain complications ensue. Inflammation of diverticula (*diverticulitis*) may occur with symptoms similar
to those of appendicitis, or there may simply be indefinite signs of
intra-abdominal inflammation. Perforation with abscess formation

occasionally occurs and rarely carcinomatous changes take place in a diverticulum.

The condition is progressive as the intestinal wall gradually gives way more and more. Careful bowel regulation may tend to prevent progress but there is no special treatment. If abscess or carcinoma develops, operation with drainage or resection is in order.

Diverticula of the small intestine and especially of the duodenum occasionally occur. There has been some dispute as to what extent they are congenital or acquired. Unless ulceration or adhesions arise in connection with them there are not likely to be any symptoms. As a rule, the condition is discovered on roentgen-ray examination.

THE RECTUM.

Most of the diseases of the rectum require surgical or other special procedures for their relief. Diagnosis, however, as a rule, can and should be made by the general practitioner or internist who sees the patient in the early stages of his trouble when treatment can be carried out most effectively. Furthermore, certain findings in the rectum may have a bearing on general or remote disease and experience has indicated that no physical examination can be considered complete until at least a digital examination of the rectum has been made. This the physician should be prepared to supplement with proctoscopy, if necessary.

The external anal region should first be inspected. Here the demonstration of bleeding hemorrhoids may give the key to an obscure case of anemia or the discovery of a fistula may clinch the diagnosis of tuberculosis. As the finger is introduced into the rectum the sphincter tone should be noted; abnormal relaxation occurs with certain spinal cord lesions and abnormal spasticity is common in mild neurasthenic states. In the rectum proper strictures or tumors should be sought for and in men the size and consistency of the prostate gland and of the seminal vesicles should be noted. In certain cases of malignant disease in the abdomen metastases occur in the cul-de-sac between rectum and bladder where they may be felt as a hard irregular ridge. This phenomenon, the rectal shelf (Blumer), may give a clue to correct diagnosis in cases otherwise obscure.

INFECTIONS OF THE RECTUM.

The rectum may be involved in any of the various types of dysentery or colitis—amebic, bacillary or ulcerative, and where such involvement is marked the local symptoms consist of great frequency and urgency of stool, and of tenesmus—a painful, spastic, burning feeling in the lower back and anal region. The extent of the rectal lesions is revealed by proctoscopy which should be done in every suspicious case both for diagnosis and prognosis. The matter has already been discussed above in the section on Ulcerative Colitis, to which the reader is referred.

Tuberculous infection of the rectum is rare. It usually occurs in association with tuberculosis of the intestine (see above) and as part of a widespread acid-fast infection. The lesions are similar to those which have already been described in connection with the bowel and at the time when the patient is seen there are usually multiple ulcers of varying size. The symptoms are those of any rectal infection, pain in back or lower abdomen, tenesmus and usually diarrhea. Diagnosis is made by recognition of tuberculosis of the bowel or of other structures, by the appearance of the ulcers and by biopsy. Tubercle bacilli may be demonstrated in scrapings, although this is usually difficult. Local applications, irrigations or cauterizations are used by surgeons and proctologists, but the general regimen of intestinal tuberculosis is most important.

Syphilis of the rectum is extremely uncommon. Primary lesions rarely occur in or about the anus. It was formerly believed that stricture of the rectum was almost always syphilitic in origin, but this view has recently been questioned, and rectal strictures are now thought to follow a variety of inflammatory processes. Gonococcal infection must be considered in connection with obscure proctitis and stricture, and solitary ulcers of doubtful origin are sometimes encountered.

TUMORS OF THE RECTUM.

Single or multiple *polyps of the rectum,* while not very common, are of importance since they may be the source of serious bleedings and they may also undergo malignant change. It is sometimes possible to extirpate them under direct inspection through the proctoscope.

Cancer of the rectum is by far the most important tumor. It occurs more frequently than cancer of any other part of the bowel, and if recognized early a fair proportion of the cases can be cured by radical operation. The tumors are usually adenocarcinomata; they may ulcerate early and develop into huge sloughing or fungating lesions or there may be sclerotic types which narrow or deform the rectum. Metastases take place early in the regional nodes and the liver may be involved even with small primary growths. Later, extensions into the sacrum or other adjacent structures and widespread metastases occur.

The early symptoms are insignificant and some of the most distressing medical tragedies are those cases of cancer of the rectum in which an early diagnosis could have been made had the physician not failed to take these minor complaints seriously. Alteration in the normal bowel habit of any sort, slight constipation or diarrhea, a feeling of discomfort or fullness in the rectum or in the anal region, or bleeding usually comes first. Any of these symptoms, especially in men over thirty-five years of age, call for rectal examination, proctoscopy and careful observation. It is little short of malpractice to ignore the complaint of bleeding, for example, and to tell the patient that it is probably just hemorrhoids. Later the situation becomes obvious when frequent bloody purulent stools are passed or when obstructive symptoms with anemia and cachexia are present.

In the early stages *physical examination* shows nothing remarkable and the condition is recognized by rectal examination. The palpating finger may encounter an irregular projecting mass or it may become engaged in a narrow orifice produced by an annular stricture. There is usually not much local pain. Proctoscopy, of course, reveals the exact state of affairs. In the late stages there are pallor and emaciation and metastatic nodules are sometimes felt in the liver. If obstruction is present there may be abdominal distention.

The *diagnosis* is usually definite. Occasionally it is necessary to rule out non-malignant ulcerations or strictures by biopsy.

The *prognosis*, on the whole, is poor although radical surgical procedures supplemented, perhaps, by radiation occasionally effect a permanent cure. It is also true that what appears to be a small localized lesion may already have given rise to metastases, whereas extensive growths which appear hopeless sometimes do not recur for several years after operation. The technical side of the surgical procedures cannot be gone into here; the operation is always serious and requires great skill and judgment. Palliative measures such as colostomy are, at times, advisable.

HEMORRHOIDS.

Hemorrhoids are, perhaps, the most common disorder of the rectum; in mild form most people are affected at one time or another. As a rule the condition is purely local, but with stasis in the pelvic vessels caused, for example, by back pressure from portal obstruction (cirrhosis of the liver) it may furnish evidence of remote trouble.

Anatomically the disturbance consists of dilatation or varicosity of the rectal (hemorrhoidal) veins. The degree of engorgement varies from time to time, depending upon general or local conditions (constipation) but in extreme cases there are permanent masses which are made up of the dilated veins together with redundant mucous membrane. Ulceration and infection with the fibrosis of chronic inflammation may be superadded and severe anemia may result from prolonged bleeding. A clinical "attack" of hemorrhoids is usually due to prolapse of the hemorrhoidal mass which becomes engaged in or protrudes through the anus. Actual strangulation with necrosis may result.

While constipation, obesity and a sedentary life are set down as the usual causes it must be admitted that many healthy, active and even athletic people are affected. The trouble tends to increase with advancing years and most of the extreme cases occur in middle-aged or elderly people. In women, the effects of childbirth—pelvic relaxation and prolapse of the viscera—often play a part.

The commonest *complaint* is a mild fullness or discomfort in the rectum with or without occasional bleeding. The symptoms are usually periodic and "attacks" with long intermissions are the rule. If the hemorrhoids prolapse there is intense continuous pain in the anus which may be almost unendurable at the time of a movement. External examination may show tags of indurated mucous membrane which sometimes present a rosette-like appearance about the anus, or one or more prolapsed veins present themselves as dusky bluish tense swellings. Further masses may be felt or seen on proctoscopic examination.

The physician is usually called on to relieve one of the periodic attacks. If there is a protruding mass it should be reduced, if possible, by gentle manipulation. The patient lies on his face and bits of ice are applied locally to shrink the congested veins. After reduction an astringent ointment should be freely applied and suppositories should be used two or three times a day until the symptoms have entirely disappeared. There are a great variety of preparations which have been said to possess virtue, of which one may mention especially the well known gall and opium suppository and the tannic acid ointment (20 per cent). Exercise, careful regulation of constipation and reduction of obesity tend to prevent recurrences.

Persistent, extreme or complicated cases present problems which are best deal with by the rectal surgeon. A variety of surgical procedures have been used with good results; an occasional annoying untoward sequel is incontinence of feces because of injury to the rectal sphincter.

DISEASES OF THE LIVER.

Introduction.—The liver may be incidentally implicated in a great variety of diseases a full description of which would carry us into every domain of medicine. It will be necessary, therefore, in the present section to restrict our discussion to those disorders in which the liver bears the brunt of the morbid process; the hepatic lesions of Hodgkin's disease and of leukemia, the changes secondary to cardiac failure, the alterations which occur in Graves' disease, or with amyloid infiltration —to give only a few examples—are dealt with elsewhere in their proper places.

The main diseases of the liver may be grouped under the headings of inflammation and tumor. The former can be further subdivided into suppurative focal hepatitis, including abscess and pylephlebitis, and non-suppurative diffuse hepatitis, acute and chronic, comprising such conditions as acute yellow atrophy, catarrhal (infectious or toxic) jaundice and, finally, cirrhosis. Metastatic cancer is by far the most common tumor; primary cancer and other neoplasms are encountered only occasionally. Syphilis of the liver will be briefly considered as well as malformations and displacements.

In recent years more and more stress has been placed on the functional pathology of the liver, and serious disturbances of protein, carbohydrate and fat metabolism are undoubtedly to be related to disorders of this organ. Failure of the liver to properly detoxicate various injurious substances or products of intermediary metabolism may also lead to clinical difficulties. These syndromes, however, are as yet ill-defined and it remains for the text-books of the future to offer an adequate chapter on this interesting subject.

Methods of Examination.—**History.**—There is usually little in the patient's story which points directly to disease of the liver; the organ can be riddled with cancer or abscesses without there being any local complaint. There may, however, be pain in the epigastric region or upper right quadrant, or the presence of a lump, or a feeling of fullness in the abdomen attracts the patient's attention. Jaundice, if present, is the most outstanding symptom; it will be considered in detail presently.

Physical Examination.—In contrast to the paucity of local symptoms the liver is readily accessible to physical examination. Changes in size and consistency as well as tumors can often be demonstrated with considerable accuracy. Jaundice is readily detectable and one should look for the spider angiomata so characteristic of cirrhosis. Finally the evidences of portal obstruction may make it obvious that disease of the liver exists.

Laboratory Tests.—For many years efforts have been made to devise tests for "liver function." It was hoped that some procedure could be perfected which would not only reveal the presence of hepatic disease or dysfunction but which would make possible a quantitative measure of the degree of damage. These efforts have been successful only in part. A detailed consideration of the problem cannot be given here but the main objection to these tests is that when they indicate extreme impairment of function the situation is usually obvious from the clinical examination alone, whereas in doubtful cases the test is also equivocal. This criticism applies especially to the various "carbohydrate tests" for liver function which in our experience are of no practical use and to a lesser extent to the dye retention tests. Of these the rose-bengal procedure is probably the best. Measurement of the blood bilirubin is of great value (see Jaundice).

Roentgen-rays.—The roentgen-ray is of especial use in gall-bladder disease (see below). The size and position of the liver can sometimes be better determined by roentgenography than by physical examination, and recently there have been attempts to visualize the organ by the intravenous injection of radio-opaque materials which are taken up by the liver. This procedure is still in an experimental stage.

JAUNDICE (ICTERUS).

Jaundice is that disorder in which, as a result of an excess of bile pigment in the blood stream, the tissues become stained a yellow or greenish-yellow color. It arises from various causes and is to be thought of as a symptom rather than as a distinct malady. Jaundice is, however, of such great importance in diseases of the liver and of the biliary tract that special discussion is in order.

To understand the mechanism of the production of jaundice one must have clearly in mind the physiology of bile pigment formation and excretion. Briefly, according to current views, bilirubin (bile pigment) is formed by cells of the reticulo-endothelial system, both in the liver (Kupffer's cells) and elsewhere, from the non-ferrugenous part of the hemoglobin molecule. This is made available by the constant wear and tear and breakdown of the red blood corpuscles. The bile pigments are *excreted* into the bile capillaries by the parenchymal (polygonal) cells of the liver which do not, however, play a part in their formation. From the intrahepatic ducts the bile passes in large part to the gall-bladder where it is concentrated by absorption of water. During digestion especially bile is ejected into the intestine; here it is reduced to stercobilin, part of which is lost with the feces and part of which is reabsorbed to be converted again to bilirubin for further excretion. In certain diseases of the liver some of the pigment reabsorbed from the bowel is put out in the urine as urobilin, presumably because the damaged liver is unable to reëxcrete it as bilirubin. Urobilinuria may therefore give a clue to impairment of liver function.

From the above résumé it is clear that hyperbilirubinemia, the precursor of clinical jaundice, may, theoretically at least, come about in various ways: (1) As a result of excessive blood destruction more pigment is formed than can be excreted even by a normal liver. (2) Damage to the liver cells may impair their ability to excrete the pigment so that it accumulates in the blood stream, and (3) as a result of occlusion of the smaller or larger bile ducts pigment after excretion into them regurgitates into the lymphatics and blood capillaries. All of these mechanisms, often in combination, are actually operative in one or another disease. In congenital hemolytic jaundice, for example, an excess of bile is excreted but, in spite of this, so much pigment is formed that not all can be put out and jaundice results. The best example of icterus due to disease of the liver parenchyma is catarrhal or infectious jaundice; at certain stages inflammatory occlusion of the small bile passages also plays a part. Finally as instances of "regurgitation" jaundice one may mention occlusion of the common duct by cancer or by stone. In practice the vast majority of cases of *intense* jaundice are due to hepatitis, stone or cancer.

In the presence of icterus the problem always comes up whether the hyperbilirubinemia is due to actual disease of the liver (and bile passages) or whether there is an extrahepatic ("hematogenous") cause. If no bile enters the duodenum one may be sure there is disease of the liver or bile passages; the presence of bile in the intestine, on the other hand, does not exclude this possibility, although it should make one consider extrahepatic causes.

Pathology.—With slight degrees of jaundice there is merely an increase of pigments in the blood. When the hyperbilirubinemia is intense or of long standing the body tissues themselves become stained; the color of the scleræ is especially striking. Pigment may actually be deposited in the cells in small granules. The urine contains bile or urobilin which seems to have an injurious effect on the kidney, since its presence is often associated with albumin and casts. The sweat as well as sputum and pathologic body fluids (pleural and peritoneal) are tinged, but not so milk, spinal fluid or lachrymal secretions. When there is occlusion of the bile ducts they become greatly distended and pigments permeate the whole liver substance, giving it an intense bottle-green color.

Clinical Features.—Slight grades of jaundice are hard to recognize clinically. The yellow color is best seen in the scleræ, which may be definitely tinged before skin discoloration is noticeable. In negroes one must depend on inspection of the eyeballs and the mucous mem-

42

branes of the mouth, especially the under surface of the tongue.   In
long-standing intense icterus the skin, at first canary yellow, tends to
assume a dusky greenish cast.   Itching is a prominent feature and the
characteristic linear scratch marks which result from the patient's
clawing are often evident. Certain other systemic effects are to be
noted. The appetite is usually in abeyance and there may be great
aversion to food, especially fat and meat. The pulse is said to be
slow, but this has not been a notable finding in our experience.   In
some cases of intense jaundice there is a tendency to bleeding; practically every factor entering into the coagulation of blood has been
incriminated and the mechanism probably varies with the underlying
disease, diminution of fibrinogen, the presence of a fibrinolytic ferment
and disturbances of calcium perhaps all playing a part at times. The
general depression of jaundice, stressed by the older writers, is undoubtedly real. The patients are often gloomy and discouraged.   The
permeation of the tissues with bile seems to exercise a general "toxic"
effect and to this the relatively high operative mortality of jaundice
cases must in part be ascribed. These patients seem to lack resistance
and they react badly to any trauma or infection. If bile fails to enter
the digestive tract, fats are poorly split and absorbed and, for this as
well as less well-defined reasons, there is often rapid loss of weight and
strength.

Diagnosis.—Jaundice is recognized clinically by inspection of skin
and scleræ and by the appearance of the urine. Slight grades are best
detected by measuring the amount of bilirubin in the blood; quantitative measurements are also of great value in following the trend of
a case. Either the icterus index or the van den Bergh test is useful
in determining whether more than the normal 0.1 to 0.5 mg. per cent
of bile pigment is present.   In our experience the type of van den Bergh
reaction (direct or indirect) has been of no help in differentiating types
of jaundice as some have claimed. With slight degrees of icterus,
regardless of cause, one gets the indirect reaction; with intense jaundice,
always the direct.

Jaundice is rarely confused with other types of pigmentation. It is
said that carotinemia, picric acid and dinitrophenol poisoning may
produce a confusing discoloration.

Prognosis and Treatment.—(See under Special Diseases.)

HEPATITIS (NON-SUPPURATIVE).

One of the main groups of liver diseases includes those cases in which
there are diffuse non-suppurative inflammatory or degenerative lesions.
The process may be violent and rapidly fatal, as in "acute yellow
atrophy," or there may be prompt and complete healing such as
occurs in most instances of hepatitis (infectious jaundice, catarrhal
jaundice). In other cases the early stages are perhaps entirely latent
and the disorder only emerges into clinical prominence in a terminal
stage (cirrhosis). It seems highly advisable in the interests of orderly
thinking to try, tentatively at least, to correlate these various pictures
as has been done so well with nephritis in which an analogous state of

affairs seems to exist. Fig. 36 will serve at any rate as a working basis for our discussion, which may be summarized as follows:

Acute hepatitis: { Acute yellow atrophy.
{ Infectious or catarrhal jaundice.
Subacute hepatitis.
Chronic hepatitis: Cirrhosis of the liver.

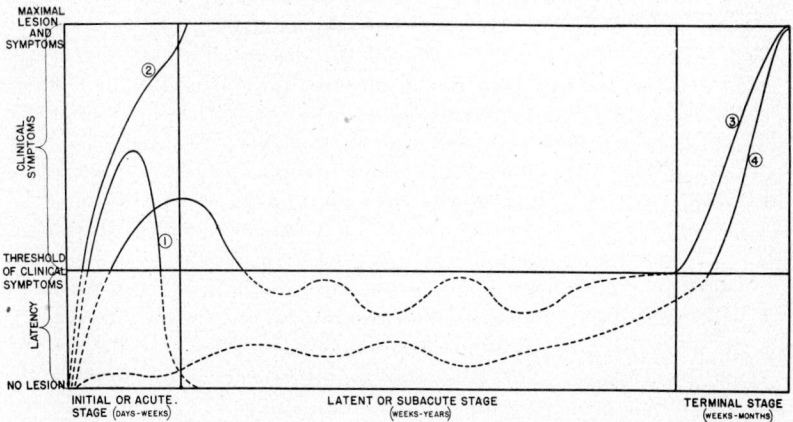

FIG. 36.—1. Acute hepatitis (toxic or infectious) with complete recovery (catarrhal or infectious jaundice). 2. Acute hepatitis (toxic or infectious) with death (including acute yellow atrophy). 3. Acute hepatitis which, after an initial stage, progresses slowly below threshold of clinical symptoms with termination, perhaps after years, with cirrhosis. The initial stage may be entirely subclinical (4). Various other possibilities suggest themselves.

Acute Hepatitis.

Acute Yellow Atrophy.—In certain cases of poisoning by chloroform, phosphorus, trinitrophenol, arsphenamine, cinchophen and other substances there is a widespread necrosis of liver cells. A similar intense hepatitis, usually ending in death within a few weeks, occurs occasionally without any demonstrable cause; this condition is spoken of as acute yellow atrophy. Syphilis, pregnancy and gastro-intestinal infections have been alleged to play a part, but the etiology is unclear.

In extreme cases the liver exhibits nothing short of a devastating lesion. Literally no normal tissue can be seen and only the framework of the lobules and the blood-vessels remains together with an occasional shadow of a liver cell or bits of detritus. The changes are best described as a necrosis. When the damage is less severe areas of more or less intact hepatic cells can be made out, and if the patient lives long enough cellular infiltration and increase of fibrous tissue take place. Grossly the liver is reduced to a fraction of its normal size, it is usually yellowish-brown in color and shows a complete disorganization of structure. There may be some nodules of relatively intact tissue surrounded by flabby shrunken areas. The spleen is sometimes slightly enlarged.

Clinical Features.—The onset is sudden, with the symptoms of a violent gastro-intestinal upset—nausea, vomiting, prostration, and sometimes severe abdominal pain. Fever is usually absent at the start but the pulse is accelerated. After a variable length of time jaundice appears. Otherwise there are no characteristic abnormalities on physical examination, although epigastric tenderness is often present. As time goes by, one can sometimes detect by percussion evidence of shrinkage of the liver. After days or weeks, toxic symptoms—restlessness, delirium, or drowsiness and coma—supervene, the temperature rises, the pulse becomes more rapid and feeble, the blood-pressure falls, there may be bleeding from the mucous membranes and death ensues. The total duration of the disease is about five or six weeks. In occasional cases portal obstruction and ascites have been observed, findings which would make one suspect that a subacute or chronic hepatitis had preceded the final violent outburst. It must be emphasized that while acute yellow atrophy probably deserves to be considered as a clinical entity, it shades off imperceptibly into the more common and less violent form of hepatitis to be considered in the next section (catarrhal jaundice). Furthermore, recovery may occasionally take place, and Goodpasture and others have reported healed lesions, which indicated a previous acute yellow atrophy in people who died later of other causes.

Laboratory Tests.—The leukocyte count is normal or moderately elevated. The urine contains bile, albumin and casts. In the terminal stages the blood urea may be elevated. The occurrence of amino-acids in the urine—leucine and tyrosine—has been emphasized in the literature, but expert chemical technic is required to demonstrate these substances. It is supposed that the liver has lost its deaminizing function. The fibrinolytic ferment of Goodpasture may be present in the blood when there is extreme hepatic insufficiency.

Treatment.—The patient should be kept in bed, and general measures to control shock and prostration are of the utmost importance. One has to cope not only with the effects of the acute liver damage but with starvation, dehydration, acidosis and sometimes impairment of renal function. If the patient can retain nourishment, small amounts of high-carbohydrate foods (liquid and soft) should be given, such as skimmed milk, gruels and fruit juices. Any considerable amount of protein (meat) and fat must for the time being be avoided. If fluids cannot be freely taken *per os*, at least 2 liters should be given daily parenterally in the form of intravenous infusions of 10 per cent glucose and subcutaneous clyses of normal saline. There is some evidence that calcium protects the liver against the toxic effects of injurious agents such as carbon tetrachloride, and 5 or 10 cc. of a 10 per cent solution of calcium chloride may be given daily by vein if no untoward reaction ensues. Insulin, too, has been advised as well as liver extract. If the patient can be tided over the disorganization of body chemistry which occurs with the acute necrosis of the liver, and provided some tissue which can regenerate remains, recovery is at least temporarily possible, although the risk of further slow deterioration (chronic hepatitis) must always be feared.

Infectious (Catarrhal) Jaundice.—There are three principal varieties of infectious jaundice: the spirochetal jaundice of the Japanese, a severe disease with high mortality-rate; epidemic infectious jaundice, a milder disorder the causal agent of which has not been determined, and, finally, sporadic cases of hepatitis, often of unknown etiology, and usually benign in their course. It is the mild variety only which concerns us here.

Etiology.—Hepatitis, mild or severe, may be caused by various poisons such as arsphenamine, cinchophen or phosphorus (see Acute Yellow Atrophy). In most cases, however, the etiology is obscure. Infection by various banal intestinal bacteria as well as vague toxic influences has been stressed but, just as with the etiology of acute nephritis, one deals largely with assumptions. The group is probably not homogeneous, and doubtless various causes operate in different cases. It is reasonable, for example, to assume that in those instances associated with acute gastro-intestinal manifestations, infection may proceed from bowel to liver *via* the bile passages or lymphatics. Syphilitic hepatitis will be discussed in a later section.

Pathology.—The postmortem descriptions are meager since the patients rarely die. Opportunity for inspection of the liver at the height of the disease occasionally occurs when laparotomy is done under a mistaken diagnosis. The organ then is seen to be swollen and firm and stained intensely green by the bile pigments. Biopsies show cloudy swelling of the parenchymal cells and compression and inflammation of the small bile ducts. The larger ducts are patent and the gall-bladder is distended. The hypothetical plug of mucus in the common duct, thought by the older writers to be responsible for the jaundice, is not found.

Symptoms.—The onset may be insidious and jaundice is noticed to the surprise of the patient or his friends while he is at work and feeling quite well. In other cases there is a preliminary period of malaise and lack of appetite, or definite acute gastro-intestinal symptoms (nausea, vomiting, diarrhea) with fever precede by a few days the appearance of icterus. Profound prostration and all the general symptoms of an acute febrile disease are not uncommon.

Physical Examination.—In severe cases the patient is obviously ill and prostrated. The tongue is heavily coated. The liver is enlarged and there is tenderness on pressure over it. The spleen is often palpable. The intensity of the jaundice varies in different cases and with the stage of the disease, but at the height there is usually an intense canary-yellow color.

Laboratory Tests.—There are no specific changes in the red cells, but the leukocytes are often reduced in number to 4000 or 5000 per c.mm. Normal or even increased white cell counts are encountered in some cases. The urine contains bile and there are usually albumin and casts. The stools may or may not contain pigments, depending on the stage of the disease. At the height of the process there is obstruction of the passage of bile into the duodenum as a result of inflammatory occlusion of the small ducts; later, even before the jaundice has cleared up, bile is poured into the bowel, sometimes in great quantities. Material obtained by means of the duodenal tube may show evidences of disease in the form of pus and epithelial cells and abnormal quantities of mucus. The degree of jaundice is best followed by the icterus index or van den Bergh test. At the height of the disease the former may give a reading of as high as 100 or more units.

Course.—The duration of the jaundice varies from two weeks to several months. In the majority of mild cases there is no great disability and often the patient resents confinement to bed. The appetite is poor and there may be positive aversion to insipid foods, especially fat. Itching of the skin is one of the most annoying symptoms. As the disorder subsides the patient feels better, appetite returns, jaundice fades and itching abates. The urine becomes lighter and the stools resume a normal color. The liver ceases to be tender and is no longer palpable and the splenic enlargement subsides. In severe cases fever continues for a variable length of time and as a result of anorexia, gastric discomfort, nausea and diarrhea, loss of weight and weakness may be quite marked and convalescence is prolonged. If visible jaundice persists for over three months there has probably been a mistake in diagnosis, although occasional cases drag on or pass into a progressive subacute or chronic hepatitis.

Chemical tests of the blood even after apparent recovery show a slight clinically undetectable hyperbilirubinemia for long periods of time, and in such circumstances one suspects that latent trouble still exists. It is possible or, indeed, probable that certain cases which begin as an ordinary catarrhal jaundice, after entering such a latent stage, may gradually progress until eventually, perhaps after years, termination comes with the clinical picture of cirrhosis. An instance in point was that of a man, aged fifty-five years, not a user of alcohol, who died in hepatic coma after an abdominal exploration which revealed an advanced cirrhosis. Ten years previously he had had an attack of "catarrhal jaundice" from which he apparently recovered completely, and he remained symptom-free for nine years. We have under observation now a man who three years ago had a mild acute hepatitis with jaundice, the icterus index reading 46. Tests of blood bilirubin have been made at almost monthly intervals ever since, and while he is apparently well the icterus index varies from 9 to 14, a definite elevation, and the edge of the liver continues to be palpable.

The usual forms of infectious or catarrhal jaundice are practically never immediately fatal, although there are all degrees of severity and an occasional patient may die—usually with the variety of the disease associated with fever and severe gastro-intestinal symptoms.

Diagnosis.—A definite diagnosis cannot be made until jaundice appears. Conditions which may lead to confusion are icterus incident to a variety of infectious diseases, and obstruction of the bile ducts especially by stone or cancer. Often time alone will tell, but jaundice in young people preceded perhaps by a gastro-intestinal upset usually turns out to be a simple hepatitis.

Treatment.—Bed rest must be ordered, even in mild cases, until the jaundice has disappeared. Feeding is often difficult because of nausea and anorexia. A simple diet, high in carbohydrate and low in fat should be offered. Fat often produces nausea and, furthermore, it is not well digested when bile is absent from the intestine. Carbohydrate, on the other hand, is thought to protect the liver from damage in various infectious or toxic states. High-protein feeding has been shown to be injurious in certain types of experimental liver injury and it seems wise to restrict meat in clinical cases of hepatitis. Any article of food within reason which will stimulate the appetite may be allowed. Water should be taken freely and the bowels, if constipated, are best regulated by mild saline purgatives such as effervescent phosphate of soda, 30 gm. daily. In very sick patients who have lost much fluid by vomiting or diarrhea, salt solution subcutaneously or intravenous glucose infusions are in order. Feeding of ox-gall or bile salts has accomplished nothing in our hands except to upset the patient still further, nor has lavage of the duodenum with magnesium sulphate proven to be of definite value. For the itching, sponging with a calamine lotion containing phenol 1 per cent, or with a saturated solution of bicarbonate of soda, may be tried. Dusting the body and bedclothes with cornstarch sometimes helps.

Subacute Hepatitis.

We preserve this heading mainly for the sake of completeness in order to emphasize the transitions which exist between acute hepatitis and the chronic end stage (cirrhosis). Every patient who has passed through an attack of catarrhal jaundice must be regarded as a potential candidate for chronic changes, as has been pointed out in the previous section, and from time to time one may actually observe the transition stages. Interesting examples have been reported by Chester Jones.

Chronic Hepatitis (Cirrhosis of the Liver).

Under this designation are included a variety of disorders of the liver featured by a destruction of parenchymal cells with the development of a fibrosis which eventually leads to disorganization of structure and interference with normal function.

Etiology.—Mallory proposes the following grouping: alcoholic cirrhosis (the most common type), pigment cirrhosis, syphilitic cirrhosis, infectious cirrhosis and toxic cirrhosis. In our experience, after syphilitic scarring and those cirrhoses which follow long-standing bile stasis and infection have been excluded, all the other cases may be thrown into one group for the purposes of the clinician. As one sees the disorder in practice the picture as a rule conforms more or less to the type described in the literature as "alcoholic," "atrophic," or "Laennec's" cirrhosis. One wonders whether in our present state of knowledge these designations add much and whether it is not simpler merely to say chronic hepatitis or cirrhosis without further qualification unless an adjective of unequivocal significance can be attached. As a matter of fact, there are probably a variety of factors which play a part in inducing these extreme forms of liver change. A history of excessive use of alcohol is so common that one cannot doubt it often plays a part; on the other hand, cirrhosis occurs in people who take no liquor. Infection of low grade has been emphasized, but at most it is a contributory factor. In brief, why these relentless inflammatory-degenerative changes proceed to ultimate destruction of the liver (*hepatitis*) is as obscure as the cause of progressive chronic *nephritis, arthritis* or *iritis*. We have already developed the concept of cirrhosis as the end-stage of a long-standing latent progressive hepatitis, in turn the outcome of an acute or at least initial process which commenced years previously, and in fact most of the cases are seen in middle life. Men are much more frequently affected than women.

Pathology.—With the "alcoholic" type the liver is small and the surface presents a finely nodular or granulated appearance. Microscopically this is readily correlated with the disorganization of structure. The normal architecture of the lobule is destroyed and there remain irregular clusters of cells, some of which have become markedly hypertrophied, lying between bands of fibrous tissue. The so-called "cirrhosis" which follows bile stasis and infection usually results, on the other hand, in some enlargement of the liver. The main histologic feature is inflammatory change about the bile ducts followed by fibrosis and scarring. In patients who survive a violent acute hepatitis, the end stage consists of a coarse type of scarring which results from the destruction of large areas of liver tissue with a nodular hypertrophy of the surviving islands. Syphilitic cirrhosis will be described later and pigment cirrhosis is discussed under hemochromatosis. The semi-mythical cirrhosis of Hanot is perhaps a variant of the "biliary" type.

When the cirrhotic process obstructs the small radicles of the portal vein there is back pressure with ascites and the portal blood, no longer able to pass freely through the liver, seeks the systemic circulation through other channels. The principal routes for such collateral circulation are (1) from portal vein through the coronary veins of the stomach to the esophageal veins and thence to the superior caval system, (2) *via* enlarged veins in the ligaments of the liver (parumbilical veins) to the superficial abdominal veins and thence up and down to both superior and inferior caval systems, (3) by anastomosis of vessels in the portal system with retroperitoneal veins (of Retzius) and (4) by anastomosis of portal branches with the hemorrhoidal veins and thence to the inferior cava. The esophageal varices, hemorrhoids and dilated superficial abdominal veins so common with cirrhosis are all indications of the enlargement of these channels.

Clinical Features.—The symptoms are the result of impairment of liver function and of mechanical difficulties due to portal obstruction. This concept is the key to the understanding of the complicated clinical pictures which are encountered with cirrhosis, since a patient with great ascites may still have plenty of functioning liver tissue and another may die in coma of hepatic insufficiency with only slight evidences of portal obstruction.

In the early stages of the disease, as we have already pointed out, symptoms may be absent. Initial complaints are swelling of the abdomen or legs (due to portal obstruction and pressure on the inferior vena cava), hematemesis or melena (usually from gastro-esophageal varices) and indigestion or diarrhea (associated with gastritis and congestion of the gastro-intestinal tract). As the disease progresses, weakness, malaise, lack of appetite, mental inadequacy, jaundice, bleeding from mucous membranes and finally stupor or coma are noted in various combinations.

Physical Examination.—The appearance is often characteristic and the diagnosis may be made at a glance. The "hepatic facies"—a bleary appearance of the face with watery, muddy, conjunctivæ and dilated venules over the nose and cheeks—is hard to describe graphically, but once seen is never forgotten; it betokens perhaps the alcoholic element in the situation. Light variable jaundice is the rule. The skin is lax as a result of malnutrition, and large spider angiomata, if present, are absolutely specific of cirrhosis. They are not to be confused with the tiny punctate telangiectases found on any skin. If ascites is present one sees the typical protuberant belly which stands out in contrast to the emaciated chest and extremities. For this striking appearance Boggs suggested the appropriate term of "arachnogastria"—spider-belly. Dilated veins about the umbilicus—the caput Medusæ of classical descriptions—is in our experience practically never seen in outspoken form; when veins are visible the flow can be shown, by stripping, to be centrifugal from the navel. In occasional cases a venous hum is heard on pressing the bell of the stethoscope over the epigastrium. The liver is, of course, best felt after removal of ascitic fluid. Its size varies, but on the whole it tends to be small. One is usually able to feel at or a little below the costal margin a very firm and sometimes irregular edge. The spleen is enlarged often to a considerable degree. Hemorrhoids (congestion of hemorrhoidal veins) are common.

Laboratory Tests.—Patients with cirrhosis are usually pale, even in the absence of gross bleeding. The anemia is typically macrocytic and the blood picture in some respects resembles that of pernicious anemia. The leukocytes are rarely elevated; there is often leukopenia. The urine may show an excess of urobilin and, if jaundice is marked, there is bilirubinuria. Diarrhea and blood in the stools are common. Gastric secretion may be deficient but there is no rule about this. The terminal hemorrhagic tendency is associated with disturbance of fibrinogen formation and with the presence of a fibrinolytic ferment in the blood which, as pointed out by Goodpasture, can be demonstrated by placing a tube of blood in the thermostat for twenty-four hours when the clot will be partly dissolved. This phenomenon, if present, always indicates maximal impairment of hepatic function. The icterus index is moderately elevated and the rose-bengal test is said to show abnormal dye retention in the blood stream. If the diet is inadequately absorbed, nutritional hypoproteinemia with general edema may result.

Course.—Symptoms may progress rapidly and the patient dies within a few months or he may go on with ups and downs for years until coma or some complication terminates the disease. Ascites rarely abates and after tapping the belly is usually full again in two to four weeks. Exacerbations of hepatitis may be associated with increase of jaundice, prostration and gastro-intestinal symptoms. When the liver parenchyma is finally largely destroyed, alterations in the coagulability of the blood (see below) result in oozing from the mucous membranes (gums, nose) and a general hemorrhagic tendency. Finally dullness, stupor and coma supervene and death comes in a state of so-called "cholemia" which superficially resembles "uremic coma." But most patients do not survive to this extremity; they die of some complication. Of these, one of the most frequent is hemorrhage from rupture of esophageal or gastric varices. Next in importance are intercurrent septic infections to which these patients are quite susceptible, or tuberculous peritonitis. Sudden thrombosis of the portal vein is a serious event. Abdominal pain, rapid increase in ascites with bloody fluid, fever and leukocytosis make one suspect this accident.

Differential Diagnosis.—Cirrhosis is confused especially with other disorders in which ascites is present such as chronic peritonitis with perihepatitis (Pick's disease), tuberculous peritonitis and peritoneal carcinosis. The long, variable course with light jaundice, the fascies, the spider angiomata, the small, hard liver and the large spleen usually suffice to make the diagnosis. The conditions usually grouped under the terms splenic anemia and Banti's disease merge imperceptibly with typical cirrhosis; until more is known of the etiology and pathogenesis, differentiation will often be impossible, if indeed these are actually different diseases.

Treatment.—The disease is incurable and the therapeutic problem is to preserve what remains of functioning tissue, to control ascites and to prevent complications. General restriction of activity and safeguarding measures must be worked out to suit the needs of the special case. Heavy physical work should be curtailed and positions involving serious responsibilities for the patient or others must be abandoned. The occurrence of any infection such as a cold or a furuncle calls for bed rest, as do the acute exacerbations of hepatitis with fever and increase of jaundice. The use of alcohol must be foregone and tea, coffee and spices should be taken in moderation. A liberal varied simple diet serves to maintain nutrition, but meat should be restricted because of the evidence of its harmfulness in experimental cirrhosis (Mann).

Ascites is one of the most stubborn and annoying symptoms. Periodic tappings at which 4 to 12 liters of fluid are removed at a sitting are the most useful measure. Sometimes the collateral circulation improves and the ascites becomes less marked. Diuretics (theocin, ammonium chloride and salyrgan) have been extensively used, but in our experience accomplish so little as to be hardly worth while; tappings must be done in any case. Operations supposed to improve collateral circulation have been advocated. The surface of the liver is abraded so as to promote vascular adhesions to the diaphragm and the omentum is sutured into the rectus muscle with the same end in view. No benefit has been seen from these procedures in our cases. Perhaps some of the newer operations designed to reverse the portal circulation through the spleen will yield better results.

Hemorrhage is treated by rest, supportive measures, large doses of iron (iron and ammonium citrate up to 6 grams daily) and transfusion.

The hemorrhagic tendency discussed above calls definitely for transfusion.

In the terminal toxemia little can be done. Transfusion, intravenous infusions of dextrose, stimulants (caffeine) and complete rest may be followed by temporary improvement.

SUPPURATIVE HEPATITIS (ABSCESS OF LIVER).

Abscesses of the liver are large or small, single or multiple. They may be of hematogenous origin in which case they are usually incidents in a general sepsis, they may result from infection through the portal vein (suppurative pylephlebitis), or the organisms come from the bowel (amebic colitis) or from other foci by means of the lymphatic path, along the bile passages or by continuity as in instances of perforation of a stomach already adherent to the liver. In the Stanford series of autopsies the following sources for liver abscess were encountered: pyemia, ulcerative endocarditis, appendicitis, rectal infections, colitis and suppurations in the biliary system. The pyogenic cocci, intestinal bacteria (streptococci and members of the colon group) are usually at fault; even when the primary necrosis is due to the amebas of dysentery secondary bacterial infection usually takes place.

Anatomically all sorts of changes are encountered. In one case the liver may be riddled with hematogenous abscesses of all sizes, in another the radicles of the portal vein, filled with yellow pus, stand out on section like the branches of a tree against the red background of hepatic tissue, and in a third a huge excavation, perhaps of long standing and well encapsulated, disgorges an immense quantity of foul material and detritus. When suppuration occurs in connection with cholangitis, stones or cancer bizarre pictures of great variety result.

From the above outline it is clear that the clinical picture must be subject to wide variations which depend upon the underlying conditions. We shall not attempt therefore to describe liver abscess occurring simply as an incident in a generalized septic infection, but shall confine discussion to those cases in which hepatic suppuration is the outstanding feature. Large (so-called solitary or tropical) abscess occurs especially in those localities where severe dysentery is prevalent. There are usually the general features of a septic infection—chills, fever and sweats with malaise, anorexia, progressive weakness, loss of weight and anemia. Symptoms pointing directly to the abscess can be absent even when it has attained large proportions, or the patient may complain of pain or a dragging full feeling in the abdomen, lower chest or back. The liver is not necessarily palpable, especially when the abscess is near the dome, in which case the enlargement tends to be upward; the signs are those of compression of the lung or of pleurisy, and a mistaken diagnosis of empyema may be made. Downward enlargement of the liver is also common; the surface is usually smooth, but it may be hard and irregular so that one suspects tumor rather than abscess. Tenderness on pressure is the rule and even when the liver cannot be felt, a sharp tap over the lower thorax elicits the telltale wince so suggestive of the presence of pus.

Liver abscess is often overlooked unless one's attention is focused on the possibility. A history of any of the usual precursors is especially important. If, for example, following an appendix operation there develop chills and fever one should always suspect septic thrombophlebitis of the portal vein with suppurative hepatitis. Or if a patient with amebic dysentery or a severe ulcerative colitis shows the general evidences of sepsis, liver abscess should be thought of. The possibility should always be considered with prolonged fevers of obscure origin since the primary focus is sometimes insignificant. Differential diagnosis from collections of pus outside the liver, such as subphrenic abscess, is often impossible.

Polymorphonuclear leukocytosis is the rule, but otherwise the laboratory gives little assistance. Most of the correct diagnoses of liver abscess are made by clinical acumen and not by technical aids. Roentgen-ray evidence of abnormal elevation of the right diaphragm, especially if successive examinations show progressive change, is helpful. The introduction of an aspirating needle for diagnostic purposes is, we believe, quite justifiable and reasonably safe, provided there is a large area of flatness at the right base. The puncture should always be made behind the anterior axillary line. Contamination of the pleura is a theoretical risk, which has never led to actual trouble in our experience. Failure to obtain pus by no means rules out the presence of abscess; even with the abdomen open, the aspirating needle of the surgeon introduced directly over the most suspicious area often fails to yield the contents of a deeply placed abscess.

Evidence of spontaneous healing of liver abscess is occasionally found at autopsy, or perforation through the diaphragm into a bronchus, a rare complication, may be followed by recovery. Progressive failure and death with the picture of sepsis is, however, the rule. Intraabdominal rupture is followed by peritonitis, usually fatal. Incision and drainage is the only effective treatment. The surgical problem is complex, and to obtain good results the services of an expert are necessary. Rest and upbuilding by means of a liberal high-vitamin diet, transfusion and the administration of iron for anemia are useful adjuvants, together with such treatment as is indicated for the underlying or associated lesions. Amebic necrosis, if recognized before advanced excavation has taken place, may be arrested by emetine and other antiamebic drugs, but resort must usually be had to operation.

SYPHILIS OF THE LIVER.

The liver is affected by syphilis in several ways. In the early stages there may be a mild diffuse hepatitis; acute yellow atrophy is said to occur also but it must be an extremely rare event. Late visceral syphilis involves the liver either in the form of a diffuse cirrhosis similar to that described in a previous section (chronic hepatitis) or there are single or multiple gummata which, on healing, lead to a very coarse type of scarring (hepar lobatum). All of these types, at least insofar as they present themselves clinically, are infrequent in general practice; even in a syphilis clinic (Moore) the diagnosis was made only 34 times among 6420 patients.

Clinical Features.—The clinical features of the hepatitis of early syphilis differ in no significant respect from non-syphilitic catarrhal jaundice. The diagnosis is based largely on the presence of other evidence of syphilis and a positive serologic test. The same statement holds in regard to diffuse syphilitic cirrhosis which is clinically indistinguishable from an ordinary atrophic cirrhosis. The scattered gummata of late syphilis, on the other hand, may present fairly definite features, and if in a syphilitic and in the presence of a positive Wassermann test one discovers a coarse lumpy enlargement of the liver perhaps with fever, jaundice or palpable spleen, one is justified in making a tentative diagnosis which becomes a certainty if the constitutional symptoms subside and the liver decreases in size after antiluetic therapy. On the subjective side there is nothing characteristic. McCrae, for example, lists the following complaints: swelling of the abdomen, pain, jaundice, shortness of breath, loss of weight and strength, edema of legs, fever and vomiting.

The most important point for the student to keep in mind is that syphilis of the liver may, on occasion, masquerade as almost any sort of acute or chronic intraäbdominal disease. We have seen it mistaken for such widely different conditions as cancer of the stomach and suppurative cholecystitis. It must be remembered on the other hand, as Wassermann himself emphasized, that a positive complement-fixation test does not make an "organ" diagnosis; even though the test is positive the patient's presenting disease is not necessarily syphilis.

Treatment.—Treatment is that of the underlying syphilitic infection (see article on Syphilis) but there are a few points which require special emphasis. In the first place it is usually safer to defer arsphenamine therapy and to begin with iodide of potash and bismuth for several weeks. Sudden destruction of large numbers of treponemas by the potent arsenicals may be followed by acute therapeutic shock with further damage to the liver. This applies especially to the late types; early benign hepatitis can be safely treated with the arsphenamines. The results, on the whole, are not brilliant and diffuse syphilitic cirrhosis has in our experience been little if at all influenced by specific therapy. The general measures already described in the section on hepatitis are applicable to the syphilitic cases as well.

NEOPLASMS OF THE LIVER.

Metastatic cancer is by far the most common tumor of the liver. Sarcoma is much less frequent. Primary cancer of the liver is a rare disease. When it does occur there is usually an underlying cirrhosis. Very occasionally one encounters other tumors such as large angiomata.

Cancer of the Liver (Secondary).—The primary growth is notably in the area drained by the portal system, especially the gastro-intestinal tract, pancreas and gall-bladder, but even remote cancers such as those of the breast or the thyroid may metastasize to the liver. In Symmers' series of 298 tumor cases there were metastases to the liver in 34 per cent, regional lymph nodes only being more frequently involved. Table 11 gives further details from the Stanford autopsy material.

TABLE 11.

Site of primary tumor.	Metastases to liver (frequency per cent).	
	At autopsy.	Recognized clinically.
Pancreas	81.0	22.0
Gall-bladder	75.0	25.0
Kidney	54.5	27.3
Stomach	40.2	19.3
Breast	38.5	0.0
Bowel	37.0	7.5
Bronchus	33.0	8.3
Rectum	28.0	9.5
Esophagus	21.0	3.0
Prostate	16.0	4.0
Uterus	10.0	0.0
Skin	8.3	8.3 (1 case)
Larynx	7.7	0.0
Tongue	7.7	0.0

Pathology.—The metastases are hematogenous except where there are extensions from neighboring viscera such as the gall-bladder. Hence there are usually multiple nodules of varying size, some of which may attain immense proportions. In extreme cases the liver practically fills the abdomen. On inspection the pale gray or yellowish masses seem to bulge from under the liver surface and on section one notes the compression of the surrounding normal tissue. Tumors reaching the surface may give rise to localized fibrinous exudate, and there is often ascites associated with cancerous implantations in the peritoneum. The centers of large nodules undergo necrosis and softening and occasionally pressure on the larger bile passages leads to jaundice.

Clinical Features.—The findings depend upon the type of primary lesion and the general distribution of the metastases. As regards the liver itself small nodules are unrecognizable; they may even attain considerable proportions before giving local symptoms. If there is any complaint it is likely to be a feeling of fullness or vague abdominal distress. Great pain is rare. The patient himself may note the increasing size of the abdomen or he may actually feel the mass. The findings on examination vary: in one case the liver is barely palpable, whereas in another it may be felt as an immense mass with a hard, irregular surface sometimes studded with large bosses. There is rarely any doubt about identity of the tumorous organ, since the general shape is preserved, it is superficial and it descends freely on inspiration. Jaundice of marked grade is rare and ascites, if present, indicates an associated peritoneal carcinosis. Fever is the rule with rapidly growing necrotic tumors. This does not necessarily indicate secondary infection even where there is great tenderness, but adhesions to adjacent organs, perforation of carcinomatous masses and abscesses, all may occur.

The course is rapidly downhill after the liver is once materially involved, the details of the picture varying with the type and distribution of the primary cancer.

Diagnosis is usually easy, but cirrhosis of the liver and other types of hepatitis, including that which occurs in association with gall stones and syphilis, as well as other hepatic enlargements, may cause confusion. A search for a primary cancer elsewhere or the demonstration of other metastases are the most important points in reaching a diagnosis.

Treatment, including radiation, is entirely ineffective. The indications are to meet urgent symptoms as they arise and to make the patient as comfortable as possible by rest and sedatives.

Primary Cancer of the Liver.—Primary cancer of the liver is a rare disease. It is encountered in less than 1 per cent of autopsies, and in Ophuls' Stanford series of 3000 cases there were only 13 instances. The growths arise from the liver tissue proper, or less often from the smaller bile ducts. They tend to spread into the blood-vessels and secondary nodules may become disseminated throughout the liver. In from 40 to 100 per cent of the cases in various series there was an underlying cirrhosis; previous liver damage thus seems to predispose to subsequent malignant change. Extrahepatic metastases may be found in the regional lymph nodes, in the lungs, bones and elsewhere.

The clinical picture resembles that of cirrhosis except in very rare cases in which the tumor arises in a liver previously normal. Progressive enlargement of the liver with gross irregularities of the surface, bloody ascitic fluid and the demonstration of metastases are the main data upon which diagnosis must be based. The condition is, however, rarely recognized during life unless the examiner has the possibility in mind. Treatment is ineffective and the problem is to meet urgent symptoms as they come up and to make the patient as comfortable as possible.

ANOMALIES OF FORM AND POSITION OF THE LIVER.

No special attention need be devoted in these days to the deformities of the liver formerly so common as a result of the tight lacing of corsets. Transposition of the liver to the left side is a rare anomaly; it occurs as part of a general *situs inversus* and has no clinical significance; except insofar as it may increase the difficulties of diagnosis of abdominal disease. If the probability is thought of, the condition is readily detected by simple physical examination which can be confirmed by the roentgen-ray. In a considerable number of healthy people the liver edge is felt at the costal margin or several inches below. As a rule this is due to a ptosis which involves other organs as well but produces no definite symptoms. Sometimes the liver is not only prolapsed but rotated forward, in which case it is often mistaken for a tumor. Finally there should be mentioned the lappets of liver attached to the gall-bladder which may descend a considerable distance when the latter organ is distended. It has been referred to as a Riedel's lobe, a useless designation.

REFERENCES.

Tests of Liver Function.

ALTHAUSEN, T. L., BISKIND, G. R., and KERR, W. J.: The Rose Bengal Test of Hepatic Function, Jour. Lab. and Clin. Med., 1933, **18**, 954.

BOLLMAN, J. L., and MANN, F. C.: Experimentally Produced Lesions of the Liver, Ann. Int. Med., 1931, **5**, 699.

BLOOMFIELD, A. L., and HURWITZ, S. H.: Tests of Hepatic Function—Clinical Use of the Carbohydrates, Bull. Johns Hopkins Hosp., 1913, **24**, 375.

GOODPASTURE, E. W.: Fibrinolysis in Chronic Hepatic Insufficiency, Bull. Johns Hopkins Hosp., 1914, **25**, 330.

HARROP, G. A., and BARRON, E. S. G.: The Use of Blood Bilirubin Curves as a Test for Liver Function, Jour. Clin. Invest., 1930, **9**, 4; 1931, **9**, 577.

McNEE, J. W., and KEEFER, C. S.: The Clinical Value of the van den Bergh Reaction, Brit. Med. Jour., 1925, **2**, 52.

Jaundice.

BARRON, E. S. G.: Bilirubinemia, Medicine, 1931, **10**, 77.

RICH, A. R.: Pathogenesis of Forms of Jaundice, Bull. Johns Hopkins Hosp., 1930, **47**, 338.

Acute Yellow Atrophy.

WILSON, J. D., and GOODPASTURE, E. W.: Yellow Atrophy of the Liver—Acute, Subacute and Healed, Arch. Int. Med., 1927, **40**, 377.

Infectious Jaundice.

JONES, C. M., and MINOT, G. R.: Infectious (Catarrhal) Jaundice, Boston Med. and Surg. Jour., 1923, **189**, 531.

Cirrhosis of the Liver.

HUGHSON, W.: Portal Cirrhosis with Ascites and Its Surgical Treatment, Arch. Surg,. 1927, **15**, 418.

MALLORY, F. B.: Hemochromatosis and Chronic Poisoning with Copper, Arch. Int. Med., 1926, **37**, 336.

SNELL, A. M.: Clinical Aspects of Portal Cirrhosis, Ann. Int. Med., 1931, **5**, 338.

Syphilis of Liver.

McCRAE, T., and CAVEN, W. R.: Tertiary Syphilis of the Liver, Am. Jour. Med. Sci., 1926, **72**, 781.

DISEASES OF THE GALL-BLADDER AND BILE DUCTS.

Diseases of the gall-bladder and bile ducts may be classified briefly under the headings of congenital deformities, inflammations (cholangitis, cholecystitis), gall stones (cholelithiasis), and neoplasms (especially cancer). Combinations of lesions such as cholelithiasis and cholecystitis, or cholecystitis, cholelithiasis and carcinoma frequently occur and, as already indicated in the previous section, disorders of the bile passages are inextricably involved with disease of the liver proper. It is only for convenience of exposition, therefore, that we discuss these items separately; a composite picture of "biliary tract disease" should really be kept in mind.

CHOLANGITIS.

Cholangitis, inflammation of the bile passages, usually occurs in association with or following some other trouble. Stone, for example, is frequently followed by infection (see above) and the various forms of hepatitis as pointed out in the previous section show inflammatory lesions in the bile passages, especially the small ducts. Hence there are no specific symptoms referable to the cholangitis itself; its presence may be inferred if the proper setting exists.

Under certain special circumstances cholangitis becomes the outstanding lesion and may be directly responsible for death. This applies notably to those cases in which, as a result of obstruction of the common duct (by stone or cancer), the dilated passages filled with stagnant bile become infected, usually by streptococci, staphylococci or colon bacilli. The entire biliary system may then become filled with pus, the walls of the passages are necrotic, abscesses develop through the liver parenchyma and perhaps, by metastasis, in other situations.

If the process is severe the picture is that of a septic infection quite similar to what has already been described under "liver abscess." There is high irregular fever with chills and sweats, loss of weight, anemia, leukocytosis, and tenderness in the hepatic region. The size of the liver varies. Jaundice is usually present.

Treatment.—Treatment is bound up with that of the underlying lesion. In severe cases with pus in the ducts the outlook is always serious and surgical interference is urgently indicated. The accessory measures discussed in connection with liver abscess, especially the forcing of fluids and intravenous glucose injections, are in order.

CHOLECYSTITIS.

Acute Cholecystitis.—Cholecystitis, like cholangitis, usually occurs in association with stone, cancer or some other antecedent lesion. At times, however, a gall-bladder supposedly normal becomes the site of an acute infection. Streptococci, staphylococci and intestinal bacteria are the usual causal agents and the path of invasion may be by the blood stream or along the lymphatics. All degrees of inflammation from a "catarrh" of the mucous membrane up to a deep-seated necrotizing process are seen. Unlike appendiceal infections which so often are followed by perforation, the gall-bladder rarely ruptures; when this accident does occur, infected bile is poured out and a fatal peritonitis usually follows. After recovery from acute cholecystitis a shrunken, fibrous gall-bladder remains.

Symptoms.—The symptoms are those of an acute septic infection: fever, often with chills and sweats, malaise, prostration, nausea and vomiting. Epigastric or abdominal pain is usually present, and on palpation there is tenderness and reflex spasm or rigidity of the abdominal wall in the gall-bladder region. Occasionally a distended gall-bladder may actually be felt. The leukocyte count is elevated to 15,000 to 25,000. Jaundice is not necessarily present.

Treatment.—Treatment varies with the nature of the underlying situation. If there is reason to believe that cholecystitis is associated with a stone impacted in the cystic duct (see article on Gall Stones) immediate operation is indicated. In uncomplicated cases one may wait, keeping the patient absolutely at rest and allowing only sips of fluids by mouth. An ice-bag should be placed over the gall-bladder region. If, in a day or two, fever and symptoms abate and the leukocyte count falls, the process will probably subside; with increasing septic manifestations and a rising leukocyte count it is wiser to operate.

43

Chronic Cholecystitis.—This, like chronic appendicitis, is an elusive entity which has been especially exploited in the surgical literature. Chronic inflammation and scarring of the gall-bladder does, of course, frequently occur, especially in patients who harbor gall stones, but it is very questionable whether the lesion is actually to blame for most of the symptoms attributed to it.

Chronic cholecystitis is alleged to cause indigestion—epigastric discomfort, gas, fullness, burning and sometimes even nausea or vomiting. It is said that a special intolerance to fat exists and that after eating greasy food the symptoms are worse. The author's experience has convinced him that so-called "gall-bladder indigestion" differs in no significant respects from indigestion due to peptic ulcer, to a neurosis or to various reflex disturbances in the abdomen. In other words, to diagnose cholecystitis from the symptoms of indigestion is entirely gratuitous. Discomfort and tenderness in the gall-bladder region are also said to occur, but similar signs can often be elicited in neurotic people with an irritable colon in whom the gall-bladder turns out to be normal.

At operation the surgeon usually is able to convince himself that a lesion actually exists, but the gall-bladders from people who obviously die of other causes often show similar changes at autopsy. The strongest argument against the syndrome of "cholecystitis and indigestion" is that cholecystectomy has led to relief of symptoms in less than one-third of the cases. In brief, unless stone is present or unless there have been previous unequivocal acute attacks, we do not believe that one is justified in making the diagnosis. In doubtful cases a normal gall-bladder visualization after ingestion of tetraiodophenolphthalein helps to rule out cholecystitis.

Treatment.—The treatment which is usually advised is either cholecystectomy or a regimen similar to that discussed under the heading of gall stones (*q. v.*).

CANCER OF THE GALL-BLADDER AND BILE DUCTS.

Cancers of the gall-bladder and bile ducts are rare conditions; in Ophuls' Stanford series each occurred about one-tenth as often as cancer of the stomach. The majority of gall-bladder cancers occur in women with gall stones and the trauma to the mucosa from the concretions is probably a predisposing factor. Cancer of the bile ducts may arise in the common or hepatic ducts or in the papilla of Vater.

The clinical features are variable. If the common duct is occluded progressive intense jaundice results and the diagnosis may be suspected. If jaundice is not present the condition is usually not recognized except at operation or autopsy. A mass due to cancerous infiltration of surrounding tissues or lymph nodes is sometimes palpable, and this, together with general failure, abdominal pain or metastases elsewhere, makes it probable that a cancer exists, although the exact location is as a rule only a guess. In any event complete surgical extirpation is impossible and symptomatic and palliative measures are all that can be done.

CHOLELITHIASIS (GALL STONES).

Cholelithiasis or gall stone disease includes those states in which concretions of various sorts are found in the gall-bladder or bile passages.

Composition and Character of the Concretions.—The study of gall stones is a fascinating chapter and it is difficult by mere description to convey an adequate picture of the variegated characteristics of these concretions. One should study an actual collection of stones or at least some good illustrations.[1] In size they vary from mere particles of gravel to masses which practically fill the gall-bladder; they may be oval or spherical, or when a number exist in close contact the surfaces are faceted. The principal ingredients are cholesterin, bile pigments and calcium together with other salts and organic material in smaller amounts. One of the most interesting things about gall stones is that they seem to be laid down in crops so that all the stones found in a certain gall-bladder usually are similar and appear to have originated at the same time. On cross-section the stones frequently show concentric layers of material of varying composition which gives an appearance not unlike the rings of a tree; these layers clearly indicate successive deposits of material. The number of stones which may be found in a single gall-bladder varies from one—usually a large oval cholesterin stone—to many, perhaps hundreds of smaller pigment concretions.

Pathogenesis of Gall Stones.—The huge literature on the pathogenesis of gall stones—clinical, experimental and speculative—has led to no generally accepted view. Briefly the factors which have been stressed are stasis of bile, infection and perversions of cholesterin metabolism. Without entering into controversial details it seems impossible to escape the fact that abnormalities in the way the body handles cholesterin play an important part; but whether the abnormality consists of excessive excretion, disturbances of the bile-concentrating mechanism or the intervention of unknown factors is not clear. It also seems logical that stagnation of bile and alteration in the reaction might promote precipitation, although arguments against such a mechanism have also been advanced. Whether stone occurs in the entire absence of infection (inflammation) is also difficult of proof; certain it is that infection often occurs in bile passages, the seat of concretions and plays an important part in the ultimate picture, although in the Stanford autopsies 62 per cent of the gall-bladders containing stones were apparently normal (Ophüls). The fact that stones are common in obese women who have passed through pregnancies has been linked with the theories of stasis and of disturbed cholesterin metabolism.

In the Stanford series gall stones were found in 7.1 per cent of all autopsies—5.86 per cent of all males and 10.65 per cent of all females. These figures are in accord with the general impression that cholelithiasis is two to four times as common in women as in men. In the age period from twenty to thirty years, the incidence was only 1.2 per

---

[1] Beautiful photographs in color of gall stones are to be found in Bethe-Bergman: Handbuch der normalen und pathologischen Physiologie, 1929, vol. 4.

cent; this steadily increased to a figure of 19.1 per cent in subjects over 70 years of age. Stones were found in the gall-bladder alone in nearly 90 per cent of the cases, in gall-bladder and ducts in something less than 10 per cent, and in the ducts alone in only 3 per cent of 206 cases.

Clinical Features.—Gall stones may exist for years without producing any definite symptoms and they are often found at autopsy as an incidental finding. Some writers, especially in the surgical literature, believe that eventually trouble always occurs; of this we are not entirely convinced. It is difficult, at any rate, to paint a composite picture and we shall discuss separately the most outstanding syndromes which are associated with cholelithiasis.

Reflex Symptoms of Gall Stones.—Organic disease of any sort in the abdomen may manifest itself by the occurrence of reflex gastric disturbances—indigestion. Such symptoms as may be set up in patients with gall stones—fullness and discomfort in the epigastrium, gas, burning and eructations—differ, however, in no essential respect from those occurring in association with peptic ulcer, chronic appendicitis or in purely neurotic conditions, and the relationship is only proved if removal of gall stones leads to relief of the trouble. In other patients there may be vague discomfort in the epigastrium or right upper quadrant, sometimes exaggerated after eating fatty food. The occurrence of symptoms of this sort in stout middle-aged women should always arouse a suspicion of cholelithiasis. Physical examination usually yields no specific findings; there may be slight tenderness on pressure below the right costal margin. Jaundice rarely occurs except in more outspoken disorders such as stone in the common duct.

Biliary Colic.—If a stone becomes impacted in the neck of the cystic duct, biliary colic results. The attacks may occur frequently or only at rare intervals. They come especially at night and the onset is usually rather abrupt. There is an intense deep-seated cramp-like or colicky pain in the epigastrium radiating more or less over the upper abdomen and often to the back and toward the right shoulder. The pain is continuous but waxes and wanes in intensity; the patient vainly seeks a comfortable position; he gets up, he lies down, he does not know what to do. Nausea is the rule and vomiting frequently occurs but brings no special relief. Unless mitigated by morphine or by other means the attack is likely to last through the night or for several hours, when the severity gradually abates. For a day or two afterward there is often prostration and slight nausea. One presumes that the colic subsides after the stone either drops back into the gall-bladder or (more rarely) is passed by way of the common duct.

Physical examination during the attack shows the objective evidence of pain and prostration. During violent bouts the face is drawn, sweat breaks out and the patient groans or grunts. The pulse may be accelerated and sometimes there is slight fever. The upper abdomen is held tensely but in contrast to peritonitis gentle pressure gives some relief and does not increase the pain.

Stone in the common duct does not usually produce the violent colic described in the preceding paragraph. The onset is often insidious, the symptoms being compounded of indigestion, upper abdominal pain of variable severity and general malaise and failure. At some time during the disease jaundice is likely to occur; it may come and go; it may be light or intense. Physical examination aside from icterus again yields little that is specific, although there may be tenderness in the upper epigastrium or a palpable liver edge. Associated low-grade infection often causes fever and leukocytosis. This is exquisitely shown in the so-called intermittent biliary fever of Charcot where there may be violent chills with a widely swinging fever of septic type, even in the absence of marked inflammation. The situation is perhaps analogous to the chill and fever which occur after mechanical manipulation of the lower urinary tract.

Gall Stones Associated with Cholecystitis and Cholangitis.—If a stone impacted in the cystic duct does not drop back into the gall-bladder the organ may become greatly dilated. Eventually the bile pigments disappear and there is an accumulation of more or less colorless watery mucoid secretion. This rare condition is spoken of as hydrops of the gall-bladder. In other cases an impacted stone compresses the cystic artery and necrosis and infection of the gall-bladder follow; instead of the colic clearing up there is increasing fever, tenderness and prostration. Unless the situation is dealt with surgically empyema of the gall-bladder followed by rupture, peritonitis and death usually ensue. This is one of the most serious incidents of cholelithiasis and should be watched for in every instance of biliary colic. Aside from such violent catastrophes insidious infections often occur with stones in the biliary passages. The most amazing pathologic consequences may result—fibrosis and obliteration of the gall-bladder, stenosis of the ducts, partial perforations with adhesions whereby stones may ulcerate through the walls of the passages and become encapsulated in the peritoneum. Occasionally stones which have passed into the bowel produce intestinal obstruction. The exact nature of such complications is rarely recognized except at operation or autopsy. They are to be kept in mind in patients with a background of gall-bladder disease when atypical symptoms arise. Diffuse cholangitis with hepatitis or actual liver abscess are exceedingly grave complications.

Diagnosis of Cholelithiasis.—Gall stones may occasionally be demonstrated in the plain roentgen-ray plate, but usually there is not enough calcium in the concretions to render them radio-opaque and cholecystography must be employed. If the dye is properly concentrated the stones stand out as radiolucent spots against the opaque background. It must always be remembered that the mere demonstration of gall stones does not prove them to be the cause of the patient's complaints. Many a gall-bladder has been removed without producing a cure and some other cause for the trouble is subsequently discovered.

Typical biliary colic is not likely to be confused with other conditions, especially if one considers the general setting of the attacks and the age and sex. Renal colic is usually distinctly unilateral and pain radiates to groin and leg rather than upward. Stone in the common duct with jaundice can readily be confused with cancerous occlusion of the bile passages and with infectious jaundice; here the essence of the diagnosis is time. Gastric crises of tabes, lead colic and spasm or obstructions of the bowel occasionally cause mistakes, and coronary occlusion, if the pain is confined to the lower sternum or epigastrium, may to some extent mimic biliary colic.

In cases complicated by infection and septic phenomena exact diagnosis is extremely difficult and here very careful analysis of the past history is especially helpful. In general it may be said that the most useful data in diagnosis of cholelithiasis are the "background," *i. e.*, age, sex and habitus, jaundice if present or definitely known to have been present, the character of the symptoms and cholecystography. Physical findings usually are of little help.

Prognosis.—Stone in the gall-bladder, if no infection follows, may be carried indefinitely without serious symptoms, but colic or the graver septic complications may come as a rude shock at any time. Common duct stone on the other hand is always serious. The concretions in this case are usually multiple and jaundice and infection are likely to complicate the picture.

Treatment.—**Medical.**—There is no method whereby gall stones can be dissolved or made to pass into the duodenum. Medical treatment is directed, therefore, toward the relief of symptoms and, if possible, the prevention of further stone formation.

During an attack of acute biliary colic the patient should be kept quiet and heat should be applied to the epigastrium—a hot bath may give some relief. As soon as the diagnosis is made morphine in full doses (gr. $\frac{1}{4}$ to $\frac{1}{2}$, hypodermically) is indicated. This is the sovereign remedy; it not only relieves the distress but tends to shorten the attack. Atropine (gr. $\frac{1}{120}$ to $\frac{1}{60}$) may be given with the morphine. For a day or two after the severe colic has subsided, rest is advisable and the diet should consist of fruit juices, cereals and thin milk. If there is any reason to believe that a pyogenic infection of the gall-bladder has supervened (high, persistent fever, leukocytosis of over 15,000 to 20,000, and tenderness over the gall-bladder region) it is wiser to operate than to risk a fatal sepsis.

Patients known to carry gall stones had better remain in the vicinity of a center where adequate surgical aid can be obtained on short notice. Excessive weight should be reduced by restriction of fats and sweets (see section on Obesity), and constipation is to be avoided. A good deal of stress has been placed on diet, but it must be admitted that many of the complicated lists which are given to patients seem to have no rational basis. It has been definitely shown that large amounts of fat either reflexly or, more probably, by means of a chemical (hormonic) mechanism stimulate the gall-bladder to contract, and in actual fact a fatty diet leads in many gall-stone patients to discomfort or even to colic. It has also been claimed on theoretical grounds that a diet high in fat or cholesterol leads to excessive excretion of cholesterol into the bile and promotes gall-stone formation, although in practice this proposition is not proved. On the other hand, if fat is well borne it may be useful in stimulating the gall-bladder to contract, thereby keeping up free drainage of bile and preventing stasis. The whole subject is confused by conflicting theories as to the formation of gall stones, and our feeling is that no very elaborate dietary prescription is usually necessary. The food should be simple and plainly cooked without high seasoning. Fats (cream, butter, egg yolk, lard, olive oil) should be restricted provided their use produces symptoms. If there is evidence of hepatitis meat should be taken sparingly. Carbohydrate can be used freely. Many patients do just as well on a simple general diet as on a prescription and avoid the mental hazard which is likely to ensue on a restrictive regimen.

Indications for Surgical Interference.—It is doubtful if interference is indicated for the first or even the second biliary colic if evidence of infection is lacking. When the attacks come frequently, operation is advisable provided the patient's condition allows. It must be recalled that stone often occurs in elderly people with hypertension, myocarditis, diabetes and other disabilities which increase the surgical hazard. Stone in the common duct should be treated surgically just as promptly as possible; if one waits the operation usually must be done later under the disadvantageous conditions of an emergency or complication. Definite infection in association with stone usually renders operation advisable, but the decision in the individual case may be extremely difficult. No simple rule can be laid down and the best judgment obtainable must be enlisted.

STENOSIS AND CONGENITAL OBLITERATION OF THE BILE PASSAGES.

Stenosis of the ducts in connection with stone and cancer is discussed elsewhere in this section. Cicatrices following inflammation, external adhesions and pressure from enlarged glands occasionally lead to obstruction of the larger ducts. The findings are those of obstructive jaundice. Parasites (flukes) in certain localities such as China are a not uncommon cause of bile duct obstruction. Congenital obliteration of the bile ducts is a very rare condition, the exact origin of which is not clear. The child shows a progressive jaundice with absence of bile from the bowel, and it usually dies within a few months.

REFERENCES.

Aschoff, L.: Lectures on Pathology, New York, 1924.

Ferguson, A. N., and Palmer, W. L.: Cholecystography: A Study of 2070 Cases, Jour. Am. Med. Assn., 1933, **100**, 809.

Graham, E. A., Cole, W. H., Copher, G. H., and Moore, S.: Diseases of the Gall-bladder and Bile Ducts, Philadelphia, Lea & Febiger, 1928.

Judd, E. S., and Baumgartner, C. J.: Malignant Lesions of the Gall-bladder, Arch. Int. Med., 1929, **44**, 735.

Mentzer, S. H.: Anomalous Bile Ducts in Man, Jour. Am. Med. Assn., 1929, **93**, 1273.

Twiss, J. R., and Greene, C. H.: Dietary and Medical Management of Diseases of the Gall-bladder, Jour. Am. Med. Assn., 1933, **101**, 1841.

Walsh, E. L., and Ivy, A. C.: Observations on the Etiology of Gall Stones, Ann. Int. Med., 1930, **4**, 134.

DISEASES OF THE PANCREAS.

Introduction.—The more important diseases of the pancreas may be classified under the headings of inflammations (acute and chronic pancreatitis, abscess) and tumors (especially cancer and cysts). Disorders of the external secretion occur mainly in connection with occlusion of the large pancreatic ducts. Derangements of the internal secretion of the islands of Langerhans (diabetes mellitus, hyperinsulinism) are dealt with elsewhere in this book. Except in the case of large tumors or cysts, the pancreas is not directly accessible to physical examination, and trouble in this organ must be inferred mainly from the evidences of disturbed secretion or from remote effects, such as the jaundice which occurs as a result of pressure on the common duct by cancer.

Deficiency of the external secretion (absence of ferments) leads to failure of digestion, especially of fats and, to a lesser extent, of meat; hence stools which contain an abnormal quantity of fat or of muscle fibers suggest pancreatic disease. The concentration of ferments in the duodenal content can be measured but the methods are difficult and unreliable and they are not to be recommended for general use.

PANCREATITIS.

Acute Pancreatitis.—Acute pancreatitis is really a violent necrosis of the gland which results from the liberation into its substance of digestive ferments. In approximately one-half the cases, impaction of a stone in the ampulla of Vater leads to a diversion of bile, usually infected, into the pancreatic ducts, and this is thought to activate the pancreatic enzymes. In other cases an accessory duct opening by itself into the duodenum may allow regurgitation of intestinal contents and ferments, but in a good many instances no anatomical reason for entry of abnormal material into the pancreatic ducts can be demonstrated. In any event the lesions consist of intense widespread necrosis of pancreatic tissue with hemorrhage. The organ may appear as a swollen bloody mass and no normal acinar tissue can any longer be recognized, even under the microscope. Escape of lipase into the peritoneal cavity leads to the classical areas of fat necrosis—small opaque whitish spots—in the omentum and other fatty tissues. Peritonitis finally results. Rich and Duff have recently described a specific form of vascular necrosis which they believe explains the hemorrhages into and about the gland. They also report the presence in autopsy material of localized duct obstructions from concretions and epithelial metaplasia which may perhaps lead to rupture of acini and escape of pancreatic juice into the gland tissues.

The condition is a rare one; it was found only nine times in the Stanford series of 3000 autopsies.

Clinical Features.—Acute pancreatitis is one of the catastrophes of medicine. The onset is usually sudden with violent general or upper abdominal pain, nausea, vomiting and prostration. There may be acute shock with feeble rapid pulse, sweating and low blood-pressure. The temperature rises, often to high levels. On examination one is usually struck by the profound collapse, but little in the way of objective findings is at first to be made out in the abdomen. Within a few hours, however, the signs of peritonitis—great tenderness and reflex rigidity—appear. Unless there is surgical interference the course is rapidly downhill and spontaneous recovery rarely takes place. There is increasing prostration and within a few days the patient dies with the picture of general peritonitis.

The leukocyte count is increased; there are no specific laboratory data.

Diagnosis.—The correct diagnosis is rarely obvious and it is only by keeping the possibility in mind that the condition is recognized clinically. Acute abdominal accidents of all sorts, such as perforated peptic ulcer, suppurative appendicitis, and acute intestinal obstruction must be excluded. The violence of the symptoms and the profound collapse should rouse one's suspicions of pancreatitis.

Treatment.—An occasional patient can be saved by prompt laparotomy with drainage. Medical therapy is of help mainly as a preliminary to operation and afterward. Measures to combat shock—morphine, intravenous glucose and subcutaneous salt solution—may help to tide one over the crisis of the disease. In those who survive the acute features of hemorrhagic pancreatitis suppuration may ensue with a fistula through which bits of pancreatic tissue are discharged, sometimes for long periods. There may be localized abscesses which require secondary operation. Rare cases have been reported in which diabetes mellitus followed recovery from acute pancreatitis.

Chronic Pancreatitis.—Chronic pancreatitis is a vague entity, as a rule not clearly recognizable during life. At autopsy a certain amount of fibrosis, usually detectable only with the microscope, is found in a good many elderly people, but it is doubtful if this leads to any clinical symptoms. Stress has recently been placed by surgeons on low-grade pancreatitis, which they claim occurs in connection with chronic biliary tract infection. It is thought that bacteria or toxic material passing by way of the lymphatics causes pancreatic damage manifest at operation as enlargement or induration of the gland. In the author's experience the whole matter is difficult of interpretation and unless there is definite evidence of disturbance of pancreatic function, which rarely is the case, the diagnosis is unjustifiable.

CANCER OF THE PANCREAS.

Cancer of the pancreas must be classed among the common neoplasms of the abdomen. In the Stanford series the frequency was about one-third that of cancer of the stomach. It occurs almost always in people over thirty years of age, especially men. Histologically the growths are said to arise either from the duct epithelium or from the acinar cells. The island cells are rarely the point of origin. There is an infiltration of the gland and the tumor is usually not of great size. Implication of the pancreatic and common bile ducts leads to important symptoms (see below). In the Stanford series the liver and regional lymph nodes were involved in over 75 per cent of the cases; other common sites for metastases are peritoneum, lung and adrenal. Deposits in bone are rare.

Clinical Features.—The early symptoms are often vague. There may be indigestion, deep-seated abdominal distress, general loss of weight and strength or anemia. If fever is present an infection may be suspected. Occasionally the first manifestation results from distant metastases. If the growth arises in the head of the pancreas, characteristic symptoms follow invasion and obliteration of the ducts at the ampulla of Vater—progressive intense jaundice (see article on Jaundice) which may be the initial symptom, and digestive disturbances due to the exclusion of bile and pancreatic juice from the duodenum. On physical examination the tumor itself is rarely palpable. The most striking finding is the icterus; in some cases it is possible on inspection and palpation to demonstrate distention of the gall-bladder which may reach the size of a large pear unless previous inflammation and fibrosis prevent it from dilating. Metastases may be detected in the lungs (roentgen-ray) or occasionally in the glands above the left clavicle. Growths arising in body or tail of the pancreas give no specific signs and are rarely correctly diagnosed.

Laboratory Findings.—Anemia is the rule; it may be severe. If bile and pancreatic juice are excluded from the intestine the stools become soft, gray and pasty from excess of undigested fat. There is a great increase of bilirubin in the blood (icterus index 100+) and bile appears in large amounts in the urine. Glycosuria is rare even with large tumors.

Course.—The course is that of any malignant tumor with progressive weakness and emaciation. Fever is common. The size and situation of the metastases lead to variations in the picture.

Diagnosis.—The possibility of cancer of the pancreas should be considered in any case of obscure abdominal disease. In patients with jaundice hepatitis and common duct stone are to be ruled out, but intense progressive icterus with complete absence of bile and pancreas ferments from the bowel is in favor of cancer.

Treatment.—Medical treatment is purely symptomatic. The roentgen-ray is useless. In the cases with jaundice, anastomosis of the gall-bladder to the stomach or duodenum (cholecystgastrostomy or duodenostomy) leads to rapid clearing of the jaundice and relief from the annoying symptoms resulting from it. Digestion and nutrition are improved by returning the bile to the duodenum in this way, and if the tumor remains localized the patient may have several years of comfort before the downhill course is resumed.

CYSTS OF THE PANCREAS.

Pancreatic "cyst" may result from the retention of fluid in a dilated duct or from cystic changes in a tumor such as an adenoma. The condition is a rare one. There are no specific symptoms and the complaints are referable to pressure on neighboring viscera. There may be indigestion or a feeling of fullness. The tumor, if palpable, presents in the upper abdomen usually to the left of the mid-line. In the two instances seen by the author the masses were mistaken respectively for spleen and left kidney. They may be smooth or nodular, stony hard or fluctuant. Pancreatic cysts are said to be fixed, but in one of his cases the mass descended freely on inspiration. The treatment is surgical. The operation should be done only by an expert because of the difficulties both of excision and of preventing subsequent fistulæ.

PANCREATIC CALCULI.

Calculi in the pancreatic ducts occurred only twice in Ophüls' series of 3000 autopsies. The stones are usually small and unproductive of symptoms but occasionally colic results. It is indistinguishable from that due to gall stones. The diagnosis is rarely made; one usually thinks of some other hollow viscus colic. Since pancreatic calculi are often radio-opaque the diagnosis can sometimes be made by the roentgen-ray. Unless the colics are violent and frequent, and unless there are evidences of pancreatitis, interference had best be avoided.

REFERENCES.

FRIEDENWALD, J., and CULLEN, T. S.: Pancreatic Cysts, Am. Jour. Med. Sci., 1926, **172**, 313.
KIEFER, E. D.: Carcinoma of the Pancreas, Arch. Int. Med., 1927, **40**, 1.
OPIE, E. L.: Diseases of the Pancreas, Philadelphia, 1903.

DISEASES OF THE PERITONEUM.

ACUTE GENERAL PERITONITIS.

The peritoneal cavity occasionally becomes infected by way of the blood stream, but in the vast majority of cases peritonitis results from perforation of an intraäbdominal viscus or by direct extension. Viscera which rupture and spill foreign material and bacteria into the peritoneal cavity are above all the appendix (acute appendicitis), the stomach and duodenum (peptic ulcer), the intestine (typhoid ulcers) and, less frequently, the gall-bladder (purulent cholecystitis) and other organs. Cancerous foci in the abdomen (stomach, colon) may become eroded and discharge material which sets up peritonitis. But even without actual rupture infection can extend from inflamed viscera to the peritoneal surfaces. This is notably so of intestinal obstruction and acute pancreatitis. In addition to the above, there should be mentioned peritonitis following surgical operation and traumatic rupture of viscera such as the urinary bladder. Peritonitis is said to result from entry of sterile irritants such as bile into the peritoneum, but infection usually plays an important part.

It is evident, therefore, that the causes of peritonitis are complex and manifold, and that the picture will be modified by the underlying condition. The anatomic changes in the peritoneal membranes are, however, always much the same. At the start of infection the surfaces are intensely hyperemic, they lose their normal moist glistening appearance and histologically there is a desquamation of the superficial cell layers. Fibrin is soon poured out and coils of intestine, viscera and omentum tend to be glued together by sticky exudate. Finally there may be an immense accumulation of pus which pours out when the abdomen is opened. The remarkable tendency which the omentum has to become plastered over areas of beginning peritonitis, as well as the sticky character of the early exudate, often results in the infection becoming localized or walled off; an abscess, which is much less serious and more amenable to therapy than a generalized infection, then develops. In some cases, for unknown reasons, this protective reaction is inadequate or in abeyance and no localization of the process occurs. Under certain conditions peritonitis is confined to the lesser peritoneal sac.

In Ophüls' series of 3000 autopsies acute suppurative peritonitis was encountered 125 times. In 10 cases only was the infection "primary." In 63, peritonitis resulted from perforation of the stomach or intestines, and in 19 by extension from various viscera. Infection during surgical operation accounted for 29 more cases, and in only 4 was peritonitis metastatic from a distant focus of infection. Almost any organism may be at fault; inasmuch as perforation of stomach, bowel and intestine are such common causes of peritonitis, colon bacilli, streptococci and other intestinal bacteria are likely to predominate in the exudate.

Clinical Features.—The symptomatology varies with the underlying condition but as regards the peritonitis itself there is a fairly typical sequence of events. The onset is sudden and the outstanding feature is severe abdominal pain. It is usually widespread but, for a time at least, may be localized in one or another part of the belly. With the pain there are prostration, nausea, vomiting and malaise, and sometimes faintness and collapse. Fever is the rule. The typical objective findings are those of shock—rapid feeble pulse with low blood-pressure, cold, clammy extremities and the pinched, anxious expression described as long ago as Hippocrates. The abdomen is exquisitely tender and on pressure there is usually a reflex tightening of the abdominal muscles. In extreme cases there is the classical "board-like" rigidity of the belly wall. The bowel is paralyzed and distended. There is rarely enough fluid to contribute materially to the abdominal distention but flatness in the flanks which shifts on change of position can occasionally be demonstrated. Absence of peristaltic gurgling is notable on auscultation; very rarely friction rubs can be heard over the liver. General peritonitis is a serious disease with high mortality and unless prompt measures are instituted the patient usually dies in a few days. Toward the end there is often a curious septic state; the patient may be abnormally alert and, intoxicated by the poisons which he has absorbed, he no longer complains of any special discomfort although the pulseless, clammy extremities, high fever and rapid, feeble heart action proclaim the imminence of death. In other cases there are flightiness or delirium or he lapses into a stupor. The leukocyte count is elevated; laboratory tests otherwise are of no help in diagnosis.

The recognition of peritonitis is usually easy; the exact diagnosis of the accident which has precipitated it is often extremely difficult and it may be impossible to tell whether rupture of a peptic ulcer, appendicitis, pancreatitis, intestinal obstruction or some other lesion has preceded the catastrophe. A careful consideration of the past history and the events immediately antecedent to the accident is of great help. In our experience the presence of general peritonitis has been overlooked until it is too late to help mainly in the cases in which rigidity of the abdominal wall is not outstanding. Extreme generalized abdominal *tenderness* with the evidence of *bowel paralysis* (failure of bowels to move, absence of peristalsis), together with the general features which have been described justify the diagnosis even when the belly is not rigid.

Treatment.—Prompt surgical intervention is imperative, although it must be admitted that the resistance of the patient must in any case play a large part in recovery. However, the repair of a perforation so that leakage of infected material ceases and the insertion of drains to the source of the trouble seem logical procedures. Accessory measures consist of absolute bed rest, good nursing and the introduction parenterally of salt solution and glucose. Two to 4 liters of fluid should be gotten in daily—500 to 1000 cc. of 10 per cent dextrose intravenously and 1 to 3 liters of saline subcutaneously. Until improvement sets in nothing except sips of water should be given by mouth; one desires to keep the abdominal contents as far as possible at rest in order to promote localization of the infection. Persistent vomiting, especially when large quantities of "fecal" material accumulate in the stomach, requires frequent lavage or continuous aspiration through a small nasal tube. The general shock is best combated by morphine, which should be used freely in doses of $\frac{1}{6}$ to $\frac{1}{3}$ grain hypodermically. For collapse one may try elevation of the foot of the bed, application of heat to the extremities, small doses of whiskey, and caffeine sodium benzoate hypodermically (gr. iii to v—0.2 to 0.32 gm.).

LOCALIZED PERITONITIS (ABSCESS)—ACUTE AND CHRONIC.

Autopsy frequently reveals adhesions and scars which remain as the legacy of localized peritonitis from which the patient has recovered. In clinical cases, also, the infected area sometimes becomes walled off between adjacent viscera or by the omentum, and an abscess results. The most common situations are in the pelvis in connection with pelvic inflammatory disease, between coils of intestine after perforation of the appendix, below the dome of the diaphragm (subphrenic abscess), in the lesser peritoneal sac from perforation of the stomach, and between viscera such as the stomach and liver (peptic ulcer, cancer of the stomach). In some cases multiple pus pockets form in various parts of the peritoneum. The picture will obviously vary with the antecedent events and with the size and situation of the abscess; no all-inclusive description can be given. The following points are of importance: The presence of general evidences of a septic infection such as fever, sweats, malaise, rapid pulse and leukocytosis, and localized abdominal pain or tenderness. Rectal and pelvic examinations are of special importance in localizing pelvic abscesses, if tenderness or the presence of a mass can be detected. Subphrenic abscess (see article on Liver Abscess) is readily confused with empyema, especially if the collection of fluid is large and if there is collateral effusion into the pleural cavity; the roentgen-ray is helpful in locating the position of the diaphragm. In general, minute attention to the history, pains-taking physical examination and, above all, clinical skill and experience are necessary in diagnosis of these conditions.

The presence of abscess may be entirely overlooked and the case masquerades as one of obscure fever, typhoid or some other infection, or a diagnosis of cancer, gall stones, or other intraäbdominal disease may be made, especially if pain or gastro-intestinal symptoms pre-dominate without much fever. The violence of the symptoms varies and it should be emphasized that some of these cases run the long course of a chronic septic infection with a lapse of months before death or recovery takes place. The abdominal abscess may be the source from which septic emboli reach other parts of the body such as the liver, lungs or brain.

Treatment.—The treatment is essentially surgical, but the decision as to when the abscess has reached an optimum degree of encapsulation requires nice judgment. No rules can be laid down. Repeated oper-ations are necessary in some cases if extension takes place or if there are multiple pus pockets.

CHRONIC ADHESIVE PERITONITIS.

Chronic adhesive peritonitis is a rare condition; it was present only 9 times in the Stanford series of 3000 autopsies. The etiology is obscure. Low-grade infection with the tubercle bacillus or other organ-isms has been claimed but not proved, and cultures from the peri-toneum yield no growth. The lesions consist of diffuse or localized areas of peritoneal thickening both of the visceral and parietal sur-faces. The affected areas have a dull gray appearance and the viscera, especially the liver, may be covered with a thick layer of fibrous tissue like the icing of a cake. Localized bands sometimes cause intestinal obstruction. The peritonitis is occasionally associated with adhesive pleuritis and pericarditis—polyserositis. The relation of this group of lesions is not clear but it is of interest that experimental pericardial injuries with adhesions may be followed by chronic peritonitis with ascites (Herrmann).

The clinical onset is usually insidious. There is a gradual swelling of the abdomen and it soon becomes evident that there is free fluid in the peritoneum. The general health is usually not seriously affected; in the cases with pericarditis cardiac symptoms may supervene. On examination ascites is the striking feature, but the signs of collateral circulation evident in cirrhosis are absent. The liver is enlarged, firm and smooth, and the spleen may be palpable. Weakness, indigestion and other vague complaints are mentioned. The ascitic fluid is clear and of low specific gravity; it has the features of a transudate. The leukocyte count is unaltered and there is no fever. The course extends over years with recurring ascites; the patient usually dies of some other disease. A mistaken diagnosis of cirrhosis of the liver is often made, even though there is no evidence of impairment of hepatic function.

Little can be done in the way of therapy except to draw off the ascitic fluid from time to time, and adjust the patient's activities to his handicap. In the cases with pericardial adhesions and symptoms of cardiac embarrassment operations designed to free the heart from its sheath of fibrous tissue have been of some help.

TUMORS OF THE PERITONEUM.

Cancer of the peritoneum comes about by extension from a primary growth in the abdomen. Small nodules, in appearance not unlike miliary tubercules, become seeded over the surface or there may be large masses of neoplastic tissue especially in the omentum, which often becomes tremendously infiltrated. Implantations may accumulate in the cul-de-sac in front of the rectum where they can be felt as a hard ridge—the so-called rectal shelf. Occasionally extensions along the lymphatics become manifest as palpable nodules in the umbilical depression. Ascites is a frequent event.

Clinically cancer of the peritoneum is inextricably bound up with the features of the underlying growth. The presence of ascites or of irregular masses on abdominal palpation should rouse suspicion. The peritoneal fluid usually is not remarkable but it may be bloody and occasionally cancer cells are demonstrated by special methods. In the rare cases of colloid cancer of the peritoneum arising from a primary growth in the stomach or ovary a curious gelatinous fluid containing bizarre masses of cancer cells may be obtained. In the differential diagnosis confusion with tuberculous peritonitis is the commonest error. Treatment is obviously of no avail, although the removal of certain ovarian tumors is occasionally followed by regression of peritoneal implantations.

Peritoneal nodules with ascites may also occur as part of a metastatic sarcomatosis.

CHAPTER XV.

DISEASES OF THE RESPIRATORY TRACT.

By JAMES ALEXANDER MILLER, M.D.

FUNCTIONAL PATHOLOGY OF PULMO-
  NARY DISEASE.
PULMONARY ATELECTASIS.
EMPHYSEMA.
  Interstitial Emphysema.
PULMONARY FIBROSIS, PNEUMOCONIO-
  SIS, PULMONARY ARTERIOSCLEROSIS.
BRONCHIECTASIS.
INFECTIONS OF THE UPPER RESPIRA-
  TORY TRACT.

ABSCESS OF THE LUNG.
GANGRENE OF THE LUNG.
PULMONARY TUBERCULOSIS.
SYPHILIS OF THE LUNG.
MYCOTIC DISEASES OF THE LUNG.
HYDATID DISEASE OF THE LUNG.
TUMORS OF THE LUNG AND PLEURA.
PLEURISIES.
AFFECTIONS OF THE MEDIASTINUM.
AFFECTIONS OF THE DIAPHRAGM.

FUNCTIONAL PATHOLOGY OF PULMONARY DISEASE.

WHILE functional pathology has made great strides in most other branches of medicine, in pulmonary disease we still continue to think of pathologic conditions in terms of tissue changes, with disregard of their effects upon function. Yet, in the lungs, structure and function are so intimately associated that perhaps in no other organ of the body does normal function depend so much on intact structure. This circumstance affords an opportunity for functional disturbances more marked than in any other organ of the body. These disturbances occur often without evident disease, but are invariably present in greater or less degree whenever pathologic conditions exist.

Recent researches have added greatly to our knowledge of these functional changes, and it is now recognized that they materially affect the clinical evidences of pulmonary disease as manifested by symptoms or by physical and roentgenologic signs, and also that they have a direct bearing upon the course and treatment of these diseases.

It seems desirable, therefore, to include in our description of various lung diseases a brief consideration of this newer knowledge the importance of which has been too little appreciated by clinicians.

Extrinsic and Intrinsic Mechanism of Breathing.—The paramount rôle of the lungs is to afford the surface for the purely physico-chemical processes of gas exchange and evaporation. The intrinsic function of the lung must therefore be to maintain the breathing surface in such a manner as to ensure smooth and optimum operation of these physico-chemical processes. Purposeful adaptation of the extent and character of the breathing surface, the optimal variations in the dimensions of the air spaces, and the self-cleansing efficiency of the breathing surface, are the components of intrinsic lung function.

This intrinsic mechanism of breathing is in turn served by the visible pulmonary and bronchial mechanisms of air and blood circulation which provide for the ventilation of the air spaces and perfusion with blood of the breathing surface. The latter may therefore properly be called the extrinsic mechanism of breathing.

Both intrinsic and extrinsic function together go to make up the mechanics of breathing which is a complex yet so well correlated function that disturbances in any of its components will involve changes in all of them. Clinically these reveal themselves to us at first by the indirect associated changes in pulmonary circulation and ventilation. Eventually disturbances in lung function lead to disturbances in the processes of gas exchange, which will reveal themselves by the blood changes and the tissue metabolic changes. Finally changes in nervous regulation of breathing may be brought about by both the disturbed mechanics as well as gas exchange.

The clinico-pathologic features of disturbed lung function can therefore be classified as follows:

1. Phenomena of disturbed mechanics of breathing.
2. Phenomena of disturbed gas exchange.
3. Phenomena of disturbed regulation.

1. Phenomena Due to Disturbed Mechanics of Breathing.—The constant circulation and ventilation in the lungs are provided for by tidal volumes of air with each respiration, and tidal volumes of blood with each heart cycle. The respiratory excursions of the lungs as carried out and regulated by the neuromuscular apparatus invested in the bronchial and chest walls and the diaphragm, serve simultaneously the promotion of pulmonary circulation and ventilation.

Any disturbance in this respiratory mechanism manifests itself therefore in simultaneous changes in pulmonary circulation as well as ventilation. Pathologic changes in the lungs usually interfere more or less with the respiratory mechanics, and therefore affected lung areas have a tendency to become immobilized, their ventilation and circulation decrease or may even cease almost entirely and simultaneously. Interference with ventilation of a lung area is soon followed by stoppage of its circulation and, *vice versa*, interference with blood supply to a lung area soon results in arrest of its ventilation.

The evidences of disturbed mechanics of respiration may be divided into those which are primarily circulatory and those which are primarily ventilatory in origin, it being understood that eventually both part functions become involved.

(a) **Circulatory Phenomena.**—(1) *Pulmonary Congestion and Edema.*— It has been estimated that the lungs hold about 20 per cent of the total circulatory blood volume of the body. All blood must pass the lungs on its way from the right to the left heart, so that the lung is one of the most blood-rich organs of the body.

Pulmonary congestion, by which is meant simple active hyperemia of the lungs, is a very common phenomenon representing the mildest degree of disturbance in respiratory mechanism. It is present as a physiologic phenomenon in physical exertion in form of the "effort lung," which is analogous to the so-called "effort heart." Exposure to

44

extremes of temperature (fever or severe cold), mechanical, traumatic, nervous, or chemical (inhalation of fumes) causes, will in first degree lead to pulmonary hyperemia. In most of these instances we are dealing simply with an exaggeration of the physiologic response reaching pathologic proportions. The transitions from physiologic to pathologic response are fluent and it is difficult to draw a sharp borderline.

The lung is a surface of evaporation from which normally about 600 to 800 cm. of moisture are evaporated daily. This fluid is derived from the blood of the alveolar capillaries, from which a constant stream of blood serum filters into the air spaces, much greater in amount than is evaporated. This physiologic filtration into the alveoli depends upon the capillary circulation, and in pulmonary hyperemia it is much increased. Under conditions of normal respiratory function the greater part of this physiologic transudate is diverted back into the alveolar capillaries by the suction of negative intrapulmonary pressure arising during every inspiration. The rest of this transudate which is not evaporated reaches the air passages, whence it is drained away by the lymphatics.

Other things being equal, the degree of pulmonary congestion will depend upon the efficiency of the respiratory mechanism, the pulmonary excursions. With adequate increase of pulmonary excursions, transmission of blood through the lungs may keep pace with hyperemia; at the same time powerful inspirations provide for adequate resuction of alveolar filtrate, and adequate expirations greatly enhance lymphatic drainage of fluid from air passages.

Pulmonary congestion reaching such a degree as to interfere with efficiency of pulmonary movements, closes a vicious circle by which blood transmission is slowed down, filtration of serum into alveoli is greatly increased while at the same time its resuction and drainage by the capillaries and lymphatics decrease. The result is flooding of air passages with serum filtrate which, in extreme cases of pulmonary edema, bubbles up into the air passages of the patient.

As a terminal phenomenon pulmonary edema is frequently the result of exaggerated compensatory effort on the part of non-involved areas of the lung when there is extensive disease involving the greater part of available lung space. In such conditions a large amount of blood is shunted into the uninvolved areas, which favors congestion there and later edema, and when the vitality of the patient fails, this explains the terminal edema of many pulmonary conditions which may thus be termed respiratory failure as opposed to heart failure, to which it is usually ascribed.

2. *Infectious Edema. Infiltration. Consolidation.*—The lungs constitute the largest surface of the body exposed to outside air; as such they become the most frequent site of foreign matter deposition and bacterial invasion, infection. Infectious invasion of the lungs is a conspicuous cause of general pulmonary congestion. The edematous imbibition of the lungs' tissues and filling out of air spaces which takes place as the first reaction to infectious invasion of lung, differs in no respect from that described above as following congestion and edema as a result of disturbed respiratory mechanism due to other causes.

In fact pulmonary processes frequently represent secondary invasion by infectious agents of lung areas subjected to congestive edematous changes from other causes.

Pulmonary infiltration represents invasion of the lung tissues and air spaces by formed elements from the blood, and reticulo-endothelial elements from the vascular system, in response to microbic infection. There are no hard and fast borderlines between infectious edema and exudate. Probably simple infectious edema is the precursor of exudative infiltration which begins in the center of the affected area but is surrounded by an area of collateral infectious edema or perifocal, zone of inflammation.

Consolidation of lung areas is frequent in infectious processes because of the abundance of cellular semiliquid elements which constitute a typical exudate, and in acute pulmonary infections infiltrations tend to be out of all proportion to the extent of the primary lesion because of the free intercommunication between lung areas by way of the vast number of air passages and the interalveolar pores of Kohn.

On the other hand, the means available to the lungs for elimination and absorption of infiltrations are enormous, as shown by the prompt resolution of extensive pneumonic lesions. The outstanding factor in this absorption is the intrinsic function of the lung with its amazing self-cleansing power. It is aided by the remobilization of the affected area, which is accomplished by reëstablishment of circulation and of ventilation, that is, of the extrinsic respiratory mechanisms.

(b) **Ventilatory Phenomena.**—1. *Atelectasis and Emphysema.*—The average individual at rest holds about 2500 cc. of air in his lungs, one-half of which, residual air, cannot be removed except with collapse of the lung, atelectasis, by opening of chest, or by interruption of tidal air supply.

Even under normal conditions distribution of the pulmonary air contents between the various lung areas is unequal, while under pathologic conditions, when the affected lung areas are excluded from normal ventilation, the differences in the air contents between various sections of the lungs become much exaggerated. Atelectasis in affected areas is compensated for by hyperdistention of intact lung areas and both atelectasis and compensatory emphysema, which are usually associated with most pulmonary conditions, are all the more pronounced the more extensive the underlying process.

The paramount factor playing a rôle in regulating the distribution of air contents between lung areas under physiologic but particularly under pathologic conditions is the intrinsic function of the lung which regulates breathing surface and air-space expansion. The next important factor is the autonomic activity of the myo-elastic elements in the walls of the air passages (bronchogenic factor) and the collateral air exchange between adjacent lung units through interalveolar pores. There is evidence to indicate that bronchospastic phenomena (an exaggeration of normal bronchoconstriction) in affected lung areas play an important rôle in the shunting away of the air supply intended for affected lung units toward intact lung units, whereby atelectasis of the former and emphysematous hyperdistention of the latter are produced. However, there is also evidence to indicate that collateral air exchange between adjacent lung units as aided by bronchial activity—which regulates intrabronchial air pressure—plays at the same time a significant rôle in the prevention of total collapse of affected but particularly of surrounding lung units, as well as in the prevention of excessive emphysematous hyperdistention of intact lung units. It is thus obvious that bronchial function and collateral ventilation which serve both atelectasis and emphysema, can also limit these either by desirable immobilization on the one hand, or by compensatory hyperfunction on the other.

Pulmonary Fibrosis.—Concluding from the above we can say that any form of pulmonary air space obliteration (atelectasis, edema, infiltration) is essentially a phenomenon involving both failure of ventilation as well as self-cleansing function. They are usually reversible and the lung areas thus affected may reëstablish their function. If the failure is permanent, pulmonary *fibrosis* is the result, as an expression of the irreversible failure of self-cleansing power. Thus nature permanently obliterates lung surface which has lost its self-cleansing power. In the polluted atmospheres of our industrial centers in the course of a lifetime considerable lung surface is lost and is being made up for by compensatory hyperfunction of other lung areas. This is particularly conspicuous in the case of workers exposed to industrial dusts.

Respiro-circulatory Failure.—Compensatory lung function is effective only if the ventilatory and circulatory facilities can keep pace with it. Beyond a certain individually feasible extent, hyperinflation of the lungs does not increase the breathing surface and the number of air spaces, but merely distends the existing air spaces, which immediately deteriorates their ventilatory and circulatory capacities. Such hyperinflation of the lungs is pathologic emphysema which so overdistends the chest and bronchi as to interfere with their movements. Such emphysema is already an expression of disturbed mechanics of breathing which becomes a source of pulmonary decompensation. Thus, individual constitutional limitations determine the extent to which increased lung function may go to still have a compensatory effect. Hyperfunction carried beyond this limit leads to decompensation which then involves both the ventilatory and circulatory functions. The end may be respiro-circulatory failure, either in the form of more acute pulmonary edema or in the form of chronic emphysema with right heart failure.

2. **Phenomena of Disturbed Gas Exchange.**—Pulmonary diseases disturb the gas exchange in proportion to the extent they interfere with intrinsic lung function and affect breathing surface maintenance and air-space ventilation. Breathing surface changes affect the extent and quality of the breathing surface through which diffusion must take place. Ventilatory disturbance goes with changes in composition of the alveolar air with which the blood must become equilibrated in contents and tensions of the gases. Most frequently the situation is such that eventually a combination of these changes develops, so that

the permeability of the diffusing membrane and the composition of alveolar air both become altered. This is in accord with the intimate relationship which exists between the different phases of intrinsic lung function.

Breathing surface changes interfere in the first place with O_2 absorption, while faulty air-space ventilation leads in the first place to CO_2 retention. Whether O_2 want or CO_2 retention will prevail depends upon which of these changes prevails in the combination. However, the opportunities for the development of O_2 want or CO_2 retention or both depend greatly upon the differences in the provisions Nature has made for the absorption of O_2 and the elimination of CO_2.

While the O_2 reserve of the body is limited to a three-minute supply, the power of the tissues to buffer CO_2 is practically unlimited. While the blood can under no circumstances take up in the lungs more than 20 volumes per cent of O_2, there is no limit to the amount of CO_2 that can be blown off in the lungs by compensatory hyperventilation. The diffusion power of O_2 is very much less than that of CO_2, and very much less breathing surface is required to prevent CO_2 retention than to prevent O_2 want. CO_2 elimination holds the key position in the regulation of the chemical reaction of the blood, and so the response to CO_2 retention is such a very immediate and striking one that dangerous CO_2 retention is observed only in terminal conditions. Oxygen want when it develops slowly is so insidious that it may remain unnoticed until it has reached very serious degrees. Indeed the dangerous potentialities of severe degrees of O_2 want will bear strong emphasis.

In favor of O_2 absorption, however, the natural provisions for the O_2 supply of the body are such that there exists a rather large pressure gradient for this gas between the tissues and the outside air. The arrangement is such that as long as at least one-half of this pressure gradient prevails, arterilization of the blood in the lungs is secured. Thus, only under conditions of very extensive breathing surface changes or serious ventilatory failure will the O_2 saturation of the arterial blood begin to be affected. On the other hand, CO_2 elimination may become affected fairly early in the presence of serious ventilatory failure such as arises for example in advanced emphysema or in asthma, particularly in patients past middle age.

The special features of disturbed gas exchange can be described from the above as follows:

Disturbed O_2 Absorption.—The mildest form of this develops even in normal individuals in exercise in form of so-called O_2 *debt* of the tissues, which is made up by hyperventilation after exercise.

Next in severity is the so-called O_2 *deficit* which develops in the tissues of patients, while their arterial blood may be still fully saturated. This O_2 deficit reveals itself in the excess O_2 such patients will absorb when they inhale O_2 at a higher concentration than that of the atmospheric air.

Hypoxemia is the term for outright O_2 want in the presence of an unsaturated state of the arterial blood as it leaves the lungs. This O_2 saturation deficit of the arterial blood varies of course with the level of O_2 pressure in the blood. Until this is not less than one-third of the atmospheric O_2 concentration, the O_2 supply of the tissues is still compatible with life. When the pressure drops below this level (50 mm. Hg.), the life of the patient is in danger, because the O_2 supply of the tissues depends in the first place upon the pressure of the gas.

Disturbed CO_2 Elimination.—Oxygen want is to begin with, usually associated with *hypocapnia, i. e.,* excess CO_2 elimination, due to the hyperventilation it produces. The combination of hypoxemia with hyperventilation is essentially a compensatory measure which enables the arterial blood to take up more O_2 in the lungs as it rids itself of more CO_2. However, in case a severe degree of hypoxemia should develop, this mode of compensation may become dangerous because hypocapnic blood also tends to hold on to its O_2 content, and this may even increase the already serious O_2 starvation of the tissues and result in insidious asphyxia.

Fortunately the situation is such that in conditions which might lead to such degrees of hypoxemia there soon comes about the tendency to turn from excess elimination of CO_2 to retention of this gas in the blood and tissues, *i. e.,* hypercapnia develops.

3. **Phenomena Due to Disturbed Regulation of Respiration.**—Regulation of breathing is invested in the respiratory center in the medulla. This center functions automatically, generating its own rhythm by integration of the multitude of stimuli reaching it from the periphery, from the tissues of the entire body and the structures of the intrinsic and extrinsic neuromuscular apparatus of breathing.

By means of a steady stream of impulses the respiratory center keeps all the striped and smooth breathing musculature in a constant state of tonus which increases in inspiration and decreases in expiration. The metabolic needs of the tissues, the chemical composition of the blood, the gas tensions in the blood and the alveoli, the pressure balance between the chest and lungs, all play the rôle of important stimuli and their precise regulation is included in the complex function of respiratory regulation.

In pulmonary affections this regulatory function manifests itself in such compensatory changes as the increased rate and depth of respiration due to anoxemia or hypercapnia, the slowing-down breathing in hypocapnia. Real disturbances in respiratory regulation are observed in connection with pulmonary diseases usually as terminal phenomena, such as periodic breathing (Cheyne-Stokes or Biot types) and shallow rapid breathing which is analogous to the gallop rhythm of the heart.

The Clinical Syndrome of Pulmonary Diseases.—Diseases of the lungs are characterized clinically by a conspicuous set of objective symptoms of functional origin, and so this is the proper place for their discussion. In the order of their frequency they are as follows:

1. **Coughing.**—This is a ventilatory phenomenon of unusual character and significance. It represents an utmost expiratory effort so abrupt, rapid, and forceful that it bursts open the adducted vocal cords. Greatly increased intrapulmonary pressure is thereby produced, carrying out an unusually large part of the lung air and everything within the bronchi is swept along with it.

In the light of recent bronchoscopic and bronchographic observations, the old conception that coughing serves exclusively the removal of bronchial secretions, is, to say the least, too narrow. To begin with, the degree of inflation of the lung area beyond the bronchus containing the secretions or obstruction, determines whether the cough will have an inward or outward promoting effect, so that in a deflated lung area cough will act to sweep air as well as bronchial contents inward. Furthermore, even in a perfectly cocainized air passage (insensitive to touch) cough is elicited by any obstruction to normal air flow, indicating that decrease in air supply constitutes a cough stimulus which serves to displace such obstruction.

The deeper air passages are insensitive to local stimulation. In pulmonary conditions accompanied by excessive suppuration, these air passages may be filled with material without inciting cough. Such patients learn to keep their body in a position in which they can have undisturbed sleep, keeping their bronchial contents below the level where they will incite cough. On rising, these secretions reach the stem bronchi, which are sensitive to local stimulation, and the characteristic morning cough and expectoration result.

Clinical Significance.—Cough as a clinical phenomenon is thus susceptible to several interpretations. At times it represents an effort at compensation for hypoinflation incidental to the pulmonary or pleural affection in question, tending to reinflate lung areas held down by painful breathing or by bronchial obstruction. More frequently it represents overstimulation of the mucous membrane of the central large air passages or upper respiratory tract (trachea, larynx, pharynx) due to an increase of contents within their lumina.

At other times cough indicates a state of hypersensitiveness of the lining tissues, particularly of the upper respiratory tract, which is usually due to their locally inflamed, hyperirritable state. Frequently enough such a local hyperirritability may be psychic in its origin. Where lung patients live together in great numbers, effects of "crowd suggestion" in their cough habits are particularly enlightening as to psychic influences upon the reflex mechanism of coughing. Such reflex cough may be elicited not only from the upper respiratory tract, but also from other organs of the body.

Undoubtedly much of the coughing serves no purpose whatsoever. Excessive coughing is always more harmful than useful. Intrabronchial spilling due to cough is now recognized as most instrumental in spreading infection, for under such conditions coughing just as frequently promotes the intrabronchial contents inward as outward. Coughing also goes with marked increase of intrathoracic pressure and increase of functional burden upon the circulation already considerably burdened in all pulmonary conditions. Finally, through straining, cough is partly responsible for such complications of pulmonary disease as hemorrhages, interstitial emphysema and pneumothorax or it may cause or aggravate an abdominal or inguinal hernia.

As a clinical symptom cough is of great interest because its distinct types frequently give hints of much diagnostic value. Some of the well distinguishable types of cough are as follows:

The dry, hacking, unproductive cough of the patient with pneumonia, or the same cough with a painful moan of the patient with pleurisy.

The dry, barking cough of the patient with larynx obstruction or inflammatory swelling of the cords, or irritation of larynx and trachea.

The bitonal cough of the patient with lower tracheal irritation or hilar obstruction (mediastinitis).

The muffled, air-cushioned, reverberating cough of the patient with emphysema, and entirely toneless cough of the senile emphysematous man.

The squeaking cough of the patient with bronchial obstruction or asthma.

The loose, hollow and throaty cough of the patient with cavitary and profusely suppurating lung processes of phthisis, bronchiectasis and abscess.

2. **Expectoration.**—Through the self-cleansing power of the lung, the normal air spaces and air passages can rid themselves of the vast amounts of serum filtrate and foreign matter. Even inflammatory products of vast amounts can be absorbed completely by the lungs' tissues, as is evident in the rapid resolution of lobar pneumonias.

In lung areas with pathologic tissue changes there is a tendency toward accumulation of serum, inflammatory products, as well as foreign matter, not only because of lack of self-cleansing power and proper drainage, but because there is drainage into these immobilized lung areas from adjacent mobile lung areas—intrabronchial spilling. This is particularly conspicuous in the dependent lung areas. Thus, in pulmonary processes associated with tissue necrosis and much suppuration, the task of ridding the air passages of their contents devolves upon the special function of expectoration.

Clinical Significance.—Efficient expectoration requires very little coughing. The autonomous activity of the bronchi, aided by ciliary movements, promotes the bronchial contents to a point near the bifurcation, whence a short hacking or rasping is usually sufficient to lift them above the larynx.

In conditions with excessive bronchial contents, patients soon learn to put their chests in such a position as to aid evacuation by gravity. In some cases patients may expectorate amounts totaling several times their own body weight during the last weeks of their lives. Obviously, such vast amounts of fluid cannot be derived from secretions and inflammatory products exclusively. As a matter of fact, the bulk of such vast amounts of sputum is the serum filtrate poured into the lung in excess under such circumstances. To this are added the mucus secreted in the bronchi and the pus derived from the lesions. In colorless sputa of thin consistency, serum prevails. In colorless tenacious sputa of thick consistency, mucus prevails. In greenish-yellow colored sputa of very thick consistency, pus prevails. In sputa containing all three elements in a great amount, serum separation into layers takes place, the pus sinking to the bottom, globular masses of muco-pus remain floating in the colorless bulk of watery serum. Admixture of blood gives sputa color varying from brownish-rusty to bright pink or red tinge.

The quantity as well as quality of the sputa of patients suffering from the various pulmonary processes has certain characteristics of clinical value. The following are some of the characteristics of sputum typical of some lung conditions.

In pneumonia it is scant, tenacious, globular, rusty in color. In pulmonary edema it is abundant, thin, frothy, colorless or pinkish from a bloody tinge. In asthma it is frothy, tenacious, colorless. In chronic bronchitis and early phthisis it is thick, muco-purulent, globular, grayish- or greenish-yellow, moderate in amounts. Abundant muco-purulent pus-colored sputa are characteristic of cavitary phthisis and early bronchiectasis. In late bronchiectasis vast amounts of three-layered sputa are the rule. In lung abscess foul-smelling, colored and abundant creamy pus prevails in the sputa. In lung gangrene the sputa are extremely fetid, highly colored and abundant, and contain pieces of tissue fragments.

In pulmonary processes going with tissue destruction, elastic tissue fragments are a usual constituent of the sputa. Search for elastic tissue fibers is frequently a helpful diagnostic procedure. It differentiates pulmonary from bronchial suppuration. The extent of tissue destruction becomes manifest in the amount of elastic fibers to be found in the sputa.

Hemoptyses.—A most important and frequent constituent of sputa is blood. The unparalleled blood richness, the unusual width of the pulmonary capillaries, and the frequency of congestive states in the lungs, more intense here than in any other organ of the body, account for the fact that lung tissue bleeds readily, and that considerable hemoptyses are possible from mere diapedesis or capillary oozing in congestive or inflammatory conditions of the lungs. In ulcerative or destructive lung processes, severe hemorrhages are prevented only by the fact of markedly reduced circulation in affected areas and thrombosis of vessels by inflammatory process. On the other hand, destructive processes frequently leave the vascular trunks of the evacuated lung tissue lying within pulmonary cavities, with damaged aneurysmatic wall liable to rupture, and frequently result in fatal hemorrhages.

The hemoptyses of very fresh or very chronic cirrhotic tuberculous lesions of pneumonia, of chronic left heart disease, of pulmonary edema, of pulmonary infarction, are usually due to capillary diapedesis or oozing in the lungs' tissues. Hemoptyses of bronchiectases, of cirrhotic extensive lung processes, are usually due to oozing from congested bronchial capillaries, less frequently from ulcerative bronchial processes in case of bronchial carcinoma. The frequent and brisk hemorrhages of phthisis, cancer, destructive processes of the lungs, usually come from erosion of smaller branches of the vascular tree of the lungs (arteries or veins). Hemorrhages from sizable pulmonary arteries are easily distinguished by the extraordinary amount and suddenness of the bleeding.

3. **Dyspnea.**—Dyspnea is an expression of disturbed, at times of failing respiratory mechanism. Its best definition is labored or distressed breathing regardless of rate or rhythm of respirations. While the problem-complex presented by dyspnea in various clinical condi-

tions of pulmonary and cardiac diseases is still unsolved, the weight of more recent evidence indicates that disturbances in alveolar ventilation and alveolar capillary circulation are the paramount factors in its pathogenesis. Under ordinary circumstances, when changes in alveolar ventilation and circulation arise gradually, the sensation of dyspnea is not produced until the greatest part of available air space has become affected.

The sensation of dyspnea depends upon sensory impulses arising within the tissue elements of the lung itself, which functionate in the respiratory mechanism. Inasmuch as gas exchange disturbances—O_2 want or CO_2 retention—lead to dyspnea, they do so by bringing about decompensation and failure of the respiratory mechanism. This is usually the result of exaggerated compensatory effort on the part of the respiratory mechanism to make up for deficient gas exchange.

Recent evidence indicates that the physical mechanism of respiration is much more sensitive than is its chemical regulation, which indicates that dyspnea is a distress signal on the part of the neuromuscular apparatus of the respiratory mechanism, signifying its functional decompensation.

4. **Cyanosis.**—Cyanosis is due to accumulation of reduced (non-oxygenated) hemoglobin in the capillaries of the skin, becoming first apparent at the body tips (lips, fingers, toes). As such it is an expression of disturbed gas exchange. Although it is O_2 missing from its chemical combination with hemoglobin, which is directly responsible for the phenomenon of cyanosis, it is clear today that other factors, too, indirectly play a significant rôle in its production.

The following are some of the well-established facts about cyanosis: When the relative amount of reduced hemoglobin in the blood of the skin capillaries rises above 5 volumes per cent (a third of its total hemoglobin content), cyanosis makes its appearance in normal individuals. (Anemic patients having lost more than two-thirds of their normal hemoglobin content can never show cyanosis, while patients having hemoglobin in excess of normal value may show cyanotic body tips even under normal conditions.) This threshold level of cyanosis corresponds to 6.5 volumes per cent of O_2 unsaturation, the normal O_2 content being 20 volumes per cent. Normally at the periphery from 3 to 5 volumes per cent of O_2 are given up to the tissues as the blood passes from the arterial to the venous side. On its return to the lungs the blood replenishes its O_2 to 20 volumes per cent, by which it becomes resaturated to 95 per cent. It would follow from this that in pulmonary affections in which the blood leaves the lungs in a state of saturation below 80 to 85 per cent, cyanosis should make its appearance at the periphery. However, this is not always the case, because circulatory conditions in the peripheral capillaries affecting CO_2 elimination from the tissues have a more telling effect upon the phenomenon of cyanosis. Peripheral circulatory stasis, permitting the loss in the capillaries of an unduly large part of the available O_2, will lead to cyanosis regardless of the level of arterial blood saturation.

Much of the problem complex presented by the phenomenon of cyanosis in the various pulmonary and cardiac conditions remains to be solved, but it is clear, however, that in most instances cyanosis represents a phenomenon in which at times the respiratory, at other times the circulatory disturbance plays the leading rôle, but that there is always present some combination of respiro-circulatory decompensation.

5. **Clubbing.**—Clubbing of the fingers and toes is a very common phenomenon in chronic respiratory and circulatory diseases. It appears to be dependent upon the unique capillary circulation in these body tips, but the exact cause of this interesting condition is not yet known. That it is associated with some disturbance of gas exchange seems probable.

6. **Polycythemia.**—The fact that polycythemia is a frequent phenomenon of subacute and chronic pulmonary affections, indicates that the tissues of the erythropoietic organs are also hypersensitive to degrees of respiratory and circulatory changes which do not manifest themselves in alterations of the physico-chemical composition of the blood, characteristic of disturbed gas exchange of definitely pathologic degrees. Polycythemia is a compensatory phenomenon for increasing the available amount of oxygen-carrying hemoglobin; the body attempts to make up with quantity for quality.

PULMONARY ATELECTASIS.

Definition.—Pulmonary atelectasis (collapse of the lung) may be defined as a functional failure resulting in deflation of the lung and immobilization in this deflated state. Atelectasis may affect individual units, or it may involve the greater part of or even the entire lung.

Classification.—The following clinical forms of pulmonary atelectasis may be distinguished:

1. More or less *localized forms of pulmonary atelectasis* are present in or about the involved lung areas in all pulmonary conditions of whatever origin, during some phase of such disease.

2. A *localized, but at the same time extensive form of pulmonary atelectasis* is present in *massive collapse* which may involve one or more lobes.

3. When pulmonary failure affects the organ as a whole, we have the most generalized form of atelectasis involving scattered lung areas *en masse* in the form of *pulmonary edema.*

Etiology.—All pathologic conditions in which interference with the normal respiratory mechanism may arise play a rôle in the etiology of pulmonary atelectasis. The most important of these are the following: *Mechanical conditions:* separation of pleural surfaces by pneumothorax, effusion; interruption of air or blood supply, bronchial or vascular occlusion; reduction of intrathoracic space, chest deformity, new-growth, cardiac hypertrophy. *Inflammatory conditions* in lung, bronchi and pleura, which includes all infectious diseases resulting from aspiration and inhalation of irritant foreign substances. *Nervous functional disturbances:* cerebrospinal lesions affecting respiration, phrenic paralysis, toxic and drug effects upon broncho-vascular innervation such as anaphylactic states and poisonings.

Pathogenesis.—Pulmonary atelectasis is not exclusively a pathologic condition. In normal respiration only a fraction of available air spaces is in function. In physiologic states of lowered activity (sleep) hypoinflation may amount to partial atelectasis in which the fraction of open alveoli is still less; the lung loses its reserve air volume.

Pathologic states of low breathing activity, hypoinflation, differ from the physiologic only in degree, not in kind, from the standpoint of lung deflation, so that fluent transitions exist between physiologic and pathologic degrees of atelectasis.

The two essential criteria of pathologic atelectasis are deflation and immobilization, but there are essential differences between various types of atelectasis and collapse as they are produced in various lung conditions.

(a) *Separation of the Lung from the Chest Wall.*—When the lung becomes separated from the chest wall by pneumothorax, or effusion in the pleural space, atelectasis arises because the expiratory forces inherent in the lungs' tissues gain the upper hand because of lack of the traction power of an expanding chest wall. The lung retracts to a point of new dynamic equilibrium between outside and inside pressure. When the air in the pleural cavity rises to an amount as to completely neutralize the traction power of the chest wall, lung retraction will amount to complete collapse.

This is equally true for conditions in which intrathoracic space is reduced by chest deformity, new growth, cardiac enlargement, or encroachment of neighboring organs.

(b) *Bronchial Occlusion.*—When the air supply to an area of an otherwise normal lung becomes interrupted, as, for example, in *bronchial occlusion*, thoracic traction gains the upper hand over the autonomic pulmonary movements. The affected lung is drawn toward the chest wall, the traction force of which is enhanced by the increased intrathoracic suction due to the fact that, one part of the lung being immobilized, less lung tissue takes part in expansion of the same extent. The functioning lung areas increase atelectasis of the affected lung area by their overexpansion at its expense.

(c) *Vascular Occlusion.*—Pulmonary infarction caused by vascular occlusion also interrupts normal ventilation, so that atelectasis and hemorrhagic exudate are associated. To this condition infection may be added which frequently involves the pleura as well as the lung.

(d) *Inflammatory Processes.*—In inflammatory conditions of the lungs and pleura we observe greater or less degrees of immobilization, which vary according to the extent of the process. Any immobilized areas may go on to fibrosis if long continued, but in those due to infection this result is particularly apt to follow.

(e) *Nervous Disturbances.*—The rôle of nervous disturbances in the disruption of the normal respiratory mechanism producing atelectasis, as, for example, in phrenic paralysis, is clear, as it is also in disturbances of nervous function affecting the cerebrospinal nerve apparatus active in breathing, as observed in diseases involving this nervous apparatus. The rôle played by disturbances in the innervation of the bronchial and vascular systems of the lungs is less certain.

Massive Collapse.—This is a clinico-pathologic entity of considerable interest which occurs mainly in association with surgical operations.

The etiology of massive collapse is still an open question. Mechanical (bronchial obstruction), infectious (pleuro-diaphragmatic inflammation) and nervous (vaso- and broncho-motor) disturbances have been considered among the theories attempting to explain massive collapse. Phenomena due to any of these causes may exist, but vary from one case to another. But the ultimate pathogenetic factor is always failure in function of the lung. This function is of the type we call vegetative; but the exact manner in which mechanical, infectious or nervous influences bring this function to a failure is still unknown.

Massive collapse has its analogy in that elusive circulatory phenomenon called shock. Indeed, it has been termed "respiratory shock" by some investigators.

Pathology.—The morphologic picture in the atelectatic lung is that of obliteration of air spaces, intense vascular congestion with edema. Atelectatic tissue frequently becomes infected because its high serum and blood contents offer good soil for microörganisms and, when it remains atelectatic for a long time, it is invaded by connective tissue proliferation which obliterates the air spaces completely and brings on a state of fibrosis known as collapse induration.

Compressed lung tissue, on the other hand, may remain in the deflated state for many years unchanged. The alveolar spaces remain free, the tissues retain enough of their elasticity to preserve their functional capacity for years, and such a lung will be able to reopen again after compression has been relieved. Thus, lungs under artificial pneumothorax compression will be able to again reinflate even after years of deflation.

The fundamental difference between atelectasis and compression lies in the fact that pulmonary circulation is interrupted in compressed lung, which prevents the congestion and resulting connective tissue hyperplasia which occur in atelectasis.

Clinical Picture.—(a) *In Atelectasis.*—As atelectasis of various lung areas is usually compensated for by emphysematous hyperexpansion and hyperfunction of unaffected areas, no evidence of respiratory embarrassment need arise, even when the atelectasis involves 50 per cent of the available air space. When the atelectasis occurs gradually, so that a sufficient time is allowed to make the necessary adjustments, there are usually no symptoms of the condition. When, however, the atelectasis occurs over large areas quickly, so that prompt compensation is impossible, or when there is a lack of adequate available lung space, as in immobility due to adhesions, then symptoms of severe respiratory decompensation arise. As the blood circulates through the atelectatic lung, but is not aërated, it returns to the arterial system in a venous state. Thus it may give rise to anoxemia, hypercapnia, dyspnea and cyanosis. These symptoms subside as pulmonary retraction becomes complete and available lung areas are able to expand and to establish compensation.

The clinical picture of pulmonary atelectasis varies greatly with the underlying pulmonary condition with which it may be associated. The symptoms of this underlying disease frequently obscure those of atelectasis, so that it is frequently not easy to recognize it.

The *physical signs* of the underlying pulmonary disease may be exaggerated to the extent of the additional atelectasis, and in the same way the roentgen-ray densities may be increased. The roentgen-ray appearance of pulmonary atelectasis, when associated with other pulmonary disease is quite similar to that of inflammatory exudate, from which it is not easy to differentiate it in the roentgenogram. But inasmuch as pulmonary atelectasis frequently disappears rapidly, the exaggeration of signs and symptoms caused by it may be transient, thus accounting for instances of rapid appearance as well as rapid clearing up of apparently new lesions; this is particularly notable in the case of pulmonary tuberculosis. The emphysema with which the atelectasis is so frequently associated may also obscure the physical signs and modify the roentgen shadows which may be caused by it.

(b) *In Massive Collapse.*—The symptoms of massive collapse usually come on suddenly with dyspnea, cyanosis, pain in the chest and, frequently, fever. These symptoms may be so severe as to be very alarming and may clear up just as rapidly within a few hours, with the patient going into a profuse sweat and beginning to cough and expectorate large quantities of frothy, colorless material. The condition rarely lasts more than thirty-six to forty-eight hours, rarely results fatally, and usually clears up entirely, although occasionally small unresolved areas of density due to unresolved lung may persist.

In the more gradual production of massive atelectasis such as is seen following bronchial occlusion from foreign bodies, tumors and pressure of calcified glands, the condition comes on more gradually and often produces no symptoms at all, excepting gradual shortness of breath.

The physical signs of massive collapse closely simulate those of acute consolidation. The affected side is immobile, with exaggerated respiratory movement of the opposite side. The heart and mediastinum are shifted *toward* the collapsed lung and the diaphragm is elevated at the same time. There is extreme negative pleural pressure which may amount to 70 mm. of mercury. The roentgen signs are those of a diffuse homogeneous shadow corresponding to the portion of the lung involved, with the characteristic shift of the heart and other mediastinal structures and the diaphragm toward the side of the lesion. The opposite lung shows increased illumination due to compensatory emphysema.

Treatment.—When the amount of atelectasis is considerable, leading to evidences of functional lung failure, stimulation by means of carbon dioxide may be indicated. This is best used in the combination of 5 per cent of CO_2 with 95 per cent of O_2, the latter to compensate for the considerable O_2 want which exists.

When, however, very marked symptoms of severe respiratory distress are present, stimulation of the respiration by CO_2 is contraindicated, as the unaffected lung areas are already overstimulated and in an extreme state of compensatory hyperfunction. Oxygen inhalation alone is therefore indicated in such conditions, and stimulation of circulation by means of adrenalin or caffeine may also be needed. Sometimes it is even desirable to relieve the distressing dyspnea by slight depression of the respiratory hyperactivity, which may be accomplished by small doses of morphine.

In the case of massive collapse, and, in fact, in the majority of cases of all forms of atelectasis, the symptoms usually subside fairly promptly with very little treatment. In the case of massive collapse, change of position, massage, inhalation of a mild irritant to excite cough, may aid in reinflating the collapsed lung areas. In extensive unilateral massive collapse, the introduction of artificial pneumothorax on the affected side, to reduce the markedly increased negative pressure in the pleura and replace the heart toward its normal position, may give marked relief.

When the massive atelectasis is due to bronchial occlusion from any cause, the treatment consists in the treatment of the cause of the obstruction, in case of foreign body by removal through the broncho-scope, in other cases, as from tumor and pressure of calcified glands, there is usually no effective method of treatment.

EMPHYSEMA.

Definition.—Emphysema is essentially a functional disease of the lung. It may be defined as a permanent and irreversible insufficiency of pulmonary retraction.

Incidence.—The normal ageing process involves a progressive physio-logic insufficiency of pulmonary retraction known as senile emphysema. When this permanent insufficiency of retraction occurs below the age of fifty years, it may be termed pathologic. This condition occurs in a very considerable number of cases much larger than clinical records would indicate, as it is often obscured by other conditions. Localized areas of permanent emphysema occur with the greatest frequency associated with other pulmonary conditions. The temporary form of emphysema known as compensatory emphysema is extremely common. This latter condition, however, is not true emphysema, although if the temporary or compensatory form persists for a long time, it may become permanent, and true emphysema results.

Pathogenesis.—In the introductory section emphysema was defined from the standpoint of functional pathology as being an expression of disturbed mechanics of breathing. As explained there, disturbance in any of the components of the correlated functions will involve changes in all of them. Thus, pulmonary retraction may become involved by any of the following disturbances:

1. **Failure of intrinsic retraction power of the lung** may in the first place be due to some constitutional inherent weakness of the lung parenchyma. In individuals so affected the elastic recoil of the lung parenchyma will give way sooner or later under the stress of function. Hereditary factors have been long believed to have a predisposing influence here, and variations in the constitutional fitness of individuals point in the same direction. The tendency is accentuated particularly in those whose work entails exertion out of proportion to their indi-vidual constitutional capacity.

The intrinsic retraction power of the lung may give out under the effect of prolonged intrapulmonary pressure brought about by air passage obstructions such as may arise as a sequel of recurrent protracted asthma, severe and prolonged spastic bronchial conditions, or very chronic obstructing conditions in the upper respiratory tract (substernal goiter).

2. **Immobilization of the bony chest wall or diaphragm** has long been known to produce emphysema. There are some workers who still hold the concept, much in vogue a generation ago, that early calcification of the rib cartilage and the resulting fixation of the rib cage is a primary cause of emphysema. A similar rôle is being attributed to fixation and straightening of the spine by calcification of the intervertebral disks. That congenital and pathologic scolioses and kyphoses with the attending distortions of the chest cage are invariably associated with a great deal of genuine emphysema in the non-compressed lung areas, has served to support these contentions. Flattening-out and immobilization of the diaphragm by subdiaphragmatic conditions which press apart the costal arches to which the diaphragm is attached, also tend to produce pulmonary emphysema. Perhaps the emphysema of individuals with constantly high intra-abdominal pressure due to conspicuous abdominal obesity and meteorism is also attributable to more or less fixation of the diaphragm. Similarly, immobilization of the diaphragm takes place in long-chested individuals with marked enteroptosis and flaccidity of the abdominal wall, leading to abnormally low pressures under the diaphragm. The tendency of such individuals to become emphysematous has also been noted.

3. **Failure of pulmonary circulation**, bringing about active or passive congestion in the lungs, is an outstanding factor in the production of pulmonary emphysema. The frequent conspicuous association of emphysema with cardiovascular disease in general, but particularly with chronic mitral diseases, chronic arteriosclerosis in the thoracic aortic segment and arteriosclerosis in the lesser circuit, has long been recognized. Frequently indeed such emphysema with its attending bronchitis and cough are the first indications of failing cardiovascular function.

Pathology.—The emphysematous lungs are large, and do not collapse when the thorax is opened. They are soft to the touch, pit on pressure, and are pale in color. Frequently bullæ or blebs are seen on their surface, particularly along the anterior borders. These may occasionally rupture, causing pneumothorax. The upper and anterior portions of the lungs are much more involved than the lower and posterior.

Microscopically, the alveolar spaces are large, communicate with each other; their walls are very thin, and many of the capillaries are obliterated, but remaining ones are dilated, so that the normal quantity of blood traverses the lung. The distention of the air spaces does not break through the interlobular septa; but as the lobules increase in size, the walls of the alveoli give way in a manner which has been described as gloved fingers being converted into a mitt.

The walls of the bronchi are usually chronically inflamed and thickened, often to a considerable degree.

Functional Pathology.—The essential functional change in emphysema is a marked increase in the residual air volume of the lungs. This at first equals, and finally exceeds the vital capacity, the vital capacity under such circumstances being gradually reduced until the individual must breathe with all his available mobile lung volume, that is, the tidal volume becomes also the vital capacity.

Since marked enlargement of the air spaces is the fundamental lesion of emphysema, while the lungs as a whole need not contain more than the normal amount of air, it is evident that the chief trouble lies in the unequal distribution of the air contents between the various lung areas. This is borne out by the fact already described, that in so-called general emphysema the upper and anterior portions are mainly affected. In localized forms of emphysema associated with other pathologic disease in the lung, the same unequal distribution prevails to a less extent. Atelectasis and fibrosis usually occur in the non-emphysematous areas, and these conditions, together with chronic inflammatory lesions, play an interchanging rôle with emphysema in many lung diseases. As pointed out in the introductory section, disturbances of bronchomotor activity such as occur in asthma and bronchitis, and in the function of collateral ventilation associated with these bronchomotor disturbances, are significant factors in the causation of this unequal air distribution.

As the condition progresses, the chest becomes more and more fixed in an inspiratory position, which is frequently intensified by calcification of the costal cartilages. The impaired mechanics of respiration, together with the difficulty of adequate ventilation, combine to cause disturbances of gas exchange, which explains the most characteristic symptom of emphysema, namely, dyspnea.

Symptoms.—Dyspnea is by far the most outstanding and characteristic symptom of emphysema. It is characterized by a marked increase of expiration time which may occupy three-fourths of the entire respiratory cycle. As the power of pulmonary retraction increasingly fails, the patient must interrupt his prolonged expiration by abrupt, snapping efforts at inspiration. Frequently the dyspnea takes on the acute form of asthma when associated with bronchitis and bronchial spasm. This is worse at night.

Cyanosis may be severe in the chronic, advanced cases due to increased venous pressure affecting the capillary circulation. In these advanced cases there are usually evidences of cardiac disturbance with dilatation and insufficiency of the right heart, associated with signs of pulmonary edema.

Associated with the dyspnea there is usually a great sense of fatigue which is intensified by exertion, and which is probably dependent upon the chronic state of anoxemia which exists.

Cough is not a characteristic symptom of emphysema *per se*, but is frequently associated with it because of the accompanying bronchitis or bronchial spasm. Polycythemia may occur in the chronic, advanced cases as a factor in compensation for O_2 deficiency.

Spontaneous pneumothorax occurs occasionally, and may even be bilateral, producing acute dyspnea and cyanosis, and sometimes

45

leading to death within a short time. Occasionally spontaneous pneumothorax causes surprisingly little disturbance, and in some instances where the chest wall is not yet reached, it appears to be followed by some improvement in the symptoms after the lung reëxpands.

Physical Signs.—The physical signs of emphysema are those of the characteristic barrel-shaped chest increased in its antero-posterior diameter and fixed in an exaggerated inspiratory position. The percussion note is hyperresonant or tympanitic, obscuring the normal dull areas over the heart and the liver and, what is often most important, obscuring the normal physical signs of other pathologic conditions such as tuberculosis and fibrosis. The breath sounds are muffled. Inspiration is short and very feeble and the expiratory sound is very prolonged and low-pitched. Because of the associated bronchitis, sibilant and sonorous râles are often heard over both chests.

Roentgenologic Signs.—These show characteristic, highly illuminated lung fields, and, as in the case of the physical signs, these may distort or obscure densities which would otherwise be easily appreciated. On the other hand, the densities which do appear show up very sharply in contrast to the highlight of the emphysema. The normal lung markings are less prominent than normally, particularly over the upper lobes; over the lower lobes they may be accentuated because of compensatory fibrosis.

Course of the Disease.—Emphysema is a very chronic disease, often lasting an entire lifetime to old age. Its presence complicates the severity of any accompanying pulmonary or cardiac disease, and frequently, in the end, cardiac insufficiency with combined pulmonary and cardiac failure terminates the picture. During the progress of the disease recurrent attacks of pulmonary edema with embarrassment of the right heart, from which the patient gradually recovers, constitute the usual picture.

Diagnosis.—The diagnosis of a characteristic advanced case of emphysema is not difficult, but less marked forms are often not recognized. There are many cases in which emphysema of the lungs plays an important rôle in the symptom-complex which may be associated with other conditions. The interchanging rôles played by emphysema, atelectasis, fibrosis and chronic inflammatory processes such as tuberculosis, have already been indicated.

Oftentimes the transitory state of pulmonary retraction insufficiency, known as compensatory emphysema, is confused with true emphysema. This latter condition may supervene, but only after the temporary disturbance has persisted such a long time as to have become permanent and irreversible.

Treatment.—The treatment of pulmonary emphysema is purely symptomatic and directed toward an effort to delay the progress of the disease and its effects. This can best be done by very strictly modifying the patient's life to avoid fatigue and overexertion and getting out of breath. Every effort should be made to diminish the likelihood of acute respiratory infections which, when they occur, should be treated with the greatest care and promptness. As these occur most often in winter, residence in a warm, mild, equable climate at low altitude during the winter months is frequently desirable.

In advanced cases with marked dyspnea and tendency to cyanosis, associated as they are with chronic anoxemia, the inhalation of O_2 at repeated intervals affords considerable relief.

Adrenalin is most useful in relieving bronchial spasm and tends to reduce the emphysematous hyperdistention by decreasing the bronchomotor element. In cases associated with bronchitis, tincture of belladonna, potassium iodide, with very small doses of morphine, are often helpful.

True emphysema itself is incurable and is usually slowly progressive in spite of all treatment.

Interstitial Emphysema.—Definition.—Interstitial emphysema is an inflation with air of the spaces in the interstitial framework of the lung.

Etiology.—The escape of air into the interstitial tissue may be due to external injuries, or wounds of the chest or of the trachea and larger bronchi. More usually, however, it follows violent cough. The conditions in which this cough is particularly apt to produce this accident are: whooping cough, bronchopneumonia in measles and influenza especially, diphtheria and miliary tuberculosis. These conditions are much more frequent in children than in adults.

Interstitial emphysema may also occur from very marked and prolonged contraction of the abdominal muscles, such as occurs in labor. This contraction causes a raising of the diaphragm, and, being associated with the closure of the glottis, it markedly increases the pressure in the lung.

Pathology.—The air escaped from the bronchi or alveoli penetrates usually first the connective tissue along the bronchi, then it may travel to the subpleural connective tissue, particularly along the anterior borders of the lung and also in the opposite direction, into the mediastinal connective tissue, from whence it escapes upward along the fascial planes into the subcutaneous tissue first in the neck and then, in extreme cases, over the entire trunk.

The air beneath the pleura may produce subpleural blebs which may rupture and cause spontaneous pneumothorax. Occasionally the condition is due to rupture of emphysematous blebs due primarily to alveolar emphysema.

Symptoms.—The principal symptom is dyspnea, which may be associated with substernal pain when the mediastinal tissue is invaded, and very considerable discomfort in the case of extreme subcutaneous emphysema. Usually the tear in the lung heals in a few days and the air is gradually absorbed. Occasionally when it is associated with bronchopneumonia, particularly in influenza, bacterial infection may invade the mediastinum, causing a suppurative mediastinitis.

The *treatment* in uncomplicated conditions is purely palliative.

PULMONARY FIBROSIS, PNEUMOCONIOSIS, PULMONARY ARTERIOSCLEROSIS.

Definition.—The conditions included in this section are all based upon a common pathologic process, namely, connective tissue hyperplasia tending to obliterate the air spaces, lymphatics and blood channels of the lungs. They are generally found associated together and even when they appear as apparently distinct conditions of recognized etiology, their etiologic factors are closely related, also, their clinical features are very similar or identical. Hence, we would be justified in discussing them as a single clinico-pathologic entity under the designation of "pulmonary fibrosis." However, to avoid confusion by a too abrupt break with tradition, they will be discussed here separately but brought together under the same heading in order to emphasize their obviously close relationship.

Incidence.—Recent investigations of occupational fibroses show that the actual incidence of pulmonary fibrosis has been much underestimated.

The air spaces of the lungs represent the largest externally exposed surface of the body and their huge capillary bed represents a filter for all pathogenic agents in the blood stream; thus the lungs are the most frequently affected organ of the body. The various forms of pulmonary fibrosis represent sequelæ of all the damages and affections of the lungs of both external and internal origin, and as such it is probably the most common pathologic lung condition.

General Etiology and Classification.—The clinico-pathologic processes by which pulmonary fibroses manifest themselves fall naturally into the three etiologic groups implied in the titles:

1. **Pulmonary Fibrosis.**—Pulmonary fibrosis (*clinical fibroses*) in the strict sense includes the fibrotic processes involving chiefly the parenchyma of the lungs and is the result of more or less well-defined clinico-pathologic lung conditions, especially the infections.

2. **Pneumoconiosis.**—Pneumoconiosis (*occupational fibroses*) includes the fibrotic processes involving primarily the lymphatics of the lungs and represents the result of considerable or prolonged exposure to industrial dust or other similar agents.

3. **Pulmonary Arteriosclerosis.**—Pulmonary arteriosclerosis (*vascular fibroses*) includes the fibrotic processes affecting primarily some part of the vascular system of the lungs, partly of known but largely of unknown etiology.

It is to be understood that the line of cleavage between the processes included in these three groups is never very sharp. The clinical fibroses include many borderline conditions to the industrial types, inasmuch as exposure to the polluted atmospheres of our cities produces the so-called "physiologic pneumoconiosis" which is an important contributory factor in the causation of occupational fibroses. Again in pneumoconioses, supervening bronchiectatic and pleuritic processes may add a purely clinico-pathologic element to the picture.

Finally, more or less vascular sclerosis is characteristic of all forms of pulmonary fibrosis, although it is only in one distinct group of conditions that this is the chief pathologic substratum of the disease.

1. Pulmonary Fibrosis (Clinical Fibroses).

Special Etiology.—In the special etiology of this condition the following factors play an outstanding rôle:

(*a*) **Repeated Inhalation of Irritating Substances.**—The inhalation of dust and fumes and the minor respiratory infections to which all who live in cities are subject, cause slight degrees of pulmonary fibrosis. As a rule they do not represent clinical disease.

(*b*) **Chronic Inflammatory Conditions of the Lungs and Pleura.**—This includes all the various chronic types of pneumonic, suppurative or granulomatous processes in the lungs, bronchi, pulmonary vessels and pleura, all of which tend in time to a greater or less degree of pulmonary fibrosis.

(*c*) **Functional Conditions of the Lungs.**—In emphysema and in the bronchial spasm of asthma, the disturbances of bronchial activity causing a shunting of the circulation to other parts of the lung lead to arteriocapillary congestion and finally to fibrosis.

Atelectasis with prolonged deflated state of the affected lung areas from any cause leads finally to obliteration of many air spaces and their capillaries by fibrosis.

Pathogenesis.—The pathologic process in pulmonary fibrosis is an overgrowth of connective tissue.

Following the various etiologic factors above described there is an interference with the self-cleansing function of the lungs, a mobilization of the large mononuclear phagocytic cells from the walls of the alveoli, which gravitate to the lymphatic system, clogging the lymphatic vessels and lymph nodes. This leads to an immobilization of larger or smaller areas of the lung, interfering with capillary circulation, and the consequent organization of the cellular elements into fibrous tissue. This effect is the same whether the condition is due to the inhalation of dust, to bacterial infection, or to interference with circulation. The large mononuclear phagocytes are the same cells whether termed "dust cells," "heart failure cells," or "macrophages," "clasmatocytes," or "monocytes," which are so important in the pathogenesis of pulmonary tuberculosis. This cellular reaction is the main factor in the early stages of fibrosis through the clogging of the lymphatic system. The effect is cumulative and slowly progressive until the increasing encroachment upon the lung alveoli and capillaries interferes with both the ventilatory and circulatory functions.

The reciprocal action which occurs between various lung areas in the presence of atelectasis and fibrosis, on the one hand, and emphysema, on the other, can be best understood by comparative study of the section on these conditions, and the principles enunciated in the introductory section.

Pathology.—The amount of fibrosis varies greatly in extent and distribution, as well as in the presence of other associated lesions.

In mild cases there is slight thickening and generally pigmentation of the pulmonary lymph nodes, and slight peribronchial or perivascular fibrosis with, however, little or no encroachment upon the alveoli or the capillaries and consequently no apparent impairment of function. The fibrosis which may be termed pathologic is of greater extent than this, and may be disseminated or localized in distribution, or nodular or diffuse in character.

The disseminated forms are usually nodular, generally bilateral, and primarily involve the hilum and the central portions of the lung areas. They may eventually extend, however, into the entire lung field, or may progress into the diffuse form.

The localized forms depend largely upon the location and extent of the preëxisting etiologic process such as pulmonary infections or atelectasis, which conditions may involve the whole or portion of any lobe, either upper or lower, but more frequently the latter. When the fibrosis is associated with emphysema which predominantly involves the upper lobes, the corresponding fibrosis appears in the lower lobes. The involved areas are firm, dense and imperfectly or entirely non-aërated due to the obliterated air spaces, and they are frequently bluish in color because of the obstructed circulation. The interlobular and interlobar septa are thickened, as is the pleura, which is also adherent. Other areas of the lung, especially those in the immediate neighborhood of the fibrosis, are usually emphysematous, and the bronchi are chronically thickened and inflamed, may be occluded, and are often dilated into true bronchiectases.

Following the tendency of all fibrotic tissue to contract, the involved portion of the lung shrinks; in the case of an entire lobe it may be to as much as one-fourth of its normal size. This leads to retraction and immobilization of the chest wall, and displacement of the mediastinum and diaphragm in the direction toward the lesion.

These extensive fibrotic lesions in the lungs have been variously termed *interstitial pneumonitis, cirrhosis of the lung*, or *chronic organizing pneumonia*. But it is less confusing to think of them all as representing a pulmonary fibrosis of varying extent and distribution.

Associated with fibrosis there are frequently other conditions such as bronchial occlusion, suppuration and bronchiectases, which materially affect the pathologic changes as well as the clinical symptoms. In cases associated with bacterial infection, this may extend to the pleura with the occurrence of pleurisy with effusion, but in uncomplicated fibrosis, the changes in the pleura are those of chronic, adhesive pleurisy. As the condition of pulmonary fibrosis advances, both ventilatory and circulatory functions of the lung gradually fail, and pulmonary edema ensues.

Symptoms.—In mild cases the symptoms may be very slight or absent. When they occur they are those of the associated slight bronchitis.

In the more marked cases, dyspnea and cough are the outstanding symptoms. Expectoration may be slight or absent in uncomplicated cases, but usually is present in variable amount and character, depending upon the bronchitis, bronchiectasis or pulmonary suppuration with which the fibrosis may be associated. Hemoptysis may occur, especially in those cases complicated with bronchiectasis. Pleuritic pain is common, but not marked. Fever occurs only in the presence of secondary infection, which, however, is common.

As the condition progresses the dyspnea increases and is accompanied by cyanosis, both of which symptoms are intensified when the attacks of pulmonary edema intervene.

Physical Signs.—In the disseminated forms the physical signs may be very slight, most usually sibilant râles due to the slight bronchitis. The physical signs of increased density are often obscured by the accompanying emphysema.

In the diffuse and in extensive localized lesions, the physical signs are those of a consolidated lung, associated with numerous moist râles over the area, or the signs may be those of a markedly thickened pleura. In such cases there is usually retraction and diminished mobility of the corresponding side of the chest, and displacement of the heart and mediastinum toward the affected side. In advanced cases, particularly those associated with dyspnea and cyanosis, clubbing of the fingers is very common, as is polycythemia.

Roentgenologic Findings.—In the early stages of pulmonary fibrosis the roentgen-ray findings are very slight. They may show slight increase of the normal markings and of the hilum shadows. In the disseminated forms the shadows are quite definite, sharply circumscribed, and are most marked around the root and in the mid-portions of the lung. As the progression of the disease is watched by means of the roentgen-ray, these shadows gradually fuse into each other, becoming more extensive and more diffuse. The uninvolved areas show the increased illumination of the accompanying emphysema.

The localized forms of fibrosis, which may involve the greater part or the whole of one lobe, particularly the lower, show a dense, homogeneous shadow with contraction of the intercostal spaces and displacement of the heart and other mediastinal contents, as well as the diaphragm, toward the lesion. Bronchograms made with the aid of lipiodol may show the presence of bronchial occlusion or of bronchiectases.

Diagnosis.—The diagnosis of pulmonary fibrosis is usually dependent upon the successful search for the underlying disease. In other cases the history of exposure to predisposing conditions, such as the excessive inhalation of dust, gives the clue. In cases of pure fibrosis not associated with other definite pulmonary disease, the diagnosis is not so difficult and is largely dependent upon the correct interpretation of the roentgen-ray film.

The most important differential diagnosis is from tuberculosis. The character and development of the symptoms, the localization of the lesions, in tuberculosis usually the upper lobe, in fibrosis usually the lower, and the careful examination of the sputum, are helpful aids to the study of the roentgenograms. It should be remembered that chronic tuberculosis is itself normally accompanied with a very marked fibrosis.

Other conditions which must be differentiated are: pulmonary abscess, bronchiectases, bronchial carcinoma, syphilis and mycotic diseases. The bronchoscopic examination is often the most helpful aid to differential diagnosis in these conditions, showing the presence or absence of bronchial obstruction, of foreign body, or carcinoma, and helping in the diagnosis of associated abscesses or bronchiectases.

As already emphasized, it is important not to remain satisfied with the diagnosis of pulmonary fibrosis without the consideration of the other possible associated pathologic conditions.

Course of the Disease.—Pulmonary fibrosis runs a very chronic course in disseminated cases. It is usually slowly progressive, with gradual increase of the pulmonary and systemic symptoms. In localized cases the course depends upon the etiologic associated lesions and the ability to treat these conditions with the aid of bronchoscopy or by surgery.

Fibrosis of the lung, excepting when it is in the form of silicosis, does not tend to develop into tuberculosis, so that the presence of fibrosis should not be considered as a predisposition to this disease.

Treatment.—Pure fibrosis of the lung is a permanent and usually progressive lesion not amenable to treatment. But as in most cases there is an underlying or associated lesion which may be treated, the treatment of these conditions is the proper procedure, whether it be abscess, bronchiectasis or bronchial occlusion. In cases with dyspnea and recurrent cyanosis, a regimen of rest and freedom from physical strain is very important, as is the prevention of acute intercurrent respiratory infections in all cases. Inhalations of O_2 may afford relief in cases with dyspnea, cyanosis and pulmonary edema.

Bronchoscopic treatment is not only helpful in diagnosis, but also for the relief of bronchial obstruction and for drainage in the case of associated pulmonary suppuration or bronchiectases.

In the extensive localized cases of pulmonary fibrosis involving the greater part or all of one lobe, advances in thoracic surgery have made possible a complete cure of some cases by radical operation. This operation is in the nature of one of the various forms of lobectomy.

2. Pneumoconiosis (Occupational Fibroses).

Special Etiology.—The pneumoconioses have been described under various names according to the supposed effects of different kinds of dust, such as *silicosis, anthracosis, siderosis, chalicosis* and *asbestosis.* Recent studies, however, appear to have demonstrated that the characteristic changes in the lung which are identified as pneumoconiosis are all actually due to the inhalation of silica dust. Less serious changes not characteristically those of pneumoconiosis may be caused by the inhalation of non-silicious dust, both inorganic or organic; for example, wood, textiles, tobacco and other organic dusts, and coal, iron, cement, brick and other similar non-silicious inorganic dusts. True pneumoconiosis depends upon the amount of silica in the particular dust inhaled, and occurs particularly in special occupations such as miners, quarriers, drillers, sand-pulverizers and sand-blasters, and in certain factory occupations such as grinders, pottery workers, asbestos workers and the makers of various commercial powders containing silica, especially scouring soaps and powders. The pneumoconioses which are apparently due to the inhalation of non-silicious dust, such as in the mining of iron, lead and other metal ores, coal, and in such occupations as steel grinding, appear to be due to the fact that these dusts contain a harmful amount of silica, or, in the case of metal grinding, to the dust arising from the abrasive substances employed, particularly sandstone. Pneumoconiosis has become an important industrial problem, not only because of the amount of physical disability resulting, but also from the standpoint of the employers' liability under the various Workmen's Compensation Laws.

Pathology.—It follows from the foregoing discussion that true pneumoconiosis is usually, if not universally, a silicosis. The changes which occur in the lungs in silicosis depend upon the same cellular reactions with clogging of the lymphatics as have already been described under clinical fibrosis. On account of the severity of the dust exposure the lesions in silicosis are much more extensive and widespread. In the most ventilated parts of the lungs—about the hili and lower lung fields—the lesions may appear conglomerated, while throughout the rest of the lungs they appear disseminated in nodular form, of more or less homogeneous distribution.

For convenience the degrees of pneumoconiosis have been divided into three stages. The first stage represents the clogging of the lymphatic vessels and the arrest of the dust-laden cells in the various lymphoid structures, with a very small amount of fibrosis. In this stage, and in the other stages also, there is a certain amount of bronchitis.

The second stage represents the increased amount of fibrosis localized in certain areas throughout the lungs where these lymphoid deposits are present. It is apt to be more marked on the right side and in the central zones of the lungs. In this stage there is a very considerable amount of fibrosis localized in these scattered areas which are rather sharply circumscribed. This second stage has been designated the nodular stage.

The third stage represents a more advanced condition in which the areas of fibrotic density are more diffuse, less sharply circumscribed from each other, and extend over a much larger total extent of the lung. The reaction in the tracheobronchial hilum nodes is more marked as the stage of disease becomes more advanced.

Associated with these characteristic fibrotic changes there is a considerable amount of bronchitis sometimes associated with bronchial spasm or asthma, and a greater or less degree of pulmonary emphysema between the areas of fibrosis. There is also in the more advanced stages a chronic thickening of the pleura due to the extension of the process into the pleural lymphatic channels, and occasionally the lesion may cause rupture of the pleura with pneumothorax. Pleural effusions rarely or never occur.

This characteristic fibrosis appears to be due to a specific action on the tissues caused by the chemical changes in silica in the presence of the alkaline fluids of the body. As the condition advances and persists for a longer time, this same specific chemical reaction creates a medium particularly favorable to the development of tuberculosis which sooner or later is the most frequent end result of silicosis. The special features presented by silicosis combined with tuberculosis will be discussed in connection with the pathologic and clinical phases of pulmonary tuberculosis.

The non-silicious dusts, both inorganic and organic, produce a chronic inflammation of the mucous membrane, that is, a bronchitis, but comparatively little fibrosis. The chronic bronchial catarrh may render the lungs more susceptible to acute respiratory infections, but produces no predisposition to tuberculosis. This is an exaggeration of the condition so generally found in all city dwellers, which is described in the section on clinical fibrosis. The difference is one of degree dependent upon the extent of the exposure to dust.

Recent studies upon the special form of silicosis called asbestosis indicate that the inhalation of asbestos, which is a silicate and does not contain free silica, may, in dust form, produce a condition similar to true silicosis. The character of the fibrosis is more diffuse and does not take on the nodular forms so common in true silicosis, but it may be very extensive, involving the greater part or even all of both lungs. Cases of asbestosis also appear to have an increased susceptibility to tuberculosis, which, however, is not as marked as in the case of true silicosis.

Symptoms.—The onset of pneumoconiosis is usually very slow, that is, over a period of years. It is only rapid in the presence of very excessive amounts of dust or of an extraordinarily high percentage of silica in the dust.

The most characteristic symptom is a slowly developing dyspnea. With this there may be little or no cough until the later stages, when cough and slight expectoration occur, particularly in the morning. In the more advanced cases there is gradual failure in health and strength, digestive disturbances, and occasionally pain due to pleuritic adhesions or to the occasional occurrence of spontaneous pneumothorax. In some cases there may be attacks of bronchial asthma.

There is no fever in uncomplicated pneumoconiosis. When it occurs it is due to coincident infection which, in the later stages, is very apt to be tuberculosis. The tuberculosis progresses more rapidly than usually and presents the usual symptoms of advancing tuberculous disease.

In the conditions due to non-silicious dust the symptoms are those of a simple bronchitis. But in the case of asbestosis there is apt to be more expectoration, which may contain the characteristic curious yellow bodies which have been designated "asbestos bodies."

Physical Signs.—The physical signs of pneumoconiosis are usually very slight, even in advanced cases. They are usually those of a general bronchitis associated with deficient lung expansion, and may be associated with the signs of emphysema. In fact, many cases present the picture of ordinary emphysema and bronchitis on physical examination.

Roentgenologic Findings.—The roentgen-ray picture of true pneumoconiosis or silicosis is very characteristic and upon it the diagnosis usually depends. In the first stage the appearance on roentgen-ray is very similar to that of a chronic bronchitis, namely, an increase of the bronchial markings and especially of the hilum markings. In some cases there may be a hazy ground-glass appearance in the central and lateral portions of the lung fields, usually more marked in the right side.

In the second stage there are evidenced very characteristic, rather sharply circumscribed densities of varying size, scattered through both lung fields, particularly on the right, and invariably more dense in the middle portions, although they may extend from apex to base.

In the third stage these densities are very much larger and more diffuse and less sharply circumscribed. They too are more marked in the middle portions of the chest and vary greatly in size, density and distribution. In both this stage and the second stage the hilum densities are markedly increased.

There may be roentgen-ray evidences of pleuritic adhesions, or more rarely of pneumothorax. In cases in which there is considerable emphysema the densities stand out more sharply in contrast against the emphysematous lung.

In the non-silicious dusts the roentgen-ray picture is very much the same as that of the first stage of silicosis, namely, increased markings and increased root shadows. In cases in which tuberculosis supervenes the tuberculosis is very apt to be first evidenced in some of the areas where the silicosis is evident, although sometimes it first shows in the apex in the usual way, giving the evidences of the various phases of tuberculosis described under that disease.

In the nodular form of silicosis associated with tuberculosis it is often not easy to differentiate with certainty the changes which are due to silicosis from those which might be due to tuberculosis.

Diagnosis.—The diagnosis of pneumoconiosis depends primarily upon the knowledge of the exposure to harmful dust over a considerable period of time. Where the occupation of the individual is known to entail such hazard, cases which would be ordinarily dismissed as those of bronchitis or emphysema should always be carefully investigated with the roentgen-ray, which usually reveals the true condition. Problems of differential diagnosis arise because of the similarity which may exist between diffuse nodular pneumoconiosis and various forms of tuberculosis. This difficulty is enhanced by the frequent association of the two. In other cases cancer of the lung may appear a possibility, either in a localized form as a bronchial carcinoma, or in the diffuse form due to secondary metastases in the lungs.

Pneumoconiosis must also be differentiated from pulmonary fibroses due to other causes, especially those which are primarily due to infections or chronic circulatory changes.

Course of the Disease.—The disease runs a slow course for many years. It is very variable in the rapidity with which the symptoms occur and also in the amount of actual pathology produced in different individuals under the same conditions. One individual may show definite pneumoconiosis in one year, which might not show in eight to ten years in the case of another individual under the same conditions. Moreover, the course is very materially influenced by the character of the dust, its intensity, the percentage of silica, and the associated lesions such as bronchitis, bronchopneumonia, and particularly tuberculosis. A very important feature is the permanency of the characteristic roentgen-ray shadows; they practically never disappear, and also the disease may continue to progress slowly even after the exposure to dust has been removed. Indeed the situation may frequently be such that even the roentgen evidence of the disease may become manifest only years after the exposure has ceased. This is due to the continuing action of the chemical disintegration of the silica. In advanced cases the amount of disability becomes very marked because of the dyspnea and progressive weakness. In the end, tuberculosis claims a very large percentage of the cases of true pneumoconiosis.

In the cases of mild pulmonary infections due to the inhalation of non-silicious dust, the picture is that of a chronic bronchitis with an increased susceptibility to colds and other respiratory infections, especially various forms of pneumonia. These conditions are not in themselves disabling.

Treatment.—The treatment of pneumoconiosis is the removal of the cause of the disease. As already indicated, this is not effective after actual pneumoconiosis has been produced. The symptoms may be relieved by palliative measures such as one might employ in any case of bronchitis, or symptomatic for various complications as may arise, such as asthma, pleurisy, and pneumothorax. In the end, the treatment of a large percentage of cases becomes that of the complicating pulmonary tuberculosis.

The only really effective treatment of pneumoconiosis is its prevention. This fact has led to markedly increasing measures to protect the workers in dusty trades from the inhalation of dust. This is done in many ways, such as blowing the dust away from the worker, moistening of the dust, protection of the worker by masks and, particularly by periodic roentgen-ray examinations, picking out early cases and eliminating them from that particular employment. In many countries and states of this country, silicosis is now recognized as an occupational hazard, and the workers in certain industries are protected under the Workmen's Compensation Laws. As the occupations in which these dust hazards occur are becoming more and more numerous, the importance of the recognition of this disease and its proper prevention, as well as the determination of employers' liability, have become modern medical problems of considerable importance.

3. Pulmonary Arteriosclerosis.

Primary and secondary forms of this are distinguished. Under the primary there are included all sclerotic processes in the lesser circulation for which no obvious cause can be demonstrated. Syphilis and rheumatic fever have been mentioned as possible etiologic factors, but for the majority of cases these could be ruled out. The secondary processes are found in association with various clinico-pathologic conditions leading to prolonged hyperemic states in the lungs. Active pulmonary arterio-capillary congestion may arise with continuous strain upon the lungs in such diseases as asthma, emphysema, tuberculosis, bronchiectasis, and in compensation for marked deformities of the chest, kyphoscoliosis. Passive pulmonary congestion is present in cases of chronic cardio-circulatory disease, as in mitral stenosis.

In the primary form the lesion is chiefly an arterio-capillary fibrosis with obliteration and angiitis of the smaller arterioles. In the secondary forms we are dealing with widespread sclerosis of the larger branches of the pulmonary artery, frequently involving even the latter.

The *clinical course* is characterized by what frequently goes now under the name of Ayerza syndrome, which includes marked cyanosis, dyspnea, cough with expectoration and occasional hemoptyses, headaches and angina hypercyanotica. The cause of the conspicuous dusky color is not so much the anoxemia as the frequently marked polyglobulia and stasis in the skin capillaries. When anoxemic cyanosis is added to it, the picture becomes that of the "cardiacos negros" of Ayerza and Arrilaga. By that time usually right-heart failure phenomena become apparent, to which most of these patients eventually succumb.

There is evidence that O_2 inhalation temporarily at least benefits these patients. When the cardiac failure symptoms make their appearance, cardiac drugs are indicated, The secondary form of the disease is one of slow evolution and frequently of rather long duration. The primary form appears frequently as a condition which leads to a fatal end within a few months or years.

BRONCHIECTASIS AND CYSTIC DISEASE OF THE LUNGS.

Definition.—This clinical entity includes all simple or destructive distention of the air passages, regardless of origin, time and circumstances of development.

Pathogenesis.—The following three main factors play a rôle in the pathogenesis of bronchiectatic and cystic disease of the lungs:

1. **Development of the Lungs and Bronchi.**—Three phases of this must be considered. Failure of terminal bud formation in the *prenatal* period results in distention, at birth, of the bronchi, and in creation of false air spaces, with subsequent pursing-up of some of these in the form of cystic structures no longer in communication with the rest of the air passages.

Intranatal failure of establishment of breathing function in some lung areas, leaving these in the atelectatic state, will also result in a similar bronchiectatic polycystic condition in the lungs, produced by distention of the larger bronchi or smaller bronchioles.

Growth of the lungs has recently been shown to continue in children up to the age of fourteen years. Various developmental or pathologic factors which may constitute an *interference with this postnatal growth* of the lungs during childhood years, are predisposing or directly leading to the development of bronchiectatic disease in later years.

2. **Lung Function and Dysfunction. The Balance of Tensions within the Chest and Lungs.**—The persistence of an infantile lung unfit to assume the adult lung function must be particularly considered here. As more fully explained in the introductory section of this article, bronchomotor activity, collateral ventilation and elimination of the normal moisture and foreign matter deposits, are the components of lung function playing a rôle in the maintenance of the tension balance within the chest and the lungs. Deficiency of these functions in

any lung area involves unequal air distribution (emphysema or atelectasis) and failure of drainage (accumulation of moisture and cough).

Thoracic traction and intrapulmonary pressure will both be increased in lung areas in which the bronchi are functionally inert. Such bronchi will be at the mercy of the mechanical forces active in inspiration as well as expiration, which will both work to distend the lumina of such bronchi having lost their control over the pressure conditions within.

Failure of drainage explains the enormous accumulation of secretions in bronchiectatic lungs and the attending incessant cough, both of which are added mechanical factors working to distend the lumina of functionally inert bronchi.

3. **Infection and Bronchial Destruction.**—Without infection and actual destruction of the bronchial wall there is no bronchiectatic disease, only bronchial dilatation which may or may not manifest itself clinically. If it does, sooner or later infectious destruction of the bronchial wall will be added. What we call *dry bronchiectasis* is such a condition in which a bronchial dilatation existed without manifesting itself clinically until bronchial wall ulceration shows itself by hemoptysis. Such a hemoptysis may functionally incapacitate the involved bronchi, open the way for infection and thus lead to real bronchiectatic disease. Every form of pulmonary pathology (pneumonia, abscess, tuberculosis, lues, cancer) involving the pulmonary interstitium and the walls of bronchi may thus lead to bronchiectasis, with the aid of the above-mentioned mechanical factors distending the bronchial lumina. Childhood diseases are especially prone to involve the interstitium of the lungs in the inflammatory process (pertussis, measles, childhood bronchopneumonias), and are well recognized as particularly important predisposing factors in the pathogenesis of bronchiectasis. Obstructions such as may arise in connection with tuberculous lymph gland enlargements, tumors, or foreign body aspirations will of course also invoke both pathologic wall destruction as well as mechanical lumen distention and produce bronchiectasis. Pathologic processes arising in the rudimentary accessory inferior lobe have recently been recognized as a fairly frequent source productive of bronchiectatic disease.

Etiology. — **The Infectious Agent and Its Source.** — The infectious process in the bronchial wall is generally a primary one. The assumption has been made that we may be dealing here with a special form of anaërobic infection. Recent evidence indicates however that the infectious agents are the microörganisms common in the infections of the upper respiratory tract, of which the anaërobes are only a part. The coexistence of chronic infections of the sinuses, tonsils, teeth with bronchiectasis, especially of the sinuses, is too frequent to be overlooked as a source of the infection of bronchi which have lost their normal defense inherent in their self-cleansing power.

Pathology.—With Schneider we must distinguish between atrophic and hyperplastic bronchiectasis. In the order of sequence the process is first a purely atrophic cylindric dilatation of the bronchus. The next stage is that of an atrophic process to which became added chronic inflammatory changes consisting of cellular infiltration in the subepithelial layer of the bronchial wall. When this has reached a marked degree we have the stage of hyperplastic bronchiectasis. The latter is due to the infectious process in the bronchial wall, appearing frequently in the form of transitory pneumonic processes which are not to be confused with chronic pulmonary processes of other etiology. The final stage of bronchiectasis is present when unequal cirrhotic shrinkage of the granulation tissue, which has gradually replaced the entire bronchial wall, leads to saccular distentions in the bronchial lumina. At this stage there is usually present considerable involvement of surrounding lung tissue, which may finally extend out to the pleura and involve it with adhesions with cirrhotic induration of the entire portion of the lung.

In bronchiectatic processes of secondary origin the localization and the character of the primary conditions (pneumonias, tuberculosis, syphilis, abscess) determine the site, the extent and the special pathologic features of the bronchiectatic lesions.

Symptoms.—In the early cases the symptoms are those of moderate cough and expectoration, exactly as one would expect in chronic bronchitis, with, however, a marked tendency to recurrences in the winter months. The most characteristic symptom, after bronchiectasis of any form becomes well developed, is persistent cough with excessive amount of expectoration which is usually foul, due to anaërobic putrefaction, and which separates into three layers on standing. With this there may be some dyspnea and in bad cases cyanosis and frequently hemoptyses, often of very considerable amount.

The constitutional symptoms may be slight, particularly during quiescent periods, but frequently exacerbations with fever are to be expected, due to the retention of secretion or the inflammatory reactions in the surrounding tissue resulting in bronchopneumonia. These exacerbations are much more frequent in the winter months and may last for weeks at a time, gradually subsiding, but with cough and expectoration persisting and often aggravated by them. Anything which tends to obstruct the emptying of the cavities by cough leads to such exacerbations. In the earlier stages the amount of cough and expectoration may be slight and often not foul, and constitutional symptoms are very slight and exacerbations evanescent. As the disease becomes more advanced, dyspnea and cyanosis occur with greater or less impairment of general health and strength.

Physical Signs.—In the bronchitic type the physical signs are those of bronchitis over both lower lobes. There may be little change in percussion or breath sounds, but there are numerous moist râles over these areas. In the more localized forms of bronchiectasis associated with extensive interstitial pneumonitis, the signs are those of consolidation of the lung and of marked thickening of the pleura, namely, marked impairment of resonance, diminished fremitus, changes in breath sounds toward the bronchial or broncho-amphoric type of breathing, with numerous very moist râles. If the condition is persistent for any length of time there is usually marked clubbing of fingers.

Course of the Disease.—The condition is a very chronic one. When well established it rarely, if ever, is cured spontaneously, and the course of the disease is marked by the exacerbations above noted with increase of all the symptoms and greater frequency of febrile attacks, the amount of sputum becoming enormous, often a pint to a quart a day, often extremely fetid, with frequent hemoptyses, increasing weakness and prostration, and the patient becoming a very obnoxious associate because of the odor of his breath and sputum. He finally becomes bed-ridden with continuous irregular temperature, and finally dies after months of such illness, usually during an exacerbation of a bronchopneumonia.

In other cases the condition remains mild, cough and expectoration are moderate, exacerbations few and not severe, and the patient may continue a fairly normal life with comparatively little disability, annoyed only by the chronic cough and expectoration.

Any acute exacerbation of the conditions of the upper air passages, which are so frequently associated with bronchiectases, leads to an aggravation of the chest symptoms. If these can be avoided, very frequently the unfavorable course of the disease may be controlled.

In the cases of "dry bronchiectases" there are usually no symptoms except periodic hemoptysis, the cause of which is often puzzling until the true condition is recognized.

Diagnosis.—It follows from what was said above about the pathogenesis of bronchiectasis that the condition is usually present long before it develops into bronchiectatic disease. To make the early diagnosis of bronchiectasis we should not wait until such clinical symptoms as chronic cough and foul expectoration present themselves. These symptoms mean advanced bronchiectatic disease associated with marked physical signs. In the bronchitic cases these are simply those of bronchitis, and when localized in the upper lobe they may simulate completely those of chronic pulmonary tuberculosis. Again, very often in either upper or lower lobe these localized cases present physical signs and symptoms very similar to those of chronic pulmonary abscess.

For the early diagnosis of bronchiectasis we must demonstrate the bronchial dilatations by the bronchographic method at a time when there exist as yet no symptoms of the disease and when even the plain roentgenogram often fails to show characteristic lesions. The roentgen plate then frequently shows only the bronchial markings to be increased, or it shows densities due to complicating bronchopneumonia or localized interstitial pneumonia.

Hemoptysis is that most frequent early symptom which should arouse our suspicion for the presence of bronchial dilatations even in absence of all other symptoms, physical or roentgenographic signs. It is a good rule in practice that every case of clear-cut hemoptysis should be given the benefit of a bronchographic study to rule out bronchiectasis.

Intrabronchial injection of lipiodol enables us to visualize the lesions in a most clear-cut manner. The bronchial cavities stand out in beautiful outlines, and the method is therefore of extreme value not only in establishing the diagnosis but in determining the location and the extent of the lesions. The method is of particular value when the bronchiectases lie behind the heart shadow, below the diaphragmatic shadow, or within a dense mass of consolidated lung. Of all lung diseases bronchiectasis is the one condition in which bronchography is of the greatest value, and its use is essential to a proper understanding of these cases.

Treatment.—The treatment of a well established bronchiectasis is most unsatisfactory and usually fails to do more than palliate the condition. Drugs are of little or no value. Change of climate, particularly to dry and mild equable climate free from the changes and exposures to infection incident to the winter climate of the temperate zone, may be of some assistance. Bronchoscopy repeated at frequent intervals helps to establish drainage, thus preventing retention of sputum and relieving to some extent the offensive odor of the sputum, and may have a favorable effect in diminishing the number and severity of exacerbations. Instillation of mild antiseptic material through the bronchoscope is also sometimes used with dubious benefit. Postural drainage such as is employed in the treatment of pulmonary abscess also helps to keep the drainage of the cavities more complete and acts similarly as, but less effectively than, the use of bronchoscopy.

In recent years various surgical procedures have been suggested for the cure of bronchiectasis, and when the lesions are limited to one lobe radical lobectomy is the ideal method of treatment. This operation is still attended with great risk. Phrenicotomy has been suggested but is not to be advocated as a rule, and other surgical procedures such as extrapleural thoracoplasty have been fairly useful in a limited number of cases. Artificial pneumothorax has been advocated but is frequently most unsatisfactory because of the presence of pleural adhesions or the fact that it interferes with proper drainage of the cavities through kinking and blocking of the bronchi and by diminishing the expulsive power of the cough. In cases of severe and repeated hemoptyses artificial pneumothorax is, however, indicated for the control of the hemorrhage.

Preventive Treatment.—Inasmuch as modern methods of examination permit the recognition of bronchial dilatations at a time before they develop into actual bronchiectatic disease, we are able to practice real prophylaxis in this disease. This consists in the first place in the correction of all conditions which predispose toward infection of the dilated bronchi, especially elimination of foci of infection in the upper respiratory tract, sinuses, teeth, and tonsils. Too much emphasis cannot be placed upon the prompt elimination of these coincident infections in individuals in whom bronchographic examination indicates already, or makes them suspicious of, the presence of bronchial dilatations. Such individuals must chiefly guard against recurrent respiratory infections. Individuals so predisposed may be required to change their place of residence for a warm dry climate such as the desert, which may help to prevent recurrent bronchitis with its threat of bronchiectasis.

INFECTIONS OF THE UPPER RESPIRATORY TRACT.

In this modern era of specialism in medicine, affections of the upper respiratory tract have come largely within the domain of the nose

46

and throat specialist. But many of these conditions are very important to the general internist. There will be no effort in this place to deal in detail with all of these conditions, but some of the more important of them will be considered particularly from the standpoint of their relationship to diseases of the chest.

Acute Coryza.—Acute coryza, the ordinary cold in the head, is one of the most common affections. It is generally localized in its manifestations and self-limited in its course. It is not, however, sufficiently appreciated how frequently it is associated with infection of the accessory nasal sinuses, particularly the ethmoids, and the person who is subject to very frequent recurrent colds usually has more or less disease of these sinuses. The inflammation of the nasal mucous membrane also is very frequently communicated to the pharynx, to the trachea and to the bronchi, so that a general inflammation of these respiratory surfaces is very often associated with the coryza. If these attacks are frequently repeated a chronic condition of inflammation of various portions of the respiratory tract may result. This condition leads to greatest susceptibility to reinfections and to permanent changes often of considerable moment.

Focal Infections.—Of the localized chronic foci of infection in the upper air passages, the sinuses, the tonsils and the roots of the teeth are the most important. They may not only lead by direct extension to inflammation of the lower respiratory tract, but may produce symptoms in other parts of the body, due either to the mobilization of the bacteria themselves, or to the toxins which they generate. These "focal infections" therefore become very important to the general practitioner. The nature of the infection may be the ordinary pyogenic bacteria, of which the streptococci are the most important. But frequently such foci, particularly in the mouth, harbor anaërobic organisms of the fuso-spirochetal type which may be of even more significance.

Facility in examination of the nasal passages, the accessory sinuses, the naso-pharynx, mouth, pharynx and larynx, should therefore be acquired by anyone wishing to become expert in the diagnosis and treatment of respiratory diseases. The conditions in the chest which are most frequently secondary to these upper respiratory infections are tracheitis, bronchitis, peribronchitis, bronchopneumonia, bronchiectasis and lung abscess. In all of these conditions a predisposing infection in the upper respiratory tract may often be detected, and its diagnosis and proper treatment are frequently essential to adequate treatment of the chest conditions.

The clearing-up of these foci of infection by proper local or operative treatment of the sinuses, by removal of infected tonsils and adenoids, extraction of infected teeth and general prophylaxis of the buccal cavity, is a procedure of prime importance which frequently must precede the treatment of the chest condition. Moreover, when these upper respiratory infections are effectively eliminated, many cases of chest disease may be entirely prevented.

Laryngitis.—**Acute Laryngitis.**—Acute laryngitis is often associated with acute coryza, but may be entirely independent of it. The voice is hoarse, or may be entirely lost. There is a sense of irritation of the larynx, a dry cough and frequently actual pain. Examination reveals a general diffuse redness and some swelling of the mucous membrane, which may be sufficient to cause slight dyspnea. There usually is little or no constitutional disturbance such as fever. The course of the disease is usually a few days and is favorably affected by rest of the voice, confinement to a room in which the air is kept moist and warm without changes in temperature, and, as is the fact in many acute conditions in the respiratory tract, exposure to changes of temperature and to outside air, particularly in cold weather, is to be avoided. Steam inhalations medicated with eucalyptus, menthol and benzoin give relief.

Chronic Laryngitis.—Following repeated acute attacks, and particularly when these are secondary to a chronic infection of the nasopharynx or sinuses, a chronic condition of laryngitis may result. This may also result from chronic irritation due to the inhalation of irritating substances or excessive use of the voice. The hoarseness is less marked than in the acute cases, and the voice retains a normal tone. There is no pain, but considerable irritability causing a hacking cough, and the mucous membrane on examination is less acutely red, but is thickened, often has a granular appearance, particularly in the interarytenoid space. In some cases there is an irregular or more localized distribution of this induration which may suggest tuberculosis. The effective treatment of this condition is the removal of the cause.

Edema of the Larynx.—Acute edematous swelling of the larynx occurs occasionally as a complication of acute or chronic laryngitis and diphtheria, as a complication of tuberculous or syphilitic laryngitis, or associated with edema elsewhere in the body, as in nephritis or in angioneurotic edema. The onset is sudden, dyspnea is intense, the voice may be entirely lost, respiration is stridulous. Examination shows acute boggy swelling of the entire larynx, particularly of the epiglottis and the ary-epiglottidean folds. If prompt relief does not follow the use of astringent applications, prompt intubation or tracheotomy may have to be employed to save life.

Tuberculous Laryngitis.—This condition may be primary, but is usually secondary to tuberculosis of the lungs. Slight huskiness of the voice is very common in pulmonary tuberculosis. When it persists and becomes a marked hoarseness, the larynx should always be examined with extreme care. The condition tends to aggravate the cough, and when ulceration occurs, there is pain which often becomes very marked. If the epiglottis is involved, the pain is most marked on deglutition; when the internal portions of the larynx are involved, particularly the cords, the pain is most marked during phonation.

The most usual sites of early lesions are the posterior commissure and the arytenoid cartilages. In the early stages the color of the mucous membrane is pale; later it becomes a marked red. The false cords are frequently involved, as are the true cords themselves, often bilaterally, but frequently localized to one side. The thickening of the tissue may cause restriction of the normal movements of the vocal cords.

When the infection is limited to the box of the larynx its course is usually slow and inclined to be benign. When, however, the arytenoid cartilages and the epiglottis are involved, the condition is often very acute and rapidly progressive with extensive ulceration, and the prognosis is definitely bad. In the earlier cases, particularly those localized to the interior of the larynx, the prognosis is by no means bad if proper treatment is instituted.

This *treatment* consists mainly in absolute rest, complete silence, with the use of pad and pencil for communication being frequently necessary, and application of bland cleansing sprays to the larynx may be helpful. In cases with pain, cocaine is frequently essential. Cauterization of the larynx in some cases by means of an electric cautery has the chief good results in skilful hands but, ordinarily, better results are obtained by a policy of non-interference and rest. Under careful control, sunlight deflected into the larynx by mirrors may be useful. If reactions occur, however, the results are disastrous. In the painful cases, injection of the inferior laryngeal nerve with alcohol has sometimes helped. Hanging of the head and swallowing fluid nourishment "uphill" is frequently useful in these painful cases.

Syphilis of the Larynx.—Syphilis of the larynx is usually seen in the tertiary stage of syphilis. Occasionally gummata are seen, but more often there is an infiltration of the entire larynx which is very apt to involve particularly the epiglottis and the ventricular bands. The color is more red than in tuberculosis and edema is more common. The ordinary antisyphilitic remedies are specific in this condition.

Cancer of the Larynx.—Primary cancer of the larynx is not infrequent. It occurs usually after the age of fifty years, and is more common in men than in women.

In its earlier forms the principal symptom is hoarseness, but as the disease progresses ulceration ensues and considerable pain results. There is often a dry cough, frequently spasmodic.

Examination of the larynx in the earlier stages shows a thickening which is more apt to be in the anterior portion of the larynx and to involve the true cord on one side. With this there is frequently impaired movement of that cord. As the disease progresses, the infiltration becomes more marked and involves the entire larynx on that side and spreads to the opposite side. Before this occurs, involvement of the regional lymph nodes in the neck usually occurs.

The course of the disease may be slow, but in other cases it is quite rapid, and early diagnosis is essential if life is to be saved. In suspicious cases a biopsy should be made to determine the nature of the condition. In early cases, surgical treatment, either partial extirpation of the larynx or, more usually, total removal of the organ, is necessary to save life.

Differential Diagnosis of Chronic Laryngeal Disease.—The problem of differential diagnosis in patients exhibiting evidence of continuing laryngitis is between a simple chronic laryngitis, a tuberculous laryngitis, syphilitic laryngitis and cancer of the larynx. The first of these conditions usually presents no difficulties, but in some cases very closely simulates some forms of tuberculous laryngitis or cancer of the larynx. The presence of association of chronic inflammatory lesions in the upper respiratory tract, the more general distribution of the laryngeal lesions, the absence of tubercle bacilli in the sputum and of evidence of any tuberculosis in the lungs and of a Wassermann reaction of the blood, usually clear up the diagnosis. But prolonged observation is frequently necessary. The first step to be taken when tuberculous laryngitis is suspected is careful examination of the lung and of the sputum for tubercle bacilli. The negative Wassermann reaction usually excludes syphilis, and only in rarer cases is the laryngeal picture such as to be confused with cancer. In syphilitic laryngitis, if the appearance of the larynx is not characteristic, the serologic examination of the blood is usually determining. In cancer of the larynx the diagnosis between it and chronic laryngitis is not always easy, and the localized form of tuberculosis may closely simulate it. The fact that tuberculosis is more often encountered in the posterior portions of the larynx and cancer in the anterior portions is frequently a very helpful feature. In any of these four chronic conditions the possibility of any of the other three should be kept in mind, and all of the differential tests and procedures should be made. Repeated observations are often necessary to reach correct conclusions.

Tracheitis.—This condition is almost always acute and is often associated with coryza. The constitutional manifestations are very mild and the characteristic symptoms are a very harsh, unproductive type of cough associated with substernal pain. Any of the respiratory microörganisms may cause this condition. The course of the disease is two or three days, unless associated with a definite bronchitis. The treatment similar to that recommended for acute laryngitis is helpful, and medication of some form of expectorant tends to increase the secretion and to diminish the harshness of the cough and the severity of the pain.

Bronchitis.—Acute Bronchitis.—This is an acute catarrhal inflammation of the bronchi which may either be limited to the larger bronchi or extend down to the smallest ramifications. It is usually associated with and is secondary to infections of the upper respiratory tract, most frequently beginning with a coryza, and any of the respiratory microorganisms may be the causative agent.

Symptoms.—The onset of the condition is usually not acute, but an ordinary cold of the head becomes associated with malaise, slight fever and cough, which at first is tight and barking in character and often paroxysmal. In some cases there is definite stricture of the bronchi with asthmatic breathing and dyspnea. The condition is usually associated with a tracheitis with its associated substernal pain. After a few days the acute symptoms subside, the cough becomes looser, expectoration of muco-purulent sputum occurs and consequent relief of all the symptoms.

Physical Signs.—The physical signs in the chest are bilateral, usually most marked over the lower lobes. There may be high-pitched sibilant or sonorous râles over both chests which, as the secretion occurs, become more moist, with fine mucous râles over both bases. The bases of the lungs are the last to clear. There is no abnormality in percussion or respiratory murmur, excepting in the asthmatic cases where the inspiratory murmur is diminished.

Course of the Disease.—A simple bronchitis usually clears up in four to five days. Where, however, it is associated with chronic infection of the upper respiratory tract, especially the sinuses, it may persist for a much longer time and clear up only to recur from time to time. In some cases the infection reaches the peribronchial tissues, and a bronchopneumonia may result. This is particularly apt to be the case in some of the infectious diseases such as measles and whooping cough and in older people who are confined to bed longer than the usual period on account of weakness.

Treatment.—In the acute stage the patient should be kept absolutely in bed, without too much access of fresh air or change of temperature. Medicated inhalations may give relief. Mustard plasters on the chest are helpful and expectorants may be of value. In cases associated with asthma, the hypodermic administration of adrenalin or ephedrin may be necessary. In recurrent cases associated with upper respiratory infections the treatment of these conditions is of major importance.

Chronic Bronchitis.—Chronic bronchitis is usually associated with some other lesion. It may be due to recurrent attacks of bronchitis, which in turn have their primary cause in the upper respiratory infection. It is more apt to be associated with pulmonary emphysema. Chronic valvular heart disease may predispose to chronic bronchitis, and it is much more apt to occur in older than in younger people. The symptoms are usually those of chronic cough and expectoration, with a definite tendency to dyspnea on exertion, especially if it is associated with heart disease or with emphysema. In the emphysematous cases there is very apt to be more or less asthmatic contraction of the bronchi, in which case the symptoms are more marked at night, as in cases of true asthma. Expectoration is usually not very profuse and is more marked in the morning. There is a definite seasonal variation in the symptoms which are worse in winter than in summer. There is very little or no fever or other constitutional disturbance.

Physical Signs.—The physical signs are similar to those of acute bronchitis, excepting that the sibilant moist râles predominate and are constant. In cases associated with emphysema or asthma the inspiratory murmur is diminished and the expiratory murmur prolonged. The signs are always bilateral and more marked in the lower lobes.

Treatment.—Where any other chronic infection is present the best treatment is the treatment of those infections. Where this is impracticable, or where there is associated emphysema or heart disease, climatic treatment is of definite importance—mild, warm climate in winter with freedom from changes in temperature and from wind and dust. Restriction of exercise is important, and fatigue and dyspnea are to be avoided. The use of ordinary expectorants in these cases is of little value. Potassium iodide is frequently helpful, and the time-honored emphysema mixture of potassium iodide, tincture of belladonna and nitroglycerin, with or without very small doses of morphine, is often helpful. In cases with asthma the use of adrenalin or ephedrin may be necessary. To a lesser extent than in acute bronchitis, medicated inhalations are of value.

Peribronchitis.—This is a clinical entity not always recognized as such, and has been variously described as "subacute bronchopneumonia," "non-tuberculous basal infection of the lung" and "peribronchitis."

Etiology.—Any of the respiratory infections may cause this condition; the pneumococcus and the influenza bacillus, however, seem to be most usually at fault. In this class of cases also the chronic infection of the sinuses or of the tonsils is very frequently the predisposing factor in the occurrence of the chest condition.

Pathology.—The typical form of this condition is a localized inflammation in an entire lobe, or a considerable portion of one. It is associated with a definite bronchitis in that portion of the lung, a thickening of the peribronchial tissue, and a slight amount of exudate in the alveoli immediately surrounding the bronchi. This inflammation is acute and may gradually become chronic, in which case there is a replacement of the exudate with fibrous tissue and, if long continued, it leads to a weakening and dilatation of the walls of the bronchus, which may result in bronchiectasis.

Symptoms.—The symptom of this condition is usually a mild febrile attack coming on rather suddenly, with cough, moderate expectoration, usually muco-purulent, and occasionally associated with very small hemoptyses. The fever usually lasts only three to four days, but the cough and expectoration and the physical signs may persist for a considerable time.

Physical Signs.—The physical signs are quite characteristic of very slight or no impairment of resonance, no change in respiratory murmur, but a profusion of small moist râles over the entire lobe involved. As the patient improves and the constitutional symptoms disappear, these signs may persist for weeks and may become chronic or even permanent. It is in these cases that bronchiectases may occur. In other cases the course is more subacute and the signs persist for a month to six weeks and then disappear. A frequent characteristic of this condition is the proneness to recur, and any respiratory infections, months or even years after the first attack, may cause a reappearance of the physical signs in their entirety.

Diagnosis.—The diagnosis is based upon the extensive nature of the lesion as revealed by physical signs, the mild and short duration of the constitutional symptoms, the persistence of the signs long after these symptoms have disappeared, and the absence of any definite radiographic picture. Tuberculosis is often suspected in these cases, but the absence of tubercle bacilli in the sputum, the slight constitutional disturbances in the presence of an obviously extensive lesion, the location of the lesion in a lower lobe, and the absence of any radiographic evidence of disease, are the principal points of differential diagnosis.

Treatment.—The treatment of this condition is simple. The constitutional symptoms subside quickly, and the persistence of the physical signs may cause anxiety as to the presence of a more serious disease,

particularly tuberculosis. Prolonged rest does not seem to be necessary, as the cases which clear up seem to do so quite as well when up
and about as when at rest. Change to a mild, equable climate in
winter may be of advantage. In the more chronic cases the clearing up
of the upper respiratory infections is of extreme importance. It is
usually in that way that the gradual production of bronchiectases may
be prevented.

Foreign Bodies in the Bronchi.—The modern development of bronchoscopy and the more general use of the roentgen-ray, have led to
the recognition of the considerable frequency with which foreign bodies
become lodged in the bronchi. These foreign bodies may be of considerable size, and consist of all sorts of objects of various shapes and
of various materials. When these materials are metal, bone, shells,
or rubber, they are radio-opaque, and the roentgen-ray is of material
assistance in recognizing their presence and their location. Other
materials such as food particles, organic fibers, or pieces of tissue, are
not radio-opaque, and the recognition of their presence depends upon
the history and the symptoms which they produce.

The inhalation of these objects is more common in childhood, due to
inexperience and accidents. They are also quite common in adult life,
due to holding foreign bodies in the mouth, the inhalation of extraneous
objects during anesthesia, the inhalation of food which accidentally
enters the respiratory tract and pieces of teeth or dental fillings.

The pathologic results of such inhalations and the symptoms they
produce depend very largely upon the character of the objects themselves and the presence or absence of secondary infection.

Pathology.—A non-irritating foreign body may produce very little
reaction other than a localized bronchitis. But more often this local
irritation leads to chronic inflammation, the formation of granulation
tissue, the partial or complete obstruction of the bronchus with the
infection of the corresponding portion of the lung, or in other cases
to a local weakening of the wall of the bronchus with formation of
ulcers or of localized bronchiectases. Bronchial occlusion leads to a
greater or less amount of pulmonary atelectasis with or without suppuration, and the formation of a lung abscess.

Symptoms.—Quite frequently inhalation of foreign bodies may produce no symptoms for a considerable length of time, often years. In
other cases there is an immediate reaction and choking and coughing,
and the history of the accident is direct and circumstantial. Cough
may persist and is often of paroxysmal character, and when secondary
infection results, which is especially apt to occur with bronchial occlusion, there may be a considerable amount of expectoration of pus,
often foul, and the association of fever, in other words the symptoms
of an abscess of the lung. In other cases the cough is less persistent,
is worse only at intervals, and there may only be recurrent hemoptyses
with little or no other expectoration. These are the cases of localized
dry bronchiectasis around the foreign body, with ulceration of the
bronchial wall.

Physical Signs.—The physical signs are very variable. They may
be entirely absent. In cases of partial obstruction one of the most

characteristic signs is a localized wheeze in a portion of the chest, which is usually more marked in expiration. If the obstruction is more complete, impairment of resonance and diminished breath sound due to localized atelectasis may be recognized. When an abscess of any size is produced the physical signs are those of that condition. Sometimes the obstruction is of a ball-valve nature which traps the air behind the obstruction, giving signs of localized emphysema with a prolongation of the expiratory murmur beyond the limit of expiratory effort, so-called "after-breathing."

Diagnosis.—The diagnosis depends mainly upon the history. Where that is absent and one of the suspicious symptoms is present, the roentgen-ray examination is often the deciding factor in an accurate diagnosis. In all cases of abscess of the lung, especially in children, the possibility of foreign bodies as its primary cause should be considered. Bronchoscopy is the surest means of accurate diagnosis, particularly when the inhaled objects are not opaque to the roentgen-ray.

Treatment.—The correct diagnosis leads to effective treatment by removal of the foreign body through the bronchoscope. In cases where the object has remained in the bronchus for a considerable time, this is not always easy, but in skilful hands it is almost always effective.

ABSCESS OF THE LUNG.

Definition.—Abscess of the lung may be defined as a localized suppuration in the parenchyma of the lung. It is usually associated with necrosis of tissue and includes what some authors consider gangrene of the lung.

Etiology.—Pulmonary abscess is caused by infection of the lung tissue with the microörganisms of suppuration. Formerly the condition was supposed to be due to the ordinary pyogenic organisms, and the anaërobic microörganisms were considered to be secondary invaders of no pathologic significance. Recent investigations have shown that in many instances the original infection is due to these anaërobes, particularly spirochetes, fusiform bacilli, and motile bacilli of the colon group. These anaërobes are the ones which are regularly found in uncleanly mouths, crypts of the tonsils and in pyorrhea, and it is they which are responsible for the characteristic necrosis of lung tissue. Pulmonary abscess is caused by the inhalation of these organisms with or without the association of the ordinary pyogenic organisms. Conditions which favor the entrance of these organisms from the upper air passages, especially operations such as tonsillectomy or tooth extraction, favor the development of abscess through the aspiration of infected blood.

The inhalation of foreign bodies is a frequent cause of pulmonary abscess, especially in children. These foreign bodies may cause partial or total occlusion of a bronchus with consequent edema in the area distal to the occlusion, and often atelectasis, which conditions offer a most favorable opportunity for bacterial infection.

Lung abscess may also be caused by infections through the blood stream. The lesion is then in the nature of an infected embolus which breaks down into suppuration. This is particularly apt to occur following operations upon a suppurative focus in any part of the body, particularly upon the head or neck.

Pathology.—It has been usually assumed that pulmonary abscess begins as a pneumonia and that the necrotic process is superimposed. This frequently occurs; but as a matter of fact in many cases the pathologic process is necrotic from the start. The area of suppuration breaks down to a small cavity and is surrounded by a zone of edema and exudate in the neighboring alveoli, often swarming with anaërobes, and in the acute stage not surrounded by any definite wall. As the process develops more and more, this area breaks down until the abscess may become of very large size with a corresponding marked increase of the collateral zone of exudate.

Very early in this process the pus breaks through into a smaller or larger bronchus and is discharged through the mouth by cough. Very occasionally this does not occur for several days, but usually it takes place within forty-eight hours. The amount of drainage which occurs through the bronchus largely determines the outcome of the process. If insufficient, the process continues to extend until a large portion of the lung may be involved. On the other hand, if drainage is effective, the pus is evacuated, the area of exudate surrounding the abscess is absorbed, and prompt resolution occurs.

In other cases the drainage is only partially effective, being insufficient to totally drain the abscess cavity, but sufficient to prevent the extension of the process. This is frequently due to swelling and granulation tissue formation in the bronchial mucous membrane, or it may be due to the imperfect communication between the abscess cavity and the lumen of the bronchus. In such cases the process becomes localized; a fibrotic wall tends to form around the area of infiltration, and what is known as chronic abscess results. Fibrosis in the affected area then occurs and with it frequently the formation of bronchiectasis.

Symptoms.—The onset of the disease is acute with a sudden rise of temperature, often with chill. Frequently pain in the chest simulates the onset of pneumonia which, in fact, often occurs. Within two or three days, however, the characteristic symptom of expectoration of pus, usually foul, occurs, and it is on this symptom that the presence of the condition is usually suspected. Fever remains high, prostration is considerable, and the amount of expectoration may increase to 20 or even 30 ounces a day, with very distressing paroxysmal cough. The expectorated pus contains many microbes, separates into three layers on standing, and it may be tinged with blood, in which case it is usually dark, chocolate-colored. Free hemorrhage, however, is quite rare in acute cases.

In the chronic cases the systemic symptoms disappear, but cough and copious purulent expectoration persist, and free hemorrhage may occur. In very extensive cases dyspnea and cyanosis may ensue because of decreased facilities for normal gas exchange.

Physical Signs.—The physical signs of early lung abscess are often very scanty. They may be absent altogether even in the presence of an abscess of considerable size. The most usual signs are impairment of percussion note and numerous fine moist râles without change in breath sounds. As the process becomes more chronic the physical signs are more abundant and they simulate those of a chronic extensive pulmonary tuberculosis with cavity. The location of the abscess may be in any lobe, but is more frequently in the right lower lobe. Clubbed fingers are a common and often early finding.

Roentgenologic Signs.—Examination by means of the roentgen-ray offers by far the most satisfactory means of diagnosis and also of following the course of the disease in pulmonary abscess.

In acute cases the characteristic roentgen-ray finding is an area of homogeneous density with frequently an area of rarefication in the center. The borders of the density are soft in outline and fuse gradually into the surrounding normal lung picture. The greater part of the density represents the area of edema and exudate already described as surrounding the central necrotic area, and the soft outlines represent the tendency of this process to invade the normal lung.

The rarefied center representing the cavity may show a very characteristic dense shadow of shifting fluid level in its dependent portion. While this picture of cavity and fluid level has frequently been characterized as pathognomonic of lung abscess, it is by no means always present. Very frequently the entire area of density is homogeneous. This may be due to the fact that no area of cavitation sufficiently large to be detected by the roentgen-ray exists, or it may be due to the fact that the cavity is completely filled with exudate.

In chronic cases the characteristic picture of cavities with fluid levels is more common, and they are often multiple. The outlines of the shadow, however, are sharply circumscribed in contrast to the surrounding lung tissue, due to the fibrous wall.

As one studies serial roentgen-ray films, which should be taken at least at weekly intervals, the tendency to absorption is evidenced by a diminution in the size of the shadow and a sharpening of the outline between it and the surrounding lung. As the process clears, the densities may entirely disappear, leaving no trace behind. In other cases slight localized densities may persist for a long time, or even permanently, representing a residual fibrosis. In the chronic cases which become associated with bronchiectasis, the outlines of the dense areas not only become sharp, but the areas themselves contract, due to fibrosis, and frequently numerous small rarefied areas may be identified, best visualized by lipiodol injections. The use of lipiodol for bronchograms in acute lung abscess with copious purulent expectoration is undesirable, as the oil fails to penetrate the affected area, but may favor the spread of the infection to other parts of the lung.

It is also by careful study of the roentgenologic findings that the indications for the most favorable time for surgical intervention may be determined.

Course of the Disease.—In the most favorable cases the acute symptoms of fever, cough and foul expectoration may last only two or three weeks and gradually subside, with complete clearing up of the symptoms within four or five weeks. More frequently the symptoms run several months even under good treatment and are very apt to be marked by remissions and exacerbations. If the expectoration of pus is blocked, fever is apt to go higher and, correspondingly, when it becomes free the temperature subsides. In many cases the acute symptoms never subside and the condition of the patient becomes extremely grave within four to six weeks after the onset. In other cases it gradually drifts into a more chronic stage with marked cough and expectoration continuing, which gradually becomes less foul; the temperature may come to normal, and the process then may remain at a standstill for many months, neither improving nor becoming worse. This represents the chronic abscess.

Diagnosis.—The diagnosis of pulmonary abscess is suspected by the characteristic expectoration of foul pus. It is corroborated by roentgen-ray examination, and the diagnosis as well as the course of the disease can much better be determined by roentgen-rays than by physical examination.

The differential diagnosis is mainly between pulmonary tuberculosis and bronchiectasis. When the abscess is chronic and situated in the upper lobe, the similarity to tuberculosis is very great. Differential diagnosis then depends upon the persistently negative sputum, the history, the onset and the course. The differential diagnosis from bronchiectasis is more difficult because chronic lung abscess is often associated with bronchiectasis. The roentgen-ray, however, is usually different, particularly if lipiodol injections are made, which are quite characteristic in bronchiectasis, but which in lung abscess fail to enter the suppurative focus on account of the obstructed bronchial lumen.

In the acute forms of lung abscess the differential diagnosis between both of these conditions is easy; in the chronic forms it often requires time and patient study.

Bronchial carcinoma also may simulate lung abscess after it becomes infected and breaks down. In fact, in older people the occurrence of a typical picture of lung abscess should always arouse the suspicion of bronchial carcinoma as the real cause of the condition.

Treatment.—It has long been recognized that cases of lung abscess may get well spontaneously within a few weeks. On the other hand, up to recent years the condition has largely been considered as a surgical one, requiring operation for external drainage.

Recent advances in the treatment have shown the possibility of very materially increasing the percentage of cases which can recover without operation, that is by adequate drainage through the bronchi. This is facilitated by strict rest in bed combined with postural drainage accomplished by inverting the patient with his head to the floor with the body tilted, so that the affected lung is uppermost. This is to be continued for five to six minutes and repeated several times a day, which enables the cough to be more effective and adequate drainage to be established.

Such conservative treatment may be persisted in for a couple of weeks, but if no definite results occur, then bronchoscopy is always indicated. Bronchoscopy has the advantage of opening up the swollen mucous membrane of the bronchus, of establishing the presence or absence of a foreign body, and of allowing better drainage and aëration of the diseased area. Properly executed, the combination of bed rest, postural drainage and bronchoscopy will cure about 50 per cent of all abscesses of the lung if begun in the earlier stages.

It is important to continue comparative rest for several weeks after all purulent expectoration has ceased and after the roentgen-ray picture appears normal. The reason for this is that residual infection may persist for some weeks, which lights up into activity again upon physical work or exercise.

Artificial pneumothorax has been suggested because of its success in pulmonary tuberculosis. In some cases it may be effective, but it is not a desirable method for general use for the reason that it may cause rupture of the abscess into the pleura with subsequent virulent empyema, or it may block the drainage from the bronchus either mechanically or by preventing the effective action of cough.

Specific treatment by intravenous injection of arsenical compounds —neoarsphenamine—has been suggested because of the predominance of spirochetes in the sputum of many of these patients. In fact, the condition has sometimes for this reason been termed "spirochetosis" or "fuso-spirochetal disease."

Occasionally this treatment seems to be of help in the earlier stages, but in the hands of most observers it has been disappointing and certainly can not be looked on as a real specific method of treatment.

Surgical Treatment.—In about one-half of all cases the conservative treatment above outlined fails, and surgery by means of thoracotomy and drainage must be employed. Surgical treatment is absolutely contraindicated during the early, very acute stages of the disease. Operation at that stage is almost certainly disastrous.

On the other hand, if conservative treatment is persisted in too long the disease becomes chronic, the abscess becomes surrounded by a thick fibrous wall, and the results of surgery are most unsatisfactory because of the more frequent occurrence of hemorrhage, of embolism, particularly to the brain, or of the persistence of a bronchial fistula which may result in fibrosis and the development of chronic localized bronchiectasis.

The problem, therefore, is to determine the correct time for operation. This can best be done by weekly roentgen-ray studies on the part of the internist, surgeon and bronchoscopist, determining the progress of the case. When this is not satisfactory, surgery becomes necessary; this is best undertaken after the acute stage is passed and before the chronic stage has been reached. In this manner it is possible by careful study of the individual case to effect a cure in between 80 to 90 per cent of all cases.

Preventive Treatment.—The appreciation of the rôle played by chronic infections of the mouth, particularly the anaërobes, in the causation of pulmonary abscesses offers the opportunity for their prevention in many cases in which surgery in the mouth is contemplated. It is very important that preceding such operations as tonsillectomy or other major operations in the mouth, and especially in the extraction of teeth, a preparatory course of prophylactic treatment to clear up these oral infections should be carried out.

During operation every precaution should be taken to prevent blood from entering the trachea. This is a more important factor than the choice between local and general anesthesia.

GANGRENE OF THE LUNG.

Definition.—By gangrene of the lung we understand a death of lung tissue *en masse*.

Gangrene of this type is rare. Its usual cause is obstruction of the blood supply to that portion of the lung, frequently by means of embolus or thrombosis.

The portion of the involved lung is dark red, soft and soggy, and foul beyond description. This gangrenous area soon breaks down into a soft fluid mass which is discharged through a bronchus, and occasionally the condition may thus clear up as in lung abscess, leaving, however, a large, permanent cavity with fibrous wall. Such a result is unusual.

Clinical Signs.—The symptoms are generally those of marked sepsis with high fever, with a persistent cough, with expectoration of large quantities of extremely foul, bloody sputum. The physical signs vary as in the case of pulmonary abscess, and may simulate those of acute pneumonia, and the roentgen-ray also varies in the same way.

The *diagnosis* between pulmonary gangrene and lung abscess depends largely on the character of the sputum and the extreme acuteness of the process with associated evidences of septicemia.

The *prognosis* of lung gangrene is very bad by any method of *treatment*. Very occasionally spontaneous recovery will occur. Usually surgery should be attempted, but the mortality is extremely high.

PULMONARY TUBERCULOSIS.

The infectious nature of pulmonary tuberculosis was suggested for ages, but this fact was not generally accepted until Villemin substantiated it, in 1865, and Koch demonstrated the tubercle bacillus, in 1882.

As an infection of the lung, pulmonary tuberculosis can be understood only if its various manifestations are interpreted in the light of knowledge of the characteristics of tuberculous infection in general. These characteristics, like those of infections due to any other pathogenic agent, are determined by the following factors: the bacillus, the infected individual, and the evolution of the disease as affected by the flux of endogenous and exogenous circumstances. Before attempting to trace the special pathogenetic factors operative in pulmonary tuberculosis we must therefore analyze the characteristics of the tuberculous infection in general.

The Tuberculous Infection in General.

1. **The Bacillus.**—The tubercle bacillus is an organism endowed with considerable powers of resistance owing to its fatty capsule. Although

highly sensitive to sunlight, the tubercle bacillus survives long under the protecting cover of particulate matter which is its chief carrier. Of the many varieties distinguished, only the human and bovine tubercle bacilli are of clinical significance.

(*a*) **Sources and Modes of Transmission.**—The source of the infection in the vast majority of cases is the excretion of this bacillus in the discharges from some other human individual. In a much smaller number of cases the source of infection is from tuberculous cattle. Bovine tuberculosis in all, however, does not account for more than 1 to 2 per cent of all cases and this percentage has been materially diminished in late years, due to the control of bovine tuberculosis in cattle and to the pasteurization of milk. The comparatively few cases due to bovine infection are transmitted almost entirely through infected milk or milk products.

The usual method of transmission is from the respiratory tract of one to that of another individual. This may take place in three ways: (1) Droplet infection, that is, the direct inhalation of moist particles of sputum, either directly or through the infection of some intermediate object; (2) through dust inhalation, the discharged bacilli usually contained in the sputum becoming dry are taken up in the form of dust and are thus easily inhaled; (3) direct smear infection. The importance of this method of infection is emphasized by some authorities, especially in the case of children who play upon the floor where direct contact with gross sputum is possible.

(*b*) **Virulence of the Bacillus as a Factor in Infection.**—From 90 to 95 per cent of all adults become infected with tubercle bacilli, but disease results in a very small percentage of these. Development of disease depends in part upon the dosage of infection, which includes the number of bacilli as well as the frequency of the repeated infections. There is reason to believe that it also depends upon variations in virulence of the tubercle bacilli themselves. Dead bacilli do not produce disease; bacilli attenuated in virulence produce very mild disease which may tend to heal promptly. Recent studies on the dissociation of bacteria have shown that tubercle bacilli as well as many other bacteria tend in their growth, whether on artificial media or in the body, to change in character under the influence of their environment. As the infection becomes more chronic and localized the bacillus changes into a less virulent form, called R-forms. On the other hand, under change of environment these may revert back into virulent or S-forms. It is quite possible that what is termed virulence is largely dependent upon these biologic characteristics of the bacilli themselves, so that as these changes occur, either spontaneously or under conditions little understood, they may determine the ease and rapidity of the development of the lesions, independently of the tissue responses.

2. **The Individual.**—There exist individual differences in susceptibility and in resistance to all infections. The resistance to any infection, including tuberculosis, may be a non-specific, natural one, or it may consist in an acquired, specific immunity, hence individual differences in susceptibility to infection may depend upon predisposing factors involving either of these two conditions.

(a) **Non-specific Predisposing Factors.**—In all Western civilized communities where tuberculous infection is still so prevalent today, tuberculosis was at one time an epidemic disease. In some non-civilized races and even in some families of civilized nations, tuberculous infection still appears in this form. The relatively low tuberculosis morbidity as compared with the prevalence of infection in civilized communities indicates that these people have acquired a great resistance and have therefore lost much of their susceptibility to tuberculous disease. This may be either an acquired or inherited natural resistance, and in those races and individuals who seem to lack this we are dealing with a natural inherited susceptibility to tuberculosis, which may be considered as a genuine predisposing factor of great importance.

Heredity.—It used to be thought that this susceptibility depended upon certain inherited types of constitution or body configuration, such as the habitus phthisicus, but these assumptions have been largely discarded and there are no known hereditary characteristics predisposing to tuberculosis. While recent studies strongly suggest that lack of natural resistance to tuberculosis goes in races and families, we must simply admit complete ignorance as to the exact manner in which this susceptibility is transmitted, and contact infection after birth far overshadows it in importance.

Congenital tuberculosis exists as far as we know only in the form of the exceptional cases of intrauterine, transplacentary, or intranatal infection. There is no evidence whatsoever of infection through the sperm of the father.

Sex and Age.—There does not appear to be any principal difference in susceptibility between the sexes or with regard to ages, although men may be more exposed to infection, and with the coming-of-age of children, acquired immunity may be expected to become an operative factor. The increased susceptibility to tuberculosis manifest in infancy, puberty and senility appears to depend upon some fundamental biologic phenomena which are not yet properly understood but which may have a great deal to do both with the age and with the sexual evolution and involution of the body.

Circumstances of Life.—The general state of health of the individual, particularly as influenced by the mode of life, hygienic conditions of surroundings, state of nutrition, habits of work and leisure, plays a rôle of considerable importance as a predisposing factor.

Trauma.—Trauma as a factor in the development of tuberculous disease has been the subject of much debate. It is of course clear that it could play no possible rôle in the infection itself. In individuals harboring a type of focus which is a potential source of reinfection, trauma with the congestive stasis it produces locally in the tissues cannot be excluded as a predisposing factor. As this amounts to mere reactivation of the disease, the evidence of such an occurrence must follow closely upon the trauma to establish a connection between the two.

Concurrent Diseases.—Certain diseases which are associated with the tuberculous infection apparently influence susceptibility, particularly *measles, whooping cough* and *influenza,* among the infectious diseases. On the contrary, diseases of the lung, as pneumonia and various other chronic lung infections, with the exception of silicosis, produce no predisposition to tuberculosis. Certain metabolic diseases, particularly *diabetes*, do appear to have a definite influence. Among the *valvular cardiac diseases*, cases with pulmonary stenosis show a high frequency of pulmonary tuberculosis, while those of mitral stenosis have a diminished incidence. It is possible that this difference is due to changes in the blood supply of the lung. During *pregnancy*, and especially during the puerperium, tuberculous disease has a definite tendency to develop. The influence of alcoholism is doubtful.

(b) **Specific Predisposing Factors.**—The immunobiologic response to tuberculous infection shows some features peculiar to itself. The "Koch phenomenon" demonstrated that lesions produced in previously inoculated animals show characteristics peculiar to reinfection with tubercle bacilli. Pirquet then demonstrated that the specific tuberculin hypersensitiveness, to which he gave the name "allergy," reveals a previous infection with the utmost certainty. It has since become well recognized that "allergy" is evidence of the specific immunobiologic response of the body to tuberculous infection. It has been found that this specific response varies greatly between different races, individuals, and varies even in the same individual from one time to another according to the combination of the same endogenous and exogenous factors which play a rôle in natural resistance, many of which are altogether unknown to us. The quantity and virulence of the bacilli and the time intervals between successive invasions have also been found to play an important rôle in the allergic response.

While the exact nature of the immunobiologic response in tuberculosis, which, in man at least, is inseparable from allergic manifestations, is still largely unknown, there is evidence that it is chiefly of the nature of a cellular reaction which eventually becomes restricted to the site of invasion and the multiplication of the bacilli. At best this immunobiologic response in tuberculous infection accomplishes only a "state of resistance to progression of the infection." There is established a balance between the bacilli and the tissues, whereby the former become isolated, made harmless, and may eventually even be destroyed. This balance may fluctuate between a real permanent resistance to the development of disease and what amounts to but a temporary control over a slumbering focus, easily upset by a change in the combination of the endogenous and exogenous factors playing a rôle in that balance.

Two unfortunate results follow from the circumstance that the immunobiologic response ends up in a tissue reaction restricted to the site of the implantation and even there is unable to destroy the bacilli. In the first place, when the local reaction happens to be so excessive as to lead to destruction of the tissue area involved, living bacilli in large quantity will be liberated within the body, exposing other tissues to invasion by contiguity or by transport through internal channels (the lymph or the blood stream, the canal systems of viscera), and secondly it follows from the character of the immunobiologic process in tuberculosis that with the invasion of bacilli at every new site, the tissue reaction must be repeated time and again, thus paradoxically

47

involving the possibility of progressive tuberculization as a result of the immunizing process.

Another paradoxic phenomenon in the immunobiologic response in tuberculosis is the fact that the balance upon which the resistance of the body is conditioned, may be present at any level of allergy. Both increased and decreased hypersensitiveness may be associated with effective resistance to disease, just as both may be associated with a critical phase in the balance of resistance. Allergy is thus merely an essential phenomenon of, and not identical with, the process by which the body resists development of tuberculous disease from infection. Because of these paradoxes there is still a lively dispute as to the exact rôle of allergy in the process by which development of tuberculous disease in the body is resisted, and some workers are convinced that allergy is a harmful rather than a protective phenomenon. There is good reason to believe that allergy is chiefly responsible for the prevention of reimplantation by inhalation, which, considering the ubiquitous nature of tubercle bacilli, must be a frequent occurrence. Its protection, however, fails under circumstances involving inhalation of large quantities of bacilli upon contact exposure and especially under the circumstances when bacilli in still larger quantities are liberated from a breaking-down focus into another as yet uninvolved part of the body.

It follows from this that the evolution of the tuberculous process is in itself one of the chief endogenous factors affecting the immunobiologic balance in the body. This creates a constant flux in the resistance to development of disease, as produced by secondary invasions, that is, implantations ("takes") in the tissues of the various organs. Thus this flux in the evolution of tuberculous disease is an essential factor in its own development.

In closing this section on the rôle of the individual factors in the tuberculous infection the situation may be summed up by saying that for the most part the individual predispositions depend upon some lack of natural resistance, but that under certain conditions changes in the allergic reaction of the individual, that is, in specific resistance, may play an important rôle in shaping the course of the infection in the individual. Undoubtedly the combination of the two factors—natural, and specific or acquired resistance—largely determines the characteristic individual response to tuberculous infection.

3. **The Evolution of Tuberculosis in the Body.**—As a disease tuberculosis shows some unique characteristics. It may appear as a most acute as well as a most chronic disease. Between these extremes it may appear in the form of a great variety of clinico-pathologic conditions quite unmatched by any other infectious disease. The natural history of the evolution of this vast disease complex is a difficult and a still largely unsolved problem. Recent progress in our knowledge has produced a definite change in the concepts which have hitherto prevailed, particularly in this country. According to this previous concept the clinico-pathologic forms of tuberculosis represent the result of two distinct and independent infections, a childhood and an adult infection, both of which are assumed to be identical—exogenous—

in origin. The first results in the childhood, the latter in the adult forms of tuberculosis, their differences in clinico-pathologic features being explained by the allergy left behind by the childhood infection. Recent evidence has, however, conclusively demonstrated that first infection leaves behind not only allergy but also reactivable foci which during later life under stress or with added exposure to infection may become the source of reinfection which now becomes definitely endogenous in origin. This concept of tuberculogenesis by endogenous reinfection explains many puzzling phenomena in the evolution of tuberculous processes. Above all it enables us to look upon tuberculosis as a single but discontinuous biologic process comparable with other infectious diseases.

The baffling variety in the manifestations of tuberculosis becomes simpler when a basic pattern of the disease is concentrated upon, consisting of a first infection followed by generalization and then finally by localization, with each of these phases manifesting fairly characteristic lesions. Upon this pattern as a background are then superimposed all of those endogenous and exogenous reinfections with their sequelæ which are often so confusing, but with the pattern clearly in mind fairly definite pathologic and clinical pictures emerge which are most helpful in the understanding of the disease.

The idea must be constantly borne in mind that all phases of the disease, from the slightest focus to the most acute overwhelming processes, are a part of an essentially systemic infection. In all systemic infections where the infection is overwhelming with no resistance, acute and rapid extension occurs by all available routes. When the infection is milder, extension occurs by the lymphohematogenous route and the generalization is fleeting in character and leads finally to localization. After localization occurs, further extension is of a special and local character, and generalization through the lymph and blood stream no longer occurs.

So it is in tuberculosis. Fulminant forms (as they appear in very young infants and individuals of aboriginal races) are seen where first infection is followed by extension of the tuberculous process both locally (by contiguity and bronchogenic spread) as well as systemically (by lymphohematogenous dissemination), so that not a single organ of the body may be left uninvolved. We see the proliferative primary complexes (as appearing in overexposed or less resistant individuals) from which the whole gamut of generalized or more or less protracted disseminations are derived. The more subacute processes may last long enough for localization phenomena to become conspicuous by the intracanalicular extensions of the processes in the various organs, as represented by the bronchogenic spread in the lungs. Finally the apparently harmless primary complexes are seen, which, although they produce no disease and apparently become obsolescent, yet persist and may lead to later disease with local or general dissemination. The more discontinuous or protractedly chronic the process becomes, the more generalization is held in abeyance and localization predominates. With localization comes a characteristic mode of local extension, and the process is then known as isolated organic phthisis which occurs chiefly in the lungs but it may be in any organ of the body.

In the systemic evolution of tuberculosis two types of foci appear to play the principal rôle. They are the lymphatic component of the primary complex, from which secondary foci arise by lymphohematogenous dissemination, and the secondary foci themselves from which localized organic phthisis may develop. Thus *endogenous reinfection* because of the persistence of tuberculous lesions in the body comes to loom large in the concept of the evolution of the disease.

Many opportunities for additional *exogenous reinfection* occur in the ordinary course of life. In the face of the increased incidence of morbidity associated with intimate prolonged exposure to infection, we must continue to consider exogenous reinfection as also a very important factor, and next to endogenous reinfection the prevalent mode of reinfection.

The exact relationship between these two modes of reinfection is unknown. It is well recognized that those individuals who harbor old stabilized foci will be easily reinfected or reactivated upon contact exposure. At the same time many patients with stabilized old foci offer a surprising resistance to contact exposure as compared with the poor resistance to reinfection shown by individuals in whom only a perfectly obsolete primary complex can be demonstrated. The impression is, that such a primary complex endows the average individual with a resistance, associated with allergy, which suffices for ordinary conditions of life but affords no protection in the case of intimate contact involving a quantitatively severe inhalation infection. A patient who holds in check a focus derived from a severe infection may be endowed with a resistance which holds up even under conditions of intimate exposure, while such a patient may not be able to control a superinfection of endogenous origin which in turn implies a quantitatively more severe infection than inhalation infection can involve under any circumstances. So that in some manner, as yet unknown to us, endogenous and exogenous reinfection seem to go hand in hand in the evolution of tuberculous disease in the body, but with either form of reinfection the dosage and the varying degrees and types of resistance appear to be the determining factors.

Pathologic Histology.—The main histomorphologic processes of tuberculosis are: tubercle formation, caseation, fibrosis, and calcification. The extent and the order of sequence of these processes depend chiefly upon the above discussed balance between infection and resistance.

Tubercle Formation.—The basic histologic unit in tuberculosis is the tubercle. When the tubercle bacilli enter the lung they usually lodge in the terminal bronchi or alveolus, and the tissue responds by an exudate of large mononuclear phagocytes which proliferate rapidly and phagocyte the bacilli as far as they are able. These mononuclear cells, which might be called defense cells, thus avoiding the discussion which is raging as to whether their origin is from so-called alveolar epithelium or from the mesenchyme, form around the invading bacilli in a concentric manner and develop into epithelioid cells, which in turn are surrounded by lymphocytes which later become surrounded by a connective tissue capsule. Giant cells develop in this tissue and in the center of the tubercle, necrosis or caseation soon occurs. If the amount of infection is large, there is also a considerable exudate of polymorphonuclear leukocytes which phagocyte the tubercle bacilli but do not destroy them. This leads to an exudative inflammation of greater or less extent. As the center of the tubercle caseates, or as the polymorphonuclear leukocytes containing live bacilli wander into neighboring structures, extension of the original infection occurs, either by direct contact or through the neighboring air passages or into the neighboring lymphatics and thus into the corresponding lymph nodes.

The amount of exudate which is set up by the infection and the corresponding intensity of reaction is very variable. It may subside quickly and become absorbed, or it may extend and caseate rapidly. Sooner if the exudative reaction is slight, and later if more marked, there usually comes a stage where the inflammation subsides and organization into fibrous tissue occurs. If the caseation has been considerable, this resulting fibrosis may not occur until a very considerable damage of tissue has resulted. In the later stages where caseation and fibrosis have occurred, lime salts are deposited from the blood serum, and calcification, and in some cases even ossification, may result.

Caseation is perhaps the most characteristic histomorphologic process produced by the special toxins of the tubercle bacilli. The poisoned cells succumb to coagulation necrosis followed by fatty degeneration which may be associated with immediate or delayed liquefaction, the tuberculous pus formation. Evacuation of this liquefied cheese leads to excavation and tissue defect.

Fibrosis may occur as a process of demarcation for the destructive changes taking place in the affected area. This fibrotic process consists of proliferation of the cells of adjacent interstitium and comes to form a capsule of dense fibrous tissue limiting the extension of the destructive process. In the more productive processes in which caseation is localized to the center of the individual tubercles, the fibrotic process consists of marked proliferation of the connective tissue elements forming the capsule of the single tubercles themselves.

Calcification.—Incrustation with calcium salts is the end result in lesions in which caseation was not followed by liquefaction and excavation. The calcium salts are deposited into the inspissated cheese which becomes thus eventually entirely petrified. Lesions that are isolated from the circulation (blood and lymph) by a thick dense fibrotic capsule are much less likely to become calcified, hence the observation of greater tendency toward calcification of primary and postprimary foci.

What happens in the case of the tubercle happens on a larger scale in all tuberculous lesions. Sometimes absorption and healing may result, but usually exudative inflammation, caseation, fibrosis and calcification are found hand in hand and side by side in all tuberculous lesions, and the destructiveness of their character again depends upon the dosage and virulence of the infection, and the defensive reaction of the tissues which depends upon the specific immuno-biologic state of the body.

Whether the tubercle bacillus always causes primarily an exudative reaction, or whether it may primarily produce sometimes a productive and sometimes an exudative reaction, is a matter of considerable debate; but, practically, the ultimate result would appear to be the same.

The specific character of the tuberculous lesion will, of course, vary somewhat, depending upon the particular organ involved; the essential characters, however, are the same, and all of these lesions can be produced by the tubercle bacillus, without the necessity of invoking the rôle of secondary pyogenic organisms to explain them.

Although the essential characteristics of the tissue reaction are the same whether the lesions are primary infections or reinfections, the predominance of the destructive lesions and the amount of allergic reaction which occurs may be definitely different in each individual case or in each individual focus.

Pathogenesis.—To the above basic pattern of evolution of the tuberculous infection in general, some special pathogenetic features must be added which govern the development of pulmonary tuberculosis in its various forms. From the systemic nature of the tuberculous infection there follows the possibility of hematogenous invasion of the lung in all phases of the disease, but also its greatest likelihood in the phase of generalization and its least likelihood in the phase of localization of the infection. From the place and function of the lungs, their structural and mechanical conditions, there follows that they represent the most exposed organ of the body, laid open to ceaseless exogenous invasion and bronchogenic extension of the infection to every part of it. This possibility too is open at every stage of the infection, but its recurrence will be of greatest significance in the localized stage of the disease.

Special local factors are also operative in the lungs, which, within the scheme of the above discussed basic evolution of the infection, favor "take" of, and determine the localization, the arrangement and evolution of the pulmonary lesions of various origins. This results in some special pathogenetic features and characteristic forms of pulmonary tuberculosis as they arise in the various phases of the infection. We can therefore speak of special local predispositions of the lung to development of pulmonary tuberculosis, as well as special pathogenetic forms of pulmonary tuberculosis.

The fact that all blood must pass the lungs before it can be returned to the greater circulation makes hematogenous invasion of the organ almost inevitable whenever tubercle bacilli reach the blood stream. Hence the simultaneous presence of pulmonary lesions in the vast majority of cases of tuberculosis of organs which can be reached only by the blood stream (bone, kidney).

Because of the extreme delicacy of the lungs' structures, hematogenous lesions upon their extension immediately obtain the air spaces, and when they break down the infectious material may reach any part of the lungs by way of the bronchi, thus making bronchogenic extension of lesions of hematogenous origin a common sequence of events.

The vastness of the inverted lung surface exposed constantly to the outside air and the constantly alternating air currents from and to the vast system of air passages converging into a single common outlet make possible constant invasion and aspiration of infectious matter from outside into all parts and from any part to any other part of the lungs.

The lungs function incessantly. Even when at standstill the lungs are expanded under negative suction. The tissues of the lungs are constantly under negative tension. There is good reason to believe that this permanent tension under which the lung tissue is kept, favors "take" of infection upon invasion by bacilli. There is also evidence to show that this same tension in the tissues of the lungs is a great handicap to the natural healing tendency of tuberculous lesions of the lungs.

The particular manner in which these local factors play a rôle in the development of special pathogenetic forms of pulmonary tuberculosis, within the basic pattern of evolution of the disease, will now be discussed in connection with the respective special forms.

The Clinico-pathologic Forms of Pulmonary Tuberculosis.

In the light of the above data with regard to the evolution of tuberculosis in general, the special pathogenesis of pulmonary tuberculosis and the pathomorphologic processes underlying it, we should now be in a position to consider a clinico-pathologic classification of the forms of pulmonary tuberculosis. From the preceding it is clear that tuberculosis should be looked upon as a systemic infection in which the lungs are the main scene of events and that therefore pulmonary tuberculosis includes clinico-pathologic conditions representing the whole gamut of evolution of the disease. A genuine practical classification of pulmonary tuberculosis has not yet been achieved for the reason that with so many fundamental questions unsolved it has not yet been possible to reduce its manifold variations to a group of clear-cut clinico-pathologic pictures. Such classifications as one finds in the literature are based exclusively on pathologic or pathogenetic principles.

The division into childhood and adult forms, in vogue chiefly in this country, is essentially a pathogenetic classification, based as it obviously is on the principle that all childhood forms are derived from the first infection, while all adult forms originate with exogenous reinfection in later life. Inasmuch as the first infection and the systemic invasion which follows it happen to take place, in the majority of cases, during childhood, while the subsequent reinfections fall necessarily into later years, it is, practically speaking, quite feasible to label these respective processes according to the age period in which they mostly appear.

In the light of recent experience it is no longer desirable to emphasize age as the line of cleavage in the pathogenesis of pulmonary tuberculosis. In the first place it is now found that more and more primary infections occur only in adolescence or later. It also is known that reinfectious forms of pulmonary tuberculosis do occur, indeed not infrequently, throughout childhood. Above all, however, it is known that forms of pulmonary tuberculosis of lymphohematogenous origin are not at all characteristic only of childhood, but that as a matter of fact much adult pulmonary tuberculosis is derived from lesions of the very same origin.

Inasmuch as it seems necessary for general guidance to include here a clinico-pathologic classification of the various forms of pulmonary tuberculosis, there offers itself as the most logical basis for such a classification the above outlined phasic evolution of tuberculosis in general, as supplemented by the special pathogenetic factors which play a rôle in the origin, and by the pathologic processes which give the character to the morphologic features of the various forms of pulmonary tuberculosis. By the integration of these factors the following classification of pulmonary tuberculosis is devised.

1. **Primary Forms of Pulmonary Tuberculosis.**—The primary tuberculous lesion represents *par excellence* an exogenous focus produced by the inhalation of bacilli. Accordingly, its site, in the overwhelming majority of cases, is likely to be in the better ventilated lower two-thirds and only less frequently in the upper third of the lung. Pathologically, the primary complex is seen most frequently in its non-progressive form as an ossified residue of the lung focus and its associated calcified lymph-glandular component at the hilum. In its progressive forms the primary complex represents a caseous-pneumonic focus and an associated more extensive hilar caseous lymph-glandular packet. The more virulent the primary complex, the more extensive the hilar component, and the huge caseous gland packets in the hilum (potato glands) are characteristic of the most virulent primary complexes seen in young children or in individuals of aboriginal races. Even in less virulent primary complexes, involvement of the paratracheal glands can frequently be followed clear up to the venous angle, indicating that the infection has reached the point of entry to the blood stream. Extensive lymph-glandular involvement reveals the process to be in the primary stage, for reinfections do not usually produce hilar components or only to a much smaller extent. The marked tendency of primary lesions to calcify is also an outstanding pathologic feature.

Of the various clinico-pathologic forms of primary pulmonary tuber-culosis, the following are the most frequent and important ones:

(*a*) *The bipolar primary complex* is characterized by its peripheral pulmonary and central hilar lymph-nodular focus, as observed in its acute stage in children and as seen in form of its calcified residues in adults. Another frequent subacute or chronic form of it is as follows:

(*b*) *Epituberculous infiltration* may correspond to an extensive perifocal infiltration of an entire lobe or a part of it, about the pulmonary focus or its lymph-glandular component. In some instances of the latter, obstruction of the bronchus of the involved lobe, due to adjacent lymph node enlargement, may be a contributory factor in the long delay of absorption of the exudate. Epituberculous infiltrations tend to clear up, even though they may persist a good many months. As a rule they do not caseate.

(c) *Caseous pneumonia* may occasionally be the result of breakdown of a caseous hilar lymph-glandular complex, when the caseous material is aspirated into the stem bronchus of the adjacent lobe. The result is extensive caseation, breakdown and destruction of a great part of the involved lobe.

The hilar glandular focus of the primary complex has the tendency to persist much longer than the pulmonary component, and it is from this persisting lesion that tubercle bacilli may reach the blood stream by way of the venous angle. The result is:

2. **Hematogenous Forms of Pulmonary Tuberculosis.**—The overwhelming majority of primary complexes being in the lungs, bacilli reaching the blood stream from such primary complexes are brought right back to the lung itself. Hence, the frequency of tuberculous lesions of hematogenous origin in the lungs, which are discussed in the literature under a great variety of names. From the clinico-pathologic standpoint the most clearcut distinction can be made between them according to the acuteness of the process with which they are associated. Accordingly, the most clearcut form of hematogenous pulmonary tuberculosis is (a) *acute miliary tuberculosis of the lung* as a part of a generalized miliary tuberculosis. The prevailing concept now is, that this form represents the result of breaking down of a caseous (generally glandular) focus and its direct inruption into the blood stream, involving a one-time or shortly repeated massive invasion of the blood stream. The very characteristic features of this form depend on this special pathogenesis as well as upon the structural peculiarities of the lungs which permit dense and perfectly homogeneous dissemination throughout both lungs by the pulmonary circulation. The histomorphologic features of its unit lesion are those of the tubercle as above described.

Another quite characteristic form of hematogenous pulmonary tuberculosis is (b) *protracted disseminated tuberculosis in the lungs.* This form comes next in severity and extent of the lesions. It most probably represents the result of repeated disseminations by the blood stream, each less massive in character than miliary. Like miliary, the lung lesions are associated with similar ones throughout the body, but unlike miliary this process presents discrete lesions which are larger and more irregular, and runs a somewhat discontinuous and prolonged course in which some of the lesions have time to coalesce and break down. This explains its chief pathologic feature, namely, the variation in size and age of the lesions and the signs of localizing tendency, as indicated by the beginning breakdown and coalescence. The result is a more or less subacute condition with unusually widespread mixed hematogenous and bronchogenic disseminations. Clinically, this form stands about midway between acute miliary tuberculosis and (c) *chronic discrete hematogenous pulmonary tuberculosis.* This form represents the result of an occasional mild blood stream invasion producing characteristic bilateral symmetrical lesions in the lungs. Mild as these processes are, they may not give rise to distinct clinical symptoms and are frequently recognized only by roentgen examination, and are very apt to be calcified.

It is a well recognized fact that hematogenous disseminations in the lungs tend to be denser toward the apices, in the tapering cone of the lung. Again, it is here that such foci tend to coalesce into larger units and persist even after the foci from all other parts of the lungs have become absorbed. Characteristic residues of past hematogenous disseminations can be demonstrated by roentgen examination throughout the lungs, but nowhere as frequently and in as clearcut manner as in the apices.

Two characteristic postmortem findings represent the pathologic substrate of this form: (1) The interstitial foci of so-called "reticular lymphangitis," appear as marked thickening of the interalveolar and interlobular septa. These are interpreted as residues of, or even fresh but very discrete, miliary disseminations, usually scattered throughout the interstitium of the lungs but particularly dense in the cortical areas of the upper third of both lungs, in a characteristic bilateral symmetric arrangement. (2) Post-primary apical foci is the collective term now applied to certain characteristic tuberculous lesions which form the link in the evolution of pulmonary tuberculosis between the lymphohematogenous pulmonary foci and chronic phthisis, as revealed by postmortem studies of the lungs of people dying from other causes than tuberculosis. Their most characteristic form is that usually seen in the upper third of the lung (Simon foci, Puhl focus) where they may be found either in form of calcified or fibrotic, apparently obsolescent lesions, or in a reactivated state.

Upon reactivation these chronic hematogenous foci in the lung progress locally and proceed to coalescence and breakdown, whereupon they obtain the lumina of the pulmonary parenchyma whence they may continue to extend by the bronchogenic route. The pathologic features of these hematogenous lesions in the reactivated state are usually described as caseous endo- and peribronchitis, with bronchiolectasis which is the characteristic initial lesion from which chronic bronchogenic tuberculosis of the lungs takes its origin. Before closing this section on the hematogenous forms of pulmonary tuberculosis we must include here another form which belongs to this group, namely, (d) *tuberculous pleurisy, with or without effusion*, as occurring in the post-primary period, unassociated with tuberculous foci in the lung parenchyma. This form is now considered to be a part of the mild chronic hematogenous disseminations and as such is interpreted as an allergic reaction out of all proportion to a discrete pleural focus, quite characteristic of the allergic hypersensitiveness of the generalization phase in which it occurs.

3. **Transitional Forms of Pulmonary Tuberculosis.**—There is much evidence available at present that perhaps the greater part of pulmonary phthises originate with a preëxisting pulmonary lesion of hematogenous origin, most probably of the chronic discrete type just described. The tendency of such lesions to be situated in the upper cone of the lungs has been explained by their being most crowded here, a circumstance which favors coalescence into larger units more difficult to

absorb. Again, the tendency for such lesions to exacerbate in later life has been explained by the fact that the tension in the lung parenchyma happens to be greatest just in this tapering-out part of the lungs. What Forlanini termed the "constant trauma" to the tissues of the lungs is greatest in the apices or just below them. There is ample evidence to show that lesions which happen to be situated in the apices are least likely to heal spontaneously or stay healed, and are most likely to proceed to coalescence, breakdown and cavitation. This is just what happens to some of the old residual apical lesions of hematogenous origin. Their exacerbation, coalescence and breakdown opens the way for local bronchogenic extension, resulting in that rather frequent process characterized by transition from hematogenous origin to bronchogenic extension, and which we consequently describe under the term *transitional pulmonary tuberculosis*. The characteristic picture of this form is that of a more or less simultaneous bilateral symmetrical process progressing by proliferation, coalescence, ulceration, cavitation and cranio-caudal extension. On the whole, this type of tuberculous process tends to be exquisitely chronic, to be frequently interrupted by long intervals of quiescence and arrest, and to become frequently stabilized for long periods at a low grade of activity.

In the pathologic aspects, evidences of transition from lymphohematogenous origin to bronchogenic extension are characteristic of most pulmonary processes developing from lesions of the postprimary or generalization stage. As soon as these lesions have obtained the air spaces, in their local progression, they continue in the form of mixed hematogenous and bronchogenic phthisis. Their pathologic features are exquisitely productive, torpid in nature and extending in characteristic bilateral symmetrical fashion, grazing down the lungs from the apices toward the base by a very slow process of coalescence and crumbling-down of previously disseminated lesions. As these productive lesions coalesce and crumble down slowly in the midst of non-reactive surroundings, cavities, exquisitely round in shape and punched-out in appearance, are produced, with hardly any cavity walls to separate them from their as yet uninvolved surrounding. The scant bacillary contents of these foci and their prevalent fibrotic tendency explain why they may persist for such long periods of low-grade activity without giving rise to bronchogenic metastases of serious extent.

However, as these processes extend and obtain the larger air passages or are complicated by hemoptyses, the bronchogenic element comes to prevail in the picture and a more rapid extension becomes possible, which will then give the process an aspect more and more like that of so-called chronic pulmonary tuberculosis.

4. **Chronic Pulmonary Phthisis.**—There is no doubt that a considerable part of cases of pulmonary tuberculosis originate with a focus set up by exogenous reinvasion, which then evolves by bronchogenic spread of the infection to other parts of the lungs. The initial lesion for this type of process also is likely to be situated in the upper third of the lung. The predisposition of the upper part of the lung for such exogenous invasion has never been adequately explained. It is prob-

able that while the apices tend to inhale bacilli rather less frequently, their ability to resist implantation must also be very considerably less than that of the rest of the lung. Once implantation has taken place, the tendency for the lesion to progress here is amply explained by the same local predisposition described above for hematogenous lesions in the apices.

Among the pathogenetic characteristics of this form, the first to be mentioned is its frequent tendency to begin more or less acutely and abruptly, appearing in the form of an infiltrative focus, and also to extend frequently in the form of periodic exacerbations of this focus or by the cropping-up of new aspiration foci in a very characteristic fashion, namely, by infraclavicular infiltration followed by broncho-genic metastases to other lung areas. The favored sites for such bron-chogenic aspirations correspond exactly to what one should expect from the observations of bronchial spilling from the respective lung areas, which frequently results in cross-spilling into the opposite lung instead of the continuous cranio-caudal extension described for the transitional form. Furthermore, this type of process is very soon complicated by cavitation, hemoptyses, or laryngeal involvement, all of which open the way for frequent very widespread disseminations of various quantities of infectious matter by the air passages. Depend-ing on the dispersion of this material, large, medium, small-grained, the lesions thus disseminated may appear as large-nodular broncho-pneumonia, or small-nodular peribronchiolar, or very finely seeded miliary-alveolar foci. The latter foci if they be widely and homogene-ously scattered may simulate the picture of hematogenous miliary tuberculosis of the lungs.

The most outstanding characteristic of this type of process is the tendency for the lesions to coalesce, break down and generally to per-sist in their progressive character, even though their evolution may be marked by periodic ups and downs associated with every exacerbation or new crop of lesions. It is this form of pulmonary tuberculosis which constitutes the bulk of our consumptives which require treatment for more or less persistently active disease.

From the pathologic standpoint the initial lesion of chronic pul-monary phthisis is a caseous endo- and peribronchitis. It is still a matter of dispute just how frequently such a lesion develops by way of exogenous reinfection, or by way of reinfection or reactivation of an older focus of endogenous origin. In its progress this lesion leads to characteristic bronchogenic metastases the extent of which depends greatly on the momentary balance between infection and resistance (allergy), but even more so on the amount of infectious matter carried over by way of intrabronchial spilling. Upon the size of these meta-stases depends the unit size of pulmonary parenchyma involved, which in turn determines the pathologic character of these lesions. The scale includes the wide range of processes from tuberculous endo- and peribronchitis, through focal bronchopneumonia and confluent broncho-pneumonia, to the most extensive caseous-pneumonic processes involv-ing an entire lobe.

Bronchogenic dissemination may also give rise to foci involving the terminal units of the lung parenchyma. It is thus well recognized now that bronchogenic dissemination into the alveoli of finely dispersed infectious matter, produced by hemorrhage or extensive laryngeal ulceration, may produce miliary foci of bronchogenic origin.

Cavities represent the most characteristic lesion of bronchogenic phthisis. They are in the nature of a tissue defect resulting from evacuation of caseated destroyed tissue, having a characteristic wall of demarcation. In the early phase this wall consists of infiltrated tissue capable of resolution, by which cavities may completely disappear. In the later stages this wall becomes a solid ring of fibrotic or cirrhotic tissue, but within, the cavity may still contain much detritus and infectious matter, making it a continuous source of bronchogenic reinfection.

The continuity of the destructive lesions is broken up by the extensive cirrhotic induration which is another characteristic morphologic feature of chronic pulmonary phthisis, indicating Nature's attempt at healing. This may come about by hyalinization of already caseated but not evacuated lesions or by hyaline degeneration of extensive fibrotic lesions. Thus, the characteristic pathologic end-picture of chronic pulmonary phthisis is represented by a heterogeneous combination of old cirrhotic shrunken lesions with their cleaned-out cavities, of more fresh confluent caseous bronchopneumonic lesions with their shaggy-walled fibro-ulcerous cavities, and recent mixed large and small-nodular scattered lesions. The oldest lesions are likely to be crowded in one or both upper lobes, while the most recent lesions will be scattered throughout the remaining lung parenchyma.

Silicosis and Tuberculosis in the Lungs.—As a subdivision of chronic pulmonary phthisis this form must be included here. It represents a process of definitely exogenous origin with bronchogenic extension of the lesions. The initial lesions arise here frequently in those areas of the lungs favored also by the first silicotic lesions, which are in the lower two-thirds and near the hilum. The picture betrays its pathogenesis by dust inhalation with its frequently homogeneous dissemination of invariably bilateral symmetrical arrangement. The picture is somewhat like that produced by hematogenous disseminations in the lungs, which, as was pointed out above, can be exquisitely simulated also by finely dispersed bronchogenic disseminations. This is particularly the case in that peculiar process which is now recognized under the term of silico-tuberculosis. The unit lesion of this (the silico-tuberculotic nodule) bears characteristics of its own, making it differ from the tubercle as well as the silicotic nodule. The prevalence of fibrotic changes is here the outstanding histomorphologic feature. The bronchogenic factor may lead to coalescence and conglomeration of the lesions and may transform the end-result into a process in which silicosis and tuberculosis are combined into a condition with characteristic special features of its own.

The Clinical Aspects and the Clinical Course of Pulmonary Tuberculosis.

It follows from the above considerations of the pathogenesis that the initial lesion from which progressive pulmonary tuberculosis originates is frequently carried over in a dormant state from the first infection in the past. Furthermore, examination, chiefly by roentgen-ray, of large numbers of people from various sections of the population as well as examination of large numbers of contacts has demonstrated that pulmonary tuberculosis may progress for a considerable time and extent without giving rise to any clinical symptoms or physical signs; or the onset may be marked by a pneumonia or grippe-like acute clinical picture in form of the so-called initial, or infraclavicular infiltration, which may quickly subside and repeat itself at intervals.

Even when manifest, the clinical picture of pulmonary tuberculosis is not easy to trace in sharp outline. Considering the varied modes of pathogenesis, one must expect that the symptoms and signs should present an infinite variety of clinical combinations, with variations in the sequence of events over a considerable period of time.

The following are therefore the fundamental concepts to bear in mind in connection with the clinical aspects of pulmonary tuberculosis:

1. In its early phases the disease may entirely escape us, when it can be detected only by roentgen-ray examination which must be resorted to in all cases of exposure as well as on mere suspicion.

2. Pulmonary tuberculosis after it becomes manifest is essentially a relapsing disease. The evidences of its activity rarely, if ever, progress uninterruptedly toward either cure or death, but their course presents a series of exacerbations alternating with periods of quiescence, which vary in duration, in character, and in severity. They seldom present the same picture in their chief manifestations, and they must be considered as a whole and in correlation with the pathologic development of which they are the clinical manifestations.

3. These clinical manifestations may be divided into two main categories: the focal, which are caused by the lesions in the lungs, of which the physical and the roentgenologic signs are the most important evidence; and the constitutional, or systemic, which are indicated by the symptoms presented.

Of the two, the constitutional symptoms are the more important both from the standpoint of the diagnosis of the disease and the proper appreciation of the course which it runs. This fact is frequently overlooked because of an over emphasis which has been placed upon the importance of the physical signs in the study of this disease.

4. Infection of the body with tubercle bacilli does not necessarily result in clinical disease. Evidence of such infection may be present in the form of slight physical signs at an apex, or of roentgenologic evidence of the primary complex, or of a positive reaction to tuberculin. These findings in themselves do not necessarily mean clinical tuberculosis and should be interpreted in connection with all the other clinical evidences, of which the constitutional symptoms are often the most important part.

The Clinical History.—With these concepts in mind it is apparent that the value of a careful clinical history cannot be overemphasized in the study of pulmonary tuberculosis. In developing such a history, the setting in which one finds the individual case should be studied. This study would include careful inquiry into the probable opportunities for infection through contact with other cases of the disease. It would also include inquiry into the hereditary and constitutional make-up of the individual and possible predisposing factors in his environment such as social and economic conditions, habits of life, or predisposing illness, all of which factors have been discussed in our consideration of the predisposition to tuberculosis.

Then the whole previous medical history of the individual should be studied, not only in regard to possible predisposing illnesses, but also to apparently slight non-disabling ailments which might be interpreted as slight previous manifestations of tuberculosis. Very often these ailments masquerade under misleading diagnoses or frequently have been almost overlooked or forgotten altogether. Inasmuch as the primary seat of tuberculosis is usually in the lungs, particular care should be taken in bringing out any symptoms referable to the respiratory tract. In compiling this history each such episode should be analysed on the basis of the same presenting symptoms as though the patient were complaining of them at the present time.

Presenting Symptoms.—Whether we are engaged in such an analysis of the past history or of the story of the present illness, certain presenting symptoms occur in tuberculosis with sufficient regularity to make their recognition very essential. These symptoms may be focal in the lung or, inasmuch as tuberculosis may first manifest itself outside of the lungs, they may be focal in some other organ, or they may be general or systemic in nature.

Focal Symptoms in the Lung.—*Cough* is the most important and the most frequent early manifestation of pulmonary tuberculosis. There are, of course, many causes of cough, and in tuberculosis it may vary from a very slight hack to a pronounced and persistent cough. In general the story of any cough that persists for three or four weeks is always in itself suspicious of the possibility of pulmonary disease, and all such cases should be kept under strict observation until the cough either disappears or is adequately explained.

Expectoration usually accompanies the cough, but not always. It may be mucoid or muco-purulent, scanty or profuse, and in the early stages, even when pulmonary tuberculosis is present, it contains tubercle bacilli only in a relatively small percentage of the cases.

Hemoptysis is also a frequent focal symptom; frequently it is the first manifestation of the disease. It often occurs in persons in apparently excellent health and in such cases is frequently unaccompanied by suspicious physical signs. In such cases its significance is often missed, and all too frequently this danger signal is dismissed as of no importance or with the diagnosis of having come from the throat. Practically all real blood spitting comes from the lungs, and in from 90 to 95 per cent of such cases is due to pulmonary tuberculosis; consequently the only safe rule is to consider tuberculosis as a very likely disease in cases of hemoptysis, until the possibility of its presence has been satisfactorily eliminated.

Pleural effusion is another chest condition which frequently ushers in the first clinical evidences of tuberculosis. The significance of this condition is discussed under pleurisies, but it should be repeated here that in a very large majority of all pleural effusions not connected with an acute infection such as pneumonia or rheumatic fever, the cause is the tubercle bacillus. All such cases should be consequently diagnosed and treated as tuberculosis even when definite evidence of an underlying pulmonary lesion is lacking.

Hoarseness of the voice is sometimes one of the earlier manifestations. This may be associated with cough or due to it, or may be independent of it. It may be associated with actual disease of the larynx, but more frequently in the earlier stages there is no evidence of laryngeal disease.

Focal Symptoms in Other Organs.—When definite tuberculosis manifests itself in any organ the possibility of a coëxisting lesion in the lung should always be borne in mind whether symptoms pointing in this direction exist or not. Ischiorectal abscess, or fistula-in-ano, or present or preëxisting tuberculous glands, or bone and joint disease, or tuberculosis of the genito-urinary tract, always present the problem not only of the correct diagnosis of the local condition, but also of the possibility of associated lung disease.

General Symptoms.—The general or systemic symptoms due to tuberculosis may occasionally come on acutely, but are usually insidious in their onset, and may continue a long time before leading to a disabling illness. Of these the most important are those of *general malaise* associated with more or less loss of strength and flesh. This is frequently most evident as *fatigability*, that is, tire without unusual exertion. These symptoms may be very indefinite, but when present are very often associated with slight afternoon *rise of temperature* and *increased pulse-rate*, for the recognition of which observation over a period of several days may be necessary. Such malaise associated with slight fever is frequently dismissed as a "touch of malaria," or, if it happens to be associated with cough, it is frequently designated as "grippe." *Night-sweats* may accompany fever, but are caused by many other conditions than tuberculosis, and when marked are usually associated with advanced rather than the earlier stages of tuberculosis.

Disturbances of the digestive tract, lack of appetite and other gastric disturbances, are quite frequent in early tuberculosis, and with this is sometimes a very definite disturbance of the nervous system which may lead to the erroneous diagnosis of neurasthenia. In young people the constitutional evidence of tuberculosis may be a secondary anemia which may be treated as such instead of recognized as a symptom of the underlying infection.

Taking all of these various symptoms together, we have a picture of the more frequent methods of onset by which tuberculosis manifests itself. Bearing in mind, however, the characteristic relapsing nature of the disease, one does not expect to find all of these symptoms at any one time, nor any one necessarily presenting itself over a continued period of time, but rather one should look for them manifesting themselves at intervals with intervening periods of apparent good health with no symptoms.

Inasmuch as these above mentioned symptoms are the more usual ones in tuberculosis, when two or three of them occur in the same patient at the same time or at intervals, the suspicion of the presence of tuberculosis becomes so much the greater, so that the pieces of evidence which are linked together in the history may be widely separated in time or in localization in the body. It is the knowledge of this evidence in the past and present history of the individual which offers frequently presumptive evidence of the presence of tuberculosis even before an examination of the patient is made.

Methods of Examination.—Three methods are available to us in the examination for pulmonary tuberculosis, namely, the roentgen, the clinical and the laboratory methods. It cannot be too strongly emphasized that all three must be employed in every suspected case. The order in which these three methods are here enumerated indicates our estimation of their comparative value from the standpoint of the diagnosis of incipient pulmonary tuberculosis. The recent development of our roentgen technic, and still more the recent revelations of the great frequency of latent progressive pulmonary tuberculosis, have advanced the roentgen method of examination definitely ahead of the two other methods of examination and it is therefore to be considered first.

Roentgen Examination.—Efficiency in this method of examination is predicated upon familiarity with enough of technical details to make proper use of it, as well as upon sufficient experience to properly interpret its results: to recognize the properties of a properly made lung film and interpret them, and to interpret what is seen by fluoroscopic examination.

Roentgen pictures are not anatomic representations *in vivo;* at best they are optical phenomena. In the case of the lung, its changing air content is responsible for phenomena of attenuation or of summation of shadows, which materially affect the portrayal of the pathologic changes within the organ. The appreciation of these facts requires much expert training, but this cannot overcome the deficiencies of the method inherent in its physical limitations which must also be appreciated.

There is no escaping the fact, that a roentgen picture of the lungs will usually reveal the presence of tuberculous foci in the lungs at a stage long before this could be detected by our methods of physical examination or would be indicated by clinical symptoms. It also should be emphasized that serial follow-up by periodic roentgen examination of the vast number of manifest cases of pulmonary tuberculosis has demonstrated the fact that the method is the most reliable indication of the course of the process. Whether the process be progressing or regressing, the roentgen evidence for the most part transcends all other evidence concerning the course of the disease.

Special Roentgenologic Forms.—As in the case of the clinico-pathologic variations the possible combinations of the roentgenographic

48

aspects of pulmonary tuberculosis are so numerous that no two pictures are quite alike. Yet it is possible to describe some common features corresponding to the forms included in our above clinico-pathologic classification, many of which rest upon a clinico-roentgenologic basis.

The roentgen features of the special forms of pulmonary tuberculosis will be discussed in detail in the section on the "Clinico-roentgenologic Course," in recognition of the fact that in practice the observation of the clinical course of the disease is in reality a serial roentgenologic as well as a clinical study.

General Physical Examination.—A complete physical examination is due to any patient who consults the physician, no matter what the ailment. Unfortunately, this, for various reasons, often is neglected, and many cases of tuberculosis as well as other conditions are consequently overlooked.

Too often also when one is suspecting pulmonary disease the examination of the rest of the body is neglected or slighted. Too much emphasis cannot be placed upon the assessment of the general condition of the patient: state of nutrition, fatigability, color, presence or absence of flushing of the face or of slight sweating, the determination of the pulse and respiratory rate, the evidence of slight dyspnea on exertion, examination for possibly enlarged lymph nodes, particularly the examination of the upper air passages for possible evidences in the larynx which might point toward tuberculosis, but particularly for evidences of chronic infection of the upper respiratory tract which might account for cough and other symptoms otherwise suspicious of tuberculosis. Examination of the abdomen may reveal an enlarged spleen, due possibly to Hodgkin's disease or leukemia or bacterial endocarditis in cases which otherwise might be suspected of having tuberculosis. Also, tuberculosis of the abdominal organs, particularly of the ileocecal region and the pelvic region in females, may be detected. Examination may furthermore reveal suspicious lesions in the bones and skin, phlyctenulæ on the conjunctiva, or chronic fistula-in-ano. Examination of the extremities gives valuable evidences as to circulation as evidenced by color, temperature or sweating; or clubbing of the fingers may lead one directly to the chest as the most likely cause.

The importance of this general examination usually lies in the early diagnosis of a complication of an already recognized pulmonary tuberculosis. But not infrequently the process is reversed and their discovery points the way to the lung condition.

Examination of the Chest.—The physical signs of pulmonary tuberculosis are as varied as the corresponding pathologic lesions. While all areas of the chest should be thoroughly examined, it should be remembered that the earlier localization of pulmonary tuberculosis is almost invariably in the upper lobe, and consequently these areas should be examined with particular care when tuberculosis is suspected.

The most common points on the chest where these signs manifest themselves first are below the clavicle, particularly in the inner or outer third of the first intercostal space or, posteriorly, in the supraspinous fossa. Less frequently these signs may first be detected above the clavicle; sometimes, particularly in children, in the antero-lateral region of the chest, just outside of the nipple, and, quite frequently, the first signs are detectable in the area corresponding to the apex of the lower lobe, namely, the interscapular space between the level of the fourth to sixth vertebral spines. This area is often only satisfactorily examined after extreme rotation of the scapula outward.

On the other hand, it should be remembered that every now and again the first detectable evidence of pulmonary tuberculosis may be in the lower lobes, in which case it is frequently in the form of an extensive disease simulating other pneumonic processes.

None of the regular methods of physical examination should be neglected. *Inspection* of the chest may show inequalities of contour or of movement, which is usually in the form of retraction and lagging on the affected side. *Palpation* may elicit increased fremitus if the densities in the lung are of sufficient extent, or the fremitus may be diminished or absent over fluid or air in the pleural cavity or over extensive pleuritic adhesions, or over emphysematous areas. Palpation may also show increased muscle spasm, particularly of the intercostals and of the sterno-cleido-mastoid and trapezius of the affected side. This is often associated with increased sense of resistance on percussion. Palpation of the trachea may show a deviation from the median line, particularly toward the affected side, due to adhesions.

Percussion of the chest may show all variations in the presence of tuberculosis. It may be normal or dull, depending upon increased density; or hyperresonant, depending upon associated emphysema; or flat over effusions or massive pleural adhesions; or amphoric, "cracked-pot," over large cavities. Percussion as well as inspection and palpation will determine the position of the heart, which may be displaced by fluid or by adhesions.

Auscultation is by far the most important and valuable method of physical examination of the chest. A systematic technic of auscultation should be developed, which consists of slightly exaggerated respiratory movement, with the lips slightly open, and a sharp cough punctuated between each respiratory act. This procedure should be repeated systematically all over each area of the chest with particular care over the suspicious areas already noted, and with special attention paid to each phase of the respiratory cycle, namely, the inspiration, the expiration and the cough, the latter both for its own sound and its effect upon possible adventitious sounds. In addition to this, the voice sounds, and particularly the whispered voice, are important.

All varieties of modified breath sounds may be heard in the various phases of tuberculosis. They may be perfectly normal in some cases, in others the inspiratory murmur may be diminished or may be slightly interrupted or granular in character. When there is much increased density of lung tissue the expiratory sound is prolonged and high-pitched, becoming bronchovesicular or purely bronchial as the lung density increases. In some cases the associated emphysema obscures all changes due to the densities caused by the tuberculous lesion. Over fluid or air in the pleural cavity, or over extensive pleural adhesions, the breath sounds may be entirely absent. In cases with cavity there may be the characteristic signs of cavity, such as cavernous or amphoric breathing, or mixed forms of these types in the form of bronchocavernous, or broncho-amphoric breath sounds. Frequently, however, cavities perfectly evident by roentgen-ray show no such modification of breath sounds. Over pneumothorax, metallic tinkle or coin sound may be evident.

The adventitious sounds which one hears over the chest in tuberculosis are very numerous and various in character, but they are of prime importance. The most important of these are the so-called fine, mucous or subcrepitant râles which are often only brought out by coughing, and are usually best heard either in cough or in inspiration immediately after the cough. Unless the lesion is extensive, these fine mucous râles are usually inaudible in quiet breathing.

In other cases the adventitious sounds have the nature of a crepitant or crackling râle, most frequently heard above the clavicles in connection with old fibrous lesions, which are frequently of no clinical significance.

As the disease extends, and particularly when caseation progresses, the fine moist râles become larger and moister, and in the presence of pneumonic consolidation may have a ringing character, or with large cavities may reverberate.

Sibilant sonorous râles are often heard due to the slight bronchitis which may associate the early invasion of the lungs with tubercles. When these are localized or persistent over an upper lobe they are of considerable significance and, although they in themselves indicate simply a bronchitis, their localization should always arouse suspicion of the possibility of underlying lung disease.

In the presence of a fibrinous pleurisy, friction sounds will be heard, particularly in the axilla or, in some cases of chronic pleural adhesions, leathery friction rubs may be present.

In general, it may be said that the perfection of the systematic method of auscultation above described and skill in the recognition of fine râles are the most important points to be emphasized in the physical diagnosis of suspected cases of tuberculosis. Of course, when the disease is advanced, the presence of disease is obvious and the problem then more often becomes one of differential diagnosis between tuberculosis and some other disease, rather than one of early diagnosis.

Laboratory and Other Special Methods of Examination.—The Sputum.—The demonstration of tubercle bacilli in the sputum is the absolute and unimpeachable evidence of the presence of pulmonary tuberculosis. Their absence, however, does not exclude the disease, for in the earlier stages tubercle bacilli are not present in the sputum in more than 35 or 40 per cent of the cases, so that a negative sputum report in a doubtful case carries very little weight.

On the other hand, when there is very evident extensive disease of the lungs associated with the expectoration of considerable sputum, then repeated negative examinations of the sputum for tubercle bacilli constitute positive evidence of very real value against the likelihood of such extensive disease being due to tuberculosis; often the sputum should be collected for twenty-four hours and examined by one of the concentration methods.

The presence of elastic fibers in the sputum indicates destruction of tissue and, while not pathognomonic of tuberculosis, in the presence of tuberculosis is an indication of caseation.

The detection of the secondary pyogenic organisms, such as streptococci, staphylococci, pneumococci, influenza bacilli, is of very little clinical value in cases of tuberculosis, and too much importance should not be placed upon their presence as a factor in the production of lesions, or particularly as a basis for specific therapeutic procedure.

Complement-fixation Test.—A test similar to that of the Wassermann reaction for syphilis has been devised for demonstration of specific tuberculous antibodies in the blood. This test has very little value as a means of diagnosis, but may be of value in prognosis, inasmuch as the reaction is usually absent in the earlier stages, is fairly regularly present during active stages, and then disappears when the disease becomes arrested.

The Blood.—Clinical examination of the blood shows usually a slight secondary anemia in well-developed pulmonary tuberculosis, with the characteristic blood picture. The study of the leukocytes may be of some value, particularly the relation of the monocytes to the lymphocytes, and the so-called monocyte-lymphocyte ratio. This ratio is normally about 3 to 7, becomes increased when the disease is more active or more progressive, and is correspondingly lower as progress is made toward arrest of the disease. Also, the polymorphonuclear count is apt to become greater as the disease is more progressive, together with a moderate increase of the total leukocyte count, so that a leukocytosis, with increased proportion of polymorphonuclears and an increased monocyte-lymphocyte ratio may be looked upon as an unfavorable blood picture, and changes in the opposite direction are corespondingly favorable. The red cell sedimentation rate is also of considerable prognostic value.

Animal Inoculations.—Animal inoculations of the various excreta or secreta suspected to contain tubercle bacilli, are frequently necessary. Guinea-pigs are usually employed for this purpose. This is particularly helpful in the examination of pleural exudates, spinal fluids and suspected urine.

Tuberculin.—Tuberculin is, as a diagnostic agent, of definite but limited value. The best method of administration of this test is the intradermal or Mantoux test. In infants under two years of age, positive reactions are of great significance. As the age of the child increases, it becomes less and less significant, for it is found that at the age of thirteen years, about 50 per cent of all children react positively, and in adult life about 90 per cent, so that the test loses its value in adults, unless it is negative. It must be borne in mind, however, that in very advanced progressive tuberculosis, the test always becomes negative and also in the presence of some other diseases, particularly measles.

Clinico-roentgenologic Course.—With the changing flux of the clinico-pathologic possibilities of pulmonary tuberculosis it is hardly to be expected that it should run a stereotyped clinical course. Indeed it is possible to trace such a course only for some individual cases which follow throughout a persistently acute or chronic course. Speaking therefore of the clinical course of pulmonary tuberculosis it is feasible only to point out those forms which more or less tend to follow an acute or chronic course. We may also outline the circumstances and the features of more or less acuteness and more or less chronicity in the clinical course of other forms which follow individually changing or alternating courses. In doing this, it will be of advantage to keep the order of our above classification.

Such a review of the course of the special forms of pulmonary tuberculosis must needs be a clinico-roentgenologic one, due to the fact that in modern practice the clinical and serial roentgenologic follow-up have become inseparably united.

1. **Primary Forms of Pulmonary Tuberculosis.**—The clinical course of these is for the most part very mild. In the overwhelming majority of people the primary complex produces hardly any symptoms or only very ephemeral ones. In very young infants or in cases of very severe infections, in individuals of aboriginal races, or in some individuals with exceptionally low resistance, the primary complex may be associated with a comparatively acute course. At other times in these cases a more or less prolonged subacute febrile course is seen, with all the symptoms of persistent infection.

The roentgen features of the fresh or old calcified bipolar primary complex are too well known to need more than mere mention. Roentgen differentiation between the features of an epituberculous infiltration frequently involving an entire lobe, and those of caseous pneumonia, is a matter of observation. Rapid breaking-down tendency reveals the latter condition. Progressive primary complexes show the roentgen evidence of more or less persistence of the pneumonic lesion but even more so of the hilar lesion. It is to be emphasized that these infiltrations are comparatively benign processes and may persist symptomless for many months. In the cases of progressive primary complex with a more or less subacute clinical course we are already dealing with systemic disease which soon leads over to other forms.

2. **Hematogenous Forms of Pulmonary Tuberculosis.**—These again may take on forms of varying degrees of acuteness or chronicity. The dramatic course of *acute miliary tuberculosis* so frequently associated with tuberculous meningitis is well known. The roentgen picture is also easily recognized by the characteristic distribution of the fine homogeneous seeding into every part of the lung fields. Genuine acute miliary tuberculosis is for the most part an overwhelmingly fatal condition. It is probable that the cases reported as having recovered from it were not genuine but belonged rather to the group of more or less subacute miliary-like disseminations, so-called *protracted disseminations* which, particularly in children, are compatible with an almost symptomless course, at least for shorter or longer intervals. Even here in the majority of cases after a more or less protracted course the end is an acute fatal dissemination, and only occasionally is healing observed. .The roentgen features of protracted disseminations are characterized by the differences in size and sharpness of outline of the lesions which are not quite as widely disseminated as those of miliary

tuberculosis. The tendency to coalesce and even to progress toward cavitation becomes manifest in the roentgen picture of some of the more protracted cases.

Another important hematogenous form we designate under the term *chronic hematogenous pulmonary tuberculosis* which usually begins as an acute clinical condition of short duration, fading out gradually into a chronic clinical process with occasional febrile exacerbations. The clinical process as a whole simulates greatly the condition of focal infection as we know it from other infections. Its clinical recognition is by no means easy and it frequently must be based solely on the roentgen evidence of discrete pulmonary disseminations usually associated with a still active hilar complex. The outstanding roentgen feature of these discrete pulmonary disseminations is the bilateral symmetrical arrangement of the lesions, with a tendency to be densest in the upper lung fields. The lower lung fields may show but indistinct discrete mottling, while toward the apices the lesions become more distinct, the nodules become harder in outline and more variable in size. Eventually the apices will show coalesced larger foci with definite signs of fibrosis and calcification, as residues of the chronic hematogenous dissemination the lesions of which have disappeared from the rest of the lungs.

Pleurisy with or without effusion is another characteristic clinical picture to be included in the hematogenous group of pulmonary tuberculosis. It is usually benign, the fluid eventually becomes absorbed, when frequently the roentgen evidence of some post-primary discrete hematogenous foci makes its appearance. The roentgen features of pleural effusion need of course no description. On the other hand, chronic pleural tuberculosis is a roentgenologic entity usually revealed by obliteration of the costophrenic sinuses, tenting of the diaphragm due to adhesions, and thickening of the pleura in the interlobar fissures or along the lateral margins.

3. **Transitional Forms of Pulmonary Tuberculosis.**—These are characterized by their almost entirely symptomless clinical course for long periods of years. Most of the tuberculous conditions of the lungs discovered accidentally, either at the occasion of contact periodic health examinations or examinations of the lungs in connection with tuberculous processes in some other part of the body, or in connection with some other suspected disease of the lungs, or following hemoptysis in an otherwise entirely symptomless patient, usually belong to this form. Even in later phases the so often remarkably slow clinical progress interrupted only at long intervals by periods of activity of more or less short duration, is an outstanding feature of this type of condition, frequently in sharp contrast with the apparently considerable extent of the lesions. The cases with extensive bilateral, so-called chronic cirrhotic (fibroid) processes are very slowly progressive and eventually die not of their tuberculosis but rather of the right heart failure due to the marked fibrotic and emphysematous changes in their lungs. Less frequently the hematogenous origin of these conditions unmasks itself by a terminal recurrence of the blood stream dissemination in a miliary-like manner. Again, frequently the transitional

character of the process asserts itself, and the course takes a turn toward a genuine phthisical process which is marked by multiple cavitation, hemorrhages and bronchial spilling. Compact broncho-pneumonic focal lesions become superimposed upon the old characteristic bilateral symmetrical nodular coalescing foci of parallel cranio-caudal progression. The end-picture and its course is that of chronic advanced phthisis.

The roentgen features of these forms are characterized by the bilateral, more or less symmetrical and disseminated arrangement of the lesions throughout both but particularly the upper lung fields. The shadows indicate the lesions to be of a productive fibrotic type. Their coalescence can be followed as they lead to characteristically punched-out symmetrical round cavities or to more or less calcified and densely cirrhotic residues of the first larger units at the apices. More distally on both sides the signs of slow progressive coalescence and breakdown are apparent in the scattered fibro-ulcerous symmetrical lesions. These together with the associated marked emphysema of the intervening lung areas and that of the lower lung fields are the roentgen features which suggest that the process belongs to the transitional forms of pulmonary tuberculosis.

4. **Chronic Pulmonary Phthisis.**—The periodically relapsing acute exacerbations, with parallel periodic extension of the lesions, superimposed upon a basically chronic course are the most outstanding characteristics of this form. The onset probably is with repeated grippe-like attacks coming at intervals of shorter or longer duration. The first of these are usually so ephemeral that they are taken for harmless colds. The patient becomes almost completely symptomless, but residues of the lung focus, usually an infiltration of greater or smaller size, remain and are certain to exacerbate again. With every recurrence the attack becomes more severe, more prolonged and productive of such more or less permanent symptoms as cough, expectoration, pains in the chest, night sweats, anorexia, loss of weight and probably hemoptysis. With every recurrence of an attack a crop of new foci are produced, or the old foci extended and new areas of the lungs on the same or the opposite side are invaded, and even greater residual lesions are left, sure to exacerbate again sooner and sooner. Spontaneous recovery thus becomes less and less likely with each repetition of the exacerbation. This course may run over a period of years during which there may be definite progression of the process or definite improvement toward arrest and healing. Rarely does any one case go in continuous fashion either to healing or to the fatal end.

In the roentgenologic course the onset is seen usually in the form of an acute infiltration, infraclavicular or otherwise, where the rest of the lungs are perfectly clear. Frequently, however, there is present already, at the time when such an infiltration is first noted, evidence of a previous infiltration in the form of hardened residual shadows of an older focus. At other times the acute infiltration shows a fresh cavity in its center, with evidence of metastatic foci showing the characteristics due to bronchial spilling. Frequently enough the process is discovered only when roentgen evidence shows already the existence of a tuberculous bronchopneumonic area, generally in one of the upper lobes, and usually with evidence of some spilling into one or all other lobes, which in turn may have the same characteristics as the source lesion if the spilling was massive, or may be but a very fine seeding if the spilling was moderate. The exquisitely miliary-like bronchogenic disseminations observed so frequently following hemorrhages and also the very widespread but less fine disseminations associated with extensive laryngeal ulcerations are very characteristic roentgenologic entities important to bear in mind constantly in connection with chronic pulmonary phthisis.

Appearance of the permanent cavity marks the turn in the clinical course. Fresh cavities appearing within an infiltration may disappear with the resolution of the infiltration, leaving behind but very small scars. Cavities developing fibrotic walls tend to become permanent, and although they may shrink markedly after a considerable length of time, they tend to make the process a more or less continuous one, even though the patient may have shorter or longer periods of quiescence during which he will be amazingly free of constitutional symptoms. However, more or less chronic cough and expectoration of bacillus-laden sputum are those inseparable symptoms of such a patient with cavity, which are instrumental in extending the process continuously until it reaches the terminal phase. It is rather an exception that a patient with an open cavity and positive sputum recovers spontaneously and completely. As a rule, unless measures are taken to collapse the cavity artificially and eliminate the source of the positive sputum, such a patient will soon be overtaken by even more acute and prolonged periodic exacerbations ending finally in a clinical picture of hectic fever, incessant cough, profuse expectoration with frequent hemoptyses, emaciation and loss of strength until the end. Less frequently even the spontaneous course is by such slow degrees that life ebbs almost imperceptibly, with the process extending until so small a fraction of normal lung tissue remains that it is amazing to see the patient alive. The average spontaneous course of chronic pulmonary phthisis is estimated between five and seven years.

The roentgen features of advanced chronic phthisis with its motley picture of cirrhotic and thick-walled cavities of all possible shape and size, mostly crowded toward the upper fields, but not infrequently to be found in almost any part of the lung fields, with its wide range of variations in the quantity, quality and arrangement of the lesions, are so manifold and so individually variable that there exist no two processes giving quite identical roentgen pictures.

Pulmonary Tuberculosis and Silicosis.—Pulmonary tuberculosis assumes somewhat unusual features when combined with silicosis. Clinically this combination may appear in three forms; the patient shows characteristic evidence of manifest extensive old pulmonary tuberculosis with a positive sputum, which has been reactivated by silicosis acquired through professional exposure of more or less short duration. The character of the process and its course are more like frank phthisis here. Then it may be that a patient with long-standing silicotic condition in his terminal phase develops added pulmonary tuberculosis with frank clinical manifestations of the latter. Finally, it may be a case of so-called genuine "silico-tuberculosis" which is called by some "infectious silicosis." In the first two forms the course of the process is determined essentially by the character of the tuberculous process. In the latter form there is a process which is clinically characterized by its equisitely chronic symptomless course and persistent absence of tubercle bacilli in the sputum, which frequently makes it almost impossible to distinguish it from pure silicosis. Increasing amount of pathologic evidence indicates that in the overwhelming majority of cases silicosis is combined with tuberculous infection productive of a process which is essentially different from both silicosis and tuberculosis.

The above three possible combinations will be reflected also in the roentgen features of the combination between silicosis and tuberculosis. Thus there may be the picture of an extensive chronic cavitary phthisical process combined with some silicotic lesions disseminated in the lower lung fields or an extensive silicotic process widely disseminated throughout both lungs with a superimposed confluent bronchopneumonic or cavitary lesion in some part of the lungs. Finally the picture of "silico-tuberculosis" simulates greatly that of bronchogenic miliary tuberculosis, except for the somewhat larger size of the nodules.

Diagnosis.—All hope of successful treatment depends largely upon the early recognition of pulmonary tuberculosis. Nevertheless, it is still true that a very considerable percentage of all cases are not so recognized and that, consequently, the results of treatment are frequently unsatisfactory.

The responsibility which rests upon the physician for making an early diagnosis is very great, although other factors enter into the problem. If the physician constantly bears in mind the insidious character of tuberculosis, its great frequency and the variety of its manifestations, many unnecessary errors may be avoided.

The principal factors to be emphasized are the points in the history already described; the appraisal of the general condition of the patient; careful physical examination, with the localization in the upper lobe particularly borne in mind; routine examination of the sputum in suspected cases, but with a recognition of the fact that in early tuberculosis the sputum is often negative. Above all, however, the insistence upon roentgen-ray examination in all suspicious cases, whether abnormal physical signs are present or not, cannot be overemphasized. In view of the recent mass observations of entirely symptomless evolution of pulmonary tuberculosis from old dormant foci, failure to make a roentgen examination of a suspected case of tuberculosis must be considered an act of negligence. All of these procedures, combined with a careful correlation of the data, usually lead to a correct diagnosis.

Differential Diagnosis.—The conditions which are to be considered here may be divided into two main groups: (1) those of which the history and symptoms are suspicious of tuberculosis but the local lesion is slight and difficult to find—a problem in physical examination; (2) those cases presenting very definite physical signs in the lungs—a problem in interpretation.

1. **Conditions in Which Suspicious Symptoms Predominate.**—Under this heading would come those cases described in our consideration of history taking, namely, definite symptoms of malaise, or asthenia; disturbances of the digestive system or of the nervous system; anemia; slight persistent fever of obscure origin, in which the differential diagnosis mainly lies between typhoid or paratyphoid fever, malaria, influenza, various types of focal infections, bacterial endocarditis; and sometimes with some disturbance of metabolism, particularly in hyperthyroidism.

When any of this group of symptoms present themselves, tuberculosis should always be borne in mind as a possibility and excluded only after most careful study.

2. **Conditions Presenting Obvious Physical Signs.**—Under this heading come first those slight apical physical signs due to slight *obsolescent healed lesions,* which in the absence of constitutional symptoms frequently have no clinical significance whatever. The other conditions which present physical signs often mistaken for tuberculosis are *emphysema and chronic bronchitis;* subacute or chronic *bronchopneumonia;* various types of *fibrosis* of the lung, especially *pneumoconiosis; abscess* of the lung; *syphilis* of the lung; *various fungus infections; tumors* of the lung, and chronic pulmonary *changes secondary to chronic cardiac disease.* All of these various conditions have been discussed from the point of view of the differential diagnosis from tuberculosis in their appropriate sections.

The general principles underlying this differential diagnosis, however, consist mainly in the predilection of tuberculosis for the upper lobe, which is not the case in any of the other conditions; the presence in almost all of these conditions of abundant sputum which is persistently negative for tubercle bacilli and, lastly, the characteristic differences on roentgenologic examination which usually exist. In some cases the differential diagnosis is by no means easy, and careful study under close observation for a period of time may be necessary.

Prognosis and Clinical Status.—In the discussion of the pathologic and clinical aspects of the disease it has been pointed out repeatedly that the progressive and regressive tendency in the evolution of the lesions is more or less characteristic. It has been particularly emphasized in connection with the transitional forms of pulmonary tuberculosis that they constitute for the most part benign clinico-pathologic conditions in which the spontaneous healing tendency and the exquisitely prolonged benign course are rather the rule. Exceptions are to be made of course of the not infrequent instances in which a recurrence of hematogenous disseminations or a transition to frank bronchogenic phthisis takes place, both of which may turn the clinical course into an acute or subacute one.

In contrast to the above, the prognosis of the course of chronic pulmonary phthisis is extremely difficult on account of the numerous factors involved. In general it depends particularly upon the extent of the disease at the time treatment is established; upon the character of the lesion, whether it is the acute exudative type, or with a tendency to a very slow progression with considerable fibrosis; the amount of constitutional symptoms, and the presence or absence of serious complications.

The most reliable basis for prognosis is the character of the response of the individual patient to proper treatment. If the response is promptly favorable, a better prognosis can immediately be given. But this, too, depends upon other important factors, particularly the duration of the treatment, which is often unduly short because of various conditions, none more important than the social and economic status of the individual, which may not only make proper treatment difficult to obtain, but exerts a constant temptation to return to normal active life prematurely.

As has already been noted, certain laboratory tests, such as the character of the leukocyte count, the blood sedimentation test, and the complement-fixation test may be of some aid. The age of the patient also is a factor, inasmuch as in older people the disease tends to a milder and more chronic course.

In general it is well to give a guarded prognosis, bearing in mind the uncertainties of the disease, for, while good results may be obtained in the large majority of cases in which proper treatment is begun early, the outcome in any individual case may be influenced by many unexpected and often unpreventable factors.

Assessment of the clinical status of our cases for comparative records requires a status classification based upon some standard basis which should enable us to designate the particular condition in which a patient is found at any given time. Many such classifications have been suggested. The one that is now most widely used and on the whole most satisfactory is that of the American Sanatorium Association. Under this system the Roman numerals I, II, III are employed to designate the extent of the lesions, and the letters A, B, C similarly to designate the amount of the constitutional impairment:

CLASSIFICATION OF LESIONS.

I. Slight infiltration limited to a small part of one lobe, with no tuberculous complications.
II. Marked infiltration with little or no evidence of cavity formation, and no serious tuberculous complications.
III. Extensive infiltration or consolidation with cavity formation or the presence of serious tuberculous complications.

CLASSIFICATION OF SYMPTOMS.

A. Slight or no constitutional symptoms.
B. No marked impairment of function, either local or constitutional.
C. Marked impairment of function, either local or constitutional or both.

Under this system the following combinations are therefore possible:

I A	II A	III A
I B	II B	III B
I C	II C	III C

For example, I C would indicate slight apical lesion with considerable constitutional involvement while, on the other hand, III A would mean extensive lesions, possibly with cavity formation, with very slight constitutional impairment. The utilization of this classification is simple and the application is obvious. It is very useful in the assessment of the condition of a patient at any one time and facilitates comparison with previous or later observations.

Classification of Comparative Condition.—In the same way, certain terms have been adopted by the National Tuberculosis Association to denote the comparative condition of patients at different periods of observation:

Apparently Cured.—All constitutional symptoms and expectoration of bacilli absent for two years under ordinary conditions of life.

Arrested.—The same situation which has lasted for a period of six months.

Apparently Arrested.—When this condition has been present for three months.

Quiescent.—Absence of constitutional symptoms. Bacilli in the sputum may be present or absent, and physical signs stationary or regressive. The foregoing conditions to have existed for at least two months.

Improved.—Some amelioration of symptoms or regression of physical signs.

Unimproved.—All essential symptoms and signs unabated or increased.

It will be noted that in the utilization of this classification the length of time that has passed during which the described conditions have existed, is the point of particular emphasis. The use of this system facilitates comparison of results of treatment by various observers.

Treatment.—The basic principles of the treatment of pulmonary tuberculosis are contained in what has been called the hygienic-dietetic method of treatment. In the forms of bronchogenic phthisis, where this is feasible the various methods of collapse or immobilization therapy must be added to the above.

1. **Hygienic-dietetic Therapy.**—Hygienic-dietetic therapy consists of a regimen of life carried out over a considerable period of time, requiring modification according to the various conditions which may arise. This regimen is composed of various factors which should be separately considered, but which, together, comprise an entity which must be adopted as a program of living.

Rest and Exercise.— *Rest* is the most essential single item in the treatment of pulmonary tuberculosis during the active stages. This should be absolute rest in bed during periods of fever, and in bed or upon a reclining-chair for a goodly portion of each day for several months in almost every case. This principle of rest must be learned by every patient if a successful result is to be obtained. It requires relaxation of mind and body, which is an art which can only be attained by patience and persistence. It is, moreover, a test of character. Peace of mind and freedom from excitement are as important as physical relaxation of the body, so that various forms of mental activity must be controlled according to their effect upon the individual patient, and worries and anxieties should be eliminated as fully as conditions will permit.

Rest may be overdone. Gain in weight, which may be a valuable index of improvement at first, is not necessarily so when it degenerates into excessive flabby fat accompanied by complete mental inertia.

After the active symptoms—as indicated particularly by temperature, pulse-rate and fatigability—have subsided, then *graduated exercise* under careful medical advice is indicated. By this means, by easy stages, a gradual progress from absolute rest to normal physical and mental activity is achieved in the course of several months.

The period of beginning exercise is often the most critical. The amount that each patient is able to do can only be accurately determined by experiment, and consequently each attempt at exercise is tentative. If, after a few minutes of slow walking, symptoms tend to recur, rest must again be enforced for a longer period, and the attempt at exercise repeated again later. One day of indiscretion in overexertion may undo the results obtained by many weeks of patient rest, and such exercise therefore must be very gradually increased and only as the condition of the patient indicates.

The progress in increased exercise proceeds through sitting up in a chair, to slow walking of specified and gradually increasing duration, to such wider activities as driving, longer walks, some form of light manual work and, later, to the lighter forms of sports: tramps, skating, horseback-riding. The process is really one of gradual training under strict supervision, so as to have the individual patient eventually become physically fit, so that in the end he may be on unlimited exercise toward the end of his cure, and then may be able to contemplate a return to regular work and normal life.

During all of this time these periods of exercise are interrupted by periods of strict rest. Usually this means staying in bed until 10 o'clock in the morning, then resting absolutely for two hours after the mid-day meal, and returning to bed at night by 9 o'clock. This allows two periods for the prescribed exercise: one in the latter part of the morning and the other in the afternoon; as a rule, the more active exercise is best taken in the morning.

This schedule of life must be maintained for a minimum of six months in early favorable cases, and in more advanced cases it is not infrequently a matter of two or three years or even more.

Nutrition and Diet.—When the patient with tuberculosis first begins his rest treatment he is usually, although not always, underweight. A good deal of stress has always been placed upon gain of weight as tangible evidence of improvement. Within limits this is true; but the gain in weight should be gradual, and the diet carefully regulated rather than forced. The days of extreme overfeeding with large quantities of milk and eggs, in addition to three regular meals, have been superseded by a more rational method of diet, which is more successful because it is less apt to disturb the digestion, and more permanent because more gradually and naturally attained.

Poor appetite and more or less indigestion are very common symptoms during the period of active disease, and rest in the open air is the best remedy for this condition, but at the same time very careful attention to the idiosyncrasies of the individual should be given, and every effort made to restore digestion to normal.

In general it has been found wise to give the usual patient three regular meals a day of a mixed diet, with the principal meal in the middle of the day. Feeding between meals is frequently undesirable and should never be given if it detracts from the appetite for the regular meals. In some cases digestion and appetite demand it and then it is not objectionable.

In other cases these regular substantial meals cannot be given, and more frequent feedings in small amounts of easily digested foods must be substituted; but as the active symptoms subside and the patient improves, the objective to be reached is that of the three regular meals which, when the patient is at rest, need not total more than 2500 calories, but when the exercise period has begun, may be increased to 4000 or even more if the appetite demands it and the digestion is good.

The care of the bowels is extremely important during this whole period, and is preferably regulated by a diet containing the proper proportion of fruits and vegetables rather than by laxatives. The vitamins contained in various fruits are important, and in some cases, particularly in those complicated with intestinal tuberculosis, vitamins in the form of cod-liver oil and tomato juice may be added to the diet with advantage.

Any symptoms of indigestion should be noted and treated promptly, as poor digestion is one of the chief obstacles to successful treatment of this disease.

Open Air and Climate.—The open-air life has become an axiom in the treatment of tuberculosis. In most cases this is more effective when the temperature of the air is cool and bracing. The favorable effect of rest in the open air upon the toxic symptoms of tuberculosis is often most striking, and the use of this agent should be begun at once in the treatment, and continued through all of its stages until it becomes a more or less fixed habit of life. The patient should, if possible, be out-of-doors during all of the daylight hours, and in the majority of the cases out-of-door sleeping is also an advantage, although not absolutely essential if plenty of air is available through open windows.

While the effect of cold air appears to be favorable in most cases, in some patients with poor circulation, especially in the advanced stages of the disease, the reaction is bad, and exposure to cold weather should not be insisted upon in such cases. Exposure to dust and wind should always be avoided. While rain and fog may be undesirable, they do not constitute a contraindication to the open-air cure.

For many cases of tuberculosis exposure of the body to sunlight has proven helpful. This form of *radiotherapy* is particularly valuable in non-pulmonary forms of tuberculosis, but patients with pulmonary tuberculosis appear to be very much more sensitive to the sun-rays, and may react unfavorably by rise of temperature, hemoptysis and restlessness, so that, as a rule, this form of therapy is only employed in pulmonary tuberculosis in exceptional instances. In all cases exposure of the head to the direct rays of the sun should be avoided at all times, and any form of radiotherapy should only be employed under careful medical supervision.

The question of *climate* has always loomed large in both medical and lay thought concerning tuberculosis. There can be no doubt that where the climate is such as to make the out-of-door life comfortable and easy, it has a very definite, favorable effect. This is particularly true during that phase of the cure when the patient is able to take more or less exercise.

There is, however, no one ideal climate. Young people with good circulation respond particularly well to cold, dry, stimulating climate, while older people, or those with poor circulation or with a tendency to nervousness, usually do better in milder, more relaxing climates. Inasmuch as the dry, cold climates are usually found in the mountains, altitude is a necessary accompaniment. It may in itself have some value, but in some cases altitude of any considerable degree is contraindicated because of cardiac disease, sleeplessness, nervousness, tendency to hemorrhage and particularly in all cases with dyspnea.

In general, it may be said that climate has come to take a somewhat secondary place as an essential in the treatment of pulmonary tuberculosis, and it should never be sought at the expense of opportunities for proper rest, suitable food and contentment of mind, but that a change of climate is often extremely helpful, and during some stage of the cure is usually a most effective adjunct to the other fundamentals of the treatment.

Environment.—More important than the question of climate itself is that of an environment suited to the individual patient. The chief factor in this is personal contentment and satisfaction. Individual tastes must be studied and every effort made to satisfy them within the limits of a strict conformity to the essentials of the cure. This applies not only to the place in which the patient takes the cure, but also to the conditions of life, whether in a sanatorium or in his own home. Unhappiness and homesickness have wrecked many well-planned cures.

Medical Supervision.—It is rare indeed that a patient can get well of pulmonary tuberculosis without regular, skilled medical supervision. The advice all too often given to "go off on a farm, live out-of-doors and eat plenty of milk and eggs" has been the undoing of many patients. In no phase of the treatment is this more important than in the supervision of the graduated exercise desired, but also is very important in the selection of the diet, the care of the digestion and in the treatment of minor symptoms which may arise. The aid of the physician is also most valuable in upholding the morale of the patient and in helping him to develop a philosophic attitude of mind toward his illness. This mental readjustment, important as it is in every chronic disease, is nowhere more so than in tuberculosis, and the physician often has splendid opportunities for developing it among his patients.

Perhaps the most valuable result of such medical supervision is the gradual education of the patient in the principles underlying the plan of treatment. Thus, a patient becomes skilled in the appreciation of his own limitations and, when he finally returns to normal life, is trained in proper habits of living, which in itself will go far to prevent relapse.

The Time Element in the Treatment.—Not only must the regimen of the cure be systematic in detail, but it must be extended liberally in time. While many cases improve rapidly, practically no case can become surely arrested in a short time. It is important that this be understood at the outset, so that necessary family and financial adjustments can be made. Inadequate provision in point of time leads to disappointment, to real hardship, and sometimes may force a premature return to work, which frequently leads to relapse. A wise policy demands provision for a little more rather than a little less time that may be estimated as necessary; thus, bitter disappointment or real tragedy may be avoided.

Sanatorium Treatment.—From what has been said concerning the importance of the regimen of the cure and medical supervision, the advantages of sanatorium care are obvious. It becomes a comparatively easy matter for a patient to fall in line when others are doing the same thing and, unconsciously, in such an institution an education in habits of life is going on, which is far-reaching in its results and very difficult to attain by more individualistic methods. In general it may be said that this training constitutes probably the chief value of sanatorium treatment, and the majority of patients are much the better for having the advantages of such training during some part of their treatment.

Home Treatment.—As opposed to sanatorium treatment, there has been a growing tendency to treat patients in their own homes rather than to submit them to the expense, inconvenience, or unhappiness of removal to some distant health resort. The basis for this change is an increased appreciation of the value of rest. It has come about, therefore, that during the acute febrile stages many cases are most satisfactorily treated in their homes, with absolute bed rest provided, and all of the other necessary conditions fulfilled. Sometimes the patient is much happier, more contented, rests better and, consequently, does better.

On the other hand, frequently the home conditions are distracting, the regular schedule of curing easily interrupted, and the temptations arising from association with only those who are well are very much greater than when all are doing the same thing, as in the sanatorium. Consequently, it may be said that bed rest at home during the acute stages is often helpful and justifiable and may even be preferable, but that continuous home treatment throughout the complete course of the cure is more often unsatisfactory, the principal defect being the lack of educational and training advantages which the sanatorium or health resort affords.

After-care.—It is an unfortunate fact that a very considerable percentage of patients who have taken a cure for tuberculosis and returned to normal life, sooner or later relapse. An analysis of these relapses shows that they are largely due to faulty methods of living or to the

49

strain of a too rapid return to regular, active life. They are therefore to a very considerable extent preventable.

The best protection against such relapse is the education of the patient which we have already emphasized. Too often, however, economic stress tempts the arrested case beyond his endurance, or a careless temperament tends to forgetfulness. For several years after successful curing of tuberculosis the patient should continue to live a very careful and, to some extent, restricted life, avoiding stress and strains, both physical and mental, taking plenty of time for sleep, for recreation and for out-of-door life.

The character of the occupation, provided it is not obviously an unfavorable one, appears to make comparatively little difference, and the widespread notion that with arrested tuberculosis a patient should only return to an out-of-door life is a fallacy. Frequently such out-of-door jobs entail hard physical exercise to which the patient is usually unaccustomed, and this physical strain does more harm than the open air can possibly do good. As a rule, it has been found that a return to the same occupation which the patient had previously is desirable. This involves less physical and mental strain, is usually more remunerative, and thus provides for the maintenance of higher standards of living.

Medical supervision at regular intervals with careful physical and roentgen-ray examinations should be maintained for several years after a patient with arrested tuberculosis returns to normal life. In this way faulty habits of living are corrected early, slight symptoms remedied, and suspicious signs of relapsing disease detected before serious harm has resulted.

2. **Collapse or Immobilization Therapy.**—Our methods of collapse therapy may be divided into non-surgical and surgical ones. The first include pneumothorax and oleothorax; the latter include the whole range of surgical procedures, from simple phrenic section to the most extensive thoracoplasty of an entire side of the chest wall. The latter include besides phrenic exairesis, apicolysis and partial thoracoplasties, also intrathoracic caustic pneumolysis as an adjuvant to pneumothorax. The principle underlying them all is the same, namely, immobilization or collapse of the affected lung. The goal aimed at is a double one: release of the affected lung from the thoracic pull associated with breathing activity, and elimination of the permanent source of bronchogenic extension afforded by the open, mostly cavitary lesions. Both of these factors have been found to be chiefly responsible for the ultimate defeat of the spontaneous healing tendency which is manifest in probably every case of chronic pulmonary tuberculosis.

These methods have obtained their most brilliant results in cases where only one lung was involved or involvement of the other lung was minimal. This circumstance makes chronic pulmonary phthisis, as defined in the above presentation, that special form of pulmonary tuberculosis in which these methods are particularly indicated and to be employed early in the disease before bilateralization of the process. The fact that transitional forms of pulmonary tuberculosis tend to be bilateral, militates against the applicability of these methods in this form. Fortunately these conditions are for the most part so benign that collapse is hardly indicated. In those instances of this form in which transition to frank phthisis takes place, this is usually associated with a marked extension, chiefly and at first only on one side, so that active collapse therapy becomes feasible. Furthermore, the modern methods of selective bilateral pneumothorax, and the combinations of pneumothorax with phrenicotomy, or apicolysis, or partial thoracoplasty on alternating sides, opened up various possibilities also for cases belonging to this form.

As a general principle it should be emphasized in connection with all these collapse procedures that hygieno-dietetic treatment should first be given a chance to see what it can accomplish. It should be particularly remembered that infiltrative processes, even if extensive, may resolve completely even after weeks or months of persistence. The clinical course and particularly the bacillary content of the sputum should be our guide rather than the extent and localization of the lesions. Excepting the occasional desperate cases of caseous pneumonic processes, as revealed by the corresponding clinical course, in which there is everything to gain and nothing to lose by an early collapse (pneumothorax), we are not justified in proceeding to active therapy before having waited a reasonable period for spontaneous resolution. Particularly in connection with cases belonging to the transitional form with a negative sputum or a sputum of scant bacillary content, and especially in absence of cavities, expectant rest treatment will be much preferable to active treatment with its many hazards of pleural infections and hardships of surgical procedures.

The successful application of the various collapse methods depends in the first place on utmost efficiency and skill in their use, but even more so on intimate familiarity with their general and special indications varying with the individual clinico-pathologic features of the case, and a thorough understanding of the limitations of the various procedures, as well as seasoned judgment in assessing the clinical condition and fitness of the individual patient.

Artificial Pneumothorax.—This is the most important of these procedures and has now come to take a very definite place in the treatment of pulmonary tuberculosis. Probably from 25 to 40 per cent of all cases are suitable for this method of treatment. This should only be carried out by those who are skilled in its use and familiar with the indications and limitations of this method of treatment.

In general it is mainly indicated in unilateral cases of disease which do not respond promptly to bed-rest treatment; in cases with cavities which do not tend to close; in hemorrhage cases, particularly if large and repeated; and in pleural effusion complicating pulmonary tuberculosis as a supplementary procedure to aspiration. It is inapplicable in many cases on account of pleural adhesions, and even more frequently it is only partly successful because of localized adhesions. In many cases, after several months of treatment, pleural effusions occur in the pneumothorax cavity, and these not infrequently become purulent and require the various methods of treatment described under tuberculous empyema.

In a very few carefully selected cases bilateral pneumothorax has been successful.

In proper hands, treatment by artificial pneumothorax is without danger, although occasional cases of death from pleural shock and air embolism have been reported; and this method of treatment has added materially to the percentage of patients with pulmonary tuberculosis in which arrest of the disease and return to active life have been obtained.

Oleothorax.—Recently mineral oil has been used in place of air to produce collapse of the lung. The chief indications are to produce reaction with adhesions when a movable mediastinum makes satisfactory collapse impossible. It has also been suggested to aid in the collapse of cavities which resist pneumothorax. Its field of usefulness is limited.

Pneumolysis.—By this term is meant a minor surgical procedure by which localized adhesions preventing proper collapse in the course of an artificial pneumothorax are severed by the aid of an instrument called the thoracoscope, similar in construction to the cystoscope.

Phrenicotomy.—This is another surgical procedure by which a section of the phrenic nerve on the affected side is resected or evulsed, in order to produce a permanent paralysis of the corresponding leaf of the diaphragm. This paralysis results in diminished movement of that side and a raising of the level of the diaphragm so as to diminish the functioning area of the lung. This method has recently become quite popular, and some cases of successful control of lesions and collapse of cavities have been reported. It is also often recommended as a preliminary procedure to a thoracoplasty. There is a general impression that the enthusiasm for this comparatively simple procedure has led to its too wide application, and judgment as to its permanent place in the treatment of pulmonary tuberculosis should still be reserved.

Apicolysis.—Apicolysis is a more major form of surgical procedure, designed to immobilize and collapse the apex of the lung through the insertion of some foreign material, such as paraffin, muscle or fat, extrapleurally between the parietal pleura and the chest wall. It is of value in a certain limited number of cases.

Thoracoplasty.—This is a major surgical procedure which has now come to have a very real place in the treatment of pulmonary tuberculosis. It should never be employed until pneumothorax has first been tried, and has its chief field of usefulness in cases where the pneumothorax is impossible or unsatisfactory on account of adhesions, or where a tuberculous empyema has resulted, or in other cases where the severity of the original disease was such that ultimate reëxpansion of the lung is deemed undesirable. In skilful hands the mortality of this operation is slight, the deformity and physical handicap much less than would be anticipated, and the results are increasingly more satisfactory.

In the consideration of all of these local methods of treatment it must be borne in mind that with them, all of the details of the regimen of cure above described should be carried out at the same time, and that these procedures are simply an aid in such cures and not a cure in themselves.

3. **Symptomatic Treatment.**—While the systematic regimen is the fundamentally important factor in the treatment of any case, symptoms will arise from time to time which demand special medical attention.

Cough.—Rest in the open-air constitutes the best treatment for cough and frequently is all that is necessary. Conscious control of the cough can be developed, and should always be encouraged. If the cough disturbs the sleep or is violent and protracted, so as to upset the stomach, sedatives must be given, but always in moderation. Codeine alone or in combination is the most reliable drug. Combinations with terpene hydrate or with a few drops of dilute hydrocyanic acid, or with a mild expectorant such as ammonium chloride or ammonium carbonate, are often helpful. Bromides are also often helpful. But all cough remedies should be prescribed in very simple form so as not to disturb the digestion. Morphine should never be given solely to relieve cough.

Digestive Disturbances.—Rest, open-air life and proper attention to diet will meet most of the indications for disturbed digestion, of which overfeeding and constipation are the most common causes. A simple stomachic bitter, of which none is better than nux vomica, often helps the appetite and the digestion. Simple remedies, such as bicarbonate of soda, rhubarb and soda mixture, milk of magnesia, pepsin, pancreatin, dilute hydrochloric acid, are all useful in some cases and are to be preferred to more complex remedies. The care of the digestion should be a matter of the utmost concern and demands constant and detailed attention.

Fever.—Absolute bed rest is the specific treatment of fever in tuberculosis. Even slight elevations of temperature coming in the afternoon cannot be disregarded, and absolute rest should be maintained until the temperature remains normal at all times of the day. Mild antipyretics sometimes may be desirable to relieve the discomfort of the fever, particularly the headache, but should be given sparingly. Sponge baths and alcohol baths are often most helpful.

Night-sweats.—These are usually the corollary of the fever, are due to the same causes, and demand the same rest treatment. Alcohol baths are particularly effective for their relief. Sometimes a little belladonna or atropine may be indicated.

Pulmonary Hemorrhage.—Slight pulmonary hemorrhages need no treatment other than absolute bed rest and the reassurance of the patient. Bed rest should be enforced for four or five days after all trace of blood has disappeared from the sputum. The diet should be cut down to liquids and the bowels kept open by laxatives. In severe or repeated hemorrhages, morphine followed by codeine is usually indicated to insure quiet and control the cough. Sometimes the hemorrhage seems to recur at a certain level of the blood pressure. In such cases control of the blood pressure by nitroglycerin or sodium nitrite may be helpful. Medication designed to increase the coagulability of the blood, such as calcium lactate, gelatin, or the hypodermic administration of normal blood serum, is of doubtful value.

More important than these are mechanical methods designed to partly immobilize the affected lung. This can be done by weights on the chest and in the axilla, but particularly by the administration of artificial pneumothorax when the bleedings are serious because of amount or of frequent repetition.

4. **Treatment of Complications.**—When symptoms of active tuberculosis recur, particularly fever, the possibility of their being due to some tuberculous complication rather than to the lung disease must always be borne in mind. When this is discovered, appropriate treatment should be immediately instituted. Among the most important conditions which demand such treatment are: *tuberculous laryngitis*, the treatment of which has been considered elsewhere, and *tuberculous enteritis*, which calls for careful regulation of the diet, frequently local radiotherapy over the abdomen, best by one of the lamps designed to produce a high percentage of ultra-violet radiation, and the ingestion of cod-liver oil and tomato juice.

The principal complications in the chest which may arise are: pleural effusions, spontaneous pneumothorax, pyopneumothorax, the treatment of which is considered elsewhere. Other extra-pulmonary forms of tuberculosis should have appropriate treatment, which is frequently surgical, but with due regard to the effect that any operative procedure may have upon the ·pulmonary lesion. Radiotherapy is often of great value, either alone or combined with surgical treatment.

5. **Specific Treatment.**—In spite of all the hopes that have been raised in the fifty years since Koch discovered the tubercle bacillus, there is still no specific treatment for pulmonary tuberculosis. All sorts of chemicals have been tried; tuberculin has been used and found wanting; vaccinations, serums and extracts of various animal organs were recommended and tried in vain. The most recent attempt at vaccination is that of Calmette with the use of the B.C.G. culture of attenuated living tubercle bacilli. This, however, is recommended only for preventive vaccination and not for treatment, and its value even as a preventive is as yet unproven. From the experience with the multitude of so-called cures for tuberculosis the medical profession can conscientiously continue to exercise considerable caution and reserve before accepting the frequent claims of the discovery of such cures.

Prevention.—Tuberculosis prophylaxis has become an essential part of the activities of public health authorities. The means used are registration, supervision and inspection of infectious cases; the segregation of dangerous cases in institutions; the examination of contacts in the families who have been exposed to infection; and a systematic effort to uncover early cases through public dispensaries; surveys of certain industries; and general education and propaganda. In addition to this, the health authorities assume the responsibility for betterment of the living conditions and working conditions which may predispose to tuberculosis. Pasteurization of milk has become almost universal and has been largely instrumental in the elimination of bovine tuberculosis from human beings.

If any conclusions at all can be drawn from our experiences of recent years with the public antituberculosis campaign, it is, that the ferreting-out of the cases in the early and latent phase of the disease, and the finding out of the potential cases harboring old reactivable lesions, in the course of contact or mass examinations of whole sections of the population, has been by far the most efficient prophylactic procedure. This bears out fully the concept promulgated in the above presentation, that pulmonary tuberculosis, in the majority of cases, originates with the lighting-up of the incompletely healed lesions of the first infection or one of its satellites. Therefore, a main objective to be attained in the prevention of tuberculosis is the task of preventing latent tuberculous infection from becoming manifest tuberculous disease.

The Rôle of the Physician in Prevention.—The time has gone by when a physician is considered to have fulfilled his entire responsibilities when he gives his best individual treatment to the patient who is ill. In the management of the individual case of tuberculosis he has in addition the responsibility for controlling the spread of the infection to other members of the family or other associates; for looking into the possibility of early tuberculosis in those who may have been exposed and for systematically examining all such contacts, particularly children.

In addition, the physician has a wider responsibility to the community as a whole; he should take an intelligent and leading part in those forces, both public and private, which are playing so important a rôle in the prevention of tuberculosis and in the improvement of general health. Only as he realizes his responsibility in this wider sphere of service does he fulfil his full responsibility both as a citizen and as a physician.

SYPHILIS OF THE LUNG.

Incidence.—The prevalence of syphilis of the lung as a pathologic entity has been a subject of considerable controversy. Previous to the bacteriologic era the clinical diagnosis of syphilis of the lung was very common, but with the discovery of the tubercle bacillus it was found that a very large percentage of these cases were really tuberculosis. Following this, for a number of years there was an increasing tendency on the part of pathologists to minimize the occurrence of syphilis in the lung, so that today this condition is widely considered a pathologic rarity. On the other hand, in recent years there has been a revival of interest in the subject, and not a few able clinicians contend that it is actually not so infrequent, but is mistaken for other conditions.

In general, however, it may be stated that pathologists still consider the condition to be an uncommon one, and available autopsy statistics up to the present appear to confirm this opinion, as they show syphilitic involvement of the lung only in 0.5 per cent of autopsies of syphilitic patients.

Pathology.—**Congenital Syphilis.**—This is a condition well recognized in new-born syphilitic children, concerning which there is no question. The lesion consists of homogeneous, smooth consolidations which may involve the lung in scattered patches or extend over considerable portions of the lung, and is sometimes called white pneumonia. The microscopic pathology is a round-cell infiltration with marked fibrosis.

Gumma.—Gummata of the lung are larger or smaller areas of sharply circumscribed infiltration which may attain considerable size, representing a syphilitic tumor. These gummata are surrounded by a dense fibrous capsule, contain spirochetes in great number and, occasionally, they may break down, forming cavities, or may empty into a bronchus, become secondarily infected, presenting the symptoms of abscess of the lung in a manner similar to other tumors of the lung.

A number of cases of small gummata disseminated throughout both lungs have been described, simulating the picture of miliary tuberculosis.

Fibrosis.—This is the usual form of pulmonary syphilis which is encountered clinically. The condition usually arises in the central portions of the lung. It presents a picture very similar to other forms of diffuse fibrosis from other causes, with marked involvement of the tracheo-bronchial glands and sclerotic changes along the lymphatics, and involving the connective tissue framework of the lung surrounding the bronchi and blood-vessels, in the interlobular septa and beneath the pleura, and it also may extend to the mediastinum.

The syphilitic processes may involve the branches of the pulmonary artery predominantly, in which case fibrosis occurs due to the resulting circulatory impairment. Associated with this fibrotic condition there is a considerable round-cell infiltration such as is the familiar picture of syphilis elsewhere in the body. These fibrotic changes may be very extensive and localized so as to present the picture of complete consolidation of a considerable portion of or an entire lobe. The lesions of proven syphilis are apt to be bilateral, but may be unilateral, and are characteristically localized in the central portions of the lung fields and around the hilum.

Symptoms.—The symptoms of pulmonary syphilis are those of fibrosis. Especially dyspnea and cough are the outstanding features. Expectoration may be considerable; hemoptyses may occur, and in cases of secondary infection the sputum may be very abundant and foul. There is often slight fever in the more advanced cases, in which case night-sweats may occur, and as the disease progresses there is considerable loss of flesh and strength.

Physical Signs.—The physical signs are those of any chronic fibrosis of the lung, depending upon the location and the extent of the lesion. They are in no way characteristically different from those which may be produced by fibrosis from other causes, from chronic fibroid tuberculosis or bronchiectasis.

Roentgenologic Examination.—The evidences of syphilis shown by the roentgen-ray are very similar to those already described under diffuse pulmonary fibrosis. In cases of gumma the picture may be that of a lung tumor, but in most instances the picture is that of a fibrosis, either nodular or more diffuse, extending out from the root of the lung with marked increase of the hilum shadows.

Diagnosis.—The diagnosis of pulmonary syphilis is usually made clinically on the basis of the evidence of one of the pulmonary lesions above described, especially the fibrotic form, associated with definite evidence of previous syphilitic infection as corroborated by the positive Wassermann reaction, or by evidence of syphilitic lesions in other organs.

The condition should always be borne in mind as a possibility whenever such lesions occur in which tuberculosis can be excluded and where a syphilitic infection can be proven. In most reported cases the diagnosis is claimed to be confirmed by the improvement or disappearance of the lesions under specific treatment. There is some doubt whether this result can be assumed as definite proof of the syphilitic nature of the pulmonary lesion, inasmuch as many non-syphilitic conditions, such as tuberculosis, abscess of the lung, have been shown to be favorably affected by specific treatment where syphilis is an associated condition.

Treatment.—The treatment of syphilis of the lung is the same as that of syphilis elsewhere; intravenous injection of arsphenamine combined often with the use of mercury and iodides. In cases of general syphilis associated with other infections, particularly tuberculosis, treatment of the associated syphilis is very important before improvement of the other condition can be expected. In pulmonary tuberculosis systemic reactions from arsphenamine injection must be avoided, so that the dosage must be materially reduced below the average or, what is often preferable, reliance placed upon the use of mercury or bismuth. The use of iodides in pulmonary tuberculosis is usually contraindicated.

MYCOTIC DISEASES OF THE LUNG.

The etiologic significance of fungus diseases of the lung is still in a confused state. The outstanding feature of these infections is the great resemblance they bear to tuberculosis both in their clinical and pathologic aspects. Some of the fungi may even appear in the form of acid-fast rods, and most of them are capable of setting up lesions not unlike those of genuine tuberculosis. To add to our difficulties, most of these fungi also exist in saprophytic form or as secondary invaders in the air passages of many normal individuals, or in patients with other pulmonary conditions, including tuberculosis. This accounts for the frequency with which these conditions are overlooked, and explains the contention of many workers in this field that these infections are much more frequent than our records would indicate. Considering the ubiquitous nature of these fungi, the relative infrequency of these conditions is surprising.

Streptothricosis and Actinomycosis.—Etiology.—It is customary to discuss these conditions as separate clinico-pathologic entities. In reality they are but various forms of infection by the same species of fungi, namely, that of genus Nocardia.

In *streptothricosis* the fungi remain in their filamentous form, the so-called agranular type of Nocardia, which sets up lesions of a more severe type with tendency to rapid generalization.

In *actinomycosis* we find in the lesion the so-called ray fungus or granular Nocardia, which is but a reaction form of the same fungus existing exclusively in the tissue lesions or their products. The actinomycotic process is usually milder in type, tending to chronicity, although acute lesions may arise here, too, and eventually generalization is the rule. Mycelia and spore formation are identical in both forms of the fungus, and in both conditions the fungus may be present in the form of acid-fast bacilli very much like Koch bacilli.

The fungus is ubiquitous. Its particular sources are grains, weeds and soil dust. Skin abrasions, carious teeth and aspiration are its most probable modes of entry.

Pathology.—The pulmonary lesions in both streptothricosis and actinomycosis appear least frequently in the form of miliary nodules simulating true tuberculosis. Chronic broncho- and pleuro-pulmonary granulomatosis, with more or less extensive necrotic suppuration and connective tissue proliferation, represents the most frequent form of the lesions.

In the more acute streptothricoses the processes usually take the form of necrotic bronchopneumonia ending up in lobar and multilobar most extensive lesions of a gangrenous character. The tendency is toward rapidly fatal generalization with pyemia and metastases, usually to the brain.

In the more chronic types of actinomycosis the typical lesion is the thoraco-pleuro-pulmonary granulomatous process in which chest wall (including ribs), pleural layers and lung parenchyma are matted up in a most intense, board-hard tissue induration characteristically tunnelled by numerous, very narrow, fistulous tracts discharging the scant, yellowish, foul pus containing the "sulphur granules."

These lesions differ from tuberculosis in one very important respect, namely, their tendency to invade neighboring structures; in this they resemble malignant growths.

Clinical Picture.—In the more chronic processes in the earlier phases of the condition, this may simulate tuberculosis of the lung in every respect. Later, extensive pulmonary lesions give an unusually flat percussion note, the characteristic smell and color, with scant pus, and finally the early and typical fistulization, suggest the diagnosis. Otherwise, unless the "yellow granules" or flakes of mycelia, appearing in unusually large amounts in scant sputa, establish the diagnosis in the internal, closed phases, the process may look so much like pulmonary tuberculosis with or without pleural suppuration that differentiation is difficult indeed.

The more acute necrotic processes, particularly in streptothricosis, will come to resemble pulmonary abscesses. Pyemia, metastatic abscesses, particularly to the brain, are more frequent in mycotic than in lung abscesses.

In serial roentgen observations the early phases of the pulmonary process are indistinguishable from tuberculous lesions, with the exception that they are much less frequently found in apices or upper lobes, but rather in the lower lobes. As the disease progresses, the changing aspects of the roentgen features will come to resemble almost any other pulmonary condition.

Diagnosis.—The positive diagnosis must depend upon the demonstration of the fungi in the sputum or in the pus from the discharging lesions. The main difficulty in differential diagnosis lies between tuberculosis and abscess of the lung. In the early and more chronic fibroid types of the disease, the similarity to tuberculosis is very close, and the correct diagnosis lies on the demonstration of the fungi on the one hand, or tubercle bacilli in the other. The cases with considerable suppuration are clinically indistinguishable from chronic lung abscess, and the diagnosis can only be made by the recovery of the fungus from the sputum.

In the later phases when secondary abscesses are formed and fistulous lesions reach the surface, the diagnosis is comparatively easy if one has the possibility of fungus disease in mind.

Course.—These fungus diseases run a very chronic course, but almost always they eventually terminate fatally. Some cases are more acute and may last only a few months. Others may last for ten or more years. In a very few chronic cases healing has been reported but it is very rare.

Treatment.—Sodium iodide in large doses has been recommended, and recently roentgen irradiation has been used, but neither of them has any real effect on the progress of the disease. Surgical intervention of the abscess cases, whether by simple aspiration or by incision and drainage, is apt to lead to a spread of the infection.

The more important of the other forms of pneumomycoses are as follows:

Yeast Diseases.—Yeast diseases of the lung are due to yeast-like bodies, such as the cases of blastomycosis observed in this country, particularly in and about Chicago, or moniliasis, several forms of which are known, one being the coccidioidal granuloma or California disease. These conditions constitute one of the obscure causes of chronic fibrosis of the lung, and should be borne in mind in such cases. Also, as in the mycoses already discussed, these bodies are present regularly in the sputa of many patients without having any pathologic significance.

Mold Diseases.—Mold diseases of the lung due to various types of mold-like filamentous fungi, such as are found in the cases of aspergillosis, are reported every now and then from various parts of this country. In the majority of these conditions aspiration is the mode by which the fungi enter the air passages, where they may be normally found in saprophytic state to become pathogenic under certain circumstances as yet unknown.

The lesions produced by the fungi vary from mild intra- or peribronchial nodule formation with more or less chronic ulcerative bronchomycosis to quite extensive granulomatous processes in the parenchyma of the lung. Even acute necrotic bronchopneumonic processes of gangrenous tendency occasionally occur.

The *clinical picture* is so mild in the majority of the cases that it belies the apparent extent of the lesions when these are demonstrable by roentgen examination as involving quite considerable lung areas. At times, however, alarming clinical symptoms may be ushered in by hemorrhages, indicating rapid progress of the occasionally fatal case. Thus the typical case of bronchomycosis takes the form of very chronic, severe bronchitis with abundant, at times blood-tinged expectoration, rarely purulent in character. Occasionally extensive pulmonary infiltration with cavitation is produced, and the conditions come to resemble fibroid or even exudative phthisis.

Diagnosis must rest upon the finding of the fungi in vast amounts in the typical frothy, non-purulent sputa with grayish-white flakes which contain the yeast bodies or mycelia of molds, and upon the absence of tubercle bacilli.

HYDATID DISEASE OF THE LUNG.

Etiology.—This is a parasitic disease due to invasion by Tænia echinococcus. This parasite lives in the human body exclusively in its larval state, *i.e.*, upon reaching the tissues the embryo proceeds to transform itself into a cyst in which it multiplies. Infestation takes place by ingestion of contaminated water, raw vegetables, or by carriage to the mouth from that of dogs or sheep which are the most frequently infested animals. The embryos pass the thin intestinal wall and reach the lung by way of blood or lymph stream. Infestation usually takes place in childhood. The lungs become involved in 20 per cent of the cases. The disease is particularly prevalent in Iceland and in Australia, but from recent reports there would appear to be a tendency to its increase in this country.

Pathology.—The cyst is usually single in the lungs, rarely are daughter cysts observed; it has an inner germinative layer upon which grow to walnut size the brood capsules producing the scolices. This layer is surrounded by an outer lamellated cuticle. No direct tissue connection exists between tissues and cyst; nutrition takes place by way of osmosis of tissue juices. The majority of cysts, upon reaching certain size, rupture. Obsolescence may occur, but is rare. In the lung, growth of cysts is more rapid because resistance of surrounding tissue is less.

Clinical Picture and Diagnosis.—These vary according to whether we are dealing with uncomplicated or complicated cyst.

Uncomplicated cyst may be latent over long periods of time, giving no evidence of its existence. Eventually it will cause some bronchial irritation, giving rise to cough, blood-tinged expectoration, pain and some dyspnea. The diagnosis rests on roentgen picture of characteristic rounded or oval shadow with very clean-cut edge. The differential diagnosis from lung tumor sometimes presents difficulties.

Complicated cyst phenomena are due to rupture of cyst. There is a history of abrupt coughing spell followed by profuse expectoration having salty taste, containing ("grape skin") fragments of cyst and small bodies (hooklets of degenerated scolices). Soon cough becomes productive of purulent material having foul odor, and constitutional symptoms of generalized sepsis follow. Phenomena of pulmonary or pleuro-pulmonary disease become manifest.

Rupture may produce profuse hemorrhage or may drown the patient with a greal deal of fluid from the large cyst. Marked anaphylactic shock is frequent upon rupture. The roentgen feature of rupture within the lung is the "pneumocyst," of rupture into the pleural cavity is sero- or pyopneumothorax. Hooklets and scolices should be found in expectorated or aspirated material. Thoracocentesis is strongly contra-indicated because of the danger of new implantation and anaphylactic shock.

The *diagnosis* rests upon finding of hooklets or scolices in sputa. The complement-fixation test of Weinberg is helpful; while not abso-lutely specific, the percentage of false reactions is negligible. The activity of antigen is most important. As it deteriorates in four to five months it must be used fresh. The *treatment* is surgical.

TUMORS OF THE LUNG AND PLEURA.

Tumors of the lung may be benign or malignant. Strictly speaking, they include only those tumors which have their origin in the bronchial wall or, more rarely, in the parenchyma of the lung itself.

In connection with these tumors it is convenient to consider also tumors of the pleura and of the mediastinum with which they may be confused and often may be associated.

Benign Tumors of the Lung.

These may be due to congenital malformations, embryonic rests and misplacements, or they may be real non-malignant neoplasms such as adenoma, fibroma, chondroma and osteoma.

Dermoid Cysts.—Of the congenital tumors the dermoid cysts are the most common and the most important for consideration. They usually have their origin in or near the mediastinum, and frequently produce no symptoms. In other cases they gradually increase in size and give symptoms because of pressure or irritation on surrounding parts. In some cases they become infected, when systemic symptoms, particularly fever, are added. In other cases they may rupture, par-ticularly into the bronchus, in which case the diagnosis of lung abscess may be erroneously made.

Diagnosis.—The diagnosis is usually made by roentgen-ray, although the differential diagnosis from other forms of tumors is not always easy, and repeated observations may be necessary, as dermoids increase in size very slowly or often not at all, while the progression of a malig-nant tumor is obvious in a few months or sometimes weeks.

Treatment.—The treatment in those cases which give no symptoms consists in leaving them alone. In cases in which symptoms of pressure or infection are present, surgical intervention is necessary, which in the hands of a skilled thoracic surgeon can usually be successfully accomplished.

Adenomata and Fibromata.—Adenomata and fibromata of the bronchial wall constitute another important class of benign tumors, largely because of the difficulty of differential diagnosis. Many of these cases give no symptoms. In others the only symptom is repeated hemoptyses, in which case tuberculosis is usually suspected. Cough may be present but is not a constant or marked symptom. Sometimes they may cause partial or complete obstruction of the bronchus with the same symptoms as occur in obstruction following malignant tumor of a bronchus.

Physical Signs.—Physical signs may be absent or they vary according to the associated pathologic conditions. Roentgen-ray examination frequently fails to reveal any abnormality in cases in which there is no obstruction. In other cases the obstruction may cause atelectasis or abscess formation with characteristic roentgen-ray appearances.

Diagnosis and Treatment.—Bronchoscopy is one of the most useful means of diagnosis and, also, frequently the tumor may be removed by this means. In cases of repeated hemoptyses where tuberculosis cannot be proven, bronchoscopy is frequently recommended as a diagnostic procedure and may be rewarded by the discovery and removal of such benign tumors.

Malignant Tumors of the Lung.

Sarcoma.—Sarcoma of the lung itself is very rare, and it is now believed that most cases so diagnosed are probably atypical carcinomata.

Carcinoma.—Incidence.—Primary cancer of the lung which, as already noted, is almost invariably bronchial carcinoma, is a quite common condition and appears to be increasing. It is found, of course, with greatest frequency in the so-called cancer age, that is, above the age of fifty years, although it may be occasionally found in quite young people. It is more frequent in males than in females.

Etiology.—The etiology of primary bronchial carcinoma has received a good deal of attention because of its increasing incidence. No accurate knowledge of the causation of the disease exists, although there does seem to be a definite relationship between it and preëxisting inflammation in the respiratory tract such as bronchitis, influenza, bronchiectasis, abscess and tuberculosis, these chronic inflammations apparently occasionally going over into carcinoma by a metaplasia of tissue.

Irritation of the bronchial mucosa caused by the inhalation of dust, smoke and gases, and of late particularly inhalation of dust containing tar, have received attention as possible causes of bronchial cancer.

Pathology.—In primary bronchial carcinoma the common site is the wall of a bronchus, usually near the hilum of the lung. The right lung is somewhat more often involved than the left, and the location may be in either upper or lower lobes with fairly equal distribution.

Histogenesis.—Considerable discussion has surrounded the question of the cellular origin of bronchial carcinoma. The generally accepted opinion at present is that the cuboidal and goblet cells lining the bronchi and the cells of the mucous glands beneath the mucous membrane are none of them concerned in the origin of cancer, but that they uniformly arise from the basal cells of the mucous membrane. Metaplasia of these basal cells is particularly apt to occur following their proliferation as the result of chronic inflammation.

Extension of the primary growth may be by direct invasion of the surrounding tissues, or by metastases to other organs, or both. Some tumors which are characteristically carcinomatous on section are clinically comparatively benign and may remain localized for several years. Others rapidly invade the surrounding lung or any other structure in their path, such as the mediastinum or the wall of the heart.

Metastases to other organs may be early or late, depending upon the type of tumor, but almost invariably occur eventually. They may take place either through the lymphatics or the blood stream, and the organs most frequently involved in these secondary metastases are the tracheo-bronchial lymph nodes, the opposite lung, the brain, the bones, the liver and the adrenals, but any organ of the body may be involved.

Histology.—The microscopic characters of these bronchial tumors are extremely variable. The following types have been described: adenocarcinoma, medullary carcinoma, "oat-cell" carcinoma and epithelioma, which may be either of a polyhedral or squamous cell variety. These types are often mixed in any individual case.

Associated Lesions.—These tumors are often very vascular and bleed easily because of their location in the wall of the bronchus. This leads to hemoptyses. As the respiratory tract offers easy access to microorganisms, infection of these tumors very frequently occurs. This leads to softening and inflammation with resulting localized pneumonia or abscess formation.

Also these tumors frequently partly or entirely obstruct the bronchus, in which case atelectasis of the corresponding portion of the lung results, which in turn becomes very easily infected, leading to suppuration.

Symptoms.—The symptoms of bronchial carcinoma are frequently very insidious. They may be due to the local lesion itself, which may produce cough, thoracic pain, expectoration of various sorts—mucoid, muco-purulent, often fetid—or frank hemoptyses; when more advanced, dyspnea and cyanosis may be present. Systemic symptoms may arise when a secondary infection occurs giving fever, chilly sensations, nausea, vomiting, weakness and loss of weight. Actual cachexia is relatively slow in manifesting itself as compared with cancer of other organs. Of all the symptoms cough, repeated small hemoptyses, and persistent pain are the most common. When these occur associated with purulent expectoration which suggests abscess, bronchial carcinoma should always be suspected in the patients of the cancer age. Dyspnea occurs rather late unless there is involvement of the pleura with considerable effusion of fluid.

Physical Signs.—The physical signs are very varied and are not pathognomonic. In early cases they may be altogether absent, and in others some metastases may be recognized before the diagnosis of the original bronchial tumor has been made.

A significant sign which is frequently present when the lesion is in an upper lobe is a peculiar flatness upon percussion, giving a sensation of greater resistance to the pleximeter finger than that found in any other condition. This is often associated with very definite tenderness on pressure.

When associated inflammatory changes are present, the physical signs may be those of impaired resonance, changed breathing and râles, just as are found in tuberculosis. When obstruction of the bronchus occurs with atelectasis, impaired resonance and diminished breath sounds may be present, together with displacement of the heart and mediastinum toward the affected side.

On account of the frequent involvement of the pleura the usual signs of pleural effusion may occur. This fluid is usually bloody, and on microscopic examination may reveal cancer cells.

Clubbing of the fingers is a very frequent finding.

Roentgenologic Signs.—The examination by roentgen-ray gives the most valuable evidence for the diagnosis. The picture varies considerably, depending upon the location and nature of the tumor and the associated lesions. There may be simply localized densities around the root of one lung, or more massive densities involving the greater part of one lobe. Sometimes there is evidence of a cavity in the center of these densities. In other cases serial examination reveals rapidly increasing densities from day to day, with displacement of the mediastinum toward the affected side due to the development of partial or complete atelectasis. This frequently goes on to involve the entire lung field, giving the typical roentgenologic picture of massive collapse. In other cases the roentgen-ray findings may be very similar to those seen in chronic tuberculosis, bronchiectasis, or pulmonary fibrosis.

Pleural effusions are frequently evident and, when extensive, may completely obscure the underlying lesions.

The densities seen on roentgen-ray in cases of bronchial carcinoma are so variable and often so little characteristic that prolonged study by means of serial roentgen-ray examinations is necessary to a satisfactory understanding of the case.

Diagnosis.—The diagnosis of primary bronchial carcinoma can usually be made during life, provided the varying characteristics of the pathologic changes are borne in mind and the age incidence is considered.

Bronchoscopic examination should always be made in cases where this condition is suspected. It is a good rule never to omit this form of examination in the presence of obvious lung disease in which tuberculosis can be excluded and when the age of the patient is over forty years. Frequently the diagnosis can be absolutely determined by biopsy made through the bronchoscope. In other cases the bronchoscopic picture is very convincing even when a satisfactory biopsy cannot be made. Sometimes, but very rarely, pieces of cancer tissue may be expectorated with the sputum and the condition identified in that way.

In cases complicated with pleural exudate it should be borne in mind that bloody pleural exudates are almost invariably due either to tuberculosis or to cancer. Frequently careful microscopic study of the pleural fluid, particularly when this is concentrated and properly fixed, will reveal characteristic cancer cells.

Differential Diagnosis.—Confusion is possible with pulmonary tuberculosis, lung abscess, bronchiectasis, dermoid cysts, aneurysm of the aorta and chronic pneumonia. Only careful consideration of the course of the disease, the roentgen-ray, bronchoscopic, and laboratory studies will lead to the correct diagnosis.

The frequency of associated inflammation with its consequent symptoms, particularly fever, must always be borne in mind.

Treatment.—There is no satisfactory treatment for bronchial carcinoma at the present time. *Medical treatment* consists in the alleviation of symptoms and the treatment of associated conditions such as pulmonary suppuration or pleural effusions. Repeated roentgen-ray treatment by means of high-voltage roentgen-rays will frequently relieve the pain, and in some cases will result in a diminution in the size of the roentgen-ray shadow and perhaps a retardation of the normal progress of the disease.

A few cases of very early bronchial carcinoma have been successfully treated by *surgical treatment*, by removal of small tumors through the bronchoscope. These cases are usually relatively benign tumors which have just begun to undergo metaplasia. Such fortunate results from bronchoscopic operation are very rare.

With the development of thoracic surgery extirpation of tumors of the lung may be attempted with less risk than formerly. Lobectomy for chronic inflammatory conditions is frequently performed and, theoretically, if the diagnosis of bronchial carcinoma could be made while the disease is still limited to one lobe of the lung, its complete removal might be contemplated. As a matter of fact, however, usually before this diagnosis is established, the tracheo-bronchial glands are involved, and a very serious operation simply is added to the other distressing symptoms. Of course, where more extended metastases have occurred even the consideration of such surgery is out of the question. It is not too much to hope, however, that improvement in early diagnosis and operative technic may, in the future, bring early bronchial carcinoma within the possibility of successful surgical treatment.

Primary Carcinoma of the Lung.—It has already been stated that primary carcinoma of the parenchyma of the lung is rare. Many authorities assert that it never occurs.

The symptoms and signs are those already described in the more frequent condition of carcinoma of the bronchus, excepting that the various complications arising from infection of the tumor and obstruction of the bronchus do not occur. Moreover, the approach by means of the bronchoscope cannot be successfully made.

Primary Carcinoma of the Pleura.—Many pathologists deny that this occurs, stating that all such apparent primary pleural tumors are really secondary to a preëxisting tumor elsewhere, particularly in the lung. The so-called endothelioma of the pleura has been generally recognized as a clinical entity, but the validity of this classification is also seriously questioned. For clinical purposes, therefore, it may be assumed that in cases in which pleural newgrowths occur, they are most apt to be secondary to lung tumors. Such cases are practically invariably associated with pleural effusion which is bloody, with the same characteristics already described in the pleural effusions secondary to bronchial carcinoma. The microscopic examination of the fluid is a very important procedure in these cases.

50

Secondary Carcinoma of the Lung.—The lung is a very frequent location for metastases from tumors occurring anywhere in the body. These tumors are usually multiple and frequently bilateral. Inasmuch as they reach the lung by the blood, or lymph stream, they have no connection with the bronchial mucous membrane and produce none of the conditions associated with bronchial carcinoma, such as infection, inflammation, suppuration and hemorrhage. The structure of these tumors may closely coincide with that of the original tumor, or it may be essentially different, so that the character of the tumor found in the lung may not accurately determine the source of the original tumor which may be difficult to find. The most usual tumors which metastasize in the lung are those of the breast, of the prostate, of the adrenals and of the stomach, but metastases from any organ may find their way there.

Symptoms.—The most common symptom of metastatic carcinoma in the lung is dyspnea, which may become extreme and is frequently associated with cyanosis. Cough is usually present but is generally unproductive, and hemoptyses rarely occur. Pain is also a much less common symptom than in primary bronchial carcinoma, unless the pleura is involved. As the disease progresses, the condition of the patient becomes very distressing from marked dyspnea and general cachexia.

Physical Signs.—The physical signs are very uncertain and irregular and are not to be counted upon very heavily in the diagnosis, excepting in the case where the pleura is involved with effusion.

The *roentgenologic pictures* of metastatic tumors of the lung are very characteristic. They consist of sharply circumscribed, rounded densities of various size, which may be single at first, but usually are multiple and bilateral, and may be crowded together in such a way as to resemble nothing so much as a heap of snowballs. When this roentgen-ray picture is once recognized in a proven case, the nature of these round shadows in a given case can hardly be mistaken.

THE PLEURA.

PLEURISIES.

Fibrinous Pleurisy.—Fibrinous pleurisy is an acute inflammation of the pleura characterized by an exudate of fibrin which covers both the visceral and parietal layers. It is very variable in extent and is usually most marked in the lower and lateral areas of the chest.

Etiology.—Such acute fibrinous pleurisy may occur occasionally as an apparently primary infection, but it is usually secondary to infections elsewhere, particularly in the underlying lung, of which tuberculosis, pneumonia and, less frequently, abscess or cancer are the most important conditions. Less frequently it may be associated with infections in more distant organs, particularly in the upper air passages, such as the sinuses, or with acute abdominal conditions. Of all these causes tuberculosis in the lung is by far the most common.

Symptoms.—The characteristic symptom is sharp, sticking pain in the side, associated with moderate fever and dry, unproductive cough.

The characteristic physical sign is a to-and-fro friction rub heard over the lower and lateral portions of the chest, with slight impairment of percussion note and diminution of respiratory murmur.

Roentgenologic Examination.—The roentgen-ray examination in uncomplicated dry pleurisy shows a very slight homogeneous density most marked in the lower lateral regions near the diaphragm. When secondary to underlying lung conditions the roentgen-ray evidence of fibrinous pleurisy is usually obscured, excepting in tuberculosis, when the roentgen-ray evidence of tuberculous lesions at an apex is frequently the clue to the nature of the pleurisy itself.

Course.—Fibrinous pleurisy frequently develops into serofibrinous pleurisy. If it does not, the symptoms last but a few days and the physical signs promptly disappear. Occasionally such fibrinous pleurisy develops into chronic pleurisy with adhesions.

Treatment.—The treatment is simple, consisting of rest in bed, strapping of the chest and, when necessary, sedatives for relief of pain. The suspicion of an underlying tuberculosis should always be borne in mind. When no other obvious cause is present, and when tuberculosis is proven or strongly suspected, treatment for that condition should be instituted.

Serofibrinous Pleurisy.—Serofibrinous pleurisy is an inflammation of the pleural membranes characterized by an exudate of fibrin and serum with a varying amount of cellular elements, usually with the lymphocytes predominating. The exudate may be very slight, or it may be so extensive as to fill the whole pleural cavity.

Etiology.—By far the great majority of so-called idiopathic pleurisies with effusion are tuberculous. They may constitute the only manifestation of this disease, but frequently are secondary to recognizable pulmonary tuberculosis. Occasionally acute pleurisy with effusion is also seen in the course of acute rheumatic fever, or rarely it may be caused by the pneumococcus or streptococcus when these infections are very mild, as usually they cause an empyema. Pleural effusion may also occur in cancer of the pleura, in which case it is usually hemorrhagic.

Symptoms.—The onset of the disease may be sudden, with acute pain in the side, or may come on very gradually, with slight dyspnea on exertion constituting the main symptom. Occasionally the pain may be localized in the abdomen, especially when the diaphragmatic pleura is involved. It is accompanied by a dry cough and a considerable amount of fever. As the amount of fluid increases, the pain subsides and the amount of dyspnea increases, frequently associated with cardiac palpitation.

Physical Signs.—There is an impairment of respiratory movement of the affected side with an obliteration of the intercostal depressions overlying the site of the fluid, absence of respiratory fremitus, and marked impairment of percussion note which is usually absolutely flat over the fluid, but may be tympanitic or Skodaic above that level.

The line of percussion dulness frequently assumes an S-curve with the height in the axilla, and may change its position with posture.

Pressure of the fluid may displace the heart and other mediastinal contents in the opposite direction to a very considerable degree, and on the right side the liver may be displaced downward.

On auscultation a friction rub may be heard in the early stages, which disappears as the fluid accumulates; the breath sounds become markedly diminished or absent, or sometimes they may have a distant, low-pitched, bronchial quality. On the left side the neighboring pericardium may be involved, causing a pleuro-pericardial friction rub. The voice sounds are usually markedly diminished, but may be intensified, and at the level of the fluid egophony is frequently heard. Above the level of the fluid the breath sounds may be exaggerated. Occasionally moist râles may be heard at or near the level of the fluid, but are usually absent.

Roentgenologic Examination.—Examination by the roentgen-ray shows a very dense shadow corresponding to the location of the fluid, which is homogeneous, may change slightly with posture, and tends to extend higher up in the lateral regions of the pulmonic fields. Displacement of the heart and trachea when present is easily corroborated by the roentgen-ray. The roentgen-ray also affords the most accurate method of determining the presence or absence of underlying lung lesions, particularly tuberculosis. These may be obscured, however, by the pleural shadow.

Blood Examination.—The leukocyte count may be normal or subnormal, is usually slightly elevated in cases of tuberculous pleurisy. In the rare cases due to pneumococcus or streptococcus it is markedly increased, with a relative increase of the polymorphonuclear cells.

Course of the Disease.—Serofibrinous pleurisies run a very variable course, usually from two to three weeks, but often considerably longer, and in rare cases the effusion may last for months, recurring after repeated removals.

In the mild cases the absorption of the fluid is complete, leaving no apparent trace behind. More frequently there is a greater or less amount of pleuritic thickening, or the condition may go over into an extensive chronic pleurisy with adhesions.

The ultimate course of pleurisy with effusion depends largely upon the treatment. Tuberculosis is the most frequent cause of this condition, but if this is not recognized and the case is treated as one of pleural effusion rather than as a manifestation of tuberculosis, active pulmonary tuberculosis is very apt to develop sooner or later. In the cases where the fluid remains in the chest a long time, the production of chronic pleural adhesions is very apt to occur, with more or less permanent mechanical interference with the respiratory movement.

Diagnosis.—The diagnosis of pleurisy with effusion is simple when it is suspected, and by means of exploratory puncture of the chest. When fluid is obtained, its cellular character and high specific gravity will distinguish it from the transudate of a hydrothorax, and its serous character will distinguish it from the pus of an empyema. When the fluid is bloody, tuberculosis or cancer is usually present.

Microscopic examination of the fluid shows a high lymphocytic count in tuberculous pleurisies, and a relatively high polymorphonuclear count in those due to pneumococcus or streptococcus. Cultures of the tuberculous effusion remain sterile, while those due to the other infections show growth of the respective microörganisms. Tubercle bacilli can rarely be demonstrated in the fluid, but injection of the tuberculous pleural exudate into guinea-pigs produces tuberculosis in about six weeks. It is a very useful test, although slow and not absolutely certain.

Other chest conditions which may simulate pleural effusions are massive pneumonia, certain types of intrapulmonary tumors, and particularly pleurisy with adhesions. On the right side occasionally subdiaphragmatic abscess, or conditions causing marked enlargement of the liver upward, may prove confusing. On the left side extensive pericardial effusions may simulate pleural effusion, a mistake which paracentesis does not necessarily correct. Careful roentgen-ray studies are of the greatest value in the differential diagnosis of these various conditions.

Treatment.—During the early stages the case is treated as is the fibrinous pleurisy, with rest, strapping of the chest and palliative remedies for the relief of pain, of which codeine is generally the most helpful.

If the amount of fluid is small, its removal by aspiration is unnecessary, unless to establish a diagnosis. But when the amount of fluid increases to a level which approaches the angle of the scapula posteriorly, sooner or later aspiration is usually desirable, and in large effusions it may be essential for the relief of dyspnea. The problem of when to aspirate and how much fluid to withdraw constitutes the nice question in the treatment of pleural effusions. If fluid is withdrawn early during the acute, febrile stage, it usually reaccumulates rapidly, and only transient relief is obtained. If, on the other hand, a large pleural exudate is allowed to remain in the chest for several weeks, even after the acute symptoms have entirely subsided, absorption of the fluid takes place very slowly, pleural thickening of often very considerable extent results, and permanent handicap of respiratory function may follow. Moreover, if the pleural effusion is secondary to an underlying acute pulmonary tuberculosis, the presence of the effusion, by immobilizing the lung, may have a beneficial effect upon the pulmonary lesion and, conversely, removal of fluid, by allowing rapid expansion of the lung, may aggravate the pulmonary lesion into greater activity. As already indicated, such an underlying pulmonary lesion is usually present, even though it may not be demonstrable by roentgen-ray or other examination. Consequently, such possible lesions should be borne in mind carefully in the treatment of pleural effusion itself.

In general it is a satisfactory procedure not to aspirate during the very acute febrile stage of the first two weeks unless such aspiration is indicated for the relief of dyspnea, and even then only sufficient fluid should be removed to accomplish that purpose. When the acuteness of the condition is subsiding, and is evidenced by a beginning fall of temperature, it is then usually the optimum time to aspirate. Only a portion of the fluid present as a rule needs to be aspirated, for example, in a chest which may be estimated to contain 3000 cc. of fluid, if 1000 or 1500 cc. is removed, and if the acuteness of the inflammation is subsiding, the remainder of the fluid frequently is absorbed very rapidly or, if not, subsequent aspirations of similar amounts may be repeated.

In cases in which definite underlying tuberculosis is recognized, it is now considered the best practice to replace part of the fluid withdrawn by air introduced at the time of aspiration, thus producing an artificial pneumothorax and converting the condition into a seropneumothorax. The advantage of this procedure is that the air keeps the underlying lung from expanding without having the irritating effect of the fluid, which so often produces chronic pleural thickening. Moreover, it offers the opportunity for later continuing the treatment of the lung lesion by artificial pneumothorax, which is usually impossible after a pleural effusion has become absorbed and the layers of the pleura became adherent.

Aspiration of the chest should be accomplished painlessly under local anesthesia; the withdrawal of fluid should be gradual and should be interrupted as soon as coughing occurs. Care should be taken not to wound the underlying lung, which may produce a pneumothorax, or in rare instances cerebral air embolism, and sometimes an annoying, but less serious, subcutaneous emphysema. If very large quantities of fluid are aspirated very rapidly, cardiac palpitation and faintness may result.

Probably the most important factor in the treatment of tuberculous pleural effusions is the recognition of their tuberculous nature even though no associated pulmonary tuberculosis may be discovered. It should be a general rule to treat all such pleurisies with effusion exactly as one would an early case of proven pulmonary tuberculosis. Treated in this way over a period of months with the ordinary rest and hygienic treatment, the immediate and ultimate results are excellent, and active pulmonary tuberculosis rarely ensues. If, on the other hand, as is so often done, cases of pleural effusion are discharged from observation a few weeks after the acute symptoms have subsided and the effusion has been absorbed, a very considerable number develop active pulmonary tuberculosis within one to three years.

Chylous and Chyloid Pleurisies.—Very occasionally a case which may be considered to be a simple one of pleural effusion reveals, on exploratory puncture of the chest, the presence of a turbid, milky fluid instead of the expected clear, amber-colored serum. In rare cases this fluid may be found to contain a very high percentage of fat, with fat droplets recognized by chemical analysis and under the microscope. This condition can only be caused by communication between the thoracic duct and the pleural cavity, and such communications may be due to various ulcerating lesions, but most frequently malignant tumors.

More often such turbid fluids are pseudochylous or chyloid in character. The turbidity is less marked in these cases than in those of true chylous pleurisies, and the percentage of fat may be very low or may be absent altogether, and the turbidity of the fluid is found to be due to cholesterol crystals, or degenerated cellular detritus. These chyloid fluids usually occur when an ordinary serofibrinous exudate has existed a very long time in the chest, and they have no further significance than that of a chronic pleurisy with effusion, that is, they are usually tuberculous.

Hemorrhagic Pleurisies.—A serofibrinous pleural effusion may contain a considerable amount of blood so as to produce a distinctly hemorrhagic fluid. When this is not due to trauma, as in the case of a penetrating wound of the chest or tearing of the lung by fractured ribs, these hemorrhagic fluids are almost invariably due either to a definite tuberculous infection of the pleura or to cancer, which latter may occasionally be primary, but is usually secondary to cancer of the lung.

Examination of these fluids with the microscope, as indicated in the sections on tuberculous pleurisy or cancer of the lung, may aid in the differential diagnosis. In other cases the diagnosis rests upon the development of the case, particularly the correct diagnosis of the underlying pulmonary lesions.

Empyema.—**Etiology.**—Empyema, or purulent pleural effusion, is usually secondary to an infection of the underlying lung, which may be acute, as in the case of pneumonia or abscess, or may be less acute, as in the case of tuberculous disease. Sometimes the empyema is caused by infection from without the chest, as in penetrating wounds, fractures of the ribs and rupture of the esophagus.

In the acute conditions the most usual infecting microörganisms are the pneumococcus and streptococcus, occasionally the typhoid or influenza bacillus or, in cases secondary to pulmonary abscess, the anaërobic organisms of the fusiform, spirochetal group. In the case of tuberculous empyema the organism is, of course, the tubercle bacillus. The infecting microörganisms in either pure or mixed cultures can usually be obtained from the pus. In the case of tuberculosis tubercle bacilli alone may be found, or they may be associated with any of the other secondary infections.

Pathology.—In the early stages of a pneumococcus or streptococcus empyema the fluid may be thin and merely turbid. In a short time, however, the pus becomes thick and may become extremely so in chronic cases. In the cases due to anaërobic infection it has a very fetid odor.

The pleural membranes are covered with a shaggy coating of fibrin which gradually becomes very thick, and in the very chronic cases it may become calcified. The empyema may erode the visceral pleura, thus communicating with the bronchi, with the expectoration of pus and the formation of a bronchial fistula, or it may erode the parietal pleura and penetrate the chest wall between the ribs.

Symptoms.—An empyema may begin in the same manner as a serofibrinous pleurisy with greater constitutional reaction and a very high leukocyte count. In other cases, particularly when secondary to pneumonia, it may either appear during the acute course of the pneumonia or after defervescence. In the latter case a secondary rise of temperature occurs with an increased leukocytosis.

The cough is usually not marked and dyspnea is only present when the effusion is of very great amount. If the bronchus is perforated there is an expectoration of pus which may simulate an abscess of the lung.

As the empyema becomes more chronic, an irregular, septic type of temperature develops. There is a marked wasting and secondary anemia and progressive weakness. Occasionally the acute symptoms may subside as the infecting organisms die out, and the pus remains encapsulated in the chest for a long time, even many years, without giving rise to serious symptoms.

Physical Signs.—The physical signs are those of fluid in the chest, already described, but in cases associated with pneumonia or with tuberculosis they are modified by the underlying lung conditions. In the case of pneumonia the appearance of small amounts of pus in the chest is often difficult to determine by physical signs. It is significant that in such cases the consolidation of the lung persists as long as there is pus in the pleural cavity, and the signs of this consolidation may obscure those of the fluid. The diagnosis should always be suspected in cases of prolonged unresolved pneumonia associated with fever, for in general such an unresolved pneumonia with fever is almost invariably due either to an empyema or to tuberculosis.

In chronic cases clubbing of the fingers is often seen.

Roentgenologic Examination.—The roentgen-ray often gives information of the greatest value, as the density of the fluid is greater even than that of the consolidated lung. The pleural shadow is apt to be higher in the axilla than is the case with serous effusion.

When the condition is suspected, exploratory puncture of the chest should always be made, and the accurate location of the fluid can often be facilitated by exploration under the fluoroscope.

Treatment.—Empyema is a surgical condition and should always be treated as such. In the acute stages of pneumonia with beginning empyema it is undesirable to operate until the very acute process has subsided somewhat and the pus has passed from the turbid to the thick stage. In cases with bronchial fistula very considerable amounts of pus may be evacuated in that way, materially relieving the symptoms, but complete cure in these cases also requires surgical intervention.

The treatment of tuberculous empyema is quite different. When no secondary organisms are found in the pus, incision and drainage are usually undesirable, as a thoracic fistula usually develops and the pus may be secondarily infected from without. If small in amount, these tuberculous effusions may be left alone, or in larger exudates, if necessary because of pressure symptoms, the fluid may be withdrawn by repeated aspirations, care being taken to disinfect the needle tract with alcohol as the needle is withdrawn to prevent tuberculous infection of the chest wall.

If secondary infections are superimposed upon the tuberculous one, surgical intervention is necessary. In some cases of tuberculous empyema, aspiration and subsequent obliteration of the pleural cavity by thoracoplasty is indicated.

Chronic Pleurisy.—A chronic pleurisy is a thickening of the pleural membranes, with adhesions of the visceral and parietal pleura of greater or less extent, which usually occur as a result of a serofibrinous pleurisy, particularly if the effusion is allowed to remain in the chest a long time so that absorption takes place very slowly. These chronic pleurisies are almost always basal and the physical signs may closely resemble those of a pleural effusion. The chest, however, is apt to be retracted and the heart and mediastinum pulled toward the affected side, and occasionally dry, leathery friction rubs may be heard.

Treatment.—The treatment of chronic pleurisy of this type is best if preventive, that is, the withdrawal of serous effusions before this chronic thickening takes place. After it has occurred it is permanent and may handicap respiratory function considerably. Breathing exercises and respiratory gymnastics may be of value in overcoming this handicap.

Localized Pleurisies.—Any of the above described types of pleurisy may be localized. In the case of dry or chronic pleurisies these localized conditions are usually secondary to a chronic pulmonary tuberculosis, in which case they are most apt to be apical. In fact, a chronic apical tuberculosis almost always produces apical pleurisy with the formation of adhesions. The recognition of this condition does not necessarily mean the diagnosis of active tuberculosis, and care should be taken to analyze the clinical symptoms before placing too much importance on the physical signs. Roentgen-ray examination is of great value in differentiating between active lesions and chronic obsolescent ones.

Encysted or sacculated pleural effusions, whether serous or purulent, particularly the latter, are frequent. These sacculations may occur in any portion of the pleura and they may be multiple. They are particularly apt to be located, however, on the lateral surface of the pleura, in which case the physical signs are localized to the axilla. In other cases they are localized on the median side of the pleura when they are termed *mediastinal pleurisies* of which the physical signs are obscure. In other cases they are localized low down in the chest upon the diaphragm; then they are designated *diaphragmatic pleurisies*.

The roentgen-ray examination is by far the most important means of diagnosis and location of these effusions, the presence of which can be corroborated by needle puncture.

A very interesting and by no means uncommon type of localized pleurisy is the *interlobar pleurisy*. This pleurisy involves the so-called esser pleural sac between the lobes of the lung. It may occur in any of the interlobar fissures, but is particularly common in the fissure between the right upper and middle lobes. These pleurisies may be fibrinous, serous, purulent or fibroid. The purulent pleurisies are usually secondary to the same conditions as those described under empyema in general, and very frequently rupture into the bronchus with the discharge of pus, in which case the differential diagnosis from lung abscess is by no means easy. The other types of interlobar pleurisy are very apt to be tuberculous.

The physical signs of interlobar effusions are by no means characteristic. They are almost always associated with signs of involvement of neighboring lung tissue and frequently signs of a localized pneumonia. The roentgen-ray is again of the greatest value and, particularly when taken in different positions so as to show lateral and oblique views of the lung fissure, leads to correct diagnosis.

The treatment of interlobar empyema must always be surgical. In other forms of interlobar pleurisy the acute condition subsides, and the treatment usually consists of that of the underlying pulmonary tuberculosis.

HYDROTHORAX.

Hydrothorax is a collection of serous fluid in one or both pleural cavities which consists of a transudate rather than an exudate, and the condition is secondary to constitutional diseases, particularly chronic heart disease and chronic nephritis. Occasionally such transudates may be caused by pressure on the pulmonary veins.

These transudates are more frequent on the right than on the left side, but are often bilateral. They are associated usually with signs of chronic, passive congestion in the lungs. In fact, it is noticeable that the basal râles of a passive congestion often persist after a considerable amount of fluid has accumulated in the pleural cavity. The signs otherwise are the same as those of pleural effusion.

The *diagnosis* rests upon the recognition of the underlying cause of the condition, and examination of the fluid shows a low specific gravity and low cell count as compared with pleural exudates.

The *treatment* likewise depends upon the treatment of the underlying disease, but removal of the fluid by aspiration is often imperative to relieve dyspnea, which may become excessive. The fluid, however, is very likely to recur.

PNEUMOTHORAX.

Definition.—Pneumothorax is a condition of air in the pleural cavity. It is frequently associated with fluid. When this fluid is serous the condition is designated hydropneumothorax; when the fluid is purulent it is called pyopneumothorax.

Etiology.—Pneumothorax may occur from a wound in the chest wall even when the lung is not punctured. The usual cause, however, is a rupture of the visceral pleura due to underlying disease of the lung. By far the most important underlying lung condition causing pneumothorax is tuberculosis. In other cases it may be due to emphysema, less commonly to the rupture of an abscess from the lung, or an erosion of a chronic cancer of the lung, or the pleural membranes may be perforated by diseases penetrating through the diaphragm, such as lung abscess or cancer of the stomach or colon. It may arise from a perforation of the esophagus, either abscess or, usually, a cancer. The cause of the pneumothorax in these cases is the collapse of the lung which occurs from the elastic retraction of that organ when air at atmospheric pressure enters the pleural cavity, which normally has a pressure 3 to 5 mm. of mercury less than that of atmospheric air, the so-called negative pleural, or Donders' pressure.

Pathology.—The presence of a pneumothorax, if it is complete, results in a collapse of the corresponding lung, with a marked shift of the heart and mediastinum toward the opposite side. In many cases, particularly those secondary to chronic disease such as tuberculosis, the pneumothorax may be sharply localized by pleuritic adhesions. Occasionally, particularly in cases of emphysema, the pneumothorax may be bilateral, and in this condition also it is very apt to be recurrent. In the cases of pneumothorax secondary to pulmonary emphysema the ordinary large lung emphysema may rupture because of the thinning of the pleural surface. In interstitial emphysema this accident occurs even more frequently.

More common, however, and less generally appreciated is the fact that in individuals who present no evidence of general emphysema, even in young people, there frequently occur localized emphysematous blebs on the surface of the lung, particularly along the anterior margin, and it is the rupture of these blebs which gives rise to a considerable number of the spontaneous pneumothoraces, which should not be confused with those secondary to pulmonary tuberculosis.

If only air escapes into the pleural cavity the pleural membrane shows no pathologic changes. The underlying collapsed lung becomes more or less atelectatic and, if the condition persists over a long period, fibrosis occurs and the lung may remain permanently incapable of reëxpansion.

The size of the opening and the character of the underlying lesions determine the extent of the pneumothorax and also its duration. If the opening is small it may be quickly sealed by fibrinous exudate, and the lung gradually reëxpands in the course of three or four weeks. If the opening is large and the underlying disease of a necrotic nature, the closure of the opening is less easy, and the condition may persist for months or even permanently. Sometimes the opening is valve-like, allowing increasing escape of air into the pleural cavity without similar escape in the opposite direction, in which case so-called "high tension pneumothorax" occurs.

Very frequently with the rupture of the lung a bacterial infection occurs, with the formation of either a hydro- or pyopneumothorax. The formation of a hydropneumothorax is more common in the course of tuberculosis, although here also secondary infections into the pleura frequently occur. In the case of perforation of suppurative conditions such as abscesses, the condition becomes immediately a pyopneumothorax, often presenting the picture of acute empyema of extremely serious nature.

Symptoms.—The symptoms of a spontaneous pneumothorax are usually very acute, with sharp pain in the affected side and acute dyspnea, cyanosis and often marked cardiac palpitation. These symptoms may be extremely severe—very marked dyspnea, cyanosis, feeble, rapid heart action, evidences of acute pulmonary edema and sometimes death within a few hours.

In other cases the onset is very insidious even when the pneumothorax is complete. Pain and dyspnea are evident but are very much like those of an acute fibrinous pleurisy with which indeed it is frequently confused, and accommodation to the condition of the chest may become established in a few days, so that the patient may go about very comfortably, pursuing his normal life. When the pneumothorax is localized the symptoms are always milder and may be extremely slight, amounting only to a stitch in the side. Such localized pneumothoraces are often overlooked. When infection occurs there is usually a febrile reaction. With the onset of the fluid the patient may be conscious of a splashing sound in his chest.

Physical Signs.—The physical signs of a complete pneumothorax are very striking. The chest is immobile on that side; the normal intercostal depressions are obliterated. The percussion note is very hyperresonant; the fremitus and the breath sounds are absent. Frequently replacing the normal breath sounds is a distant, tinkling, amphoric type of breathing which may not be continuous, but interrupted with the metallic tinkling sound. This tinkling sound is best brought out by auscultating the chest when tapped with a coin on the opposite side, giving a very characteristic echoing, tinkling sound. When fluid is present, shaking of the body produces the pathognomonic succussion splash. In the upright position this fluid gives rise to the usual signs of exudate in the lower portion of the chest, but it moves very readily with the change of position. When the fluid is considerable in amount the entire anterior chest may be flat on percussion, which changes on lying down to a hyperresonant, tympanitic note. Examination of the heart and mediastinum shows marked displacement toward the opposite side of the chest, and there may be a very marked disturbance of cardiac action as evidenced by tachycardia or arrhythmias.

In the case of localized pneumothoraces, the signs may be entirely obscured by those of the underlying lung lesions, but careful examination will usually disclose a localized area of hyperresonance and diminished breathing, to which attention is directed by the pain of which the patient is apt to complain. Fluid may accumulate in these smaller pneumothoraces also, the signs of which may or may not be appreciable, depending upon the amount of fluid and the size of the pneumothorax cavity.

Roentgenologic Examination.—The roentgen-ray picture is extremely characteristic and is often the means of diagnosis, particularly in localized pneumothoraces. The pneumothorax cavity shows an area of markedly increased illumination with absence of the normal pulmonary markings. If the pneumothorax is complete it shows a sharp line of demarcation between the pneumothorax cavity and the collapsed lung, and brings out sharply the displacement of the heart, trachea and other mediastinal viscera. In the presence of fluid this also is obvious, and its free movability is evidenced by the rippling of the surface of the fluid with the slightest motion of the body.

In the case of localized pneumothoraces the same picture presents itself. It often can best be brought out, when the pneumothoraces are small, by roentgen-ray pictures taken in various planes. In the case of emphysema, sometimes the projecting emphysematous bleb may be seen on the surface of the collapsed lung.

Diagnosis.—Complete pneumothorax should usually be diagnosed without difficulty, but cases with gradual onset and mild symptoms may be hastily mistaken for a simple pleurisy. When suspected, the very characteristic physical signs and the displacement of the heart make the diagnosis easy.

In localized pneumothoraces the diagnosis is not so simple and often is not made unless the frequency with which they may occur in chronic pulmonary tuberculosis is appreciated. In such cases chest pains should always be considered with this possibility in mind.

A very large pulmonary cavity may closely simulate the physical signs of pneumothorax, and when the cavity contains fluid there may even be a succussion splash and coin sound. The differential diagnosis between such a cavity and a localized pneumothorax is by no means always easy. Also the rarer condition of a diaphragmatic hernia may simulate a pneumothorax closely.

Treatment.—The treatment of the acute symptoms of a complete pneumothorax is largely symptomatic: sedatives for the relief of pain, cardiac stimulations if necessary and O_2 inhalations if cyanosis and tendency to pulmonary edema are present. In cases of high-tension pneumothorax, the acute symptoms can only be relieved by removal of the air by thoracic puncture and, in order that this relief may be more permanent, a small cannula fitted with a valve, which will allow free escape of air outward but not in the opposite direction, may be of great service. In other cases of simple pneumothorax, rest in bed in time usually results in absorption of the air and reëxpansion of the lung.

In cases of hydropneumothorax, aspiration of the fluid may be indicated. This is usually best deferred until the lungs show signs of beginning reëxpansion indicating closing of the pleural opening. In pyopneumothorax the treatment depends entirely upon the character of the pus, the indications being the same as those in ordinary simple empyema. In cases of tuberculosis, and when there is no secondary infection of the pleura, the cases are usually best left alone entirely, without even aspiration unless dyspnea demands it.

In cases secondary to pulmonary emphysema, fluid is not apt to be present, and the lung usually reëxpands in a shorter time than is the case in tuberculosis. The recognition of the frequency of this condition due to rupture of localized emphysematous blebs in young people is very important, as the condition is usually diagnosed as probably tuberculous while, if the proper cause is recognized, the unnecessarily long treatment for a presumed tuberculosis is avoided.

THE MEDIASTINUM.

Anatomic Considerations.—The mediastinum is a portion of the body rather rarely the site of disease. But when disease in that locality is present it is apt to be of an important nature, to the appreciation of which the knowledge of the anatomy of the region is essential.

Anatomically the mediastinum lies between the median layers of the pleura of each lung and is divided into four sections. The *anterior* mediastinum is a very small space lying in front of the heart and beneath the sternum. It contains the thymus gland or its remnants, a few lymphatic glands contained in real areolar tissue. The *middle* mediastinum contains the heart and the pericardium. The *superior* mediastinum is the space that extends from the arch of the aorta to the upper region of the thorax and extends in the antero-posterior direction from the sternum to the spinal column. This region is in particular relation to the trachea with the peritracheal lymphatic glands on each side. It contains the great arteries and veins, the thoracic duct, the esophagus and the main nerve trunks of the sympathetic system, the vagi and the phrenic nerves. These structures are loosely surrounded also by areolar connective tissue. The *posterior* mediastinum is the most important from the standpoint of the pathologic conditions and is continuous with the posterior portion of the superior mediastinum; it extends behind the heart downward to the diaphragm. This space serves primarily for the transmission of important structures which traverse it, namely, the descending aorta, the two main bronchi to each lung arising from the bifurcation of the trachea, the superior and inferior venæ cavæ, the thoracic duct, the esophagus, and the sympathetic, vagus and phrenic nerves. The main localized structures in the posterior mediastinum are the lymph nodes, which are of considerable number and size and the principal ones of which are the group known as the tracheo-bronchial lymph nodes.

Methods of Examination.—The situation of the mediastinum does not lend itself readily to the usual methods of physical examination of the chest. In the anterior mediastinum abnormal densities may give increased dulness to percussion over the manubrium and to each side of the sternum. To a less extent the same change may be evidenced in similar conditions of the superior mediastinum. Physical examination of the posterior mediastinum is difficult and unsatisfactory. Lesions of considerable size may give impairment of percussion note in the interscapular regions of the chest, and there may be intensification of the respiratory murmur on auscultation, the most significant of which is the D'Espine sign, which is best brought out by the increased whisper over the spines of the thoracic vertebræ. Roentgen-ray examination is by far the most satisfactory method for the study of the mediastinal regions. Frequently, films taken in the lateral and diagonal, as well as in the ordinary antero-posterior plane, are important.

Symptoms.—The most important symptoms of mediastinal conditions are evidenced by the pressure which they exert upon the various important structures which this region contains. This may result in pain, sometimes in dyspnea, but the valuable diagnostic pressure signs are those on the *superior vena cava* resulting in engorgement and edema of the head, neck and arms; occasionally on the *inferior vena cava* resulting in distention of the abdomen with ascites, enlargement of the liver, and edema of the lower extremities; or pressure on the *esophagus* giving symptoms of difficulty in swallowing with or without actual dysphagia, this condition being best checked by the observation of barium swallowed at the time of a fluoroscopic roentgen-ray examination; or pressure on the *trachea* and *bronchi*, especially the right, which is more accessible, causing more or less dyspnea and, particularly in the case of the bronchi, greater or less atelectasis of the corresponding lung with corresponding physical signs. Pressure on the *recurrent laryngeal nerve* which loops around the aortic arch may give paralysis of the left vocal cord. Pressure on the *vagi or sympathetic nerves* may give changes in the size and reaction of the pupils; pressure on the *phrenic nerves* rarely, if ever, produces sufficient disturbance to cause paralysis of either leaf of the diaphragm. Pressure on the *bones*, particularly the *spinal column*, may give intense boring pain characteristically worse at night. Pressure on the *main arteries* is usually not sufficient to give any physical signs or symptoms. Cough is frequently produced by any condition in the mediastinum and is of reflex, unproductive, paroxysmal character, and varies considerably with the size and location of the lesion.

TUMORS OF THE MEDIASTINUM.

Benign Tumors.—Tumors of the mediastinum are relatively frequent. They may be benign, of which the lipomata and dermoid cysts are the most common. *Teratoma* is a frequent form of dermoid. These dermoid cysts appear in young adult life, run a very slow course, and usually are recognized by the gradual appearance of pressure symptoms which should lead to careful roentgen-ray examination. Differential diagnosis between a dermoid tumor and a malignant tumor, especially sarcoma, is not always easy and is best determined by prolonged observation of the case and serial roentgen-ray examinations.

Many of these dermoids require no treatment, but when pressure demands it, they are satisfactorily amenable to radical surgical treatment. They occasionally become infected, in which case an abscess results which demands prompt surgery.

Malignant Tumors.—Sarcoma.—Sarcoma of the mediastinum is by far the most common of the malignant tumors. They more frequently occur in young adult life and give origin to the gradual development of the symptoms above outlined, and show very definite localized sharply circumscribed densities on the roentgen-ray, extending to one or the other side or both of the normal mediastinum shadow. They are apt to develop fairly rapidly, giving increasing symptoms and showing increased size on serial roentgen-rays. Surgical removal of these sarcomata is rarely, if ever, feasible, but these tumors respond very satisfactorily and promptly to deep roentgen-ray therapy, which is an important point in the differential diagnosis between them and carcinoma or dermoid cysts. Unfortunately these results are not permanent and the disease eventually progresses to eventual death, with often distressing symptoms of pain, dyspnea, cyanosis and marked pressure symptoms.

Carcinoma.—Primary carcinoma of the mediastinum is comparatively rare. When it occurs it is usually in the older age groups, progresses more slowly than sarcoma and does not react favorably to deep roentgen-ray therapy. The pressure and other symptoms are quite similar to those produced by other tumors. Secondary carcinomata are more common, but the presence of these is usually masked by the symptoms of the primary condition, particularly carcinomata of the lung which quite frequently secondarily involve the mediastinum either by metastases to the tracheo-bronchial lymph nodes or by direct extension.

INFLAMMATORY PROCESSES OF THE MEDIASTINUM.

Tracheo-bronchial Lymphadenitis.—Acute, subacute and chronic enlargement of the tracheo-bronchial group of lymph nodes is very common. It is particularly apt to follow acute infections of the upper respiratory tract, and is frequently associated with acute bronchitis. When this lymphatic engorgement is considerable it gives rise to characteristic paroxysmal, unproductive cough, rarely to other pressure symptoms, and develops no abnormal physical signs. The roentgen-ray examination of the chest shows these engorgements as very marked increase of the normal hilum shadow which varies considerably in size according to the severity of the infection.

Acute Mediastinitis.—Acute mediastinitis is an inflammation of the areolar tissue of the mediastinum, usually secondary to infection of the tracheo-bronchial lymph nodes, or it may be secondary to acute pneumonia. It is associated with substernal pain, paroxysmal cough and fever. This condition may subside fairly promptly. Occasionally there may be an exudate of serum into the mediastinal space which prolongs the condition and may give rise to moderate pressure symptoms.

Empyema of the Mediastinum.—Occasionally an acute mediastinitis due to any of the respiratory bacterial infections may break down into a localized collection of pus. This, however, is comparatively rare. The differential diagnosis between this condition and sacculated mediastinal empyema of the pleural cavity is not always easy. Both conditions call for prompt surgical treatment. The localization of the process can usually be made by the roentgen-ray taken in various planes and corroborated by exploratory aspiration.

Chronic Mediastinitis.—Most chronic infections of the mediastinum are due to tuberculosis and occasionally to syphilis. In the case of tuberculosis the primary lesion is the involvement of the tracheo-bronchial lymph nodes, which is extremely common in tuberculosis, particularly in children. This usually gives no symptoms, but occasionally gives rise to the same paroxysmal cough as noted in the case of simple lymphadenitis from which it is differentiated by the presence of characteristic calcareous deposits seen in the roentgen-ray in the case of tuberculosis, by the tuberculin test in children, and by the presence or absence of associated tuberculous lesions, particularly in the lung.

Such tuberculous glands may caseate and occasionally give rise to tuberculous empyema of the mediastinum. The *treatment* of this condition is that of tuberculosis in general. In the case of tuberculous empyema of the mediastinum it is usually best not to attempt surgical treatment, which is apt to lead to infection with secondary organisms and to a chronic fistula.

Syphilitic Mediastinitis.—Syphilitic mediastinitis is associated with syphilis elsewhere, particularly when the aorta is involved, and usually the evidence of aortitis or actual aneurysm obscures the evidence of mediastinal involvement. Occasionally, however, this condition may be more marked and give rise to pressure symptoms. The treatment is the same as for syphilis elsewhere.

Other Conditions.—The involvement of the mediastinal lymph nodes, which frequently takes place in Hodgkin's disease and in lymphatic leukemia, gives rise to a picture very similar to that already noted in connection with primary conditions in the mediastinum. Often there is no essential difference in the symptoms, physical signs and roentgen-ray picture between these conditions and sarcoma of the mediastinum, and frequently extensive tuberculous tracheobronchial nodes may also present very similar pictures. The differential diagnosis between these conditions offers problems of interest and frequently of considerable difficulty. They can only be solved accurately by careful study and often by consideration of evidences of disease in other parts of the body, such as the characteristic blood count of leukemia, the enlargement of the spleen and other lymph nodes in Hodgkin's disease, or the association of other tuberculous lesions in the case of the tuberculous lymph nodes.

Emphysema of the Mediastinum.—Rarely the areolar tissue of the mediastinum may become infiltrated with air which arises from rupture of a bronchus or from other causes of interstitial emphysema, the air extending along the connective tissue surrounding the bronchi into the mediastinum, distending this loose tissue, and then through the mediastinum up into the neck where it follows the lines of the deep fasciæ, and may extend over the entire body as a subcutaneous emphysema. The usual causes of this condition are trauma or very excessive attacks of coughing, particularly in whooping cough in children, or pulmonary emphysema in older persons. It may follow tracheotomy.

THE DIAPHRAGM.

Introduction.—The diaphragm is the musculo-tendinous partition which is situated between the abdominal and thoracic cavities. Embryologically the diaphragm develops from the membranes which are formed to separate the pericardial space from the two pleural cavities, on the one hand, and the peritoneal cavity on the other. Eventually the partitioning of the thoracic and abdominal cavities is brought about by changes in position and coalescence of corresponding segments of the membranes. It is this development of the diaphragm from segments which is responsible for the congenital as well as some of the acquired defects in its continuity which give rise to herniation. These conditions result in partial or total functional failure of the diaphragm, which gives rise to the clinical phenomena of diaphragmatic relaxation. Similar functional disturbances arise in conditions in which the phrenic nerve or its central nervous connections are involved.

51

The normal function of the diaphragm consists in maintaining the static and dynamic mechanical balance between the two large internal (thoracic and abdominal) cavities of the body. The diaphragm is kept in a state of permanent tonus which increases with inspiration and diminishes with expiration. Upon this basic tonus there are superimposed the active as well as the passive movements of the diaphragm. The active movements may be brought about by reflexes as well as by volition. The passive movements are due to pressure fluctuations in the thoracic and abdominal cavities, in the production of which the thoracic and abdominal musculature, pulmonary and gastro-intestinal functions play the paramount rôle.

The function of the diaphragm is so correlated with the mechanical conditions and the organic functions in the two cavities partitioned off by it that the greater the pressure differences the greater is its tonus. The amplitude of diaphragmatic excursions depends upon the pressure fluctuations between the two cavities, which are greatest with mean pressure differences and tend to decrease when the difference between the pressures in the two cavities is too high or too low. This explains the tense diaphragm high up in the chest of hypersthenic individuals, and the low placed diaphragm of hyposthenic individuals with enteroptosis.

By its function the diaphragm aids the generation of negative pressure in the chest and serves the physiologic fluctuation of pressures in the chest as well as in the abdomen, which are conditions essential for normal respiro-circulatory as well as gastro-intestinal function.

Dysfunction of the Diaphragm.—This manifests itself in abnormal position of the diaphragm. The position which it takes under normal as well as pathologic conditions depends, in the first place, upon its own tonus which overcomes both the positive intra-abdominal and the negative intrathoracic pressures. Since the tonus changes in the diaphragm depend upon the pressure differences between the thoracic and abdominal cavities, this difference will have its influence upon the position of the diaphragm. When it loses its tonus, its position will come to depend altogether upon these differences in the pressure in the two cavities. The toneless diaphragm will be sucked up into the chest with every inspiration and left to flop back in every expiration (paradoxical movements in diaphragmatic palsy). It may, on the other hand, be pushed down into the abdomen by increased intrathoracic pressure such as occurs in pulmonary emphysema, pneumothorax, or pleural effusions.

Elevation of the diaphragm will thus be observed under the following circumstances: (1) in the presence of increased abdominal pressure, as in ascites or meteorism. This is particularly the case if the abdominal pressure increases abruptly, while slow increase of abdominal pressure, such as occurs in pregnancy or abdominal tumors, may be compensated for a long time by elevation of the lower ribs and increase of the diaphragmatic tonus; (2) in the presence of increased thoracic pull such as is exerted by retractive processes in the lungs and pleura, or pulmonary collapse; (3) in the presence of reduced diaphragmatic tonus such as occurs in relaxation of the diaphragm, whether congenital or acquired, or in phrenic nerve palsy.

The most frequent form of elevation of the diaphragm due to reduced tonus is that arising in paralysis of the phrenic nerve which is now so frequently produced artificially as a method of treatment in various pulmonary diseases, particularly tuberculosis.

Descent of the diaphragm, on the other hand, will be observed under the following circumstances: (1) decreased thoracic suction as occurs in some cases of emphysema, of asthma, and in pleural effusion; (2) decreased abdominal pressure such as is seen in general visceroptosis; (3) increased diaphragmatic tonus associated with diaphragmatic spasm in such nervous disorders as hiccough, encephalitis, tetanus, and in some cases of poliomyelitis.

ORGANIC DISEASES OF THE DIAPHRAGM.

Hernias.—For convenience the condition known as eventration of the diaphragm is included under the general classification of hernias which may be classified as follows:

1. **False Hernias.**—(*a*) Congenital perforating defects of all layers of the diaphragm, or absence of an entire leaf. (*b*) Traumatic perforating rupture of all layers.

2. **Genuine Hernias.**—These are non-perforating defects which involve the muscular or tendinous layer, but leave intact the pleural and peritoneal covering. They may be (*a*) congenital, or (*b*) acquired.

3. **Eventration of the Diaphragm.**—This may be a diffuse relaxation of the entire organ, or merely a circumscribed diverticulum.

Inclusion of eventration with hernias is justified because they are frequently indistinguishable clinically and, furthermore, because in some cases the diaphragmatic layer may be so thin that there exist transitions from genuine hernia to eventration, which make distinction between them a matter of fine histological technic but of no practical significance.

Diagnosis.—The diagnosis of this condition is, practically speaking, a roentgenologic one. It is frequently quite impossible to determine, however, even by the roentgen-ray, whether we are dealing with genuine or with false hernia, or with eventration.

Symptoms.—When the defect is small or only a part of the stomach protruding, there may be only mild occasional digestive disturbances, and the patient may go through life without serious inconvenience. When a small part of the stomach protrudes centrally the symptoms may be vomiting, dysphagia, or cardiac symptoms suggesting nervous instability. When the aperture is large there may be dyspnea, marked indigestion, abdominal distention, cyanosis, cough and sometimes shoulder pains. In about 15 per cent of the cases of diaphragmatic hernia the clinical picture of acute intestinal obstruction arises. But, on the other hand, very extensive hernias may exist without symptoms and be discovered accidentally.

Physical Signs.—These may vary from total absence of any evidence to the most fantastic clinical picture. There may exist abundance of physical signs in the chest, which are characteristically very inconstant and may differ at any two examinations, varying also according to the position of the patient and the period of the day, particularly before and after eating. Depending upon the amount of the food taken, the extent of the hernia and the lung compression, the physical signs may vary from flatness to tympany on percussion, from absence of breath sounds to exaggerated metallic breath sounds. Metallic borborygmi, as evidence of the intestines being high up in the chest, is a pathognomonic sign. Dextrocardia is very frequent, and if other causes can be excluded should suggest the diagnosis.

Hernias of the diaphragm are almost invariably in the left side. The principal difficulty in differential diagnosis is from pneumothorax or hydropneumothorax.

Roentgenologic Signs.—The roentgenologic evidence obtained by a contrast meal is conclusive. Slight hernias may not be visualized. Sometimes a well-rounded regular archline of double contour may be evidence of the diaphragm and permit the diagnosis of eventration as against that of hernia. The contour of the part of the diaphragm, a hernia ring and, above this, a pear- or bologna-shaped hernia may be seen protruding into the chest, with the irregular borderline separating the lung from the intestines. Fluoroscopic study may reveal paradoxic movements indicating relaxation of the diaphragm, but extensive eventration may be immobile just as an extensive hernia, and differentiation will be impossible.

It should be emphasized that eventrations are much more frequent than is generally realized, and that they need not be congenital in nature. A great variety of clinical conditions may lead to degenerative and atrophic processes in the diaphragm with subsequent relaxation of the left leaf while the right leaf is kept in place by its hepatic support.

Distressing forms of diaphragmatic relaxation may occasionally follow evulsion of the left phrenic nerve. It is also worthy of notice that the recent increase of motor accidents has materially increased the incidence of acquired diaphragmatic hernias through weak spots of the stomach in predisposed individuals.

Inflammatory Processes (Diaphragmitis).—The diaphragm is not infrequently involved in inflammatory processes of adjacent structures. This is due to its rich lymph supply which is closely connected with the lymphatic systems above and below the diaphragm. In this way thoracic and abdominal infections may lead to suppuration in the diaphragmatic tissues with pocketing of pus above or below the diaphragm, or with occasional perforation of all layers with free communication from one cavity to the other. A frequent form of this condition is subphrenic abscess.

It is also to be remembered that the normal openings of the diaphragm may permit the extension of infections from one side to the other. This is particularly important in connection with suppurative conditions of the mediastinum which may extend down into the retroperitoneal space.

In passing it must be noted that trichinosis frequently has its site of predilection in the muscles of the diaphragm.

Treatment.—The treatment of the various diaphragmatic conditions is mainly surgical. Often hernias require no treatment, and frequently even surgical treatment is unsatisfactory.

REFERENCES.

Text-books on Diseases of the Lungs in general.

VON BERGMANN, G., and STAEHELIN, R.: Handbuch der Inneren Medizin, vol. **2**, pt. 2; one volume on lungs, clinical; Berlin, Julius Springer, 1930.

THANHAUSER, S. J.: Diseases of the Lungs, in G. von Bergmann's, *et al.*, Lehrbuch der Inneren Medizin, vol. **1**, Berlin, Julius Springer, 1931.

HENKE, F., and LUBARSCH, O.: Handbuch der speziellen Pathologie, vol. **3**, pts. 1, 2, 3; three volumes on lung pathology; Berlin, Julius Springer, 1928, 1930, 1931.

SPECIAL SECTIONS.

Pulmonary Atelectasis:
HENDERSON, Y.: Physiology of Atelectasis, Jour. Am. Med. Assn., 1929, **93**, 96.

VAN ALLEN, C. M., *et al.*: Obstructive Pulmonary Atelectasis; Problems of Pathogenesis and Clinical Management, Arch. Surg., 1930, **21**, 1195; Jour. Clin. Invest., 1931, **10**, 559.

Pulmonary Fibrosis, Pneumoconiosis, Pulmonary Arteriosclerosis:
LEMON, W. S.: Pulmonary Fibrosis; Experiments of Short Duration, Am. Jour. Med. Sci., 1932, **183**, 153.

PANCOAST, H. K., and PENDERGRASS, E. P.: Review of Pneumoconiosis; Further Roentgenological and Pathological Studies, Am. Jour. Roentgenol., 1931, **26**, 556.

POLICARD, A.: Introduction Histophysiologique à l'Étude des Pneumoconioses, Arch. Med. Chir. de l'Appareil Respiratoire, 1930, **5**, 1.

Emphysema:
WILSON, H. G.: University of Toronto Med. Bull., 1927, **8**, 9.

Interstitial Emphysema:
MILLER, W. S.: Human Pleura Pulmonalis; Its Relation to Blebs and Bullæ of Emphysema, Am. Jour. Roentgenol. and Rad. Ther., 1926, **15**, 399.

Bronchiectasis:
BALLON, H., SINGER, J. J., and GRAHAM, E. A.: Bronchiectasis, Jour. Thoracic Surg., 1932, vols. **2**, **3**, **4**.

MILLER, J. A.: The Pathogenesis of Bronchiectasis, Jour. Thoracic Surg., 1934, **3**, 246.

Abscess of the Lung:
KLINE, B. S.: The Pathology of Bronchiectasis and Lung Abscess, Am. Rev. Tuberc., 1931, **24**, 626.

CLERF, L. H.: The Bronchoscopic Treatment of Bronchiectasis and Lung Abscess, Am. Rev. Tuberc., 1931, **24**, 605.

HARRINGTON, S. W.: Surgical Treatment of Bronchiectasis and Lung Abscess, Am. Rev. Tuberc., 1931, **24**, 612.

LAMBERT, A. V. S., and MILLER, J. A.: Abscess of the Lung, Arch. Surg., 1924, **8**, 446.

MILLER, J. A., and LAMBERT, A. V. S.: The Treatment of Abscess of the Lung, Am. Jour. Med. Sci., 1926, **171**, 81.

Pulmonary Tuberculosis:
BRAEUNING, H., and REDEKER, F.: Tuberkulose Bibliothek, vols. **38**, **39**, Leipzig, J. A. Barth, 1931.

DUKEN, J.: Erg. d. Inn. Med. u. Kinderh., 1931, **39**, 344.

MILLER, J. A.: Hematogenous Pulmonary Tuberculosis, Am. Rev. Tuberc., 1934, **29**, 489.

NEUMANN, W.: Klinik d. Tuberkulose d. Erwachsenen, 2d ed., Berlin, Julius Springer, 1930.

Cancer of the Lung:
FRIED, B. M.: Primary Carcinoma of the Lung, Baltimore, Williams & Wilkins Company, 1932.

MILLER, J. A., and JONES, O. R.: Primary Carcinoma of the Lung, Am. Rev. Tuberc., 1930, **21**, 1.

Affections of the Mediastinum:
LAMBERT, A. V. S., and BERRY, F.: The Mediastinum, Arch. Surg., 1927, **14**, 261.

CHAPTER XVI.

DISEASES OF THE ENDOCRINE GLANDS.

By J. H. MEANS, M.D.

INTRODUCTION.
THE THYROID GLAND.
  Endemic Goiter.
  Sporadic Colloid Goiter.
  Nodular Goiter.
  Exophthalmic Goiter.
  The Heart in Thyrotoxicosis.
  Myxedema.
  Cretinism.
    Juvenile Myxedema.
  Malignant Disease of the Thyroid Gland.
  Thyroiditis.
  Developmental Anomalies.
  Hypometabolism Without Myxedema.
  Thyroid Problems of Pregnancy.
THE PARATHYROID GLANDS.
  Hypoparathyroidism.
  Hyperparathyroidism.
    Osteitis Fibrosa Cystica Generalisata.

THE ADRENAL GLANDS.
  Addison's Disease.
  Hyperfunction of the Adrenal Medulla.
  Hyperfunction of the Adrenal Cortex.
  Other Diseases of the Adrenals.
THE PITUITARY GLAND.
  Acromegaly.
  Gigantism.
  Simmonds' Disease.
  Hypophyseal Dwarfism.
  Fröhlich's Syndrome.
THE PANCREAS.
THE FEMALE GONADS.
  Hyperfunctional States.
  Hypofunctional States.
  Amenorrhea.
  Functional Uterine Bleeding.
THE MALE GONADS.
  Hyperfunctional States.
  Hypofunctional States.
THE PINEAL BODY.
THE THYMUS BODY.

Introduction.—The glands of internal secretion through the regulatory substances which they produce and deliver to the circulation, the so-called autacoids or hormones, take part in every activity of the body. The science of endocrinology, as though itself influenced by a hormone of some sort, is in process of active growth. In no field of medicine, lately, has new knowledge more rapidly been gained and consequently in no field has speculation been more rife. The charlatan finds it a realm quite after his own heart, and many is the fraudulent endocrine preparation that a gullible profession has prescribed and a faithful public consumed.

It is very necessary, therefore, for the practitioner to distinguish sharply between fact and fancy in matters endocrine, and to be able to do this he must know not only sufficient of the functions of the several glands to recognize the syndromes which derangements in them produce, but also what remedial agents of proven value are available and when they should be used. New evidence in the field should be constantly searched for, but when found, should be scrutinized with thoroughness and caution.

The several glands with which we are concerned are the pituitary, pineal, thyroid, parathyroids, adrenals, islands of the pancreas and the gonads. Of these, the thyroid, parathyroids, pancreatic islands and male gonads, so far as known, have the function of secreting a single autacoid each. The pituitary, adrenals and female gonads certainly secrete at least two each. The pituitary probably secretes six or more. The thymus body, which is also included in this chapter, is an organ of less well-known function. The most recent evidence, however, suggests that it properly belongs in the endocrine category.

Of the several identified autacoids, thyroxin, epinephrin, insulin and the female sex hormone have been obtained in pure crystalline form. Thyroxin and epinephrin have been synthesized and their precise chemical structure is known. The female sex hormone, theelin, has not been synthesized but its chemical structure is known. The others are biologically but not chemically known. It should be mentioned at this point that the accepted endocrine glands are by no means the sole producers of internal secretions. Important autacoids arise from quite other sources, for example, secretin produced by the intestinal mucosa which activates the flow of pancreatic juice and the recently discovered sympathins of Cannon, substances apparently produced by the smooth muscle of the pilomotor apparatus of the cat and also by that of the intestine, bladder and uterus. One of these is given off from smooth muscle which is incited to contract by sympathetic impulses, the other from smooth muscle inhibited by such impulses. Escaping from its cells of origin the former is carried by the blood stream and is capable of causing contraction in distant smooth muscle organs, the latter analogously affects smooth muscle organs which relax.

On the experimental side, the functions of the endocrine organs have been learned through observation of the effects of extirpation and of the administration of substances derived from the glands. These principles apply to each of the glands. On the clinical side, important information has been gathered through observing the effects of endocrine disease.

The diseases of the endocrine glands taken as a whole may be said to consist in hyperfunction and hypofunction with their anatomic counterparts of hypertrophy or hyperplasia on the one hand and of atrophy and congenital absence on the other, together with inflammation and new-growth. Any of the glands, theoretically at least, may become over- or underactive, and any may be the seat of inflammation or new-growth. Furthermore, any of them also may produce local manifestations, neighborhood symptoms, by increase in their size. Not all of the theoretically possible morbid processes of each and every gland have as yet been found in the shape of clinical disease. Physiologic knowledge is, however, leading from time to time to additions to the list. The recent recognition of hyperparathyroidism and hyperinsulinism as clinical entities are cases in point. Hyperfunction associated with tumor is of particular interest. Hyperfunctioning adenomata have been found in most of the glands. Indeed, clinical evidence suggesting an excessive supply of the hormone of any particular gland should lead to a search for a tumor of the said gland.

In treatment also certain principles apply to the endocrine glands in common. In the case of underfunction one seeks to provide an extraneous supply of the hormone which is lacking. This is called substitution, opo- or organotherapy. Successful substitution therapy for hypothyroidism was discovered in 1891. Others have been subsequently added from time to time, as will be related in the sections on the individual glands. The use of insulin in diabetes mellitus, cortin in Addison's disease and the female sex hormone in certain ovarian disturbances represents recent and dramatic advances in this field. It should be noted in this connection that while the active principle of the thyroid is readily absorbed from the gastro-intestinal tract, most of the others are not but require parenteral administration.

Transplantation or grafting of endocrine tissue has also been practised in an attempt to restore a lost function. Although grafts of some of the glands will live and function for a time, permanent restoration of function by this means has seldom if ever been secured. The grafts do not renew themselves and consequently in time their parenchyma disappears. Transplantation in the case of any of the glands is not a therapeutic method which has come into common use.

The principles involved in the treatment of overfunction are chiefly extirpation and irradiation. Partial resection of the hyperfunctioning gland has been a remarkably successful therapy in the case of the thyroid and also in the case of hyperfunctioning adenomata of several of the other glands, such as the pituitary, parathyroids, adrenal cortex, adrenal medulla and the pancreatic island tissue. Attempts at reduction in the secretory activity of endocrine glands by means of irradiation (roentgen-ray or radium) have met with some success in the case of the thyroid, pituitary and gonads. Continuous depression in the function of any one gland through the administration of the active principle of another, having an antagonistic action, is perhaps theoretically possible but has not yet met with any general practical success.

Each endocrine gland doubtless influences most or all of the others. The pituitary, for example, controls the gonads and has an important influence over the thyroid, pancreas, adrenals and probably the parathyroids as well; indeed, it may in a sense be considered as the master gland. Important, too, is the interrelation of adrenal medulla, pancreatic islands and pituitary, in carbohydrate metabolism and that of pituitary, adrenal cortex and gonads in the attainment of puberty and the maintenance of sexual activity. Taken as a whole, the system may be considered to be presiding over metabolism, growth, differentiation and reproduction; and disturbances in any phase of this function will be manifest by alteration in any of these processes. Nevertheless, as we find such disturbances in the clinic it generally turns out that one gland seems chiefly at fault. There has been much loose talk of polyglandular syndromes. Such terminology is generally a cloak to ignorance of the real pathology in the given case. In the sections which follow, the diseases of each gland will be considered separately, and it is the author's belief that, for the present at least, given an endocrine syndrome, the clinician should make it his duty to discover the chiefly offending gland and plan his treatment to correct the error in that particular gland. Guesswork diagnosis of polyglandular disorders and shotgun endocrine therapy, designed to treat the same, have no place in intelligent medical practice. If one wishes to make a therapeutic test, a single agent should be employed at a time and its effect noted and carefully controlled. Any other practice leads but to confusion. Many biologically assayed endocrine preparations are now available. None other should be used either for diagnosis or treatment.

From the point of view of frequency, thyroid disorders far outnumber all the rest, and since the functions of the thyroid and parathyroids are probably simpler and better understood than those of any of the others, these will be considered first.

REFERENCES.

BARKER, L. F.: Endocrinology and Metabolism, 5 vols., New York, Appleton, 1922.
BAUER, J.: Innere Sekretion: Ihre Physiologie, Pathologie und Klinik, Berlin, Springer, 1929.
CANNON, W. B., and BACQ, Z. M.: A Hormone Produced by Sympathetic Action on Smooth Muscle, Am. Jour. Physiol., 1931, **96**, 392.
FALTA, W.: Die Erkrankungen der Blutdrüsen, 2d ed., Vienna, Springer, 1928.
TRENDELENBURG, P.: Die Hormone: Ihre Physiologie und Pharmacologie, Berlin, Springer, 1929.

THE THYROID GLAND.

The symptoms produced by thyroid disorders are directly traceable to over- (hyperthyroidism) or under- (hypothyroidism) function of the gland, or to regional affection produced by alteration in its size, that is to say, to an excess or shortage of the thyroid hormone throughout the body, or to pressure locally from a thyroid which has become enlarged. These three categories of symptoms may conveniently be considered before the clinical entities of thyroid diseases are discussed. The constitutional symptoms can be directly related to the known physiologic action of the hormone thyroxin and the pressure symptoms to the regional anatomy of the neck and mediastinum.

Function.—The sole function of the thyroid, so far as known, is the manufacture and storage of the iodine-containing hormone, thyroxin, and the action of that hormone seems to be essentially that of "maintaining," as Marine has said, "a higher level of metabolism than would otherwise obtain," or as Plummer has claimed, that of a catalytic agent accelerating metabolism in all cells of the body. That is to say, its action is fundamentally calorigenic. Although oxidation does not cease at once in the cells of a thyroidectomized animal, nevertheless it proceeds at a slower rate than when a supply of thyroxin is available. Concomitant with this lowered rate of oxidation there is a retardation in tissue growth and, in some species at least, in tissue differentiation. When an excess of hormone is present the level of metabolism is raised above that found in the normal animal. Thyroxin also has an action on mineral metabolism, particularly of calcium and phosphorus, the loss of these elements from their depots being accelerated when thyroxin supply increases. The work of Salter and others suggests that the mode of action of thyroxin upon cells is by increasing the activity of their enzymes. Thyroxin was obtained in pure crystalline form by Kendall in 1915 and synthesized by Barger and Harington in 1927. Normal function of the thyroid seems to be dependent on the pituitary. Removal of the pituitary impairs the histologic structure and physiologic activity of the thyroid, and administration of active preparations of the anterior pituitary have been shown by Schockaert and others to cause hyperplasia and hyperactivity of the thyroid.

Symptoms of Hyperfunction.—The symptoms of the hyperthyroid state are, in the first place, those dependent upon an increased outgo of heat from the body. If extra heat is produced, the body must likewise get rid of it if fever is to be avoided. The chief channels of heat loss are through vaporization of water from lungs and skin, and by radiation and conduction from the surface of the body. We find, therefore, increased sweating and flushing of the skin. More water is evaporated; more blood is taken to the surface where it can lose heat. This flushing gives rise to a characteristic sensation of warmth. To meet the demands of increased metabolism, increased flow of blood is required resulting in tachycardia, increased pulse pressure and often the symptoms of dyspnea and palpitation. Increased catabolism brings about loss of weight. To offset this we often find increased appetite and, to offset the increased water loss, increased thirst. The excess of hormone also brings about an increased irritability of the nervous system shown symptomatically by the central in emotional instability and increased fatigability, and by the vegetative in vasomotor instability and increased peristaltic activity. The bowels tend to become looser in hyperthyroid states; if constipated before, they become regular; if regular before, there may develop diarrhea. The skeletal muscles become asthenic and balance of opposing groups is disturbed, giving tremor. Any of these manifestations might occur in hyperthyroidism induced by ingestion of the gland. They are the manifestations of hyperthyroidism *per se*. In spontaneous disorders of the thyroid gland, there are other manifestations of which the causation is less easy to understand. The term thyrotoxicosis is therefore preferable to hyperthyroidism since it commits us to less. A toxic state dependent on the thyroid is all that it implies. Thyrotoxic states are hyperthyroid states but they may be something more. Of what more they may be, however, precisely nothing is positively known.

Symptoms of Hypofunction.—The symptoms of the hypothyroid state are in the main the opposite of those of the hyper. Less heat is eliminated, so the skin is cold and dry. The patient in consequence feels cold instead of hot. Weight is gained, though appetite is poor. Circulatory activity is reduced. The pulse tends to be slow, the pulse pressure low. Instead of being irritable the patient becomes mentally dull and lethargic. The acuity of special senses, particularly hearing, is decreased. Peristaltic activity is reduced and constipation results. Also under conditions of complete or nearly complete thyroxin lack,

certain gross changes in water balance and distribution of body water
and deposit protein characteristically ensue. Water is held back in
tissue cells and sometimes in tissue spaces as well, so that non-pitting
edema and sometimes also pitting edema may be found. Plasma
volume is decreased, plasma protein and spinal fluid protein are
increased. All of these abnormalities rapidly pass off when thyroxin
is supplied. Therefore, one of the striking actions of thyroid when
administered to persons with thyroid lack is the production of marked
diuresis during the period in which the restoration of water distribution
to normal is being brought about. Under the influence of the hormone
the pathologically stored fluid moves from tissues to plasma and from
plasma to urine until normal relations are established.

Symptoms of Pressure by an Enlarged Thyroid.—The symptoms which
may arise from pressure by a thyroid sufficiently enlarged from any
cause are, in order of their frequency, sensation of choking or stridor
from narrowing of the trachea, hoarseness or aphonia from vocal cord
paralysis, dysphagia from encroachment upon the esophagus, and
irritative cough due to direct pressure upon the larynx.

Etiology and Classification of Clinical Thyroid Disorders.—A strictly
etiologic classification is impossible since in several types of disorders
the etiology is unknown, nor is a strictly anatomic classification satisfactory. An enlargement of the thyroid from any cause may be called
a goiter. Goiters are of various sorts and may be divided into groups
from a number of different angles. They may be separated, for
example, into diffuse or nodular, into non-toxic or toxic, into benign
or malignant, into non-inflammatory or inflammatory, into endemic or
sporadic. These are all characteristics of a goiter which, in any given
case, we wish to know. Fortunately, however, we do not find clinically
every possible combination of these several variables and, for the purposes of text-book description, a few common types will suffice. We
also encounter conditions in which the thyroid is diseased but not
enlarged, the atrophies or developmental abnormalities, for example.
It should be borne in mind that the types of thyroid disorders are not
necessarily static and that in any given case there may be a progression
from one type to another as the disease develops. In the discussion of
types which follows, the classification used is purely one of convenience.
The separation is into types which present rather well-defined problems
of diagnosis and treatment.

Methods of Examination.—The history and physical examination
in persons suspected of having thyroid disease should include a search
for all the clinical evidences of over- and underfunction of the thyroid
and of pressure. The local examination of goiters is important. The
thyroid being attached to the trachea ascends with deglutition and
can be distinguished from other neck tumors by this characteristic.
Consistency, contour and configuration should all be determined.
Palpable thrills and bruits should be searched for. In palpating a
goiter it is well to stand behind the seated patient and feel with the
tips of the fingers of both hands. The patient may take a mouthful of
water and be directed to swallow when desired. The larynx may be
displaced laterally from in front with one hand and the lobe thus dis-

located felt from behind the sterno-cleido-mastoid muscle between the finger tips and the thumb of the other. When the patient swallows, a deeply situated small nodule may thus become readily palpable. Smooth fluctuant or soft nodules should be transilluminated. Cysts containing transparent fluid may thus be shown. They may appear like hydrocele.

Since paralysis of vocal cords is an important pressure phenomenon, routine laryngoscopy should be done in all persons with goiters.

Roentgen-ray examination of several sorts is indicated, of the neck and chest to outline the lower border of a goiter and to disclose evidence of compression or dislocation of the trachea, and of the heart to determine its shape and size in the presence of thyrotoxicosis or hypothyroidism. Electrocardiography is valuable in disturbed cardiac function of thyrotoxicosis and in myxedema.

Basal metabolic rate determination is desirable in every person suspected of having any sort of thyroid disorder. Often a series of determinations is important in order to determine levels or trends. Metabolic rates are expressed as per cent variations above or below certain standard figures. At the Massachusetts General Hospital, the Russell Sage Institute Standards have always been used. The metabolic rates mentioned in the following pages are deviations from those standards.

Finally there is the examination of thyroid tissue removed at operation. Enlargements of the gland may be due to increase in parenchyma, in colloid, in vascularity, or in interstitial tissue. The precise anatomic nature of any particular goiter may not be learned until it is examined microscopically.

ENDEMIC GOITER.

A type of goiter, the incidence of which seems determined by geographic factors. Certain regions of the earth are goitrigenous; others are not. For the most part, the goitrigenous are either mountainous or old glacial areas. In the United States, the most highly goitrigenous areas are the northwest and the region about the Great Lakes. The states of Idaho, Oregon, Washington, Montana, Utah, Wyoming, Wisconsin and Michigan are highly goitrigenous; those of North Dakota, Minnesota, West Virginia, Illinois, Iowa, Indiana, Nevada, Ohio, Colorado, California, Pennsylvania, South Dakota, Missouri and Virginia are moderately goitrigenous. The other states are either slightly goitrigenous or have little or nothing justifying the name of endemic. The ailment is found in females more often than in males. In mildly goitrigenous areas the ratio may be one male to eight females. As the endemic increases in severity the difference in incidence between the sexes declines.

Etiology.—The etiology of endemic goiter is without much doubt deficiency, relative or absolute, in the organism's supply of iodine. It has been shown that the iodine of ground water in the United States bears a fairly close inverse ratio to the incidence of goiter, also that endemic goiter can be largely prevented by the simple expedient of providing iodine. Other factors may indirectly play a rôle. Infections may interfere with the absorption of iodine and the deficiency may be intrinsic instead of extrinsic. Also it has been suggested that the amount of sunlight is important, perhaps because it affects the iodine content of vegetables or because it may exercise some actual inhibitory influence upon the factors which tend to produce hyperplasia. Furthermore, Marine has recently shown that vegetables such as cabbage contain a positive goitrigenous agent, the action of which, however, is inhibited by iodine and also perhaps by other substances contained in cabbage. Marine believes that this substance acts by interfering with tissue oxidations (it is a cyanide) and that this calls forth a compensatory hyperplasia on the part of the thyroid.

Character of the Goiter and Course of the Disease.—According to Marine, the thyroid first responds to iodine starvation by diffuse hyperplasia. The enlargement due to this response becomes manifest in endemic goiter regions usually coincidentally with the increased metabolic activity of puberty. At least this is true in the United States. In such regions as Switzerland, more highly goitrigenous than any areas in the United States, congenital goiters and goiters in young children are often seen. The hyperplasia is followed by increased accumulation of colloid in all the follicles and the gland becomes what can properly be called a colloid goiter. Such glands may persist without much change in size for many years. They are accompanied usually by no symptoms of either hyper- or hypothyroidism nor do they produce any sort of ill health. They may give rise to pressure symptoms if caught behind the sternum. After the age of thirty years these goiters are apt to become irregular, to take on a nodular feel. This may be due to irregularities of regression or growth, the formation of cysts and also sometimes to the development of adenomata, that is to say benign new-growths arising from thyroid parenchyma.

Diagnosis.—The diagnosis depends upon the features described above. Differential diagnosis is simply from other forms of goiter. The absence of evidence of increased function, and the form and feel of the gland itself are the chief points. The entire gland is involved and in the simple colloid stage the enlargement is symmetrical, or very nearly so. The feel is smooth and soft, softer than any of the other sorts of goiter about to be described. The outlines of the colloid gland are difficult to map out. This is a point of value in differential diagnosis.

Prophylaxis.—The prophylaxis of endemic goiter by iodine administration has proved eminently successful. Two general principles have been followed: one of wholesale iodinization of entire communities by putting iodine in the public water supply or by the general sale of iodinized table salt; the other, that of giving iodine not to the whole population but only to school children under puberty and to pregnant and lactating women. The last-mentioned method has probably the most to commend it. An adequate dose for prophylaxis has been proved to be $\frac{1}{6}$ grain (10 mg.) per week. This can be given in tablet form. Several such tablets are on the market.

Treatment.—The treatment depends upon the stage the goiter has reached and will be considered in the sections which follow.

SPORADIC COLLOID GOITER.

Symptomatically and morphologically identical with endemic goiter but lacking the endemic distribution. The etiology is obscure. Like the endemic form, it appears most often at puberty. If due to iodine lack it must be of an intrinsic variety, for there is no shortage in ingested iodine.

Treatment.—The treatment of simple colloid goiter, whether endemic or sporadic, by non-surgical methods is unsatisfactory. Iodine may be tried but only occasionally does much good. The dosage should be larger than for prophylaxis, perhaps $\frac{1}{3}$ to $\frac{1}{2}$ grain (20 to 30 mg.) per week. In cases which exhibit a reduction in metabolic rate, thyroid may be given cautiously. One and a half grains (0.1 gram) of U. S. P. thyroid once a day is sufficient for a beginning. A diffuse colloid goiter is unlikely to require operation. When goiters require surgery simply on account of size, they generally have progressed beyond the stage of diffuse colloid goiter and have taken on nodular change or cystic degeneration.

NODULAR GOITER.

The term simply implies a goiter which instead of being smooth is irregular in outline. Irregularities may be due to a variety of causes. Lumping the cases together and calling them nodular goiter, therefore, may be thoroughly unscientific, but since it is often impossible to determine the nature of nodules until the tissue is seen under the microscope, the diagnosis seems to be as exact as is usually, at the present time, clinically possible.

In some instances nodules undoubtedly represent benign new growth of thyroid parenchyma. To these the term adenoma has been widely applied, and to the glands which harbor them, adenomatous goiter. However, certain modern work seems to throw doubt on the correctness of considering all these masses true tumors. Some of them have the histology of adult, some of embryonic thyroid tissue. The latter perhaps are true tumors; some of the former may rather be involution bodies. Nodules also may be due to cystic degeneration of the gland and to malignant new-growths.

Course of the Disease.—Nodules may appear in the thyroid at any age but they are seen most frequently after the age of thirty years. In endemic goiter regions they very frequently develop in glands previously the seat of simple colloid enlargement. They may similarly develop in cases of sporadic colloid goiter in the fourth decade or later. Also they not infrequently make their appearance in glands not previously enlarged. Their growth may be continuous or intermittent. They often remain the same size for a period of many years.

Extensive nodulation of the thyroid may exist for years with no evident disturbance in the gland's function. Nevertheless there is a tendency, as patients with nodular (single or multiple) goiter grow older, for a gradually increasing thyrotoxicosis to make its appearance. In cases of this type the term toxic adenoma or adenomatous goiter with hyperthyroidism has frequently been applied. The patients are chiefly past forty years. According to Plummer, 3 patients out of every 5 with nodular goiter who live to sixty years of age will develop hyperthyroidism. It is possible that the hyperfunction in some cases is actually due directly to the activity of an adenoma; in others it may result from a more diffuse type of hyperplasia. Malignant degeneration of nodular goiters develops in some cases and the production of pressure in either benign or malignant types may be an important complication.

Treatment.—Surgical removal is the only satisfactory treatment for nodular goiter. The chief question in these cases is to decide whethèr treatment is needed at all. The existence of thyrotoxicosis or the suspicion of malignancy is a clear-cut indication for thyroidectomy. So, too, is evidence of pressure. In the case of nodular goiter which is doing none of these things, resection may be advocated as wise prophylactic surgery, prevention of the aforementioned unfavorable developments. The hardest decision is in the case of rather small nodules which are doing no apparent harm and which it is known may never do so. In these, a policy of watchful waiting may be justifiable.

In the case of large nodules or multiple nodules, the operation of so-called subtotal thyroidectomy should be done. In that of single discrete nodules with or without thyrotoxicosis, resection of the nodules alone has often been done. The belief is growing, however, that with thyrotoxicosis present, even though the nodule is single, a subtotal thyroidectomy should be done for the reason that with the more conservative operation, regrowth of thyroid tissue and return of thyrotoxicosis are not uncommon.

It is not wise to use iodine in the non-toxic nodular goiter. It does no good and there is some evidence to suggest that it may precipitate hyperfunction. When thyrotoxicosis is present it may be given prior to operation, and sometimes causes a temporary amelioration of symptoms. The dosage used should be the same as in exophthalmic goiter. (See below.)

Intrathoracic Goiter.—Goiters, nearly always of the nodular variety, may be located partially or completely within the thorax. On account of the unusual position, they present a special problem both in diagnosis and in treatment. The symptomatology, if there be any, is that of upper mediastinal pressure. In diagnosis the roentgen-ray is of vast importance. The existence of such goiters may be demonstrable by no other method. The special problem therapeutically is one of surgical technic.

EXOPHTHALMIC GOITER.

Synonyms.—Parry's disease; Graves' disease; Basedow's disease; diffuse toxic goiter; diffuse goiter with hyperthyroidism.

The disease which goes by these names constitutes a fairly definite clinical entity and distinctly special therapeutic problem. It is characterized by diffuse hypertrophy and hyperplasia of the thyroid, together with hyperfunction of that organ with resulting elevated metabolism and the constitutional disturbances that such hypermetabolism entails, also by gross disturbance in the function of the vegetative nervous system with a peculiar train of ophthalmic abnormalities in consequence. What causes the thyroid to hyperfunctionate in this disease is unknown. Other glands have been blamed, the adrenal and the pituitary. The evidence incriminating them is, however, confusing and fragmentary.

Diagnosis.—This depends upon finding the symptoms and signs of hyperthyroidism (*q.v.*) a diffuse enlargement of the thyroid together with the well known eye signs—exophthalmos, staring appearance of the eyes, lid lag, wide palpebral fissure, poor converging power and failure to wrinkle the forehead on upward rotation of the eyeballs. Puffiness of the eyelids is also frequently encountered. Among the hyperthyroid manifestations, a fine tremor of the tongue and extremities is a noteworthy characteristic. So too is violent heart action. Increased irritability and emotional instability are very common. Sometimes what amounts to an actual toxic psychosis is present. Diarrhea is common and, in the periods of greatest intoxication, vomiting. Catamenia may be scant or suppressed. In any given case some of these features may be lacking and yet the diagnosis be certain. Thus some cases lack the eye signs, others the goiter. In determining the presence or absence or, if present, the degree of hyperthyroidism, the determination of the basal metabolism is very helpful.

The differential diagnosis is chiefly from other forms of goiter, especially colloid goiter with some complicating conditions, cardiovascular disease, tuberculosis, psychoneuroses that may give symptoms simulating those of hyperthyroidism.

The goiter is usually smooth and rather firm, much firmer than the colloid gland. This is a point of diagnostic importance. It may be symmetrical or one lobe (usually the right) may be a little larger than the other. Sometimes the gland is nodular. Not infrequently the pyramidal lobe can be felt as a rather firm projection extending upward from the isthmus. It is interesting to note that when the exophthalmos is symmetrical, as is not infrequent, it is more often the left eye that is more prominent. Over the gland, especially the upper poles, a palpable thrill may be felt and with the stethoscope a systolic *bruit* can nearly always be heard. These signs are probably evidence of increased blood flow through the gland, and are practically pathognomonic of hyperfunction. The rapid amelioration of symptoms and fall in metabolic and pulse-rates, which characteristically occur in exophthalmic goiter and not in other diseases upon the administration of iodine, constitute diagnostic evidence of primary importance. In cases where the picture is not fully developed a trial of iodine for diagnostic purposes is often very helpful.

Course of the Disease.—It is seen most frequently in the third and fourth decades but it may occur at any time between early childhood and old age. It is more frequent in females than males, the difference between the incidence in the two sexes apparently being less in goitrigenous than in non-goitrigenous areas. Of its true incidence but little is known, of its etiology nothing. It is common in goitrigenous as well as non-goitrigenous regions. Some writers believe that hereditary and constitutional factors are important in causation, but these aspects of the problem are still rather nebulous. The onset may be abrupt, even fulminating, a matter of a few days following a psychic trauma, or very insidious without obvious inciting cause. Spontaneous remission and relapse are not infrequent and spontaneous recovery can occur. Untreated, the disease may run a course of several years.

One of the characteristics of the disease is the tendency toward sudden *crises* of intensified thyrotoxicosis. These may occur spontaneously or be precipitated by operation. The picture in crisis or storm, as it is sometimes called, is that of marked increase in the severity of the symptoms of hyperthyroidism, together with fever, nausea and vomiting from which result dehydration and acidosis, also marked tachycardia and prostration. Crises are responsible for the majority of the deaths from the disease.

There are some interesting differences in the picture of the disease seen in men from that in women. The subjective phenomena are less marked in men, particularly the nervous phenomena. Men with severe exophthalmic goiter will often admit of no symptoms at all. The tachycardia is relatively less in men and instead the increased blood flow is met more by increased systolic discharge shown by a widening of the pulse pressure.

The Iodine Response.—As pointed out by Plummer in 1923, iodine in this disease has a very remarkable and one might almost say specific effect. If a sufficient dose is used this consists in a rapid improvement in the toxic symptoms and a fall in the pulse and basal metabolic rates. The magnitude of the fall in the basal metabolic rate is of the order of 40 points from levels in the +60's and +70's, 30 points from the +40's and +50's, and 20 points from the +20's and +30's. The fall in pulse-rate is essentially similar. The changes are noticeable in a day or two and complete in about ten days. The irritability decreases or disappears. Emotional stability is in large measure regained. Patients who have been subject to uncontrollable crying and beset by fears become cheerful and serene. The heart action becomes quieter, the profuse sweating subsides and the flushing and feeling of warmth disappears. The goiter usually becomes harder and smaller, and sometimes the thrill and bruit disappear. These changes are to be interpreted as colloid storage and decreased blood flow through the gland. The eye signs generally are not very much changed.

It is the writer's belief that the effect of iodine is to diminish the intensity of the thyrotoxicosis at any one time and not at all to alter the duration of the disease. Patients kept continually on iodine throughout the course of their disease seem to run a milder course, but not a shorter course, than they would without the drug. Kept continuously on iodine, patients may grow worse, but this seems not to be because iodine has lost its effect for, if the drug is omitted, the patients become still worse.

The form of iodine or the portal of entry to the body seems to matter not at all. The indication is simply to give enough to produce the maximum effect.

Treatment.—The most effective treatment and the one productive of the quickest and most lasting cures is that of subtotal thyroidectomy

52

done when the patient is fully under the influence of iodine. The iodine remission makes it possible to do this operation with very little risk and in one stage. The intensity of the intoxication is greatly decreased and the likelihood of postoperative crises, which in pre-iodine days often proved fatal, is very slight. The operative mortality in the hands of good surgeons under present-day conditions is less than 1 per cent, whereas before iodine it was often over 5 per cent. Roentgen-ray and radium, though effective in some cases, are on the whole slower and less certain in their effect. In many instances these forms of treatment make patients better but do not make them well, resembling in this respect the less radical resections that were done in pre-iodine days. The time to operate is as soon after the diagnosis is made as full iodinization is obtained, except with such patients who, on the continued use of iodine, are getting worse. With these a delay until a period of spontaneous improvement sets in is desirable. When operation has been decided upon, iodine in the dosage of saturated solution of potassium iodide, 3 to 6 minims (0.2 to 0.4 cc.) once daily should be given for ten days and the patient kept in bed. Smaller doses may be effective but are not recommended for routine care. The iodine should be continued on the day of operation and thereafter for two or three weeks. If, upon omission, any toxic symptoms recur it should be resumed. In fact, after operation it should be continued, no matter how long, until such time as the patient will remain free from symptoms without its use. Mild residual toxic symptoms following operation are usually controlled completely by 2 to 5 minims (0.15 to 0.3 cc.) once daily of 20 per cent solution of potassium iodide. Contraindications to operative treatment are practically non-existent. Cardiac insufficiency is added indication for operative treatment; so is a complicating diabetes mellitus. Acute infections, especially respiratory, may necessitate a brief postponement. Chronic tonsillar or sinus infection, we have found, is better treated radically after the goiter is out than before.

At the Massachusetts General Hospital since the advent of iodine, the results of such a program have been in round numbers, as follows: About 4 out of 5 patients are promptly and satisfactorily relieved of their thyrotoxicosis. About 1 out of 5 has persistent thyrotoxicosis but in one-half of these it is controllable by iodine and finally disappears. In the others, further surgical or roentgen-ray treatment has been needed. In about 1 in 100, a condition of hypothyroidism requiring continued substitution therapy with thyroid has developed. Sometimes too much parathyroid tissue is removed with resultant tetany. (For further discussion, see Parathyroid Gland.) A thermal response usually occurs following operation with an average temperature of 101.5° F. on the third day and passing off by the sixth day. This fever requires no special treatment. Postoperative pneumonia is rarer than after abdominal surgery.

When a toxic crisis or storm is precipitated by operation, or when it comes on spontaneously, for that matter, it should be treated with large quantities of fluid—glucose solution intravenously and saline or tap water by rectum. Iodine must be given in doses of at least 15 min-

ims (1 cc.) of saturated solution of potassium iodide daily, by rectum
if there is vomiting. If the temperature becomes alarmingly high some
form of hydrotherapy, cold packs or even ice packs, may be required.
Morphine and digitalis are of very little value. If cyanosis is present,
an oxygen tent or chamber should be used.

Whether purely medical treatment is ever justifiable in exophthalmic goiter is open to debate. Undoubtedly certain cases are destined
to run a mild course and could be carried through on iodine alone without coming to harm, but there is no way of distinguishing them in
advance. Sometimes patients are seen years after the onset of the
disease, in whom there exists a mild chronic thyrotoxicosis of fairly
constant intensity. In these cases iodine may abolish all the symptoms
and if so it is legitimate to keep up its administration indefinitely.
Such cases, however, are rare.

Treatment by irradiation either with roentgen-ray or by radium
has had a wide vogue. It undoubtedly produces good results in some
of the cases. It is not to be recommended at the present time, for
it offers less certainty and less rapidity of cure than subtotal thyroidectomy done under full iodine control.

Of drugs other than iodine in the treatment of exophthalmic goiter,
little need be said. There are none of any great importance except
those indicated by complications, digitalis for cardiac decompensation,
quinidine for auricular fibrillation or insulin for diabetes, which sometimes coëxist. Quinine hydrobromide and ergot preparations which
have been used in the past have nothing to recommend them now.
Phenobarbital may be used for its sedative action but some thyrotoxics
are hypersensitive to the drug.

Prolonged rest figures large in text-books but there is no good excuse
for recommending it today. It is true that with long rest in bed some
improvement will take place, but to advise such dilatory tactics when
a treatment is available that in a vast majority of cases will bring about
restoration to full activity in a few weeks is hardly sound practice.
On both humane and on economic grounds the program which offers
quickest and most complete restoration to health, provided it does
not entail too great risk, is the one of choice.

Sequelæ of Operation and Irradiation and Their Treatment.—Either
hypo- or hyperthyroidism may occur after thyroidectomy or irradiation
for exophthalmic goiter. A study of these residuals in the thyroid
clinic of the Massachusetts General Hospital disclosed that there are
several different types of hypometabolism to be found under such
circumstances. There are those in which clinical myxedema is present
and those in which it is absent. Of the former some are temporary,
some prove permanent. When evidence of myxedema (*q. v.*) is present,
thyroid should be given (more than thyroid, U. S. P., 3 grains [0.2 gram]
once daily is seldom necessary). However, if thyroid is administered
it is well to discontinue it from time to time in order to determine if
continuance of such therapy is indicated. In the group of hypometabolism without clinical myxedema, there are two varieties—those
cases in which the condition is temporary and those in which it is
permanent. The latter appear to be in other respects quite normal

individuals. Sometimes these low rates of metabolism are observed only when the patient is taking iodine. In such patients the rate rises on omission of the drug. This phenomenon is to be interpreted as mild residual thyrotoxicosis controllable by iodine.

The incidence of all forms of hypometabolism following treatment for exophthalmic goiter in the series studied at the Massachusetts General Hospital was in the neighborhood of 27 per cent of the cases treated, but in these only one-sixth had clinical myxedema. Of those with myxedema, the ratio of temporary to permanent forms was as 3 to 8. The incidence of permanent myxedema following subtotal thyroidectomy seems to be about 1 per cent, and after irradiation treatment, about 4 per cent. The incidence of permanent low metabolic rate without clinical evidence of hypothyroidism was about 9 per cent of the cases treated. These patients usually showed rates above −25 per cent, those with myxedema below.

The indications for treatment in these conditions are thyroid when clinical myxedema is present but with omission from time to time, as noted above, to discover whether the condition is permanent. Hypometabolism without myxedema is not a condition which requires any treatment *per se*. It may merely represent a return to what is the normal state for the particular person. (See Hypometabolism without Myxedema.)

Persistence or return of thyrotoxicosis after roentgen-ray treatment is very common. In fact, at the Massachusetts General Hospital, the experience was that in only about one-third of the patients could the thyrotoxicosis be considered abolished. In another one-third it was diminished and in another one-third it was unaffected. After subtotal thyroidectomy the incidence of postoperative thyrotoxicosis at the Massachusetts General Hospital has been about 20 per cent. In most instances this seems to be a persistence of the disease rather than a true recurrence. True recurrence with growth of a new goiter after the disease had apparently been cured occurred in but 2 per cent.

Persistent thyrotoxicosis after operation is usually mild and usually amenable to treatment by iodine alone. After a period of months or even years it will be found, by omitting iodine, to have disappeared. Its duration probably represents the natural duration of the disease. The disease has run its full natural course, but in milder form because of the operative removal of a large portion of the gland. The dosage of iodine required to control these residual types is not usually over 3 minims (0.2 cc.) of 20 per cent potassium iodide solution per day.

When there is true recurrence with regrowth of goiter, roentgen-ray treatment may be tried, but further thyroidectomy is the method of choice.

THE HEART IN THYROTOXICOSIS.

The terms "thyroid heart disease" and "thyrocardiac" are often heard. One certainly encounters myocardial insufficiency which can be cured by abolition of thyrotoxicosis. Whether this disease ought to be ranked as a form of heart disease in itself is open to question.

It seems likely that thyrotoxicosis alone does not produce congestive failure. Violent heart action is a characteristic finding, but hypertrophy is unusual even though the thyrotoxicosis is of long standing. One patient observed by the writer was known to have been thyrotoxic for seventeen years, yet the heart was normal by physical, roentgenographic and electrocardiographic examination.

It is probable that only when the burden of thyrotoxicosis is placed upon a heart already damaged, as for example by rheumatic infection, sclerosis or hypertension, that congestive failure occurs. When it does, the picture is that of congestive failure from any cause plus that of thyrotoxicosis. Congestive failure is seen more frequently in the older group of thyrotoxic patients, namely, those with the most sclerosis. In these sometimes the picture of thyrotoxicosis is so shadowed by that of congestive failure as to be missed entirely. These are the cases which have been described as thyrotoxicosis masquerading as heart disease.

The type of thyrotoxicosis, whether of the typical Graves' type or of the type without eye signs and with nodular goiter, seems to make little difference in determining the incidence of these cardiac complications. It is rather the age and previous condition of the cardiovascular apparatus which counts. (See also Thyrotoxic Heart Disease, in Diseases of the Heart, p. 394.)

MYXEDEMA.

Synonym.—Gull's disease.

A state of profound hypothyroidism due to under- or absent function of the thyroid gland regardless of its cause will lead eventually to the clinical picture known as myxedema. The characteristics of this picture are the symptoms and signs of hypometabolism which have been described earlier. In the fully developed stage of the disease the appearance of the patient is unmistakable. The bloated, expressionless face with yellowish and pallid tint, the coarse and scant hair of scalp and eyebrows, the thick clumsy tongue, the slow speech, the hoarse voice, the swollen squarish hands, the indurated subcutaneous tissues, the coarse, thickened, cold, dry skin are among the features which make it so.

Hypothyroidism, when it occurs spontaneously, is probably always a permanent condition. After thyroidectomy for toxic goiter, as noted in an earlier section, it may be temporary. The spontaneous variety is encountered at any age as in the form of *infantile myxedema* or *cretinism, childhood* or *juvenile myxedema* and *adult myxedema*. In nongoitrigenous regions the thyroid is invariably atrophic. In goitrigenous regions, fully developed hypothyroidism with resulting myxedema may occur in persons with goiters. The clinical picture of hypothyroidism is influenced by the age at onset, for if this be before growth is completed, we have certain developmental defects in addition to the picture of myxedema *per se*. (See Cretinism.) The picture when it develops after thyroidectomy, the cachexia strumipriva of Kocher, is in no wise different from spontaneous myxedema of adults as described by Gull.

Spontaneous myxedema of adults is seen most often in the third, fourth and fifth decades and is very much more frequent in women than in men. Its cause is quite unknown. The pathology in the gland is that of atrophy of the parenchyma and fibrosis. The onset is very insidious. Often years pass before the symptoms attain sufficient prominence to bring the patient to the doctor and then perhaps a few years more before the doctor makes the correct diagnosis. Untreated, so the older literature shows, the disease runs a course of about ten years, ending in death from cachexia if not from intercurrent disease.

Diagnosis.—The diagnosis is of the utmost importance for it is a calamity to fail to recognize an otherwise fatal disease for which we possess a perfectly satisfactory treatment. Diagnosis should be simple and depends upon the discovery of the clinical features mentioned above plus the confirmatory evidence of a greatly lowered basal metabolic rate. In full-blown, untreated myxedema, the metabolism is invariably depressed to 30 per cent below standard. Usually it is from 35 per cent to 45 per cent below. Equally low rates are occasionally found in other conditions than myxedema, chiefly in malnutrition and other forms of cachexia. They are conditions, however, which do not closely resemble myxedema in their clinical features.

Of the symptoms which may lead to an early recognition of the disease may be mentioned an increased tendency to put on weight in spite of declining appetite, a gradually increasing constipation, impairment in memory, especially for recent events, chilliness, drowsiness, weakness and decrease in sweating. Progressive diminution in acuity of hearing may be an early symptom. The presence of any of these should suggest the possibility of hypothyroidism and indicate the desirability of a metabolic rate determination. Other symptoms often encountered in myxedema are paresthesiæ and indefinite pains in the arms and legs, menorrhagia and dizziness.

The differential diagnosis is chiefly from chronic nephritis, pernicious anemia and from non-myxedematous hypometabolic states. The features which chronic nephritis may possess in common with myxedema are chiefly the pale, puffy face, edema of the extremities, weakness, anorexia, anemia and enlargement of the heart. Albuminuria may occur in myxedema and clear up under treatment. Hypertension is present in a considerable number of patients with myxedema probably because myxedema seems to accelerate the process of arterial decay. The presence of anemia, hypertension and albuminuria would greatly increase the resemblance of myxedema to chronic nephritis.

The points in common between myxedema and pernicious anemia which seem to lead to confusion are pallor, yellow color, weakness, numbness and tingling of the extremities, edema, chilliness and tongue symptoms. The tongue symptoms, of course, are not alike in kind. The tongue in pernicious anemia is sore and atrophic. In myxedema it is enlarged and clumsy but not sore. Until recently we had thought that there was no real excuse for confusing these maladies, but the discovery of several patients who undoubtedly were suffering coincidentally from both made us change this view. At present, we believe that the indication in the case of either is to consider the possibility of the coëxistence of the other. In pernicious anemia we determine the basal metabolism; in myxedema we study the blood smear and analyze the gastric juice. There is generally achlorhydria in pernicious anemia and often in myxedema. The finding of acid, however, might be helpful.

The Response to Thyroid.—When a patient with myxedema is given thyroid, an important series of phenomena rapidly takes place. The most fundamental is a rapid rise in rate of metabolism with resulting disappearance of the symptoms of hypothyroidism. The patient feels warmer and more alert. A profound rearrangement of body water leads to a disappearance of the bloated look. A copious diuresis takes place. The migration of water is from the tissues to the plasma and from the plasma out through the kidneys. With this loss of water there is of necessity a marked loss of weight. It has been shown that in myxedema the volume of the plasma is reduced and that under thyroid it returns to a normal value. Also it has been shown that the blood flow is retarded in myxedema and that under thyroid it accelerates. This is shown clinically by increased frequency of the pulse and widening of the pulse pressure. The bowels act more freely and the growth of tissues is accelerated as shown by a faster growth of hair, nails and desquamation of the thickened skin. In women who have myxedema before the menopause, the catamenia are characteristically increased. Under thyroid they tend to become normal.

Treatment.—The treatment consists in giving sufficient thyroid to keep the patient symptom-free, preferably the minimum amount that will accomplish this purpose. A single intravenous injection of 10 mg. of thyroxin will produce a rise of about 40 points in the basal metabolism, the peak being reached in about five days, with coincident disappearance of signs and symptoms. After such a single injection, it requires somewhere in the neighborhood of eighty-five days for the patient again to sink to his previous state.

The injection of such doses of thyroxin, however, is not without danger. Severe reactions, taking the form of fever, cramp-like pain, muscle tenderness, nausea and vomiting may occur. These symptoms may last for several days. For this reason and because of the general objection to drugs that have to be given intravenously (thyroxin does have to be so administered because it gives local reactions when given subcutaneously and is very uncertain in action when given by mouth) and for the further reason that thyroid by mouth is entirely efficacious, it may be fairly said that thyroxin has no place in the routine treatment of myxedema.

The method of choice is the oral administration of thyroid, U. S. P., in doses of 3 grains (0.2 gram) once daily. In the course of ten days to two weeks, a maximum effect should be obtained. The dose can then be cut in half for a maintenance ration. If no symptoms recur, it may be maintained on that for a permanent ration. If symptoms recur it should be raised not more than half a grain at a time. The object of treatment should be to keep the patient free of symptoms with the smallest dose that will do this. Patients with myxedema will require treatment for the rest of their lives. It is essential therefore for the doctor to check their condition at least two or three times a year.

In carrying out such treatment it should always be borne in mind that the patient with myxedema may be made thyrotoxic by too much thyroid. Any symptoms suggestive of this indicate cessation of treatment until they have disappeared and then resumption with a smaller dose.

A persistent tachycardia without other signs of hyperthyroidism is alone an indication for smaller dosage of thyroid.

The heart in myxedema needs special mention. It is practically always enlarged, though this is often demonstrable only by roentgen-ray. This enlargement seems due to a state of hypotonus and to edema of the myocardium. Under thyroid the enlargement disappears as the tone improves. The *T*-wave of the electrocardiogram is inverted or absent in the untreated stage of the disease. Under thyroid it returns to a normal upright position. Cases are reported in the literature of myxedematous cardiac hypotonia so great as to give frank congestive failure. In our experience this is rare. However, even in these, digitalis has little effect and thyroid is clearly the drug these patients need.

Another aspect of the heart in myxedema is the production of angina pectoris or anginoid pain by increasing its work too fast. These patients are often sclerotic, and if their hearts are suddenly called upon to double their work, coronary insufficiency may result. The doctor therefore should always have patients under close observation during the inauguration of thyroid therapy and should inquire frequently for precordial distress or pain. It is easier to avoid these with guarded oral administration of thyroid than with intravenous thyroxin which constitutes another objection to the use of the latter drug.

The Blood in Myxedema.—A mild to moderate secondary anemia is the rule. Usually under thyroid alone this will gradually disappear. It is, however, the last of the myxedema signs to do so. If hypochromia is marked it is well to try iron in addition. A good form is iron and ammonium citrate, U. S. P., a teaspoonful of the crystals three times a day dissolved in milk or orange juice.

If the blood picture is that of pernicious anemia, liver extract should be given along with thyroid.

Morphine in myxedema is contraindicated during the untreated stage. This was shown by Lund and Benedict in 1929, but is insufficiently known to the profession. Patients with myxedema have a greatly lowered tolerance to this drug. It has the effect of deepening the cachectic state to a degree that may be fatal. There is no objection to giving it in the properly treated case.

The Psyche in Myxedema.—The usual condition is retardation and memory defect. Occasionally disorientation, confusion and excitability occur. Ordinarily the restoration to normal under thyroid is prompt. We have, however, seen the mental changes persist for some weeks after the other manifestations of the disease have gone, and then clear up suddenly for no apparent reason. It has impressed us that the persons acquiring myxedema for the most part belong to a certain type. In bodily habitus, they are of the "pyknic" type, short-necked, broad-shouldered and plump. In disposition they are cheerful and serene. One is constantly impressed in observing, after their myxedema has been thawed by thyroid, what delightful people they turn out to be.

CRETINISM.

Synonym.—Infantile myxedema.

Cretinism is a condition due to congenital hypothyroidism. The cretin differs from the adult with myxedema in that his hypothyroidism exerts its morbid influence during the period of growth. In addition to the symptoms and signs of hypothyroidism *per se*, which are always present to some degree, there is retarded development both of body and mind. The former takes the form of dwarfism of a type in which the bodily proportions of the new-born infant are preserved. The head is relatively large, the extremities short. The tongue is so large that the mouth is held open. The face is for the most part expressionless, though cretins are capable of a rather comical grimace when amused. The belly is prominent, nearly always with umbilical hernia. As in adult myxedema, the voice is characteristically hoarse.

Endemic cretinism is found in the more severely goitrigenous regions such as Switzerland, among the children of goitrous parents. It is doubtful if any true endemic cretinism exists in the United States. Endemic cretins usually have goiters.

Sporadic cretins, the type met in this country, are born usually of apparently healthy parents. As a rule they have no goiter. The cause of their athyreosis is unknown. The onset is insidious; as a rule symptoms begin about the third month. They probably have underactive thyroids from birth, but for that length of time the influence of a supply of maternal thyroxin keeps them symptom-free.

In cretinism, in contrast to myxedema of adults, the lack of thyroid function is not always complete. Not infrequently partial or mild cretinism is encountered. Such patients possess some functioning thyroid tissue but not enough to secure normal development. The end-result of spontaneous adult myxedema, when not treated by thyroid, in which the lack of function becomes complete is death in hypothyroid cachexia. Partial cretinism, on the other hand, even though untreated, is not inconsistent with normal life span, the patients possessing good health but showing the characteristic dwarfism and varying degrees of imbecility.

Diagnosis.—The diagnosis depends upon the discovery of the features mentioned above, plus the confirmatory evidence of a lowered basal metabolic rate. Since the sooner the disease is discovered the more successful will be the treatment, it is very important to make the diagnosis early. The ideal time is in early infancy before the complete classic picture has developed. Early signs which suggest the diagnosis in the first few months of life are a heavy expression and pig-like appearance to the eyes, a yellow tint to the mesial aspect of the cheeks and a hoarse cry. If physicians caring for new-born babies will think of cretinism when such evidence is presented, a certain amount of unnecessary imbecility will be prevented. It is much more difficult to find laboratories equipped to make metabolism tests on infants than on adults. Nevertheless the early diagnosis of cretinism is so important that every attempt should be made to find one that is so equipped.

Treatment.—The treatment of cretinism with thyroid in infancy and early childhood is highly successful. If started directly after the first signs of the condition appear and maintained throughout life, completely normal development, mental and physical, should be possible. Treatment started after well-defined retardation of development has occurred is never completely successful. When applied first in the second decade or later, it is apt to be disappointing. The first year of life is a period of very rapid growth of the brain. Retardation at this period cannot subsequently be overcome by thyroid therapy. With the older cretins, therefore, the mental improvement is often so slight as to be hardly worth seeking. Furthermore, these older cretins, like patients with acquired myxedema, are readily made thyrotoxic by excessive dosage.

The dosage of thyroid (U.S.P.) required at different ages is approximately as follows:

Age.	Dosage, grains daily.
2– 4 months	$\frac{1}{10}$
4– 8 "	$\frac{2}{10}$
8–12 "	$\frac{2}{10}$ to $\frac{3}{10}$
12–24 "	$\frac{3}{10}$ to $\frac{6}{10}$
2– 4 years	$\frac{1}{2}$ to 1
4–12 "	1 to 2

After the child attains a normal status the dose can often be reduced.

Juvenile Myxedema.—In contrast to true cretinism in which the hypothyroidism is congenital, children are found who like adults acquire myxedema after a period of normal development. The mental and physical state of such patients and the prospect of restoration to complete health by thyroid therapy is related to the degree of develment attained before the hypothyroidism supervened. Myxedema acquired in late childhood should give nearly as good results as that of adult life.

There is nothing about the symptomatology of juvenile myxedema that requires special comment. It is essentially similar to that of adults. The same applies to treatment.

MALIGNANT DISEASE OF THE THYROID GLAND.

Malignant disease is found in about 2 per cent of all goiters removed at operation. From 60 per cent to 70 per cent of the cases are in women. It is most frequent in the fourth, fifth and sixth decades. The most significant etiologic factor is the tendency of malignant disease of the thyroid to develop in preëxisting goiter. Coller has gone so far as to brand colloid goiter a precancerous lesion, it being the precursor in many instances of adenomatous goiter and adenomatous goiter of adenocarcinoma. It is almost unheard of for cancer to develop in the hyperplastic goiter of Graves' disease.

The great majority of malignant tumors of the thyroid are of epithelial origin, and for the most part belong under the general heading of adenocarcinoma. The histologic picture is extremely diverse. Some tumors show solid masses of cells, but the majority show a tendency to form alveoli. Dense scirrhous forms are sometimes found. Certain adenocarcinomata are encapsulated like benign adenomata. Occasionally we find papillary cystadenomata. These tend to become papillary adenocarcinomata of low grade malignancy. Extension of malignant growth of the thyroid may be by direct invasion of contiguous structures, downward by lymphatics or veins toward the mediastinum, upward toward the submaxillary nodes or posteriorly to the region between the trachea and esophagus. Metastasis is chiefly to regional lymph nodes, next in frequency to lungs and mediastinum. Bone metastases are frequent also.

The microscopic appearance of some metastases even in bone is indistinguishable from normal thyroid tissue.

The symptomatology of thyroid malignancy is essentially that of pressure. Gross alteration of the gland's function, either increase or decrease, very seldom occurs.

The course of thyroid malignancy is very variable. It may be fulminating, leading to death in a few months. This is often the case in those growths not preceded by benign thyroid enlargement. In other cases the rate of growth is very slow with little tendency to invasion and metastasis. Death may occur from general dissemination or from local pressure on trachea or esophagus.

Diagnosis.—The diagnosis, clinically, depends upon hardness and rapidity of growth. Rapidly increasing signs of pressure are very suggestive and evidence of fixation to adjacent structures, muscles or skin, practically pathognomonic. Differential diagnosis is chiefly from thyroiditis (*q.v.*) and from other malignant diseases of the neck.

Treatment.—The method of choice is operative removal. When the growth has not extended beyond the gland capsule and is confined to one lobe, radical cure is possible, or there may be no local recurrence but later metastasis. When invasion has taken place, complete removal is still possible by sacrificing the overlying muscles and other non-essential adnexa.

Operations for malignant goiter should be followed by roentgen-ray treatment and inoperable growths may be treated by this method alone. Thyroid malignancy often responds well to irradiation, the primary tumor better than metastases; but irradiation should not replace surgery even when only partial resection is possible. Papillary adenocarcinoma is especially amenable to treatment in these ways.

THYROIDITIS.

Inflammation of the thyroid, or thyroiditis, is rare, less than 1 per cent of all the cases of thyroid disease admitted to hospital. It may be acute or chronic. It may appear in persons with previously normal thyroids or in persons with preceding goiter.

Acute Thyroiditis.—In the acute form there is enlargement of the gland, tenderness and pain. Swallowing is often painful and obstructive symptoms may arise. Constitutional manifestations such as fever and leukocytosis may be present. The whole process may clear up in ten days, or go on to suppuration. The non-suppurative cases require nothing in the way of treatment beyond ice-collar, sedatives and the measures applicable to any acute infection. If suppuration occurs, incision and drainage are indicated. Thyroiditis arising in nodular goiter is the more likely to suppurate. Suppuration is dangerous because there may be extension into mediastinum or perforation into trachea or esophagus.

Chronic Thyroiditis.—Chronic thyroiditis may follow acute thyroiditis. It is a chronic fibrosing process leading sometimes to myxedema. Resection may be undertaken on account of the tumor or for persistent pain. When this is done myxedema is likely to follow. This, however, is easily relieved by thyroid. Microscopically a certain amount of interstitial thyroiditis is found in some of the glands removed from patients with exophthalmic goiter.

A special form of thyroiditis, so-called ligneous, has been described by Riedel (Riedel's struma). It is characterized by extreme hardness of the gland and its adherence to adjacent structures. It usually occurs in persons under forty years of age. Obstructive symptoms arise from the constricting action of the goiter. Operation has to be done on that account. Differential diagnosis is from malignant disease. It is difficult and may only be possible by microscopic examination of the tissue.

Another special form of thyroiditis is that described by Hashimoto. Four cases of this type have recently been reported by Graham and McCullagh. The picture is that of a diffuse hard enlargement of the thyroid with pressure symptoms. This struma does not adhere to neighboring structures as does Riedel's. The histology is peculiar. There is fibrosis of the gland together with lymphocytic infiltration and hyperplasia of lymphoid tissue. This type of struma is seen chiefly in women past forty years of age.

Tuberculosis and *syphilis of the thyroid gland* have been described but are extremely rare. There is a form of thyroiditis occurring in an insect-borne trypanosomiasis, Chagas disease, in South America.

DEVELOPMENTAL ANOMALIES OF THE THYROID GLAND.

In the embryo, the thyroid gland develops from an invagination of the anterior wall of the primitive pharynx, which descends as a cellular stalk to the neck, there to give rise to epithelial strands which become the thyroid gland. The connection with the pharynx, the thyroglossal duct, normally disappears. Imperfection in the development gives rise to certain anomalies which present problems in diagnosis and treatment.

The thyroglossal duct may persist and give rise to a thyroglossal cyst. These are found in the median line between the isthmus of the thyroid gland and the hyoid bone. They may become infected and rupture spontaneously or require incision. When this happens, a sinus results which can only be got rid of by complete removal of the cyst.

Aberrant thyroid tissue may be found in the region of the foramen cecum (lingual goiter), along the course of the thyroglossal duct (pyramidal lobe), or in the neck lateral to the usual thyroid, or in the mediastinum. Lateral aberrants are particularly important clinically as they seem to be especially likely foci of malignancy.

HYPOMETABOLISM WITHOUT MYXEDEMA.

It is becoming increasingly evident that a considerable number of persons presenting no clinical evidence of myxedema have basal metabolic rates well below the usually accepted range of normal. Some authors believe that these persons have a deficiency of thyroid function in spite of the absence of myxedema. Some of them doubtless have just that, which, and also for want of a better place, is sufficient excuse for grouping the lot under diseases of the thyroid. Nevertheless in many of them the thyroid probably has little if anything to do with the low metabolism. The reduction in metabolic rate in these cases is for the most part not greater than 20 per cent below standard, whereas in untreated myxedema the reduction is of the order of 35 per cent to 40 per cent below standard.

Some of the people exhibiting hypometabolism seem to be entirely healthy. Their hypometabolism is to be regarded as physiologic. It is lower than the usual, that is to say the standard, but is not to be considered pathologic for the individuals in question. It consequently requires treatment no more than does red hair or an habitual respiration rate of 6 per minute.

On the other hand, a considerable number of persons with non-myxedematous hypometabolism do have symptoms of one sort or another. There is, for example, a group of ptotic, neurotic individuals, chiefly women, suffering also from constipation and dysmenorrhea. Some of these are helped by thyroid, especially their constipation, others are not. A considerable number of very thin girls are seen nowadays and many of these prove to have hypometabolism. Many of them, paradoxically enough, will gain weight on thyroid. Although it raises their metabolism, it also increases their appetites and consequently improves their state of nutrition. A certain number of arthritics have low metabolism and, in some of these, thyroid seems to relieve the joint symptoms. There is a group of obese patients with low metabolism and in these it is proper to use thyroid to aid in weight reduction. Sometimes Ménière's syndrome is accompanied by hypometabolism and relieved by thyroid.

In general, regarding treatment of hypometabolism, it may be said that if symptoms of any sort exist which can conceivably be related to the hypometabolism, it is legitimate and reasonable to try the effect of thyroid therapy. This should be undertaken, however, with the understanding that it may prove useless and that, if it does, it will be abandoned.

THE THYROID PROBLEMS OF PREGNANCY.

It is important to the developing fetus that the mother shall have no diminution of thyroid function during pregnancy. The thyroid gland of the pregnant woman ordinarily undergoes a slight enlargement which doubtless is indication of increased function. Also the metabolic rate physiologically increases during pregnancy until it reaches about +15 per cent to +20 per cent in the fourth to sixth month.

If it be discovered that this physiologic increase is not taking place and particularly if there be symptoms suggestive of thyroid hypofunction, thyroid therapy should be begun and continued through pregnancy. Small doses, 1 to 2 grains daily, should suffice.

In women with goiters but without evidence of underfunction, it is well to give small doses of iodine, 20 per cent solution of potassium iodide, 2 minims (0.15 cc.) per week, throughout pregnancy.

A certain number of habitually aborting women are found who present low metabolic rates. Some of these will go through normal pregnancy if put on thyroid. Also sterile women with low rates have been described who became fertile when placed on thyroid.

Thyrotoxicosis and Pregnancy.—Thyrotoxic patients may become pregnant or pregnant ones become thyrotoxic. In either event, the indication for treatment is clear, namely, the usual treatment of toxic goiter, subtotal thyroidectomy after thorough iodinization. These patients stand operation well and the pregnancy usually is unaffected. If left untreated, they often miscarry and the thyrotoxicosis may be aggravated.

The physician is often asked whether previous exophthalmic goiter makes pregnancy inadvisable. The answer may be given unequivocally that it does not, provided the thyrotoxicosis has been completely abolished.

REFERENCES.

HARINGTON, C. R., and BARGER, G.: Chemistry of Thyroxine: Constitution and Synthesis of Thyroxine, Biochem. Jour., 1927, **21**, 169.

MARINE, D.: Etiology and Prevention of Simple Goiter, Medicine, 1924, **5**, 453.

MEANS, J. H., and RICHARDSON, E. P.: Diseases of the Thyroid, Oxford Monographs on Diagnosis and Treatment, New York, Oxford Press, 1929.

RIENHOFF, W. F., JR.: A New Conception of Some Morbid Changes Occurring in Diseases of the Thyroid Gland Based on Experimental Studies of the Normal Gland and the Thyroid in Exophthalmic Goiter, Medicine, 1931, **10**, 257.

SCHOCKAERT, J. A.: Enlargement and Hyperplasia of the Thyroids in the Young Duck from the Injection of Anterior Pituitary, Am. Jour. Anat., 1932, **49**, 379.

THE PARATHYROID GLANDS.

The parathyroid glands, usually four in number, rest upon the posterior aspect of the capsule of the thyroid or are embedded in its substance. They are very small, usually about 6 x 3 x 2 mm. in size. Their number is sometimes as high as twelve or as low as one. Their blood supply is very rich.

Function.—In spite of their small size, the parathyroids, unlike for example the adrenal medulla, and like the adrenal cortex, are necessary to life. Their function has to do chiefly, or perhaps solely, with the metabolism of calcium and phosphorus.

Complete parathyroidectomy gives rise to the following changes: (1) fall in serum calcium; (2) fall in urinary calcium excretion; (3) rise in serum phosphorus; (4) fall in urinary phosphorus excretion. Coincident with these biochemical changes there develops a state of hyperirritability of the nervous system, with the symptom-complex known as tetany. Complete parathyroidectomy in dogs, if untreated, leads to death in ten days or less. In addition to the convulsive state there is rapid emaciation and fall in temperature. It has been shown that a parathyroidectomized animal, however, can be kept alive for long periods if vigorously treated by administration of calcium salts.

In 1924 Collip obtained an extract from the parathyroids which will prevent or relieve tetany in parathyroidectomized animals. Study of this substance in normal humans has shown that it produces biochemical changes precisely opposite to those occasioned by parathyroidectomy, namely: (1) rise in serum calcium; (2) rise in urinary calcium excretion; (3) fall in serum phosphorus; (4) rise in urinary phosphorus excretion. Collip has shown that animals can be rapidly killed by excessive dosage with this extract. The serum calcium steadily mounts and later, after its initial fall, the serum phosphorus. Coincident with this the animal has vomiting, bloody diarrhea and respiratory distress. Blood volume diminishes; blood viscosity increases. The circulation gradually fails; the kidneys shut down and the animal passes into collapse.

Albright and Ellsworth, on the basis of their observations of the effect of the extract in man, have advanced the hypothesis that the primary action of its active principle is upon the rate of excretion of phosphorus. Increased excretion of phosphorus causes a fall in serum phosphorus. This brings about an unsaturation of the blood with calcium phosphate, which is met by a mobilization of calcium phosphate from the bones with resulting increase in serum calcium.

The function of the parathyroids, then, so far as known at present, is to manufacture a hormone which is present in Collip's extract, which has the actions upon calcium and phosphorus metabolism which have just been numerated. In light of the knowledge gained from the study of this hormone, it becomes apparent that there are conditions to be found clinically that represent the effect both of its presence in excess and of its shortage.

HYPOPARATHYROIDISM.

Synonym.—Parathyroid tetany.

A case of proven idiopathic hypoparathyroidism has been reported by Albright and Ellsworth. Such a condition may be regarded as the counterpart, in the case of the thyroid, of spontaneous myxedema.

Hypoparathyroidism, however, is most frequently encountered clinically in patients who have undergone thyroidectomies in which parathyroid tissue by accident has likewise been removed. The symptomatology in the idiopathic and postoperative varieties is the same, namely tetany, and the biochemistry is the same as that already described in the section on parathyroid function. The duration of the hypoparathyroid state in Albright's and Ellsworth's case was five years, at the time the patient came under observation, and in the postoperative cases the symptoms may continue over a period of years. In some cases of parathyroid tetany following thyroidectomy the hypofunction is temporary. In these, the blood supply of the glands may have been temporarily interrupted or sufficient parathyroid tissue remains eventually to supply, after hyperplasia has taken place, an adequate amount of hormone.

Tetany.—This syndrome, which constitutes the symptomatology of hypoparathyroidism but which may also result from other conditions in which there is calcium deficiency, such as rachitis, osteomalacia, sprue and other chronic diarrheas, is quite peculiar. The most characteristic manifestation is a sharp flexion of the wrist and ankle joints known as carpopedal spasm. The sequence of phenomena in developing tetany is frequently first irritability then paresthesiæ, muscle twitchings and cramps, and finally convulsions. Sometimes there are attacks of stridor which have been mistaken for asthma. The patient in the hypoparathyroid state may develop any of these phenomena on slight provocation.

Three signs are common to all forms of tetany: Chvostek's, which consists in twitching of the mouth and face upon tapping in the region of the facial nerve; Trousseau's, which is the production of carpal or pedal spasm by the constriction of the extremity above; and Erb's, which consists in increased electrical excitability of motor nerves.

Diagnosis of Parathyroid Tetany.—This is made first by the recognition of tetany from the phenomena just described and then by its separation from other forms of tetany. Tetany following thyroidectomy may be assumed at once to be of parathyroid origin. Tetany occurring otherwise is usually of some other origin. To make a diagnosis of idiopathic parathyroid tetany it would be necessary to demonstrate the biochemical changes characteristic of hypoparathyroidism. In the blood these would be low calcium and high phosphorus. In the tetany of rickets, calcium and phosphorus would both be low and in other forms of tetany they would probably be normal.

Treatment of Hypoparathyroidism.—The treatment consists in first securing an adequate intake of calcium. For acute phenomena calcium chloride may be given intravenously 5 to 10 cc. of 10 per cent solution. This can be repeated in several hours if necessary. Later on, oral administration may be substituted, as 10 cc. of a 30 per cent solution of anhydrous calcium chloride three times a day. This drug tends to produce an acidosis which in itself inhibits tetany; it also tends to raise the blood calcium. In cases of mild degree calcium in the form of a quart of milk a day, perhaps with calcium lactate, 5 grams, three times a day in addition, may be sufficient.

When calcium therapy alone does not suffice Collip's active principle, to which the name parathormone has been given, may be used in addition. The usual dosage is from 10 to 100 units of this substance given daily intramuscularly.

There are certain objections to the continued use of parathormone. It is expensive. It may produce painful local reactions. If given in conjunction with high calcium intake there is always some risk of hypercalcemia. Finally it has been found that when given continuously to a patient with hypoparathyroidism its efficacy gradually diminishes. In chronic cases, if given in very small doses such as 5 units per day, this difficulty may be avoided. It does not provide us with a totally adequate substitution therapy for permanent hypoparathyroidism in the way that thyroid does in myxedema. However, in certain cases we are obliged to use it, and in treating sudden severe phenomena resisting calcium it might be life-saving.

Viosterol, together with a high calcium intake, may suffice in certain cases. Also in the chronic case, thyroid may contribute some benefit, raising blood calcium by drawing on calcium stores.

HYPERPARATHYROIDISM.

Occasionally hyperparathyroidism results from the hyperfunctioning of diffusely hyperplastic parathyroids just as does the thyrotoxicosis of exophthalmic goiter result from the hyperfunctioning of a diffusely hyperplastic thyroid. In most of the reported cases, however, the hyperparathyroidism has been produced by the hyperfunctioning of a parathyroid tumor, such hyperparathyroidism being the counterpart of the hyperthyroidism produced by a hyperfunctioning thyroid adenoma. In a number of reported cases removal of such parathyroid tumors has abolished the evidence of parathyroid hyperfunction.

The morbid physiology of spontaneous hyperparathyroidism is no different from that following the administration to normal people of parathyroid hormone (*q.v.*). There is hypercalcemia, increased excretion of calcium by the kidneys and consequent loss of calcium from the skeleton, which if long continued often gives rise to a characteristic syndrome known as—

Osteitis Fibrosa Cystica Generalisata.—The picture in this condition is that of a progressive and deforming chronic bone disease. Spontaneous fractures are common. Bowing of the legs and kyphosis of the spine frequently occur. The contour of bones becomes markedly irregular; large bony swellings may be found in any part of the skeleton. Bony tumor of the jaw or epulis may be an initial manifestation. The patient may lose considerably in stature. Roentgen-ray examination shows marked generalized decalcification of bones, with numerous deformities in consequence. There are also numerous tumors and bone cysts of varying sizes with marked thinning of the bone cortex. The disease may occur at any age, and is about three times as common in females as in males. It may last for a number of years. If those afflicted do not die of intercurrent disease, they ultimately die of suffocation resulting from inability to lift the decalcified bony thorax. In many of the women the disease begins following pregnancy. It has been suggested that the parathyroid hyperplasia which may be physio-

53

logic in pregnancy may continue thereafter with the production of a hyperfunctioning adenoma.

Patients with chronic hyperparathyroidism also present polydipsia and polyuria due, in all probability, to the increased call of calcium and phosphorus for elimination, and kidney stones and gravel in the urine due to the increased output of these elements. There is loss of weight which is not apparent because it is mineral loss. Weakness, hypotonia of muscles and relaxation of ligaments are also common and the opposite of what is found in tetany. Some secondary anemia usually occurs.

Other Clinical Types.—It has been pointed out by Albright, Aub and Bauer that not always does hyperparathyroidism present the picture of classic osteitis fibrosa cystica. In some cases, for example, the bony changes are insignificant and extensive calcification of the kidneys (nephrocalcinosis) is the major lesion. In this type there may be actual renal insufficiency with the symptoms of Bright's disease. An osteoporotic form without bone cysts may be mentioned, and those in which urinary calculi constitute the presenting lesion.

Diagnosis of Hyperparathyroidism.—This depends upon the clinical finding of osteitis fibrosa cystica, or one of the other clinical pictures mentioned, and the chemical demonstration of increased blood calcium, decreased blood phosphorus and increased loss of calcium in the urine.

The differential diagnosis is from other bone diseases which may bear a clinical resemblance, e. g., osteoporosis, osteomalacia, Paget's disease or osteitis deformans, and multiple myeloma, also from other types of urinary calculi and from diabetes insipidus, Bright's disease, and other diseases accompanied by polyuria. Metastatic bone neoplasms might occasionally come up for differentiation. In none of these would the characteristic biochemical findings of hyperparathyroidism be present. In osteomalacia serum calcium and phosphorus would both be low. In multiple myeloma blood calcium may be high but phosphorus will not be low. In the other diseases just mentioned they would probably be normal. The roentgen-ray pictures are also quite different.

Treatment of Hyperparathyroidism.—The most successful treatment so far has been the removal of hyperfunctioning parathyroid tumor tissue or subtotal parathyroidectomy in the cases with diffuse hyperplasia. To a certain extent the decalcification can be prevented or diminished by diet high in both calcium and phosphorus. This can be accomplished by giving calcium glycerophosphate, 1 tablespoonful five times a day in a quart of milk.

REFERENCES.

ALBRIGHT, F., AUB, J. C., and BAUER, W.: Hyperparathyroidism a Common and Polymorphic Condition, Jour. Am. Med. Assn., 1934, 102, 1276.
ALBRIGHT, F., and ELLSWORTH, R.: Studies on the Physiology of the Parathyroid Glands, Jour. Clin. Invest., 1929, 7, 183.
COLLIP, J. B.: The Parathyroid Glands, Medicine, 1926, 5, 1; also published in The Harvey Lectures, Series XXI, Baltimore, Williams & Wilkins Company, 1927.
MACCALLUM, W. G., and VOEGTLIN, C.: On the Relation of Tetany to the Parathyroid Glands and Calcium Metabolism, Jour. Exper. Med., 1909, 11, 118.

THE ADRENAL GLANDS.

The paired adrenal or suprarenal capsules consist of two parts, medulla and cortex, which, although in close proximity, have as far as known totally different functions and are of different embryonic origin. The medulla, being derived from sympathetic ganglionic tissue, is consequently of ectodermal origin; the cortex, being derived from the cœlomic endothelium, is of mesodermal origin.

Function of the Adrenal Medulla.—The medulla, made up of cells of sympathetic nervous origin, but at the same time to be regarded as gland cells, is a part of the so-called chromaffin system to which the carotid bodies and the paraganglionic bodies also belong. Its sole function, so far as known at present is the secretion of the hormone epinephrin, a substance having a varied and striking physiologic action. This hormone was crystallized by Takamine in 1901 and synthesized by Stolz in 1906. The rate of secretion of the hormone, as Cannon has shown, is powerfully influenced by the nervous system. States of violent emotion, such as fear and rage, also pain and asphyxia, greatly increase its output.

The action of epinephrin is difficult to describe for the reason that in high concentration it may act differently than in low. It also may act differently in one species than in another and in any one species its action will vary with the preëxisting state of the organism. The effects to be noted after the injection of epinephrin are the same as those which follow stimulation of the sympathetic nerve fibers. In fact, epinephrin acts upon the neuromotor junctions of the sympathetic system and gives the same result therefore as stimulation of its fibers. There is constriction of certain arteries, especially those which supply the abdominal viscera, no effect on others and possibly dilatation of yet others. The smooth muscle of the intestinal tract and bronchial tract is relaxed. Intestinal peristalsis is inhibited. Liver glycogen is converted into glucose and delivered to the blood stream, thus producing hyperglycemia and glycosuria.

The rate of general metabolism is raised. In other words epinephrin has a calorigenic action as does thyroxin. It is a much more rapid one, however. After the injection into a human subject of 10 mg. of thyroxin the peak of the calorigenic response is reached in from three to five days and the effect takes much longer than that to wear off. After the injection of 0.625 mg. of epinephrin, the calorigenic peak is reached in about thirty minutes and the effect wears off in from one and one-half to two hours more.

In the human, after the injection of such a dose of epinephrin, there are symptoms such as consciousness of heart beat, throbbing in the head, unrest in the chest, increased irritability, sweating and breathlessness. Sometimes full-blown angina pectoris is produced. The pulse-rate, pulse pressure, systolic pressure and pulmonary ventilation all increase essentially parallel to the metabolic rate. The diastolic pressure falls.

This behavior of the blood pressure in the human, the widening of pulse pressure and falling of diastolic pressure, can hardly be interpreted on the basis of a total vasomotor effect of vasoconstriction. Rather is it due to a marked increase in total blood flow, which can be demonstrated by minute volume observations. The mass movement of blood in man is markedly augmented by epinephrin, the increase being not parallel to, but relatively far greater than the increase in metabolism. The stroke volume of the heart is increased and with this comes the increase in pulse pressure. Direct application of epinephrin to the heart causes great increase in force of contraction.

Finally epinephrin has the remarkable property of directly combating most of the untoward effects of anaphylaxis.

The effect of deprivation of the organism of epinephrin has been determined by Cannon and his co-workers in connection with their studies of complete sympathectomy. Sympathectomized animals show none of the evidences of discharge of epinephrin upon provocation which produces such evidence in normal animals. In other words there is no evidence that the denervated adrenals secrete epinephrin. Yet sympathectomized cats can live sheltered lives apparently as well as normal cats. So, too, can cats in which removal of one adrenal and demedullation of the other has been done in addition to total sympathectomy. The hormone epinephrin therefore is not necessary to normal existence under certain conditions of external environment.

The function of epinephrin appears to be chiefly concerned with the stimulation of the sympathetic nervous system and in this way the preparation of the organism rapidly and efficiently to adjust its internal organization to meet alterations threatened by sudden change imposed by the external environment, a process to which Cannon has given the name of homeostasis.

The secretion of epinephrin, therefore, at least in amounts necessary to play a part in homeostasis, is certainly intermittent. Whether during quiet life any secretion takes place is unknown. If there is, according to Hoskins, it is below the threshold necessary to stimulate the sympathetic nervous system.

Function of the Adrenal Cortex.—The cortex, in striking contrast to the medulla, is necessary to life. Animals, as has been already stated, may live indefinitely, apparently healthily, with no medullary tissue. Deprived of all cortical tissue, on the other hand, they promptly die. Yet what the action of the active principle or principles produced by the cortex may be is largely unknown. Hartman, and also Swingle and Pfiffner, have obtained cortical extracts free from epinephrin and toxic substances which will keep completely adrenalectomized animals alive for an indefinite period. That of Swingle and Pfiffner is now on the market under the trade name of eschatin (Parke, Davis & Co.). A possible instance of the effect of an excessive secretion of the active principle of the cortex is to be found in the case of certain new-growths of cortical tissue. The effect seems to be solely on the genitalia and the secondary sex characters. The female takes on the characters of the male, and in the male, masculinity is intensified.

The symptomatology attendant upon disturbed function of the adrenals can be discussed to best advantage in connection with the description of the various clinical pictures known to be associated with disease of these glands.

ADDISON'S DISEASE.

This malady was first described by Addison in 1855 and was recognized by him to be due to disease of the adrenal glands. He identified as among its cardinal manifestations asthenia, feeble heart action, irritability of the stomach and pigmentation; in fact, but little of importance has been added to our knowledge of the disease since his original description.

Etiology.—The symptoms and signs of the disease are clearly due to destruction of adrenal tissue by disease and since the full clinical picture has been observed in cases with anatomically normal medulla it is now thought that destruction of the cortex is chiefly, if not solely, responsible for its production. Only lesions which involve both adrenals can produce the picture.

A recent study by Guttman of 566 cases reported in the literature provides excellent statistical information concerning etiology, duration and incidence. In 60 per cent the destructive lesion of the adrenals was tuberculous; in 16 per cent it was primary atrophy. In the remainder there were such conditions as amyloid disease, new-growths, vascular lesions, syphilis, fatty degeneration and pyogenic infections. Bilateral metastatic tumors of the adrenals are not uncommon, but rarely if ever produce Addison's disease, probably because they do not completely destroy the cortical tissue.

The incidence may be accurately inferred from the death reports, since the disease is invariably fatal. For the years 1923 and 1924 the death-rate was 0.4 per 100,000 population for the registration area of the United States. The general death-rate for 1923 was 12.3 per 1000 and for 1924 11.8 per 1000, and that from all forms of tuberculosis was 93.6 per 100,000 in 1923 and 90.4 per 100,000 for 1924.

The peak of the age incidence is in the fourth decade of life, although the disease has been reported at all ages from childhood to senescence. The atrophic form of the disease is more common in females than in males.

Course of the Disease.—The onset of Addison's disease is variable. Sometimes it is very insidious with pigmentation for a considerable time the only manifestation; in other cases there is a rather rapid development of asthenia, with but little pigmentation. A history of tuberculous adenitis in the past is common. Generalized or active tuberculosis elsewhere in the body occurs but is rare during the course of Addison's disease. The course may be progressively downward or there may be definite remissions and relapses. Sometimes the patient's condition remains stationary for several months, then suddenly enters a period of active progression. There is a strong tendency to rather sudden crises of prostration and collapse, during which the picture is that of vasomotor shock, vomiting and dehydration. It has been shown that loss of sodium and chloride plays a very important rôle in the production of these crises. Both adrenalectomized animals and patients with Addison's disease eliminate a large portion of the sodium chloride they ingest, and, unless this loss is offset by an excessive salt intake, the drainage leads to disaster. It is to be presumed that the cortical hormone is either directly concerned with salt metabolism or indirectly through an action on the kidney. Death may occur during crisis or the patient may improve and return at least to his condition prior to the crisis. Sudden death may also occur at any time without obvious cause. As in diabetes, intercurrent infection tends to aggravate the disease.

It has been observed that those patients who develop early pigmentation run a more chronic course than those with early asthenia. Severe diarrhea and vomiting indicate a rapid downward course. The average duration of the disease in the former has been given as forty-three months and the latter as seven months. It has also been observed that in the tuberculous variety the course is shorter, average thirteen months, than in the atrophic variety, average thirty-four months. Very few patients live over five years.

Pathology.—The tuberculous variety is usually secondary to tuberculosis elsewhere, chiefly in the lungs, which has often healed and escaped recognition clinically. The infection of the adrenals is presumably blood-borne. The medulla appears more susceptible than the cortex and is usually completely destroyed. Remains of the cortex can be made out in most cases. Cases are found at autopsy in which there has been bilateral destruction of the medullas of both adrenals without any clinical evidence of Addison's disease.

The tuberculous process invariably involves both adrenals, though often one gland shows more recent and less extensive involvement than its mate. The explanation has been offered for the bilateral involvement that sensitization of one organ to the tubercle bacillus or its products follows upon infection of the other.

In the atrophic variety the pathologic picture is one of slow necrosis involving the cortical cells and leading finally to their disappearance. Partial function may be maintained by small surviving nodules of cortical cells. The cause of the atrophy is as unknown as is that of the thyroid in myxedema.

Symptoms.—Associated with the weak heart action described by Addison, there is often a marked hypotension with low pulse pressure. This, however, is not invariably present and cannot be regarded as an essential part of the syndrome. It was formerly thought to be a manifestation of hypofunction of the medulla. In the light of present knowledge this seems unlikely, since complete destruction of the medulla may occur without fall in pressure. It is of a sort which is greatly influenced by posture, in the upright position systolic, diastolic and pulse pressure all being considerably lower than in the recumbent. In the upright position, too, the pulse-rate is accelerated. Rowntree and Snell find the usual systolic pressure in Addison's disease to be between 90 and 100. Systolic pressure below 70 indicates a critical condition. Attacks of severe dyspnea sometimes occur.

The pigmentation is of considerable interest. It may be the first sign of the disease. It is the normal skin pigment melanin but is deposited in excess of what is normal for the individual. The color is essentially brownish. It varies greatly in intensity and distribution. The exposed parts tend to be the most highly pigmented. All skin folds tend to become deeply pigmented. This is well seen in the creases of the palms of the hands, axillæ and groins. Scars of any sort are likely to become deeply pigmented. Black freckles are sometimes seen. The distribution may be very patchy or it may tend to evenness, so that as it gradually deepens the white person may come to resemble the negro. A characteristic of some importance is the pigmentation of the mucous membrane. This is seen best in the oral cavity where it usually takes the form of brownish spots of varying size scattered over the gums, palate and inner aspect of the cheeks. Areas that have been traumatized by teeth are especially apt to become pigmented. Occasionally cases of apparently true Addison's disease have been found with no pigmentation.

It has been suggested that the pigmentation represents a faulty synthesis of epinephrin. A certain precursor of epinephrin is also a precursor of melanin. When, because of destruction of the adrenals, epinephrin ceases to be formed this precursor collects in the skin and is converted into melanin. One objection to this theory is that pigmentation may occur when the medulla is intact, but that could be explained on the supposition that some product of the cortex is necessary to the synthesis of epinephrin by the medulla.

There is usually progressive wasting, but this is not always the case. Temperature is normal or low unless active tuberculosis is present outside the adrenals.

The gastro-intestinal symptoms consist in anorexia, sometimes extreme, nausea, vomiting, occasionally diarrhea. In the terminal stages vomiting may be intense. It is often present in the crises and contributes to the dehydration.

The asthenia is both physical and mental. Marked increase in fatigability is characteristic. The increased fatigability of muscle can be shown graphically by ergographic tracings. These serve as one of the few quantitative methods of measuring the severity of the morbid state. Apathy and sometimes other mental symptoms occur. Convulsions and coma have been observed, particularly in the more acute cases and sudden exercise may produce syncope. All these phenomena are probably related to hypoglycemia. Diminution in hearing and vision have been described. Speech may become weak and slow. In the later stages even talking is hard work.

Menstruation may be either excessive or scant. In the male, decrease in sexual desire and power usually occurs. Women, however, may become pregnant when well advanced in the disease and, when they do, rather remarkably improve. Improvement may last through lactation. Temporary improvement in symptoms has been noted during menstruation. In pregnancy the improvement occurs before the fetal adrenals are formed. During pregnancy there is a physiologic hypertrophy of the adrenal cortex. In Addison's disease pregnancy may call forth added function of the cortex which remains, or it is possible that the corpus luteum may to a certain extent be able to take on the function of the lost cortex. It has also been suggested that the pituitary hyperplasia of pregnancy is responsible for the improvement.

In brief, then, present evidence lends weight chiefly to the theory that the syndrome described by Addison is largely if not entirely the result of lost cortical function with loss of chloride and sodium playing an important rôle in the mechanism. It differs from that resulting from experimental removal of the glands, in that the destruction is gradual, so that only toward the end does the lack of cortical function become complete. In the tuberculous variety there is the added effect of active tuberculosis, although this does not greatly modify the picture, provided it is active in the adrenal glands alone.

Diagnosis.—This depends upon the finding of the clinical features described. Pigmentation and asthenia are usually the first to give the clue. On account of the former, differential diagnosis is from other pigmented states, arsenic poisoning, hemochromatosis, vitiligo and other forms of tuberculous disease. In these other forms of pathologic pigmentation the mucous membranes are seldom involved. On account of wasting, weakness and gastro-intestinal symptoms, as well as the pigmentation, abdominal cancer must be ruled out. On account of the muscle fatigability, myasthenia gravis and other myasthenias may come up for differential diagnosis.

Of laboratory tests the blood sugar is often low and sugar tolerance is often high. The basal metabolism is usually moderately depressed but none of these findings are of great diagnostic importance. In the tuberculous form calcification of the adrenals can often be demonstrated by roentgen-ray.

Treatment.—Substitution therapy by means of cortin is now possible (in the average case 1 or 2 cc. of "eschatin" once daily subcutaneously). The commercial extract is still very expensive. The rôle of salt is very important. With a low salt intake more cortin is required to maintain life than when the supply of salt is abundant. In the average case something like 10 grams of sodium chloride daily in addition to the salt of the diet is desirable. Patients may be carried for considerable periods on high salt alone without cortin. In these it may be necessary to give cortin only intermittently. No rule can be laid down. The individual case must be studied.

Patients with Addison's disease are hypersensitive to cold, and avoidance of chilling is important.

If crisis or collapse occurs patients should be kept absolutely still. They bear transportation badly and are likely to die suddenly at any time particularly if disturbed. On account of the vomiting fluids are withheld by mouth. Large doses of cortin (perhaps 20 cc. of eschatin intravenously) together with forced intravenous saline and glucose, and keeping the patient warm are the agents imperatively indicated.

HYPERFUNCTION OF THE ADRENAL MEDULLA.

So far as the writer is aware, authentic instances of hyperfunction of the adrenal medulla have been met with only in association with tumors. It has been suggested that ordinary essential hypertension is caused by persistent hyperfunction of the adrenal medulla, but this theory lacks proof and is no more tenable than the view that vasomotor shock is due to adrenal insufficiency.

Tumors of the adrenal medulla, however, have been described which almost certainly have been productive of medullary hyperfunction. Patients suffering from such tumors have paroxysmal attacks of symptoms bearing a striking resemblance to those which follow the injection of epinephrin. Sudden marked elevations in blood pressure are characteristic and, along with these, as in the case reported by Pincoffs, violent heart action, oppression in the chest, feeling of apprehension, throbbing in the head and sensation of heat. In a similar case reported by C. H. Mayo, in which the tumor was called a retroperitoneal malignant blastoma, there was in addition nausea and vomiting, headache and, in the more severe attacks, actual acute pulmonary edema.

The removal of the tumors in both Mayo's and Pincoffs' cases entirely relieved the symptoms. The intermittent or paroxysmal character of the symptoms in both these suggests that these tumors pour forth epinephrin intermittently in a fashion similar to that in which Cannon believes the normal medulla functions. The tumor removed in Pincoffs' case had a high epinephrin content.

HYPERFUNCTION OF THE ADRENAL CORTEX.

Changes in the genitalia and secondary sex characters are the only manifestations that we can as yet safely consider as hormonic in nature and attributable to hyperfunction of the adrenal cortex. The changes are in either sex usually in the direction of increased masculinity, although in certain female children it may cause precocious menstruation. The syndrome has been called by Gallais "le syndrome génito-surrénal."

The female child may be born with, or acquire, pseudohermaphroditism. There is early development of the secondary sex characters of the male (virilism). The male child shows precocious puberty and sexual precocity, not, however, increase in spermatogenesis.

Cortical tumors in women, with sexual changes, have been reported by a number of writers. The one of Gordon Holmes may be taken as a fair illustration. He summarized the findings as follows: "The case . . . is that of a young woman in whom a large slowly growing tumour of the right suprarenal body was associated with changes in the sexual organs (atrophy of the uterus, overgrowth of clitoris), disturbances of the sexual functions (cessation of menstruation for nine years), alteration in the secondary sexual characters (growth of hair, atrophy of mammæ, change in the distribution of fat, and masculine appearance in limbs) and psychical changes (loss of erotic feelings, lack of modesty), all of which symptoms disappeared within a relatively short time after the removal of the tumour and left the patient again an apparently normal woman." The histology of the tumor bore a very close resemblance to normal cortical tissue.

The chief importance of recognizing adrenal virilism is because of the possibility of its cure by the removal of a tumor.

OTHER DISEASES OF THE ADRENAL GLANDS.

A variety of tumors of both cortex and medulla, benign and malignant, are recognized by pathologists. These may or may not be accompanied by hormonic manifestations. They are all rare.

The so-called hypernephroma of the kidney, which is by no means rare, was in the past supposed to arise from adrenal tissue. There is now some doubt as to the correctness of this view and certainly these tumours never produce evidence of increased medullary or cortical function.

Hemorrhage into the adrenals may occur in new-born infants from the trauma of labor. In older children and adults it is very rare. Bilateral hemorrhage into the adrenals sometimes causes hyperpyrexia and has been given as a cause of sudden death.

REFERENCES.

HARTMAN, F. A., BROWNELL, K. A., HARTMAN, W. E., DEAN, G. A., and MAC-ARTHUR, C. G.: The Hormone of the Adrenal Cortex, Am. Jour. Physiol., 1928, **86**, 358.

LOEB, R. F.: Chemical Changes in the Blood in Addison's Disease, Science, 1932, **76**, 420.

LOEB, R.F., ATCHLEY, D. W., BENEDICT, E. M., and LELAND, J.: Jour. Exp. Med., 1933, **57**, 775.

ROWNTREE, L. G., and SNELL, A. M.: Clinical Study of Addison's Disease, Philadelphia, W. B. Saunders Company, 1931.

SWINGLE, W. W., and PFIFFNER, J. J.: Studies on the Adrenal Cortex, Am. Jour. Physiol., 1931, **96**, 153, 165, 180.

THE PITUITARY GLANDS.

The pituitary gland, or hypophysis, possesses two lobes anatomically and embryologically distinct, one of which probably produces four active principles, the other at least two. The anterior lobe, derived from the oral ectoderm, has a glandular structure somewhat resembling the thyroid. It possesses three types of cells with different staining properties, acidophilic and basophilic, which probably have different secretory functions, also certain chromophobe cells which may have no secretory function. The posterior, derived from the brain, is made up of ependymal and neuroglia cells and bears but little resemblance to other glandular structures. In this respect it is somewhat akin to the adrenal medulla.

The anterior lobe of the gland is necessary to life. Thus it has been shown by Cushing and others that experimental removal of the whole gland, or of the anterior lobe, rapidly causes death. Removal of the posterior lobe only, however, causes little in the way of symptoms. Partial removal of the anterior lobe causes obesity and sexual infantilism. These relationships remind us of the adrenal where the glandular cortex is necessary to life and the nervous medulla is not.

The clinical manifestations of pituitary disease can be divided into the hormonic, that is to say those produced by over or under supply of one or more of the several active principles, and neighborhood, that is to say those produced mechanically by enlargement of, or pressure upon, the gland in its narrow quarters within the skull. Owing to the multiplicity of hormones, the supply of which is by no means always increased or decreased in parallel fashion, it is misleading to speak of hyper- or hypofunction of the gland as a whole as hyper- or hypopituitarism in the way we do of the thyroid or parathyroid glands, which so far as known produce a single hormone.

The Anterior Lobe Hormones.—The presence in the anterior lobe of a principle promoting growth in general, with the production therefore of giants, has been proved by various investigators in various ways. Uhlenhuth (1921) showed that feeding anterior lobe to salamanders produced gigantism. Evans and Long (1921) produced giant rats by injecting an emulsion of anterior lobe. While in these species the effect is on growth of essentially all tissues with the production of oversized but well-proportioned animals, in other species the growth may be disproportionate. Thus Putnam and his collaborators have shown that in the dog, an animal in which the bony epiphyses become closed in contrast to the rat in which they do not, the injection of an anterior lobe extract produces not only gigantism but also specific enlargement of "acral parts" and in fact an experimental syndrome altogether similar to human acromegaly (*q. v.*).

Separable from the growth-promoting hormone is the sex hormone. It is sex non-specific. That is to say, the hormone obtained from the pituitaries of either male or female animal will activate the gonads of both sexes. By stimulating the gonads to produce their hormones it influences the entire reproductive system. It has no action, therefore, in gonadectomized animals. It brings about the sexual development occurring in either sex at puberty. The attainment of sexual maturity is impossible in its absence. Its action is to be distinguished from that of the adrenal cortex hormone, which produces changes in the direction of increased masculinity in either sex. It has been shown that the pituitary sex hormone does not require any intermediary action by the adrenal cortex, or any other gland outside the gonads themselves. The sex hormone has been shown by Zondek actually to be two hormones which he has called Prolan A and Prolan B. The action of these will be discussed in the Section on the Female Gonads (*q. v.*).

In addition to its growth-promoting and sex functions, the anterior lobe also exerts a calorigenic action resembling thyroxin and has been claimed in addition to intensify the specific dynamic action of foodstuffs. In the animals of Putnam *et al.*, cited above, injected with anterior lobe extracts, the thyroids became hyperplastic and took on a histologic appearance much like that in human exophthalmic goiter. It seems probable that the calorigenic action of the anterior pituitary depends upon the mediation of the thyroid, in fact the principle involved may be looked upon as a thyrotropic hormone of the anterior pituitary.

In addition there are a number of other recently discovered anterior pituitary actions which may be termed insulo-tropic, diabeto-tropic, adreno-tropic and parathyro-tropic. An extract which directly stimulates lactation, prolactin, has been obtained by Riddle. It would not be sound to interpret all these actions as indication of separate hormones at the present time.

The Posterior Lobe Hormones.—Posterior lobe extract is essentially a drug and appears as such in the U. S. Pharmacopœia under the name Liquor Pituitarii. This preparation contains at least two active principles. It is widely used in medical practice for its pharmacologic action in symptomatic treatment, and in this rôle it does not further concern us. Its use resembles more that of epinephrin than any other of the internal secretions. The only instance of its use in pituitary disease is in the case of *diabetes insipidus*. This disease is the only one definitely attributed to the posterior lobe of the pituitary and it is not absolutely clear that even this should be. Also it is not clear whether the use of posterior lobe extract in this disease for its antidiuretic action is to be considered true substitution therapy, in the sense for example that thyroxin is in myxedema.

In 1928 Kamm *et al.* were able to separate, in highly pure form, two active posterior lobe principles. One, which they called alpha-hypophamine, causes contraction of the uterus and the smooth muscle of the bowel (also called oxytocin or pitocen). The other, which they called beta-hypophamine (also called vasopressin or pitressin), raises blood pressure and has a diuretic-antidiuretic action.

The posterior pituitary is also concerned in fat metabolism. An injection of whole lobe extract causes a fall in blood fat.

Symptoms.—The neighborhood symptoms, that is, those resulting mechanically from enlargement of the gland, are chiefly headache, usually bitemporal, and primary optic atrophy with consequent restriction of the visual fields, usually bitemporal hemianopsia. Mental dullness may result from encroachment of a pituitary growth on the frontal lobe. Sometimes there are fits, especially of the uncinate type. Evidence of general increased intracranial pressure such as choked disks is rare.

Of the endocrine or hormonic manifestations some can readily be attributed to over or under supply of one of the known hormones. Others are less easy of interpretation. It should be recalled that the effects of the same hormone may be different, if the excess or shortage occurs during the growth period, from what they are in the adult. Also clinical pictures may be complicated by an alternation of periods of oversecretion and undersecretion with certain features of one lasting over into the effective period of the other. Some of the more important hormonic signs are as follows:

Excess of growth hormone during the growth period gives rise to overgrowth of all bones as well as soft parts, with gigantism of about normal proportions. When the excess begins in adult life, there is not gigantism but merely overgrowth of the acral, short and flat bones only. The jaw becomes large (prognathism); the bony prominences increase; the bones of hands and feet become wide and dense with terminal tufting and exostoses. Both upper and lower teeth become separated owing to growth of jaw bones. There is also thickening of soft parts over head, hands and feet, and enlargement of the viscera.

Shortage of the growth hormone during the growth period gives rise to dwarfism. This may be proportionate or the extremities may be relatively shorter than the trunk. Shortage beginning in adult life would give less striking changes. Slender, tapering fingers and genu valgum may be attributed to it.

Excess of the pituitary sex hormone may be responsible for certain cases of sexual precocity in either sex. Shortage during the growth period produces genital infantilism and prevents development of the secondary sex characters. In the adult female, shortage produces amenorrhea; in the male, impotence; and in both sexes, sterility.

The hormonic signs of the posterior lobe are less easy to identify. Polyuria may be taken to be due to a shortage of beta-hypophamine. At any rate it is sometimes most remarkably controlled by the use of posterior lobe extract (so-called pituitrin). Lowered sugar tolerance and glycosuria may be the result of a posterior lobe hyperfunction of some sort, and high sugar tolerance of posterior lobe hypofunction.

Pituitary hypermetabolism, seen chiefly in association with acromegaly and gigantism, is believed by some writers to be due to a posterior lobe hyperfunction. It is more likely due to true hyperthyroidism induced by the thyrotropic action of the anterior lobe of the pituitary. So, too, is the hypometabolism seen in the syndromes of insufficiency of growth and sex hormone more likely an anterior than a posterior lobe hypofunction.

The mechanism of pituitary adiposity, which has the characteristic of being chiefly about the pelvic girdle and not at all in the face or extremities, is not clear. It may be related to the supply of the calorigenic principle of the anterior lobe or to the fat regulating action of the posterior lobe.

Methods of Examination.—In case of suspected pituitary disease, examination first of all consists in careful search for all the hormonic manifestations that have been enumerated. The history should include careful inquiry into urinary output, menstrual phenomena, libido and sexual power, headache, and visual disturbances.

The roentgen-ray gives important evidence chiefly as to the shape and size of the sella turcica which is enlarged in acromegaly and often reduced in size in certain other pituitary dystrophies. Changes in the skeleton due to excess of the growth hormone may also be first picked up radiologically. Exostoses, especially of the terminal phalanges, with shirt stud appearance, are characteristic.

Examination of the fields of vision by perimetry is very important. In any pituitary disease associated with enlargement of the gland there may be limitation. The characteristic type is that of blindness of the nasal sides of the retina, that is to say, bitemporal hemianopsia. Ophthalmoscopy should be done to detect choking of the disks.

Metabolic studies such as that of sugar tolerance and basal metabolic rate are indicated.

ACROMEGALY.

This syndrome in the light of modern knowledge is to be regarded as primarily due to hyperfunction of the anterior lobe of the pituitary and its most striking manifestation, overgrowth of the acral parts of the skeleton, the chest and flat bones, the bony prominences, is unquestionably due to an excess of the growth hormone.

The anatomic findings in the pituitary are those of hyperplasia or actual adenomatous tumor of the acidophilic cells of the anterior lobe.

Diagnosis.—The diagnosis rests solely on the recognition of the characteristic change in bodily habitus. The lower jaw becomes enlarged and protrudes (prognathism), the brows become prominent. The teeth become separated owing to growth of the maxillæ. The hands and feet become enlarged owing to growth of all the small bones and the spine often develops a forward bending. The soft parts also are thickened. The nose and lips become enlarged and the skin becomes coarse. The fingers are very wide with blunt ends. The picture in its full development is unmistakable. By roentgen-ray the sella turcica is found enlarged. The frontal sinuses are often huge. Diagnosis must include an estimate of the probability of tumor. This is judged from the intensity of the neighborhood symptoms.

Differential diagnosis is from other bony diseases such as Paget's and occasionally from a very marked grade of chronic pulmonary osteoarthropathy. The resemblance to either of them is superficial. In neither of these are the changes in the bones of the face characteristic of acromegaly present.

Course of the Disease.—The onset is usually between twenty and forty years and the sexes are afflicted in about equal numbers. The characteristic habitus may attain its development in a few months. During this phase there are apt to be associated symptoms such as headache, menstrual irregularities and decreased sexual power and desire. The growth hormone seems to be produced by the eosinophilic cells; the sex hormone very likely by the basophilic cells of the anterior lobe. The proliferation of the former in acromegaly may encroach upon the latter so that coincidentally with the excess production of growth hormone there is decreased production of sex hormone. Asthenia and loss of strength are common. If tumor is present neighborhood symptoms may develop at this time. There also may be evidence of posterior lobe involvement, as polyuria or glycosuria, these being due to posterior lobe hypofunction, possibly caused by encroachment upon the posterior lobe by an enlarged anterior lobe. It is during this stage that the basal metabolism is increased and sometimes one finds thyroid fullness together with the manifestations characteristic of hyperthyroidism.

In women, a number of cases begin at pregnancy and indeed it is possible to discover very slight changes of habitus suggestive of acromegaly in many women after pregnancy. Erdheim first described hypertrophy of the pituitary as a feature of normal pregnancy and it seems likely that, coincident with the extra supply of the sex hormone which undoubtedly is put forth by the pituitary during pregnancy, there is in some women some excess of growth hormone put forth as well.

In the cases unassociated with tumor, after a certain period, months to a few years, an inactive stage is reached. The acromegalic habitus, at least that directly dependent on bony change, remains for the duration of life. The soft part changes may recede. The condition may remain stationary for years, and is not inconsistent with good health and does not necessarily shorten life.

Treatment.—In cases associated with tumor, the treatment is surgical decompression or resection. In those accompanied by simple hyperplasia the roentgen-ray offers some prospect of converting the hyperfunction into a hypofunction. If this were applied very early in the active stage it might arrest the development of the bony changes. In those cases in which phenomena of posterior lobe hypofunction are present, polyuria for example, substitution therapy in the shape of posterior lobe extracts may offer much. Posterior lobe extract has a profound antidiuretic effect in diabetes insipidus to which polyuria associated with acromegaly is akin. Pituitary glycosuria which may accompany acromegaly is to be regarded as a posterior lobe hyperfunction of some sort. It would only require treatment if it had assumed the characteristics of diabetes mellitus, and then should be treated as that malady is.

When, in the early stages of the disease, the thyroid is enlarged and the metabolic rate elevated, a response to iodine may be secured entirely comparable to that in exophthalmic goiter. Iodine should be tried in acromegaly whenever the symptoms of hyperthyroidism are present.

In the later stages of acromegaly, when the picture is rather that of anterior lobe underfunction, the use of one of the new preparations containing the sex hormone offers something.

GIGANTISM.

Gigantism is undoubtedly due to hyperfunction of the anterior lobe of the pituitary, with the production of an excess of the growth hormone during childhood before the union of the epiphyses. Not only is growth accelerated by the excess of growth hormone but also the period of growth is extended because an associated decrease in production of sex hormone, as in acromegaly (*q. v.*) with sexual infantilism, delays the union of the epiphyses. Under such circumstances the increased growth of the various tissues and organs is parallel, thus giving proportionate gigantism. If the hyperfunction persists after union of the epiphyses the acromegalic habitus may be superimposed upon the gigantic.

Gigantism is not infrequently associated with pituitary tumor and consequently accompanied by neighborhood symptoms.

Giants are apt to be weakly and of inferior intelligence. They seldom live beyond forty years.

In treatment both surgery and roentgen-ray offer something, particularly in the cases associated with tumor.

SIMMONDS' DISEASE.

This rare syndrome, cachexia hypophyseopriva, first described in 1914, is a type of cachexia associated with atrophy of the anterior lobe of the pituitary, supervening in adult life in either sex. It represents the effect, presumably, of complete deprivation in adult life of all the anterior lobe hormones.

Symptoms.—The picture is that of progressive emaciation, asthenia and cachexia. There is loss of teeth and pubic and axillary hair, and the appearance of smallness and premature senility. There is amenorrhea and sterility in the female, impotence and loss of sexual desire in the male. The disease may progress for several years, often with gradually developing psychosis and ending in coma and death. There are certain points of resemblance to myxedema, dislike of cold, subnormal temperature and hypometabolism. The fluid accumulation of myxedema is absent and the facies therefore completely different. The diseases are comparable in their causation, myxedema being a cachexia due to lack of thyroid tissue, Simmonds' disease being a cachexia due to loss of the anterior pituitary. Simmonds' disease might also be likened to Addison's, in which there is destruction of the adrenal cortex, and it must be differentiated from both of these in diagnosis.

Simmonds' disease, also, is in many respects the opposite of acromegaly, just as myxedema is the opposite of thyrotoxicosis. Farquharson and Graham, who have recently reported 3 cases, give the following comparison:

"In acromegaly there is great increase in size of the features and organs: an appearance of bigness; huge organs; a general splanchnomegaly. In Simmonds' disease, on the other hand, there is a marked smallness everywhere and a microsplanchnia. In acromegaly the metabolic rate tends to be increased; in Simmonds' disease it is greatly lowered. Acromegalics tend to have a high blood sugar, to be diabetic; patients with pituitary cachexia tend to have a low blood sugar, to suffer from hypoglycemia. In the former there is an overgrowth of hair during the active stage; in the latter there is loss of hair. The one tends to have increased pigmentation; the other, a loss of skin pigment, giving rise to marked pallor. Acromegaly is a disturbance of metabolism due to hyperplasia of the eosinophilic cells of the anterior lobe; Simmonds' disease is a disturbance resulting from almost complete destruction of the anterior lobe."

Treatment.—The treatment logically would be by substitution with an anterior pituitary preparation containing all of the hormones. No startling results have been reported as yet from such treatment, but it is only very recently that really potent extracts have been available.

HYPOPHYSEAL DWARFISM.

This is a type of dwarfism due to lack of development or destructive lesions of the anterior lobe. The hormonal deficiency is effective during the growth period and is presumably one of both growth and sex hormones. It cannot be complete for no cachexia ensues. As excess of the growth hormone during the growth period gives gigantism so does an insufficient supply give dwarfism. Furthermore, these dwarfs are of the well-proportioned type. Sexual infantilism is present and due presumably to the lack of sex hormone.

Since the epiphyses remain open, slow growth may be possible through life, and as these dwarfs grow older they may take on the appearance of premature senility, associated at the same time with sexual infantilism, a condition known as progeria. The syndrome must be differentiated from physiologic, rachitic, achondroplastic and cretinous dwarfism.

It would be reasonable to use active anterior pituitary preparations in these drawfs as in cases of Simmonds' disease.

FRÖHLICH'S SYNDROME.

Synonym.—Dystrophia adiposogenitalis.

The precise disturbance in hormonic physiology present in this syndrome cannot be stated with certainty. The picture differs from Simmonds' disease in lacking the cachexia. Instead there is obesity but associated as in hypophyseal dwarfism with sexual infantilism.

The endocrine situation is probably that of both an anterior and posterior lobe hypofunction. In the anterior lobe the deficiency is probably more of the sex hormone than of the growth hormone. The exact mechanism in the causation of the obesity is not clear. It probably is due to a posterior lobe underfunction. In contrast to the hypophyseal cachexias the supply of anterior lobe hormone is probably reduced rather than absent. Increased sugar tolerance frequently met with is probably a posterior lobe phenomenon.

The typical syndrome of Fröhlich develops during childhood or adolescence. But a hypofunction coming on in adult life may give a similar picture. Cushing has shown that symptoms of this sort may be associated with chromophobe adenoma of the anterior lobe. In the adult type, the obesity is of the characteristic pituitary type, that is, most marked about the pelvic girdle. Amenorrhea comes on in women and impotence and loss of desire in men. The type beginning in childhood may be outgrown and normal adult status be attained. The mistake should not be made of prescribing organotherapy for every fat boy with genitalia appearing small because of the surrounding fat. Such boys usually become normal at puberty without any treatment.

The hypofunction in true Fröhlich's disease may be a result of tumor or cyst of the pituitary itself or may be due to pressure on the gland by a suprasellar cyst.

Diagnosis.—The picture of obesity, genital infantilism, lack of development of secondary sex characters, unchanged voice in the male, short extremities, genu valgum, in its fully developed form is unmistakable. In mild grades the finding of increased sugar tolerance and lowered basal metabolic rate is suggestive.

The diagnosis of the presence or absence of tumor depends upon an evaluation of the neighborhood symptoms.

Treatment.—If tumor is present, resection or decompression may be possible. For the endocrine symptoms substitution therapy is undoubtedly possible. In the past, organotherapy, even with simple dried preparations of the whole gland, given by mouth has been claimed to have produced some improvement. With the more potent extracts rapidly becoming available, good results should be had before long.

54

CUSHING'S SYNDROME.

Cushing has recently called attention to a syndrome associated with tumors of the basophilic cells of the anterior lobe. It is characterized chiefly by obesity of the pituitary type, hypertrichosis, decreased sexual activity, hypertension and osteoporosis.

The symptomatology bears some resemblance to that of adrenal cortex hyperfunction. This is understandable on the basis of the known adreno-tropic action of the pituitary. The osteoporosis may be likewise interpreted as due to parathyroid hyperfunction resulting from para-thyro-tropic action of the anterior lobe.

REFERENCES.

CREW, F. A. E., and WIESNER, B. P.: On the Existence of a Fourth Hormone Thyreotrophic in Nature of the Anterior Pituitary, Brit. Med. Jour., 1930, i, 777.

CUSHING, H.: The Pituitary Body and Its Disorders, Philadelphia, J. B. Lippincott Company, 1912.

———— The Basophil Adenomas of the Pituitary Body and Their Clinical Manifestations, Bull. Johns Hopkins Hosp., 1932, **50**, 137.

CUSHING, H., and DAVIDOFF, L. M.: Pathologic Findings in Four Autopsied Cases of Acromegaly with a Discussion of Their Significance, Monographs of the Rockefeller Institute, No. 22, April, 1927.

EVANS, H. M.: Function of the Anterior Hypophysis, The Harvey Lectures, Series XIX, Philadelphia, J. B. Lippincott Company, 1925.

UHLENHUTH, E.: Experimental Production of Gigantism by Feeding Anterior Lobe of Hypophysis, Jour. Gen. Physiol., 1921, **3**, 347.

THE PANCREAS.

The pancreatic islets produce the hormone insulin isolated by Banting and Best in 1921. The syndrome produced by hypoinsulinism is diabetes mellitus. This disease, together with the physiologic action of the hormone, is discussed in the chapter on Diseases of Metabolism (*q. v.*).

There remains for mention here the rare condition of *hyperinsulinism* which has been proved in a few reported cases to be due to the hyperfunctioning of an islet tissue tumor.

The characteristic symptom which should lead to the diagnosis is periodic syncope with associated symptoms giving precisely the picture of an insulin reaction. If the blood sugar is determined during such a seizure, a marked hypoglycemia will be found.

The spontaneous attacks like those occurring after insulin injections are most likely to occur when the taking of food has been delayed. Candy or other sugar may abort them.

In an individual with such a picture an exploratory laparotomy is indicated. In the cases reported, removal of the tumor has been followed by complete relief of symptoms.

REFERENCE.

WILDER, R. M., *et al.*: Carcinoma of the Islands of the Pancreas: Hyperinsulinism and Hypoglycemia, Jour. Am. Med. Assn., 1927, **89**, 348.

THE FEMALE GONADS.

The physiology of the ovaries is perhaps the most complex of any of the endocrine organs. Besides their obvious function of producing ova, the ovaries manufacture certainly two, and perhaps more, internal secretions which have the function of maintaining the menstrual cycle and of making possible the establishment of pregnancy. The internal secretion of the ovary is also necessary to the development of the secondary sex characteristics and the attainment of sexual maturity. Removal of the ovaries prior to puberty leads to the development of an undifferentiated sexless type of adult, while after puberty it leads to those changes which normally take place at the menopause.

The Ovarian Hormones.—In 1922 Allen and Doisy demonstrated beyond doubt that the ovary produces an internal secretion which will bring about changes in the uterus and vagina of spayed rats characteristic of œstrus. In 1928 they isolated this body in pure crystalline form. This hormone, known as theelin, or the female sex hormone, is present in the fluid of the ripening Graafian follicle. It has to do with the building up of the endometrium which follows menstruation. After the rupture of the follicle the corpus luteum develops and it in turn produces a hormone called progestin by Corner—and lutin by Zondek—since it seems to sensitize and prepare the endometrium for the reception of the fertilized ovum. If no ovum is fertilized, the corpus luteum involutes and the uterine edifice disintegrates, which constitutes the phenomenon of menstruation. It would seem that so long as the corpus luteum functions menstruation cannot take place.

These two hormones, however, are not alone sufficient to maintain the female sex functions. They are dependent upon the sex hormones of the pituitary, the Prolan A and B of Zondek. The ovary is incapable of functioning until activated by these pituitary hormones. Prolan A promotes the secretion of theelin and Prolan B that of lutin, and of these probably B is necessary to ovulation. On the other hand, the pituitary hormones in the absence of the ovary have no effect on the female reproduction apparatus (although they may promote lactation). In the intact organism the synergistic action of pituitary and ovary is necessary to sex function.

It is likely that in the light of this newer hormonology, disorders in the female sex functions will be better understood and better treated. Many menstrual disturbances will be recognized as primarily endocrine in origin, and organotherapy used with a clearly defined objective. Organotherapy in the past has been empiric and disappointing in its results; but that is because truly active preparations have been non-existent until very recently. With the active preparations now available and the tests for the hormones that are being devised, all this is likely to be changed. The test for the anterior pituitary hormone, which was devised by Aschheim and Zondek and has subsequently undergone various modifications, serves as a test for pregnancy, since this hormone only appears in detectable quantities in the urine during pregnancy. It depends upon the production of ovulation and of corpora hæmorrhagica and lutea either in immature animals or in species like the rabbit which do not ovulate without copulation. As a matter of fact, it is as yet undetermined whether the hormone which appears in the urine of pregnant women is actually derived from the anterior pituitary or whether it may originate in the placenta and stimulate the pituitary to produce its hormone. Tests for theelin in various body fluids, such as urine and blood, have been devised which depend upon the production of œstrus in castrated female animals.

In the consideration of diseases which follows, only those are included which seem to depend chiefly on disturbances in the internal secretion of the ovary. Other diseases of the female generative tract do not come within the scope of the present section.

HYPERFUNCTIONAL STATES.

Precocious puberty, that is to say, early development of the secondary sex characters and early establishment of menstruation, is seen in association with adrenal cortex tumors and primary tumors of the ovary. There are also cases without tumor which probably represent primary hypergonadism. The logical treatment in primary gonadal hyperfunction would seem to be roentgen radiation or, failing success with that, partial oöphorectomy and, in cases with tumor, removal of tumor. Such children must be protected against sex violation.

Hyperfunction in the adult may also occur as a secondary result of the hyperfunction of other glands, perhaps the pituitary, possibly the thyroid.

HYPOFUNCTIONAL STATES.

Absent or underfunction of the ovaries before puberty, like castration, leads to female eunuchism. Menstruation does not occur and the secondary sex characters and sexual desire fail to develop.

Such conditions may be due apparently to primary hypogonadism or may be secondary to hypofunction of the anterior pituitary as in Fröhlich's syndrome or in hypophyseal dwarfism.

In the normal adult woman the sexual functions may fail prematurely owing to ovarian disease or to acquired disease of the other endocrine glands just mentioned. Bilateral oöphorectomy producing premature menopause is the commonest hypofunctional state of all.

Treatment.—Organotherapy offers something in some of these disorders. In primary hypogonadism and certainly in the secondary form attributable to the pituitary, concentrates of the hormone contained in the urine of pregnant women, now obtainable commercially under the name of "prolan," and others, are worth trying. If the ovaries are out the pituitary has no action. Under these circumstances theelin could be tried. When the thyroid appears at fault thyroid therapy may be very helpful.

The menopause constitutes a physiologic hypofunction and it has been found that its unpleasant symptoms, especially hot flashes, are diminished by ovarian preparations containing theelin. However, such drugs as phenobarbital often have an equally good effect.

AMENORRHEA.

Cessation of menstruation due to endocrine causes rather than local disease of the pelvic organs is very common. Its precise endocrine physiology is not clear. Probably there are many types. Failure of ovulation on the one hand or persistence of the corpus luteum on the other might lead to it. It is, of course, a part of the picture of any of the secondary ovarian hypofunctions mentioned in the preceding section. Many amenorrheas seem to be due to purely psychic causes. Others are secondary to a wide variety of kinds of chronic ill health. Just what these represent in terms of ovarian function is probably unknown. It would be logical in any of them to try the effect of "prolan" or theelin.

FUNCTIONAL UTERINE BLEEDING.

There are probably several varieties of purely functional uterine bleeding. Shaw has described four. His Type I deserves special mention. It is more often seen in women approaching the menopause in which several months of amenorrhea are followed by prolonged continuous bleeding, metrorrhagia. Shaw has found in these cases that the uterus is large, the endometrium hyperplastic but without evidence of secretory activity. One of the ovaries in these cases showed a big follicle cyst. The interpretation is that the dysfunction is originally due to failure of ovulation. The follicle does not rupture but becomes a cyst. No corpus luteum is formed, hence no lutin. The final edifice of the endometrium is not built and no menstruation takes place. This accounts for the period of amenorrhea. The endometrium finally undergoes thrombosis and breakdown, giving metrorrhagia, but this is not true menstruation. "Prolan" cures these cases.

Another type of functional uterine bleeding is that of too frequent catamenia due to too frequent ovulation. The corpus luteum is not lasting long enough and one may stimulate it with "prolan" to produce more lutin.

REFERENCES.

ALLEN, E., and DOISY, E. A.: An Ovarian Hormone, Jour. Am. Med. Assn., 1923, **81**, 819.

GRAVES, W. P.: Female Sex Hormonology, Philadelphia, W. B. Saunders Company, 1931.

SMITH, P. E., and ENGLE, E. T.: Induction of Precocious Sexual Maturity in the Mouse by Daily Pituitary Homeo and Heterotransplants, Proc. Soc. Exper. Biol. and Med., 1927, **24**, 561.

ZONDEK, B.: Hormone des Ovariums und des Hypophysenvorderlappens, Berlin, Springer, 1931.

ZONDEK, B., and ASCHHEIM, S.: Der Scheidenzyklus der Weissen Maus als Testobject zum Nachweis des Ovarialhormons, Klin. Wchnschr., 1926, **5**, 979.

THE MALE GONADS.

Like the female, the male gonads have not only the obvious function of producing germ cells, but also that of elaborating an internal secretion, the male sex hormone.

This hormone is necessary to the development of the secondary sex characters and the attainment of sexual maturity. Its secretion is motivated as in the case of the ovarian hormones, by the sex hormone of the anterior pituitary. Without the pituitary hormone there is no secretion of male sex hormone and consequently no sexual development. Some progress in the isolation of the male sex hormone is being made by McCullagh.

HYPERFUNCTIONAL STATES.

Precocious puberty in the male may apparently be due to primary hypergonadism or associated with tumors of the testicle, or it may be secondary to adrenal cortex or pineal hyperfunction. Hypergonadism may arise in the adult from any of these causes. Actual pathologic increase in sexual power must be distinguished from mere increase in libido which may be purely psychic.

Treatment.—When a tumor is present it should be removed. In cases without tumor irradiation may be tried.

HYPOFUNCTIONAL STATES.

Sexual infantilism in the male may result from primary hypogonadism due to atrophy or developmental failure of the glands. Bilateral cryptorchidism, that is to say, undescent of the testicles, is a not infrequent cause.

Hypofunction may also be secondary to hypofunction of other glands as, for example, the thyroid or pituitary.

Eunuchoidism, which is the somatic picture seen in males deprived of the male sex hormone during the growth period, is that of a neutral or sexless individual, having the voice of the child, the hair distribution of the female and the other secondary characters of either sex. Such individuals are impotent and devoid of sexual feeling.

Hypogonadism coming on in adult life produces less striking changes. Impotence with or without lack of desire is the rule. However, individuals completely castrated in adult life sometimes retain sexual power for long periods.

Treatment.—Reports are to be found of the relief of hypogonadal symptoms by testicular transplants. Ligation of the vasa deferentia which has the effect of causing the spermatogenic elements of the testicle to atrophy and the interstitial to hypertrophy has also been recommended (Steinach operation).

Substitution therapy offers something, particularly with the newer potent extracts. If the condition is secondary to pituitary or thyroid hypofunction, treatment with the hormones of these glands may be effective.

THE PINEAL BODY.

Synonym.—Epiphysis.

Very little is known of the endocrinology of this structure. Like the thymus it involutes after childhood and often becomes calcified. It is familiar to roentgenologists as a small dense shadow seen in the lateral plate about 4 cm. behind and 2 cm. above the tip of the posterior clinoid process. Tumors of the pineal have been reported and associated with some of them there has been sexual precocity which has been believed to be a pineal hormonic sign. Other hormonic signs accompanying such tumors are probably due to pressure upon the pituitary. Diagnosis of pineal tumor has seldom been made during life. It must be made from neighborhood, not hormonic signs. It is a problem of intracranial localization.

THE THYMUS BODY.

Very little is known of the function of the thymus. Indeed, it has never been conclusively proved that it is to be looked upon as an endocrine gland. However, some very recent work by Rowntree, Clark and Hanson gives weighty evidence that it does properly belong in that category. These investigators, giving thymus extract to successive generations of white rats, find a remarkable acceleration in the rate of maturation of the organism. Growth and differentiation are both greatly speeded up, but giants are not produced as would be the case with the pituitary growth hormone. When adult size is reached, growth ceases, but this size is reached more quickly than in the untreated controls. The significance of this work remains to be evaluated, but it is proper to mention it, even in a text-book, as indicative of the direction endocrine research is taking.

The thymus is relatively at its greatest size in the newborn infant, but attains its maximum weight at puberty after which it rapidly involutes and in the adult it normally is atrophic.

Types of Thymic Disorder.—Tumors, thymomata, both benign and malignant, are rare. Simple hyperplasia and persistence after the period when involution should occur are more frequently encountered. Hyperplasia of the thymus associated with splenomegaly and generalized lymphoid hyperplasia is a well recognized clinical syndrome going under the name of status thymicolymphaticus. It is believed, in some mysterious way, to predispose the individual to sudden death. Recent work seems to throw considerable doubt on this traditional belief. For some reason, also not understood, persistent thymus is usually found in exophthalmic goiter and in myasthenia gravis.

Thymus symptomatology is essentially that of mediastinal pressure. This may take the form of intermittent attacks of stridulous dyspnea, *thymic asthma*, or in the case particularly of tumors, of persistent stridor together with dysphagia, disturbed cardiac function due to sympathetic or vagal pressure, dilatation of neck and arm veins and cyanosis. On physical examination increased substernal dullness may be made out and by roentgen-ray a characteristic mediastinal shadow.

The lesser grades of enlargement may be demonstrable by roentgen-ray only and, therefore, whenever enlargement is suspected, roentgen-ray examination becomes imperative.

Treatment.—Under irradiation with roentgen-rays the thymus involutes. This treatment is applicable to all thymus enlargements.

CHAPTER XVII.

DISEASES OF THE BLOOD.

By CYRUS C. STURGIS, M.D.

INTRODUCTION.
CHRONIC SECONDARY ANEMIA.
IDIOPATHIC MICROCYTIC ANEMIA.
PERNICIOUS ANEMIA.
APLASTIC ANEMIA.
CHRONIC HEMOLYTIC JAUNDICE.
CHLOROSIS.
SICKLE-CELL ANEMIA.
PURPURA.
   Idiopathic Thrombocytopenic Purpura.
   Secondary or Symptomatic Thrombocytopenic Purpura.

PURPURA—(Continued).
   Idiopathic Non-thrombocytopenic Purpura.
HEMOPHILIA.
LEUKEMIA.
   Chronic Myelogenous Leukemia.
   Chronic Lymphatic Leukemia.
   Aleukemic Leukemia.
   Acute Leukemia.
   Monocytic Leukemia.
AGRANULOCYTIC ANGINA.
HODGKIN'S DISEASE.
SPLENIC ANEMIA.
POLYCYTHEMIA RUBRA VERA.

Introduction.—Incidence.—It is difficult to estimate accurately the incidence of the various types of blood diseases which are encountered in the practice of medicine, but undoubtedly chronic secondary anemia is the condition most frequently observed. This is true because so many different conditions are responsible for this variety of anemia. Chronic blood loss due to uterine disorders, hemorrhoids, bleeding peptic ulcer, neoplasm, improper diet and almost any chronic long-continued disease may cause a secondary anemia. Various other anemias, such as pernicious anemia, which have been considered somewhat rare in the past, have appeared to be more common within recent years. This is probably because the condition is now recognized with greater accuracy, due to improved diagnostic methods and a more widespread knowledge concerning the disease.

Apparently various blood diseases fluctuate greatly in frequency as the result of unknown causes. One of the mysteries of medicine is why a disease such as chlorosis which was so common in the past has now almost completely disappeared. Within the past few years at least two blood diseases appeared to be increasing in frequency—idiopathic microcytic anemia, which occurs for no obvious cause in women of middle age, is now a relatively common disease, and agranulocytic angina has only recently been recognized as an increasingly common clinical entity.

The Mechanism of the Production of the Anemias.—In health the number of formed elements of the peripheral blood, the red blood cells, white blood cells and platelets, are maintained at a constant level with great exactness. In the case of the red blood cells and probably the white blood cells and platelets, this is accomplished because in any given period of time the same number of red blood cells are delivered from the bone-marrow to the circulation as are destroyed. If blood is lost by hemorrhage, by a failure of the marrow to produce mature red blood cells at a normal rate, or because of an abnormal increase in blood destruction, this delicate balance which maintains the peripheral blood at a constant level is upset, and an anemia develops. An excellent example of an anemia due to decreased blood production is seen in aplastic anemia where there is an actual destruction of a large part of the bone-marrow with a resultant decreased efficiency. An anemia, which is probably due solely to an increased destruction of red blood cells, is seen in chronic hemolytic jaundice. In this condition it is possible to demonstrate that the red blood cells have an increased fragility and this explains, in part at least, why they are destroyed more easily.

In all types of anemia an attempt should be made to form an opinion as to whether the cause is due to blood loss, to increased destruction, decreased production or a combination of these three factors. Evidences of increased blood destruction are poikilocytosis, hyperbilirubinemia and fever. With an increase in the amount of bilirubin of the serum, there develops an icteric tint to the skin and conjunctivæ which is apparent in the various hemolytic anemias. As bilirubin is derived from hemoglobin, it has been assumed that this is a rough index of the amount of blood destruction. This is undoubtedly true in some instances, but in certain anemias, such as pernicious anemia, it must be admitted that an excess of bilirubin in the serum may mean nothing more than a failure to use all of this material in the formation of red blood cells. Decreased blood production is indicated by a lack of evidence of bone-marrow activity. This is shown by an absence of the immature forms of red blood cells, such as reticulocytes, normoblasts, megaloblasts and cells showing polychromatophilia.

The diseases which concern the number of white blood cells, excluding infections, are not numerous but they do occur as seen in the various leukemias. This statement applies also to the blood platelets, but in the thrombocytopenic purpuras the essential lesion is a marked reduction in these elements of the blood. It is interesting to note that all three formed elements of the blood are subject to alterations in numbers, there being either an increase or decrease in various diseases. For example, the red cells are diminished in the anemias and increased in polycythemia. The white blood cells are increased in the leukemias and decreased in agranulocytic angina. The platelets are diminished in some types of purpura but there is no disease where the essential change is an increase in the number of platelets, although this may occur following hemorrhage, after splenectomy, and sometimes in the leukemias. In most diseases of the blood, although the fundamental change is in the number of any one of the three formed elements, there is almost always an associated change in the other two.

Symptoms in Diseases of the Blood.—In almost all diseases of the blood there are important symptoms and signs which are due to an associated anemia. These manifestations are common to all anemias, regardless of the cause, and their severity is directly proportional to the reduction in the hemoglobin of the peripheral blood. Evidences of an anemia are pallor, dyspnea, palpitation, weakness, fatigability, vertigo, fainting attacks and sometimes edema of the ankles. Pallor as observed in the face is not always indicative of an anemia, as the color of an individual's skin is not entirely dependent on the amount of hemoglobin of the blood, but is also concerned with the distribution of the skin capillaries, natural pigmentation, sunburn, artificial coloring and excessive fatigue. These factors may lead to an incorrect conclusion concerning the presence or absence of an anemia when judging from a patient's appearance. More reliable information may be obtained by noting the color of the mucous membranes and, as Duke has recently emphasized, the palms of the hands.

Dyspnea and palpitation on exertion are almost invariably associated with pronounced anemia, although rarely is the anemia so severe as to cause these symptoms to appear when the patient is at complete rest. These complaints are due to the diminished capacity of the blood to carry oxygen to the tissues. When exercise demands an increased amount of oxygen, the air breathed and the circulatory rate is increased unduly with the production of these symptoms.

Weakness is the most constant complaint associated with anemia and may be of such extreme grade as to confine the patient to bed. This is attributed to an inability of the cardio-respiratory apparatus to deliver sufficient oxygen to the tissue for the necessary combustion incident to muscular exertion.

Edema of the ankles is not infrequently observed in the severe anemias, but its cause is undetermined. That it can be due entirely to the anemia is evidenced by the fact that it disappears if the blood returns to normal. Various theories have been suggested to explain the mechanism of its production. It has been ascribed to an associated myocardial weakness, changes in the capillary walls as a result of nutritional disturbances which render them more permeable to fluid, and decreased osmotic pressure in the capillaries as a result of a reduction in the plasma proteins.

Vertigo and faintness are considered to be due to anoxemia of the brain.

Importance of an Accurate Diagnosis.—An accurate diagnosis is absolutely essential in the management of the various blood diseases, for the treatment and prognosis differs greatly in the various types. For example, liver extract and ventriculin have a specific action in pernicious anemia, but this form of treatment is of no value in the treatment of chronic secondary anemia. On the other hand, iron has a specific effect in various types of secondary anemia but is useless in pernicious anemia. An erroneous diagnosis may likewise result in an incorrect prognosis. If the diagnosis of aleukemic leukemia is confused with pernicious anemia, a serious error in the prognosis would result for leukemia is an invariably fatal disease, whereas pernicious anemia is amenable to treatment and can be controlled.

CHRONIC SECONDARY ANEMIA (CHRONIC MICROCYTIC ANEMIA).

Introduction.—The term secondary anemia was originally introduced to include those anemias which were due to a recognizable cause in contrast to the primary anemias whose etiology was unknown. For some years, however, it has been customary to include in the group of secondary anemias those in which the color index is low, despite the fact that their cause is not known. The anemias which will be described under the heading of Chronic Secondary Anemia in this article include those which are either secondary to a known cause or those with a low color index, or those which meet both qualifications. In most instances a large percentage of the red blood cells are below normal in size and, therefore, the term chronic microcytic anemia is appropriate.

Anemia Due to Blood Loss.—Evidences of acute blood loss due to trauma, bleeding peptic ulcer, ruptured extra-uterine pregnancy, and many other causes, are tachycardia, sweating, subnormal temperature, pallor, hypotension and rapid shallow breathing. With the return of the blood volume to normal, the acute symptoms subside and only those remain which are associated with the anemia. An immediate examination of the hemoglobin and red blood cells following an acute hemorrhage does not give an accurate idea of the amount of blood lost as there is a concentration of the blood due to a diminution of the total volume. Following the restoration of the blood volume to normal, there is a dilution of the blood and consequently the hemoglobin falls and the red blood cell count diminishes. As a result of the loss of blood the bone-marrow is stimulated to an increased activity, but as the red blood cells regenerate more rapidly than the hemoglobin, the color index falls. The earliest changes in the blood following an acute hemorrhage are a leukocytosis varying from 15,000 to 20,000 per c.mm. and an increase in the number of blood platelets. This may occur within a few hours after the hemorrhage. Evidence of active regeneration of blood is seen in an increase in the number of reticulocytes, which may reach 15 to 20 per cent, and the appearance of nucleated red blood cells and cells showing diffuse and punctate basophilia.

Chronic Hemorrhage.—This most frequently occurs as a result of bleeding hemorrhoids, uterine disorders, peptic ulcer, repeated epistaxis, or malignancy of the gastro-intestinal tract. Constant loss of blood over a period of months may produce a profound anemia. The symptoms in such a patient are: (1) those due to the anemia and (2) those peculiar to the condition which accounts for the loss of blood. The symptoms of a chronic anemia are weakness, pallor, dyspnea, palpitation, vertigo, faintness and occasionally edema of the ankles. The characteristic findings in the blood are a reduction in the red blood cell count and hemoglobin of the peripheral blood with a color index which is usually low, and moderate anisocytosis and poikilocytosis. A majority of cells are below the average size. The white blood cells, as well as the platelets, may be normal or decreased in number.

Anemia Associated With Cancer.—The anemia associated with neoplasms may be due to mechanical blood loss (as bleeding from gastric carcinoma), to a myelophthisic anemia associated with metastases to the bone-marrow, and possibly due to a diminished blood formation resulting from a toxic action on the bone-marrow. An additional factor in the causation may be an inability to ingest and assimilate a proper diet. The blood picture usually resembles that due to chronic blood loss but occasionally there may be a true macrocytic anemia.

Anemia Due to Infection.—Almost any type of acute or chronic infection may cause an anemia. In acute septicemia there is a rapidly developing anemia which may reach a severe grade. This may be of the hemolytic type as suggested by an increase in bilirubin of the blood plasma and the development of a distinct yellowish tint to the skin and conjunctivæ. Almost any type of chronic infection may cause a moderate degree of anemia. Anemia of this kind may be seen in chronic arthritis, any prolonged pyogenic infection as osteomyelitis or lung abscess, tuberculous infections, especially of the intestines, and many others. Various parasitic infections, such as uncinariasis, malaria and amebic dysentery, may be associated with this type of anemia.

Anemia Associated With Disturbances of the Ductless Glands.—There is not infrequently an anemia associated with myxedema and Addison's disease. This probably results from a lack of secretion of the thyroid gland and the adrenals. The anemia of myxedema is not usually severe unless there is a coëxisting pernicious anemia, which occurs rarely. The blood may in some instances resemble the picture seen in pernicious anemia with the exception that the red blood cells are more frequently round instead of oval. It is an anemia due to diminished blood formation. There may be a moderate anemia observed in Addison's disease, but this is rarely an important feature of the syndrome.

Myelophthisic Anemia.—This is a type of anemia which is due to an invasion of the bone-marrow with a malignant growth or a leukemic infiltration. As a result, the red blood cell forming tissue is displaced from the marrow and a diminished production of red blood cells results. As blood destruction occurs at the normal rate, an anemia develops. This variety of anemia is seen in some patients with cancer, Hodgkin's disease and leukemia of any type.

Other Causes of Chronic Secondary Anemia.—There are many other causes of chronic secondary anemia which will be only briefly enumerated. An anemia is frequently observed in chronic parenchymatous nephritis. It is usually moderate in extent and is due chiefly to a diminished blood production rather than the frequently associated hematuria. Anemia may be due also to various poisons such as mercury, lead, arsenic and benzol. There is considerable evidence that the ingestion of an improper diet may cause a definite secondary anemia. This appears in patients who have difficulty in eating on account of cardiospasm or other conditions, or those who have existed over a period of years on a very peculiar diet, lacking in iron or essential vitamins, as a result of personal whims. A nutritional anemia is more frequently observed in women due to the presence of the menstrual cycle and pregnancy, and in growing children. Occasionally a patient with some other type of anemia, as pernicious anemia, may develop an associated nutritional anemia which alters the characteristic blood picture of the original disease. A total fast of several weeks' duration does not cause anemia in a normal person.

IDIOPATHIC MICROCYTIC ANEMIA.

Definition.—An anemia usually occurring in women of middle age, characterized by asthenia, vague gastro-intestinal complaints, decreased resistance to infection and a favorable response to iron medication.

Etiology.—This type of anemia has not received the emphasis to which it is entitled, as it occurs rather frequently. To overlook the condition and omit the proper treatment is regrettable for the response to iron medication is very striking. It is entirely possible that the condition is a new clinical entity as it has been only in recent years that the attention of the profession has been directed to it. The etiology is unknown, although probably the cause is concerned with the metabolism of iron. One view regards the cause as an iron starvation resulting from defective absorption. It occurs in women, sometimes in early adult life, but most frequently between the ages of thirty and fifty years.

Symptoms.—The onset is usually insidious, and the length of time the disease has been present is difficult to determine. Often it has undoubtedly been active for several years before a physician is consulted. The patients' chief complaints are usually vague and commonly consist of asthenia, mild chronic indigestion, low resistance to respiratory infections and emotional instability. The menstrual periods may be scanty but menorrhagia of a serious degree may be present at times. In some patients there are attacks of recurrent glossitis as in pernicious anemia. When these patients complain of dysphagia in addition to the other symptoms, the condition is then spoken of as the Plummer-Vinson syndrome. Physical examination shows a variable degree of pallor, moderate undernutrition, and frequently oral sepsis, which is probably not related etiologically to the disease. An important point in the physical examination is to exclude other conditions which might cause a similar anemia. In some cases there may be an acute glossitis with a tongue which appears intensely reddened, while other patients may have no symptoms referable to the tongue, but there may be atrophy of the papillæ which gives the dorsum a smoothed-out appearance. A number of these patients have a peculiar concavity of the finger nails, koilonychia ("spoon nails"), which usually affects the nails of several fingers.

Blood.—There may be a reduction in both the red blood cells and hemoglobin of the peripheral blood. Characteristically, however, there is a greater reduction in the hemoglobin than the red blood cell count, which gives a color index in the vicinity of 0.5. There is a definite degree of achromia and slight anisocytosis and poikilocytosis. The white blood cells and platelets are normal.

Gastric Analysis.—In most patients there is a complete lack of hydrochloric acid in the gastric contents. In some patients acid is present, but in reduced amounts.

Prognosis.—The outlook in the chronic secondary anemias depends entirely on the underlying cause of the condition. In the idiopathic microcytic anemia of women, the course is chronic with exacerbations, especially during pregnancies. When adequate iron therapy is employed the results are striking. Usually within a few weeks the blood returns to normal and there is a marked improvement in the patient's general condition. Iron should be continued over a long period or the patient kept under observation as there is a tendency to recurrence.

Treatment of Chronic Secondary Anemia.—The essential requirement in the treatment of many cases of secondary anemia is to remove or control the underlying cause if this is known. Until this is done, it is too much to expect that various measures calculated to overcome the anemia will be completely effective. Each patient with chronic secondary anemia, therefore, should be studied thoroughly in an attempt to discover the cause and apply the proper corrective measures, if this is possible. If the anemia is secondary to bleeding, this must be checked. Various infections, if present, should be eliminated. Caution should be used in ascribing the anemia to various septic foci such as teeth and tonsils, and there should be reasonable assurance that such foci are the cause of the anemia before they are removed. The patients' dietary habits should be investigated and corrected if it is likely that an improper diet plays a rôle in the production of the anemia. In such conditions as Hodgkin's disease and the leukemias the associated myelophthisic anemia can only be improved by the use of roentgen-ray therapy and radium. In many cases of chronic secondary anemia it is beneficial to administer iron, especially if the anemia is the idiopathic microcytic type. L. J. Witts has very aptly stated: "Few facts in medicine are so unanimously believed by the expert, so strongly backed by evidence, and so little known to the profession, as the absolute necessity of *very large* doses of iron in the treatment of these chronic anemias." Poor results in the past have been due, in many instances, to an inadequate dosage. Ferric ammonium citrate may be given in a 50 per cent solution in doses amounting to 4 to 6 grams (60 to 90 grains) daily, or reduced iron, 0.5 to 1 gram ($7\frac{1}{2}$ to 15 grains) in capsules, three times daily. These are very much larger doses than those which are usually recommended in text-books, but satisfactory results will not be obtained unless these amounts are given. Large doses are well tolerated and rarely cause digestive disturbances, contrary to the usual belief. Apparently the parenteral administration of iron is unnecessary and the addition of copper is not required because all of the pharmaceutical preparations of iron are grossly contaminated with this element.

Transfusions.—This form of treatment may be used but ordinarily it is not indicated. If given in the secondary anemias due to cancer, it can give at the most only temporary improvement. In the anemia secondary to bleeding it should be employed only if the patient's life is in danger from acute hemorrhage, or to sustain the patient until a therapeutic agent such as iron can become effective. When bleeding has stopped, and a severe anemia exists, it will cause the blood to return to normal more quickly, but it is doubtful if it is wise to employ this method of treatment routinely.

REFERENCES.

MEULENGRACHT, E.: Large Doses of Iron in the Different Kinds of Anemia in a Medical Department, Acta med. scand., Stockholm, 1926, **58**, 594.

MILLS, EDWARD S.: Idiopathic Hypochromemia, Am. Jour. Med. Sci., 1931, **182**, 554.

MINOT, G. R., and HEATH, C. W.: The Response of the Reticulocytes to Iron, Am. Jour. Med. Sci., 1932, **183**, 110.

WITTS, L. J.: Achlorhydria and Anemia, Practitioner, 1930, **124**, 348.

PERNICIOUS ANEMIA.

Synonyms.—Addisonian anemia; Progressive pernicious anemia; Addison-Biermer anemia.

Definition.—Pernicious anemia is a disease of unknown etiology, most frequently occurring during middle life or later, usually characterized by a marked reduction in the red blood cells and the hemoglobin of the peripheral blood, probably always associated with an achlorhydria and frequently complicated by degenerative changes in the posterior and lateral columns of the spinal cord. When untreated, it progresses slowly, usually with remissions, to a fatal termination.

History.—The disease was first described as a distinct clinical entity by Thomas Addison of Guy's Hospital in 1849 and later in 1855. Widespread interest in the condition was not aroused until the publications of Biermer in 1867 and 1872. Important contributions concerning the bone-marrow have been made by William Pepper (1875), Cohnheim (1876), Zadek (1921) and Peabody (1929). The fundamental relationship between the stomach and pernicious anemia has been emphasized by the remarkable and epoch-making experiments of W. B. Castle (1929). There was no satisfactory treatment of the disease until Minot and Murphy introduced the liver diet (1926). This was followed by the development of an effective liver extract by Minot and Cohn (1927) and by the introduction of desiccated defatted hog stomach as a potent therapeutic agent by Sturgis and Isaacs (1929).

Etiology.—Pernicious anemia is a relatively common disease in North America, for of every 1000 patients admitted to a general hospital there are 3 or 4 with the disease. The apparent increase in the incidence of the condition is due undoubtedly to more accurate methods of diagnosis.

There is no question that the disease has a greater incidence in certain races than in others. It is observed frequently in the United States, Canada, England, Scotland, Ireland and the countries of northern Europe, whereas it is rarely seen in natives of the tropics, China, South America and among negroes.

Symptoms develop most frequently between forty and sixty-five years of age. If a group of patients with pernicious anemia are considered according to their age and the number of individuals living at the various ages, however, the highest incidence is between sixty-five and seventy years. True pernicious anemia probably never occurs in young children, but the onset may occasionally be during the second decade of life. It is not rare in individuals between twenty and thirty years of age. The two sexes are affected with equal frequency. The hereditary occurrence of pernicious anemia is now an established fact. Not only are outspoken cases of pernicious anemia observed in the same family but a number of the other immediate relatives may have achylia gastrica, recurrent glossitis or minor changes in the blood, suggesting an early or incomplete type of pernicious anemia.

The cause of pernicious anemia which is most generally accepted at present may be stated as follows: There is thought to be a predisposing inherited constitution of which the most important factor is an inability to derive from ingested food in the stomach an unidentified substance which controls the maturation or development of red blood cells in the bone-marrow. This is due to the lack of the intrinsic factor of Castle, which is apparently secreted by the gastric mucosa. As a result, a decreased number of red blood cells are released in the peripheral blood. As blood destruction proceeds at a normal or possibly an increased rate, the total red blood cell count of the peripheral blood must fall and an anemia develop. As yet there is no satisfactory explanation of the pathologic changes which occur constantly in the gastro-intestinal tract and the nervous system. The blood picture of pernicious anemia may arise following widespread liver damage which results in a failure of this organ to store the unidentified substance and thereby release it as needed to control the maturation of the red blood cells. Also this type of anemia may develop if there are intestinal anastomoses and an inability to absorb the substance from the intestines. The present tendency is to ascribe the central nervous system lesions to "toxic influences."

Pathology.—No single pathologic change is recognized as characteristic of pernicious anemia. The most constant anatomic findings are: the anemia; widespread fatty degeneration of many parenchymatous viscera and the muscles; hyperplastic changes in the bone-marrow with the megaloblast as the predominating cell; and focal degenerative changes in the white matter of the spinal cord. It was recognized many years ago by Hunter that the liver, kidneys and spleen may contain deposits of hemosiderin, an iron containing pigment which is derived from hemoglobin. Peabody, by means of biopsies, observed that during relapse the essential histologic lesion in the bone-marrow is a proliferation of megaloblasts which results in a hyperplastic but functionally inefficient marrow, as these cells fail to differentiate toward mature erythrocytes. During a remission there is a great relative increase of normoblasts and mature red blood cells in the marrow, whereas the megaloblasts are rare.

Symptoms.—These may be divided into three groups, depending on whether they are referable to the anemia, the gastro-intestinal tract or the nervous system. In a very large percentage of patients there are usually manifestations of varying degree, representing each group.

The symptoms which are due to the anemia are weakness, pallor, dyspnea, palpitation and sometimes edema of the ankles. Those associated with the gastro-intestinal system are anorexia, recurrent attacks of glossitis, nausea, vomiting and either constipation or diarrhea or an alternation of the two. The most common manifestations indicating involvement of the nervous system are numbness of the hands and feet, spasticity of the muscles of the lower extremities, ataxia and loss of control of the sphincter of the bladder. The history of the average case is one of gradually developing weakness in a person of middle age, which becomes progressively worse until it is completely incapacitating. Coincident with the development of this symptom, pallor with a yellowish tint, dyspnea and palpitation on exertion, and sometimes edema of the ankles are observed. About 81 per cent of the patients complain of numbness and tingling of the hands and feet. Recurring attacks of sore tongue occur in more than one-half of the patients and occasionally it is the initial and outstanding symptom. This complaint varies in intensity from a mild burning discomfort to a serious degree of involvement which may interfere markedly with the ingestion of food. As the anemia becomes pronounced, nausea, vomiting, fever and delirium may appear.

Physical examination of a patient with pernicious anemia usually reveals a fairly well-nourished individual, although there is commonly a loss of 10 to 20 pounds in body weight during the illness. There is often a pronounced pallor with an associated yellow tint, which gives the so-called lemon-yellow or grapefruit appearance to the skin and conjunctivæ. The hair is usually partly or completely gray and the eyes are most frequently colored the lighter shades, such as gray, green or blue. Not infrequently the tongue, over the dorsum, has a smooth appearance due to atrophy of the papillæ. In some instances it may be a fiery red as a result of the associated glossitis. Rarely is the tongue coated during the period of severe anemia. The lungs are usually normal and the heart shows no conspicuous changes except that frequently a soft systolic (so-called hemic) murmur is present, and there may be borderline enlargement of the left ventricle. The spleen and liver are rarely palpable. Not infrequently the abdomen is distended, which may be a troublesome symptom, especially in patients with spinal cord involvement. A slight to moderate edema may be present in patients when the red blood cell count is below 2,000,000 per c.mm. When the anemia becomes severe a hemorrhagic tendency may develop, as evidenced by petechiæ and ecchymoses, retinal hemorrhages, epistaxis and bleeding from other sources. Objective evidence of degenerative changes in the posterior and lateral columns of the spinal cord are commonly encountered. Those due to posterior column involvement are loss of vibratory sense and the sense of position of the lower extremities while those due to changes in the lateral columns are spastic paraplegia, exaggerated knee jerks and a bilateral positive Babinski sign.

Fever is commonly associated with pernicious anemia when the red blood cell count falls to a low level. This disappears when the anemia becomes less. In some instances the fever may be due to a

55

cystitis which is associated with a loss of control of the sphincters of the bladder and a residual urine which becomes infected.

The Blood.—The red blood cell count in pernicious anemia during a relapse is usually below 2,000,000 per c.mm. and it may fall to below 500,000 red blood cells per c.mm. During a spontaneous remission the count may reach normal, but it is usually between 3,000,000 and 4,000,000 cells per c.mm. In therapeutically induced remissions the red blood cell count is almost always above 4,000,000 per c.mm. and in some instances it may reach 6,000,000. The hemoglobin shows a drop which is less than the red blood cell count, and as a result the color index is 1 or greater. A high color index is a constant finding in uncomplicated pernicious anemia. A normal or reduced white blood cell count is characteristic of pernicious anemia during a relapse. It is exceedingly rare to observe a leukocytosis, even with an active infection, when the red blood cell count is low. The most characteristic finding when a stained blood film is examined is the presence of large, round or oval red blood cells which are well filled with hemoglobin. These macrocytes, as they are called, may make up 25 to 30 per cent of all the red blood cells. In addition there are a variable number of small red blood cells, microcytes, which may measure only 3 or 4 microns in diameter. Poikilocytosis, or irregularity in shape of the red blood cells, is almost always present when the anemia is pronounced. Various forms of immature red blood cells may be present, such as normoblasts, megaloblasts, cells showing diffuse basophilia or stippling, and less frequently Howell-Jolly bodies and Cabot's ring forms. With a special vital stain, such as cresyl blue, reticulocytes may be demonstrated. It should be emphasized that immature red blood cells in the peripheral blood are not essential to the diagnosis of pernicious anemia. They appear only when the patient is improving and the red blood cell count is rising. There is practically always a reduction in the number of platelets.

Other Laboratory Tests.—*Gastric Analysis.*—One of the most important laboratory procedures from the standpoint of diagnosis is an examination of the gastric contents for hydrochloric acid. In our series of several hundred cases at the Simpson Memorial Institute in whom a fractional gastric analysis was done, there was a complete absence of hydrochloric acid in every single case and a uniformly low total acidity. Three to 5 specimens were removed in each instance, and in many of the patients the analysis followed the injection of 1 mg. of histamine intramuscularly. Not only does the achlorhydria exist at the time the clinical manifestations of pernicious anemia are apparent, but it is now well established that it may be present many years prior to their appearance and probably exists since birth. It is known also that the absence of free hydrochloric acid persists when the blood returns to normal and when the patient is free from symptoms either as a result of a spontaneous or therapeutically induced remission. The facts regarding the achlorhydria of pernicious anemia are so well established that the presence of free hydrochloric acid in the gastric contents of a patient who is suspected of having pernicious anemia casts serious doubt upon the diagnosis, regardless of other convincing evidence of the disease. In addition to the lack of free hydrochloric acid, pepsinogen (the precursor of pepsin) is rarely, if ever, present in the gastric contents.

Hyperbilirubinemia.—It is well established that the bilirubin content of the blood serum is always increased when the red blood cell count is low, and that it falls as the red cell count rises. While it may not be accepted that the amount of bilirubin in the serum is an index of the degree of blood destruction, nevertheless it is a fairly good index of the course of the disease and as an aid to diagnosis. There are two clinical methods for estimating the bilirubin in the blood serum. These are the van den Bergh reaction and the icterus index. The upper limit of normal for the former test is 0.7 mg. of bilirubin per 100 cc. of serum, whereas the normal limits of the icterus index are expressed in the arbitrary figures 4 to 6. In pernicious anemia during relapse the icterus index averages between 20 and 25 and the van den Bergh reaction often gives a reading varying from 1 to 2 mg. per 100 cc. of blood, although occasionally higher figures are noted.

Cell Measurements.—The Price-Jones procedure consists in measuring the diameter of 250 red blood cells and charting the results according to the percentage of cells of various diameters. In pernicious anemia when the red blood cell count is low, a characteristic curve is formed. The greatest percentage of cells measure between 9 and 9.5 microns, but there is also a great variation in the size of the cells which may range from 3.5 to 14 microns. While the measurement curve which is typical of pernicious anemia may be seen in a few other types of anemia, it is totally different from the cell measurements which are observed in the blood of patients with many of the secondary types.

It is claimed by some that a superior method of demonstrating the increased cell size in pernicious anemia is by determining the volume index or the mean corpuscular volume of the erythrocytes.

Diagnosis.—Usually the diagnosis of pernicious anemia is not difficult. If an adult complains of the usual symptoms of an anemia such as weakness, pallor, dyspnea, palpitation and slight edema of the ankles, and there is a yellowish tint to the skin and conjunctivæ, the most likely diagnosis is pernicious anemia. If additional complaints include numbness of the hands and feet and recurrent attacks of glossitis, and an achlorhydria is present, the diagnosis is almost certain. Other findings which are helpful in the diagnosis are the characteristic blood picture, hyperbilirubinemia, a history of remissions and findings suggesting subacute combined degeneration of the spinal cord. There are at least three conditions which have a blood picture resembling pernicious anemia. They are the anemia of Dibothriocephalus latus infestation, some anemias of pregnancy and sprue. The tapeworm anemia can only be differentiated by finding the ova or segments of the worm in the stool. Sprue may be differentiated because emaciation is usually a prominent part of the clinical picture, the nervous system is not involved, achlorhydria may or may not be present, and the bilirubin content of the blood serum is not increased. The severe anemia of pregnancy may resemble pernicious anemia but differs from it because the patient usually recovers following transfusions, the therapeutic use of liver or desiccated stomach and delivery of the fetus. The glossitis and neurologic changes are not present in this condition.

Other conditions which sometimes must be differentiated from pernicious anemia are malignancy of the stomach, colon or pancreas, myxedema, nephritis and aleukemic leukemia. Usually following a careful study, including the important laboratory methods and the therapeutic test with the use of liver or stomach, there is no difficulty in recognizing the correct diagnosis. It has been emphasized recently that a macrocytic anemia, resembling pernicious anemia, may be present in patients who have widespread liver damage, as is observed in cirrhosis of the liver.

Prognosis and Course.—The average length of life of a patient with pernicious anemia, before the modern methods of treatment were introduced, was given as two or three years from the time of the appearance of the earliest symptoms. During the course of the disease, in untreated patients, there usually occur one to three or four spontaneous remissions, at which times the blood improves remarkably, the patient gains strength and may feel perfectly well for a period of three to six months to several years. Invariably, however, there is a recurrence of the condition, which results fatally unless the proper treatment is given. Following the introduction of liver and stomach therapy, the outlook has been completely changed. Although these substances are not a cure for the disease, they are successful in controlling the anemia. A less favorable prognosis should always be given in patients who show extensive spinal cord damage.

Treatment.—The essential part of the modern treatment of pernicious anemia is to administer adequate amounts of liver, either cooked or uncooked, a potent liver extract or ventriculin (desiccated, defatted hog stomach) until the blood reaches normal. Following this, sufficient amounts of one of these substances must be given regularly in order to maintain the blood at a normal level. The initial dosage, calculated to cause the blood to increase at the rate of about 400,000 red blood cells per c.mm. per week is as follows: liver, ½ pound daily; liver extract, the amount derived from 500 to 600 grams of fresh liver daily, or ventriculin, 10 grams daily for each 1,000,000 deficit in the red blood cell count. The liver extract or ventriculin may be given dissolved or suspended in water, orange or tomato juice or ginger ale.

The first evidence of improvement is seen within three to six days after the treatment has been begun. The earliest effect is a remarkable increase in the patient's appetite and rapid disappearance of the gastro-intestinal complaints. The temperature and pulse-rate fall to normal, the patient gains strength and, in uncomplicated cases, is usually able to resume a normal life within four to six weeks. The earliest change in the blood is an increase in the percentage of immature red blood cells or reticulocytes, which is usually 1 per cent or less during a relapse. This reticulocyte response is in the form of a curve beginning after three to six days of treatment, reaching a peak on the seventh to the ninth day, and returning to normal by the fifteenth day. The height of the peak varies inversely with the level of the red blood cells just prior to treatment. The red blood cell count may not change during the first two weeks, despite striking clinical evidence of improvement. Following this, there is a rapid increase, so that the average increase per week from the beginning of the treatment until the blood reaches normal is about 400,000 per c.mm. per week.

After the red blood cell count has reached normal the average maintenance dose required to keep it at this level is as follows: liver, $\frac{1}{4}$ pound, five or six times a week; liver extract, the amount derived from 300 grams of fresh liver, five days a week; ventriculin, 10 grams, six days a week. These are the average initial and maintenance doses, which may not be sufficient for all patients. The only safe method of regulating the treatment is to give a sufficient quantity which will cause a satisfactory increase in the red blood cell count, and then a maintenance dose which will keep the red blood cells within normal limits. Additional medication, such as iron, arsenic or dilute hydrochloric acid is apparently unnecessary. In some patients when the red blood cell count is extremely low, it may be wise to give one or two transfusions which will sustain the patient during the next forty-eight hours, at which time the liver or stomach therapy will become effective.

Recently, Castle and others have reported satisfactory results from the intravenous and intramuscular injection of liver extract which has been specially prepared for this purpose. There are now several preparations available on the market which can be administered by these methods. The results are satisfactory, but unpleasant reactions may follow the intravenous injections of some preparations. Within the past few years Roger Morris has reported that the intramuscular injection of concentrated swine gastric juice produces a remarkable increase in the reticulocytes and the red blood cells. This product, addisin, is not available for general use at present.

The treatment of the neurologic complications is less satisfactory than the treatment of the anemia. With the disappearance of the anemia, the minor neurologic manifestations may become less prominent or disappear entirely. It is now thought that the nervous system manifestations will be arrested or show improvement if the red blood cell count is maintained at a high level of normal. Ungley has recommended that fresh brain, finely ground, $\frac{1}{4}$ pound, two to four times a day, be given in grape juice. Various physiotherapy measures, such as the application of light, heat and the use of massage may be useful.

REFERENCES.

CORNELL, BEAUMONT, S.: Pernicious Anemia, Durham, N. C., Duke Univ. Press, 1927.

DAVIDSON, L. S. P., and GULLAND, G. L.: Pernicious Anemia, St. Louis, C. V. Mosby Company, 1930.

EVANS, FRANK A.: Pernicious Anemia, 1st ed., Baltimore, Williams & Wilkins Company, 1926.

ISAACS, RAPHAEL, STURGIS, CYRUS C., and SMITH, MILLARD: Treatment of Pernicious Anemia, Jour. Am. Med. Assn., 1928, **91**, 1687.

MINOT, G. R., and MURPHY, W. P.: Treatment of Pernicious Anemia by a Special Diet, Jour. Am. Med. Assn., 1926, **87**, 480.

MORRIS, R. S., SCHIFF, L., FOULGER, J. H., RICH, M. L., and SHERMAN, J. E.: Treatment of Pernicious Anemia: Effect of a Single Injection of Concentrated Gastric Juice (Addisin), Jour. Am. Med. Assn., 1933, **100**, 171.

STURGIS, CYRUS, C., and ISAACS, RAPHAEL: Clinical and Experimental Observations on the Treatment of Pernicious Anemia with Desiccated Stomach and with Liver Extract, Ann. Int. Med., 1931, **5**, 139.

APLASTIC ANEMIA.

Definition.—Aplastic anemia is a disease in which, from an unknown cause, the bone-marrow ceases to function with the result that there is marked decrease in the red blood cells, white blood cells and platelets of the peripheral blood. The course is usually rapidly downward, with a fatal termination, often within a few months, but occasionally brief spontaneous remissions may prolong the patient's life.

History.—This is a disease which has been recognized only in comparatively recent years, having first been described by Ehrlich in 1888.

Etiology.—There are two varieties, primary and secondary, which differ from each other only that in one a cause for the condition is recognized, whereas in the other it is unknown. Aplastic anemia may arise secondary to sepsis, various infectious diseases, as a result of arsphenamine injections, and from certain poisons such as benzol. Pathologic changes are punctate hemorrhages in practically all subserous and subperitoneal surfaces and fatty degeneration of the bone-marrow.

Symptoms.—The condition occurs most frequently in young adults and equally in the two sexes. There is often a rapidly developing pallor, a marked hemorrhagic tendency with bleeding from the mucous membranes into the skin and subcutaneous tissues. Fever frequently occurs. The condition may prove fatal within a few weeks or there may be a short remission and the patient survive as long as a year and a half.

Blood Picture.—There is a striking reduction in the red blood cells, hemoglobin, white blood cells and platelets. The red blood cell count often falls below 1,000,000 per c.mm. and the white blood cell count to only a few hundred per c.mm. The platelets may disappear almost entirely from the peripheral blood. The red blood cells appear surprisingly normal. There is rarely poikilocytosis or anisocytosis and each cell appears to contain the normal amount of hemoglobin. Nucleated red blood cells and various forms of polychromatophilia are usually not observed.

Treatment.—There is no curative treatment. In the secondary type an attempt should be made to determine the primary condition and eliminate or control it if possible. Repeated blood transfusions may give some temporary relief and control for a time the hemorrhagic tendency.

REFERENCES.

LARRABEE, RALPH C.: Aplastic Anemia and Related Conditions, Jour. Am. Med. Assn., 1920, **75**, 1632.

MUSSER, J. H., JR.: Study of a Case of Aplastic Anemia, Arch. Int. Med., 1914, **14**, 275.

SCHNEIDER, J. P.: Aplastic Anemia, Am. Jour. Med. Sci., 1918, **156**, 799.

CHRONIC HEMOLYTIC JAUNDICE.

Synonyms.—Chronic acholuric jaundice; Chronic familial jaundice; Hemolytic splenomegaly..

Definition.—A form of chronic jaundice associated with a diminished resistance of the red blood cells to hypotonic salt solution, an anemia and an enlarged spleen. There is both a congenital and acquired variety, the former occurring more frequently.

History.—The first accurate description of the disease was published by Minkowski in 1900, although imperfect accounts of the congenital form had been given prior to that time. The malady was first recognized in America by Tileston and Griffin in 1910. Chauffard in 1907 established the fact that the red blood cells have an increased fragility, and a year later reported the presence of large numbers of reticulocytes in the peripheral blood.

Etiology.—The cause of both types is obscure but it is probably closely related or the same in both varieties. In the congenital type there may be a history of the disease in several previous generations, or several cases may occur simultaneously in the same family. It is transmitted by the two sexes and occurs equally in both. The jaundice is undoubtedly accounted for by an increased hemolysis which in turn is probably partially due to an increased fragility of the red blood cells. The enlarged spleen has been thought to result simply from the increased number of red blood cells destroyed there. The relationship of the spleen must be of greater importance than this, however, for following splenectomy the jaundice and anemia disappear, although the increased fragility of the red blood cells may persist. The acquired symptomatic type, which is associated with a secondary lues, malaria, pregnancy and various infections, is a different disease and will not be considered here.

Pathology.—There is marked congestion of the spleen which involves the pulp but not the sinuses. The endothelial cells of the spleen, liver, bone-marrow and lymph nodes (reticulo-endothelial system) show evidence of activity as indicated by phagocytosis of red blood cells and pigment. The bone-marrow is hyperplastic as is seen in many severe anemias. About one-half of the patients show evidence of gall stones.

Symptoms.—The clinical picture is essentially the same in the two varieties, although the course is said to be more severe in the acquired form. In the congenital type jaundice is present at birth or appears during childhood, and remains throughout life. It is never intense, and is often present only to a very slight degree. The urine does not contain bile but it is present in the stools. The spleen is usually moderately enlarged but may reach very large proportions.

Blood Examination.—There is usually a red blood cell count which varies between 2,000,000 and 3,500,000 per c.mm.; the average hemoglobin content varies between 40 and 70 per cent. The color index is most frequently about 1. The average size of the cells is decreased, but macrocytes may be seen. There is some anisocytosis, but poikilocytosis is not common. Nucleated red blood cells and polychromatophilic cells are commonly present. The reticulocytes are frequently increased to between 10 and 15 per cent and in some patients there may be a very much greater increase. There is usually a decreased resistance of the red blood cells to hypotonic salt solution. Normal red blood cells show beginning hemolysis at 0.44 to 0.48 per cent and it is complete at 0.3. In hemolytic jaundice hemolysis may begin at 0.6 per cent and be complete at 0.4 per cent.

Prognosis and Course of the Disease.—Often these patients live for years without serious symptoms and they may reach an advanced age. It is characteristic, however, for exacerbations of symptoms to occur, the so-called "crises," at which time there is persistent vomiting, fever and abdominal pain. Associated with this, there is an increase in the jaundice and a rapid development of a severe anemia. A frequent complication is an associated cholelithiasis with typical attacks of biliary colic.

Treatment.—The ordinary therapeutic agents such as iron and arsenic are of no value in the treatment of the disease. If the patient's condition is serious enough, splenectomy should be considered, as this usually produces remarkable results. Within a very short time after the operation, the jaundice disappears, the blood returns rapidly to normal and all symptoms subside. This procedure is more successful if performed early in the course of the disease.

REFERENCES.

MEULENGRACHT, E.: Der chronische hereditäre hämolytische Ikterus, Leipzig, Dr. Werner Klinkhardt Verlag, 1922.

TILESTON, WILDER: Hemolytic Jaundice, Medicine, 1922, 1, 355.

CHLOROSIS.

Definition.—This condition has been described as one of obscure origin, occurring in young girls, characterized by an anemia with a low color index, which is curable by iron.

History.—Under various names, chlorosis has been described by ancient authors, but there were no accurate clinical studies of the disease until those of Hoffmann and Duncan (1731). The name "chlorosis" was given to the disease by Jean Vavandal in 1620. "Hayem was the first to place the disease on a sound pathological basis." (Sir Clifford Allbutt.)

Etiology.—It is a disease limited to the female sex and usually having the onset between the ages of fourteen and seventeen years. Recurrences are said to be common, extending into the third decade. In many respects it resembles the chronic microcytic anemia of middle-aged women, which is now relatively common, although there is a sharp difference in the age incidence of the two conditions.

One of the mysteries of medicine is why a disease so common as this several decades ago has now almost completely disappeared.

Symptoms.—The prominent signs are those of any anemia: pallor, dyspnea, palpitation and weakness. The pallor has been described as having a greenish-yellow tint. Gastric distress is common and there is poor appetite, with a craving for certain foods such as acids.

Blood.—The characteristic feature is a reduction in hemoglobin, which may be marked, with a red blood cell count which is usually normal or only slightly decreased. Thayer reports 63 cases with a red blood cell count averaging about 4,000,000 per c.mm. and an average hemoglobin of 42 per cent.

Treatment.—Iron is specific in this condition, although it should be administered over a period of several months and the patient observed for recurrences. Ferric ammonium citrate may be given in a 50 per cent solution in doses of 4 to 6 grams (60 to 90 grains), daily, or ferrum reductum 0.5 gram ($7\frac{1}{2}$ grains) to 1 gram (15 grains), three times daily.

REFERENCE.

ALLBUTT, SIR CLIFFORD: Chlorosis, System of Medicine (Clifford Allbutt and H. D. Rollston), 1909, **5**, 679.

SICKLE-CELL ANEMIA.

Definition.—This condition is an anemia probably due to a congenital defect in blood formation, limited almost exclusively to the negro race, and is characterized by the appearance of a considerable number of sickle-shaped red blood cells in the peripheral blood, a moderate anemia, attacks of abdominal pain with nausea and vomiting, recurrent leg ulcers and cardio-vascular disturbances.

History.—J. B. Herrick's classical report in 1910 established this disease as a clinical entity characterized by the association of elliptical or sickle-shaped red blood cells with a severe anemia and certain clinical manifestations. It is probable that Dresbach had observed the same condition in 1904, but his report is incomplete. The name "sickle-cell anemia" was suggested by Mason in 1922. Sydenstricker and his associates have demonstrated in recent years that the disease is not uncommon.

Etiology.—The disease probably exists from birth as it is usually seen in children, although it is observed at all ages. It is familial and probably congenital. The condition is characterized by periods of activity and quiescence. During the latent period the blood may show no changes when the ordinary methods of examination are employed, except a moderate anemia. If a preparation of fresh blood, placed on a cover-slip and sealed with petrolatum, is allowed to stand at room temperature for a number of hours, a very great majority of the cells will assume the characteristic sickle shape (latent sickling). During the active stage of the disease this typical shape is noted in many of the red blood cells, when an ordinary blood film is made in the usual manner.

Symptoms.—The active symptoms of the disease are vague attacks of abdominal pain, nausea, vomiting and moderate jaundice. Additional symptoms are headache, malaise and pain in the muscles and joints which are usually associated with a moderate febrile reaction. Remarkable features of the disease are the leg ulcers and the cardiac involvement. Characteristically the ulcers occur about the ankles, average 1 to 3 cm. in diameter, and have sharp edges with a "punched-out" appearance, similar to luetic ulcers. In a fair proportion of patients there is definite cardiac hypertrophy and not infrequently symptoms of chronic cardiac failure. With the history of recurrent attacks of painful joints in a young person, and an enlarged heart and an apical systolic murmur, the incorrect diagnosis of rheumatic mitral insufficiency is sometimes made. Early in the disease the spleen and liver become moderately enlarged.

Treatment and Prognosis.—No specific remedy is known. Liver and ventriculin are ineffective. The only treatment indicated is general hygienic measures, possibly blood transfusions, treatment of cardiac failure, if present, by the usual measures, and the local treatment of the leg ulcers. There is no convincing evidence that splenectomy is beneficial, although this has been tried in a few cases. The patients often are underdeveloped and emaciated. The periods of activity may be prolonged and frequent, which result in a serious handicap to their activities. On the other hand, apparently there may be long latent periods and the patient suffers but slight inconvenience from the disease.

REFERENCES.

HERRICK, J. B.: Peculiar Elongated and Sickle-shaped Red Blood Corpuscles in a Case of a Severe Anemia, Arch. Int. Med., 1910, **6**, 517.
STEINBERG, BERNARD: Sickle-cell Anemia, Arch. Path., 1930, **9**, 877.
SYDENSTRICKER, V. P.: Sickle-cell Anemia, South. Med. Jour., 1924, **17**, 177.
——— Further Observations on Sickle-cell Anemia, Jour. Am. Med. Assn., 1924, **83**, 12.

PURPURA.

Definition.—Purpura is a symptom produced by the extravasation of blood into the skin, subcutaneous tissues and mucous membranes. The discoloration of the skin is at first light red in color, is not raised, does not disappear on pressure and varies in size from a pin-point (petechiæ) to much larger areas (ecchymoses). The purpuric areas gradually undergo an evolution in color from bright red to a dark greenish-brown and finally to a light brown before disappearing.

History.—Purpura was the name given by the ancients to the eruption of certain infectious diseases, such as measles and scarlet fever, as well as hemorrhages into the skin. The name *Morbus maculosus* was first used by Werlhof. *Peliosis rheumatica* was the term introduced by Schönlein to describe the purpuric condition associated with arthritis. Denys, a Belgian histologist, first observed that the platelets were diminished in the blood in certain types of purpura and this was confirmed by Hayem (1890) and Ehrlich (1898). Hayem also made the original observation that the clot did not retract and express serum in some types of purpura.

Classification.—Purpura is observed in a very large number of conditions. In some it is the outstanding clinical feature while in others it is of incidental importance. The classification of Leschke, somewhat modified, is given below. The criteria used in grouping the purpuras are as follows: Is the condition present without recognizable cause (idiopathic or essential purpura) or is it secondary to a known disease (secondary or symptomatic purpura)? A further division is made into the purpuras associated with a decrease in blood platelets (thrombocytopenic purpura) and those in which there is no demonstrable abnormality of the peripheral blood (non-thrombocytopenic purpura). With the above criteria in mind, the following classification may be given as one of practical clinical value which is probably as satisfactory as our present knowledge permits:

I. Thrombocytopenic purpura (decreased platelets, delayed bleeding-time, non-retractile clot, tourniquet test positive).

    (*a*) Idiopathic thrombocytopenic purpura (Werlhof's disease).

    (*b*) Secondary thrombocytopenic purpura (associated with aplastic anemia, benzol poisoning, excessive irradiation, myelophthisic anemia, snake poisoning.)

II. Non-thrombocytopenic purpura (platelets normal, no disturbance in bleeding-time, tourniquet test negative).

    (*a*) Idiopathic purpura (the allergic group including the purpura of Schönlein and Henoch and various erythemas).

    (*b*) Symptomatic group (purpura simplex, purpura of infection, various chronic diseases, cachexia, scurvy.)

Idiopathic Thrombocytopenic Purpura (Werlhof's Disease).—Definition.—A disease of unknown etiology, characterized by purpura, spontaneous bleeding from the mucous membranes, a diminution in the number of platelets of the peripheral blood, a prolongation of the bleeding-time and the inability of the blood to form a retractile clot.

Etiology and Pathology.—The condition occurs with equal frequency in the two sexes and is most commonly observed in children or young adults. The severity of the spontaneous bleeding is roughly proportional to the reduction in platelets, although there may be striking exceptions to this statement. The cause of the decreased number of platelets is unknown but it has been suggested that it may be due to the action of an unidentified toxin on the giant cells of the marrow or possibly to an increased destruction of platelets. The bleeding is not due solely to the diminution in platelets as it may not be present when the platelet count is extremely low. It has been held by some that there is capillary damage, as the production of congestion of the arm by a tourniquet results in the appearance of petechiæ. The bone-marrow does not show characteristic changes; there does not appear to be a reduction in the number of megakaryocytes. The only constant finding on postmortem examination is evidence of extensive capillary hemorrhage which may be present in any organ of the body.

Symptoms.—The disease may be divided into the acute and chronic types, the latter being much more common. In the chronic form the symptoms may persist for a long period of time and then disappear permanently; or the attack may be present for a few weeks to several months and then, after an interval of health for a few months to many years, it may recur. The disease may be present intermittently for years.

Purpuric lesions associated with bleeding from the mucous membranes, usually of the nose or mouth, without obvious cause, constitute the chief clinical evidences of this form of purpura. The purpuric eruption varies greatly in extent from a few scattered lesions the size of a pin-point to large ecchymoses. The skin lesions are red at first, do not disappear on pressure, appear superficial and are not raised or indurated. They begin to fade within a few days and go through the various color changes observed in the familiar "black and blue" spot due to trauma. Similar lesions occur in the various mucous membranes of the body.

The bleeding from mucous membranes varies from a slight oozing to hemorrhages so extensive as to result in a severe secondary anemia. The bleeding is usually from the nose and next in frequency from the mouth, but may occur from the gastro-intestinal tract, the uterus, the urinary tract and into various organs of the body, including the brain, which may be the immediate cause of death. Pulmonary hemorrhage is rare. Fever ranging from 100° to 102° F. is not infrequently present in the acute cases and when the anemia is severe. It is rarely seen in the mild cases or in the chronic forms of the disease unless the bleeding is intensive or some complication exists. The spleen may be enlarged in the chronic cases but this is not a common finding.

The Blood.—Characteristic findings are present which are highly important from the standpoint of diagnosis. They are: (1) a reduction in the number of platelets, (2) a delayed bleeding-time, (3) non-retractility of the blood clot, and (4) a normal clotting-time.

The blood platelets are usually reduced from a normal average number of 300,000 per c.mm. to 60,000 per c.mm. or less when active bleeding is present. Counts as low as 5000 to 10,000 per c.mm. have been reported. The bleeding-time as determined by noting the length of time required for a puncture wound of the ear to stop bleeding is characteristically prolonged. Normally when blood is taken up from the wound on filter paper once a minute the bleeding persists for not longer than three to four minutes. If the bleeding-time persists for over ten minutes it is considered to be prolonged. In some cases it may continue for hours. The coagulation-time is normal but the clot when formed does not retract and express serum as it does normally.

Additional data concerning the tendency to bleed may be derived from the tourniquet test. This procedure consists in applying a tourniquet (a blood-pressure cuff may be used) and making sufficient pressure to obstruct the venous return but not the arterial flow. In thrombocytopenic purpura, petechiæ or ecchymoses usually appear below the location of the tourniquet in from three to ten minutes.

The other changes which are found in the blood depend upon the amount of bleeding and are of the usual type seen following hemorrhage—a color index below 1, slight anisocytosis and poikilocytosis and a slight leukocytosis with an increase in the polymorphonuclear neutrophil cells. Occasionally normoblasts, cells showing diffuse polychromatophilia and stippling are seen and staining with cresyl blue usually shows an increase in the number of reticulocytes when a definite anemia is present.

Prognosis.—The severity of the disease varies widely. The symptoms may be exceedingly mild and persist for only a few days, or the condition may be fulminating and terminate fatally within forty-eight hours. Other cases have a moderately severe course with symptoms which persist for several months. There is a definite tendency for the disease to recur but there is no way of predicting accurately that this will or will not occur.

Treatment.—Transfusion by either the direct or indirect method will often control the hemorrhage. Unless the patient shows an associated spontaneous improvement at the time, the effect is transient and it is assumed to be due to the introduction of platelets with the transfused blood. It is a valuable therapeutic measure, however, and several transfusions are indicated in purpura when bleeding is serious. It is of value not only in stopping the hemorrhage but also in overcoming the secondary anemia which may be present. One or more transfusions should always be given prior to splenectomy when the bleeding-time is prolonged.

Splenectomy.—It has been determined in recent years that removal of the spleen is a valuable therapeutic measure in patients with the chronic form of the disease. This radical form of treatment should not be employed except in those patients who are seriously incapacitated by the disease and in those in whom blood transfusions have failed to give relief. A great majority of these patients have a dramatic recovery following splenectomy and apparently the results are permanent, although additional data bearing on this point are necessary before a final statement can be made. The operation is contraindicated in the acute form of the disease on account of the high operative mortality. Following splenectomy the platelets may return to normal in some patients coincident with the cessation of bleeding, but in other cases the bleeding may cease although the platelet count remains low.

Other Forms of Treatment.—The use of the ultra-violet light has been said to increase the platelets and thereby influence the course of the disease favorably, but all observers are not in agreement concerning the efficacy of this form of treatment. Other therapeutic measures such as aromatic sulphuric acid (1 to 2 cc.), three times daily, or oil of turpentine (1 cc.), three or four times daily, or calcium lactate (1 gram), three or four times daily, have been recommended but apparently are of little value. A high-protein, high-vitamin diet and viosterol are said to be of value in the treatment of this disease, but there is no conclusive evidence in support of this view.

Secondary or Symptomatic Thrombocytopenic Purpura.—This type of the disease presents the clinical picture of bleeding from the mucous membranes, purpura and a reduction in the number of circulating blood platelets, which is secondary to a known disease. The reduction of the platelets and production of this syndrome is due to various causes, depending upon the disease to which it is secondary. In leukemia the giant cells, the progenitors of the platelets, are reduced in number as a result of the leukemic infiltration of the marrow. In pernicious anemia this same situation occurs on account of the hyperplastic red blood-cell-forming elements of the marrow. In aplastic anemia there is a destruction of all elements of the marrow, including the giant cells, due to the action of some unknown toxin. Likewise excessive irradiation with radium and the roentgen-rays and such poisons as benzol and arsphenamine produce an aplasia of the marrow with a destruction of giant cells and a diminution of the platelets in the peripheral blood. The clinical picture need not be given in detail here; it consists of the symptoms of idiopathic thrombocytopenic purpura with the additional symptoms and signs which are associated with the primary disease.

Idiopathic Non-thrombocytopenic Purpura (Allergic Purpura).—Definition.—A purpura which is probably evidence of a true allergic condition and characterized by purpuric spots, sometimes associated with joint involvement and visceral manifestations.

Etiology and Pathology.—In this condition the blood is normal with reference to bleeding-time, clotting-time, retractibility of the clot and the number of platelets. The *symptoms* vary widely and may include arthritis (*Schönlein's purpura*), attacks of intestinal pain with or without hemorrhage from the bowel (*Henoch's purpura*) and such varied skin manifestations as purpura, urticaria and erythematous lesions. The onset is characterized by fever, malaise, anorexia and headache. The various symptoms arise from a common pathologic change and the nature of the symptoms depends upon the location of the lesion. The change is a focal disturbance in the small blood-vessels which results in congestion, exudation and hemorrhage. The disease has been considered as allergic in nature because it resembles serum sickness in some instances and also because it can be demonstrated in some patients that they are sensitive to various types of protein which induce the attacks.

Prognosis and Treatment.—The condition is rarely fatal and usually subsides within several weeks, although recurrences are common. The most important step in the treatment is to determine from the history and by appropriate tests if the attacks are due to a specific protein and, if so, proper treatment should be given. If there is evidence of urticaria this may be controlled by the use of adrenalin hydrochloride, 0.5 cc., 1 to 1000 solution, subcutaneously.

Symptomatic Non-thrombocytopenic Purpura.—In a very large group of diseases there may appear a purpura secondary to a recognized disease which is not associated with changes in the blood. This condition is seen in any type of infection and is observed in some as the characteristic skin lesion (epidemic cerebrospinal meningitis). It may also appear in chronic nephritis, any cachectic state and following the use of a number of drugs (iodide, quinine, atropine).

REFERENCES.

ALEXANDER, H. L., and EYERMANN, C. H.: Allergic Purpura, Jour. Am. Med. Assn., 1929, **92**, 2092.

BRILL, N. E., and ROSENTHAL, N.: Treatment by Splenectomy of Essential Thrombocytopenia (Purpura Hæmorrhagica), Arch. Int. Med., 1923, **30**, 939.

CHRISTIAN, H. A.: Purpura and Allied Conditions, Oxford Medicine, 1920, **2**, 781.

ROSENTHAL, N.: The Blood Picture in Purpura, Jour. Lab. and Clin. Med., 1928, **13**, 303.

HEMOPHILIA.

Definition.—This condition is an hereditary anomaly of the blood characterized by a delayed coagulation-time, which results in a tendency to excessive hemorrhage. It appears only in males and is transmitted only by females.

History.—There is little evidence to indicate that the ancients were familiar with the condition, although reference was made in the early part of the twelfth century to males in certain families who bled excessively. In 1874 Fordyce observed a hemorrhagic tendency in several members of the same family. The first comprehensive description of the disease was by John C. Otto in 1803, who made a careful study of a family of "bleeders" in Plymouth, N. H. The name "hemophilia" was given by Schönlein. The most complete monograph concerning the subject is the one written by Bulloch and Feldes in 1915.

Etiology.—The cause of the delayed coagulation-time is unknown, but it appears to be related to a qualitative deficiency in prothrombin, an antecedent of thrombin. One view is that there is a qualitative change in the blood platelets which results in a delayed release of prothrombin. There is no doubt that the condition is hereditary and may be transmitted through many generations by females, although the active disease appears only in males. Some believe it is limited to the Teutonic race. There are no pathologic changes associated with the condition except the delayed coagulation-time and the results of bleeding into various tissues of the body.

Symptoms.—The outstanding symptom in hemophilia is the abnormal tendency to excessive bleeding from minor injuries to the skin, from the mucous membranes or into the joints. The symptoms usually appear in early childhood as the result of a minor operation, such as circumcision, from injury to the gums due to eruption of the teeth or from insignificant wounds of the skin. Extraction of a tooth is a frequent cause of prolonged hemorrhage which may prove fatal. Profuse epistaxis is common. Spontaneous bleeding may occur into the skin and subcutaneous tissue or muscles forming ecchymoses or hematomas. A serious and not infrequent complication is hemorrhage into the joints which may result in a permanent deformity. The knee- and elbow-joints are most frequently involved. Bleeding may occur into body cavities or the various viscera. Hematuria is not rare. Physical examination usually shows no abnormalities unless it is the evidence of anemia from a recent hemorrhage, ecchymosis or joint involvement.

Blood Examination.—The blood is normal in every respect with the exception of a delayed coagulation-time, unless there has been a recent hemorrhage which results in the picture of a secondary anemia. The coagulation-time varies from day to day, and may range from thirty minutes to a number of hours. The clot, when formed, retracts and appears normal. Bleeding-time as determined by a pin-prick of the lobe of the ear or the finger is not prolonged. The blood findings differ from thrombocytopenic purpura as in this condition the platelets are diminished, the coagulation-time is normal, although the clot does not retract, and the bleeding-time is prolonged.

Prognosis and Treatment.—Cephalin when added to hemophiliac blood causes a prompt clotting, and is valuable in controlling the bleeding in these patients. Jay McLean recommends the application of surgical gauze which has been impregnated with a cephalin solution. The ordinary measures which are used in the control of hemorrhage, such as the cautery, ferric chloride and the application of adrenalin may be given a trial, but the results are not always satisfactory.

The production of an anaphylactic reaction has been recommended as a measure which will shorten the coagulation-time and stop bleeding. Patients who are non-sensitive may be given 2 to 4 cc. of horse or other serum subcutaneously, and after a ten-day interval when sensitiveness develops, another subcutaneous injection of 0.2 cc. may be given. Following this, the coagulation-time may diminish and remain so for several weeks. Repeated small injections may be given in the hope that excessive bleeding will be prevented.

In all patients when the bleeding does not yield to simple measures, a blood transfusion of either whole or citrated blood should be given. This promptly causes the bleeding to cease and hastens convalescence by replacing the blood which has been lost. The effect, however, is temporary, as the clotting-time again becomes prolonged to its original level after about three days. By the use of repeated transfusions, patients with hemophilia can be carried safely through operations. In even such minor procedures as the extraction of a tooth, these patients should be carefully prepared and observed to prevent excessive loss of blood and perhaps a fatal hemorrhage. Since the introduction of blood transfusions as a method of controlling the bleeding, the outlook is much better. In many, however, the joint deformity is a handicap and may cause them to be incapacitated.

Birch has recently suggested that ovarian therapy might be valuable in the control of this disease, but further experience has shown little value in this form of therapy.

REFERENCES.

BIRCH, C. L.: Hemophilia, Jour. Am. Med. Assn., 1932, **99**, 1566.
BULLOCH, W., and FELDES, P.: Hemophilia Memoirs, No. 12, Eugenic Laboratory, Univ. of London, 1911
HOWELL, W. H., and CEKADA, E. B.: The Cause of Delayed Clotting of Hemophilic Blood, Am. Jour. Physiol., 1926, **78**, 500.
McLEAN, J.: Hemophilia, Oxford Med., 1920, **2**, 799, New York, Oxford Univ. Press.

LEUKEMIA.

Synonyms.—Leukocythemia; Leukanemia.

Definition.—Leukemia is a fatal disease, characterized by a marked hyperplasia of the white blood-cell-forming tissue throughout the body. When fully developed there is usually a striking increase in the white blood cells of the peripheral blood, many of which may be abnormal forms. It is this latter change which differentiates it from a leukocytosis.

History.—The earliest descriptions of leukemia were by Hughes Bennett and Craigie, who wrote concerning this disease in 1845, both articles appearing in the same number of the Edinburgh Medical Journal. The condition was called "leukocythemia." It was recognized that the liver and spleen were enlarged and the white cells of the blood were greatly increased. Virchow independently and almost simultaneously described a similar condition which he called "leukemia." He classified the disease into the splenic and lymphatic varieties. Neuman, in 1870, described a third type, the myelogenous, which was characterized by changes in the bone-marrow. It was not until 1891 that

Ehrlich, who introduced the differential staining of white blood cells, recognized that the two main types of the disease were the lymphatic and myelogenous varieties.

Classification.—The leukemias may be arranged conveniently according to the following types:

1. Chronic myelogenous leukemia.
2. Chronic lymphatic leukemia.
3. Aleukemic leukemia.
4. The acute leukemias.
5. Monocytic leukemia.

Etiology.—The cause of leukemia is unknown but the prevailing view considers the condition as neoplastic in nature. A minority, however, regard it as due to an infection, chiefly on the basis that it can be transmitted to fowls by a filtrate which has been passed through a Berkefeld filter and because the acute leukemias resemble an acute sepsis from a clinical standpoint.

Any type of leukemia may occur at any age but there is a definite relationship between the greatest incidence of the several varieties of leukemia and the different age groups. Chronic myelogenous leukemia is most frequently observed between the ages of thirty-five and forty-five years, while the greatest incidence for chronic lymphatic leukemia is between the ages of forty-five and fifty-five years. The acute leukemias occur most frequently before the age of twenty-five years. Leukemia probably occurs more frequently in children than previous reports indicate, as undoubtedly in some instances the condition has not been recognized.

Chronic Myelogenous Leukemia.—Pathology.—The important and characteristic pathologic findings are observed in the spleen and bone-marrow. Other changes are due to the associated anemia and to microscopic leukemic infiltrations in the various viscera. The spleen usually is greatly enlarged and firm. There is a striking proliferation of the fibrous tissue and a loss of the normal splenic architecture as a result of the remarkable collection of myeloid cells of all types. The bone-marrow contains very little gross fat and appears pinkish gray. This is due to the great accumulation of myeloid cells, chiefly myelocytes or myeloblasts, which almost completely replace the erythroblastic tissue.

Symptoms.—The onset of the disease is so insidious that it is difficult to determine the duration of the illness. The earliest symptoms are often those which are attributed to the associated anemia, such as weakness, pallor, dyspnea and palpitation. Others first complain of a dragging dull pain in the upper left quadrant, or their attention is attracted to the bulging in the abdomen due to the splenic enlargement. Undoubtedly in many cases the changes in the white cells of the peripheral blood are present for some time before the patient is aware of symptoms. Additional complaints are those arising from the increased basal metabolism which is frequently present in these patients. These symptoms are tolerance of cold, increased sweating, tachycardia, loss of weight, and fever. As the disease progresses, the manifestations of the anemia become more striking and dominate the

56

clinical picture. Often excessive sweating and fever develop and the patient becomes so weak that bed rest is necessary. Toward the end of the disease it is common to have hemorrhages into the skin and from the mucous membranes. Death usually results from an intercurrent infection or, less commonly, from hemorrhage.

The characteristic findings on physical examination are the objective evidences of an anemia and the presence of an enormously enlarged spleen. There is pallor which may be extreme, evidence of considerable loss of weight and sometimes edema of the ankles. Characteristically there is no glandular enlargement. In some instances this may be observed but it is usually not generalized or prominent. The spleen may be enormously enlarged and fill the greater portion of the abdomen. It is firm and may or may not be tender, depending upon the degree of perisplenitis. The skin rarely shows leukemic infiltrations, but in the advanced stages there may be petechial spots. When the disease is well developed there may be an irregular type of fever.

Basal Metabolic Rate.—In untreated patients this is elevated, with few exceptions, above the normal limits, although in some instances this is slight. It is not uncommon to observe an increase between +35 and +50. In general, the degree of elevation depends on the severity of the leukemic process and is of value in indicating the prognosis.

Blood Examination.—Three characteristic changes occur in the typical cases: (1) a moderately severe anemia, (2) a striking increase in the total number of white blood cells, (3) a large percentage of polymorphonuclear neutrophils and immature granulocytes. The anemia is myelophthisic in type and is usually moderately advanced when the patient is first seen, often being in the vicinity of 2,500,000 red blood cells per c.mm., with a slightly greater proportionate decrease in the hemoglobin content which gives a color index somewhat below 1. The total white blood cell count varies between 100,000 and 500,000 or more per c.mm. As many as 90 to 95 per cent of the cells may be of the granulocyte variety. Neutrophilic, eosinophilic and basophilic myelocytes are present in variable numbers. Neutrophilic myelocytes vary from a few per cent to as high as 35 to 40 per cent, whereas the other two types are usually present in much smaller numbers. Myeloblasts are frequently present, but usually do not comprise more than 2 or 3 per cent of all white blood cells in the chronic type of leukemia. The blood platelets are usually normal or slightly reduced in the early stages of the disease. An extreme reduction may be seen in the advanced stages and may be associated with various types of hemorrhages. As the condition progresses and the anemia becomes severe, it is common to observe in the peripheral blood various types of immature red blood cells, such as normoblasts, stippled cells and those showing diffuse basophilia and stippling.

Chronic Lymphatic Leukemia.—**Pathology.**—The pathologic findings are characteristic and consist of a widespread lymphoid infiltration throughout lymphatic tissue and many organs of the body. There is a generalized enlargement of all of the lymph glands which are discrete and vary in size from a pea to a small lemon. The normal structure of the lymph gland is unrecognizable, due to the extensive infiltration with lymphocytes. The spleen is always moderately enlarged but does not reach the size which it does in chronic myelogenous leukemia. This organ is likewise altered completely in histologic appearance due to the lymphocytic infiltration. The yellow marrow of the bone is replaced by a grayish-red cellular tissue which is composed of lymphoid cells. The liver, kidneys, many other viscera and the solitary follicle and patches of the intestine likewise show an infiltration of lymphocytes.

Symptoms.—The early symptoms are mild and vague and, as a rule, do not cause the patient to consult a physician for several months. The earliest evidence of the disease is not infrequently the appearance of an enlarged, painless lymph gland, or the patient may first note the symptoms which are due to a gradually developing secondary anemia, namely, weakness, pallor, loss of weight, dyspnea and palpitation. As the disease progresses, the clinical picture is one of generalized lymph gland enlargement associated with an increasingly severe anemia. Hemorrhages into the skin or from the mucous membranes may occur but usually are not extensive.

Physical examination usually reveals an extensive and widespread enlargement of the lymph glands which is especially noticeable in the cervical, axillary and inguinal regions. The glands vary in size from a pea to several centimeters in diameter; they are firm, non-tender and are not adherent to each other or to the skin.

The spleen shows moderate enlargement but rarely reaches the size seen in chronic myelogenous leukemia. The liver edge is usually palpable several finger breadths below the costal margin. It is not uncommon to observe leukemic infiltrations of the skin in this type of leukemia. They are usually localized, but the entire skin may show the characteristic roughness and thickening.

The Blood.—The white blood cell count is usually elevated but rarely over 200,000 per c.mm., and not infrequently it is below 100,000 per c.mm. Over 90 per cent of the cells resemble the normal small lymphocyte very closely. There are usually a few lymphoblasts which measure from 10 to 15 microns in diameter, and have a very large, light-staining nucleus with wavy outlines. There are usually some lymphocytes which have such a slender rim of cytoplasm that it is almost invisible. The Rieder cell type of small lymphocyte with a notched nucleus is commonly seen in this condition. The red blood cells and hemoglobin are reduced in amount, and a moderate degree of anisocytosis and poikilocytosis is present. As the condition becomes more advanced normoblasts, megaloblasts and other forms of immature red blood cells are observed.

Treatment of Leukemia.—The therapy of the leukemias consists of: (1) symptomatic treatment to attempt the control of various symptoms as they arise, (2) the use of irradiation in the form of roentgen-rays or radium, and (3) various measures to combat the anemia. There is no treatment which is recognized as curative. The application of the roentgen-rays over the spleen frequently induces a remission in the course of the disease and may produce remarkable temporary results. Roentgen-ray therapy should be used carefully and only when the patient's clinical condition demands it. After a variable number of exposures, all patients become refractory to treatment and further improvement is not to be expected. This form of treatment should be carefully controlled by frequent blood examination and therapy discontinued when the white blood cell count falls below 30,000 per c.mm. Arsenic in the form of Fowler's solution, pushed to the tolerance of the patient, sometimes produces satisfactory results, especially in the myelogenous type. Blood transfusions are · useful when the anemia becomes severe and it is the only form of treatment which produces even slight temporary improvement in the acute leukemias. Roentgen-ray therapy is contraindicated in the latter condition as it not only fails to cause improvement but may do actual harm. The benzol form of treatment is now rarely used as it is too difficult to control. Various measures such as iron, liver and ventriculin are of little or no avail in the treatment of the anemia.

Aleukemic Leukemia.—This form of leukemia is important, chiefly because it is so often confused with other diseases. The acute form is frequently incorrectly regarded as a thrombopenic purpura and the chronic form as Banti's disease or pernicious anemia. It may exist as a chronic or acute myelogenous or lymphatic form and differs only from the usual types by the blood examination, which shows a normal or subnormal white blood cell count. In almost all cases, however, there are pathologic white blood cells, such as myeloblasts, myelocytes or lymphoblasts present in the peripheral blood. It is almost always a phase of chronic leukemia. The condition may be differentiated from pernicious anemia by the following points: in aleukemic leukemia there may be free hydrochloric acid present in the gastric contents; there is no history of glossitis or evidence of neurologic involvement; the response to liver or stomach therapy is negligible; the blood bilirubin is not increased, and poikilocytosis, if present, is very moderate. The condition is a fatal one, as no form of treatment is effective. Blood transfusions exert only a very temporary beneficial effect.

Acute Leukemia.—The acute leukemias may be of either the lymphatic or myelogenous type, but the clinical picture and course of the disease are identical. In many instances it is difficult to identify the variety, and the clinician must be satisfied with the diagnosis of acute leukemia. It was previously thought that most patients had the acute lymphatic type, but more recent studies have indicated that the acute myelogenous type is not rare.

Symptoms.—This condition is most frequently observed in patients under twenty-five years of age. The onset is usually abrupt, although it may be preceded by some type of infection, such as a tonsillitis. The initial symptoms are those which are commonly seen in a severe acute infection, namely, high fever, malaise, headache and prostration. Associated with this is a rapidly developing anemia. There may be nothing distinctive about the early clinical picture to indicate the correct diagnosis. The combination, however, of the symptoms of a fulminating infection with a rapidly developing pallor should at once suggest a blood examination which should indicate the diagnosis. As the condition progresses, other manifestations of the disease appear. A hemorrhagic tendency develops with ecchymoses and petechiæ and bleeding occurs from the various mucous membranes. In addition, the gums become swollen and reddened and this may progress until there are areas of necrosis about the mouth and throat. While there is usually lymph gland enlargement in the neck, due to the mouth condition, there is slight, if any, generalized lymph gland enlargement. The spleen may be palpable but it never attains the size seen in the chronic forms of leukemia.

The Blood.—Examination usually shows a severe anemia, the red blood cell count often being in the vicinity of 1,000,000 per c.mm. and the hemoglobin from 20 to 30 per cent. The white blood cell count is usually not greatly elevated, the average being between 15,000 and 30,000 per c.mm. Examination of a stained film shows the red blood cells to be fairly well filled with hemoglobin; there is moderate variation in size and shape, and usually immature red blood cells, such as normoblasts, megaloblasts and cells showing polychromatophilia are seen. A very large percentage of the white blood cells are immature in type. In many instances the predominating cell is large, measuring 15 to 18 microns in diameter, and has a faint blue cytoplasm which does not contain granules. The nucleus is relatively large, has wavy outlines and the chromatin is in loose strands. It is often impossible to say if this cell is a myeloblast or a lymphoblast. It is sometimes possible to trace all variations of granulocytes from this primitive form through the myelocyte series to the mature polymorphonuclear leukocytes. When this is possible, it indicates a diagnosis of acute myelogenous leukemia. At other times, the predominating type of mature cell unquestionably belongs to the lymphocyte series and the diagnosis of acute lymphatic leukemia may be made. Often, however, when there are no mature forms of white blood cells present, it is impossible to recognize the variety of leukemia.

Prognosis and Treatment.—Acute leukemia is a disease with very high mortality, as the usual course is progressively downward with a fatal issue within a few weeks to a few months. Occasionally there are brief remissions or the patient may develop a subacute type of the disease and live for a longer period. Spontaneous recoveries have been reported but they are exceedingly rare. There is no satisfactory treatment of acute leukemia. Symptomatic therapy should be used, and blood transfusions may cause transient improvement. Roentgen-ray therapy is contraindicated.

Monocytic Leukemia.—Within recent years it has been recognized that a true monocytic leukemia may occur as a separate clinical entity, which varies from the other types of leukemia only in that the predominating white blood cell in the peripheral blood is a true monocyte. In a patient recently observed, a male, aged fifty-five years, there was a history of intermittent fever and chills, general malaise, weakness, dyspnea and pallor. Physical examination showed emaciation, pallor and gingivitis which later developed into a necrotic stomatitis. There was no glandular enlargement and the liver and spleen were not palpable. Blood examination showed: red blood cell count, 2,300,000 per c.mm.; hemoglobin, 50 per cent; white blood cell count, 50,000 per c.mm. Eighty per cent of the white blood cells were typical monocytes. The symptoms and course of the disease resemble the other types of leukemia with the exception that the course is usually rapid, with a fatal termination within a few weeks to a few months. Occasionally the patient may survive for a period of several years.

REFERENCES.

DAMESHEK, W.: Acute Monocytic (Histiocytic) Leukemia, Arch. Int. Med., 1930, **66**, 718.
GORDON, A. H.: Aleukemic Leukemia, Trans. Assn. Am. Phys., 1929, **44**, 305.
ISAACS, RAPHAEL: Blood Changes in the Leukemias and Lymphomata and Their Bearing on Roentgen Therapy, Am. Jour. Roentgenol. and Rad. Ther., 1930, **24**, 648.
MINOT, G. R., BUCKMAN, T. E., and ISAACS, R.: Chronic Myelogenous Leukemia, Age Incidence, Duration and Benefit Derived from Irradiation, Jour. Am. Med. Assn., 1924, **82**, 1489.
MINOT, G. R., and ISAACS, R.: Lymphatic Leukemia: Age Incidence, Duration and Benefit Derived from Irradiation, Boston Med. and Surg. Jour., 1924, **191**, 1.

AGRANULOCYTIC ANGINA.

Synonyms.—Agranulocytosis; Idiopathic malignant neutropenia.

Definition.—Agranulocytic angina is a disease of unknown etiology, characterized by a remarkable reduction in the polymorphonuclear cells of the peripheral blood, ulcerative lesions in the mouth, throat, rectum or vagina, and often chills and fever.

Agranulocytosis may be classified as follows:

I. Primary Agranulocytosis.—(a) **Acute (Schultz Type).**—In this variety of the disease the onset is usually abrupt. The process is sometimes mild in intensity and the patient may not appear severely ill, but not infrequently the course resembles a fulminating infection with a fatal termination within a few days.

(b) **Chronic Recurring Agranulocytosis.**—A patient with this type of the disease may have many attacks with the characteristic manifestations which may be very mild, resembling an upper respiratory infection, or may have a rapidly fatal course during one of the exacerbations.

II. Secondary Agranulocytosis.—This condition differs entirely from the primary variety, but has in common with it the diminution in leukocytes of the peripheral blood and sometimes lesions of the mucous membranes. It is observed in the following conditions:

1. Chemical poisoning (arsenic, benzol);
2. Following irradiation;
3. In various infections (typhoid fever, pneumonia);
4. In certain blood diseases (pernicious anemia, aleukemic leukemia, aplastic anemia).

History.—Schultz, in 1922, emphasized the importance of the syndrome which he described as a new clinical entity. The disease had undoubtedly been described before by various observers, among them being Philip King Brown, of San Francisco, who described a typical case in 1902.

Etiology.—It has been held by some that the condition is an exhaustion of the bone-marrow, as the result of infection. Damaging evidence against this view is the observation that the leukopenia precedes evidence of sepsis. Infection with an organism which has a special affinity for the granulocytic tissue, infection of the bone-marrow itself, chemical poisoning of the marrow and a congenital hemapoietic insufficiency, have all been suggested as causes of the disease. One of the most important observations concerning the etiology of the disease was made by Madison and Squier in 1933, when they suggested that amidopyrine might be the precipitating cause of this condition in some patients, but certainly not in all.

Symptoms.—The onset may be abrupt with high fever, chills, sore throat and extreme prostration. Delirium may appear early. Characteristically there is an associated ulcerative lesion involving the mucous membranes. This usually occurs about the mouth or throat but may involve the rectum or vagina. Jaundice may develop in some instances. The severity of the condition varies from symptoms suggesting a mild upper respiratory condition to a severe illness which terminates fatally within a few days. Some of the patients with this disease give a history of taking amidopyrine or compounds containing this drug prior to the onset of their illness. Recently Thompson has suggested that in women an attack frequently begins a few days prior to the onset of the menstrual period and he believes that there may be some relationship between the disease and ovarian function.

Blood.—The striking feature is a pronounced leukopenia which may progress to such an extent that the polymorphonuclear neutrophil cells completely disappear from the peripheral blood. The reduction at first is only in the granulocytes but later the lymphocytes and monocytes are also diminished. There is no alteration in the red blood cells unless the illness is prolonged and then an anemia with a low color index may develop. The platelets are usually normal or increased except when the illness is prolonged, and they may then become diminished.

Prognosis and Treatment.—The mortality in this disease has been high, especially in the untreated patients with the acute type of the condition, averaging about 75 per cent. Some patients recover from their initial attack only to succumb to the second or third exacerbation.

Many types of therapy have been used in attempting to control the disease, including blood transfusions, injection of convalescent serum, foreign protein injections, minimal doses of roentgen-ray, intravenous injections of adenin sulphate or guanin hydrochloride, intramuscular or intravenous injections of liver extract, and the intramuscular injection of pentnucleotide (formerly nucleotide K-96). While there is some difference of opinion concerning the effectiveness of the different forms of therapy, injections of pentnucleotide are probably the most effective treatment available at the present time. The method of administration is as follows: 10 cc. of the solution, containing 0.7 gram of the drug, should be injected into the gluteal muscles, twice daily, until the white blood cell count is normal. One injection of 10 cc. should be given thereafter until the leukocyte count has been normal for three or four days. In patients who are desperately ill, the original and subsequent dosage may be doubled. If there is no improvement with the pentnucleotide therapy, repeated small blood transfusions (200 to 250 cc.) should be given.

All patients with this disease should be warned against taking amidopyrine alone or in combination with other drugs, as this may precipitate an attack of the disease.

REFERENCES.

BROWN, P. K.: A Fatal Case of Acute Primary Infectious Pharyngitis with Extreme Leukopenia, Am. Med., 1902, **3**, 649.

KASTLIN, G. J.: Agranulocytic Angina, Am. Jour. Med. Sci., 1927, **173**, 799.

MADISON, F. W., and SQUIER, T. L.: The Etiology of Primary Granulocytopenia (Agranulocytic Angina), Jour. Am. Med. Assn., 1934, **102**, 755.

ROBERTS, S. R., and KRACKE, R. R.: Agranulocytosis: Report of a Case, Jour. Am. Med. Assn., 1930, **95**, 780.

THOMPSON, W. P.: Observations on the Possible Relation Between Agranulocytosis and Menstruation, with Further Studies on a Case of Cyclic Neutropenia, New England Jour. Med., 1934, **210**, 176.

HODGKIN'S DISEASE.

Synonyms.—Pseudoleukemia; Lymphoblastoma; Malignant lymphoma.

Definition.—A disease characterized by specific changes, probably of a neoplastic nature, in the lymph glands and lymphoid tissue of the body, an anemia, a varied symptomatology and a fatal course.

History.—The disease was first described by Hodgkin in 1832, but the earliest complete description appears to have been given by Wunderlich in 1858. He not only described the changes in the lymph nodes and spleen but also mentions the severe associated anemia and differentiated it from the leukemias by noting the absence of an increased number of white cells in the blood. In 1865 Wilkes applied the name of "Hodgkin's disease" to the syndrome. In 1870 Murchinson and Sanderson published a complete description of the disease, with historic notes to date.

Etiology.—It is well recognized that the disease occurs about twice as frequently in males as in females. It may develop at any age but the largest number of patients are young adults between the ages of twenty and thirty years. The cause has been attributed to various types of chronic infections, including tuberculosis, but it is now considered to be neoplastic in origin by a great majority of students of the disease.

Pathology.—There is usually a widespread involvement of both the superficial and deep lymph glands, including the cervical, axillary, inguinal, mediastinal and abdominal glands. In size they vary from that of a pea to an orange. They are round, smooth, hard or soft, depending on the stage of the disease, and loosely held together with connective tissue. The glands are never firmly adherent to each other unless there has been a secondary infection. The characteristic microscopic picture is one of lymphoid hyperplasia with active proliferation of the germinal centers, and the endothelial and reticular cells. Multinuclear giant cells and eosinophils are frequently observed. As the process advances there is an increase in connective tissue until the cellular part of the tumor is reduced to small areas, lying between bands of fibrous tissue. While the condition primarily involves the lymph glands, almost any organ of the body containing lymphatic tissue may develop the characteristic changes. The process is noted commonly in the spleen and less frequently in the liver and kidneys. The bone-marrow may be infiltrated with lymphoid cells which in large part replace the erythroblastic tissue.

Symptoms.—The most frequent initial symptom is a painless unilateral enlargement of a cervical lymph gland, although the primary glandular enlargement may be in the axilla or inguinal regions, or in the abdomen. The glandular enlargement often rapidly spreads to the other side of the neck and other superficial lymph glands. Examination of the gland usually shows that it is firm, freely movable, not adherent to the skin or other glands and non-tender.

As the disease progresses, certain constitutional symptoms appear. Such complaints as weakness, loss of weight, pallor, dyspnea and palpitation are due entirely or in part to the associated myelophthisic anemia. Not infrequently a moderate amount of fever is present during some stage of the illness. A striking variety of the disease shows febrile periods persisting for two or three weeks, alternating with afebrile periods of a week or ten days' duration (Pel-Epstein type).

A very large variety of symptoms may result from the pressure of the enlarged glands upon nerves, blood- or lymph-vessels or various organs. Enlarged glands in the mediastinum may cause the clinical picture of a mediastinal tumor with dyspnea, cyanosis, distention of the veins of the neck and edema of the face. The trachea may be compressed and deviated. Dysphagia is not uncommon and pressure on the recurrent laryngeal nerves may result in aphonia.

Abdominal symptoms are common and are the initial ones of the disease in some patients. Abdominal pain, simulating gall-bladder disease or peptic ulcer, is not uncommon. Additional symptoms are diarrhea or constipation, distention and diffuse abdominal tenderness. Pain in the back, either with or without erosion of the spine, is occasionally a prominent symptom. A spastic paraplegia has been known to occur from invasion or compression of the spinal cord. Pain in the legs is a common symptom late in the disease but it may occur early.

An extreme degree of pruritus may be an early and annoying symptom, which sometimes constitutes the patient's chief complaint. In some patients there may be a generalized brownish pigmentation, or the discoloration may be irregularly distributed, giving a mottled appearance. Occasionally there may be an actual infiltration of the skin, producing small nodules.

Diagnosis.—The presence of a painless, enlarged lymph gland, appearing without obvious cause, should at once suggest the possibility of Hodgkin's disease. In all such cases a small gland should immediately be excised and examined microscopically by a competent pathologist. The patient should be carefully examined for evidence of other glandular enlargement, including roentgenograms of the chest to determine the presence or absence of enlargement of the mediastinal glands. In some patients the clinical picture may be that of chills and fever without obvious cause. In such patients there is usually enlargement of the superficial lymph glands, but this may not occur until late in the disease. Other patients have splenomegaly and a secondary anemia without glandular enlargement which suggests the possibility of Banti's disease.

The blood changes are not sufficiently constant or characteristic to be of great aid in the diagnosis. There is usually a moderate secondary anemia of the myelophthisic type when the disease is well established. The only rather constant additional change in the blood is a relative and absolute increase in the polymorphonuclear cells which usually occurs when the condition is advanced but may be seen in the earlier stages. An eosinophilia, usually of moderate extent, may be observed.

Prognosis.—The average patient with Hodgkin's disease lives for only two or three years after the earliest symptoms are noted. Recoveries are unknown although rare cases are reported who have survived for ten to fifteen years.

Treatment.—Radical excision of the glands has been advised in the past, but there are few advocates of this form of therapy at present. Roentgen-ray treatment is undoubtedly of great service, although there is no evidence that the life of the patient is prolonged. It does, however, alleviate symptoms, diminish the size of the glands and improve the patient's sense of well-being. Roentgen-ray therapy should be given only when the patient's symptoms demand it, as eventually after a certain number of treatments the patients become refractory to this form of therapy.

REFERENCES.

MINOT, G. R., and ISAACS, R.: Lymphoblastoma; Aspects Concerning Abdominal Lesions, Especially Their Production of Early Symptoms, Am. Jour. Med. Sci., 1926, **172**, 157.
MINOT, G. R., and ISAACS, R.: Lymphoblastoma (Malignant Lymphoma). Age and Sex Incidence, Duration of Disease, and the Effect of Roentgen-ray Irradiation and Surgery, Jour. Am. Med. Assn., 1926, **86**, 1185.
ZIEGLER, KURT: Die Hodgkinsche Krankheit. Verlag von Gustav Fischer, Jena, 1911.

SPLENIC ANEMIA.

Synonym.—Banti's disease.

Definition.—Splenic anemia is a chronic disease, primary in the spleen, of obscure origin and characterized by splenomegaly, an anemia with a low color index and a leukopenia. In the later stages of the disease cirrhotic changes occur in the liver, and, following this, ascites and jaundice develop.

History.—Although the disease had previously been mentioned, it was not until 1883 that Banti gave the first systematic and adequate description of it. This report was almost unnoticed and the syndrome did not receive widespread attention until the author's second report in 1894. The condition, to which subsequent writers have attached his name, he described as characterized by splenomegaly and cirrhosis of the liver.

Etiology.—The cause of the condition is unknown. By some it is considered as the result of the action of some toxin or bacteria on the spleen but there is no proof in support of these views. Others regard it as a clinical syndrome which may be due to a number of causes. Examination of the spleen shows a varying degree of fibrosis which is not distinctive of this disease.

Symptoms.—The condition usually appears in young adult life and is equally common in the two sexes. Banti described three stages, but the intermediary stage is brief and is usually not recognized. The important stages are the initial or preascitic and the cirrhotic. The initial stage is characterized by a gradually increasing weakness, pallor and a mild discomfort in the upper left quadrant of the abdomen. This frequently leads to an examination which reveals an enlarged, non-tender spleen. During this stage there may be hemorrhage from the gastro-intestinal tract which may vary from occult blood in the stool to massive bleeding which leads to a fatal outcome. The bleeding is associated with esophageal varices. Examination of the blood at this stage usually shows a moderately advanced anemia with a low color index and a leukopenia. The third or cirrhotic stage is characterized by recurrent ascites, occasional jaundice and progressive emaciation.

Treatment.—Splenectomy usually gives good results when employed in the earliest stages and is even recommended by some in the cirrhotic stage. This radical measure should not be performed until syphilis involving the spleen and Hodgkin's disease have been eliminated as possible diagnoses. Even in the presence of negative serologic tests for syphilis, it is usually wise to order large doses of iodides, and if this produces no change in the spleen, to apply one or two therapeutic exposures of the roentgen-rays to rule out the possibility of Hodgkin's disease. Fairly good results may be expected from splenectomy. Spontaneous recovery is unknown, death usually occurring within a few years.

REFERENCES.

KRUMBHAAR, E. B.: A Classification and Analysis of Clinical Types of Splenomegaly Accompanied by Anemia, Am. Jour. Med. Sci., 1915, **150**, 227.

PEARCE, R. M., KRUMBHAAR, E. B., and FRAZIER, C. H.: The Spleen and Anemia, Philadelphia, J. B. Lippincott Company, 1917.

POLYCYTHEMIA RUBRA VERA (ERYTHREMIA).

Synonym.—Vaquez's disease; Osler's disease.

Definition.—Polycythemia rubra vera is a rare disease of unknown etiology, characterized by an increase in the hemoglobin content and red blood cell count of the peripheral blood, symptoms which are largely referable to the nervous system, splenomegaly and usually cyanosis.

History.—The syndrome was first described by Vaquez in 1892. About ten years later Osler and others directed attention toward the disease and suggested that the condition resulted from a primary hyperplasia of the erythroblastic bone-marrow.

Etiology.—The condition occurs at any age and in both sexes, but is most frequently seen between the ages of forty and fifty years. The cause is unknown. One view regards it as due to an increased activity of the erythroblastic tissue in the bone-marrow of a neoplastic nature. Harrop assumes that there is an obstruction to the pulmonary diffusion of oxygen which causes a lowered oxygen tension in the marrow and this stimulates an excessive erythrocyte production. As a result of the increased red blood cell count the blood develops an increased viscosity which diminishes the flow. The diminished flow, together with lowered oxygen tension of the blood, produces an anoxemia which manifests itself in the brain and nervous tissues.

Pathology.—The bone-marrow is increased in amount, due to hyperplasia of the red cells, white cells and megakaryocytes. There is marked engorgement of all organs. The spleen is enlarged, due to hyperplasia of the pulp and distention with blood. Degenerative changes in the vascular system may be present.

Symptoms.—The increase in the red blood cell count and hemoglobin undoubtedly precedes the appearance of symptoms, probably for a considerable period of time. The most common complaints are referable to the nervous system and they are the ones which cause the patient to seek medical advice. Dull, mild, irregularly occurring generalized headache and vertigo are the most frequent symptoms. Other evidences of the disease are inability to concentrate, slow mental reactions, memory loss, nervousness, irritability, tinnitus, blurring of vision, hemianopsis, diplopia and paresthesia. Cerebral thrombosis may occur. A peculiar red cyanosis, most marked in the face and ears, is typical of the condition. It is not always present, as the depth of the color is independent to a certain extent of the red blood cell count and appears to depend upon the state of the capillaries. The spleen is palpable and may be enlarged down to the umbilicus. Not infrequently a dull aching pain in the upper left quadrant is associated with the splenomegaly. The basal metabolic rate is usually moderately increased, averaging between +15 and +20, but higher readings than these are sometimes obtained.

Blood Picture.—The red blood cell count averages between 7,000,000 and 12,000,000 per c.mm., and the hemoglobin between 115 and 150 per cent. The red cells usually show some variation from normal, although it may be nothing more than a slight irregularity in size or shape. There is almost always some evidence of immaturity of the red blood cells as indicated by the presence of cells with polychromatophilia and blasts. Achromia is sometimes marked and the color index may be less than one. The white blood cell count is usually elevated, the count averaging about 15,000 per c.mm., with an increase in the percentage of the granulocytes. In some instances immature white blood cells are present. The platelets are often increased. Minot has emphasized that some of these patients may eventually develop an anemia.

Treatment.—There are at least two forms of treatment which may be of benefit. Good results have been reported by irradiation of the long bones. This type of therapy should be given in the form of repeated large doses. The treatment should be controlled by blood examinations in order to avert undue depression of the white blood-cell-forming tissue. The benefit induced by the roentgen-ray is transient and eventually the patient becomes refractory to it.

Phenylhydrazine hydrochloride is useful in the treatment of erythremia as it acts to increase blood destruction and thereby reduces the red blood cell count and hemoglobin percentage to normal. The drug should be administered with extreme caution as it is toxic and has a cumulative effect. The daily dose by mouth is 0.1 to 0.2 gram in capsules. The effect should be carefully gauged by frequent blood examinations. When the red blood cells and hemoglobin approach normal or after 1 to 3 grams have been taken, it should be discontinued for one week to note if a cumulative effect occurs. The presence of a considerable number of immature red blood cells or a decided increase in the leukocytes is an indication to stop the treatment. Having produced a satisfactory result, smaller doses should be given at intervals to maintain the effect. The average maintenance dose is between 0.05 and 0.3 gram a week, but this should be determined by careful observation in each individual patient. The condition is a chronic and eventually fatal disease with periods of remissions and exacerbations. The average duration of the illness is between four and five years, but some patients with the disease have been reported as surviving for a much longer period of time. Venesection, with the removal of 500 cc. of blood, may give some temporary relief. Iodine is said by some to be of benefit and may be given a trial in the form of Lugol's solution, 5 drops, three times daily. Stone and his associates recommend that acetylphenylhydrazine be used instead of phenylhydrazine hydrochloride, as they consider that it is less toxic and that the dosage may be more easily regulated. Forkner has recently advocated the use of potassium arsenite (Fowler's solution) as a means of inducing a remission in the course of the disease.

REFERENCES.

FORKNER, C. E., McNAIR, T. F., and WU, S. C.: Treatment of Polycythemia Vera (Erythremia), With Solution of Potassium Arsenite, Arch. Int. Med., 1933, **51**, 616.

HARROP, G. A., JR.: Polycythemia, Medicine, 1928, **7**, 291.

LONG, P. H.: The Effect of Phenylhydrazine Derivatives in the Treatment of Polycythemia, Jour. Clin. Invest., 1926, **2**, 315.

PARKES-WEBER, F.: Polycythemia, Erythrocytosis and Erythremia (Vaquez-Osler Disease), London, H. K. Lewis & Co., Ltd., 1921.

STONE, C. T., HARRIS, T. H., and BODANSKY, M.: The Treatment of Polycythemia Vera, Jour. Am. Med. Assn., 1933, **101**, 495.

CHAPTER XVIII.

DISEASES OF THE SPLEEN AND THE RETICULO-ENDOTHELIAL SYSTEM.

By EDWARD B. KRUMBHAAR, M.D.

THE SPLEEN.
  Diagnosis of Splenomegaly.
  Anomalies.
  Atrophy.
  Movable Spleens.
  Congestion and Acute Splenic
    Tumor.
  Abscess.
  Infarction and Necrosis.
  Amyloid Degeneration.
  Thrombosis of the Splenic Vein.
  Cirrhotic Splenomegaly.
  Chronic Infectious Splenomegalies.

THE SPLEEN—(*Continued*).
  Syphilis of the Spleen.
  Tuberculosis of the Spleen.
  Malaria of the Spleen.
  Cysts.
  Neoplasms.
RETICULO-ENDOTHELIAL SYSTEM.
  Aleukemic Reticulosis.
  Gaucher's Disease.
  Niemann-Pick's Disease.
  Hand-Christian's Syndrome.
  Xanthomatosis.

As the spleen is an important member of the reticulo-endothelial system, and shares much of its pathology with the other members, it is appropriate to consider their diseases together.

THE SPLEEN.

The peculiar anatomy and complex physiology of the spleen make it unusually important for the clinician to be conversant with its peculiar histologic structure, its unique circulatory arrangement, its reservoir function, the part it plays with other members of the reticulo-endothelial system in disposing of effete erythrocytes and protecting against infections and neoplasms, its regulation of and direct action in blood cell formation, and so on. For further details on these physiologic points the reader is referred to *The Spleen and Anemia* (J. B. Lippincott Company, 1917) and the author's article in *Physiological Reviews* (1926, **6**, 160).

More frequently than any other organ of the body, the spleen is found postmortem to be altered by disease; in 10,000 recent autopsies at the Philadelphia General Hospital it was found to be sufficiently changed to appear in the anatomic diagnosis in over 95 per cent. Most of these, however, were cases of secondary involvement, often of relative unimportance, while its primary diseases are few. For various conditions in which the spleen is importantly concerned, such as the leukemias, Hodgkin's disease, polycythemia, pernicious anemia, the two forms of hemolytic jaundice and Banti's disease (splenic anemia), the reader is referred to other portions of this book.

Diagnosis of Splenomegaly.—As most disorders of the spleen are accompanied by an enlargement, usually palpable or even extending

(894)

to the brim of the pelvis, the diagnosis of the kind of splenomegaly becomes important. Identification of the organ is usually possible on account of its situation beneath the left diaphragm with an outlinable dulness on percussion, and its characteristic lower margin often with recognizable notches. Rendering opaque to roentgen-ray (*e. g.*, thorotrast) is as yet seldom, if ever, to be recommended. The enlargement may be due to such acute infections as typhoid, the paratyphoids, acute and subacute endocarditis (especially the latter), septicemia, poliomyelitis, diphtheria (slight), Weil's disease and epidemic catarrhal jaundice, Oroya, Malta, trench and relapsing fever; among the protozoan diseases to the malarias, kala-azar, tropical splenomegaly, Rocky Mountain spotted fever; in chronic infections to syphilis, tuberculosis and Hodgkin's disease. Mechanical obstruction to the circulation may produce enlargement in such conditions as cirrhosis of the liver, a thrombosis of splenic or portal vein, congestive heart failure or a movable spleen. It is said that in aortic regurgitation the enlarged organ may pulsate. While primary neoplasms are extremely rare, secondary involvement may produce a palpable spleen and cysts and amyloid infiltration must also be taken into account. Of the primary blood diseases pernicious anemia, the leukemias, hemolytic jaundice, von Jaksch's disease, erythroblastic anemia, splenic anemia and polycythemia, all give moderate to extreme enlargement. Exophthalmic goiter may be accompanied by enlargement, at times considerable. Of the primary diseases of the reticulo-endothelial system, Gaucher's, Niemann's and Hand-Christian's syndromes and aleukemic reticulosis will be considered in detail later.

Anomalies.—The spleen is not infrequently found completely absent, usually associated with other anomalies. It may be divided into splenunculi, or more often accessory spleens are found which share the fortunes of the larger organ and should, therefore, be removed when splenectomy is indicated. Various anomalies of size and shape need not be considered, as they are of slight clinical importance.

Atrophy.—As an organ rich in lymphoid material, the spleen normally becomes atrophic with increasing age (to 70 grams or even less). This should be distinguished from the rare, chronic interstitial splenitis. Atrophy occurs early in undernutrition as in war edema and Sweet's experimental atrophy after removal of the external function of the pancreas, and is also found secondary to chronic congestion, advanced arteriosclerosis or to local pressure, while in some cases of sickle-cell anemia marked fibrosis and atrophy have been reported (Musser and original observations). It is normally small in negroes.

Movable Spleens (Floating Spleen, Lien Mobile).—Movable spleens have been found in any part of the abdomen, and recently we found one at autopsy in the pleural cavity, having penetrated a diaphragm traumatically ruptured several years previously. *Symptoms* may be absent or part of a complex of a general visceroptosis. Sometimes they are referred chiefly to some other organ disturbed by its malposition, especially if adhesions have occurred. The characteristic notches are useful in *diagnosis*, together with the absence of normal dulness and occasionally ability to return the organ to its normal bed.

Treatment is desirable both on general grounds and to prevent torsion. General treatment for visceroptosis is usually indicated, and if mechanical supports prove useless, an operation may be necessary (splenopexy, splenectomy or packing with gauze to promote adhesions).

Torsion, a not infrequent complication of movable spleen, causes acute abdominal symptoms demanding immediate laparotomy. Sudden pain, shock, enlargement of the spleen and often fever and vomiting are characteristic, though diagnosis obviously may be very difficult.

Congestion and Acute Splenic Tumor.—In various infections and intoxications active congestion of the spleen results, while the passive congestion of chronic heart disease is a frequent occurrence. The latter in the course of time becomes sufficiently fibrosed to constitute "cyanotic induration," a smooth, hard, rounded spleen that should not present difficulties of diagnosis. The "acute splenic tumor" of infectious diseases is the commonest lesion of this organ, being a combination of active hyperemia with a hyperplasia of both lymphoid and reticulo-endothelial elements. As previously mentioned, it is found in most acute infections and may reach sufficient size to cause diagnostic difficulties.

Abscess.—Abscess is relatively rare, usually hematogenous or the result of a septic infarct, but may follow the lesions produced by severe infectious disease or occur by extension from neighboring suppuration. The *symptoms* are usually masked by the primary disorder, unless a perisplenitis or a rupture with general peritonitis occurs. Local pain and tenderness, perhaps with a friction rub, then accompany the usual signs and symptoms of a severe suppuration. One can hardly expect to elicit fluctuation. The abscess may rupture into the pleura, peritoneum, colon or stomach. The *prognosis* is grave. The operative mortality is in the neighborhood of 20 per cent—less for typhoid abscesses, more for traumatic. *Treatment*—when diagnosed, laparotomy is, of course, indicated. As the diagnosis is rarely established before adhesions to neighboring structures have occurred, or secondary abscesses formed, splenotomy is often safer than splenectomy (especially if the abscess is found to be progressing in a thoracic direction) and has been found to be attended by lower mortality.

Infarction and Necrosis.—Splenic infarction, the result of endocarditis, septicemia or atheroma of the aorta, usually occurs without being recognized clinically. If the embolus is sterile the simple anemic infarct is eventually replaced by fibrosis. Occasionally a fresh hemorrhagic infarct may be found postmortem. The rarer infected embolus causes a septic infarct which, like the abscess, is largely masked by the parent condition. The *symptoms* are then like those of abscess. The *treatment* is that of the underlying condition, except for surgical relief of suppuration, when present. The peculiar multiple necroses of Feitis (Fleckmilz), whether or not sequels of siderosis, are of but slight clinical importance.

Amyloid Degeneration (Waxy Degeneration, Lardaceous Disease).— This lesion, the spleen being the commonest site of amyloid disease, is most often associated with chronic tuberculosis, next with chronic suppurative disease, slow malignant tumors, syphilis and cardio-renal disease, in decreasing frequency. The "sago spleen," that is, the follicular type, causes little or no general enlargement and is of interest chiefly to the pathologist. In the diffuse form (bacony spleen) the palpable enlargement may be sufficient to cause discomfort (especially when lying on the right side) and possibly pain and tenderness. The *diagnosis, prognosis* and *treatment* are those of the underlying condition, except when the great weight requires mechanical support.

Thrombosis of the Splenic Vein.—Thrombosis of the splenic vein, either partial or complete, may produce symptoms lasting for years and distinguishable with difficulty or not at all from Banti's disease or other forms of chronic splenomegaly.

Symptoms and Diagnosis.—In acute thrombosis sudden abdominal pain, shock and painful enlargement of the spleen, perhaps with gastric hemorrhage, is suggestive. The addition of ascites indicates portal involvement, and diarrhea with or without blood suggests involvement of the mesenteric vein. In the chronic variety the above symptoms in milder and recurrent form, together with a tendency to jaundice, anemia and leukopenia and a spleen palpable in spite of ascites, give a picture that presents obvious difficulties, especially when the symptoms are less pronounced. A tendency toward exacerbations may be of diagnostic help. If identified either before or during laparotomy, splenectomy should be performed.

Cirrhotic Splenomegaly.—Often a prominent and early manifestation of Laennec's cirrhosis, this condition must be differentiated from other splenomegalies chiefly by the accurate history which brings out the priority of the hepatic lesions. The smooth, firm, congested spleen resembles that of congestive heart failure. Its removal has in some cases been attended by an improvement which raises interesting speculations as to the relation of the spleen, or possibly the portal system, to the cirrhotic process. (See Eppinger, "Die hepatolienalen Erkrankungen.")

Chronic Infectious Splenomegalies.—Space permits consideration only of three chief varieties; further details to be found in other appropriate chapters.

Syphilis of the Spleen.—Syphilis of the spleen may occur either in the congenital or acquired forms of the disease, in the former case signs being manifested in the first few months of life. It appears much more frequently as an enlargement due to diffuse fibrosis (spirochetes rare or absent) than as single or multiple gummata. The *diagnosis* depends on the accompanying signs of syphilis, together with an otherwise unexplained palpable spleen and tendency to jaundice and ascites. The possibility of the enlargement being due to syphilitic amyloid disease must, of course, be considered. *Treatment*—as a "backwater" where the virus is protected, the condition is frequently extremely resistant to specific treatment. In such cases splenectomy has not only produced immediate improvement but permitted the treatment of the general condition to become more efficacious than before.

Tuberculosis of the Spleen.—Tuberculosis of the spleen, usually a minor involvement secondary to a more important focus elsewhere and manifested in miliary or multiple conglomerate forms, may on

57

rare occasions assume a stellar rôle. In this case the marked enlargement, often a single large mass designated as a "tuberculoma," may
produce a palpable spleen which constitutes the chief problem in the
case. This "primary" type (*i. e.*, less, or no, significant tuberculous
lesions elsewhere) according to Winternitz may attack either sex at
any age (usually twenty to forty years). In the majority, the painful,
somewhat tender, enlarged organ was found associated with chronic
digestive and respiratory disturbances, weakness, fever and emaciation.
There is a peculiar and unexplained tendency to polycythemia. *Splenectomy* has proved a satisfactory form of treatment for such cases, for
reasons similar to those described in the paragraph on syphilis.

Malaria of the Spleen.—The huge stone-like spleen of chronic
malaria (ague-cake) has been for centuries the most important form of
splenomegaly until malaria came under the control of specific treatment
in recent times. The tremendous fibroses, often calcified, and masses of
pigment are characteristic *pathologic* features. The *symptoms* are those
common to splenomegaly with the specific signs of malaria in the blood,
which should be sufficient for *diagnosis*. *Treatment*—splenectomy for
those cases that do not respond to quinine must be considered, but
should be approached with greater caution than when elsewhere
recommended, on account of the numerous and complex adhesions
which greatly increase the difficulty of removal. The survivors of
this operation are usually greatly improved.

"Siderotic Splenomegaly" (Gandi-Nanta).—This, thought by some
to be a mycosis, may be mentioned here, although the marked fibrosis
with iron and calcium deposits apparently has a varied etiology
(Banti's disease, hemolytic jaundice, tuberculosis and, especially,
sickle-cell anemia).

Cysts.—Cysts of the spleen may be *simple* (traumatic, infolded peritoneum, dilated lymph spaces, breaking down of hematomata and
infarcts), parasitic (echinococcus) and neoplastic (dermoid, lymphangioma). If large enough to attract notice, a fluctuating mass may
be palpable and perhaps tenderness, discomfort and a dragging sensation produced. *Diagnosis* may be made by tapping, though there is
a slight danger of spreading a parasite, or better, made by splenectomy
which is here easily accomplished. *Treatment*—partial resection is
seldom indicated. In the non-parasitic forms various mechanical
supports may suffice; splenectomy, if required, is easily accomplished.

Neoplasms.—Primary forms (sarcoma, lymphosarcoma and retothelial sarcoma) are extremely rare, whereas secondary metastases are
probably commoner than is usually recognized. Benign fibromata
and angiomata are of little significance. In our series of 23 secondary
cases, arriving both by extension and by metastasis through blood
and lymph channels, the primary site was commonest in the breast,
then in the skin (malignant melanoma) and next in the pancreas and
the stomach. *Diagnosis* is usually too late to be of practical value,
although a few primary tumors have not recurred after removal. The
traditional signs of pain and a growing mass in the left abdomen with
increasing anemia and emaciation are suggestive when present.

THE RETICULO-ENDOTHELIAL SYSTEM.

Since this system was first named by Aschoff, in 1913, the concept has proved so useful in advancing knowledge of the various conditions concerned with it (phagocytosis of bacteria, cells and débris; production of antibodies; metabolic changes, etc.) that it has amply proved its worth in spite of the considerations, largely theoretical, which continue to be raised against it. It is usually regarded as including those cells of the spleen, liver, bone-marrow, lymph nodes, adrenal, lungs and other parts of the body that are particularly concerned with phagocytosis of particulate matter such as already mentioned and the inclusion of vital dyes that reach them in the colloidal state. The cells are regarded as being derived both from special types of endothelium and from the fixed and wandering histiocytes of the reticulum. Ordinary vascular endothelium shares but little or not at all in this function. The so-called large mononuclear and transitional cells (monocytes) of the blood stream are regarded as members of this system that have entered the circulation. The system is capable of progressive hyperplasia, sometimes to an extreme degree. This feature has partly obscured the experimental results of so-called "blockage" of the system with various colloidal substances, because the blockage itself— never being complete or permanent—induces a rapid hyperplasia, that is, more or less unblockage, of the system.

Under physiologic conditions the cells of this system (histiocytes) are concerned with the disposal of broken-down erythrocytes through phagocytosis of fragments disintegrated in the blood stream. Within the histiocyte it is assumed that the hemoglobin is split up into: (1) bilirubin, which is passed through the liver cells and excreted through the bile; (2) iron, which at least in part is transferred to the bone-marrow in building up new red cells; (3) globin, the fate of which has not been even outlined. Under conditions of excessive blood destruction one or more whole red blood cells, or leukocytes, may be taken up by these cells. It has been definitely shown that bilirubin can be formed outside of the liver (Mann, Rich and others) and presumably it is the Kupffer cells of this system that perform this service within the liver. Diseases of the reticulo-endothelial system may at the moment be conveniently classified into those: (1) *With hyperplastic changes manifest in tissues and blood:* (a) primary (monocytic leukemia or leukemic reticulosis); (b) secondary (infectious mononucleosis, to be differentiated from the acute lymphocytosis of Cabot). (2) *With hyperplastic changes manifest in tissues only:* (a) aleukemic reticulosis; (b) neoplastic (reticulum cell or retothelial sarcoma or histiocytoma). (3) *With predominant lipoid metabolic changes:* (a) primary (Gaucher's, Niemann-Pick's, Hand-Christian's diseases, xanthomatosis); (b) secondary (diabetic lipemia, cholesterolosis). (4) *Of unknown nature* (Hodgkin's disease). Of these monocytic leukemia, infectious mononucleosis and Hodgkin's disease are treated elsewhere in this book. The third group has been well discussed in recent reviews by Rowland, Moreau and Pick.

Aleukemic Reticulosis (Reticulo-endotheliosis).—An acute or sub-acute systemic hyperplasia of cells of the reticulo-endothelial system, characterized by lymph nodal and splenic enlargement, febrile course, progressive anemia, leukopenia and thrombocytopenia, and fatal termination. It may be first manifest by swelling of cervical or other lymph nodes (less often of the spleen) or may be announced by fever of septic type followed by weakness, prostration, emaciation and occasionally jaundice of low grade. The anemia is of the so-called "replacement" type, with progressive decrease in *all* of the formed elements of the blood; there is usually a relative lymphocytosis but absolute lymphopenia, occasionally an absolute monocytosis of insignificant degree. Differential diagnosis from tuberculosis, aleukemic lymphadenosis, aleukemic myelosis, lymphosarcoma, agranulocytosis and Hodgkin's disease depends finally on lymph node or bone-marrow biopsy; differentiation from Hodgkin's disease may be very difficult. There is replacement of lymphoid tissue of the node with complete destruction of architecture through proliferation of both reticular and endothelial elements; these are large, pleomorphic (round to stellate) cells with basophilic polychromatic vacuolated cytoplasm, often exhibiting phagocytic properties, or with "long, delicate, cytoplasmic processes" (Custer); nuclei are vesicular with from one to three nucleoli. Giant cells are characteristic (Reed or Langhans varieties), with cell infiltration of other viscera, notably liver and kidney. The treatment of this newly described clinical entity is still symptomatic with attempt to remove foci of infection; irradiation appears to be of no particular value.

Gaucher's Disease (Large Cell Splenomegaly).—This is a rare disease of obscure nature, characterized by marked splenomegaly, anemia of great chronicity and a familial tendency. The pathognomonic large foam cells are found not only in the spleen but also in the liver, lymph nodes, bone-marrow and other parts of the reticulo-endothelial system. It is probably a congenital and familial metabolic disorder concerned with deposition of complex lipoproteins.

Pathology.—The huge, smooth, firm spleen (averaging 3 to 4 kilos) is usually pale red with a cut surface that is granular with yellow or grayish-red irregular spots divided by darker red bands. Histologically throughout both the red pulp and the sinusoids are found the characteristic, large (20 to 60 microns), pale, round or spindle-shaped cells, often arranged in alveoli. Their nuclei are small, eccentric and relatively dense, the capacious cytoplasm staining faintly with eosin and showing wavy fibrils with Mallory's aniline blue. The included substance has been identified as kerasin, a cerebroside not soluble in absolute alcohol and *not* giving the characteristic fat stains but *positive for iron.* Similar cells are found in the lymph nodes and bone-marrow, either diffusely scattered or in clumps. In the liver, which may be considerably enlarged, they are confined to the sinuses (Kupffer's cells).

Symptoms.—The disease begins insidiously in infancy or childhood and pursues a very chronic course. Eventually the large spleen causes discomfort in the left abdomen with pain perhaps radiating down the left leg. The anemia is never very severe (low limit of hemoglobin, 50 per cent) and a definite leukopenia is usually found. The tendency to hemorrhage is less marked than in Banti's disease. Brownish pigmentation of the skin and a peculiar yellowish, wedge-shaped thickening of the conjunctiva, usually on both sides of the cornea, is helpful in diagnosis (indirect illumination may be required). Skeletal changes, due to the presence of the characteristic cells in the bone, have been observed both roentgenologically and at autopsy.

Death usually occurs from intercurrent infection after some years of more or less ill-health.

Diagnosis.—Though made only with certainty on examination of pathologic material (splenic puncture to be considered), a positive family history, chronic marked splenomegaly starting in a young person, moderate anemia, leukopenia, conjunctival thickening, skin pigmentation and possibly bony lesions should suggest this disease. Smears of pathologic material should show the large vacuolated cells, positive for iron but negative for fat stains.

Treatment.—Splenectomy is the only procedure that has proved of value. While improvement in those who survive the operation has almost always been striking, it is to be presumed that the disease continues independently in the other organs of the reticulo-endothelial system. Blood transfusion may be useful in preparing the patient for the surgical risk.

Niemann-Pick's Disease (Lipoid Histiocytosis).—First described by Niemann, in 1914, this disease was separated from Gaucher's by Ludwig Pick chiefly, through the earlier onset, more acutely fatal course and the positive reaction of the cells to fat stain.

It is a disease of infancy characterized by the accumulations of lipoid cells in the reticulo-endothelial system associated with splenomegaly, retarded development, gastro-intestinal symptoms and lymphatic leukocytosis. No causative agent has thus far been demonstrated; the majority of cases have been found in Jewish females. Though probably commoner than Gaucher's disease, fewer cases have thus far been studied. The chief signs have been the greatly enlarged spleen and palpable liver, slight anemia with increased resistance of erythrocytes and a leukocytosis reaching as high as 40,000. At autopsy or splenic puncture the characteristic lipoid-containing cells are found especially prominent in the spleen, lymph nodes, thymus, lung, liver sinuses, adrenal, kidney and bone-marrow. The cells, of the same size and general appearance as those of Gaucher's disease, are thought to contain a phosphatid which causes a positive, though sometimes atypical, reaction with lipoid stains and is negative for iron.

Symptoms and Diagnosis.—Gastro-intestinal disturbances, usually the first signs of the disease, may be found within the first few months of life. Retarded development, poor nutrition, anemia and edema supervene, often with a brownish pigmentation of the skin. A protuberant abdomen (enlargement of the liver as well as the spleen) calls attention to the splenomegaly which, however, must be differentiated from early Gaucher's and Banti's disease and von Jaksch's anemia.

The *prognosis* is bad, the course of the disease being acute. Death usually results from intercurrent infection before the third year is attained. No *treatment* of any value has been suggested. The few cases in which splenectomy has been attempted have not been successful.

Hand-Christian's Syndrome.—The picture of exophthalmos, diabetes insipidus and yellowish softened areas in the cranium was first described by A. Hand, in 1893, but not generally recognized until after Christian's description, in 1919, since which time a surprising number of cases have been described in this category.

The syndrome is manifest in childhood but no racial predisposition has been demonstrated nor has the relative importance of trauma, infection, dietary faults or congenital predisposition been evaluated.

Pathology.—As in the previous two diseases, apparently a disturbance of lipoid metabolism here accumulates abnormal lipoids in the cells of the reticulo-endothelial system. These respond to fat stains but have given variable results with the microchemical tests with iron. The striking bony defects (skull, pelvic girdle, vertebra), which are easily seen in the roentgen-ray picture and at autopsy, are found to contain gummy or cheesy masses made up of degenerated lipoid-containing histiocytes. The destructive changes at the base of the skull, often involving the pituitary gland, are responsible for the diabetes insipidus, which may be marked. There is often hemorrhage at the site of the bone lesion and pathologic fractures have been observed. The characteristic cells are found in increased numbers throughout the reticulo-endothelial system and in addition the parenchymal cells of liver, kidney and mucous membranes may show lipoid changes. Old lesions in the bones, especially hemorrhage, may produce an osteitis fibrosa or cholesterol and calcium depositions.

Symptoms.—The insidious onset with under-development, sometimes amounting to actual dwarfism, is usually manifested in the second or third year. Exophthalmos, usually unilateral, due to involvement of the orbital bones is almost uniformly found, while otorrhea from involvement of the middle ear and mastoid is less frequent. The blood changes are not characteristic. Tender gums and carious teeth have been reported. The course of the disease is midway in gravity between that of Gaucher's and Niemann-Pick's disease, with both of which it obviously has points of resemblance. For differential diagnosis see table in Nelson's system.

The retarded development together with the exophthalmos, diabetes insipidus and bony defects, when elicited, should make *diagnosis* easy. The microchemical staining of the characteristic cells shows so many atypicalities that, like the few chemical studies so far available, they should not be too greatly relied upon for diagnosis.

No specific *treatment* has been evolved. Dietary regulations seem rational, especially restricting the fats with liberal allowance of proteins and greens. Rowland advocates desiccated thyroid and anterior lobe of the pituitary. Good general hygiene is, of course, to be maintained.

Xanthomatosis.—Several clinical syndromes, all associated with orange or yellowish lipoid depositions in cells of the reticulo-endothelial system, may be grouped under this term. Recognized varieties are xanthelasma, the xanthoma palpebrarum of elderly people, the cutaneous xanthoma multiplex, xanthoma diabeticorum, xanthomyeloma of tendon sheaths and joints and generalized visceral xanthomatosis, of which last we have recently studied a case with marked hypercholesterolemia (760 mg.). (By xanthosarcoma is meant a collection of lipoid-containing neoplastic cells.) In early stages accumulations of lipoid-containing histiocytes are constantly found; though the usual sequence of increasing fibrosis may eventually mask or obliterate this picture. The lipoid material is usually doubly refractile, positive to fat stains in frozen sections and alcohol soluble. Hypercholesterolemia is frequent and similar visceral changes can be produced experimentally (Anitschkow) though clinically an exciting factor, such as trauma, hepatic disease or constitutional predisposition, seems necessary for the production of lesions. *Treatment*—minor disturbances require no treatment; unsightly nodules are easily removed surgically, or diminish during insulin treatment in the diabetic cases. Restriction of fats may influence the hyperlipoidemia. When the visceral types have progressed to sclerosis, the general prognosis may be poor and less benefit may be expected from dietary regulation.

REFERENCES.

ASCHOFF, L.: Ein Beitrag zur Lehre von den Makrophagen, Verhandl. d. deutsch. path. Gesellsch., 1913, **16**, 107.

———— Das reticulo-endotheliale System, Ergebn. d. inn. Med. u. Kinderh., 1925, **26**, 1.

———— Lectures in Pathology, New York, Paul B. Hoeber, Inc., 1924.

CHRISTIAN, H. A.: Contributions to Medical and Biological Research, New York, Paul B. Hoeber, Inc., 1919, **1**, 390.

EPPINGER, H.: Die hepatolienalen Erkrankungen, Berlin, Julius Springer, 1920.

FOWLER, R. H.: Cysts of Spleen. Ann. Surg., 1924, **80**, 58.

HAND, A.: Proc. Phila. Path. Soc., 1891–1893, **16**, 282.

KRUMBHAAR, E. B.: The Spleen and Anemia, Philadelphia, J. B. Lippincott Company, 1917.

———— Functions of Spleen, Physiol. Rev., 1926, **6**, 160.

KRUMBHAAR, E. B., and CUSTER, R. P.: Nelson's Loose Leaf System of Medicine, 1932, **3**, 319.

LANDAU, M.: Zur Physiologie des Cholesterinstoffwechsels, Ber. d. Naturforsch. Gesellsch. z. Freiburg, I. B., 1913, **20**, 74.

MOREAU, J.: La Dysostose Hypophysaire, Arch. Fr.-Belges de Chir., Spec. Suppl., 1931.

NIEMANN, A.: Ein unbekanntes Krankheitsbild, Jahrb. f. Kinderh., 1914, **79**, 1.

PEARCE, R. M., KRUMBHAAR, E. B., and FRAZIER, CHAS.: The Spleen and Anemia, Philadelphia, J. B. Lippincott Company, 1917.

PICK, L.: Gaucher's Splenomegaly, Med. Klinik, 1924, **20**, 1399.

ROWLAND, R. S.: Xanthomatosis and Reticulo-endothelial System; Correlation of Unidentified Group of Cases Described as Defects in Membranous Bones, Exophthalmos and Diabetes Insipidus, Arch. Int. Med., 1928, **42**, 611.

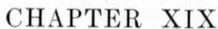

CHAPTER XIX.

DISEASES OF THE LOCOMOTOR SYSTEM.

By ROBERT GRANT TORREY, M.D.

THE JOINTS.
  Chronic Arthritis.
  Arthritis Deformans.
    Atrophic Type.
    Hypertrophic Type.
  Spondylitis Deformans.
  Acute Arthritis.
THE BURSÆ.
  Bursitis.
THE BONES.
  Congenital Defects of Bone Structure.
  Achondroplasia.
  Hereditary Deforming Achondroplasia.
  Osteopsathyrosis.
  Oxycephaly.
  Bone Defects Not Congenital.

THE BONES—(Continued).
  Osteitis Fibrosa Cystica.
  Osteomalacia.
  Osteitis Deformans.
  Defects in Membranous Bones, Exophthalmos and Diabetes Insipidus.
  Neoplastic Bone Disease.
  Sarcoma.
  Multiple Myeloma.
  Metastatic Carcinoma.
THE MUSCLES.
  Diseases of the Voluntary Muscles.
  Myositis.
  Myalgia.
FIBROSITIS.
  Panniculitis.

THE JOINTS.

CHRONIC ARTHRITIS.

THERE is great difficulty in presenting the subject of arthritis for consideration on account of the confusion in classification and terminology. The early writings on this subject are at variance, much confusion and little agreement being found in comparing the works of many authors. The description and classification offered by authors of the Middle Ages are no less at variance than those of the eighteenth and nineteenth centuries, and the last few decades have failed to clarify our classifications and descriptions of this disease. The terms chronic arthritis, gout, arthritis deformans, rheumatic gout, rheumatoid arthritis, osteoarthritis, infectious arthritis, atrophic and hypertrophic arthritis are variously employed and greatly confused.

According to the older ideas of etiology the terms rheumatism, catarrh and gout all signified determination of a humor from its normal site to the joints or to neighboring structures where its presence excited disturbance. The later use of the term "rheumatism" to designate rheumatic fever, a definite infectious disease with acute manifestations involving the joints, and with permanent or progressive cardiac involvement, has tended to limit the term rheumatism in its significance and to further confuse the understanding of the terminology of chronic joint affections.

The recognition of gout as a separate disease was made clear by Sydenham in the seventeenth century, and from 1800 on there is in general some accord in the writings on gout as to the limitations in classification and the gross pathologic features. The humoral concept as to etiology is not far removed from the present understanding of gout as a result of disturbed metabolism.

Rheumatic fever, or acute rheumatism, has been gradually withdrawn from the field of chronic joint disease. In this disease, as a rule, the cardiac involvement is important and the arthritis only troublesome. The close attention focused on the subject was prompted by the gravity of rheumatic heart disease, and this phase of the disease is the one which is now the subject of most of the research on rheumatism.

Chronic rheumatism as a result of rheumatic fever doubtless does occur as a joint disease, but the degree of frequency is questionable. It seems probable that chronic rheumatism with extensive fibrositis of muscular and periarticular structures and with subcutaneous nodules is of not infrequent occurrence in England though seen less often in the United States.

Removing rheumatic fever from consideration there is left a group of chronic joint conditions which are jumbled in confusion. There is no satisfactory etiologic classification for many of them. *Chronic infectious arthritis* is a term used loosely to cover a large group of joint conditions of unknown or doubtful etiology and is unsatisfactory as usually employed. We know too little regarding the pathogenesis of these arthritides properly to assign them as infectious or not infectious. The responsibility of infection in its etiology is assumed, often without sufficient basis, and after a succession of operations for the removal of teeth, tonsils, gall-bladder, appendix, opening of sinuses and removal of septa, bowel irrigations and the administrations of autogenous vaccines made from cultures from various sources, it dawns upon the patient that he is not improving, and upon the physician that there may be factors other than possible or potential foci of infection which operate in the production of the disease.

A great group of the chronic arthritis cases, however, may properly be classed as chronic infectious arthritis. This does not mean that the responsible infecting organism is present in the joint or in the surrounding tissue. It means that the joint inflammation is a response to invasion of the infective organism somewhere in the body, a response evoked by circulating toxins to which the joint tissues are sensitive. It is often difficult to demonstrate the foci which are to blame but frequently the eradication of an obviously malign septic area will cause a prompt and permanent clearing up of joint involvement.

Classifications based on pathologic features seem more simple and more satisfactory in that the demonstrable pathologic changes are much more definite than the theoretical causative factors; thus arthritis deformans of the atrophic and hypertrophic types (Goldthwait) is described, or rheumatoid arthritis and osteoarthritis.

Another commonly employed inclusive term is chronic non-suppurative arthritis, which is classed as proliferative or degenerative in its tendencies (Nichols and Richardson).

Another classification is based on the type of tissue involved and includes osteoarthritis and fibrositis of joint structures as well as other tissues. Fibrositis is considered as the main factor in many conditions involving muscles, tendons, sheaths, ligaments, nerves and synovial structures, and by this view much arthritis shows principally as a fibrositis of the joint and periarticular structures. This view brings many of these classifications of arthritis more nearly into accord with the recent development of thought regarding rheumatic fever and arthritis as expressed by Swift, Coburn, Small and others, laying stress on the individual reaction to focal infection as the factor determining what course the disease will pursue.

It is clear that no simple system of classification can be entirely satisfactory in covering these cases which are confusing as to etiology and which, unless autopsy material can be carefully scrutinized, are often obscure in their pathologic changes.

Let us consider the polyarticular and usually symmetrical types of chronic arthritis which are included in the term *arthritis deformans* of the *atrophic* and *hypertrophic* types. This is in part a satisfactory term in that it is an accurate description as to the deformity of the joints. As applied to rheumatoid or infectious arthritis, the atrophic types, it is wholly accurate in its description, "a deforming joint inflammation." Exception is taken, however, to its inclusiveness in bringing in the hypertrophic types of this group or so-called osteoarthritis, it now being held that this group of cases should not be termed inflammatory but degenerative conditions.

The term *rheumatoid arthritis* is descriptive in differentiating a chronic symmetrical polyarthritis with involvement of the periarticular structures from an osteoarthritis (the hypertrophic type, in which the involvement is primarily of the bone). Rheumatoid arthritis is the atrophic type of arthritis deformans, proliferative, non-suppurative arthritis, and includes most infectious arthritis.

Still's disease is infectious arthritis or rheumatoid arthritis occurring in the young. Probably most cases described under this name are identical with rheumatoid arthritis.

The *hypertrophic* type of *arthritis deformans*, or *osteoarthritis*, is quite a different condition. As has been said, it seems primarily a degenerative process, is frequently due to trauma or strain and there is doubt whether infection plays an important rôle in its production, though it is frequently held responsible. Age, failure of local blood supply and lowered general metabolism are often factors in the development, as are static or postural faults, foot strain, spinal curvature. This condition may be generally distributed throughout many joints and show a symmetrical distribution, but it does not tend to such arrangement typically as does the rheumatoid type.

Some chronic changes in joints are due to microörganisms within the joint and may be termed *septic joints*. This is truly infectious arthritis but this term is not used to cover these cases. This class is typified by infection of the joint by the tubercle bacillus, gonococcus, typhoid bacillus, or certain strains of streptococci. These arthritides should be considered as surgical conditions.

Certain joint affections are clearly and indubitably *trophic*, as the Charcot joint occurring in diseases of the central nervous system.

Others show trophic disturbance as a factor in their development and distribution even though there appears to be an infectious element concerned and even though the joint changes result in a fibrositis of the periarticular structures.

Apart from acute attacks of podagra there are found chronic joint changes due to gout. These show characteristic changes and may clearly be classified as cases of *metabolic joint disease*. It is difficult, however, to place properly the joint affections which seem to depend on focal infection but also may be caused or aggravated by the depressed metabolic state of hypothyroidism and which improve or disappear on the administration of thyroid substance. The conditions of definite septic, trophic and metabolic joint affections may be set apart from generalized chronic arthritis. They are, as a rule, fairly typical and usually involve one or only a few joints.

Classification of Chronic Arthritides.

1. **Arthritis Deformans.**
    - (*a*) Atrophic type; or rheumatoid arthritis, or chronic non-suppurative arthritis, proliferative type, characterized by symmetrical multiple involvement with atrophy of tissues, contractures, fibrosis, small joints usually involved.

      In this group, or closely allied to it, are found also— chronic infectious arthritis, rheumatic gout, Still's disease, chronic rheumatism.
    - (*b*) Hypertrophic type; or chronic non-suppurative arthritis, degenerative type, osteoarthritis. Primarily a bony degeneration with repair, monarticular, few joints, or multiple and generally distributed, particularly large joints. Atrophy of periarticular structures may be entirely lacking.
2. **Metabolic Joint Disease.**—Chronic gouty arthritis, menopausal arthritis.
3. **Trophic Joint Disease.**—Charcot joint.
4. **Septic Joints.**—Tuberculosis, gonococcus, typhoid, some streptococcic joints.
5. **Miscellaneous Types.**—Spondylitis, Heberden's nodes, pulmonary arthropathy, recurrent hydrarthrosis. (To be considered separately.)

The above classification may perhaps be thought to be too inclusive in the groupings of the atrophic type of arthritis deformans, but there is so much question and speculation regarding the etiologic factors in this group that primary division of these cases on an etiologic basis is unsatisfactory. Any classification of arthritis at the present day can be considered but a temporary makeshift.

It must be noted that as with many chronic diseases requiring classification and subdivision, the various classes or types overlap and merge in certain cases, and in arthritis deformans we may find hypertrophic and atrophic joint changes in the same individual, or we may find a chronic septic joint which seems to act as a focus of infection and produces a generalized chronic infectious arthritis.

ARTHRITIS DEFORMANS.

Atrophic Type.

Synonyms.—Rheumatoid arthritis; Infectious arthritis; Chronic non-suppurative arthritis (proliferative type).

As has been said, this group or type has certain characteristics but merges with osteoarthritis or the hypertrophic type through hypertrophic involvement of the spinal column, sacro-iliac synchrondroses and not infrequently of the hip-joints in otherwise typical cases of atrophic arthritis. Chronic infectious arthritis, undoubted from the etiologic standpoint, gives the picture of rheumatoid arthritis.

Rheumatoid arthritis most often makes its appearance during the third to fifth decades and more frequently in women than in men. Probably twice as many women as men are affected.

It occurs with great frequency in the temperate zones, the geographic distribution of this disease being the same as that of rheumatic fever. Great Britain, the Netherlands, Germany and France show it as frequently as do the northern United States. In tropical and subtropical climates these diseases are infrequent.

Predisposing causes are exposure, fatigue and exhaustion, physical and emotional shock, as grief and worry. The onset may follow any exhausting disease.

Etiology.—Rheumatoid arthritis is probably infectious in origin in most cases and may represent a sensitivity to a type or many types of bacterial infection. It would seem that a wide range of organisms is capable of exerting antigenic action in provoking exacerbations of activity in the affected joints. Whether all of these organisms, particularly the Gram-positive cocci, which have antigenic properties in this condition, are capable of producing the disease originally is not clear. Cecil describes a particular strain of streptococcus which he recovers from blood culture by an elaborate technic. He states that this organism is found in practically all cases of rheumatoid (atrophic) arthritis and in no cases of osteoarthritis, and considers it causal. Crowe, on the other hand, states that rheumatism, fibrositis and osteoarthritis are streptococcic diseases while rheumatoid arthritis and Still's disease are staphylococcic, show a certain strain of staphylococci (termed by him Micrococcus deformans) in the urine and that the serum of these patients shows agglutinin reaction with this strain.

The presence of infective foci can be demonstrated in most cases of early rheumatoid arthritis. Most frequently the tonsils, often apical tooth infection, not infrequently the prostate and often the paranasal sinuses are found to be infected. Too frequently there is found to be no improvement when infection of these foci is apparently eradicated, and objection to consideration of these foci as significant is often made on the grounds that such focal infection may be found in almost anyone if investigation is sufficiently searching. Typical rheumatoid arthritis may often be seen to develop rapidly in cases of infection with retention of pus, as in empyema, in the chest and to improve spectacularly when adequate drainage is established. This is clearly an infectious arthritis; it bears all the signs of a rheumatoid arthritis.

In considering the question of a specific organism as causal there is a wide field to be traversed. Cultures from joints from lymph glands in adjacent areas, which are assumed to drain the joint structures (Forkner, Shands and Poston), from the blood stream (Cecil) and from chronic foci of infection in other parts of the body have been studied. The intestinal contents and the urine have been used as the source of cultures thought to be specific (Crowe). The conclusions drawn by individual investigators have shown wide variance, and there is practically no unanimity on this question. The assurance with which various investigators state their conclusions and the wide range of difference in the findings indicate that they cannot all be right in their theories. If this disease were as simple as many explanations make it appear there should be no lack of confirmation of much of the work on its bacteriology which is still unsupported by other investigators. It is impossible to escape the conviction that focal infection lies back of the onset of this disease. While the demonstration of a single and specific organism as responsible has been claimed repeatedly, all of these observations lack confirmation by independent observers.

Certain diseases which seem to be manifestations of streptococcic infection are particularly variable in their occurrence, course, severity and complications. They seem influenced by climate, by season, by age, race, and by many indeterminate factors. Epidemics of scarlet fever may show a disease of such mildness as to be trivial. In the South this may be the rule. At other times or in sporadic cases the disease may show a malign severity. Rheumatic fever may be trivial in certain climates, even in children, and deadly in others. Epidemics at different times may differ in the same locality as to the characteristics of the disease prevailing in each epidemic. Climatic differences certainly affect the incidence and the course of the rheumatic diseases. Age and sex affect the course of the disease. Rheumatic fever and rheumatoid arthritis in Arizona are very different diseases as regards course and prognosis from rheumatic fever and rheumatoid arthritis in England.

Pathogenesis.—Rheumatoid arthritis is probably a manifestation of sensitivity or allergy to some bacterial infection. Focal infection seems to be a primary factor. Individual susceptibility must be present. The individual susceptibility or the virulence of the infection is subject to alteration by climatic conditions. Rheumatoid arthritis bears a close resemblance to rheumatic fever and might indeed be due to the same infection. It is probable that in those parts of the earth where rheumatic diseases are prevalent almost everyone is infected with the organisms which cause rheumatism and arthritis, but most of the population escapes the disease.

The same infection will act differently in different individuals. There is a strong nervous system factor in the development of rheumatoid arthritis. The chief characteristics of the disease are symmetry of involvement, inflammation, particularly of the joints and periarticular structures, atrophy of many structures, contractures and fibrosis of varying degree. Involvement of the nervous system is indicated by the absolute symmetry of involvement noted in many instances; this symmetry of arrangement applying not only to inflammation but also to circulatory disturbances, an appearance like Raynaud's disease being frequently seen, to atrophy of corresponding muscle groups and skin areas, and to the deformities resulting from atrophy, contracture and fibrosis in various joints. There are many indications of severe disturbances of the sympathetic nervous system in this disease and suspicion that cord effects may play a part. Atrophy is often seen to precede the arthritis in these cases, and a symmetrical local circulatory disturbance giving the picture of Raynaud's syndrome is a common accompaniment and sometimes a forerunner of the inflammatory changes in the hands. The conclusion cannot be escaped that the distribution of the lesions and course of the disease are determined by trophic and nervous influences, and that a toxin or antigen operates both centrally and locally.

Trophic effects of nervous or circulatory influences are seen in the tendency to development of the joint and tissue changes characteristic of rheumatoid arthritis on the affected side in a hemiplegic while the other side shows no such changes, and in the development of typical arthritic atrophy and contractures in one extremity following peripheral nerve injury in that limb. In the event of generalized arthritis the changes may be similar and symmetrical, but much more severe on the side of the nerve injury.

Pemberton has reported a low sugar tolerance in this disease and assumes a lowered metabolic activity in the region of the affected joint, as judged by measurements of oxygen in the blood supply. Reports on basal metabolic rates in arthritis are variable and the margin of error in these determinations is a wide one.

From information thus far collected the process of production of this disease appears to depend on tissue responses to toxic or antigenic influences from a bacterial source, probably from a micrococcus of relatively low virulence and not actively hemolytic. The local inflammation may be an allergic response, may be toxic, but probably is not the result of actual infection in the joint.

The nature and degree of tissue response is conditioned by many factors of nervous and circulatory control of the local trophic state. An organic or functional nervous system damage may be the most important factor in determining the distribution and course of the disease.

Local desensitization of the joint structures and general desensitization to toxic or allergic processes in various tissues must be taken into account in summing up the disease picture in its beginnings, and in its progress the varying degree of tendency toward atrophy, contracture and fibrosis will determine the nature of the resulting deformities and disability.

Pathology.—Description of the pathologic changes found early in the disease are rather scanty and are limited to observation of subjects who die from intercurrent disease or to tissue specimens secured in operations on affected joints.

The synovial membranes are thickened and inflamed. There is probably some villous hypertrophy followed by atrophy and thinning of the membranes. The cartilages show absorption and fibrous replacement. Changes in the bony structures are well shown by roentgenograms. Areas of decalcification will be seen toward the ends of the bones and actual loss of tissue may be very marked.

The joint cavity early contains excess fluid which may be turbid or, in very active cases, hemorrhagic. The periarticular structures show active inflammatory changes and early fibrosis. Later changes are dense fibrosis of all the soft tissues and increasing atrophy of the bone. There may be ossification in the remnants of cartilaginous tissue and bony ankylosis of the affected bony surfaces in the larger joints. In the spinal column these ossifications are particularly frequent and not only the cartilages but also the ligaments may take part in the bony change (spondylitis deformans).

There is marked blood-vessel obliteration in the soft tissues in and about the joint, loss of fat and atrophy of skin and muscle tissue. The muscle fibers show degenerative changes with loss of striation and increase in nuclei. There is much fibrous tissue found in and between the muscle bundles.

Symptoms and Course.—The onset of this condition may be acute with marked constitutional symptoms or may be gradual and insidious. In its beginning it may resemble an attack of rheumatic fever and be distinguishable from that disease only as it progresses so that symmetry in its distribution and development become evident. Fever may be high at the onset, the pulse rapid, a moderate leukocytosis observed, enlargement of the spleen and other signs denoting an acute infection may be noted. On the other hand, there may be slight pain, stiffness and swelling in a number of joints, disappearing and recurring repeatedly, becoming more severe and finally becoming persistent.

Inflammation in the joints produces a characteristic swelling of the periarticular tissues, giving a rounded appearance. In the acutely involved joints there is redness and heat and extreme tenderness and pain. In the gradually advancing cases the joints may seldom show redness though tenderness may be acute.

The joints most frequently involved are the smaller joints of the extremities, the ankles and wrists, then elbows and shoulders, and not infrequently the articulation of the jaw. The spine and the sacro-iliac joints often join in the process so that practically every joint of the body is crippled at some time. Some of these clear up and are restored to usefulness; others have their function destroyed by the sequelæ of the inflammatory stage. The temperature shows variable elevations during the inflammatory stages. The pulse shows a rather rapid rate, which is persistent. There is a slight leukocytosis showing increase during the inflammatory exacerbations. Fibrous subcutaneous nodules may be found which are moderately tender. The sedimentation rate is increased during these crises. There is marked loss of weight, and poor general nutrition is evident.

The characteristic atrophy may appear with the swelling of the joints, may be delayed or in some cases may even precede the joint involvement.   Atrophy is seen in certain muscle groups, as a rule symmetrically distributed.   The wasting of the muscles, loss of subcutaneous fat and thinning of the skin accentuate the swelling of periarticular and joint structures.

Following atrophy contractures make their appearance, and here again symmetry will be seen, often to a striking degree.

In the hands the ulnar deviation of the fingers is often noted very early.   Contractures of the fingers usually show sharp flexion of some of the terminal phalanges and often overextension in some of the middle joints.   The hamstring muscles usually show contraction early and the resulting flexion of the knee is difficult to overcome and constitutes one of the chief causes of disability.   The elbows are limited in extension and may be sharply flexed by contracture of the biceps.   An early sign of trouble is limitation in supination of the hand, it being sharply checked as the palm reaches the vertical plane.   In an extreme case the hands may be clenched except for a single extended, distorted finger, the wrists flexed and the elbows flexed at an acute angle, the feet twisted and the knees drawn up against the body.

At this stage the picture is pitiable.   The atrophy of the muscles is extreme and atrophy of the bones is such that the fingers are shortened and may seem almost boneless, or contractures and atrophy may be so extreme that total dislocation of many joints has taken place.

There may be little inflammation and little pain in the advanced stages of the disease, but joint function is largely destroyed by atrophy, contracture and fibrosis.   The degree of fibrosis is very variable.   It may be so extreme as to dominate the picture in cases which otherwise seem rather mild.   It fixes a deformity which except for this fixation would seem capable of satisfactory correction.   The fibrosis binds firmly all contiguous inflamed structures, tendons, ligaments, synovial membranes and periosteum into a firm unit.

The advanced stages of rheumatoid arthritis may be true to type with advanced atrophy and absorption of the bones and soft tissues, symmetrical contractures and moderate fibrosis accounting for the ankylosis and deformity seen, or there may be late ossification in some of the fibrous tissues and bony ankylosis of exposed surfaces in the joints.

Ossifying changes are noted particularly in the vertebral column and in the hips, sometimes in the knees and elbows, seldom in the smaller joints.   In the vertebral column it is frequent and it is quite usual to see a spondylitis with characteristic osteoarthritic changes in a case of otherwise uncomplicated arthritis of the rheumatoid type.

As has been said, atrophy may even precede the arthritis in these cases.   The writer recalls the case of a carpenter who was admitted to the wards of the Philadelphia General Hospital with a rapidly advancing case of rheumatoid arthritis.   Atrophy of many muscle groups was far advanced at the time of admission while a generalized arthritis was in its early stages.   He stated that for six months before there was any joint pain he had noticed weakness of the extremities which became so marked that he had to stop work because he could not hold a hammer or use a saw.   He also showed a well-marked Raynaud syndrome.

There are many degrees of involvement other than those showing typical distribution and course. There may be involvement of one or a few joints with varying degrees of atrophy or hypertrophic villous change and periarticular proliferation. There may be mixed cases as, for instance, a case recently seen where both sacro-iliac joints showed acute inflammation probably due to gonococcus infection of the prostate. In this case there were signs of sciatic neuritis on either side and an arthritis of the rheumatoid type involving the knees, ankles and feet, apparently determined by the sciatic nerve damage.

The characteristic features of the disease are the onset, usually with fever and general symptoms, the gradually developing symmetry in involvement—inflammatory, fibrotic, contractile and atrophic—the recurrence of inflammatory exacerbations and gradual increase in the crippling permanent changes consequent, with later a tendency to lessening of acute inflammatory phases and of the attendant pain and tenderness.

Diagnosis.—The diagnosis of rheumatoid arthritis is in part a question of the width of the limits of this group of arthritic diseases. Considering this diagnosis to apply to the great group of the atrophic types of generalized arthritis, including those of obviously infectious origin, the task is more simple than it would be were the limits more narrow.

In *rheumatic fever* the onset is usually abrupt, the temperature and constitutional symptoms more marked, the age in primary attacks apt to be younger, the tendency to cardiac involvement and pericarditis is marked and the response to salicylates is usually striking. The joints clear up without marked remaining effects, atrophy of the muscles is less in acute cases and the distribution is not symmetrical, but is apt to be irregularly distributed without pattern or order.

In *gonorrheal rheumatism* few joints are affected, local infection may be demonstrated and there is lack of symmetry in distribution.

Scleroderma may closely resemble rheumatoid arthritis but careful examination will distinguish these conditions.

In the muscular dystrophies, and in spastic involvements due to birth injuries or to encephalitis, the resemblance to rheumatoid arthritis is superficial.

Prognosis.—If these attacks are dependent on a focus of infection which can be satisfactorily eradicated, and if this can be attacked early in the disease a prompt and apparently complete arrest of the arthritis may result. Sometimes the removal of infected tonsils, the drainage of an antrum or the removal of infected teeth, or the effectual drainage of an empyema of the chest will produce a remarkable result, but these procedures are too often disappointing. In many cases the intestinal tract may be the seat of an infection by an organism to which the patient is sensitive, and at other times repeated acute respiratory infections, for which no adequate cause can be found, will on each occasion seem to evoke a fresh attack of inflammatory response in the joints. In judging the outcome of these cases one must be guided more by the complicating results than by the degree of inflammation. Atrophy, contractures and fibrosis are the permanent destructive agents as regards function of the joints, and the early appearance of these

58

complications is an unfavorable sign. Extensive spondylitis is unfavorable, as is marked jaw involvement.

Loss of weight is a good gauge of the activity of the disease, and the weight should be carefully watched during the active stages. Permanently crippled patients often gain or even become obese after the inflammatory symptoms have disappeared. The sedimentation rate is said to be a guide to activity of the inflammatory stages. Small employs this test as a guide to treatment, observing it at weekly intervals. Crowe advocates charting the weight at every treatment as an indication of the trend of the activity of the inflammatory process. If infective foci can be found and eradicated at an early stage of the disease, and if contractures and atrophy are not advanced, the outlook for practically complete relief may be fairly good.

In cases where atrophy is rapid and early, and particularly where fibrotic response to inflammation is marked and contractures are severe, the outlook for restoration of more than a minimal degree of joint function is poor.

Treatment.—The treatment of rheumatoid arthritis should be undertaken systematically and pursued with patient attention to many details. Focal infection must be sought for and suspicious foci eradicated, or drainage provided for such foci where possible. Intestinal stasis must be avoided. These patients are under *par* in their general physique and nutrition, and fatigue, strain and overwork must be guarded against, and adequate rest, sometimes continuous rest for long periods of time, provided for. Gain in weight in undernourished patients is usually a sign of improvement and loss of weight a bad sign.

More specific treatment is an effort to desensitize the tissues to the antigenic effects of infection, and many methods have been used to prevent the active inflammatory exacerbations by these methods. Among drugs salicylates and cinchophen appear to have the property of reducing tissue sensitivity and preventing these responses. Salicylate of soda or acetylsalicylic acid may be used with benefit in full dosage during acute exacerbations. Salicylates seem safe and relatively free from disagreeable or dangerous effects. Cinchophen is advocated for this purpose, but question is raised as to its safety, there having been reports of liver damage through its use. Cincophen and amidopyrin and their compounds probably should not be used.

Among other methods of desensitization the earliest to gain vogue was the use of bacterins, or so-called vaccines, in some form. Great care must be exercised in the use of such preparations. It is often seen that strikingly favorable results are obtained at first with the use of vaccines to which the patient later becomes intolerant, and instead of desensitizing the tissues it appears that the tissues become sensitized to the vaccine.

Crowe, in England, has reported excellent results on a large series of patients treated with vaccines, autogenous or stock preparations, prepared in an elaborate manner; and Burbank, in New York, reports favorably on this form of treatment. They both employ extremely small doses and carefully avoid provoking any local, focal or general reaction.

Small uses the water-soluble extract of a culture of non-hemolytic streptococcus in very high dilution and reports reactions from unbelievably minute fractions. He terms his preparation a soluble antigen and believes that it represents a specific polysaccharid and that this fraction rather than the protein portion determines the local reaction and sensitivity. Cecil uses an autogenous vaccine in most cases.

The tendency in treatment by these methods has been toward smaller and smaller dosage and avoidance of any untoward reaction either immediate or delayed. The ordinary stock vaccines as prepared and sold carry directions for use providing for dosage which is far too large for safe use with sensitive individuals.

Non-specific methods of desensitization include various forms of intravenous "shock therapy," such as typhoid bacterin, in doses of from 25,000,000 upward, colloidal metals, colloidal sulphur and other chemical agents. In most cases there is an immediate febrile reaction, often with chill, and a leukocytosis. Following this there may be a surprisingly rapid but temporary subsidence of the acutely inflammatory signs in the joints. These methods, termed "protein-shock therapy" or non-specific protein therapy, have been largely abandoned in chronic conditions. Advocated by Miller and Lusk and by Jobling and Petersen, in 1916, they were widely employed for a time. Although they seem to hold useful possibilities, it appears that these methods have not been subsequently improved and developed sufficiently to continue in general use.

Intramuscular injections of various substances are used in the production of a non-specific desensitization, as colloidal sulphur, which gives a severe local reaction, casein or sterilized milk, Coley's toxin (a streptococcus product) and many other preparations. Good results may be obtained with any of these preparations but there are many difficulties attendant on their use and there is always the danger of producing intolerance to the substance and of producing unfavorable results with lowered resistance of the patient.

Climatic Treatment.—A favorable dry southern climate may do wonders for the arthritic (New Mexico, Arizona, southwest Texas).

Baths and spa treatments are designed to correct the sequelæ of the inflammatory changes and to restore tone to the tissues and function to the joints.

Treatment of Contractures, Atrophy, Fibrosis and Ankylosis.—Orthopedic measures must be employed. Joints which are painful must be rested, but advantage should be taken of all intervals to institute systematic exercise of muscle groups to overcome atrophy, and extension and passive motion to prevent or correct contractures and adhesions. Massage is necessary and a skilled physiotherapist can accomplish much in improving the condition of the joints, even in the late stages of this disease. Contractures at times demand surgical intervention. Correction of kyphosis increases respiratory volume, diaphragm and visceral mobility, greatly aiding the circulation and general condition.

Iodides in small dosage may reduce the tendency to fibrosis.

Section of sympathetic tracts or ganglionectomy is advocated by Rowntree and Adson, who report good results in some cases.

The diet in rheumatoid arthritis must be nourishing, easily digested and rich in vitamins. Pemberton advocates a low carbohydrate intake. Careful attention to the bowels and to digestion, with such tonics as are found to improve the general state of nutrition, is demanded. Splanchnoptosis should be corrected.

Hypertrophic Type.

Synonyms.—Osteoarthritis; Degenerative arthritis.

This disease occurs in middle-aged or elderly persons who, as a rule, show other degenerative changes. It may follow joint inflammation, more often trauma; it may be generalized, affecting many joints. The cartilages and bones show the principal evidences of attack. There is relatively little involvement of the periarticular structures and little atrophy. Contrasted with subjects of rheumatoid arthritis there is observed neither the poor general nutrition nor the extensive atrophy of skin and muscle seen in the other type. Pain is not acute when the joint is at rest, and there may be surprisingly little pain at any time. Deformity is caused by the bony changes due to absorption and hypertrophy with lipping and spur formation. There may be complete ankylosis of a joint, but this is usually not caused by bony union but by interlocking of spurs and outgrowths and some external fibrosis.

Etiology.—There is probably no specific infective agent in the production of this disease. It is not an inflammatory process but is the result of many factors; perhaps often some infection plays a part, but advancing age of the tissues, vascular degeneration with failing blood supply, trauma of weight-bearing joints and loss of tone in supporting muscles, faulty posture, strain of occupation, loss of elasticity in cartilage, each of these factors may contribute its separate insult and aid in breaking down the resistance.

The spine is a frequent seat of osteoarthritis even when other joints are not involved, and a hip-joint may show advanced changes when there is no other joint involvement (*morbus coxæ senilis*).

Pathology.—The changes are very characteristic. The external appearance of the joint may show relatively little abnormality or there may be marked deformity with irregular swelling due to bony enlargement, or a tense swelling due to effusion. There may be angulation or ankylosis. The skin may show little change. The synovial membranes will show some thickening, hypertrophy and degeneration of the fringes. The cartilages may be entirely absorbed, particularly in the central portions, and replaced by fibrous or even bony tissue. The ends of the bones show porosities and dense irregular areas of new bone formation producing a marked distortion. Knobs and spurs are produced by this bony overgrowth. On the joint surfaces the new bone will be ground and polished to a smooth surface but on the margins and portions not in contact these growths persist. Fragments of bone or of cartilage may form loose bodies in the joint cavity.

Particular forms and distribution of osteoarthritis include:

Hip-joint disease of the aged: This may involve one or both hips. There is apt to be considerable atrophy of the thigh and leg muscles and possibly nerve involvement. Effusion in the joints and bursa may be marked.

Climacteric arthritis of the knees is a frequent form of arthritis occurring particularly in rather obese women at or about the time of the menopause. It may be rather mild and capable of correction. This is due to metabolic disturbance.

Hypertrophic spondylitis, nerve root pressure, may cause severe pains and disability.

Heberden's nodes are swellings which represent an early osteoarthritis of the terminal phalangeal joints. They are usually symmetrical and painless. They sometimes represent osteoperiosteal nodes and sometimes are cystic swellings connecting with the joint cavity and lined with synovial membrane. They have little clinical significance unless advanced in degree and accompanied by angulation and fixation of the joints.

Diagnosis.—Generalized osteoarthritis may resemble rheumatoid arthritis to some extent but there should be little difficulty in distinguishing them. Osteoarthritis is a gradually advancing degenerative disease and lacks the acute inflammatory exacerbations of rheumatoid arthritis—the rapid pulse, periods of fever, the atrophy and wasting of the tissues and bulbous, tender swellings of the joints, which are characteristic of this latter condition.

Treatment.—Salicylates seem to have little effect, though sometimes they may be serviceable in allaying pain and controlling periods of soreness in the joint. Acetylsalicylic acid is a favorite form of salicylate for this purpose. Small doses of thyroid gland seem useful in many cases. Iodides are probably of distinct service. Small doses should be used for an extended period of time. Arsenic and iron are recommended in this condition. Avoidance of chilling and fatigue is important. Hydrotherapeutic measures and bakings or sweats, particularly systematic treatment at a well-organized spa, with massage, exercise and baths, are valuable, and a warm dry climate is of great value. Under good conditions well-regulated exercises which do not entail prolonged weight-bearing on the joints are valuable in preventing stiffness or ankylosis.

Vaccines, antigens or foreign proteins may be of use, though many observers who employ them in rheumatoid arthritis have discarded them in this condition.

Focal infections should be attended to and the diet selected to avoid a tendency to obesity, while furnishing adequate nutrition.

Pulmonary Hypertrophic Osteoarthropathy.—A clubbing of the fingers and toes with a tendency to mild osteoarthritis in the digits, and in advanced cases involving the bones entering into the wrist and ankle articulations, secondary to other disease usually of the lungs and particularly marked in bronchiectasis and in phthisis with cavity.

Other Forms of Arthritis.—**Gonorrheal Rheumatism.**—This condition appears as an *acute septic joint,* a destructive lesion leading to obliteration of the joint cavity with ankylosis and marked contractures and fibrosis; as *chronic hydrops of a joint* either with gradual onset or as a sequel of an acute inflammatory joint; or as an *acute arthritis* of several joints showing painful and tender swelling with all the signs of an infectious arthritis of the atrophic type. A septic joint produced by gonococcus infection may be the apparent focus causing a more generalized infectious arthritis, or a chronic prostatitis of gonococcal or mixed infection may be the source of the trouble. Tendon sheath involvement and bursitis of the heel or osteoperiostitis of the os calcis are not uncommon.

Treatment.—Salicylates are not, as a rule, effective in gonococcal arthritis. Some form of intravenous shock therapy, vaccine therapy, or injections in the tissues producing a systemic reaction are measures which seem the most satisfactory. Excellent results are reported with Pregl's iodine, 5 cc. being injected directly into each lobe of the prostate through the rectal wall. Prostatitis and vesiculitis should be treated and the joint complication should be treated as infectious arthritis or septic joint of other types.

Chronic Septic Joints.—Characterized by tissue destruction, usually with pus formation, and due to the action of the organism in the joint itself. These are subjects for surgical consideration, and include tuberculosis of the joint, chronic gonorrheal joints, typhoid spine and certain streptococcic joints.

Trophic Joints.—The Charcot joint occurring in tabes dorsalis is the best example of this condition. Hypertrophy and atrophy of the bone go on together producing great distortion and deformity. The condition is usually painless. Crepitation is present to a marked degree and there is usually distention by effusion. The knee is most commonly affected and shows hyperextension and abnormal lateral motion. Ankylosis does not occur.

Arthritis due to neuritis, or in connection with hemiplegia or chronic encephalitis, may be of varying types.

Chronic Syphilitic Arthritis.—Whether due to congenital or acquired syphilis, arthritis from this cause does not present any distinctive type of joint pathology. Active or latent syphilis may retard the clearing up of an acute arthritis rendering it in effect a chronic process.

Metabolic Arthritis.—Chronic gouty arthritis is an osteoarthritis with characteristic features. Other signs of gout will be found. There will probably be a history of acute gout, and chalky uratic deposits will be found which are exposed or nearing the surface. The roentgenray will show gouty deposits replacing bone structure in the vicinity of affected joints.

Climacteric Arthritis.—Climacteric arthritis of the knees was mentioned under the subject of osteoarthritis. This condition may respond well to treatment by thyroid substance in doses carefully increased.

Intermittent Hydrarthrosis.—Intermittent hydrarthrosis shows periodic recurrences of effusion into the affected joints. This condition usually involves one or both knees but other joints may be affected. The fluid is apt to be somewhat turbid and the cellular content is variable. Pain is not severe unless distention of the joint is extreme. The cause of this condition is obscure, not infectious, and is possibly comparable to angioneurotic edema. The acute attack usually clears up after a few days but shortly recurs. Many cases clear up spontaneously and permanently. No specific treatment has been established as of value.

SPONDYLITIS DEFORMANS.

Synonyms.—Spondylose rhizomélique (Marie); Poker spine; Marie-Strümpell disease.

Spondylitis, considered by McCrae as a form of arthritis deformans, was thought by others (Marie, v. Bechterew, Strümpell) to be a distinct disease. There is early in the disease a fixation of spinal segments by bony ankylosis and by ossification of the ligaments which may be very complete. The ribs become fixed, the chest flattened and the entire spine may be totally rigid. There is frequent involvement of the hips and shoulders (rhizomélique) though often these joints escape. Nerve root pressure is a source of trouble, though in many cases there is a surprising freedom from any nerve pressure symptoms. Many of these cases are probably infectious in origin, but opinions as to etiology differ widely. Considerable relief is accomplished by orthopedic methods and physiotherapy aimed at improving the position or flexibility of the spine and freeing the ribs to some extent.

ACUTE ARTHRITIS.

Acute arthritis, which may be septic, toxic or allergic, includes the arthritis of rheumatic fever, of scarlet fever, in those epidemics in which arthritis is prevalent, and some types of meningococcic and gonorrheal arthritis. An acute arthritis with a tendency to become chronic may appear in the course of pulmonary tuberculosis, the Poncet type of "tuberculous rheumatism," which is distinct from the septic tuberculous joint. Syphilis in the early stages frequently shows very troublesome acute arthritis.

The arthritis of serum sickness, which is a common example of allergic arthritis, comes on from five to nine days after the injection of serum. It may involve many joints, is accompanied with fever and bears a close resemblance to an attack of rheumatic fever. Other manifestations of an allergic reaction accompany the attack.

All of these conditions receive consideration elsewhere as complications in the discussion of the various diseases with which they are associated.

THE BURSÆ.

BURSITIS.

Bursitis as an acute or chronic affection may occur in any of many sites; particularly troublesome is *subdeltoid bursitis*, which is often bilateral. Other frequent sites of painful inflammation are the olecranon bursa ("tennis elbow") and the prepatellar bursa ("housemaid's knee"). Subdeltoid bursitis has been very well described by Codman and by Carnett. It is a surgical condition, is to be differentiated from brachial neuritis and arthritis of the shoulder. Pain may be excruciating on extension of the arm; tenderness is localized to the region of the bursa. Constitutional symptoms are slight. Referred nerve pains are not well defined and muscle atrophy and sensory disturbances are slight. Roentgen-ray study should include both shoulders and is apt to show calcification in the bursa on either side. Paradoxically it may be found that while calcification is present on both sides, it is much less dense on the side on which symptoms are present. It seems that calcification of the bursa may be present without causing symptoms, that it is apt to be bilateral and that when inflammation occurs there is a tendency for the calcium to be absorbed, less remaining in the inflamed bursa than in the other one.

With the exception of the subdeltoid affection and of the sub-Achilles bursitis, which is a common complication of gonorrheal infection, bursitis is usually traumatic. In the subdeltoid location it is probably, as a rule, a degenerative process with superimposed trauma from erosion of the tissues by calcified matter or inflammation originating from a focal infection.

Search should be made for foci of tuberculous or streptococcic infection elsewhere, and if practicable such foci should be eradicated. Rest of the arm and shoulder muscles is necessary.

Opiates may be necessary in acute bouts of pain. The salicylates may have a favorable effect on the inflammatory process.

Heat locally may relieve pain and may hasten absorption of the calcifications. Diathermy has been recommended in this condition. Radiation by roentgen-ray might be tried. The condition may be self-limiting and subside, and if the pain can be kept within tolerable limits by medication and local measures a satisfactory clearing up of the condition may occur. Recourse to surgical intervention is frequently required in this condition.

THE BONES.

CONGENITAL DEFECTS OF BONE STRUCTURE.

1. **Achondroplasia; Chondrodystrophia.**—A common cause of dwarfism, characterized by faults in the cartilages of the epiphyses preventing lengthening of the bones. The growth of flat or membranous bones is undisturbed. This growth disturbance results in an individual with extremely short legs and arms, comparatively large head, broad face, short broad nose, short divergent fingers (trident hand), contracted pelvis, apparent lordosis and waddling gait. Mentality and sexual characteristics are normal. Thyroid gland has been used in attempting to treat this condition but without effect.

2. **Hereditary Deforming Chondrodysplasia.**—A rare disease showing multiple cartilaginous and bony exostoses at the diaphyses of the long bones. This disease is not progressive after puberty and the disturbances are the result of pressure and mechanical interference with joint function.

3. **Osteopsathyrosis; Osteogenesis Imperfecta; Lobstein's Disease; Fragilitas Ossium.**—A congenital defect of bone formation. The bones are delicate and fragile, the cortex thin and the marrow cavity enlarged. Fractures of the bones occur on slight strain or injury. Death usually takes place in infancy. Improvement may take place after maturity is reached. Calcium metabolism is disturbed and cod-liver oil, calcium and phosphorus are recommended in the treatment of this condition.

Oxycephaly or Steeple Head.—A congenital defect with premature union of cranial sutures limiting growth of the skull except in the upward direction, resulting in a tall, pointed skull with marked exophthalmos. Cranial nerve disturbance results from pressure, and optic atrophy is apt to occur.

BONE DEFECTS NOT CONGENITAL.

Osteitis Fibrosa Cystica (von Recklinghausen's Disease).—In this condition multiple areas in the bones undergo absorption with fibrous tissue replacement and cyst formation. The periosteum is not involved. Fracture or bending of the long bones is frequent. The course is chronic, beginning in adolescence or early adult life. This condition seems allied to osteomalacia, and similar to, if not identical with, the result of hyperparathyroidism observed in cases of adenoma of this gland. In the latter condition the bone absorption is checked on the removal of the adenoma. On the other hand, benign giant-cell tumors which closely resemble those of cystic neoplastic bone disease are found. Blood calcium is high and the phosphorus content low (Quick and Hunsberger).

Cases of adenoma of the parathyroid may show symptoms of muscular weakness, gastric distress, sweating and thirst for long periods of time before bone absorption and cyst formation is evident. There is a return of blood calcium and phosphorus to normal and tendency to repair of bone defects after removal of the parathyroid tumor. Tetany may supervene and require treatment after removal of the parathyroid (Shallow). Albright, Aub and Bauer, in a report of 17 cases of hyperparathyroidism due to adenoma, consider cystic disease of the bones as only one phase of hyperparathyroidism. Other manifestations are thirst and polyuria, due to rapid excretion of phosphates and calcium salts, lassitude and muscle hypotonia, due to hypercalcemia, and a fairly constant tendency to urinary calculi. Plasma phosphotase is elevated in proportion to the degree of bone involvement.

Osteomalacia.—This disease occurs in women after repeated pregnancies, but may appear under other conditions. There is a rapid absorption of calcium from the bones, causing softening of the whole bony structure. Great deformity results, particularly from fractures and bending. Fractures heal by union of uncalcified tissue.

There is a marked increase in the excretion of calcium derived from the bones; the blood calcium content is apt to be normal or low, and the blood phosphorus low. There seems to be a lack of vitamin D in at least some of these cases, particularly those due to poor nutrition (hunger osteomalacia occurring in Austria during the World War), and there is probably an endocrine disturbance in which the parathyroid glands play a part.

The onset is insidious, serious deformities of the bones occurring before attention is called to their weakened condition. The course is chronic. Improvement may take place under treatment with vitamin D, phosphorus, calcium and ultra-violet light.

Osteitis Deformans (Paget's Disease).—This disease described by Paget, in 1877, is characterized by a thickening of the bones of the skull, the long bones of the limbs, and of the vertebræ. Other bones may be affected. Coincident with the thickening of the cortex of the bone there is evidence by roentgen-ray examination of an irregular absorption, giving a mottled appearance to the bone shadow. The head may become greatly enlarged; the tibiæ bow forward and the femora curve outward. There is a gradual reduction of height, bowing of legs and spine and an increasing awkwardness of gait. The jaw and face do not enlarge with the cranium. The result of these skeletal changes makes advanced Paget's disease recognizable at a glance. Pain in the extremities and headache are early symptoms. Early characteristic bone changes are often discovered by roentgen-ray search for the cause of these symptoms.

Defects in Membranous Bones, Exophthalmos and Diabetes Insipidus (Christian's Syndrome).—This developmental defect usually associated with dwarfism was described by Hand in 1893 and Christian in 1919.

Since then Griffith, Grosh and several others have reported cases. Rowland discusses this condition exhaustively and concludes that the primary factor is a lipoid disturbance with xanthomatous infiltration of the reticulo-endothelial cells and deposits in the brain and bones.

NEOPLASTIC BONE DISEASE.

Sarcoma of the Bones (Osteogenic Sarcoma).—Sarcoma of the bones may be derived from the marrow or from the periosteum. Some of these tumors show rapid growth and an extreme degree of malignancy while others are relatively benign.

The giant-cell sarcoma of the "epulis" type appearing toward the end of one of the long bones is of the benign type. A shell of new bone forms on the periphery of the tumor mass while the central portion of the tumor is soft and almost cystic. This condition may closely resemble osteitis fibrosa cystica and in contrast to the malignant types of sarcoma should be treated conservatively.

Multiple Myeloma.—Multiple myeloma is characterized by the diffuse distribution of punched-out, sharply outlined rarefactions as shown by the roentgen-ray. All the bones of the body may be attacked. Bence-Jones albumose is found in the urine in many cases. The prognosis is unfavorable. Anemia and cachexia become progressive.

Metastatic Carcinoma.—Metastatic carcinoma of the bones is a condition frequently to be found as a result of carcinoma of the breast in women and of the prostate in men. It may become evident years after a breast removal, and in men there may be found a widespread carcinomatosis of the bones secondary to a prostatic malignant focus so small as to be difficult of recognition.

The spine, pelvic bones and bones of the shoulder girdle and the skull may on roentgen-ray study show multiple areas of absorption before symptoms are noticed.

Pain from nerve pressure, or pathologic fracture, is the usual complaint leading to recognition of this condition.

THE MUSCLES.

DISEASES OF THE VOLUNTARY MUSCLES.

Myositis.—Myositis Ossificans Progressiva.—A progressive, wasting deforming and crippling disease involving the skeletal muscles and ligamentary structures, showing generalized inflammation, atrophy, fibrosis and ossification.

Many subjects of this rare disease, which causes increasing articular and tendinous ankylosis, wasting and bony transformation of the soft parts, have been exhibited in circus exhibitions and popular "museums" as ossified men.

This condition probably starts as a myositis with later fibrous change, but by some observers is considered as primarily an inflammation of the connective tissues, an intramuscular fibrositis with later true bone formation.

Traumatic Myositis Fibrosa or Localized Myositis Ossificans.—The result of fibrous change in injured muscle. If the injury involves both muscle and bony structures there may be an ossification of the fibrous tissue.

Primary Suppurative Myositis.—An acute infection of a number of muscles with tendency to suppuration. The causative organism appears to be a strain of Streptococcus aureus. There may be large solitary abscesses or a diffuse purulent infiltration. Though this disease may be rapidly fatal, Miyake reports 33 cases with only 1 death.

Dermatomyositis.— *Non-suppurative Myositis.*—An acute or chronic disease characterized by inflammation of various muscles with edema and dermatitis. There is a gradual onset, febrile course and grave prognosis. Out of 28 cases collected by Steiner, 17 were fatal. Suppuration is absent or is limited to occasional miliary abscesses. Various micrococci have been recovered from the muscles in this disease (Fox).

Myositis Fibrosa.—Batten described an unusual chronic disease showing successive involvement of various muscle groups by painless swelling going on to muscle atrophy and fibrous tissue replacement. Constitutional and inflammatory symptoms are slight.

Polymyositis Hæmorrhagica.—This condition resembles dermatomyositis but shows hemorrhages into the muscles and cardiac muscle involvement.

A peculiar form of *myositis with abscess formation*, occurring in influenza, not infrequently resulting in rupture of the muscle, is a sharply localized condition, apt to occur in one of the rectus abdominus or pectoralis major muscles. Pain and swelling attract attention. Spontaneous rupture of the rectus may occur. There is usually formation of an abscess in the muscle, the pus from which is apt to be sterile on culture.

Myalgia (Muscular Rheumatism, Myositis).—The common form of myositis or muscular rheumatism, of which lumbago is a good example, is probably a fibrositis of muscle sheaths and of the intramuscular fasciculi.

A frequent cause of pain in the lumbar muscles is *sacro-iliac strain*, and this condition should be ruled out in all cases of lumbago, but the most common cause is fibrositis. The condition may be acute, chronic or recurrent. It usually occurs in acute exacerbations with sudden onset of pain, and showing little febrile reaction and relatively little tenderness except to deep pressure. There may be localized spots of extreme tenderness and these are apt to be marked by indurated nodules.

There must be taken into consideration an underlying tendency to this trouble and an exciting cause. Focal infection or "constitutional fault" is usually the underlying cause. The exciting agent may be acute strain, chill or a toxic factor, as an acute respiratory tract infection or a gouty flare-up.

The pain of lumbago may be slight or may be agonizing in its intensity. The muscles will be felt to be contracted, firm and rigid, possibly softening or yielding under massage and manipulation. The temperature may be normal or only slightly elevated and the pulse will be more than a little disturbed in its rate only if pain is excessive.

This pain with muscle spasm often comes on acutely following strain or exposure. It is usually unilateral and of variable extent. The pain which is situated in the lumbar muscle is frequently increased by nerve root pain occasioned by the clamping together of the vertebræ on one side of the spinal column. The spinal column curves with a concavity toward the affected side. The suddenness of onset of acute pain, lack of constitutional symptoms and slight tenderness are characteristic of this syndrome.

Diagnosis.—Renal calculus with colic shows radiation of pain toward the groin or genitalia, urinary frequency and hematuria.

Sacro-iliac strain causes painful spasm of the lumbar muscles and is one of the commonest causes of lumbar myalgia. There is distinct relief by fixation of the pelvis by a firm belt below the iliac crests. It is apt to be associated with sciatica. Pain is elicited in certain positions of the body. Tenderness is often present over the sacro-iliac synchondrosis.

Pressure *of fibroid tumor*—the presence of the tumor is easily determined by examination. *Cancer of the prostate with bone metastasis*—the bony changes are shown by roentgen-ray even though the carcinoma is difficult of recognition by digital examination. *Osteoarthritis* of the spine will be revealed by roentgen-ray examination.

Treatment of Lumbago.—Acetylsalicylic acid and acetphenetidin, neo-cinchophen and salicylates are useful, as are mustard plasters or other counterirritants locally, cupping, massage, vibration, heat applied by infra-red ray or diathermy or by the old-fashioned method of ironing with a hot flatiron. Acupuncture is said to give relief. Radiation by the roentgen-ray may be beneficial.

Focal infection should be sought for and eradicated and gouty tendency corrected. Thyroid gland (0.015 gram) with cinchophen (0.5 gram) may be of service and the reactions resulting from foreign protein injections may be serviceable in terminating an acute attack.

Trapezius Myositis.—This is an extremely common affection at the present time, at least in those localities where chronic upper respiratory affections are prevalent and persistent. It may depend largely on chronic ethmoiditis. It is characterized by pain in the trapezius muscle on one or both sides, noticeable on turning the head or extending the neck. The pain in the muscle is not severe as a rule but there may be exacerbations in which some pain is referred back of the shoulder and to the occipital region. With fatigue of the muscles of the neck, an occipital headache is apt to develop which seems due to an occipital neuralgia.

On examination a rigidity of the trapezius muscle will be noted and tender nodules or indurations will be found on deep pressure. There will probably be noted some slight enlargement of the glands of the posterior cervical chains. The insertion of the trapezius muscle shows tenderness with radiation of pain to the occipital region on pressure.

In fibrositis there is apt to be pain, particularly at the tendinous insertion of various muscles, and in the case of the trapezius there seems to be a neuralgia which is characteristic and wider in its distribution than the tenderness and pains which are localized at the insertion of this muscle. The lesser occipital nerve penetrates this muscle just short of its insertion and the great occipital nerve lies close to it. Either of these nerves may be included in an inflammatory process or subject to traction.

This type of occipital headache, due to trapezius myositis, was referred to by Cabot as "indurative headache." He cited Redinger and other writers in discussing it. This affection will be found to have been a common one during the past decade. Its *treatment* depends primarily on the free drainage of the ethmoid cells and other paranasal sinuses. This may be accomplished by the use of ephedrine in the nose. A watery solution of ephedrine sulphate, 2 to 5 per cent, 4 or 5 drops in each nostril, is satisfactory, or this may be applied by a swab through the nose to the posterior pharyngeal wall. The ephedrine should be used routinely two or three times daily, or oftener if symptoms of blockage are noted. General measures include the use of salicylates and small doses of iodide.

If shrinkage of the nose tissues by ephedrine or other local applications is not effective, exposure to the roentgen-ray in very mild doses may be satisfactory. A total of one erythema dose divided into five or six applications by cross-firing through the ethmoid region is harmless and very effective.

Local measures are important and very helpful. Massage and manipulation are useful and very successful in relieving the stiffness of the muscle and in dispersing the indurations which can be felt in the trapezius muscle. These measures are more effective if heat is first applied. Heat in itself as a hot pack or in the form of diathermy is useful. Vibratory massage which may be applied by an ordinary and inexpensive vibrator can be easily given.

Fibrositis.—As shown by Stockman and Llewellyn and Jones, fibrositis is an important factor in disease of the locomotor system. Stockman's definition of this condition is "a condition of chronic inflammation."

It is a common condition involving the fibrous tissue of muscle sheaths and bundles, tendons, ligaments, the trabeculæ of subcutaneous fatty tissue, synovial and periosteal structures. This inflammatory change is apt to have its origin in an acute or chronic infectious process and to be subject to repeated exacerbations of activity with increasing fibrous tissue proliferation. This condition accounts for many features of chronic arthritis, chronic or recurrent muscular rheumatism, peripheral neuritis, lumbago, sciatica, neuralgia and torticollis.

A generalized fibrositis may have its start in an attack of acute rheumatism or rheumatic fever or in some other infection. There are probably many factors which may be concerned in its further development: heredity or gouty tendency or diathesis, occupational or environmental handicaps, exposure or fatigue and improper feeding. Digestive and metabolic faults may play a part, and, most important, chronic focal infections or repeated acute respiratory infections.

It can be seen that the great group of arthritic conditions classed as atrophic, comprising rheumatoid arthritis, chronic rheumatism and infectious arthritis, have so much in common that repetition may be avoided by considering certain factors in the etiology and pathogenesis of these conditions together with fibrositis of the muscles and other structures, or chronic non-articular rheumatism.

All of these conditions have certain characteristics in common with chronic infection. As demonstrated by Swift, there is a close analogy between the chronic infections of tuberculosis, syphilis and rheumatic fever.

In comparing tuberculosis and rheumatism both show lesions which are infective, due to the effect of the presence of the organism and to tissue and cell response thereto. Other characteristic effects are due to the effects of circulating toxins acting on susceptible tissues and may be destructive in their effect and may stir up active tissue proliferation. Beside these actions there is another type of tissue response which is that of sensitivity or allergy and which is very striking in rheumatism.

Sensitivity seems to determine acute attacks of inflammation with exudative rather than proliferative changes, the latter being more probably a toxic response. As in hay fever one person may walk through a field of pollinating ragweed or goldenrod without a resulting symptom while another who is sensitive cannot approach this area without exhibiting violent reactions in nasal and conjunctival inflam-

matory response; so one individual may have a coryza or acute tonsillitis caused by a streptococcic infection and show only a local disturbance and a trivial constitutional reaction due to an acute toxemia,
while another in whom certain tissues are sensitive will show a severe
reaction in fibrous tissue in different parts of the body, which reaction
is termed rheumatism, myositis, neuritis, fibrositis or arthritis.

This reaction is seen much more in adults than in children. The
rheumatic child is a subject of rheumatic fever. Different tissues are
sensitive, or, to put it more accurately, more important structures are
involved.

In the case of the child we find the vulnerable tissue of most importance to be primarily the endothelial cells of the arterioles, and the
structural damage which is permanent is found to surround the vessels
which have suffered blockage through endothelial damage. The combination of arteriolar block in vessels which are practically end-arteries,
as in the heart, and toxic alteration in surrounding structures with
accompanying proliferative changes accounts for the permanent damage
which is found in this condition. It is not clear whether an infection
which in an adult, whose tissue resistance to toxemia is greater, results
in sensitivity reactions in fibrous structures, producing muscular rheumatism, arthritis and other manifestations of fibrositis, may not be
the same infection which in a child would have produced rheumatic
fever with its destructive lesions.

In considering rheumatic conditions the very careful observations
of Pappenheimer and von Glahn indicate clearly that in rheumatic
fever the pathologic unit or primary lesion lies in the endothelium
of the arteriole and in the inflammatory reaction surrounding it. This
is toxic.

The observations of Stockman and others show fibrositis to be the
essential lesion of many chronic rheumatic disorders of the adult.
This is a sensitivity reaction.

In the consideration of diseases of the locomotor system dependent
on infectious foci, it will be seen that there are many points of approach.

Given sensitive fibrous structures it is probable that the toxemia
resultant from infection by any one organism can furnish the activating
agent or antigen capable of producing an attack. We may consider
together from this point of view many types of arthritis, of so-called
muscular rheumatism and neuritis (probably in most cases strictly
speaking this is a perineuritis with inflammation and adhesions of the
perineural sheath), periosteal inflammation and many other lesions.

Panniculitis is a special form of fibrositis. This is a chronic inflammation of the fibrous reticulum of the panniculus adiposus, well described by Stockman. It is frequently confused with arthritis. It
commonly appears in tender, rounded swellings at the lateral aspects
of the knees- and ankle-joints. These have the appearance of bursal
collections or of lipomata. Associated with these swellings there may
be noted a sensitiveness or tenderness of the subcutaneous tissues of
other parts of the limb and some degree of fixation of the skin to the
underlying tissue. This condition is common in adults, and is seen
more in women than in men. It may yield to massage and application
of heat. Iodides and thyroid gland are useful in its treatment.

REFERENCES.

ALBRIGHT, F., AUB, J. C., and BAUER, W.: Hyperparathyroidism, Jour. Am. Med. Assn., 1934, 102, 1276.

BATTEN, F. E.: A Case of Myositis Fibrosa with Pathologic Examination, Trans. Clin. Soc., London, 1904, 37, 226.

BURBANK, R., and CHRISTENSEN, B. E.: Specific Vaccine Treatment of 1000 Cases of Chronic Arthritis, with Results and Clinical Observations, Bone and Joint Surg., 1931, 13, 246.

CECIL, R. L., NICHOLLS, E. E., and STAINSBY, W. J.: Bacteriology of Blood and Joints in Rheumatic Fever, Arch. Int. Med., 1929, 43, 571.

COBURN, A. F.: The Factors of Infection in the Rheumatic State, Baltimore, Williams & Wilkins Company, 1931, p. 288.

CODMAN, E. R.: Med. Comm. Massachusetts Med. Soc., Boston, 1908, 31, 277.

CROWE, H. W.: Handbook of the Vaccine Treatment of Chronic Rheumatic Diseases, Oxford Univ. Press, 1931.

FORKNER, C. E., SHANDS, A. R., and POSTON, M. A.: Synovial Fluid in Chronic Arthritis: Bacteriology and Cytology, Arch. Int. Med., 1928, 42, 5.

FOX, H.: Acute Polymyositis, Am. Jour. Med. Sci., 1913, 165, 879.

GOLDTHWAIT, J. E., PAINTER, C. F., and OSGOOD, R. B.: Diseases of Bones and Joints, Boston, W. M. Leonard, 1910, p. 685.

LLEWELLYN, R. L. J., and JONES, A. B.: Fibrositis, London, Rebman, 1916.

McCRAE, T.: Osler's Modern Medicine, 3d ed., Philadelphia, Lea & Febiger, 1927, vol. 6.

MIYAKE, H.: Beiträge zur Kenntnis des Bothriocephalus linguloides, Mitt. a. d. Grenzgeb. d. Med. u. Chir., 1904, 13, 145.

NICHOLS, E. H., and RICHARDSON, F. L.: Arthritis Deformans, Jour. Med. Res., 1909, 21, 149.

PAPPENHEIMER, A. M., and VON GLAHN, W. C.: Studies in Pathology of Rheumatic Fever: Two Cases Presenting Unusual Cardiovascular Lesions, Am. Jour. Path., 1927, 3, 583.

PEMBERTON, R., HENDRIX, B. M., and CROUTER, C. Y.: Studies in Arthritis: The Blood Gases and Blood Flow, Jour. Metab. Res., 1922, 2, 299.

QUICK, A. J., and HUNSBERGER, A. J.: Hyperparathyroidism: Clinical Picture in Far-advanced Stage, Jour. Am. Med. Assn., 1931, 96, 745.

ROWLAND, R. S.: Xanthomatosis and Reticulo-endothelial System: Correlation of Unidentified Group of Cases Described as Defects in Membranous Bones, Exophthalmos and Diabetes Insipidus, Arch. Int. Med., 1928, 42, 5.

ROWNTREE, L. G., and ADSON, A. W.: Polyarthritis: Further Studies on Effects of Sympathetic Ganglionectomy and Ramisectomy, Jour. Am. Med. Assn., 1929, 93, 179.

SMALL, J. C.: Rôle of Streptococci in Rheumatic Diseases, Jour. Lab. and Clin. Med., 1929, 14, 1144.

———— Biologic Products of Streptococcus Cardioarthritidis and Latest Developments in Technic of Their Therapeutic Applications, Jour. Lab. and Clin. Med., 1930, 15, 1093.

STEINER, W. R.: Osler's Modern Medicine, 3d ed., Philadelphia, Lea & Febiger, 1927, vol. 5.

STOCKMAN, R.: Rheumatism and Arthritis, Edinburgh, W. Green & Son, Ltd., 1920.

SWIFT, H. F.: Rheumatic Fever, Jour. Am. Med. Assn., 1929, 92, 2071.

PART III.

DISEASES OF NUTRITION—ALLERGY— METABOLISM—PHYSICAL AND CHEMICAL AGENTS.

CHAPTER XX.

DISEASES OF NUTRITION.

By JOHN H. MUSSER, M.D.

DEFICIENCY DISEASES.	RICKETS.
Avitaminoses.	PELLAGRA.
BERIBERI.	SPRUE.
SCURVY.	

DEFICIENCY DISEASES—AVITAMINOSES.

Introduction.—The term "nutritional diseases" is applied to a group of disorders which are dependent upon either an insufficient amount of, or lack of, certain types of food substances in the dietary, or else upon certain disorders which arise on account of the inability of the body properly to absorb or to make use of these food elements. The term might properly be applied, as well, to the disease, pernicious anemia, which has its genesis in the failure of the stomach to elaborate from food a substance which can stimulate erythropoiesis. The nutritional diseases are frequently considered to be solely those diseases which arise on account of an inadequate ingestion or utilization of the vitamins. Hence the expressions "vitamin disease" or "avitaminosis," are occasionally used to define particular types of disorders dependent upon vitamin lack. The name, "deficiency disease," implies a diet deficient in any one of a number of important food elements, and is more comprehensive nomenclature. The synonym, nutritional disease, has been used in order to take the opportunity of presenting succinctly and briefly some facts concerning improper dietary which may lead to disease because of the lack of certain food elements other than the important vitamins.

Normal Diet.—In order properly to maintain health the normal diet should contain: (1) a certain amount of carbohydrate, fat and protein. These dietary constituents represent tissue builders and energy providers. It is possible to live on a diet containing protein alone, and the absence of carbohydrate and fat from the dietary will not produce disease. (2) Fluid (water) is essential to life. (3) The body is made up of organic substances, as well as large or relatively minute amounts of certain minerals. These latter elements include iodine, potassium,

59

sodium, iron, copper, manganese, calcium, phosphorus, lithium and some half dozen other elements. (4) Lastly, the diet should contain those rather nebulous substances known as vitamins, proof of whose existence until recently was only demonstrable by experimental biologic tests.

In theory, deficiency of any of the important food elements may produce abnormal physical, chemical or metabolic expressions. Actually, because many of the mineral elements are needed by the organism in such minute quantities and are found so widely dispersed throughout Nature, an adequate amount is always ingested in the food of man or animal. Deficiency in certain of the above cited food factors, however, produces distinct clinical disturbances which are readily recognized for the most part. The nutritional elements, then, that may be lacking include:

1. Fluid.
2. Protein.
3. Minerals and inorganic elements:
    (*a*) Iodine.
    (*b*) Calcium.
    (*c*) Phosphorus.
    (*d*) Sodium.
    (*e*) Iron (copper, manganese, germanium).
4. Vitamins.

Water.—Water is essential to life, and the daily intake of fluid in the healthy animal is adequate under all circumstances if the water is available. Fluid acts (1) as a medium for body chemical changes; (2) as a solvent for lipoids, colloids and electrolytes; (3) as a carrier of nutritive and waste elements; (4) as a medium which is of great importance in heat regulation. Fluid intake may be inadequate in the instance of sickness, notably of a febrile type, or in the care of small children. Anhydremia is a very real cause for the development of unhappiness and bodily disorders occurring in patients whose sensibilities are obtunded by disease or who have lost much body fluid through vomiting, severe diarrhea, marked polyuria or as a result of fever. To these patients water must be supplied in quantities from 1200 to 1800 cc. a day as physiologic saline solution, best combined with 5 per cent glucose solution and, depending upon the fluid loss, should be given either intravenously, by hypodermoclysis, by rectal instillation, or through a permanent duodenal tube, assuming, of course, that the patient is unable to take fluid by mouth. Water intoxication is of academic rather than practical importance, except in the condition colloquially spoken of as "heat cramps." In this condition the body electrolytes are lost through excessive sweating. If no water is taken, or a solution of salt and water is drunk, painful muscular cramps do not occur, but if large quantities of water are imbibed, tissue electrolytes are markedly diluted and painful tonic spasms occur, chiefly of the most used peripheral muscles. In the experimental animal, water given to excess produces polyuria, diarrhea, nausea, vomiting, marked restlessness going on to ataxia and convulsions, with ultimate coma and death.

Protein Requirements.—The amount of protein needed by the body for maintenance and growth varies from $\frac{1}{2}$ gram to 2 grams per kilo of body weight, depending in part upon the age of a given individual, the growing child needing a much greater protein intake than the aged. Protein is the most important constituent of the body tissues. Loss of, or inadequate ingestion of, protein produces a negative nitrogen balance, with wasting of body tissue as the reserve store of muscle or other tissue is called upon. Nitrogen equilibrium, or a positive nitrogen balance, must be maintained by a sufficient daily ration of protein in order to preserve health. The value of protein as a food depends upon its contained amino-acids. Certain of the amino-acids must be present in the protein. If these are lacking in a given protein it is termed incomplete. Complete proteins are found in food substances of an animal nature: milk, eggs, muscle or organ meats. Vegetable proteins, usually incomplete proteins, supplement one another so that even on a so-called meat-free diet, if mixed, the various amino-acids in vegetable proteins are present in amounts sufficient to insure proper nutrition.

Marked protein reduction expresses itself most spectacularly in the development of edema. Patients who for some reason or another are placed upon a diet extremely low in proteins may develop an edema which is most pronounced. This edema depends upon the reduction in plasma protein, with the consequent loss of colloids necessary to maintain osmotic pressure so to hold fluid that it will remain in the vessels rather than the tissues as a whole.

Mineral Elements.—The mineral requirements of the body are of importance because these substances help to regulate body neutrality and to maintain osmotic pressure of the body fluids; they form an important part of the cell structure and they make up the greater part of the osseous system. Most of the mineral elements are sufficiently widely distributed in Nature so that the body chemistry never suffers from an inadequate amount of these substances. Sodium, for example, is present in most all food substances. On the other hand, the minimum requirement of certain of the elements is often so deficient that there result skeletal changes, nutritional anemias, acidosis from insufficient base or some other type of disorder. The importance of the mineral requirement of the body and the various factors that play a part in the utilization of minerals are too broad subjects to be discussed in detail. Only the outstanding features of insufficient mineral intake can be accentuated here.

Iodine.—Iodine is an element that is necessary for the body, largely for proper functioning of the thyroid gland. Insufficient iodine intake produces the goiter of adolescence (a type of deficiency disease which will be discussed under diseases of the thyroid gland—*q. v.*). Iodine is found in largest amounts in sea food, lettuce and green, leafy vegetables, provided they have not been grown in a soil which lacks iodine.

Sodium Chloride.—Common table salt plays a most important rôle in the maintenance of acid-base equilibrium. Salt is taken by the average civilized man in quantities far surpassing the daily requirements. Indeed, the interest of the physician lies primarily in reducing the salt content of the food in certain diseases, notably nephritis, in order to eliminate the harmful sodium element which is combined with chloride in ordinary table salt and which is eliminated with difficulty by diseased kidneys.

Calcium.—Calcium is one of the minerals the daily intake of which is often insufficient in amount. This statement applies particularly to growing children to whom calcium must be given in quantities of at least 1 to $1\frac{1}{2}$ grams a day. Of all foods, milk contains the largest percentage of calcium and should be fed to the growing child freely. A liter of milk a day is advisable. Many factors enter into the utilization of calcium. Suffice it here to mention the rôle played by the parathyroid hormone in calcium metabolism and to speak briefly of the disturbance of the calcium-phosphorus ratio which may be found in rickets which in turn depends upon an absence of vitamin D or an insufficient amount of viosterol which contains the ultra-violet rays of midday sunshine. *Phosphorus* is another element that may be present in the diet in inadequate quantities or which may not be metabolized properly on account of the presence of rickets. Phosphorus occurs in largest quantities in the yolk of egg. It is also found in milk and in whole wheat and beans.

Iron.—Iron is an element which is needed by the average adult in quantities of approximately 15 mg. per day. Iron is of primary importance in the maintenance of body hemoglobin, yet so complex is the whole problem of utilization of iron by the body that the mere ingestion of sufficient quantities of iron is sometimes insufficient to prevent the development of the so-called nutritional anemias. Other factors play an important rôle. Utilization of iron depends upon sufficient vitamin intake; particularly interesting is the recent information concerning the supplementary action of copper, manganese and germanium in making iron available for the synthetization of hemoglobin. These factors of course are of primary importance but, unless an adequate supply of iron is supplied to the body, vitamins or other minerals may be in excess and there may still be an anemia. Iron is found in largest quantities in the internal organs, in lean meats and leafy vegetables, notably spinach.

The Vitamins.—A broad and general discussion of the vitamins will precede a more detailed discussion of the important vitamin deficiencies—beriberi, scurvy, rickets, pellagra—which warrant a relatively detailed exposition.

The nomenclature which will be employed is the one in common use in this country at the present time, the vitamins being labelled A, B, C, D, E and G. The English employ somewhat different terminology and further subdivisions, especially of B. In American literature there is a growing tendency to discard the term vitamin G, as this vitamin has been shown to be definitely related to vitamin B, and to use instead the symbol B_2 or B_2G in referring to the antianemic, pellagra-preventing vitamin, and B_1 for the antineuritic vitamin. For the present in view of the continued state of flux of knowledge of vitamins it would seem advisable to continue with the older terminology. The vitamins are also distinguished at times by their degree of solubility in various solvents, such as water or fat. The vitamins in general may be said to be widespread throughout Nature and it is only under exceptional circumstances that the outstanding manifestations of vitamin deficiency occur. There do occur, however, various conditions of ill health, *latent avitaminoses,* which may be attributed to an insufficient or minimal intake of these substances. In theory, an individual may be obtaining from his diet a sufficient amount of, for example, vitamin C to prevent scurvy as a typical manifestation of inadequacy of vitamin C, but at the same time not receiving enough of the substance to prevent mental sluggishness or dental caries. An ample amount of the vitamins is spoken of as the optimal requirement, and in the feeding of infants, children or even adults this factor must be taken into consideration. Lack of sufficient amount of vitamin C is responsible for many irregular, relatively vague and indefinite types of ill health which can be only touched upon in a discussion of the specific vitamins.

Vitamin A.—Vitamin A occurs in Nature in the following foods: cod-liver oil, cream, egg-yolk, and the yellow plants (carrots, corn, squash) which contain much carotene, which is the provitamin, converted in the liver into vitamin A. It is found also in the green plants, liver and whole milk products. The international unit standard of vitamin A is one-thousandth of a milligram of crystalline carotene.

A marked deficiency of vitamin A is responsible for *xerophthalmia,* a condition characterized by keratinization of the ocular and the para-ocular glandular epithelium with subsequent tendency to infection and ultimate loss of sight. The condition of night blindness, *nyctalopia,* is also attributable to inadequacy of vitamin A. Some recent work would indicate that an insufficient ration of vitamin A may be responsible also for susceptibility to infection, stunted growth, and urinary calculi, as well as anorexia, diarrhea, and irregular, vague, indefinite digestive disturbances. Recently a peculiar dermatosis involving the cutaneous epithelium has been described in Uganda prisoners suffering from nyctalopia, xerophthalmia and other features of vitamin A deficiency. Particularly intriguing is the further work of Mellanby, who, though his work has not been confirmed, apparently demonstrated susceptibility to infection when vitamin A was inadequate, and that vitamin A inadequacy may also be responsible for sclerotic changes which are observed in subacute combined sclerosis and which may be also the causative factor when such changes occur in pernicious anemia. Sterility occurs in experimental animals, when vitamin A is deficient, from failure of ovulation. The histopathology of vitamin A deficiency has been thoroughly studied by Wolback and Howe. There occurs as the important and fundamental feature of vitamin A deficiency keratinization of lining and glandular epithelium, explaining the sterility that occurs as a result of cornification of the uterine endometrium or the xerophthalmia which depends upon the keratinization of the conjunctival epithelium and the epithelium of the para-ocular glands or the tendency to infection when the epithelial barriers are weakened or broken down.

Vitamin B.—This particular vitamin has been subdivided into numerous subheads, as B_1, B_2 and so on. Space will not permit, however, more than a generalization concerning this particular vitamin which occurs notably in the pericarp of grain, in animal organs, in egg-yolk, in milk, and in green vegetables. The outstanding clinical expression of vitamin B deficiency is very characteristic; beriberi will be discussed more in detail. Want of this particular vitamin is also responsible for loss of appetite, digestive disturbances, atonic constipation, enlargement of the parenchymatous organs of the body, sterility and for various types of nervous disorders. The digestive disturbances may be explained on the basis of the observations of Webster and Armour who found that for the normal activity of the gastric glands vitamin B complex must be present in the body. Of particular interest are the degenerative changes which occur in the heart which are responsible for some of the symptoms of beriberi. In addition to the pathologic changes which occur in the heart, degenerative changes also occur in the gastro-intestinal tract and multiple neuritis develops which involves the motor, secretory and sensory nerves. Minot holds that the so-called alcoholic neuritis is nothing more nor less than a neuritis due to vitamin B deficiency, dependent upon inadequacy of this substance in the diet of the drunkard or inability to absorb it from the gastro-intestinal tract.

Vitamin C.—Vitamin C occurs in Nature in large quantities in the citrus fruits and the tomato, likewise a fruit. It occurs in many other fruits and green leafy vegetables, and is present in sufficient quantities in raw meat to prevent the development of the outstanding clinical expression of this particular avitaminosis, namely scurvy. In addition to scurvy it is responsible, when deficient in the diet, for poor health in babies; in adolescents, for mental sluggishness; and in any age period for tendency to hemorrhage and general physical weakness. Anemia is a common end-result of the hemorrhages, while the decalcification of bone and the decay of teeth exhibited by patients inadequately fed vitamin C is explained by the pathology of the disorder. The essential pathology of vitamin C deficiency consists of diffuse hemorrhages and fragile bones and, according to Bessey, depletion of fat and cholesterol from the cortex of the adrenal.

Vitamin C has been shown to be a hexuronic acid, now called ascorbic acid, which has been prepared in crystalline form. The adrenal cortex contains considerable quantities of hexuronic acid.

Vitamin D.—This is one of the most interesting of all the vitamins. Vitamin D seems to have for its general action the regulation of calcium-phosphorus metabolism and the prevention of rickets, tetany or osteomalacia. The vitamin is found in cod-liver oil in large quantities. It occurs in milk and in egg-yolk. Particularly thought-stimulating is the question of the relationship of ultra-violet rays of sunlight to vitamin D and the interchangeability of the two as antirachitic agents. One of the really great contributions to medicine in the last few years is the development of viosterol, an ultra-violet irradiated ergosterol, with an antirachitic potency immeasurably greater than that of cod-liver oil, 0.0001 mg. curing rickets in the rat. Likewise, it has been shown that various food substances may be irradiated and become highly potent vitamin D agents. Very recently a crystalline substance has been isolated from viosterol, by Askew and associates, which has per milligram the potency of 40,000 vitamin D units. In addition to the deficiency expressions already mentioned, rickets, osteomalacia and tetany, inadequate intake of this particular vitamin results in caries of the teeth, malformations and deformities of bone, and general muscular, nervous and bodily asthenia.

Hyperavitaminosis is a term used to describe toxic symptoms that arise presumably from excessive intake of vitamins. Thus in the experimental animal when fed large quantities of viosterol there occur loss of weight, muscular weakness, apathy, hypercalcemia and bone lesions comparable to osteitis fibrosa cystica. Similar reactions may have occurred in infants given vitamin D and ultra-violet irradiations to excess, but it is doubtful. Clausen has shown that when blood carotinoid is increased, susceptibility to infection likewise increases, indicating an injurious effect from an overabundance of carotene (vitamin A).

Rickets will be discussed somewhat more in detail. *Infantile tetany* is characterized by intermittent spasm of certain muscle groups here and there in the body, often occurring spontaneously without any apparent stimulus. *Osteomalacia* and softening of the bone, in adults, are still other manifestations of disturbance of unusual metabolism induced by vitamin D inadequacy. The changes that take place in the skeletal system are explained by the pathology of vitamin D deficiency, namely, an imperfect calcification of the bone with an overproduction of osteoid tissue.

Vitamin E.—Vitamin E occurs in animal food, glandular organs especially, and in yeast, the seeds and green leaves of plants. It is sometimes spoken of as the antisterility vitamin because deficiency occasions a sterility which in the female depends upon fetal death due to resorption after implantation, while in the male there occurs degeneration of the germinal epithelium in the testes.

Vitamin G.—This vitamin, sometimes referred to as the P-P (pellagra-preventive) factor bears a close relationship to vitamin B and is sometimes designated as B_2 or B_2G or G (B_2). It occurs in yeast, liver and lean meat, milk and eggs. Either the actual vitamin G (B_2), or a major component of it, is flavine, the natural water-soluble pigment found in milk, eggs and muscle. A deficiency of this vitamin is very generally presumed to cause pellagra in man and black-tongue in animals. Vitamin G, usually always referred to in this connection as B_2, contains the extrinsic factor which is capable of preventing or, when developed, curing pernicious anemia and sprue, according to Castle, but contrary to the observations of Miller and Rhoads, who find that liver extract does not contain sufficient vitamin B_2G to maintain normal growth. From this they deduce that the extrinsic antianemia factor and vitamin B_2G are not identical. The fundamental pathologic changes are the epithelial surface lesions of the gastrointestinal tract, degenerative processes of the cord and brain and skin injury.

BERIBERI.

Definition.—Beriberi may be defined as a nutritional disorder probably due to a deficiency in the diet of vitamin B and characterized by polyneuritis, edema and cardiac insufficiency.

History.—McCollum says that beriberi was already known to the Chinese about 2600 B.C. Takaki, Surgeon General of the Japanese Navy, was the first observer definitely to show that the disease depended upon inadequacy of the ration and to show the relationship of beriberi to polished rice and a rice diet. Takaki and others believed that it depended upon insufficient protein. Two years later (1889) Eijkmann demonstrated the relationship of polyneuritis of fowls to white rice. Subsequent information concerning our knowledge of beriberi is due to the studies of such investigators as Grijns, Fletcher, Funk, McCarrison, Veeder, McCollum and others.

Etiology.—The evidence that beriberi is dependent entirely upon diet deficient in vitamin B is by no means conclusive. Yet the weight of evidence would seem to indicate reasonably definitely that such is the case. Other ideas and theories concerning the cause of beriberi seem to depend fundamentally on a nutritional disturbance as the basis of the genesis of the disease, although such nutritional disturbances may not be the primary or active agent. Thus a deficiency of phosphorus in the diet, or an infectious genesis (Matsumura) of the disease dependent upon improper dietary, has been invoked to explain the mechanism of production of beriberi. Another factor which is undoubtedly responsible for the production of one of the manifestations of beriberi, edema, is dependent largely, if not entirely, upon protein want. Evidence confirming this statement is found in the epidemics of dropsy that occurred during the World War, or during times of famine, and most definite proof has been obtained in several cases of edema from protein want in which we found the plasma protein figures (normal 5.6 to 7.6 grams per 100 cc.) were well below those above which edema does not occur (5 grams) and in which there was as well an inversion of the serum albumin-globulin ratio. On the other hand Keefer maintains that the edema of beriberi is dependent upon failure of the heart "embarrassed by the deficiency of vitamin."

Incidence.—Beriberi is by no means a common disturbance but it is quite possible that many mild cases pass unrecognized as it is not customary to label as beriberi digestive disturbances, sterility, loss of vigor or other symptoms due to vitamin B deficiency when neuritis and edema are not present. So-called epidemics have occurred from time to time when, for one reason or another, there have been periods of food shortage. Until the time the pathogenesis of the disease was determined, beriberi was extremely common in rice-eating countries of the world and it is said still to be a serious cause of disease in China, the East Indies and the Malay peninsula, and in Arctica where the diet is largely fish. In southern Louisiana beriberi cases are observed from time to time. Among the poor population of this section of the country beriberi is spoken of as *maladie des jambes*. These people at certain times of the year live upon a woefully inadequate diet; a diet composed almost exclusively of polished boiled rice, or rice cooked with bacon grease, riz sauce, which not only does not supply the nutritional needs for the antineuritic vitamin B, but also lacks an adequate protein ration. The disease occurs from time to time in institutions, jails, hospitals and eleemosynary homes, not that an insufficient amount of food is given to the inmates but on account of monotony in the articles of food fed the inmates.

Beriberi may be produced readily in certain experimental animals. Fowls will exhibit a polyneuritis following an exclusive diet of polished rice. The addition of unpolished rice or the pericarp of rice to the diet causes the neuritis to disappear most remarkably and rapidly. In the cock the depletion period is approximately seven days. In man the depletion period is approximately three to four months.

The disease occurs commonly with equal frequency in both sexes. Infants are prone to develop abortive symptoms when fed on a diet of skimmed milk and cereals. Any racial predilection for beriberi depends entirely on the dietary habits of the race.

Pathology.—The clinical diverseness of the symptoms arising from degenerative changes in the nervous system is explained at autopsy by the varied degrees of degeneration of the peripheral nerves which may show merely a slight degeneration of an occasional nerve fiber to practically complete destruction of the nerve trunk. In severe cases there may be also degenerative changes in the anterior horn cells and spinal ganglion, while it is said that pronounced degeneration of the brain cells may occur. The second important pathologic criterion in the recognition of beriberi is changes in the heart musculature. This organ is very generally hypertrophied and at death there is a concomitant dilatation. The cardiac musculature shows pronounced toxic degeneration. Particularly interesting are the sudden deaths that occur in this disease, attributed almost invariably to the heart but which may depend instead upon bilateral vagal degeneration. The pathologic changes that occur in the muscular system, because of their resemblance to the changes that take place in the myocardium, suggest the possibility that the myocardial degeneration may be dependent upon degenerative nervous influences entirely. McCarrison has reported in the experimental animal degenerative changes in glandular structures of the body notably, but also the parenchymatous organs of the gastro-intestinal tract.

In the moist type of beriberi edema is invariably present. Certain of the body cavities may escape the transudation of fluid into them but this seems to be more or less a matter of chance. Edema of the subcutaneous tissues is widespread and diffuse.

Symptoms.—Two types of beriberi are generally recognized: (1) *dry beriberi*, and (2) *wet beriberi*. The symptoms of the disease may come on acutely, sometimes recognized and spoken of as *acute beriberi*, or they may be relatively rapid in onset, *subacute beriberi*, or more likely they will be definitely insidious with gradual developing peripheral pains, a certain amount of malaise, gastro-intestinal disturbances and sometimes dyspnea on exertion. Wet beriberi, characterized by general edema, may be preceded by the dry type or it may appear suddenly and out of a clear sky.

Dry beriberi is accompanied by the usual symptoms of a polyneuritis. The severity of pain often bears a definite relationship to the onset. In mild attacks of the disease the development may be so insidious and the pain so slight that the disease may escape detection for a long period. The neuritis is associated with the usual paresthesias of any neuritis such as tingling of the feet and hands which may progress to severe neuritic pains and to motor disturbances so that, in the advanced cases, hand-drop and foot-drop are quite common. The course of the disease in these patients may go along for months, at times improving, at times getting worse. The *physical examination* discloses an absence of tendon reflexes, atrophy of the muscles of the extremities and frequently cardiac enlargement. At times death occurs suddenly as exemplified by a husky-appearing young negro prisoner in a parish prison who, while being transferred to the hospital in an ambulance apparently not suffering from any cardiac manifestations, died suddenly. Other expressions of cardiac disease besides sudden death include enlargement of the heart, dyspnea on exertion, and pitting edema of the legs.

The cranial nerves are usually not involved and consequently pupillary changes are not observed, an important diagnostic criterion, because in severe beriberi lack of coördination and ataxia with loss of reflexes give the impression of tabes dorsalis.

Wet beriberi is associated with marked edema. This edema may be so extensive that the patient appears to be fat and well-nourished, whereas when the edema clears up, the individual is found to be emaciated to a high degree. It should be accentuated that the extreme edema of wet beriberi is probably dependent largely upon reduction in plasma protein although the symptom, edema, may be in part the result of cardiac failure. The subjective and objective symptoms that these patients present are those which arise under any circumstance if there is pericardial effusion, pleural effusion, ascites or peripheral edema from any cause.

The subsequent course of the patient with either of the two types of beriberi is interesting. The patients who have outstanding anasarca frequently have only the mild type of beriberi; disappearance of the edema on high protein diet is spectacular. Patients with the more severe forms of neuritis, even when fed on adequate diet, may take many weeks to recover. The atrophied muscles may gradually regain their tone and the tendon reflexes may slowly reappear; sometimes such a happy result does not occur, fortunately this is rare. In one of our patients there developed a permanent atrophy of the extensor muscles of the wrist and of the feet. The wrist- and foot-drop did not improve to any very great extent, despite the use of electricity and physiotherapy, although the sensory nerve disturbances completely disappeared.

Laboratory Examinations.—The blood shows moderate anemia but there is nothing characteristic about the blood picture itself. The urine may show albumin and casts and, of course, when there is general anasarca the specific gravity is high and the twenty-four-hour excretion is low. Electrocardiographic findings of heart involvement are: small complexes, negative *T*-waves in Leads I and III, slight moderate left ventricular predominance and some slurring of the ventricular complexes (Herrmann). These observations suggest that even in the milder cases definite myocardial changes are present.

Complications.—These are of no moment and do not seem to bear any direct relationship to the disease other than the fact that infections may occur in an individual much debilitated by the disease. The alimentary tract disturbances of vitamin B deficiency, chronic indefinite indigestion, and the sterility of women as a result of cessation of the œstrous cycle, are exhibitions of the disease and not complications.

Diagnosis.—Differentiation of beriberi from primary cardiac disease is at times difficult. Muscle tenderness, reflex changes and absence of signs of congestive failure will suggest the diagnosis of beriberi. Despite the gross evidence of heart disease as exemplified by cardiac hypertrophy as well as systolic (functional) murmurs, failure to find edema of the lungs and congestion of the liver seem to indicate that the heart involvement is not as serious as most writers would indicate. It would certainly appear that the spectacular and sudden heart deaths might depend very much more on vagal degeneration than upon primary disease of the heart. This would appear to be substantiated by the fact that there have been observed patients who have died suddenly, apparently from cardiac causes, without evidences of congestive failure other than edema. The ataxia, absent reflexes and pains in the legs may suggest syphilis of the central nervous system, but the pupillary changes of tabes are absent and areas of anesthesia are common. The blood Wassermann and spinal fluid examination will definitely differentiate the two conditions. The peripheral neuritis of lead, arsenic or alcohol may be differentiated largely upon the basis of the history. Necessarily it is the dry type of beriberi only that suggests a toxic neuritis as a cause of the symptoms. Scurvy may roughly simulate or coëxist with beriberi but the absence of bleeding from the gums and hemorrhages elsewhere will exclude this particular nutritional deficiency disorder. Vedder suggests that the following diagnostic procedures be carried out where it is believed that rudimentary beriberi is present: (1) slight pressure on the muscles of the calf of the leg causes pain; (2) determine the presence of anesthesia with a pin over the anterior surface of the leg; (3) note any modification in the patellar reflexes toward diminution of the tendon reflexes; (4) have the patient squat upon his heels and note the ability to rise without the use of the hands and without this procedure causing pain.

Prognosis.—The mortality in beriberi varies considerably. The average death-rate is from 2 to 5 per cent, but this may be considerably increased if in outbreaks of the disease proper prophylactic measures are not employed. Under any circumstance the heart should be guarded by physical rest over a long period of time because of the possibility of sudden death even in cases which apparently are quite mild.

Treatment.—*Prophylaxis.*—The prevention of beriberi consists in giving an adequate diet to those to whom a regular fixed ration is issued. In this way prison, camp and ship epidemics of the disease are prevented. Instruction should be given to people who supply their own dietary; they must be educated to eat an "optimum" diet which should contain adequate amounts of eggs, vegetables and legumes, fruits, wheat germ and glandular organs. Vitamin B is found so widespread in Nature that it is only under exceptional circumstances, as war or famine or extreme poverty, that the dietetic habits of a nation or a community are so unusual that beriberi is likely to develop among the citizenry. If economic considerations are paramount in such places then the inhabitants should be warned to have their rice unmilled and their bread made from the whole wheat flour if these two particular cereals compose the bulk of the diet.

The actual *treatment* of beriberi consists in feeding the types of food that have been suggested in the prophylaxis of the disease, accentuating again the importance of a high protein (150 grams) diet in the presence of wet beriberi. In patients who exhibit cardiac symptoms, digitalis is indicated as well as prolonged rest in bed. For the neuritis after the subsidence of the acute symptoms strychnine is the drug of choice. To the drug therapy should be added, when available, galvanism, massage and in some instances, if contractures have developed, passive exercise.

Infantile beriberi will not be discussed here. Suffice it to say that this is the type of the disease which occurs in sucklings whose mothers have beriberi. The cardiac symptoms and the edema are the most outstanding clinical manifestations.

SCURVY.

Synonyms.—Scorbutus; Infantile scurvy; Barlow's disease.

Definition.—Scurvy is a nutritional disease due to a deficiency of vitamin C, characterized by a tendency to hemorrhage, sponginess of the gums and certain characteristic pathologic bone changes.

History.—The story of scurvy is one of ancient lineage. Hippocrates refers to scurvy, and Pliny the Elder in his remarkable "Natural History of the First Century after Christ" also gives a description of the disease. From this time on the disease was very generally recognized as one likely to attack armies, such as the Crusaders, or to occur among the soldiers besieging medieval cities and among those in these cities. After the discovery of the Americas, when sailing vessels were frequently many months on the high seas, the disease was first recognized as being a disorder which was likely to develop in sailors on long cruises. The relationship of the disease to dietary inadequacy was originally appreciated by James Lind, the father of naval hygiene in England, whose treatise on scurvy (1754) is a medical classic. Through the influence of Lind and Sir Gilbert Blane the British Admiralty issued an order in 1795 requiring the issuing of rations of lemon juice to the sailors. Some seventy years later the British Board of Trade issued a similar order to the mercantile marine. The relatively recent work of Holst and Frölich (1907) should be mentioned as a real advance in our knowledge of the pathogenesis of scurvy; likewise, the name of Barlow (1894) who definitely established the etiology of infantile scurvy should be noted. *Infantile scurvy* is a disorder of only the last century. Artificial feeding is responsible for the development of this disorder and artificial feeding was not employed until a comparatively short time ago. During the World War scurvy appeared in the British Armies at Mesopotamia and in Asia. The Russian troops in Poland had a severe epidemic of the disease during the World War.

Pathogenesis.—Various explanations have been advanced to explain the genesis of scurvy. These theories are only of historic interest; it has been definitely proved by experimental and clinical work that the disease is dependent upon a deficiency of vitamin C in the diet and any further discussion of the cause of scurvy should revolve about the question of the best method and the best type of food to prevent the disease. Vitamin C, as already indicated, is found notably in fresh fruits such as lemons, oranges, limes and tomatoes. Lime juice in the past has been recorded as a specific in the prevention of the disease, but the antiscorbutic property of lime is undoubtedly much less than that of orange, lemon or tomato. Besides these fruits most fresh vegetables contain vitamin C to a high degree. Vitamin C is soluble in water but is rapidly destroyed by oxidation. It follows that most of the methods of preparing vegetables for preservation over long periods of time are faulty because, due to oxidation processes, such vegetables are lacking in vitamin C. Fortunately in the canning of tomatoes the vitamin is destroyed to a very slight degree, so that canned tomatoes afford a cheap and accessible source of vitamin C. Meat has been held to be inadequate in vitamin C. Stefansson has lived for a year on a diet exclusively of meat without the development of scurvy. Apparently the antiscorbutic element is destroyed by heating the meat, and if it is merely lightly cooked on the outside or eaten raw it retains its antiscorbutic properties.

Incidence.—Scurvy in the adult nowadays is a rare disease. The disease did occur during the World War but this was largely due to misplaced confidence in dried vegetables. Even Arctic explorers who are away for long periods of time from their base of supplies, scientifically provide for the possible occurrence of scurvy among their men; witness the dried beans that Byrd took with him into the Antarctic, which, when germinated, could supply adequate quantities of vitamin C to his men. Infantile scurvy, on the other hand, is relatively common, but even this form of scurvy is becoming rare since doctors have taught mothers the importance of giving orange juice or tomato juice to their babies even before they are weaned and have stressed to the nursing mothers the importance of their taking in their diet sufficient amount of fresh vegetables and fruits to supply the suckling with vitamin C.

Etiology.—The deprivation period, when there is a total lack of vitamin C, is about six weeks. A very small amount of vitamin C may prevent the development of scurvy for many months.

Age, sex, race, previous condition of health and so on are of no importance in the etiology of scurvy except within the limitations mentioned above. The husky adult male on a diet deficient in this specific vitamin is as likely to develop scurvy as the sickly old woman or the babe in arms.

Pathology.—The essential features of the postmortem examination are the tendency to hemorrhage and the changes in the bones. Hemorrhages may occur any place within the body but occur most frequently in the subcutaneous tissues and under the periosteum of the long bones. Hemorrhagic effusions may be found in any or all of the

various serous cavities, but notably the joints. Additional features
that may be noted after death are swollen, edematous and hemorrhagic
gums and the histologic changes in the testes of degeneration of the
germinal epithelium.

Fragility of the bones is marked. Explanation of this lies in the
lesions which are found chiefly at the costochondral junction which
produces pronounced changes in the cartilage column. The "Truem-
merfeld" zone is characteristic of scurvy and is the zone of broken down
bone trabeculæ next to the line of junction with the cartilage. Below
this area is the "Geruestmark" zone, made up of regularly constructed
fibrillar tissue on the groundwork of gelatinous-like material, through
which are scattered occasional thin, bony trabeculæ. Subperiosteal
hemorrhages are also common findings. These bony changes are
particularly prone to occur in infantile scurvy (Wolbach and Howe).

Symptoms.—In the adult, scurvy usually manifests itself first by a
loss of physical tone. The patient with incipient scurvy tires easily
and quickly. Effort is accomplished with difficulty and he is prone
to become dyspneic on slight exertion. Frequently pains in the joints
and muscles are complained of, suggesting so-called rheumatism. As
the disease progresses the gums become swollen, sore and bleed on the
slightest trauma. Sometimes hemorrhage of the gums appears to be
spontaneous. With the development of these spontaneous hemorrhages,
hemorrhages appear elsewhere on the body as petechiæ or even as
ecchymoses in the muscles, particularly in the muscles of the calf,
giving rise to the brawny, painful swellings of the so-called scurvy
sclerosis. Hemorrhages elsewhere in the body may account for other
symptoms. Retinal hemorrhage is an example, as are the common subperiosteal hemorrhages with extremely painful swellings over the long
bones. In the very advanced cases the mouth condition is truly horrible; the gums may become so swollen as to conceal the teeth; the
patient drools bloody saliva and the fetor of the breath is nauseating.
The teeth may fall out and necrosis of the jaw take place. Sometimes
hemorrhages in other portions of the body are prominent symptoms.
Epistaxis may be severe and bloody diarrhea may develop. Hematuria
may occur which, with edema of the extremities and the face, suggests
the development of hemorrhagic nephritis. As the disease progresses
and the mouth infection becomes increasingly severe, a low-grade fever
is common.

A patient with scurvy may die as a result of hemorrhage. At times
a rather sudden shock-hemorrhage syndrome develops from which
the patient does not rally. Equally likely it is that death may occur
from secondary infection, notably bronchopneumonia.

Infantile Scurvy (Barlow's Disease).—Hess writes that in children
between the ages of six and eighteen months, fed an inadequate diet,
scurvy may develop in one of three forms: (1) acute, (2) subacute and
(3) latent. The *acute* type is characterized by the rapid development
of symptoms in a poorly nourished infant. Characteristically, pathologic changes occur involving the distal end of the femur so that the
child lies with the thigh inverted and flexed on the abdomen and gives

evidence of excruciating pain when this portion of the anatomy is touched or handled.

Subacute infantile scurvy expresses itself by failure to gain weight, alterations in the disposition of the child, poor health and tendency to bleed, particularly in the margins of the gums, as well as susceptibility to pyogenic infection.

Latent infantile scurvy is assumed to be present when a child is undernourished, pale, refuses more than a modicum of food and lacks normal vigor. All of these symptoms promptly disappear when a child is given orange juice or tomato juice.

Complications.—Hemorrhages into the serous cavities or into the orbit or elsewhere are often classified as complications, but really represent true expressions of the disease. The likelihood of secondary infection occurring in scurvy is well recognized. Particularly prone is the patient with scurvy to develop pulmonary complications, notably pneumonia.

Diagnosis.—In the majority of instances there is not much difficulty in recognizing scurvy. This is especially true when a clear-cut history of diet inadequacy is obtained. In occasional instances, however, such a story is not easy to elicit; in hospitals from time to time are seen patients with the disease who have lived upon an abnormal diet due to some peculiar idiosyncrasies in their feeding habits which only close questioning will discover. Such cases are rare, however. The disease bears a close resemblance to thrombopenic purpura. In this latter disease there occurs a well marked thrombopenia which is not the case in scurvy. In children the disease may resemble congenital syphilis and may often be associated with rickets. The diagnosis as a rule is not difficult and the syphilitic infection may be recognized by the Wassermann reaction. The rare resemblance of rickets and scurvy may require a dietary test to substantiate the diagnosis. Syphilitic osteitis as well as osteomyelitis from any cause may be simulated by scurvy. In the first instance the Wassermann reaction is useful for differentiation, bearing in mind that infantile scurvy may occur in a congenitally syphilitic child without the usual stigmata of the disease. In the latter instance frequently in order to distinguish between the two conditions a dietary test or roentgen-ray examination is necessary. Bromer lays stress upon the ground-glass appearance of the shaft of the bone near the diathesis and broadening of the thickened zone of temporary calcification at the end of the shaft and the dense ring around the epiphyseal zone of ossification. In advanced cases he writes that separation of the epiphysis may be observed.

The *laboratory examinations* are of some importance in the aid of the diagnosis of scurvy principally because in all instances of unexplained hemorrhage the platelets should be counted. They are found in normal numbers in scurvy, reduced in purpura. The persistency and extent of hemorrhage bear a direct relation to the degree of secondary anemia. Although the color index is reasonably low most of the time, it may be 1+ or more. Leukocytosis does not develop except after extensive hemorrhage or when secondary infection occurs. Bleeding- and coagulation-time are normal. The urine gives no diagnostic information except for the presence of hematuria. ·

Prognosis.—Orange juice and tomato juice are specifics for scurvy. Consequently if the disease is recognized the patient recovers sometimes most spectacularly with the administration of vitamin C in these or other forms. The spontaneous fractures which occur from time to time in the course of the disease quickly heal. Once in a while a hemarthrosis leaves a permanently disabled joint. Hemorrhage into the orbit may cause a loss of the eye. If the disease is unrecognized, hemorrhage, shock-hemorrhage and secondary infections are the chief causes of death.

Treatment.—*Prophylaxis.*—The average dietary of an adult contains a sufficient amount of vitamin C to prevent the development of scurvy even under exceptional circumstances. This vitamin is widespread in foods and there is very little likelihood of the adult getting amounts insufficient to prevent the disease. Where large bodies of men are grouped together and it is necessary to feed them upon a monotonous diet scurvy may develop, but dietitians are well acquainted with the necessity of giving antiscorbutic foods to such groups. To children the optimum of the antiscorbutic element should be given and they should be given it even before breast nursing is stopped, from a teaspoonful to a tablespoonful of orange juice daily or 1 to 2 tablespoonfuls of tomato juice. These liquids should be further diluted in 30 to 60 cc. of water and slightly sweetened; little babies enjoy and delight in orange juice or tomato juice so prepared. One or the other of these two antiscorbutic substances should be kept up until the child is old enough to take fresh fruits and vegetables regularly with its meals. *Curative treatment* consists in giving orange, lemon or tomato juice. Lime juice is not to be depended upon. The response to the treatment is magnificent. Treatment for the gums is rarely necessary and if a spontaneous, or non-spontaneous, fracture occurs it must be treated as any fracture. On account of the danger of infection hemorrhagic effusion should not be handled surgically.

RICKETS.

Definition.—Rickets is a common nutritional disturbance of infancy and childhood characterized by certain bony changes and produced by deficiency of vitamin D.

Incidence.—Glisson first described the disease in 1650, but it is only in comparatively recent years, with the accretion of people in large numbers in urban surroundings that the disorder has become so prevalent as it apparently is in most of our large cities. It has been said that 50 per cent of all the city children suffer from incipient to frank rickets. The disease is essentially one of the temperate zone, yet asymptomatic rickets is extremely common in New Orleans, a subtropical city. It is said to be rare in the tropics where, on account of atmospheric warmth the children are out of doors most of the time, and likewise it is uncommon to see it in children of the far north. The explanation for this apparent discrepancy, where six months of the year children are not exposed to sunlight, lies in the character of the diet of such children. Nursing is continued for a long period of time by mothers who eat fish oils which contain much vitamin D, and when the children are fed by other means they likewise are given some rich oily diet. In the cities the darker pigmented negro children are most susceptible to the disease.

Rickets shows a distinct seasonal variation. During the summer months the incidence of the disease is small, but when the fall months and colder weather come on, new cases begin to appear and reach the highest percentage in the early spring. Children that are born in the spring and who die from some intercurrent infection in the fall rarely show signs of the disease, whereas the contrary is true of children born in the fall.

The incidence of rickets is greatest among children between the ages of six and eighteen months, but it is not uncommon to see it develop as early as the third month of life and it may be met with in children two, three or four years of age (late rickets).

Pathogenesis.—There has been an immense increase in the knowledge of rickets in the past few years, but there are still many facts concerning the development of the disorder which as yet have not been explained. A host of causes have been ascribed to rickets, but from the welter of incomplete knowledge there has come definite evidence that the disease depends upon deficiency of vitamin D in the diet, or an absence of radiant energy, which, apparently through irradiation, activates the cholesterol of the skin to provide vitamin D, which has the property of rendering effectual metabolism of calcium and phosphorus. The vitamin apparently brings about the optimum ratio of calcium and phosphorus in the blood and promotes increased absorption of these two minerals from the intestine. Where the diet is inadequate in vitamin D the blood phosphate becomes lower and the characteristic metabolic feature of rickets, a disturbance of calcium-phosphorus ratio, takes place: the normal phosphorus content of the blood (5 mg.) falls below 3 mg. per 100 cc. of blood. The presence of adequate vitamin D, sunlight, or artificial ultra-violet rays prevents not only this metabolic disturbance but prevents also other general symptoms of rickets which cannot be explained on the basis of alteration in calcium-phosphorus. These factors, lack of vitamin D and sunlight, seem to be the solely responsible agents for the development of the disease. Poor hygiene seems to play no rôle; the factor of bad hygiene is instrumental only because a child may, through ignorance, be improperly fed or kept in the house too much of the day. The dietary inadequacy explains why rickets is many times more frequently encountered in children fed artificial mixtures than it is in the breast-fed child. It has been shown that the milk of cows not exposed to sunlight contains small quantities of vitamin D. This may explain the occurrence of rickets in breast-fed children whose mothers are receiving an inadequate supply of a vitamin or who are confined to the house. In older children diets may be incomplete, as only a minimal amount of the vitamin may be given to these children.

Improper metabolization of calcium and phosphorus through the

60

agency of vitamin D is responsible for bone changes that occur in the disease. It has been suggested that the osteoid hyperplasia that occurs, notably at the end of the long bones, is dependent upon deposition of calcium with improper supply of phosphorus.

Vitamin D, as already mentioned, occurs in Nature in largest amounts in cod-liver oil. It occurs in other oils and the recent important contributions of Hess, and Steenbock, have shown that the anti-rachitic properties of vitamin D may be transferred to other foods through ultra-violet irradiation. The most potent type of such a substance is found in irradiated ergosterol (marketed in the form of viosterol), which is capable in doses of one ten-millionth of a gram of preventing rickets in the experimental animal. It is said to be the most powerful therapeutic agent known.

Pathology.—The child with rickets who dies does not usually die as a result of the disease but from some intercurrent condition. There is consequently no characteristic morbid change which would identify rickets as the causative factor of death or as the contributing cause except those changes which show in the osseous system. The general appearance of such a child corresponds to the description of the child with rickets that is given under symptoms and shows the gross bony changes that take place in the head, thorax and the shafts of the long bones. Closer examination of the bones shows them to be exceedingly soft on account of the decrease in the amount of mineral matter which they contain. The imperfect calcification is accompanied by increase in the osteoid tissue which is next to the cartilage. The cartilaginous zone is irregular in shape and broad. The line of ossification in turn is decidedly irregular and imperfectly marked in contradistinction to the usual clear-cut, straight line of ossification. The diaphysis is thickened and widened and the lines of ossification in the medullary spaces are abnormally broad. As a result of the imperfect calcification, resorption of bone, together with the production of the excessive osteoid tissue, accounts for the abnormalities that are found in the bony tissue. The weight of the body and the pull of the muscles alter the contour and shape of the long bones. The excessive osteoid tissue is responsible for the thickened diaphyses, particularly exaggerated at the junction of the ribs with the sternum and the ends of the long bones. The thickening and thinning of the bone that takes place may be noted also in the flat bones and it is responsible for the unusual cranial abnormalities.

Symptoms.—The onset of clinical rickets is gradual and slow. Among the initial symptoms that deserve to be accentuated are the marked fretfulness and irritability of the child, who is content to lie quietly without moving around. During the night time it is restless, throws itself to and fro in the bed, wakes constantly and sweats excessively on the head and around the neck. Probably the most characteristic feature is the protestation of the child when it is moved about or fondled. The weakness of the muscles exemplifies itself best in the apparent inability of the younger child to learn to walk. Digestive symptoms are common and may take almost any form. Delayed dentition is an almost invariable concomitant of rickets,

The *physical examination* of the irritable, hyposthenic, but quite possibly overnourished child reveals the cause of the symptoms if the case is at all advanced. The head is oversized, square in contour, fontanels remain open and there may be palpated areas of softness. The thorax may show the characteristic deformity, but usually the chicken-breast form of abnormalities of the sternum are slow in development and do not appear until the child is reasonably well matured. The rachitic rosary may be felt and often may be seen. This consists of a series of beads at the costochondral junction extending from the first rib downward. A horizontal furrow following the insertion of the diaphragm (Harrison's groove) indicates the deformity that is produced by the powerful diaphragmatic muscles pulling on softened ribs. The spine may show some deformity, though usually none, but if any, it is likely to be kyphosis of the middle spinal regions. The long bones manifest the effect of the improper calcification. They will be deformed and when the child has learned to walk, bow legs, knock knees and flat feet are the usual findings. Such deformities may be the residuals of rickets and are not one of the suggestive evidences of the early disease, but marked enlargement of the epiphysis, particularly at the wrist and the ankles, is a reasonably early physical observation.

The child is heavy on his feet; the abdomen is found to be large and protuberant, spoken of always as the "pot belly" of rickets. Other bones of the body may also show deformities, but they are not as obvious as those already mentioned. The flattened, rachitic-shaped pelvis may not be obvious, especially on palpation, but in later life is a frequent cause of dystocia. The child is usually reasonably well nourished; in fact at times there may be a spurious robustness because of excessive fatness in a child who is unable or unwilling to use the muscles.

The *course* of rickets is prolonged, lasting for a year or two unless active measures are taken to control the disease, in which circumstance the acute symptoms are ameliorated in a few months. It is during the acute phases of the disease that the tendency to respiratory tract infection makes the child likely to develop the complicating disorder which may produce death. One of the remarkable features of the disease is the failure of the bony deformities to remain. Most of these changes ultimately disappear spontaneously or become comparatively slight.

Complications.—The child with rickets may show abnormal nerve irritability, causing an associated tetany with the usual signs of this disorder. Other characteristic evidences of nervous irritability, which may not depend upon a calcium deficiency, include croup and head knocking. The child with rickets is likewise susceptible to respiratory tract infections so that bronchitis is common and it is not unusual for it ultimately to become a bronchopneumonia, which is the most frequent of the contributary causes of death. The hydrocephalus that accompanies rickets, and that has been mentioned in the examination of the child, usually is not an extreme hydrocephalus and is of no unusual moment. Fractures of the long bones are common. Generally they are of the so-called "green stick" type. Scurvy may be present in the rachitic child, but it is not a true complication, the two conditions depending upon diverse pathogenic agencies, but which, for obvious reasons, may both be present in the improperly nourished child.

Diagnosis.—The diagnosis of rickets does not rest entirely upon the physical examination. The cross, irritable, sickly child with painful muscles suggests the disease before skeletal changes occur. Definite confirmatory evidence of the disease is obtained from examination of the blood and examination of the long bones by the roentgen-ray. The plasma inorganic phosphate is diminished from the normal of 4 to 5 mg. per 100 cc. to 3.5 to 2.5 mg. The calcium content of the blood is but slightly reduced or normal except in those cases of rickets in which there is an associated tetany, in which case there is a hypocalcemia and PO_4 may be normal or elevated.

The roentgen-ray examination discloses a most important characteristic deviation from normal which appears first in the lower epiphysis of the femur, the ulna and the radius: the epiphyseal line becomes broad, concave and irregular and the end of the diaphysis is broad, ragged and cupped. The whole bone shows the failure of proper calcification, and consequently is less dense than normal.

Treatment.—The perfection of a potent remedy in the prevention and cure of rickets makes possible a very limited discussion of the treatment of the disease. It is no longer necessary to incorporate a long series of drugs, biologic preparations and special physical methods for the control of rickets and its cure, now that viosterol is available. A few drops of this potent substance has done away with the necessity of employing direct ultra-violet irradiations, irradiated milk or irradiated food. Viosterol is given as a preventive measure once a day in doses of 8 to 10 drops. Some pediatricians recommend that it be given in the winter months; others that it should be given the year around until the child has been placed upon a mixed diet. If the child was a premature infant the dose should be doubled, and if rickets has already developed the same or somewhat larger doses should be administered. The dosage is given in drops as the preparation is now on the market, put up with standard droppers, 3 drops being equivalent to a minim. Viosterol[1] in oil 250 D is a standardized preparation of radiated ergosterol dissolved in vegetable oil. It is standardized according to the Alumni Research Foundation of the University of Wisconsin under the Steenbock patent by comparing it with a potent cod-liver oil containing in each 0.075 gram one rat unit of vitamin D; that is the amount of vitamin D which is capable of producing calcium deposits in the distal end of the radius and ulna of rachitic rats. The antirachitic potency is expressed in terms of units of vitamin D.

Other methods of treatment may be of slight contributory value, such as massage to increase muscle tone, or iron to overcome the concomitant anemia. If there are marked orthopedic deformities these may be greatly helped at times by a competent orthopedic surgeon.

[1] In some cases it is advisable to give the nursing mother viosterol, more particularly if she is living a quiet and secluded life.

PELLAGRA.

Definition.—Pellagra may be defined as a disease, presumably due to some nutritional fault, characterized by disturbance of the entire alimentary tract, dermic lesions and degenerative changes in the brain and spinal cord.

History.—Pellagra has been recognized for many years in Europe, more particularly in Italy. The first adequate description of the disease was by a Spaniard, Casal, who, in 1735, wrote of a Spanish patient who suffered with *mal de la rosa*. Frapolli, an Italian, who lived in the late eighteenth century, is responsible for the name of the disease, pellagra, or rough skin. It is generally said that Marzari, in the early nineteenth century, advanced the hypothesis that the disease was dependent upon the eating of maize, subsequently altered by the Italians to spoiled maize. The disease generally is supposed not to have been recognized in this country until 1906, yet it undoubtedly existed extensively prior to this date, as investigations have been made which indicate that doctors in the South, who subsequently recognized pellagra, knew and appreciated that they had seen a disease before this time whose nomenclature was unknown to them, but which was undoubtedly pellagra. As a matter of fact, sporadic cases were reported in Massachusetts and New York in 1864. A South Carolina physician, studying the clinical records of the South Carolina State Hospital for Insane and gathering other data, concluded that the disease "had been continuously present in South Carolina at least since 1828."

Incidence.—Pellagra is said to be a disease which is rapidly disappearing in this country. Statistics do not bear out such a statement. According to the latest available mortality statistics (1930) of the United States Public Health Service, there occurred 7086 deaths from this disease, many more than were caused by other diseases listed as communicable excepting tuberculosis, pneumonia and influenza. In Georgia, in 1929, there were 878 pellagra deaths; in Alabama 677, and in Louisiana 285. Further evidence of the importance of pellagra is afforded by the figures of the United States Public Health Service, in collaboration with the State Board of Health in Louisiana, which showed that for a period of six weeks in 1931 pellagra led all other reportable diseases in that state. Surveys which have been made in pellagrous districts indicate that it is only the more severe cases that come to the attention of the physician. It is estimated that approximately not more than 10 to 15 per cent of pellagrins receive medical attention; not that these patients are not substandard in health and do not require the services of a doctor, but because of their economic status in life it is only when they are extremely sick that they feel they can afford medical care.

Undoubtedly pellagra represents a disease which is one of the very real problems of public health; a disease which is extremely prevalent in the South; which may be relatively frequent in the North, although unrecognized because of the unusual manifestations; and a disease which increases in incidence always following, and during, periods of economic depression.

Etiology.—Pellagra is essentially a disease which develops among people economically and educationally below the average of the general population. Age incidence is greatest in those between the ages of twenty and forty years; women are more frequently attacked than men, and of the two races in this country the colored is more likely to be attacked than the white. The occupation of the pellagrous person is of no particular moment, but for the obvious reason that the social status of those who are pellagrins is low, the type of occupation is very generally that properly classified as labor.

The season of the year is significant; the greater number of cases occurring when winter breaks, so that the monthly rate is greatest in the spring months; the farther south the earlier in the spring does the disease occur. There is wont to be an exacerbation in the incidence of the diseases in the fall months.

Pathogenesis.—Innumerable theories have been advanced as to the genesis of the pathologic changes that take place in this disease. Most of these theories and ideas have been discarded. There remain three concepts, one or another of which is generally accepted as explaining the development of the disease: (1) as suggested originally by Goldberger, pellagra may depend upon some disturbance of nutrition, a disturbance which may be the result of a diet inadequate in the so-called pellagra-preventive factor; (2) a nutritional disease which renders the patient who lives upon a monotonous diet more prone to a presumably specific infection; and (3) a photodynamic hypothesis has also been advanced. Alcohol plays a more important rôle in the genesis of pellagra in the North than it does in the South. Its rôle seems to be either to destroy the pellagra-preventing factor in the gastro-intestinal tract or so to alter the latter tract that it is incapable of assimilating the P–P factor. McCollum summarizes the present-day concept of the etiology of pellagra by writing that the disease is probably produced by faulty diet; that it is caused by a deficiency of vitamin G has not been thoroughly substantiated, certainly not thoroughly enough absolutely to maintain Goldberger's idea. Joblin's theory of the importance of light sensitization certainly is more worthy of further attention than it has received in the past. Harris writes that flavine may be identical with the P-P substance of vitamin G (B_2) and that flavine may be destroyed by the action of bright sun-light, either in the food substance itself or *in vivo* in patients exposed to it. It has also been suggested that there may be a new factor, vitamin H, to account for the antidermatitis constituent of the vitamin B complex.

Pathology.—Although the pathologist is unable specifically to point out any distinctive pathologic findings in a person dead of pellagra, nevertheless such pathologic changes as occur are so unlike those that occur in any other disease that the postmortem diagnosis is readily made. There exists an intense and pronounced inflammatory reaction in the entire alimentary tract from the tongue to the rectum. Denton does not believe that the changes in the alimentary tract are purely inflammatory; he does hold that the lesions are confined to epithelial surfaces. In the description of the skin lesions Denton pictures the following stages: the stage of injury (fibrolytic); the stage of reaction (dermatitic); repair, stage of erythema; the stage of atrophy. The mucous membranes of the alimentary tract may show ecchymoses and hemorrhages. In women there is a concomitant vaginitis. The nervous lesions are those of degeneration, involving the ganglion cells of the brain and cord and quite frequently as well the posterior and posterio-lateral columns of the cord, the cervical and dorsal regions being chiefly affected.

Symptoms.—Pellagra exhibits a characteristically progressive seasonal course. The disease usually will start one year and the attack will be relatively mild. In subsequent springs it may become progressively worse, although the first attack is generally the most severe. Occasionally the symptoms start *acutely*, usually *de novo*, but often in a patient who has had previous attacks. Acute pellagra is characterized by fever, extreme prostration, severe diarrhea, and is associated with hallucinations and sometimes mania, going on in a short time to death. More regularly the chronic form occurs without the acute, rather fulminating symptoms.

The prodromal symptoms are vague and indefinite. There is a certain amount of psychic depression and physical weakness with at times a tendency to diarrhea. After two or three weeks of these symptoms the full-fledged attack may develop. This expresses itself by involvement of the alimentary tract, the skin and often the nervous system.

Alimentary Tract.—The sore tongue is one of the first symptoms of actual involvement of the alimentary tract. With this stomatitis there occurs salivation and often dysphasia. The appetite is lost and nausea, epigastric discomfort and belching of gas are common. The diarrhea varies from two or three loose movements a day to a severe bloody diarrhea at frequent intervals. As the disease wanes and blooms forth again, constipation may alternate with the diarrhea. Guthrie has shown in the Charity Hospital patients that absence of free hydrochloric acid is a common finding.

The appearance of the tongue is of diagnostic import. It is an atrophic, smooth, glistening, clean, often fiery red organ which may present shallow ulcers on the tip and lateral margins.

Skin.—The first dermic manifestations resemble closely sunburn. The exposed portions of the body, notably the backs of the hands, the skin over the cheek bones and the neck in women who do not wear collars, become bright red and slightly swollen; these particular areas burn or sting and the skin feels constricted. The margins of the skin lesion are definitely delineated and elevated. In this stage of reaction there may be a period of exaggerated augmentation of the skin symptoms. Blisters and bullæ may develop on the skin, which when they rupture exude a seropurulent material. This hyperreaction may not happen, but if it does occur the subsequent sequence of events with the skin is the same. Gradually the skin becomes dry and desiccated, rather markedly pigmented and covered with a darkish-gray to black keratinous layer. With proper care and diet the crusting of the skin disappears and the underlying skin is shown as rather dusky red and thick in consistency. After several years of relatively mild attacks, the skin of the exposed portions of the body may become thickened and permanently pigmented. Eventually atrophy of the skin may take place. The beautiful symmetry of the skin lesions and their limitations to the portions of the epidermis struck by light rays is most typical.

The V-shaped dermatitis of the neck, the rash on the dorsum of the hands extending down to the tips of the fingers, and the lesions on the ankles and feet of those who do not wear stockings, and the sharp limitation of these lesions at the shoe line, are most characteristic.

Pellagra is said at times to occur without any skin manifestations, *pellagra sine eruptione.* Such a possibility is important because of the difficulty in diagnosis which must often wait upon the development of the skin lesions.

Nervous System.—Nervous disorders are common. The patient is often accused of being neurasthenic. They are irritable and subject to periods of depression. Ultimately they develop a profound mental depression associated with change of disposition and, in the acute cases, well-marked hallucinations. In about 10 per cent of instances these patients become permanently demented. Cord symptoms are shown by the exaggeration or disappearance of patellar reflexes, depending upon the location of the principal pathologic changes in the spinal cord; well-developed disturbances in sensation are common and frequently there develops a paralysis of the sphincters.

Diagnosis.—The red, glazed tongue, the lesions on the exposed skin, the story of diarrhea and of mental depression, present a picture which makes for no difficulty in the diagnosis of the disorder. The triad of symptoms sometimes spoken of as the three D's—dermatitis, dementia and diarrhea—rarely occurs in combination in any other disease. Pellagra is said to resemble other deficiency diseases, especially scurvy, and sometimes the diarrhea suggests the possibility of sprue, but such possibilities should be reckoned as clinical curiosities rather than accepted difficulties.

Prognosis.—The prognosis of pellagra with adequate treatment is usually good. The advanced case or the acute forms present such severe manifestations that the prognosis is extremely poor. These patients may be brought into the hospital and given a diet high in vitamin G and yet get progressively worse and ultimately die. In such instances it has been suggested that on account of the changes of the mucous membranes of the intestinal tract it was impossible for the patient to utilize systemically vitamin G which is present locally in the intestinal tract. The high death-rate of this disease is mentioned on page 949. Disturbing features which make the prognosis particularly bad are inability to eat on account of severe stomatitis, extreme diarrhea, advanced mental deterioration, and acute erythematous skin lesions. Death is usually the result of the extreme cachexia and exhaustion which usually develop in the more acute cases or the chronically continued cases.

Treatment.—*Prophylaxis.*—The prevention of pellagra depends upon methods of educating the uneducated rural poor. They should be taught the advantages of having their own gardens, their cow and their pig, modifying their diet from one in which day in and day out only three or four articles of food are ever eaten and they should be taught the advantages of canning foods such as the tomato.

The *curative treatment* consists, first, of putting the patient to bed in the acute phases of the disease. The so-called specific high vitamin diet, which includes brewer's yeast, is sometimes an impossible adjunct to the treatment because of the discomfort the patients have while taking such food. They should be encouraged, however, to ingest plenty of milk, vegetable purées, soft boiled and poached eggs and tomato juice until the acute alimentary tract pathologic and functional disturbances have improved. Then the patients may be fed on glandular organs, lean meat, green vegetables, yeast and a few fruits. There is no specific drug therapy for pellagra. It is customary to give dilute hydrochloric acid (4 cc.) because of sub- or anacidity. Iron or arsenic is given to combat the not particularly pronounced secondary anemia and strychnine may be given to stimulate the appetite. Bismuth alone, or with paregoric, is as satisfactory an intestinal sedative as any that may be given. The bismuth must be given in relatively large doses (2 to 4 grams). Wet boric acid compresses are adjuvants to the treatment which gives comfort when the dermic irritation is pronounced, while Turner has had excellent results with 1 per cent butesin picrate ointment. Cold cream is soothing when the skin is dry and fissured. Dakin's solution is comforting to the membranes of the mouth. For the associated vaginitis in women, boric acid or weak potassium permanganate douches should be given once or twice a day.

SPRUE.

Synonyms.—Psilosis; Cochin-China diarrhea; Aphthæ tropicæ.

Definition.—Sprue is an endemic disease of tropical and subtropical localities characterized by sore mouth, characteristic diarrhea and hyperchromic anemia, pronounced emaciation, with a tendency to relapses and remissions.

Historical.—In 1766 Hillary observed in the island of Barbados a peculiar diarrhea to which he applied the name "aphthoides chronica" and which apparently was sprue. In 1880 Manson, in China, and Van der Burg independently in Java described a type of dysentery to which the latter writer gave the Dutch name of "spruw" which Manson anglicized later on to sprue. Since this time there have been numerous contributions to the subject of this disease. Ashford, working in Puerto Rico, has written extensively on the subject and has contributed many thoughtful communications. Castle, in 1932, presented a theory to explain the causation of sprue.

Incidence.—Sprue is a common disease in southern Asia from the Pacific borders to India. It is particularly prevalent in the Malaya Archipelago and Ceylon. The Western Hemisphere is not exempt from the disease but only an occasional case is observed. In the southern Gulf states the disease is rare but cases do occur from time to time in individuals who have spent their entire life in this section of the country. The disease is rare on the continents of Africa and of South America and virtually unheard of in Europe except when imported.

Etiology.—Where the disease is endemic the lighter skinned natives are said to be more prone to be attacked, which statement tends to be substantiated by the observation that the light skinned Anglo-Saxon who comes into a tropical country where the disease is present is quite likely to develop the disease if he lives there for any considerable length of time. Women are affected more frequently than men and it is usually those in middle life who get the disease. Predisposing factors such as previous disease, unhealthy surroundings, alcohol, and overwork may have a certain contributing influence on the development of sprue.

Pathogenesis.—A variety of hypotheses have been advanced to explain this disease, no one of which has been substantiated. The most generally recognized theory that sprue was dependent upon yeast-like organisms in the intestinal tract was first advanced by Kohlbrügge who found yeast cells on the tongue, in the esophagus and stools. This work was confirmed by others, notably by Ashford in Puerto Rico in 1914. Ashford found Monilia psilosis in the stools of 87 per per cent of his patients as contrasted with 1.5 per cent of the people living in endemic areas. He has postulated the theory that excessive carbohydrate diet exhausted the pancreas, preparing the intestines for the infection by the monilia. In view of Castle's observations it might be more appropriate to suggest that diarrhea, with the inflammatory and atrophic changes that occur in the mucous membranes of the intestine, predisposes to the implantation and growth of this fungus. There can be no question but that it is present in the great majority of stools of individuals who have this disease. On the other hand, Castle could find no significant correlation between sprue and monilia infestation. Castle, appreciating that both pernicious anemia and sprue are associated with a macrocytic type of anemia, studied 100 cases in Puerto Rico. He found that in many of these cases there was a lack of an extrinsic factor, possibly vitamin B_2, in the diet or a lack of the intrinsic factor in the gastric juice as occurs in pernicious anemia. In some severe cases an added factor was inability to absorb from the gastro-intestinal tract hemopoietic substances. Supplying this deficiency to the sprue patient effected a clinical cure. These observations would tend to substantiate Castle's contention that the disease is a "conditioned deficiency" and that it is entirely likely that pernicious anemia and sprue are different expressions of the same fundamental physiologic process. Further substantiation is the occurrence of glossitis in rats fed a diet deficient in vitamin B (Hutter, Middleton and Steenboch). The clinical evidence of endocrine dysfunction may be explained upon the basis of general tissue atony in association with the extreme emaciation of the body. This has been an explanation, in part, for the fatty stools which are so frequently observed in sprue; in this case it is presumed that the external pancreatic secretion rather than the internal is at fault, but the stools show normal fat digestion, so that failure or inability to absorb fat is probably the true explanation. Calcium deficiency, which is sometimes severe enough to produce tetany, is probably due either to parathyroid dysfunction or else due to the inability of the intestines to absorb and the body to utilize ingested calcium. Scott, assuming that sprue was in part the result of disturbance in calcium metabolism, administered parathyroid and calcium lactate with excellent therapeutic results.

Pathology.—Biopsy of the sternal bone-marrow shows megaloblastic marrow much like that seen in pernicious anemia (Castle). At death the pathologic findings are in no way characteristic. Extreme emaciation is present, with the disappearance of practically all body fat. The pathologic changes that occur are confined almost entirely to the alimentary tract. The liver and pancreas are reduced in size. The tongue is smooth, atrophic, and usually covered with a light fungous film which may also involve the esophagus. The intestinal walls are remarkably thin, the ileum particularly being almost transparent and markedly distended. Chronic inflammatory changes in the ileum, patchy in distribution, are described, notably in the submucosa.

Symptoms.—The symptoms of sprue usually begin slowly and gradually. At first there may be noticed merely a condition of dyspepsia which has exacerbations and remissions. During these attacks of dyspepsia the bowel movements have a tendency to become increased in number. Usually there is a slight diarrhea in the morning and possibly two or three soft stools before noon and then no further action. In the remission between these initial symptoms the patient may be constipated. At this time there may be, as well, change in the disposition, which might broadly be called nervousness and which usually leans toward the side of pessimism. There may be some loss of weight and very often anorexia. In women disorders of menstruation are common. Then gradually or abruptly the more typical symptoms of sprue take place. The tongue becomes distinctly sore and painful so that sometimes it interferes with ingestion of food. Coincidentally the stools take on the characteristic appearance of those which are associated with sprue. There is decided increase in frequency of bowel movement; the stools become bulky, pale, filled with bubbles (foamy), acid in reaction and extremely malodorous. There may be considerable discomfort with each passage due to rectal irritation from the highly acid stool rather than to tenesmus. The patient usually at this time begins to lose weight very rapidly and rather marked constitutional symptoms develop. As the advanced states of the disease approach, and these may occur in as short a time as a year or it may be ten or fifteen years before they appear, the patient becomes dull, apathetic and immune to slight disturbing stimuli. The diarrhea becomes almost incessant. At this time the expressions of tetany may develop. The patient, slowly or rapidly as the case may be, keeps on going downhill until death occurs.

The Physical Examination.—In the early stages of sprue the examination of the patient shows little deviation from the normal. When the terminal symptoms have developed then the appearance of the patient is in a certain sense quite characteristic. Usually there is a lemon-yellowish color to the skin, emaciation is extreme, the abdomen is distended rather markedly and liver dulness is presumed to be decreased. There is usually no fever. The appearance of the tongue during the acute stages of the disease is extremely typical. Minute vesicles, appearing in crops, develop on the tip or sides of the tongue and sometimes the mucosa of the lips and cheeks. They break in a couple of days and leave distinctive aphthous ulcers which are extremely painful. These aphthæ may disappear suddenly to recur again and again. Gradually there develops an atrophy of the filiform papillæ with the fungiform papillæ projecting outward, red and inflamed. Ultimately the tongue becomes wasted, smooth, shiny and atrophic, with the papillæ almost entirely erased.

Laboratory Examination.—The two most important laboratory findings in sprue are a macrocytic anemia and the characteristic stool. The latter has been described in part. The pallor of the stool is due to a reduction of hydrobilirubin to leukobilin (Manson-Bahr). The increased quantity of the movement is the result of an excessive amount of fat which may make up as much as 50 per cent of the dried feces.

The blood picture in the average advanced case is so like that of pernicious anemia that it is impossible for an expert hematologist to differentiate, from the blood smear, the two conditions. The outstanding feature, of course, is the increase in size of the average red cell. The Price-Jones curve shows the average diameter of the cells to be well above normal, up to 9 or 10 microns, with a considerable number of cells considerably larger than this. The color index at this time is high and the mean corpuscular volume is well above normal. The red count at this time may be as low as 1,000,000 to 1,500,000 cells per c.mm., with hemoglobin correspondingly higher, so that the color index is above 1. Improvement in the condition of the patient is accompanied by a return of the blood picture toward normal. The cells become smaller as the red count increases. The red cells exhibit other features common to pernicious anemia, such as poikilocytosis, punctate basophilia and so on. The white count shows a leukopenia the degree of which also bears some relationship to the severity of the anemia.

The gastric contents usually show a reduced acidity and at times an achylia. The urine shows nothing of moment. The blood chemistry shows calcium figures to be below normal, serum bilirubin may be increased, cholesterol diminished.

Diagnosis.—Pellagra may to a certain extent simulate sprue, but pellagra without skin lesions is practically undiagnosable and therefore one must await the appearance of characteristic stools of sprue before attempting to make a diagnosis. When the skin lesions of pellagra are present there is not likely to be any confusion between the two conditions. Pernicious anemia, insofar as the blood picture goes, cannot be differentiated from the anemia of sprue, but in pernicious anemia the weight is usually maintained, there is a practically invariable absence of free hydrochloric acid from the gastric contents and no typical stools. Neurologic findings of pernicious anemia are extremely rare in sprue.

Stomatitis from any cause might possibly suggest sprue but it is unlikely that confusion should occur. With pancreatic insufficiency the large fatty stools of this condition may suggest sprue, but in this latter condition the ratio of unsaponified-saponified fat is normal and fatty acids are in excess of neutral fat; nor is there a macrocytic anemia with a high color index in pancreatic disease.

Prognosis.—It is impossible to make any definite statements with regard to the prognosis of this condition of sprue in patients who are adequately treated with liver. When death occurs it may be due to the severe anemia, to inanition or to an intercurrent infection.

Treatment.—The treatment of sprue has been as varied as have
been the theories to explain the causation of the condition. Most of
the forms of treatment are based upon the hypotheses that have to
do with the causation of the disease. As the condition seems to be
due to a dietary defect, most of these forms of treatment can be
omitted. The most satisfactory approach for the relief of the patient
is to control the diet and to give liver extract. The diet which is to
be suggested is rather exotic and as with all such diets the patient must
be encouraged to carry out the treatment conscientiously over a considerable period of time. All carbohydrates are withdrawn from the
dietary except the carbohydrate of bananas. Bananas should be
eaten in large quantities, a dozen to two dozen a day. The bananas
should be soft, with speckled skins indicating that they are ripe and
not the greenish-yellow bananas commonly eaten. This banana diet
is supplemented by protein given in the form of meat lightly cooked,
from which all fat has been removed. This meat may be given in
quantities up to a pound daily; liver, sweetbread and kidney are of
particular value. All other articles of food are interdicted. It may
be a struggle to get patients to take bananas, but as their condition
improves they are found to take them in larger and larger quantities.
On this diet patients have been seen who have more than doubled and
in one instance tripled the weight with which they entered the hospital.
Small quantities of skimmed milk may be given but no other liquids
except water. After the patients have had a cessation of the diarrhea
and a return of the stools to normal they may gradually modify the
diet by adding green vegetables and fruits. Other types of carbohydrates and fats should be forbidden the patient for a long period—
for at least six months, and then tried out tentatively. In the severe
expressions of the disease the patient should be in bed and at absolute
rest.

The result of administering liver extract is extremely satisfactory.
The dose is the equivalent of 300 to 500 grams of fresh liver if the
anemia is severe. Castle says that there is produced promptly a
reticulocyte crisis with a striking improvement in the blood in many
cases when liver is given by mouth. Because of the fact that the liver
extract may not be absorbed in the severely sick patients, it is best
in these patients to institute treatment by the hypodermic injection
of liver extract, subsequently changing to extract by mouth. In some
cases the macrocytic type of anemia changes after treatment with liver
extract to a microcytic. In these cases iron and ammonium citrate
may be given in doses of a teaspoonful three times a day. Castle con-
tends that prompt symptomatic relief occurs in nearly all cases of
sprue following the giving of liver extract. It would seem wise, however, to enforce the dietary régime outlined above until a larger number
of patients have been reported upon who have been treated with liver
extract alone. In patients with symptoms of tetany or with a marked
hypocalcemia one or another of the parathyroid preparations may be
given intramuscularly, supplemented by calcium gluconate, 5 grams
(75 grains) three times a day.

REFERENCES.

ASHFORD, BAILEY K.: A Clinical Investigation of Tropical Sprue, Am. Jour. Med. Sci., 1923, **165**, 157.

BROWNING, ETHEL: The Vitamines, Baltimore, Williams & Wilkins Company, 1931.

CASTLE, W. B., and RHOADS, C. P.: Observations on the Etiology and Treatment of Sprue in Puerto Rico, Trans. Assn. Am. Phys., 1932, **47**, 245.

CLAUSEN, S. W.: Limits of the Anti-infective Value of Provitamin A (Carotene), Jour. Am. Med. Assn., 1933, **101**, 1384.

DENTON, J.: Pathology of Pellagra, Am. Jour. Trop. Med., 1925, **5**, 173.

FUNCK, C.: The Vitamines, Baltimore, Williams & Wilkins Company, 1922.

HARRIS, LESLIE J.: Vitamins. In Annual Review of Biochemistry, Vol. III, Stanford University Press, 1934, p. 247.

HESS, A.: Tetany and Osteomalacia, Lea & Febiger, 1929.

KEEFER, C. S.: Beriberi Heart, Arch. Int. Med., 1930, **45**, 1.

MCCARRISON, R.: Studies in Deficiency Disease, Oxford Med. Pub., 1921.

MCCOLLUM, E. V.: Newer Knowledge of Nutrition: The Use of Food for the Preservation of Vitality and Health, New York, The Macmillan Company, 1929.

MACKIE, T. T.: Nontropical Sprue, Med. Clin. N. America, July, 1933, p. 165.

MANSON-BAHR, P. H.: Sprue, Practice of Medicine in the Tropics, Vol. III, ed. by W. Byam and R. G. Archibald, London, Henry Frowde and Hodder & Stoughton, p. 2248.

MELLANBY, E.: Diseases Produced and Prevented by Certain Food Constituents, Jour. Am. Med. Assn., 1931, **96**, 325.

MILLER, D. K., and RHOADS, C. P.: Vitamin B, and B_2G Content of Liver Extract and Brewers' Yeast Concentrate, Jour. Exper. Med., 1934, **59**, 315.

MUSSER, J. H.: Clinical Manifestations of Sprue and Relation of the Disease to Pernicious Anemia, Med. Clin. N. America, January, 1926, p. 895.

TURNER, R. H.: The Pathologic Physiology of Pellagra, Jour. Clin. Invest., 1931, **10**, 61.

WOLBACH, S. B., and HOWE, P. R.: Vitamin A Deficiency in Guinea-pig, Arch. Path. and Lab. Med., 1928, **5**, 239.

CHAPTER XXI.

DISEASES OF ALLERGY.

By ROBERT A. COOKE, M.D.

ALLERGY.
ASTHMA.
ALLERGIC CORYZA.
SERUM SICKNESS.

SERUM SHOCK.
URTICARIA AND ANGIONEUROTIC
    EDEMA.
OTHER ALLERGIES.

Introduction.—In a work of this kind it is necessary to be brief, and moot questions, of which there are many, cannot be fully discussed. The term "allergy" was coined by von Pirquet to connote the "altered reactivity" of man to second or later injections of horse serum, but because it is brief and euphonious the word has been adopted and extended beyond its original application and may be used synonymously with hypersensitiveness to include all those specific reactions, whether artificially or spontaneously developed, that have been qualitatively altered from the normal of the species as a result of the stimulation or development of certain cellular activities.

All forms of life respond to a first and to a repeated stimulus by a reaction that is typical for the form so stimulated, and this holds true whether that form be unicellular or multicellular and vertebrate or invertebrate, and whether the stimulus be physical, chemical, thermal or otherwise, so long as the stimulus does not initiate new cellular activities. Such reactions may vary in degree, they do not vary in kind; the response to repeated and identical stimuli being the same as that to the first. Such reactions are not allergic, for they are not qualitatively altered upon a repetition of the stimulus.

On the other hand, in the vertebrate group, to which we may confine ourselves because the opportunity for study has been greater, the primary application of certain stimuli, *e. g.*, protein, gives no apparent reaction, but it initiates cellular activities as a result of which the second application or later applications of the same stimuli may be followed by a manifestly altered reaction that has been induced by the first and is specific. This, of course, implies the presence of a special mechanism (antibody) by which the reaction is mediated between the specific substance, or allergen, and the sensitized cell, and such antibody is demonstrable in many cases but must be postulated for others.

That there are many different forms of reaction included under the term "allergy" will be evidenced by a study of the subject from the standpoints of its etiology, pathology and immunology, hence the varied clinical manifestations of allergy.

Etiology.—Induced or Physiologic Allergy.—Allergy may be induced by the stimulation of cellular antibody on proper contact with an

(959)

exciting agent. For example, the first injection of horse serum in normal man shows no immediate reaction, but it does initiate a cellular activity that later may produce serum sickness. A repetition of the injection may give, depending on its size and on the interval, anaphylactic shock or immediate urticaria or perhaps only a shortened incubation period of the serum sickness. As a matter of fact, serum disease is nothing more nor less than an incident in the development of the anaphylactic sensitization of man. Again, the intradermal injection of tuberculin in normal man gives no reaction, but such an injection in the tuberculous individual gives an inflammatory reaction—an allergic reaction—because the skin cells have been sensitized by the absorption of tubercle. Here we have the evidence of a specific reaction qualitatively altered from the normal and induced by the absorption of tubercle. Another example of allergy is found in the dermatitis produced by poison oak and poison ivy and primula. It has been shown that the irritant is soluble in absolute alcohol, chloroform and other oil solvents, and is presumably an oil. In 1922 Spain showed that 65 per cent of patients over eight years of age gave positive reactions to such an extract of ivy oil. Eighteen infants under eighteen months were negative to a similar extract. Heinbecker tested 65 Esquimos of all ages, none of whom were previously exposed, and all were negative. Low produced on himself and other adults a typical rash from primula on the second application. The first application three weeks prior was negative. Straus tested 118 infants, one to four days old, and confirmed the earlier findings that infants were primarily not susceptible to ivy extract. Forty-eight infants were retested with the same extract after an interval of two to four weeks and 73 per cent gave positive reactions.

In these three examples cited, serum, tuberculin and ivy oil, we have illustrations of allergic reactions in man that were specifically stimulated by previous contact. Serum disease under proper conditions occurs in 90 per cent, 75 per cent of new-born infants were sensitized to ivy oil, and a tuberculin reaction is found in practically all cases of tuberculosis. Now since upon proper stimulation the majority of normal humans respond identically and specifically to the respective stimuli, we must regard such responses of man as normal and, while immunologically these three types of reaction have no relation to one another, we may properly group them together as *physiologic* or *normal* types of artificially induced allergic reaction because they can be readily produced on proper contact in the majority of the species man.

Spontaneous, Hereditary or Pathologic Allergy.—In contrast with the readily induced forms, we have in man a number of clinical allergies as asthma, hay fever, eczema, urticaria and others. They spontaneously occur in but a small per cent of the species man, they cannot be artificially induced in normal man by contact and yet they are dependent upon a special antibody mechanism which in many instances can be readily demonstrated.

What can be said as to their cause? Hereditary factors have been shown to be important in the pathogenesis but the conditions are not directly inherited. How, then, is the mechanism initiated and what determines the allergen for the particular case? For the initiation of the mechanism the hypothesis of contact stimulation is tenable solely because it conforms with the only knowledge we now have regarding antibody production and because it is difficult to disprove previous contact in any particular case. Some support to this contact theory is afforded by the fact that 70 per cent of the clinical reactions of infants are caused by the foods with which they may be in contact during and after intra-uterine life. Certainly unusual and excessive contact is not required. Our records show one child who had a severe allergic reaction to egg the first time it was eaten. Since this child had never tasted breast milk its only contact was during gestation. Several of our aspirin-sensitive cases have insisted that their asthmatic reaction to aspirin occurred with the first dose. The horse serum-sensitive asthmatics have certainly not been sensitized by previous injections of horse serum, for in only the exceptional case is a history of previous injection obtained, the great majority of serum accidents in man occurring with the first injection. The history of previous horse serum injection in an asthmatic reacting to horse serum is unfortunately taken as conclusive evidence of artificially induced sensitization. The fallacy of such an argument is seen in the following case record: A girl, aged sixteen years, received a therapeutic dose of diphtheria antitoxin at the age of twelve years. There was no reaction. At the age of fourteen she developed asthma. When tested two years later she gave an immediate urticarial reaction to horse serum, but she was also just as sensitive to horse dander and much more sensitive to rabbit serum and rabbit dander. If we cannot conceive of these reactions to rabbit protein as induced by horse serum, then it is not logical to conceive of the horse serum sensitization as anaphylactically induced. But absolute proof of absence of prior contact is difficult to obtain for most cases.

To say that hereditary factors have rendered an individual susceptible to easy sensitization is certainly far from true. Vander Veer and the writer pointed out, in 1916, that asthmatics not sensitive to horse serum who had received therapeutic horse serum injections were no more readily rendered skin-sensitive than normal man and none were asthmatically sensitive.

It must be assumed there are factors that predetermine the allergen for any particular case and factors determining what the clinical expression of the allergy shall be. The average individual has contacts with hundreds of possible allergens. That in one case it should be mustard instead of milk or cottonseed instead of dog dander is inexplicable, or that it should be one or several allergens instead of hundreds is not explained by the theory of contact in a person readily sensitized. Another peculiar feature of these sensitizations is their duration even in the absence of continued contact, whereas the induced allergies tend to disappear unless stimulated by at least an occasional contact. All we can say then at this time is that if contact be necessary to the development of an allergy, a very slight one may suffice to set off a variable and self-perpetuating mechanism of reaction to an allergen

61

that is predetermined by nature or inheritance, for other contacts great and small are ineffective.

Pathology.—Inflammatory.—One form of the allergic reaction is frankly inflammatory, as, for example, the tuberculin reaction. In certain instances, as hyperplastic rhinitis and sinusitis, there is a special type of non-suppurative reaction characterized by edema, round-cell infiltration and eosinophil cells. Reasons for our belief in the infective nature of this form of allergy are given in the section on allergic coryza.

Edema and Hyperemia.—The usual reaction as seen in asthma, hay fever and urticaria is one of edema and hyperemia, though either may exist alone. When the edema occurs in the deeper tissues it is called angioneurotic edema.

Exudative.—This type of reaction is seen in the dermatitis of ivy poisoning and in eczema.

Hemorrhagic.—Certain of the non-thrombocytopenic purpuras (Henoch's) have been shown to be due to the ingestion of protein foods, such as beef and milk.

We will not go further now into the tissue changes involved. It is necessary to recognize that these different histologic changes may be induced by an allergic reaction in man.

Practically all the tissues of the body, but especially those of the skin and mucous membrane, may react allergically with one or another of these histologic changes, depending upon the type of allergy, the particular allergen and the area sensitized. Clinical evidences depend upon the combination of these factors that happen to exist. For example, in asthma there is the hereditary type of allergy to many different substances, air-borne and ingested, and the histologic form is one of edema and hyperemia with a sensitization of the skin and mucous membrane of the respiratory tract. In eczema there is an exudative reaction involving the skin. The urticarial and the angioneurotic edema may, as we shall see, involve many tissues, and the symptoms depend upon the area and structure involved.

Immunology.—The induced serum allergy of man is regarded as the prototype of asthma, hay fever, urticaria and angioneurotic edema. There is today considerable difference of opinion among allergists and immunologists as to their identity or non-identity. Let us compare the physiologic serum sickness and the subsequent sensitization (anaphylaxis) with the hereditary allergy (asthma) to horse serum.

The parenteral injection of horse serum in normal man sets up cellular activities which manifest themselves in the production of precipitins, skin-sensitizing antibodies and smooth muscle-sensitizing antibodies. The skin-sensitizing bodies, originally demonstrated by Prausnitz and Kuster, have the capacity of specifically sensitizing the skin of normal man. When a small amount of serum, 0.05 cc. or less, from a sensitized man is introduced into, not under, the skin of a normal non-sensitive man, that skin area will shortly thereafter react with an immediate urticarial wheal to the injection of the allergen to which the skin of the sensitive man reacts. The smooth muscle-sensitizing antibody of such a serum may be demonstrated experimentally in the guinea-pig by means of the Dale reaction. It has been shown by the writer with Spain and confirmed by de Besch that these antibodies, the skin-sensitizing and the smooth muscle-sensitizing bodies, are not identical. One may be present without the other. As stated above, the three so-called immune bodies—precipitin, skin- and muscle-sensitizing bodies—are often demonstrable after the injection of horse serum in normal man and they last for a period of a few weeks or months. The skin-sensitizing body may exceptionally last for a few years.

On the contrary, the asthmatic who is found by test to be sensitive to horse serum has become so without any known previous contact with such serum. Further, the asthmatic naturally sensitive to horse serum has never yet been shown to have precipitins or smooth muscle-sensitizing bodies, while skin-sensitizing bodies are present in many times greater amount than are found in normal man after receiving large amounts of serum by injection. And more than this, the naturally sensitive asthmatic maintains this high degree of reactivity for periods measured by decades rather than by weeks or months.

The argument of desensitization formerly advanced as showing a difference between these two types of sensitization to serum, the natural and the artificial, is not now tenable, as experimental anaphylactic desensitization concerns itself solely with the smooth muscle antibody. Nothing is known regarding the neutralization of skin-sensitizing antibodies which may be, but are not regularly, produced in the animal, are apparently not factors in experimental shock but are the important factors in the reaction of the asthmatic man. Careful observations of the "anaphylactic" phenomena of man are naturally impossible on account of the great dangers inherent in such tests, but the records in the literature on accidental reactions in man following second serum injection show that anaphylactic shock, as apart from asthma, may occur in man as in the guinea-pig, though this is rare. The vast majority of deaths following serum injection in man have occurred with the first injection, and such cases therefore belong with the asthmatic in the pathologic or spontaneous group, not the induced physiologic group.

Another point of difference lies in the fact that a spontaneous sensitization-producing asthma can and does occur to such non-protein substances as quinine and aspirin, tincture of delphinium, oil of cassia, wintergreen, peppermint and rose. The final point of difference may be mentioned. Certain allergies have been spoken of as normal or physiologic because they are readily produced in the majority of the species. The factor of heredity plays no part in these artificially induced sensitizations. In the clinical allergies, asthma, coryza, eczema, however, heredity appears to be an important factor.

From this it is obvious that the only point of identity between induced serum sensitiveness and the naturally serum-sensitive asthmatic is the presence of skin-sensitizing antibodies, hence, certain clinical symptoms (urticaria) are identical. In other important respects they differ. But it is on this analogy alone that the argument for the identity of asthma and anaphylaxis rests.

All allergies, whether they be artificially induced or of the spontaneous type, depend for their reactions upon some special antibody. The induced reaction following injection of horse serum (serum sickness) depends upon certain antibodies demonstrable in the serum and present also in the cells. For the tuberculin reaction no antibodies are demonstrable in the serum and we assume therefore that they are purely intracellular. The same holds true for the reaction to the oil of ivy.

Let us consider further the mechanism of the reaction in the group of hereditary allergies. There are two types of reaction, the *immediate* and the *delayed*.

Immediate Type.—Cases of hay fever, when the skin is tested with the proper pollen extract, give within five or ten minutes a positive urticarial wheal. A drop of the extract applied to the conjunctiva produces redness and itching within the same time. Upon exposure to the proper pollen in the air, symptoms follow immediately upon absorption. Cases of asthma skin-tested with danders, pollens or foods, give, if sensitive, similar immediate skin and eye reactions to the test. The clinical symptoms also develop very rapidly after contact is established with the proper allergen. Such cases of allergy belong in a special group determined by the *immediateness* of the reaction. The time factor is important. These are the cases with circulating skin-sensitizing antibody demonstrable in the serum by the method of passive transfer mentioned above. It is in this group that the diagnostic skin tests are of value.

There are a few important exceptions. Cases of asthma sensitive to aspirin and certain other drugs will develop symptoms within twenty minutes of the ingestion of a minimal dose of aspirin or immediately after a skin-test dose. Unless they have immediate symptoms of urticaria with asthma, which is very rare (we have record of but one such case), the skin test with aspirin is negative. We also have the record of a single such case sensitive to fish as well as aspirin. Antibodies have not been demonstrated in the serum of such cases by passive transfer. The mechanism of this immediate reaction is not known. They are mentioned merely to emphasize the fact that all cases of immediate clinical reaction are not skin-sensitive, but up to the present time the sensitizations to quinine and aspirin and certain essential oils are the only well-recognized exceptions to the rule.

Delayed Type.—In contrast to these immediate clinical reactions, we have a group of allergies in which symptoms appear from several hours to several days after contact with the cause. These we designate as *delayed* reactions. The clinical manifestations of these cases are urticaria, angioneurotic edema, migraine, eczema and occasionally asthma and coryza. The cutaneous tests with the specific allergen are always negative and passive transfer is not effected and so antibody is not demonstrable. At the present time these cases can be diagnosed only by clinical observation and clinical test. Such cases might be regarded as analogous to serum sickness with its delayed appearance of from eight to ten days after injection, but if this were so then skin tests should be positive after the reaction just as in serum sickness, but they are not, even though the clinical reaction is urticaria. The mechanism of these reactions is not understood. We may hypothesize but we cannot explain. To cite a typical case: a school teacher, aged thirty-two years, had suffered from a severe and generalized urticaria for six months. There was no antecedent allergy and she herself had none, past or present, except that for which she sought relief. Intradermal tests were all negative. A careful history disclosed the fact that shortly before the onset of trouble she began to eat chocolate daily and had continued to the present. It was stopped. In two days the urticaria lessened markedly and was gone entirely in two weeks. For test purposes the usual amount of chocolate was eaten. In twenty-six hours a typical attack occurred and lasted three days. A number of trials were made. The incubation period was always between twenty-four and twenty-six hours. The cutaneous reaction was never positive, either immediately or later. This delay in the reaction does not mean merely that these cases are of a low degree of sensitivity; when the clinical reaction does occur it may be of great severity.

A common form of the delayed reaction in asthma is seen in cases of infective origin secondary to sinus or other focal infection. Infection is a cause of asthma in nearly one-third of all cases. Provided the proper organism is used for vaccine injection, asthma may be produced, the attack beginning as a rule in twenty-four to seventy-two hours and lasting several days. The immediate urticarial wheal with vaccine (which rarely occurs), as well as the not uncommon delayed inflammatory reaction (tuberculin type), cannot be regarded as diagnostic of an infective asthma, as both are often negative when symptomatic asthma has been induced by the test. So also may they be positive with vaccines not giving asthma.

It is not purposed to discuss in detail other forms of bacterial allergy, except to say that there is a growing feeling today that much of the symptomatology of infectious disease is due to a sensitization reaction to the infecting organism or its products. Krause and others maintain this view of tuberculosis. The typhoid-Maillein reaction is allergic and analogous to tuberculin. Stevens and Dochez have given very good reasons for believing that the rash of scarlet fever is an allergic reaction to streptococcus. Tillett and Francis have demonstrated in the skin both an immediate urticarial reaction and a delayed inflammatory reaction to different fractions of the pneumococcus. All these reactions of infections are physiologic or normal because they occur in the majority of the species, but asthma is a different form of allergic response occurring in but a very small per cent of individuals with an infective focus. Why this is so we do not know. The hereditary factor is found and appears as the only known force that determines the result for the individual.

It is now seen that there are, immunologically speaking, different kinds of allergy. Some have demonstrable antibodies and some have not. Some develop symptoms immediately upon contact and some are delayed for days. Some are physiologically induced and normal responses for the species, others develop spontaneously and are subject to hereditary influences. Histologically they are inflammatory, hyper-emic, edematous and exudative. Many of the body tissues may be involved in the reaction and hence the protean evidences of allergic reactions in general.

Diagnosis.—We are concerned only with a discussion of the specific diagnosis of allergy, but from what has been said it is evident that skin tests alone cannot make a diagnosis of cause in all cases. It must be borne in mind that with the tests we should seek to duplicate the essential characteristics of the clinical reaction. Lack of regard for this principle has flooded medical literature with a mass of misinforma-tion. One should not expect to diagnose the cause of eczema which is a delayed exudative allergy by means of the intradermal tests, which, if positive, is an immediate reaction of edema.

Cutaneous Tests.—In the *scratch method* a tiny area of skin is abraded and to it is applied the allergen in liquid or powder form; if the latter, a solvent is added. In the *intradermal method* a solution of the allergen is injected in small amount, 0.01 to 0.02 cc., in the most superficial layer of skin by means of a syringe, using a small (26-gauge) needle. In making tests, sterile solutions of proper strength must be used, and too many tests should not be made at one time. This test is more delicate than the scratch but is also more prone to occasion general reactions.

For the study of poison ivy we devised a *patch test*, which is applicable to the study of contact dermatitis. When the proper allergen is used the clinical lesion in miniature is reproduced. About 0.02 cc. of the solution is put on a small piece of blotting paper and held to the skin by a square of adhesive tape. These tests usually remain on for one to two days. Substances in dry form may be similarly applied.

Ophthalmic Tests.—A drop of the solution is placed on the con-junctiva. The reaction develops in about five minutes. It reproduces the clinical lesion of itching, redness and tearing. It is useful in deter-mining the presence or absence of mucous membrane allergy. It rarely exists without skin reaction, but it helps to establish the importance of a positive skin test, as it indicates a more general systemic sensitization.

The allergens used for test are prepared in many ways: the powder forms are supposed not to deteriorate and are prepared by precipita-tion from extracts or solutions. Aqueous extracts are usually prepared in an alkaline saline solution. At present there is no generally accepted method of standardization. In some cases glycerin to 50 per cent is added to aqueous extracts as a preservative and such are useful in scratch tests.

It has been shown recently that the pollen allergen in asthma and hay fever is protein; hence the most logical and uniform method of standardization of extracts is by protein nitrogen content. Based upon practical experience the minimal required dose of 0.00001 mg. protein nitrogen is called *one unit;* 0.001 mg. equals 100 units; 0.1 mg. equals 10,000 units.

Interpretation of Tests.—Readings are made in ten to twenty minutes. Only these immediate reactions are important. Occasionally one sees reactions after twelve to twenty-four hours that were immediately negative. There is no known significance to such reactions.

If *negative* there is no wheal and no redness. When the reaction is *slight* there is a little erythema and wheal. When there is a definite round wheal with erythema the reaction is classed as *moderate*. If after a test there is an increasing wheal with pseudopod extensions and definite erythema, the reaction is *marked*. When a test is positive it does not necessarily indicate clinical sensitiveness, but in the great majority of cases it is of value. To be of clinical significance it must be shown that a patient has contact with the reacting allergen. A goodly amount of common sense is required in evaluating positive tests.

Constitutional Reactions.—Both test and therapeutic injection may give rise to general reaction. Occasionally an injection may be given directly into a blood-vessel and the reaction is due to the rapidity with which it is taken up, but ordinarily it is to be regarded as an overdose. Practically all symptoms begin within a half-hour and the sooner they appear after injection the more severe and serious is the resulting reaction. Death may be produced and is due to asphyxia from bronchial obstruction.

The symptoms of general reaction start with tingling and itching of the skin with general hyperemia, then urticaria and edema with nasal and ocular irritation, cough and asthma. A reaction should be recognized at once and treatment instituted. The *treatment* of these reactions is as follows: a tourniquet is placed tightly above the injection— for this reason injections should be given preferably in the extremities—epinephrin is given at once, in doses of 0.3 to 0.5 cc., and the injection site should be infiltrated with epinephrin to delay absorption. If the reaction is very severe intravenous injection of epinephrin, 1 cc., may be indicated and should be repeated as often as necessary. Morphine, by hypodermic, may be required. Atropine and nitroglycerin and amyl nitrite are of little use. Oxygen inhalations are beneficial if cyanosis exists. Strophanthin intravenously is necessary if cardiac dilatation results. The tourniquet and drugs should always be at hand for anyone giving these injections.

REFERENCES.

Cooke, R. A.: Studies in Specific Hypersensitiveness; Constitutional Reactions: Dangers of Diagnostic Cutaneous Test and Therapeutic Injection of Allergens, Jour. Immunol., 1922, **7**, 119.

Cooke, R. A., and Spain, W. C.: Studies in Hypersensitiveness; Comparative Study of Antibodies Occurring in Anaphylaxis, Serum Disease and Naturally Sensitive Man, Jour. Immunol., 1020, **17**, 295.

Cooke, R. A., and Stull, A.: The Preparation and Standardization of Pollen Extract for the Treatment of Hay Fever, Jour. Allergy, 1933, **4**, 87.

Cooke, R. A., and Vander Veer, A., Jr.: Human Sensitization, Jour. Immunol., 1916, **1**, 218.

Frances, Thomas, Jr., and Tillett, W. S.: Cutaneous Reactions in Pneumonia. The Development of Antibodies Following the Intradermal Injection of Type-specific Polysaccharide, Jour. Exp. Med., 1930, **52**, 573.

Low, R. Cranston: Anaphylaxis and Sensitization, Edinburgh, W. Green & Son, 1924, p. 190.

Spain, W. C., and Cooke, R. A.: Specific Hypersentiveness; Familial Occurrence of Hay Fever and Bronchial Asthma, Jour. Immunol., 1924, **9**, 521.

STULL, A., COOKE, R. A., and CHOBOT, R.: Allergically Active Substance in Ragweed Pollen: Chemical and Biological Study, Jour. Biol. Chem., 1931, **92**, 569.

VON PIRQUET, C. F., and SCHICK, B.: Die Serumkrankheit, Leipzig and Vienna, Franz Deuticke, 1905.

ASTHMA.

Introduction.—With the recognition of the reaction called "anaphylaxis" by Richet, in 1898, and the discovery by Theobald Smith, in 1903, that non-toxic proteins could produce the same phenomenon, there followed a period of intensive experimental study of this phenomenon. In 1906 Wolff-Eisner suggested that clinical hay fever might be anaphylactic, and Gillette (1908) in a study of the reported deaths from diphtheria antitoxin made this inference with regard to asthma, but he called attention to the important fact that practically all of these serious reactions had occurred with the *first* serum injection. In 1910 Meltzer made the suggestion that asthma might be explained as a reaction of anaphylactic sensitization. Cooke and Vander Veer (1916), reporting their studies on the sensitizations of man, observed that hereditary influences were important, that artificial sensitization of the allergic man was not easily accomplished even though multiple sensitization was found in 42 per cent of the cases and that the clinical immunity obtained by pollen injection in hay fever was not due to an anaphylactic desensitization. The occurrence of drug sensitization was also noted in the group. Such facts together with those noted by Gillette in serum shock led Coca (1920) to question the fundamental identity of anaphylaxis and asthma. Coca and the writer later attempted a reclassification of hypersensitiveness and the word "atopy" was coined to differentiate the spontaneous allergies of man, but since, as we have seen in the section on allergy, all these hereditary allergies are not immunologically identical, such terminology seems superfluous unless used to identify a special group such as the immediate, skin-sensitive and hereditary one.

Asthma belongs in the group of allergies that cannot be artificially induced. It is the expression of a natural or spontaneously developed sensitization with a hereditary background and may be either an *immediate* or a *delayed* reaction or both. This distinction is important, as the former is practically synonymous with the skin-sensitive group and the latter with the infective types.

Definition.—Asthma is a condition of dyspnea due to an obstruction, the result of an allergic reaction in bronchi and bronchioles. It occurs in acute attacks, or the condition may be subacute or chronic.

Incidence.—There are no reliable data on its frequency but asthma is common. All ages are affected and the sexes about equally so.

Etiology.—In all its types asthma is fundamentally the expression of an allergic reaction. Some reactions are of the immediate type in which antibodies are demonstrable in the skin by the direct skin test and in the serum by the method of passive transfer of sensitiveness to normal skin. That this is allergy and what is positively known as the cause of such allergy was discussed in the previous section.

That asthma caused by infection is allergy is not so readily susceptible of proof, for it is a delayed reaction without demonstrable reacting bodies. The facts supporting this idea are these:

1. Clinical allergy is found in the antecedents with about the same frequency as in the immediate skin-sensitive group.

2. Other allergies of the skin-sensitive type are found in about 30 per cent of the infective asthmas.

3. Eosinophilia may be regarded as an evidence of allergy, and this is more often present in the nasal and bronchial secretion and blood of infective than of the other type of asthma.

4. The attack of asthma may be reproduced by injection of 0.1 cc. of 0.001 per cent suspension of the proper organism in a vaccine.

5. Drainage or removal of an infected focus in the upper respiratory tract relieves asthma, temporarily at least, with sufficient frequency to show its causal bearing.

The Cause of the Dyspnea.—Breathing is obstructed by narrowing of the bronchial lumen by edema of the mucous membranes alone or by a thickening of the entire wall of the bronchi. Usually there is also plugging of the lumen by exudates which may become so tough, tenacious and inspissated as to form casts of the finer tubes. The dyspnea of secondary emphysema is not considered here. Bronchial spasm is always given as a cause of obstruction in bronchial asthma. With the demonstration of the bronchial spasm in experimental ana-phylaxis of the guinea-pig, this obvious guess as to one of the possible contributing causes of a mechanical narrowing seemed to be on firmer footing. But as stated in the section on Allergy, the more recent immunologic studies have entirely failed to demonstrate the presence of the muscle-sensitizing antibodies in asthma, hence muscle spasm in the anaphylactic sense cannot occur. To be sure, there is increased thickness of the muscle layer of the bronchial tree, but this is no greater in asthma than it is in simple chronic bronchitis in which dyspnea of asthmatic type is conspicuously absent. In asthma of the immediate skin-sensitive type then, as from pollen or dander, the dyspnea is caused by the edema of the lining mucous membrane which is a functional reaction analogous to the edema of the positive skin test. In acute asthma of the delayed (infective) type so often seen in children, we have no knowledge based upon pathologic examination of tissue. The bronchial reaction is probably analogous to that seen in the nasal membrane. In chronic asthma of the infective type from which most of the autopsy data has been obtained the obstruction of the lumen is due to a thickening of the entire wall of the larger and smaller tubes and to the exudate in their lumen.

Predisposing.—The only important factor contributing to the genesis of asthma is an antecedent allergy.

Exciting Causes of Asthma.—It seems probable that any organic and some inorganic soluble compounds might elicit an allergic reaction. The number of substances known to have produced an asthmatic attack is continually increasing. Some substances are much more common causes than others and this does not depend upon the fact that they are commonest among our contacts.　It may depend upon the molecular conformation.

Allergens may be absorbed from the air through the respiratory tract, from the alimentary tract (foods or drugs), from any parenteral injection and from various foci of infection.　A more detailed list is given under the section on Allergic Coryza.　In infective asthma the infection may be primary and localized to the bronchi in about 10 per cent of the cases.　In the others, primary foci are in sinuses and tonsils. Hemolytic streptococcus, viridans, staphylococcus, both aureus and hemolytic, pneumococcus and Micrococcus catarrhalis are the commoner organisms.

In the asthma of infants acute respiratory infections and foods are the most important causes.　In children and young adults the airborne substances are the usual factors.　Asthma beginning after the age of forty years is usually caused by infection secondary to foci of the upper respiratory tract.

Non-specific Causes.—Among a host of causes frequently given as exciting causes of asthma are: mental and psychic stimulation, sexual excitement, exercise, exposure to cold, overeating and the inhalation of mustard gas, sulphur dioxide, chlorine and ammonia.　To be sure, any or all of these things may produce an attack but only *in those who have asthma*.　They are not fundamental causes.　We might with quite equal propriety speak of effort as a cause of angina pectoris. Reflex and neurotic asthma may be similarly regarded.

Asthma and the Autonomic System.—Imbalance of this nervous system is evident in asthma, particularly by vascular hypotonia. But since the symptoms of vagotonia persist in asthmatics without relation to the attacks, there is no evident causal relationship.　It seems more plausible to assume that vagotonia is merely a concomitant constitutional state.　The whole question of autonomic disturbance, endocrine alterations and disturbances of the acid-base balance in their possible relations to asthma is only to be considered as future knowledge lends it importance.　At present the studies have thrown no special light.

Organic Pathology.—In those serum-sensitive cases dying of asthma (asphyxia) after serum therapy, pulmonary emphysema, cardiac dilatation and edema are the only findings.

In chronic asthma the *lungs* show emphysema.　Hypertrophy and dilatation of the *heart* may exist.　The *bronchi* and *bronchioli* show marked thickening of the entire wall, the submucosa and the subepithelial layers being particularly involved.　The lumina are often extensively blocked with tenacious mucopus; eosinophilic infiltration both of the wall and of the exudate is conspicuous.

Pathologic changes of *nasal membranes* and *sinuses* are common. These are usually hyperplastic, but suppurative conditions may exist. Chronic inflammation of the tonsils and lymphoid hyperplasia of the pharynx are frequent.

Functional Pathology.—In one immunologic type of asthma there is demonstrable antibody in the skin and in the serum.　These hereditary cases develop spontaneously, cannot be artificially produced and have the clinical reaction immediately upon contact with the proper allergen. A very few of this group, such as those sensitive to aspirin, do not have demonstrable antibody. In the delayed reaction group no characteristic immune bodies have been demonstrated. Practically always these cases are due to infection but in rare cases food may be a factor. Of 688 cases of all ages recently analyzed, 51 per cent belonged to the skin-sensitive group alone, 34 per cent were caused by infection alone and in 15 per cent asthma was caused by infection as well as air-borne or ingested substances. Other functional changes, such as vascular hypotension, dermographia, hyperidrosis, disturbances of gastric and intestinal motility and secretion are not uncommon. Essentially these are the evidences of dysfunction of the autonomic system.

Symptoms.—The picture of asthmatics in a severe attack is characteristic. They sit bolt upright in bed or chair or leaning forward on folded arms with shoulders elevated and fixed by firm support to elbows or hands, thus keeping the chest in a position of partial expansion and the accessory muscles of respiration most effectively ready. Diaphragmatic breathing is impossible. The inspiratory effort is short, spasmodic and accompanied by throwing back the head. Expiration is prolonged, the muscles slowly squeezing the air from the chest. Cough is often used as an expiratory aid. Breathing is accompanied by loud whistling and wheezing sounds and bubbling râles that can be heard at some distance. It is a distressing picture to watch. The physical effort is so severe that these patients are often drenched in sweat. From such a condition some cases may within a few minutes be restored to an apparently normal state by an injection of epinephrin.

Cough is always present and is loose or dry, depending on the amount of bronchial exudate and the degree of obstruction. The characteristic *sputum* of asthma consists of macroscopic (Curschman) spirals of clear mucoid but it may be purulent.

Pain in the back and along the line of the diaphragm is common and is due to muscle fatigue.

Physical Signs.—The respiratory murmur is much diminished or absent and replaced by sibilant and sonorous sounds and râles of all sorts. These chests have been well described by the term "music-box." Certain signs, as increased resonance, are due to associated emphysema. Heart sounds may be diminished or inaudible.

Laboratory Findings.—The sputum contains Charcot-Leyden crystals and eosinophil cells in practically all cases during the attack, whether it be mucoid or purulent. The sinus discharge if present also shows abundant eosinophil cells. An eosinophilia of the blood is much less frequent and is found as frequently in cases of infective origin as in those belonging to the skin-sensitive group.

Blood pressure is frequently low. The systolic pressure may be elevated in an attack as a result of effort.

Complications.—Other allergies, such as eczema, are common. Emphysema is usually present with the attack. It is most important in older patients with long-standing asthma. Bronchitis is seen in practically all cases of infective asthma. Pneumonia and bronchopneumonia are frequent. Sinusitis is often a cause but it may coëxist and have no relation to the asthma.

Diagnosis.—The diagnosis of asthma is usually easy, but the essential diagnosis of the exciting cause requires time and study, for in many cases there may be several or many factors. The history and physical examination, the laboratory aids and the cutaneous tests are important.

The history should include data on allergies in the family and in the patient. It should trace the development of the trouble, the conditions under which, and the places where, it occurs. Special contacts at home and at work must be sought. The presence or absence of associated conditions of infective origin, such as neuritis and arthritis, may aid.

Physical examination must be complete and include a careful search for foci of infection in the upper respiratory tract.

Laboratory examinations include roentgenograms of chest and sinuses, a study of bronchial and nasal secretions and blood for eosinophils. In cases of infective origin bacteriologic studies are necessary. Sputum, blood and urine examinations should be complete.

The cutaneous and possibly ophthalmic tests are required as described under Allergy. The important air-borne substances and foods should always be tried, for even negative results have value.

Clinical Tests.—These are often necessary to establish and confirm the suspected importance of information afforded by positive cutaneous tests. If a patient with persistent asthma at home clears readily in forty-eight hours in a hospital ward, we have evidence at once of an important factor in the home. If a patient is suspected of having asthma from certain foods, the use of and abstinence from such articles will soon establish the presence or absence of a causal relationship. These clinical environmental or contact tests are of real importance.

Differential Diagnosis.—The many conditions which may cause dyspnea must be excluded. Especially are we concerned with pneumothorax, pleural effusions and fibroid changes of the lung, tuberculosis, silicosis, bronchiectasis, cardiac and renal disease, bronchial and mediastinal growths, especially those of the thymus, aortic aneurysm and foreign bodies.

Prognosis.—This is difficult. We must remember that the asthmatic constitution is inborn and ingrained and a "cure" of asthma at one period of life does not prevent its re-occurrence at a later period from another cause. Once an asthmatic always an asthmatic quite correctly expresses the situation if we use the words to apply to the constitutional state. For this reason physicians and laity must be taught that the asthmatic, like the tuberculous, should be under general supervision at intervals through life. On the whole the results of treatment are satisfactory, but to get good results the patient must give complete coöperation under competent medical direction. Asthmatics may be kept symptom-free but the ability to do this depends on the character and number of the causes. The prognosis is distinctly better the shorter the period of asthma in all cases due to infection.

Treatment.—1. *Symptomatic* (during an acute attack). Measures for relief of dyspnea are indicated: epinephrin, 1 to 1000, 0.2 to 1 cc.

(3 to 15 minims) often gives instant relief. It may be repeated as often as needed. Ephedrin has been disappointing. It is useful only for mild attacks. The dose is 0.2 to 1 cc. of the standard solution of 3 per cent or its equivalent in tablet form. Morphine sulphate, $\frac{1}{8}$ to $\frac{1}{4}$ grain (7 to 15 mg.), is required for severe cases. Aspirin must be used with care in asthma. It helps some cases but should be prescribed only for those who know it to be harmless. Antipyrin, 5 to 10 grains (0.3 to 0.6 gm.), may be similarly used. In children syrup of ipecac to produce vomiting will occasionally help. The various asthma powders and pastils on the market may be burned and inhaled with success. A few breaths of chloroform may be tried but always with care. Other drugs, such as belladonna, atropine, benzylbenzoate and nitroglycerin have relatively little practical use.

2. *General Measures.*—The stomach must not be overloaded and the bowel must be kept freely open. Climatic change is of little value except in the few cases of children with recurring bronchitis, when a warm, dry or moist climate may help. It is of no value in those cases of the infective type with established foci of infection. Our cases of this type are worse in the dry Southwest than in the moister sections of the country. Often a so-called climatic benefit is nothing more than an environmental one.

3. *Drugs.*—Sodium iodide, 0.3 gram (5 grains) or more, three times a day, may give surprising results in a few cases and should be tried. In children syrup hydriodic acid, 5 to 10 cc. (1 to 2 drams), two or three times a day, is more readily taken. We have seen no benefit from intravenous calcium therapy.

4. *Specific Treatment.*—This is successful only when based upon an absolutely accurate diagnosis of all causes.

Pollen asthma is treated as though it were simple hay fever. (See Seasonal Coryza.)

Asthma due to other substances absorbed by inhalation is preferably treated by the elimination of the exciting cause. It may be treated by injection of an extract of the exciting agent, and such treatments must be continued for a long time. (See Perennial Treatment of Hay Fever.)

When asthma is due to certain foods or drugs these should be eliminated. In exceptional cases injections may be required.

5. *Treatment of Infective Asthma.*—The management of these cases is usually difficult. Even in those with isolated attacks foci of infection are often found in the upper respiratory tract. These should be removed when possible during a latent period. Autogenous vaccine injections are preferable to stock preparations. If the vaccine is efficient it may produce attacks and hence should be given with great care. Cases with lymphoid hyperplasia not surgically removable may be benefited by roentgen-ray therapy of the pharynx and naso-pharynx.

Chronic asthma of infective origin is usually the result of persistent foci in the upper respiratory tract. Infected teeth, especially when in relation to the antra, should be removed. Infected tonsils and adenoids must be removed. The greatest difficulty occurs in cases with suppurative or hyperplastic sinusitis. Permanent antral windows have not proven very efficient. In our clinic better results have been obtained with the more radical types of operative procedure.

Vaccine therapy is indicated, using autogenous strains. A fair number of these cases do well if it can be shown that they are really sensitive to the preparation used. Extreme care is then needed. One frequently must begin with 0.0001 or 0.001 per cent suspensions.

The chronic cases often show evidences of sepsis which requires attention. Diet and rest are important. Best results are obtained in those that can be hospitalized for proper periods of time.

6. *Pre-asthmatic Care.*—Immense good may be accomplished in those cases with but suggestive symptoms of asthma and an hereditary background. If these cases can be kept free of respiratory infection in their early years they may never become truly asthmatic. The early removal of infected foci is here indicated. The contacts with important causative factors should be reduced to a minimum.

REFERENCES.

Coca, A. F.: Hypersensitiveness, Tice's Practice of Medicine, Hagerstown, Md., W. F. Prior & Co., 1920, 1, 107.

Coca, A. F., and Cooke, R. A.: On the Classification of the Phenomena of Hypersensitiveness, Jour. Immunol., 1923, 8, 163.

Cooke, R. A.: Infective Asthma: Indication of Its Allergic Nature, Am. Jour. Med. Sci., 1932, 183, 309.

Cooke, R. A., and Vander Veer, A., Jr.: Human Sensitization, Jour. Immunol., 1916, 1, 201.

Gillette, H. F.: Untoward Results from Diphtheria Antitoxin with Special Reference to Its Relation to Asthma, Ther. Gaz., March, 1909.

Huber, H. L., and Koessler, K. K.: The Pathology of Bronchial Asthma, Arch. Int. Med., 1922, 30, 689.

Kistner, F. B.: Histopathology and Bacteriology of Sinusitis, Arch. Otol., 1931, 13, 225.

Kuntz, Albert: The Autonomic Nervous System, Philadelphia, Lea & Febiger, 1934.

Meltzer, S. J.: Bronchial Asthma as a Phenomenon of Anaphylaxis, Jour. Am. Med. Assn., 1910, 55, 1021.

Otto, R.: Das Theobald Smitsche Phänomen der Serumüberempfindlichkeit, Leuthold Gedenkschr., 1906, 1, 153.

Portier, P., and Richet, Charles: De l'action anaphylactique de certains venins, Compt. rend. Soc. de biol., 1902, 54, 170.

Wolff-Eisner, A.: Das Heufiber, sein Wesen und seine Behandlung, Munich, Lehmann, 1906.

ALLERGIC CORYZA (HAY FEVER).

Coryza of an allergic nature may be acute or chronic, and seasonal or perennial; pathologically it is manifest as a purely functional vasomotor reaction or as an organic lesion with hyperplasia of the nasal and sinus mucous membranes; immunologically it may belong in the class of immediate reaction with serum and skin antibodies, or it is of the delayed type, in which case antibody cannot be demonstrated. For practical purposes we will consider this group under the headings of seasonal coryza or hay fever proper, non-seasonal or perennial coryza and the nasal infections of allergic nature.

Seasonal Coryza.—**Synonyms.**—Hay fever; Pollinosis; Vasomotor rhinitis.

Definition.—Hay fever is an allergic reaction of the immediate type with sensitization of the skin and mucous membrane of the upper respiratory tract and eye and demonstrable antibody in the serum The reaction is purely vasomotor and caused by the absorption of pollen.

History.—Hay fever was first described by Bostock in 1819. Elliotson attributed it to pollen in 1831. Blakely, a hay fever sufferer, experimented on himself in 1873 and produced an extra-seasonal attack with pollen extract. Dunbar believed the pollen contained a tox-albumin and he produced a so-called antitoxic serum by injecting horses with pollen extract. The serum was sold under the name *"polentin."* Results were unsatisfactory. With the development of ideas on anaphylaxis, Wolff-Eisner (1906) first suggested the possibility that hay fever was an anaphylactic phenomenon. Freeman and Noon (1911) were the first to publish results of treatment of hay fever with pollen extracts. In 1913 Clowes reported on the specific reactions of hay fever cases. Cooke in 1915 reported 144 cases treated with pollen extracts. Since this time the procedures have been widely extended and the early results confirmed.

Etiology.—Seasonal hay fever is caused largely by certain air-borne pollens, but recently it has been shown by Parlato and others that emanations of the sandfly, moth, butterfly and other insects seasonally abundant may cause typical coryza reactions. Contact with such trees as spruce and balsam has also been known to produce attacks. The period of the attack and the pollens causing it depend upon the location. In the warm and dry southwestern part of the United States some pollens are present almost the entire year. In the major portion of the United States, however, there are well-defined types. The spring type, from March to the end of May, is caused by the pollens of such trees as birch, ash, oak, elm, poplar, beech, alder, hazel and hickory. The summer type, from the middle of May to the middle of July, is caused by the various grass pollens and less often by plantain and sorrel. The fall, or late type, is due to the pollens of ragweed. In the proper localities hay fever may also be caused by sage, mountain cedar, careless weed and various other pollens. As a matter of fact, various pollens not air-borne, such as goldenrod, sunflower, cosmos and other members of the compositæ family, may produce attacks if the contact be sufficiently intimate.

Incidence.—It has never been possible accurately to estimate the incidence of hay fever. It is much more prevalent in the United States and Canada than in Europe, as ragweed does not grow in England or on the Continent. Both sexes are equally susceptible. The age of maximum liability is from twenty-five to thirty years, but the condition does exist in infancy and cases are known to have developed after the age of sixty-five years.

Pathogenesis.—The presence of any form of allergy in the antecedents, but especially the presence of hay fever, is of importance in the pathogenesis of this allergy.

Uncomplicated seasonal coryza is a purely functional vasomotor disturbance caused by a sensitization reaction of the mucous membrane of the nose, pharynx and eye. The reaction begins almost immediately after contact with the allergen and is characterized by edema and hyperemia of the tissues. Circulating antibodies are present in the serum and the skin is also reactive. This latter fact makes the diagostic skin tests possible.

Pathology.—Organic change is not a part of hay fever itself, but the vasomotor changes do seem to predispose to infection of the sinuses, especially in those over forty years of age. Such infections may be of the suppurative type but more commonly they lead to the hyperplastic and polypoid changes of the nasal and sinus membranes.

Symptoms.—These are localized in the sensitized area, the nose and and eye. The intensity of the symptoms is not seemingly dependent upon the degree of sensitivity. The attacks are usually paroxysmal and vary not only from day to day but from hour to hour. There is itching, tearing and redness of the eyes and photophobia. Nasal breathing is more or less obstructed. There are paroxysms of sneezing and a thin watery nasal discharge. Often there is itching of the roof of the mouth, the throat and deep in the ears. The skin of the face, especially about the nose, may itch but show no eruption. The clinical picture is very typical and characterized especially by the precise seasonal periodicity. The duration of the attack depends on the sensitizations of the individual, hence we see cases of the spring, summer or fall type singly or any combination of these.

Complications.—*Multiple Allergies.*—Cases of hay fever are very prone to other allergies. It may be a perennial coryza or asthma or take such forms as urticaria, eczema, migraine and angioneurotic edema.

Infection.—Nasal and sinus infections are common. Not infrequently these infections become chronic and lead to the hyperplastic changes to be described. Occasionally one sees hay fever that does not end with the season as expected, the symptoms being continued by a sinus infection.

Asthma.—When the bronchial membranes are also sensitized to the pollen, a strictly seasonal asthma begins soon after the coryza and terminates with it. This is the case in 15 per cent of all cases of hay fever. At times an asthmatic attack begins at the close or shortly after the hay fever season and in such cases is usually due to a sinus infection.

Diagnosis.—A careful history of the usual date of onset and offset of symptoms is of value in selecting the pollen or pollens to which an individual may be sensitive. The determination of the specific sensitization is then made by the cutaneous test and, when in doubt, by the ophthalmic test as previously described. The intradermal test, on account of its greater accuracy, is undoubtedly the method of choice over the scratch test. In view of the fact that there is no generally accepted method of standardizing extracts, one should adopt the suggestions of the commercial firm supplying the extract to be used; but accurate testing should be done to determine which pollen extract should be used.

It has now been determined that the pollens of the Gramineæ are biologically identical, that is, a person reactive to the extract of one grass pollen will react to all. Likewise a person reacting to one form of ragweed will react to the others. For the tree pollens the same cannot be said. They must be individually tested as far as genus pollen is concerned.

Hay fever cases vary greatly in the degree of sensitivity. Those that are exquisitely sensitive cannot safely receive the treatment doses required for the less sensitive. For this reason we attempt to determine the constitutional sensitiveness by testing the reactivity of the skin to graduated doses of the pollen extract, using solutions containing 10, 100 and 1000 units of protein nitrogen per cubic centimeter and designated as Solutions 1, 2 and 3, respectively.

Cases which give a "marked" reaction to the usual intradermal test dose ($\frac{1}{50}$ cc.) of Solution 1 and with Solution 2 a "marked plus" reaction (the body of the wheal is 1 inch or more in diameter) are exquisitely sensitive and are called Class A. Class B cases are "moderate" to Solution 1, "marked" to Solution 2 and "marked plus" to Solution 3. The less sensitive Class C cases give "moderate" reactions to Solution 2 and "marked" to Solution 3. Of course these distinctions are more or less artificial, as cases have no sharp dividing line, but in general this titration of the degree of sensitiveness has practical value in deciding dosage but it is not absolute.

Prognosis.—The coryzal symptoms are satisfactorily controlled but not eliminated in from 80 to 90 per cent of all cases. It is difficult to carry a case through an entire season without some minor symptoms. One-half of the cases with pollen asthma obtain complete freedom from asthma, though some nasal symptoms occur. From 3 to 5 per cent of cases treated are complete failures.

Treatment.—*Residential.*—Patients with spring and summer types of hay fever and sensitive to pollens of trees and grasses have little chance of avoiding pollen except upon the ocean. Those with autumnal hay fever from ragweed may avoid contact in the Maine woods, the White Mountains, southern California, the Canadian provinces of New Brunswick and Nova Scotia and in Europe.

Medicinal.—Cocaine as a nasal spray will lessen the symptoms but cannot be advised except in a rare and urgent case. Epinephrin and ephedrin sprays will temporarily relieve nasal obstruction, but as a rule they do more harm than good.

Specific Treatment.—That protection may be obtained by the injection of proper pollen extracts is a well-established fact. It is not understood as yet, however, what the mechanism of protection is, for cases treated by injection are almost as reactive to the test solutions at the end of the course of injections as they were before injections were begun. Therefore it cannot be desensitization.

(*a*) *Prophylactic.*—Injections are begun six to twelve weeks before the onset of symptoms and continued at weekly intervals to and through the season. The doses are gradually increased. The reaction at the site of injection should not last over thirty-six to forty-eight hours. The scheme of dosage is given with the purchased extracts.

Shotgun mixtures of extract should not be used. The protection afforded is temporary.

(b) *Phylactic.*—When patients apply for treatment shortly before or during the season treatment may still be used with considerable benefit. After testing to determine the sensitivity and its degree, small doses may be given, at first every day, then every few days, slowly increasing the dose and the interval and continuing injections throughout the period of the attack.

(c) *Perennial Treatment.*—When injections have been increased gradually by the prophylactic method to a proper maximum for any given patient, this same dose is continued at intervals of three to four weeks throughout the year. This method, first applied to the cases of perennial hay fever and asthma with the object of producing eventually what might be called a "cure," has in the past few years been satisfactorily applied to the seasonal cases. Since pollen extracts slowly deteriorate it is wise not to use those over a year old. With this perennial treatment care must be used in changing from an old extract to the new. This can be done by beginning with a considerably reduced dose. This treatment has the advantage that it reduces the number of injections required and it affords greater protection. It is too soon to speak authoritatively regarding its ability to effect a cure but results are encouraging.

Constitutional Reactions.—These are a very real danger inherent in the method of treatment. The symptoms and the treatment are given under the section on Allergy. Some physicians have resorted to the use of epinephrin and the tourniquet for each injection. This we feel is unnecessary and unwise, for the use of epinephrin tends to inhibit the local reaction which we have reason to believe is important in the development of the protective factors which the injection seeks to stimulate. Patients should remain under observation twenty to thirty minutes after each injection.

Perennial Coryza.—(Vasomotor rhinitis.)

Definition.—Clinically, immunologically and pathologically these coryzas are identical with the seasonal type. They differ only in that they are not due to pollens and hence not characterized by seasonal periodicity. Attacks occur whenever contact is established with the specific allergen.

Etiology.—Substances causing this reaction may be grouped according to the usual channel of absorption:

1. Upper respiratory tract: pulverized and particulate air-borne substances.
    (a) Animal origin: danders of all animals and birds.
    (b) Vegetable origin: seed of all cereals, cotton and kapok, flax and castor bean, orris, pyrethrum, house dust and dust of hay and straw, molds.
2. Alimentary tract:
    (a) Food: egg, milk, chocolate, nuts, fish, shellfish, celery, asparagus, bean, buckwheat.
    (b) Drugs: aspirin, quinine, ipecac, papain, senna, iodine, morphine and essential oils as wintergreen, peppermint and rose.

The great majority of these perennial cases are caused by air-borne substances. House dust is the most common because the most ubiquitous. What the actual excitant is in this dust we do not know. Most of the contacts are made in the home from household pets, substances used in bedding and upholstered furniture and cosmetics. In other cases contact is occupational, as with cooks, bakers, millers, farmers, furriers and those in many special trades where the dust consists of organic matter.

Diagnosis.—Skin tests are carried out as previously described with extracts of the various substances mentioned. Positive tests are important only when it can be shown that contact is established with the reacting substance. For this reason the history must contain a careful list of home and occupational contacts.

Treatment.—The proper management of these cases is an avoidance of the cause. If this cannot be done, specific treatment may be used and the same principles apply as in the treatment of the seasonal cases. When injections have been increased to a point providing symptomatic freedom, the perennial treatment is indicated and usually has to be continued for from one to two years.

Infective Rhinitis.—**Synonyms.**—Vasomotor rhinitis; Hyperplastic rhinitis and sinusitis. The term "coryza" is not used as ocular symptoms are practically never present. We are speaking here only of those forms that are allergic, namely, vasomotor rhinitis and hyperplastic rhinitis and sinusitis, including polyposis.

Vasomotor rhinitis may be seen as a result of a suppurative sinusitis or it may be seen in the exacerbation of infection of a hyperplastic condition. In a recent study of these cases by Grove and the writer, we were led to conclude that they represent a true allergy for the following reasons:

1. An antecedent history of allergy is often present.

2. Other allergies are present in a large proportion (30 per cent) of all cases.

3. Histologically the tissues show edema, many round cells and eosinophil cells. The nasal discharge and blood also show many eosinophil cells, which are regarded as an allergic response.

We believe that the hyperplastic changes are solely the result of infection because:

1. The tissue cultures are quite regularly positive (90 per cent), the tissue organisms being usually different from those of the antral discharge and hence not surface contaminations.

2. Exacerbations of infection produce nasal signs and symptoms quite typical of hay fever. Autogenous tissue culture vaccine may, on injection, produce the same effect.

3. Cases with hyperplasia, though often complicated by allergies of the immediate skin-sensitive type, are certainly not always so associated. Cases of seasonal and non-seasonal coryza may exist for years without hyperplasia unless associated with complicating and recurring infections.

In short, we believe the hyperplastic conditions to be the result of infection, which takes this special form because of the peculiar constitutional allergic capacity of the individual rather than because of any quality inherent in the infecting organism.

Treatment.—The local treatment is so purely for the rhinologist that it need not be discussed here. Autogenous vaccines from tissue may be of some use, especially when asthma is associated.

REFERENCES.

COOKE, R. A.: The Treatment of Hay Fever by Active Immunization, Laryngoscope, 1915, **25**, 108.

KISTNER, F. B.: Histopathology and Bacteriology of Sinusitis, with Comments on Postoperative Repair, Arch. Otolaryngol., 1931, **13**, 225.

NOON, L.: Prophylactic Inoculation Against Hay Fever, Lancet, 1911, **1**, 1572.

OTHER ALLERGIES.

Serum Sickness.—This condition did not present itself as a real medical problem until 1890, following the discovery by Behring of diphtheria antitoxin.

Definition.—Serum sickness may be defined as an allergy characterized chiefly by an itching urticarial eruption and appearing about ten days after the parenteral injection of a foreign protein.

Incidence.—Using whole serum for diphtheria antitoxin, it was found that serum disease occurred in about 10 per cent of the cases. The later discovery and use of the refined globulin fraction did not materially decrease this percentage. With the introduction of antipneumococcus serum used in much larger volumes, often several hundred cubic centimeters, the incidence increased to 90 per cent. Age and sex have no effect upon the incidence, but the Negro and Indian are not affected as frequently as the Caucasian.

Immunology.—The injection of a foreign protein stimulates cellular activity which results in the formation of at least three demonstrable and different antibodies, namely, precipitin, skin-sensitizing and muscle-sensitizing antibodies. This is the same group of immune bodies found in the experimentally sensitized or anaphylactic animal, though in animals the skin-sensitizing bodies are not as readily produced. If the injected man be normal, no reaction follows immediately as there are no reacting bodies, but these are gradually produced during the latent or incubation period. However, when antibody has reached sufficient concentration, symptoms begin, provided the foreign protein is still available within the body. In man the symptoms of serum disease are essentially caused by the reaction or union of skin-sensitizing antibodies with antigen. The incubation period varies. In those injected for the first time it is from seven to twenty days (average ten days). In those previously injected it may be shortened to one or two days. Positive skin tests are obtained as soon as the rash has subsided, and persist for several months.

Symptoms.—The attack varies greatly in intensity and lasts from one to seven days. There is erythema, itching and urticaria and, less often, edema. Purpura is rare. Temperature occurs in about one-third of the cases. It rarely rises to 103° or 104° F. The lymph nodes may enlarge as well as the spleen. Joint manifestations with pain, tenderness, redness and swelling are not uncommon. Leukocytosis may occur, especially in children, and eosinophilia is unusual. Occasionally there are gastro-intestinal symptoms with vomiting, diarrhea and pain. Suppression of urine has been recorded, as well as cerebral symptoms of headache, stupor and edema of the optic nerve. The attack may be very distressing but is not serious. No fatalities are recorded from serum disease and there are no sequelæ. Relapses are not uncommon when whole serum has been used. The first attack is explained as due to the globulin fraction and the later one to albumin. The interval between attacks is usually several days.

Treatment.—Treatment is symptomatic and palliative. Alkaline skin lotions or weak phenol solutions may be used. Epinephrin, 0.5 to 1 cc., will give temporary relief. Ephedrin by mouth is not very effective. Morphine is rarely indicated.

Serum Shock.—Coincident with the widespread use of diphtheria antitoxin there was noted with increasing frequency the reports of serious accidents, often fatal, developing immediately after the serum injections. Hubner and Johannsen showed this was due to the serum and not its antitoxin content. In 1908 Gillette collected a number of cases from the literature and first called attention to the fact that these reactions occurred in those who had never received serum before. This was the time of the development of anaphylaxis. Space will not permit a résumé of the entire subject; we can only explain the subject in the light of our present knowledge. Man may be sensitized by foreign protein injections just as the animal may be. Serum disease is an incident in the developing sensitization of man and it persists for a variable time but is rarely permanent. If reinjected at the proper time (ten days) shock symptoms may develop according to the few careful case reports in the literature, but serum studies have not been made on these cases and whether they die from bronchial spasm (muscle-sensitizing bodies) as the guinea-pig, from edema of the bronchial mucosa (skin-sensitizing bodies) as in asthma, or from some other mechanism, we do not know, but the possibility of this typical anaphylactic shock in man must be recognized. Man also may be sensitized by such doses of serum as those contained in toxin-antitoxin mixtures, hence the recent use of toxoid for active immunization against diphtheria. But these artificially induced sensitizations are mild and temporary and are relatively unimportant, according to Park.

It is the natural, spontaneous and hereditary sensitizations, especially in cases of asthma, that have caused practically all of the serious and fatal serum accidents. As stated before, these cases give no history of previous injection and the reason for the sensitization is unknown. Most of these reactions have occurred with horse serum, but there are as many cases naturally sensitive to serum of rabbit, beef, goat and sheep, so the use of these sera will not avoid the danger of serum shock. Since serum is so frequently used, the reinjection problem is ever arising. Accidents are avoidable by a procedure applicable to all cases and for all sera.

How to Avoid Serum Shock.—1. *History.*—Before giving serum one should inquire about allergy, especially asthma and hay fever, in antecedents, sisters and brothers or children.   Personal history of previous serum or toxin-antitoxin injections should include dates, symptoms and amounts when possible, also any past or present allergies, especially asthma and hay fever.

2. *Tests.*—Tests should always be done to determine sensitization and its degree.   A positive test should make one cautious.   Preferably one should use dilutions of the serum that is to be used in therapy. Skin test, with serum in dilution of 1 to 100 and 1 to 10.   If *negative* in twenty minutes, proceed with injection but always carefully and first subcutaneously in patients with asthma.   If *positive*, do eyetest with dilutions of 1 to 100 and 1 to 10.

3. *Procedure (When Skin Tests Are Positive).*—A tourniquet, epinephrin and morphine should be at hand.   Always begin injections *subcutaneously* and in the arm so that the tourniquet may be applied. If very sensitive, begin with 0.1 cc. of 1 to 100 dilution of the antitoxin. In the absence of general reaction the injections may be repeated every fifteen to twenty minutes, increasing to 0.5 and then to 1 cc. if there is no local reaction.   Then use 1 to 10 dilution, increasing in the same way, and finally use the concentrated serum to 1 cc. subcutaneously. If this is tolerated, give *intravenously*—in very sensitive cases one one-hundredth of the last subcutaneous dose, if less sensitive one-tenth of that dose.   Such injections may be increased every twenty to thirty minutes with varying rapidity, depending on any general reaction up to the requirement of therapy.   *Intraspinous* therapy should be used only after the intravenous procedure.

4. *Treatment.*—Whenever a constitutional reaction begins epinephrin should be freely given.

It is probable that no difficulty will be experienced with those cases artificially sensitized.   In spontaneously sensitive cases with marked skin and eye test to 1 to 100 dilutions, it is probable that no effective therapeutic dose will be achieved.

Urticaria; Angioneurotic Edema.— *Urticaria* is a superficial, edematous and itching eruption of the skin.   The attack may be short or it may last for months and years, depending upon the contact with the exciting cause.   Eruptions usually come and go in spells through the day.   Dermographia and angioneurotic edema are often associated.

Angioneurotic edema is a deeper subcutaneous swelling and the skin overlying is often red, burning and itching.   This condition, described by Quincke in 1882, was considered a neurosis.   Swellings occur in any part of the body and when the glottis is involved may be serious and fatal.   The abdominal type is important, as most of these cases sooner or later are operated on for obstruction, appendicitis, volvulus or strangulated herniæ.   A careful history will usually make diagnosis possible.

Immunology.—These conditions occasionally may be an immediate reaction, in which case skin and serum antibodies are present, and skin test may discover the cause.   But in 80 to 90 per cent of all cases they are delayed reactions and skin tests are negative.   Unlike serum disease, the tests never are positive even during and shortly after the attack.

Etiology.—The possible causes are the same for both conditions. External contacts may be a cause. Our records show cases due to orris root, feathers, animal danders or saliva and the factor in house dust. Ingested substances are more important. Any food, but especially fish, shellfish, chocolate, strawberries, milk, egg, beans, nuts and cereals may be responsible. Among the drugs, aspirin, codeine, quinine, iodine, arsenic, rhubarb, coal-tar products and the barbital compounds are important. Chronic foci of infection, especially of the suppurative type, should not be overlooked in seeking for a cause.

Skin tests are of value in but a small percentage of cases. The clinical procedure of trial and error, using and withdrawing certain foods or classes of foods, especially after all unnecessary and suspicious contacts have been eliminated, will ultimately determine the offending antigen.

Treatment.—Symptomatic treatment is given under Serum Disease. Epinephrin may have no effect on angioneurotic edema. Specific treatment is rarely indicated. Causative factors should be eliminated when found. Non-specific treatment: calcium, parathyroid, viosterol, peptone and many other drugs frequently advised are of little value. Autoserotherapy has seemed to accomplish results in a few cases.

Other Allergies.—There are many other clinical expressions of allergy, a complete description of which seems hardly indicated in a text-book of this kind, they deal so strictly with the specialties of medicine. Many of the dermatoses are contact allergies, and certain lesions, such as eczema, the erythemas, pruritus, pompholyx, purpura, prurigo and lichen, may be caused by a sensitization. Certain cases of "indigestion," colitis, recurrent vomiting, epilepsy and migraine may be allergic.

The object of mentioning these conditions is to give the student an idea of the protean aspects of the allergic reactions in man, many of which today are still but superficially understood.

REFERENCES.

MACKENZIE, G. M., and HANGER, F. M.: Serum Disease and Serum Accidents, Jour. Am. Med. Assn., 1930, **94**, 260.

PARK, W. H.: Human Hypersensitiveness to Whole Horse Serum or Serum Globulins Following Diphtheria Toxin-antitoxin Injections: Its Importance, Jour. Immunol., 1924, **9**, 17.

QUINCKE, H.: Ueber akutes umschriebenes Hautödem, Monatsch. f. prakt. Dermat., 1882, **1**, 129.

VON PIRQUET, C. F., and SCHICK, B.: Die Serumkrankheit, Leipzig and Vienna, Franz Deuticke, 1905.

GENERAL REFERENCES.

COCA, A. F., WALZER, M., and THOMMEN, A. A.: Asthma and Hay Fever, Pt. I, Springfield, Ill., Charles C Thomas, 1931, 851 pp.

LONGCOPE, W. T.: The Susceptibility of Man to Foreign Proteins, Am. Jour. Med. Sci., 1916, **152**, 625.

LOW, R. C.: Anaphylaxis and Sensitization, Edinburgh, W. Green & Son., 1924, 190 pp.

RACKEMANN, F. M.: Clinical Allergy, New York, Macmillan Company, 1931, 617 pp.

ZINSSER, H.: Infection and Resistance, 3d ed., New York, Macmillan Company, 1923.

CHAPTER XXII.

DISEASES OF METABOLISM.

By RUSSELL M. WILDER, M.D.

Gout.	Obesity.
Diabetes Mellitus.	Lipomatosis.
Hyperinsulinism.	Diabetes Insipidus.
Acidosis.	Hemochromatosis.
Alkalosis.	Ochronosis.

THE chemical transformations of the combustible materials of the animal organism and its ingested food, the degradation of potential energy resulting from the reactions involved in these transformations, the exchanges of non-combustible inorganic materials, the maintenance of physiologic equilibria, these constitute metabolism.

The energy of the animal organism is derived principally from the three major food factors. The energy equivalent of these, as first determined by Rubner, approximates 4.1 large calories for each gram of protein, 4.1 for carbohydrate and 9.3 for fat. The round figures 4, 4 and 9 are equally suitable for all clinical purposes. The term which expresses the sum of the heat liberated by animal oxidations is total metabolism. Influenced mainly by the mass of the organism and the physical work performed, this consists of three components: a quota of energy required to maintain the biologic activities that continue when the organism as a whole is at rest (basal metabolism), a quota demanded for the performance of work, and one attributed to the stimulation of metabolism by food (the specific dynamic action of food). The energy exchanges involved depend on chemical reactions, which in turn are governed or regulated by catalyzers and nerves.

The subject of metabolism also deals with the receipt and expenditure of non-combustible materials. Bone continually loses calcium, phosphorus and magnesium, and replaces this loss with new supplies. Sodium, potassium, iron and other elements are constantly in flux, and the part played by these and that of protein in maintaining balances of acid and base, and other ionic relationships, is of major importance.

The diseases of metabolism are disorders of the mechanisms involved in the regulation of exchanges of energy and material and in the maintenance of physiologic equilibria. Their pathogenesis is based, in part, on disturbances of glands of internal secretion, whereby possibly the nature of catalyzers is altered or the supply of normal catalyzers is either increased or diminished to an abnormal degree, in part on deficiencies in certain nervous centers or mechanisms, in part on deficiencies or excesses of any of the food factors, including salts and vitamins, and probably also in part on such less tangible influences as heredity and constitution. An overproduction of thyroxin accel-

(984)

erates oxidative phenomena and thus elevates the rate of energy exchange; the opposing state of hypothyroidism is responsible for cretinism and myxedema. The parathyroid glands play a very important if not a dominant part in the metabolism of calcium and phosphorus; the islet mechanism of the pancreas furnishes a substance, insulin, that is necessary for the utilization of carbohydrates. Functional disturbances and actual lesions of the subthalamic regions of the brain underlie cases of diabetes insipidus and obesity, and the influence of heredity is everywhere in evidence.

The present chapter covers only a part of this large field, with major emphasis on diabetes, obesity and gout, whereas the diseases of all organs of internal secretion, except the pancreas, receive separate consideration under "Diseases of the Endocrine Glands," and deficiency diseases are considered in yet another section. This classification is purely a matter of convenience. The characteristic feature of disease of metabolism is disturbance of regulation in processes of growth and maintenance.

GOUT.

Synonym.—Podagra.

Definition.—Gout is a disease of unknown etiology, characterized by abnormal metabolism of purines, whereby the uric acid content of the tissue fluids is eventually elevated. At variable stages, usually late, salts of uric acid are deposited as tophi in particularly affected parts of the body. It is generally a recurring affection, with complete remissions at first, and successive exacerbations of swollen, painful, excruciatingly tender joints, accompanied by fever and general malaise; it may ultimately lead to chronic arthritis.

History.—Gout was known to the ancients of Egypt and Greece. It is not clear that any sharp distinction was made by them between it and other varieties of arthritis. Hippocrates mentioned the paroxysmal attacks in his aphorisms, and Galen gave a clear description of gouty tophi. Sydenham (1624–1689), whom Garrod later called the Hippocrates of English medicine, was the first to distinguish sharply between gout and other rheumatic affections, and his studies combined with those of Garrod, two centuries later, form the basis of our present conception of this disease. Wollaston, in 1787, found that the "chalk stones," tophi, of gout were composed of urates, and Garrod that the blood in gout contained an excess of uric acid.

Incidence.—The incidence of gout has varied tremendously in different countries and in different times. The disease was common in Rome at the height of her power and is rare today in Italy. Like diabetes, it almost disappeared in Germany during the period of privation of the World War and its immediate aftermath. It has always prevailed in England and is said to be less common in America. It is probable that more discriminating search would reveal many more instances of it than are commonly recorded. Thus, of 100 cases of gout reported recently by Hench, only 12 were recognized before the admission of the patients to the Mayo Clinic, although in the large majority characteristic symptoms had been present for years and tophi were found in 44. In the last three years, 250 new cases have been seen, representing an incidence of about 2 per 1000 of all new registrations.

Pathologic Physiology.—Contemporary opinion places abnormal purine metabolism in a secondary position in the etiology of gout, a result rather than a cause. It is nevertheless so prominent a feature that no description of gout can be complete that fails to give special consideration to the possible sources of the accumulations of uric acid that characterize the affection.

Urates are formed in the normal catabolism of the complex proteins of cell nuclei. These proteins, called nucleins, were isolated from pus by Miescher, a pupil of Hoppe-Seyler. They consist of nucleic acid combined with protein. The hydrolytic products of nucleic acid were identified by Kossel and his pupils as phosphoric acid, sugar and pyrimidine and purine bases. The significance of the pyrimidines is still completely obscure. The purines, adenine and guanine, undergo deaminization and oxidation to hypoxanthine and xanthine, respectively, and from these in turn, by further oxidation, comes·uric acid, $C_5N_4H_4O_3$. The hydrolyses and oxidations are performed in the liver by virtue of specific ferments.

The older investigators, using Garrod's primitive analytic methods, could find no uric acid in the blood except in gout, but modern technics reveal from 2 to 4 mg. for each 100 cc. The content of muscles is about the same as that of the blood; that of the parenchymatous organs, namely, the liver, spleen, thymus and pancreas, from three to four times as great. The total content of the tissues of a normal human body has been determined to be something less than 1.5 grams, of which one-half is in the muscles (Gudzent). Similar data for bodies of patients with gout seem not to be available, but the combined weight of the tophi removed from a single patient was 245 grams, and the blood often gives from two to three or four times the minimal normal values for uric acid.

Etiology.—The accumulation of urate in gout is susceptible of explanation either by excessive production of uric acid or by delay in the rate of its destruction or excretion. The theory of excessive production has been pretty generally discarded, because accumulation of the uric acid in patients with gout was never found to be associated with increased excretion or accumulation of phosphates, such as would be demanded by accelerated destruction of nuclear proteins. On the other hand, the possibility of some source of uric acid other than nucleoprotein has not been excluded. It is significant, in this connection, that the uric acid of the excreta of birds and reptiles is mainly derived by synthesis in the liver from urea and lactic acid. Were some such synthesis possible in man, urates would accumulate without accompanying phosphates. This probably is incapable of demonstration, but it is conceivable that certain persons with gout possess some such primordial metabolism somewhat as a vestigial characteristic or throw-back.

Mammalia, with the exception of the higher primates, possess the power of converting uric acid into allantoin and 90 per cent or more of their purine excretion is in the form of allantoin. The advantage of this is the much greater solubility of allantoin. Uric acid is extremely insoluble. Man, inasmuch as he is handicapped in this respect, may be regarded as always potentially gouty. Recent investigations of Folin, Berglund and Derick seem to indicate that uric acid is destroyed in man by some other means than by conversion to allantoin. When uric acid was injected by vein it rapidly disappeared from the blood; none of it was found in the tissues, with the exception of the kidneys, and only 50 per cent appeared in the urine. Also, when purines were fed, only 25 or 50 per cent could be recovered in the urine. These experiments are technically above reproach, but their interpretation is confused by the fact that purines in the intestinal tract are rapidly destroyed by bacterial action so that there is no way of determining how much ingested purine is absorbed or, in the case of parenteral administration of uric acid, how much may have been excreted into the bowel and there disintegrated. The possibility that man, as a species, is especially predisposed to gout because of the lack of specific uricolytic ferment is thus still a matter of conjecture.

The uric acid of the urine of normal persons who are on a diet free of purine (endogenous purine metabolism) is from 0.3 to 0.6 gram a day; in gout it is often lower. Thus, some retention may occur. This is usually true only in cases in which there is accompanying renal injury.

Heredity.—Garrod stated that the incidence of heredity in gout was 50 per cent; Gudzent's estimate is 33 per cent, and many French authors place it as high as 90 to 100 per cent. Williamson, however, found gouty antecedents in only 12 per cent of his patients, and the experience at the Mayo Clinic indicates that it is very unusual to elicit a history of gout in the parents or relatives of the patient. If both parents are affected, the most rigorous dietetic and hygienic measures will not prevent the appearance of gout in the offspring (Braun and Lecorche). The rather frequent association in the same families of gout, obesity and diabetes is of conjectural significance.

Age and Sex.—Gout is a disease of all ages, from infancy to senility. It is rare, however, before the third decade of life and most common in the fourth and fifth decades. Men are much more frequently affected than women. In our experience, less than 3 per cent of all cases affected are women.

Meat and Drink.—Next in importance etiologically is food and drink. Gout has been considered to be a disease of the affluent and self-indulgent, affecting especially heavy meat eaters and those who partake freely of the stronger alcoholic beverages. This is not always the case. Many gouty patients are frugal eaters. "Poor man's gout" is said to occur among heavy beer drinkers. The majority of the patients with gout seen in the Mayo Clinic had never indulged in alcohol of any kind. The greater prevalence of gout in men has been attributed to their indulging, more than women, in alcoholic drink—an unlikely explanation for our cases. However, certain wines such as port, Burgundy and champagne are especially likely to precipitate the paroxysmal attacks of the disease.

Lead.—The part played by lead, mentioned in all the older literature in England, seems to be of little importance in the gout met with in Germany and America (Minkowski, Grafe, Pratt).

Pathology.—The most significant feature of gout is the tophus, originally described by Galen. Tophi are rare at the time of the initial attack, but usually develop in the subsequent course of the disease. They are knotty swellings of varying dimensions, occasionally attaining the size of masses 4 cm. in diameter. They occur by predilection in the cartilages of the ear, the olecranon and prepatellar bursæ, and in joints, and may develop insidiously without pain or rapidly, with evidence of acute inflammation at the time of a paroxysm. They sometimes produce pressure necrosis of the overlying skin, with resulting rupture and discharge of their content; chronic fistulas thus result.

The content of a tophus is a white, chalky, crumbly, or milky mass, which, with the microscope, is seen to be crystalline. A chemical analysis of Marchand (quoted by Grafe) gave the following percentages:

Sodium urate	34.20	Sodium chloride	14.12
Calcium urate	2.12	Organic substances	35.53
Ammonium carbonate	7.86	Water	6.80

In older tophi the urates may be largely replaced by carbonates, but so-called calcium gout, a rare condition of metastatic calcification, bears no relationship to uric acid gout.

Less characteristic than the tophi are the joint changes in chronic gout. They cause, as a rule, surprisingly little disability in the intervals between paroxysms, but are nevertheless difficult to distinguish clinically from those of other forms of chronic arthritis. A feature in favor of gout is asymmetrical distribution of lesions. In doubtful cases, puncture of a swollen joint may reveal urates, but of greater value diagnostically is a roentgenogram. The gouty process first involves the cartilages of the joint, but later advances into the ends of the bone, where necrosis occurs with replacement by urates. Such portions, actually tophi, appear rarefied on roentgenogram and, as their edges are smooth, have the appearance of being made by a curet or punch (punched-out areas). They are large enough at times to resemble cysts, with the bone actually bulging around them. This picture, if well developed, is very diagnostic, but it appears usually only in cases of long standing, and interpretation may be confused by the smaller, less regular rarefied areas which are seen at times in deforming arthritis from other causes.

Symptoms.—Premonitory symptoms of acute gout, such as malaise, depression and indigestion, usually precede the attack by a day or two. They are followed by pain in a joint which develops rapidly and which often starts in the night. The metatarso-phalangeal joint of the great toe is involved in the majority of cases, hence the name "podagra." After it, in decreasing frequency, come the other joints of the foot, the knee, the joints of the hand, the shoulder, the vertebræ, or others. The rule is for one joint only to be involved, but polyarticular attacks occur, or the inflammation in one joint having subsided, another may be involved. The tissues surrounding the affected joint are hot and swollen, deep bluish-red, and excruciatingly tender. The overlying veins are distended and tortuous. Chilling, moderate fever, and a slight leukocytosis accompany the attack as well as subjective disturbances such as exhaustion, irritability, headache, anorexia, thirst and constipation. The classical attack is of short duration. After two or three days of severe inflammation the process gradually subsides, and clears up completely within one or two weeks, leaving no discomfort or residual abnormality.

A single episode, as described, may be the only manifestation of the disease, but in chronic gout the rule is that successive attacks follow each other at shorter or longer intervals, of weeks, months, or even years, with complete remissions at first between attacks but leading ultimately to chronic disturbances, tophi, gouty arthritis, nephritis and the other complications mentioned later. In some cases the paroxysmal attacks are rare and very mild, and the disease escapes recognition until the chronic abnormalities develop.

Complications.—Chronic nephritis accompanies almost all cases of chronic gout. Deposits of urates are sometimes found in necrotic portions of these kidneys, and renal stone is a rather frequent occurrence. Arteriosclerosis and hypertension are very common. Gudzent reported atheromatosis of the larger vessels in 100 per cent of 78 cases, in which necropsy was performed. Gout is not infrequently seen in combination with bronchial asthma, and some authorities regard it as an allergic disease. No definite conclusions as to this are as yet permissible. The same may be said of the so-called gastro-intestinal equivalents. The liver has been thought to be peculiarly involved in the disease. It is often moderately enlarged and tender, but reveals, on examination, no specifically characteristic abnormality. In the central nervous system there is nothing unusual, although migraine, depression and various types of neurosis and psychosis are prevalent in the gouty. A uric acid center in the upper part of the medulla oblongata, irritation of which leads to hyperuricemia and uraturia, is reported by Brugsch. Chronic lesions of the eyes, iritis, scleritis and conjunctivitis, were noted by Garrod, who ascribed them to deposits of urates. Deposits can actually be seen in the cornea, appearing with the slit-lamp as fine crystals. Eczematous abnormalities of the skin, which respond favorably to treatment of gout, are common in the gouty. They have been attributed to the increased concentration of uric acid in the sweat (Adler).

Diagnosis.—Classical gout, with periodic swelling and pain of the great toe, is hardly to be confused with any other disease, but when another joint is the one affected, or if no history of previous attacks is available, the examiner may be placed in doubt. Acute suppurative inflammations of joints are usually associated with lymphangitis and lymphadenitis, but distinction here may be difficult, and may have to await response to treatment. Acute rheumatic fever is, as a rule, a polyarticular affection of the young, and gout a monoarticular affection of the middle aged, but monoarticular rheumatism is not uncommon, and gout may be polyarticular. The association of endocarditis in a case of recurring arthritis speaks for rheumatism; associated nephritis or renal stones for gout. Acute infectious arthritis rarely subsides without leaving joint residues, even after the first attack, whereas a characteristic of gout is to subside without leaving such residues

(Hench, *et al.*).   Metastatic arthritis in gonorrhea, pneumonia and other infections must be excluded.   In doubtful cases treatment with the tincture or other preparations of colchicum may be enlightening. The response of gout to colchicum is usually promptly satisfactory, whereas the effect of this drug in other articular affections is slight.

The diagnostic value of the determination of uric acid in the blood has been disappointing.   Occasionally individuals in apparent health give relatively elevated values for uric acid (4 to 5.5 mg. in each 100 cc.), whereas in 28 per cent of 100 proved cases of gout, normal values were obtained.   Also high values for uric acid are to be expected in leukemia, pneumonia and nephritis.   The blood plasma and not the whole blood should be examined, or Folin's newer whole blood filtrate in which the corpuscles are prevented from laking.   Substances in the corpuscles react with phosphomolybdate, to intensify the blue color produced by uric acid.

The frequency of the various forms of arthritis deformans, and the infrequency of true, chronic gout, make gout a less likely diagnosis in most cases of chronic arthritis.   However, in clinics devoted to arthritic affections, where more discriminating diagnosis prevails, the incidence of gout may run as high as 5 or 7 per cent of all patients with joint disease.   The diagnosis must depend, to a large extent, on a history of previous acute attacks, and the completeness of early remissions. The punched-out defects of the bones, visible roentgenologically, are very significant, but appear too infrequently, in early cases, to be very helpful.   Identification of tophi is not complete without microscopic or chemical analysis of their content.

Treatment.—*Prophylactic.*—A patient who has had one attack of gout, or one with a family history of the disease, should lead an abstemious life in the matter of food and alcoholic drink.   He should scrupulously avoid obesity, and be cautious of indulgence in meats rich in purines, such as liver and sweetbreads.   Regular exercise is desirable, but fatigue, either physical or nervous, is provocative of attacks.

Drugs.—The treatment of the acute attack demands immobilization of the affected joint.   If the patient has fever, rest in bed is indicated; otherwise, rest in a reclining chair, with suitable elevation and protection of the joint.   Packing in cotton wool, and either hot or cold applications, are used.   A hypodermic injection of morphine is often necessary for immediate relief of pain.   The specific remedies are two: colchicum and cinchophen.   Their derivatives, also, are used.   The former is a time-honored drug.   Its active principle, the alkaloid colchicine, is given in doses of 1 mg. four or five times for the first day or two, less frequently thereafter.   It is highly toxic in larger doses.   The official tincture of colchicum is used in a dose of 2 cc. (30 min.) three or four times daily.   Cinchophen (trade name, atophan) has recently been replaced by neocinchophen (trade name, tolysin) which is better tolerated and thought to be less toxic.   A few cases of atrophy of the liver have resulted from injudicious use of cinchophen, and one has been reported as resulting from the use of neocinchophen.   The benefit from these substances is two-fold; they produce analgesia, and in addition they increase renal excretion of uric acid.   The effect on excretion is short-lived, even when large doses are used, but if an interval of a few days is allowed to elapse the effect is again evident. In view of this peculiarity, it is customary, in the treatment of chronic gout, to give neocinchophen in doses of 1 gram (15 grains) three or four times daily for one or two days of the week, and tincture of colchicum for the remaining five days if necessary because of pain, repeating this practice week by week as seems expedient, but only under continuous supervision. Weintraud advised, wisely, that administration of cinchophen be accompanied by administration of alkali to prevent possible deposition of urates in acid urine in the stage of their increased excretion. He suggested 15 grams of sodium bicarbonate on the first day and 5 to 10 grams on succeeding days. It is also advantageous to insist on the patient taking 10 or 12 glasses of water daily. That the use of preparations of cinchophen and neocinchophen is attended with great danger is shown by Weir and Comfort, who have collected 117 cases of toxic cirrhosis with 61 deaths attributed to doses ranging from 54 grains (3.6 grams) given in five weeks to 7200 grains (480 grams) given in four months. When one of these or any drug containing the quinoline radical is used it should be given intermittently. A full diet rich in carbohydrate should be a part of the treatment, and administration of the drug should be stopped at the first signs of toxicity, such as anorexia, nausea, weakness, vomiting, malaise, pruritus or urticaria.

Diet.—Regulation of the diet is of primary importance. Obesity is to be combated, and the intake of purines must be rigidly restricted. This mainly involves the forbidding of meats, fish, fowl, beans, peas, lentils, mushrooms and such gravies and sauces as contain the juices or extracts of meats. Eggs, milk, cheese, butter, lard and all of the cereals, green vegetables and fruits are permissible. Tea, coffee and cocoa contain small amounts of methylated purines which are not formers of uric acid. These beverages are therefore allowed. Alcoholic beverages of all kinds are interdicted.

The mineral waters of the various European spas are reputed to be especially effective in the treatment of gout, but scientifically valid evidence has never been submitted to indicate that any of them possess uricolytic or other unusual properties.

REFERENCES.

Folin, O., Berglund, H., and Derick, C.: The Uric Acid Problem, Jour. Biol. Chem., 1924, **60**, 361.

Grafe, E.: Die Krankheiten des Stoffwechsels und ihre Behandlung, Berlin, Julius Springer, 1931, 519 pp.

Gudzent, F.: Gicht und Rheumatismus, Berlin, Julius Springer, 1928, 189 pp.

Hench, P. S., Vanzant, F. R., and Monland, Ruben: Basis for Early Differential Diagnosis of Gout; Clinic Comparison of 100 Cases Each of Gout, Rheumatic Fever and Infectious Arthritis, Trans. Assn. Am. Phys., 1928, **43**, 217.

Llewellyn, R. L. J.: Gout, with a Section on Ocular Disease in the Gouty, by W. M. Beaumont, St. Louis, C. V. Mosby & Co., 1921, 469 pp.

Pratt, J. H.: Gout, Nelson Loose Leaf Medicine, 1923, **3**, 37.

DIABETES MELLITUS.

Definition.—Diabetes mellitus is a primary disorder of carbohydrate metabolism the result of inadequacy in the supply of the pancreatic hormone, insulin. It is characterized by diminished capacity to utilize glucose, diminished stores of glycogen of the liver, excessive accumulation of glucose in the blood and the presence of glucose in the urine. Severe untreated cases are inevitably complicated by ketosis and acidosis.

History.—The disease was well known to the ancients, although not clearly distinguished by them from diabetes insipidus. Its name implies reference to a characteristic clinical symptom, namely, polyuria. The saccharine taste of urine of diabetic patients was described by Thomas Willis (1621–1675). The reducing power of the urine and the attributing of this to a fermentable sugar were the contributions of Dobson (1775). The polarimetric method for determining sugar was discovered by Biot (1833) and the first quantitative copper reduction method, that of Fehling, came in 1850.

Modern conceptions of the disease are mainly based on the discovery of the glycogen function of the liver by Claude Bernard (1848), the discovery that diabetes is provoked in dogs and certain other animals by ablation of the pancreas by von Mehring and Minkowski (1889), the important studies on acidosis of the Naunyn school, the elucidation of the metabolism of protein, fat and carbohydrate by C. Voit and his pupils, among whom the most distinguished were Rubner, Magnus Levy, F. Müller and Graham Lusk, and the discovery of insulin by Banting, Best, Collip and Macleod.

Incidence.—The records of ten years in the Mayo Clinic reveal the presence of diabetes in 1 of every 96 new patients registering, or an incidence of 1.04 per cent. Joslin estimated that 2 per cent of the entire population has diabetes. Mortality statistics indicate that deaths from the disease are on the increase, and that even the introduction of insulin has had little effect in reducing mortality except among the younger patients. This is attributable in large part to inadequate treatment, but is also accounted for by an increased longevity of the population as a whole, whereby a considerably greater number of persons attain an age when the liability to degenerative disorders, including diabetes, is high. The incidence in the United States is greater than that in England or the continent of Europe, and much greater than that in Japan. That this is due to the relative affluence of these respective countries is inferred from the fact that the death-rate from diabetes declined appreciably during the years of war to return to prewar and higher levels afterward.

The age incidence varies slightly with statistics from different sources. In general, however, the disease is less common among children and young adults, and is most common in the fifth and sixth decades. Recent statistics reveal a rapidly increasing incidence of diabetes in the decades after the fourth, especially in women.

Etiology.—Some anatomic abnormality can frequently be found in the islands of Langerhans of elderly subjects, but this is usually not true among children and young adults and in many such cases recourse must be had to the conception of inherited predisposition or inferiority in order to explain the functional inadequacy of the pancreas noted.

Heredity.—That heredity plays a prominent part is strongly suggested by a number of facts: (1) all the more recent observers report diabetes in the families of from 20 to 25 per cent of their cases, a valuation which is unquestionably minimal; (2) when inquiry as to heredity is extended to cover other endocrine and metabolic conditions the figures double and, as von Noorden has suggested, an inheritance of metabolic inferiority might well be expected to strike at one organ in one individual and at another in his next of kin; (3) a striking predilection for diabetes exists in certain inborn groups or races, such as the Jews and high caste Hindus; this is inadequately explained by habits of eating, or by physical indolence, and (4) in cases of uniovular or identical twins the appearance of diabetes in one is followed by its development in the other.

Given the inferiority or predilection the disease will manifest itself or remain dormant, depending on the intensity of the heredity and the severity of the metabolic overload or strain. When it develops in childhood it is usually of great intensity; in adult life it is generally characterized by mildness and chronicity.

Obesity.—Obesity is regarded by many authorities as significant in the etiology of diabetes, but to my mind it is clearly a secondary factor, a metabolic strain which will promote the development of diabetes in predisposed persons, but is without much influence in the absence of predisposition. Also obesity is itself a disease with a pronounced hereditary or constitutional background and its frequent association with diabetes is rather to be expected on that score alone. This skepticism of the significance in diabetes of obesity *per se* is not to be interpreted as a denial of the significance of overeating as a provocative cause of diabetes or as disparaging the attempt to limit the growing incidence of diabetes by the campaign directed at obesity. The remarkable decline in the mortality from diabetes of the years of enforced moderation exacted by the World War is encouragement of the belief that more sensible eating habits would prevent many cases.

Infectious Diseases.—There is no conclusive evidence that infections play a strong part in precipitating diabetes. Some cases follow closely after infectious diseases and in them such an influence may have been exerted, but the incidence of this is not more than 15 per cent, which is all the more surprising in view of the injurious consequence of infections in existing diabetes. Mumps sometimes causes pancreatitis accompanied by glycosuria, but this usually disappears when the disease has run its course. It is believed by many, from the rather high coincidence of diabetes and gall stones, that chronic infections of the biliary tract, involving the pancreatic duct, lower the functional capacity of the islets and lead to diabetes among persons who are predisposed thereto by heredity.

Nervous Affections.—The famous piqûre experiment of Claude Bernard, whereby injury to the floor of the fourth ventricle was shown to provoke glycosuria when glycogen reserves of the liver were adequate, clarifies the significance of the diabetic conditions that happen clinically with fractures of the skull and tumors of the brain. The glycosuria in almost all cerebral cases is transitory, probably dependent on

63

adequate stores of glycogen, and is therefore not the equivalent of diabetes mellitus. That emotional strain or nervous shock will aggravate existing diabetes is well known, but that much true diabetes is initiated by such nervous influences is made unlikely by the experiences of the World War. All authorities are agreed that the incidence of diabetes was very much less among the soldiers than among the civil population of comparable age, despite the exposure of the former to emotional strain of the most violent kind.

Hypophysis.—The rôle of the hypophysis in diabetes has been the subject of much recent study. The incidence of diabetes is high in acromegaly and among the hormones separated from extracts of the anterior lobe of the hypophysis is one which is reputed to possess diabetogenic activity. Hypophysectomized dogs have been depancreated without the production of diabetes, and such animals develop an intense glycosuria when injected with the diabetogenic hypophyseal hormone. Such observations strongly suggest a regulatory influence of the hypophysis in carbohydrate metabolism, but the work is quite new and its interpretation at present is hazardous.

Suprarenal.—That injection of epinephrin provokes glycosuria has long been known. Patients with Addison's disease (hypo-suprarenalism) may have abnormally low blood-sugar levels and an increased tolerance for glucose injected by vein, while those suffering with the suprareno-cortical syndrome (hyper-suprarenalism) frequently have diabetes either frankly or mildly.

Thyroid.—The incidence of frank diabetes in patients with hyperthyroidism is not very high, although when hyperthyroidism develops in a patient previously diabetic it invariably intensifies the pre-existing disturbance. Writers of authority have assumed that the thyroid secretion inhibited the pancreas. Other explanations are more probable. It may be that hyperthyroidism effects a conditioning of the liver so that more insulin is required to stabilize the hepatic glycogen. Or possibly the accelerated combustion that results from hyperthyroidism produces a more rapid decay (combustion) of what insulin is provided.

Pathology.—Primary abnormalities are to be looked for in the pancreas but these are so trivial, in most cases, that were it not for von Mehring and Minkowski's experiment and Banting's subsequent discovery, we would still be disputing whether the pancreas had anything to do with diabetes. Macroscopically, some atrophy is noticeable in many cases, but this is not so marked that the size of the organ falls below that rather wide range of the weight of the normal pancreas. Microscopically, one may find nothing abnormal and in the severest cases of the disease in children this is particularly likely to be the case. Otherwise the lesions, although more common in diabetes, are such as may be found in the pancreas of persons without diabetes. They include lymphocytic infiltration, interacinar and interlobar pancreatitis, sclerosis of the islands of Langerhans, hyaline degeneration of the islands, and fatty degeneration of acinar and island parenchyma. An exception is the so-called hydropic degeneration of the islands of Langerhans which is a specifically diabetic abnormality, a vacuolization of the cells associated with pyknosis of their nuclei, leading to complete dissolution of structure, and ultimately to disappearance of entire islets. The process is not associated with inflammatory reaction and the vanished cells do not leave scar tissue to mark their previous situation. The lesion results from functional overstrain, as shown by Allen, and in its earlier stages is reversible. It is a result of diabetes rather than a primary affection.

The insulin-producing cell of the normal islands is the *beta* cell, which contains granules with specific staining properties. Evidence for this existed in the paucity of such granules in diabetes; proof of it came with the recognition by Bensley that islet tumors causing spontaneous hyperinsulinism are composed of cells with this specific granulation (see Hyperinsulinism, p. 1011).

Of less importance in the genesis of diabetes, but significant diagnostically, are the glycogen deposits in the kidneys, especially in the epithelial cells of the loops of Henle. Also of special interest are those rare cases of hemochromatosis, in which condition the deposit of hemosiderin and other pigments of the blood causes extensive cirrhosis of the pancreas and thus leads to diabetes (see Hemochromatosis, p. 1024).

Pathologic Physiology.—Tolerance.—Since the primary abnormality of diabetes is a diminished capacity to utilize glucose, a quantitative measurement of the intensity of the condition can only be obtained by comparative observation of rates of supply and disposal of this sugar. The sources of supply are two: an exogenous inflow from the intestinal tract, which originates in the carbohydrates of the food, or is made in the liver from amino-acids of alimentary origin, and an endogenous portion manufactured in the liver from amino-acids derived from the breakdown of the proteins of the tissues. The glycerol fraction of fat, a relatively small item, is conventionally included in such estimates. The possibility of a source of sugar in the fatty acid fraction of fat, either the fat of food or endogenous fat, is undecided but improbable.

The disposal of glucose occurs by storage as glycogen, in the liver, muscle and other tissue, by reduction to fat and storage as such, or by oxidation, and so great is the tolerance of the normal organism that the entire supply is utilized even when abnormally large amounts of sugars are taken by mouth. The urine in health contains some glucose (S. R. Benedict) and the amount of this is increased after meals containing carbohydrate, but these quantities are so minute as to require microchemic methods for their detection and do not affect the present thesis. In the diabetic condition glucose accumulates in the blood stream (hyperglycemia) and is excreted by the kidneys in relatively large quantities (glycosuria). The amount in grams utilized in a given period (the tolerance) is the difference between grams of supply and grams excreted. Accurately to measure supply one must have the following data: the gram weights of carbohydrate and fat of the food, and the grams of nitrogen in the twenty-four hour collection of urine. The glucose in the first is readily calculated on the assumption that all of the carbohydrate and one-tenth by weight of the fat is converted into sugar. The glucose from protein (exogenous and endogenous) is determined from the nitrogen found in the urine; each gram of nitrogen represents 3.65 grams of glucose. In case great loss of weight has not occurred it is reasonably safe to assume that the patient is in nitrogen balance; the determination of urinary nitrogen may then be dispensed with and the supply of glucose estimated from the food by Woodyatt's formula $G = C + 0.58P + 0.10F$. G represents grams of glucose; C, grams of carbohydrate; P, grams of protein, and F, grams of fat in the food. Subtraction of the grams of sugar in the urine or output from the grams supplied gives a measure of tolerance for twenty-four hours. This may be reasonably good, 200 or 300 grams a day, or very poor, depending on the intensity of the disease. In case of complete diabetes the urine contains all the exogenous and metabolic glucose supplied.

D/N Ratio.—By dextrose-nitrogen ratio is meant the proportion of glucose to nitrogen in the urine. In the presence of complete diabetes of man, when carbohydrate is not taken as food, and stores of glycogen in the liver are exhausted, 3.65 grams of glucose appear in the urine for each gram of nitrogen (D/N ratio 3.65). In experimental diabetes produced by phlorizin poisoning the same proportions prevail. In pancreatectomized dogs the ratio is 2.8/1. These are average figures but the variations are not great and the phenomenon is the basis for the assumption that 58 per cent of protein metabolized is converted into glucose (1 gram of nitrogen represents 6.25 grams of protein; 3.65 grams of sugar is 58 per cent of 6.25).

Lusk termed the dextrose-nitrogen ratio of 3.65 the "fatal ratio," but it has been observed in a number of cases, with subsequent recovery of more or less tolerance and prolongation of life. Tolerance fluctuates considerably in all cases of diabetes and patients with a moderately intense form of the disease are probably rendered completely diabetic by any severe infection. In the pre-insulin era such infections were usually fatal; now that tolerance can be raised by injecting commercial insulin the danger of low dextrose-nitrogen ratios is avoided.

Total Metabolism and Respiratory Quotient.—The basal metabolic rate in diabetes falls, as a rule, within the physiologic range of plus or minus 15 per cent of the normal standard. Low rates were common in the days of treatment by fasting and subnutrition, while relatively high rates were sometimes seen in cases with severe acidosis, when as a result of rapid emaciation an unusually large amount of protein was being catabolized. The amount of nitrogen in the urine sometimes reached 20 or 30 grams a day. The condition was termed azoturia.

The respiratory quotient in the intensely diabetic state is instructively low. This quotient is obtained by dividing the liters of carbon dioxide in the expiration of a given period by the liters of oxygen absorbed (CO_2/O_2). Suitable corrections are made for the original carbon dioxide content of the inspired air, for temperature, barometric pressure, and so forth. If the metabolism consists exclusively of carbohydrate, the respiratory quotient (R. Q.) is unity, as is evident from the equation $C_6H_{12}O_6 + 6O_2$ is $6H_2O + 6CO_2$. For each molecule of O_2 absorbed one of CO_2 is formed, and since the molecules of all gases occupy the same volume, or exert the same pressures, the two volumes, that of CO_2 and that of O_2 are equal. The quotient in the case of fat is 0.70, indicating relatively more oxygen taken from the air for combustion; that of protein gives an intermediate value of about 0.80. The amount of protein in a metabolizing mixture of combustibles can be determined separately from the knowledge of the amount of nitrogen in the urine of the period of observation and with this information at hand a correction can be made for protein to give a so-called non-protein respiratory quotient. From the value of the latter, one obtains, with tables prepared by Zuntz, a close estimate of what proportion of the metabolism is coming from the burning of carbohydrate and what is due to fat. The non-protein respiratory quotient of normal persons, on a mixed diet, is between 0.80 and 0.90 after a fourteen-to sixteen-hour fast, but in diabetes, depending on the severity of the disease, it is lower; in severe diabetes it is close to that of pure fat, 0.70 and no amount of carbohydrate added to the food will raise it. This is interpreted as indicating the inability of the diabetic organism to oxidize glucose, and although some doubt is still attached to the validity of this interpretation, it has thus far withstood all assaults. The theory of Geelmuyden, von Voorden, Macleod and others, that diabetes is due rather to the production of sugar from fatty acids than to inability of the organism to oxidize sugar meets serious opposition on the score of observed respiratory quotients. The oxygen content of the glucose molecule is considerably greater than that of fatty acids, as is evident from their respective formulas ($C_6H_{12}O_6$, glucose; $C_{17}H_{33}$-COOH, stearic acid) and if sugar formed from fat were excreted in the urine, as the theories of neoglucogenesis demand, the respiratory quotient would fall below 0.70. This is not encountered. Quotients of 0.67 and 0.68 do occur, but such relatively slight lowering can be explained by the formation and excretion of aceto-acetic and betahydroxybutyric acid.

Specific Dynamic Action.—The metabolic stimulation of foods, greatest in the case of protein or amino-acids, least in that of fat, is not different in the diabetic organism from that observed in the non-diabetic organism. It is of unusual interest that the amino-acid alanin, although quantitatively converted to glucose and excreted as such, continues to behave as a specific dynamic agent. Equally interesting is the fact that, when glucose is given by mouth or vein to a totally diabetic animal, it raises the metabolic rate although its excretion may be nearly quantitative and its effect on the respiratory quotient nil.

Ketogenesis.—"The fats burn in the fire of the carbohydrate." This classic statement of Rosenfeld refers to the fact that the metabolism of fatty acids is imperfectly performed if the organism is insufficiently supplied with carbohydrate or, as in diabetes, is unable to utilize what it has. The fats in metabolism are first hydrolized (saponified) thus freeing long chains of carbon atoms, fatty acids which, according to Knoop's theory of beta oxidation, are then attacked at their beta carbons and disintegrated, two links at a time, until they reach the four-carbon-link stage of butyric acid ($CH_3.CH_2.CH_2.COOH$). The process thus far is unaltered in diabetes, but now oxidizing glucose, or it may be the presence of sufficient glycogen, is necessary for the continuation of oxidation and, in diabetes, incompletely oxidized derivatives of butyric acid accumulate like soot from a smoking lamp chimney (Woodyatt). The derivatives aceto-acetic acid ($CH_3.CO.CH_2.COOH$) betahydroxybutyric acid ($CH_3.CHOH.CH_2.COOH$) and acetone ($CH_3.CO.CH_3$) are excreted in the urine. Acetone to some extent passes into the expired air and imparts a characteristic fruity odor to the breath. These three substances are referred to collectively as the *ketone bodies;* their formation is termed *ketogenesis* and the state of their existence *ketosis*.

The degree of ketosis seems to bear a quantitative relationship to the deficiency of carbohydrate. Work of Shaffer and others indicates that the utilization of 2 molecules of fatty acid demands 1 molecule of glucose and experiments indicate that, when these proportions are exceeded, the excess of fat may be quantitatively recovered as ketone. In terms of grams of fat and carbohydrate the proportions are about 4 of the former to 1 of the latter. Protein contains amino-acids that are ketogenic and others, such as glycine and alanin, that are converted to glucose and thus become ketolytic. The latter predominate so that in health a diet of fat and protein will yield sufficient glucose to prevent extreme grades of ketosis. If one is desirous of producing ketosis for therapeutic purposes, as in epilepsy, it becomes necessary to reduce the carbohydrate allowance with extreme rigidity (to not more than 10 or 20 grams). Thus there is no need for concern on the score of dietary ketosis with diets which contain at least 50 or 60 grams of carbohydrate. This statement applies without respect to the fat content of such diets, provided sugar is not escaping in the urine. In severe diabetes, when not only glucose from the starches and sugars from food, but also that derived from protein is lost, there remains nothing to prevent wholesale conversion of fat to ketone, and the formation of enormous quantities of aceto-acetic and betahydroxybutyric acids. The accumulation of these throws a strain of the severest kind on acid-base regulation, with resulting uncompensated acidosis (see Acidosis, p. 1012).

Blood Sugar.—The average blood sugar, in normal individuals, after a fast of fourteen to sixteen hours, ranges from 80 to 120 mg. for each 100 cc. Most of the reducing power is due to glucose, but a fraction results from non-fermenting material. Methods which avoid or minimize the non-fermenting fraction, as is true in the case of latest Folin technic, give lower values with a range from 60 to 100. A normal rise of from 30 to 40 mg. occurs after meals, but so long as this does not exceed the so-called threshold value there is no significant outflow through the kidneys. The level at which glycosuria becomes macrochemical (*the threshold*) varies from individual to individual and is probably hereditary in character (Faber). Its usual level is about 170. The condition of low threshold results either in continuous or in cyclic, postprandial renal glycosuria (normoglycemia glycosuria).

The *blood-sugar level* in diabetes depends to a large extent on previous treatment. If the disease is controlled, either by satisfactory dietary measures or by these and insulin, normal blood sugars are to be expected; also in mild cases hyperglycemia may only occur after meals. Such cases are detected by the so-called glucose tolerance test in which from 50 to 100 grams of glucose, dissolved in water, are given orally and determinations of sugar in the urine and blood are made before and at half-hour to hour intervals for three or four hours. The normal individual reacts by a sharp elevation of 30 or 40 mg. of blood sugar, with a peak reached in from twenty to forty minutes and a subsequent fall to the fasting value within two or two and a half hours. At no time does macrochemical sugar appear in the urine. In mild diabetes with a normal fasting level, the elevation after the glucose meal amounts to 70 mg. or more, the peak is reached late, often not until the second hour, and the subsequent decline is retarded. In renal glycosuria the blood sugar reaction is that of the normal, but the urine contains sugar.

It should be emphasized that this test is not designed to give quantitative information as to the severity or intensity of diabetes. It merely permits distinction of the mild case of diabetes mellitus from the benign forms of glycosuria and, therefore, should not be used in cases of diabetes mellitus with high fasting blood sugars. The overload of sugar indeed may do some injury in severe diabetes, and the presence of a high fasting blood sugar alone establishes the diagnosis in such cases.

The height of the fasting blood sugar in diabetes mellitus, although considerably affected by previous treatment, bears some relationship to the severity of the disease, as is illustrated by the following data of Gray assembled from 210 of Joslin's fatal cases:

TABLE 12.—RELATIONSHIP BETWEEN LEVEL OF BLOOD SUGAR AND LONGEVITY.[1]
(AFTER GRAY.)

Fasting blood sugar, mg. per cent.	Cases.	Average level of life from the day of examination, years.
0.40 to 0.57	10	0.66
0.37 to 0.39	48	1.13
0.20 to 0.29	90	1.23
Under 0.20	62	1.81

Blood Fat.—The lipids of the blood in health include: (1) the glycerol-triesters of stearic and oleic acids; (2) lecithin, a glycerol-triester in which two hydroxyl groups are replaced by fatty acids and the third with cholin; (3) cholesterin, an unsaturated secondary alcohol, and (4) cholesterin ester, a compound of cholesterin and fatty acid. The total lipid in normal blood, after fifteen hours' fasting, approximates 0.6 gram for each 100 cc. It is increased irregularly after meals. In the diabetic condition, with metabolism largely restricted to fat, as indicated by the lowered respiratory quotient, it is not surprising to find the blood fats increased and, in fact, the more intense the diabetic process and particularly the greater the ketosis, the more pronounced becomes the lipemia. In diabetic acidosis venous blood contains more fat than arterial blood and it may be inferred that the fat stream is

---

[1] These figures were obtained in the era before insulin was available for treatment; that similar observations made today would give quite different results is self-evident.

directed from the tissues to the liver. With higher grades of lipemia, of 2 per cent or more, the plasma is turbid or chocolate colored, and fat separates out on standing as an overlayer of cream. Treatment with insulin controls this condition as effectively as it does hyperglycemia.

Insulin.—That the antidiabetic hormone is prepared by the islets of Langerhans is evidenced by: (1) the development of severe diabetes on ablation of the pancreas (von Mehring and Minkowski); (2) the preparation of antidiabetic pancreatic extracts (Banting and his associates); (3) the fact that islet tissue is anatomically distinct in certain fishes and that extracts of such specialized tissue are indistinguishable in their antidiabetic action from pancreatic extracts (Macleod), and (4) that tumors of islet origin, identified by the characteristic staining of their *beta* cells, produce insulin.

Commercial insulin is now prepared by a number of firms in America and abroad. Its manufacture is controlled by the Insulin Committee of the University of Toronto and the Research Council of Great Britain. The insulin unit has been defined by the League of Nations as possessing the activity of 0.125 mg. of the standard dry preparation in the possession of the Insulin Committee of Toronto. Commercial preparations are marketed in sterile aqueous solutions containing from 10 to 100 or 200 units to the cubic centimeter. They are inactive orally, but stable and dependable for subcutaneous use. Appropriate doses of insulin restore the diabetic metabolism to normal; glycosuria, hyperglycemia and hyperlipemia are arrested; glucose is again deposited in the liver, its oxidation is promoted and ketogenesis is abolished. In doses exceeding its requirement insulin depresses the blood sugar to deeply subnormal values and produces the insulin reaction (*insulin shock*) with attendant loss of consciousness and convulsions. In normal animals it likewise provokes hypoglycemia with characteristic symptoms. This was made use of in the original physiologic standardization (Collip). The unit was then defined as that amount of insulin which would bring about depression of blood sugar to 0.045 per cent within four hours in a 200-gram rabbit previously fasted for twenty-four hours. The clinical unit represented at first a third of this rabbit dose but was later strengthened 40 per cent. The hypoglycemia resulting from overaction of insulin is attended by the liberation of epinephrin, temporary elevation of metabolism (calorigenic action of epinephrin?) and discharge of glycogen from the liver.

The mechanism of the action of insulin is still a matter of conjecture and dispute. Present evidence appears to indicate that insulin acts both in the liver and the muscles and that, in appropriate dosage, it promotes the synthesis of glycogen and the preferential oxidation of glucose in all tissues. Whether it accomplishes this by some chemical action on glucose, by way of preparation of the glucose molecule, or by action on the protoplasmic material of the cell, is as yet wholly obscure.

Symptoms and Signs.—In adult life the onset of diabetes is usually insidious; in youth the full clinical picture may develop suddenly so that one can date the onset of the disease to a certain day. Illustrative of the latter type of onset is the case of a girl, aged seven years, whose urine was being examined every day because of chronic pyelitis. The urinalyses had never revealed sugar, and on the morning of the day diabetic symptoms began reduction was not obtained. Bed wetting and polyuria appeared that night and the urine of the following morning was strongly reducing. The subsequent course was typically that of diabetes of potential severity so that two years later, despite rigid treatment and a diet containing 100 grams of carbohydrate, control demanded an insulin dose of 24 units.

The more typical manifestations of diabetes are polyuria, polydipsia, polyphagia, loss of weight and strength, glycosuria and hyperglycemia. Other less constant abnormalities are pruritus, disturbance of vision, xanthosis, xanthomatosis and hyperlipemia. Pruritus, particularly pruritus of the genital organs of women, is often an extreme annoyance and, in cases in which its cause has not been recognized, has led to suicide and insanity. It resists all treatment not directed at the metabolic abnormality but responds promptly to local remedies or disappears spontaneously as soon as glycosuria is controlled. The more usual disturbances of vision are due to changes in the refractive media of the eyes, particularly the lens, the result of fluctuation of the glucose content of the tissue fluids. Such disturbances are most common during the period of initial treatment with diet and insulin, when the excess of sugar is being rapidly removed, but they also occur in cases of diabetes of acute onset when sugar is rapidly accumulating. In either case they are transitory and it is of practical importance to postpone refraction of the eyes for the fitting of glasses as a readjustment occurs spontaneously. *Xanthosis* is a yellowish coloring of the skin due to the accumulation of the carotinoid pigments of vegetable food. It is seen in other conditions but is likely to be more pronounced in diabetes. The blood stream is similarly pigmented (xanthemia, carotinemia). It is not harmful but when strikingly developed may give rise to the erroneous suspicion of jaundice. In contrast to jaundice the scleræ are rarely discolored. Slight hyperemia of the cheeks developing on a mild degree of xanthosis gives a "peaches and cream" complexion which can be misinterpreted, by the uninitiated, as the bloom of health. Xanthomas, including those of the eyelids (*xanthelasma*), are not peculiar to diabetes. They develop in association with hyperlipemia.

Course of the Disease.—Cases of diabetes may be divided into two types, the potentially severe and the potentially mild. The diabetes of young persons usually falls in the former category; that of patients who are past the third decade in the latter, but exceptions and transitions occur so that such classification cannot be made on the basis of age alone. However, in the era before the discovery of insulin, the cases of children and young adults advanced rapidly in severity and usually proved fatal in from two to four years despite most careful treatment for the diabetes, whereas the large majority of cases of older individuals developed insidiously and progressed with great chronicity. Even with indifferent treatment serious consequences are escaped in some of these chronic cases for ten, twenty or thirty years. The greatest contribution of insulin is to diabetic children, formerly doomed to early death but now alive and strong presumably for a normal lifetime.

Complications.—Acidosis.—The most serious complication of diabetes mellitus and the one formerly responsible for the deaths of from 40 to 60 per cent of all patients is acidosis. The disturbed metabolism of fat in an organism unable to utilize carbohydrate and the resulting accumulation of aceto-acetic acid, betahydroxybutyric acid and acetone has been described (p. 998). If the process is a gradual one and time is given for the complete mobilization of the mechanisms for regulating acid-base balance (see Acidosis, p. 1012), and for other accommodations the nature of which is obscure, it is possible for it to assume considerable proportions and be maintained for months or even years without fatal consequence. This is the condition of chronic diabetic acidosis that was a common occurrence in the era before commercial insulin became available. Patients with such acidosis might excrete 60 grams or more of betahydroxybutyric acid a day. They complained not infrequently of paresthesia and dull ache along the distribution of the peripheral nerves. The pains were shooting, and as the tendon reflexes were also diminished or absent the clinical picture resembled tabes dorsalis and was designated "diabetic tabes." This form of diabetic *neuritis* responds rapidly to treatment and disappears when the metabolic abnormalities are corrected.

On the other hand, with rapidly developing intense ketosis, such as is seen with severe diabetes of childhood or results from some complicating infection or from discontinuing insulin injection in any case of potential severity, intense uncompensated acidosis results which may be fatal in twenty-four to forty-eight hours.

The symptoms of acidosis are considered under the topic Acidosis (see p. 1012). The hyperpnea (*Kussmaul breathing*), the strong fruity odor of the breath, the bright red lips and cheeks, the desiccation of the skin and tongue, and the soft eyeballs make a picture which is not difficult to recognize. In the end-stages the pulse may become weak and irregular and the skin cold and clammy, as in surgical shock. Death may result from heart failure before consciousness is lost, but is usually delayed until diabetic coma has fully developed and respiratory failure ensues.

Furuncles and Carbuncles.—These conditions are common complications in untreated diabetes and it is the duty of the physician to suspect diabetes and investigate the urine of all such patients. Occasionally sugar will be found which later disappears completely, leaving no trace of diabetes (sapremic glycosuria) but even then potential diabetes cannot be excluded.

Pulmonary Tuberculosis.—This is a serious complication but not nearly as common today as formerly. The records of 3793 consecutive cases of diabetes at the Mayo Clinic showed active tuberculosis in only 37. Roentgenograms of the thorax were obtained in nearly all cases of diabetes seen during this period.

Other Metabolic Diseases.—The occurrence of more than one disease of metabolism in the same patient is observed with sufficient frequency to give rise to the belief that individuals may possess, by inheritance, a general metabolic inferiority. Obesity is frequently associated with diabetes. Gout is unusual but high values of uric acid in the blood are seen rather frequently. The incidence of acromegaly is distinctly high. That of hyperthyroidism must receive further critical consideration. Earlier studies at the Mayo Clinic indicated that only 3 per cent of patients with diabetes also suffered from hyperthyroidism, but recent observations suggest that the coincidence of these diseases may occur with a somewhat greater frequency.

Affections of the Eyes.—True diabetic cataract of young patients is extremely rare. The writer has seen only 4 cases. Senile cataract is disproportionately abundant in the older diabetic population. The picture of diabetic retinitis is so characteristic as to be diagnostic, but is hardly ever seen except in cases of arterial disease. It is therefore doubtful whether the diabetes or the vascular disease is to be held responsible.

Arterial Disease.—The association of diabetes with hypertension is high, that with atherosclerosis still higher. This, indeed, with the resulting pathologic changes in the heart (myocardial disease), kidneys (arteriosclerosis), brain and extremities (neuritis and gangrene) is responsible today for almost one-half of the deaths from diabetes. But whether diabetes causes or stimulates the development of the arterial disease or, as Weichselbaum suggested, the latter provokes the former by favoring sclerosis and hyalinization of the islands of Langerhans, or whether the inherited predisposition for the one is likely to accompany an inheritance for the other, is as yet unknown.

Diagnosis.—A fasting blood sugar of 140 mg. for each 100 cc. determined by the Folin-Wu or similar methods is usually diagnostic of diabetes mellitus. If diabetic symptoms are present further evidence is not required. In the absence of other symptoms further investigation is indicated. Glycosuria *per se* is not conclusive. Reducing substances other than glucose may appear in the urine, including other sugars such as pentose, fructose, galactose and lactose as well as the non-saccharine substances, homogentisic acid and glycuronates. The identification of these is described in the manuals of laboratory diagnosis. Glucose itself is excreted by otherwise normal individuals with low renal thresholds. As all of these non-diabetic conditions are entirely benign it is important not to confuse them with diabetes mellitus, because to do so is to subject the patient to unnecessary anxiety and useless, indeed often harmful therapy; their recognition is greatly facilitated by a tolerance test. It should be remembered that early cases of true diabetes and later cases under satisfactory treatment may have normal blood sugars and sugar-free urine.

Treatment.—The immediate objective in the treatment of diabetes is the restoration of normal carbohydrate metabolism, without the sacrifice of nutrition. This can be accomplished in mild cases by readjustment of the diet so that the total supply of sugar (carbohydrate) is limited to the patient's capacity for its utilization. In the more severe forms of the disease it necessitates the administration of insulin.

The decision as to what treatment is required should be withheld until a careful estimate has been made of the intensity of the disease, that is, a quantitative measurement of tolerance. A period of observation in a hospital is highly desirable for the purpose, but may be dispensed with provided the physician will assume the entire task, which, in hospital, can be shared with nurses, dietitians and technicians. The immediate requisites are: (1) a food scale, preferably one provided with an adjustable dial and weighing in grams; (2) tables of food values: these can be obtained from the firms manufacturing insulin or will be found in any of the numerous manuals on diabetes prepared for the joint use of patient and physician; (3) test-tubes, a test-tube rack and a supply of Benedict's solution for qualitative analysis of single specimens of urine, and (4) a 10 per cent aqueous solution of ferric chloride for the qualitative testing of the urine for aceto-acetic acid. Facilities should be available to the physician for the quantitative determination of sugar in blood and urine. The archaic procedure of estimating the severity of a case by the specific gravity of the urine or the number of drops of urine required to turn some alkaline copper reagent is to be condemned. What is required for the tolerance estimate is the total output of glucose for each twenty-four hour period for comparison with a measured supply of food. Determinations of blood sugar are helpful for diagnosis and later insulin adjustments, but provide an inadequate indication of severity.

The Observation Diet. — A satisfactory procedure in starting the treatment of a new case is to give an "observation diet" composed of a weighed amount of food that has a predetermined glucose equivalent. The diet shown below of 102 grams of carbohydrate, 60 grams of protein and 53 grams of fat is such that the mild case becomes sugar-free after three or four days, an indication that future treatment can be arranged by qualitative dieting and that the use of food scales and insulin is, at least temporarily, obviated. The moderately severe and the severe cases will continue to excrete sugar on this diet and, at least, temporarily will require weighed diets and insulin. The grams of sugar excreted under such controlled circumstances are some measure of severity. The diabetes of childhood is almost always potentially severe and even when the disease at its onset seems relatively mild it is well to start at once with careful treatment, weighed diets and small doses of insulin. A sample diet order and menus for such an observation diet follow:

SAMPLE MENUS FOR OBSERVATION DIET.

Carbohydrate, 102 grams; Protein, 60 grams; Fat, 53 grams; "G," 142 grams.

Breakfast.	Gm		Gm.
Fruit, 10 per cent, orange	100	Bread	30
Bread	30	Meat, lean	50
Bacon (cooked)	25		
Egg	1	*Supper.*	
Cream, 20 per cent	50		
		Vegetable, 5 per cent, string-beans	100
Dinner.		Vegetable, 5 per cent, cabbage	100
		Fruit, 10 per cent, orange	100
Vegetable, 5 per cent, tomato	100	Bread	30
Vegetable, 5 per cent, spinach	100	Milk	200
Fruit, 10 per cent, orange	100	Meat, lean	50

Qualitative Management.—Cases of adults of proved mildness may be treated by simple restriction of foods rich in carbohydrates according to the following plan. The patients should be cautioned, however, about the danger of later exacerbation, from infectious complications or other causes, and should be instructed in the technic of Benedict's qualitative test for sugar and urged to make one such test each day, preferably of a single specimen of urine passed at the time of retiring.

Qualitative Diet (for Cases of Mild Diabetes Not Requiring Insulin).— Sugars and sweets of all kinds, such as candies, pastries, cakes, cookies, pies, puddings, ice creams, custards, jellies and honey, are to be avoided entirely. Desserts of junket, custard or ice cream sweetened with saccharine are permissible.

Cereal grains and their products, such as flour, rice, rice flour, potato and potato flour, corn and corn meal and foods made with these, such as breads of all kinds, biscuits, crackers, dumplings, spaghetti, macaroni and breakfast foods, are to be used sparingly, in amounts not to exceed the equivalent of one thin slice of bread ($\frac{2}{3}$ ounce) at a meal.

Meats of all kinds including fowl and fish are to be eaten sparingly, in an amount not to exceed $3\frac{1}{3}$ ounces daily. Cheese is in a category with meat.

Milk should be taken in an amount of one glass a day.

Eggs should be taken in an amount not to exceed two a day.

Butter and cream are permissible as desired and should be taken in sufficient amount to compensate for the restriction placed on sugar, starches and meats. They may be added to vegetables in cooking or the butter may be eaten with the bread allowance, the cream taken as a beverage or added to other beverages.

Vegetables of the 5 and 10 per cent groups are permissible as desired. Sauces, other than pure butter sauce, are to be avoided. Fruits of the 5 and 10 per cent groups are permissible in moderation, one portion twice daily. Fruits canned or preserved with sugar are not allowed. Special brands of fruits canned without the addition of sugar may be used in place of fresh fruits.

Nuts are permissible in an amount not to exceed the equivalent of 10 half walnut meats daily.

Unsweetened coffee and tea are permissible in moderation (may be sweetened with saccharine). Drinks sweetened with sugar, such as ginger ale, Coca-Cola and root beer are to be avoided. Dry wines are permissible; beer, near beer and sweet wines are not.

Lists of vegetables and fruits according to the approximate carbohydrate content are given in Table No. 13, p. 1006. This classification prepared by Dr. Frank N. Allan follows closely one first made by Dr. E. P. Joslin.

Quantitative Management.—A measured control of food intake is indicated when the preliminary tolerance determination indicates moderate or severe diabetes, or when qualitative management proves inadequate, and in all cases of children. All food is weighed, the daily intake of glucose-forming substances is held constant and insulin is given in the dosage necessary to maintain continuous control of glycosuria. It is relatively simple to accomplish this in the hospital, but treatment must later continue in the home and, therefore, the patient must receive satisfactory training not only in the planning of his menus but also in the technic of administering insulin. Successful treatment is impossible without his intelligent coöperation, and in order to secure it a systematic course of instruction is necessary.

TABLE 13.

Vegetables.

5 per cent. (only 3 per cent available).	10 per cent (only 6 per cent available).	15 per cent.	20 per cent.
Cucumbers	Pumpkins	Green peas	Potatoes
Lettuce	Turnips	Artichokes	Shelled beans
Spinach	Kohl-rabi	Parsnips	Canned lima beans
Asparagus	Squash		Hominy
Endive	Beets		Boiled rice
Sauerkraut	Carrots		Macaroni
Beet greens	Onions		Corn
Dandelion greens	Rutabagas		
Swiss chard	French artichokes		
Celery			
Tomatoes			
Brussels sprouts			
Watercress			
Cauliflower			
Eggplant			
Cabbage			
Radishes			
String beans			
Mushrooms			
Summer squash			

Fruits.

5 per cent.	10 per cent.	15 per cent.	20 per cent.
Rhubarb (fresh)	Grapefruit	Apples	Plums
Apricots (canned without sugar)	Lemons	Pears	Bananas
Cherries	Oranges	Apricots	Prunes
Red (canned without sugar)	Cranberries	Blueberries	Grapes
White (canned without sugar)	Strawberries	Cherries	
Loganberries (canned without sugar)	Blackberries	Currants	
Blackberries (canned without sugar)	Gooseberries	Raspberries	
Peaches (canned without sugar)	Peaches	Huckleberries	
Rasperries (canned without sugar)	Pineapple		
Strawberries (canned without sugar)	Watermelon		
	Pineapple (canned without sugar)		
	Pears (canned without sugar)		
	White grapes (canned without sugar)		

The Maintenance Diet.—There are wide differences of opinion as to the best maintenance diet. Some authorities believe that diabetic patients should receive approximately the same proportions of carbohydrate and fat as are customary in the diets of normal persons, with full advantage taken of the possibilities for substitution treatment that the availability of commercial insulin permits. Others, with whom the writer is aligned, object to this on several grounds and continue to find advantage in moderate restriction of carbohydrate. There is no disagreement on the following essentials: calories must be adequate to meet the metabolic demands of satisfactory nutrition and must not exceed these. Protein should be sufficient in amount and of the proper biologic quality but should not be excessive, for adults 0.6 to 1 gram for each kilogram of body weight, for children 1.5 to 2 grams for each kilogram. Vitamins, salts, particularly calcium and iron, should be provided liberally. If these conditions are fulfilled the patient will be maintained in excellent nutritional condition irrespective of whether the bulk of the calories is provided by fat or carbohydrate. There is general agreement also that satisfactory treatment demands control of glycosuria. This the writer finds much more difficult to accomplish when diets contain large quotas of protein and carbohydrate, as recommended by Geyelin, Porges, Sansum and others.[1]

Insulin.—The grams of glucose by which the tolerance will be raised by a given dose of insulin varies with different individuals and depends to some extent on the qualitative construction of the diet. With lower carbohydrate diets in which the bulk of the calories is in the form of fat, 1 insulin unit provides for from 1 to 2 grams of glucose and in moderately severe and severe cases the dosage will vary from 20 to 60 units a day. With diets relatively richer in carbohydrate the glucose equivalent for the unit is from 3 to 4 grams of glucose, but as the amount of carbohydrate is also large, the dose often exceeds 100 to 200 units a day.

Insulin is administered subcutaneously and, since the effectiveness of an injection is exhausted within from six to eight hours, the total amount for the day is usually divided and given fifteen or twenty minutes before meals. It is important to vary the site of injection, as otherwise the tissue becomes indurated and absorption irregular. The patient should be taught how to measure his dosage and make the injections himself and, of course, the necessity for scrupulous attention to sterility must be impressed on him.

With a constant diet the insulin requirement may not vary for weeks or months at a time, but an intervening infectious complication, even a mild cold in the head, usually lowers tolerance and necessitates larger doses. Spontaneous improvement in tolerance also occurs and therefore the patient should learn to make the qualitative test for sugar in the urine, should perform these tests before each injection and should raise or lower the dose of insulin depending on the results of such tests. Alteration of the individual dose by more than 5 units at a time is rarely desirable. The patient must be warned of the danger of omitting the injections when the urine contains sugar, even if anorexia or nausea compels the partial or complete omission of meals.

Reaction.—Insulin in excess of requirement lowers the blood sugar excessively and brings about a characteristic group of symptoms with which physician and patient should be fully familiar. A sense of anxiety and tenseness, followed by tremor, drowsiness, sweating and intense hunger are the signals of reaction and indications for small doses of sugar. It is well to insist on the patient's having at hand some cubes of table sugar and to instruct him to take, for these emergencies, 1 or 2 cubes of sugar or a small glass of orange juice (100 grams). This antidote is immediately effective unless the overdose

---

[1] For the author's method of planning diets for cases of severity the reader is referred to the fifth edition of the "Primer for Diabetic Patients," W. B. Saunders Company, Philadelphia.

has been a large one. If the reaction proceeds, mental confusion follows, associated with diplopia, sensory and motor aphasia, epileptiform convulsions and finally complete loss of consciousness. Such later stages are treated by giving a single subcutaneous injection of 0.5 cc. of 1 to 1000 solution of epinephrin (to children 0.25 cc.) followed immediately by glucose. In the absence of facilities for intravenous medication, 500 cc. of 5 per cent glucose (or corn syrup) should be administered as an enema, and at the same time a spoonful of granulated table sugar is placed in the mouth between teeth and cheek. If ampules of sterile 50 per cent glucose solution are at hand, 10 or 20 cc. of such solution is slowly injected intravenously. It is not wise to overdo the treatment of these reactions. They are rarely serious, even when resulting in profound coma, and. 15 or 20 grams of glucose is usually all that is necessary for complete restoration. The danger is greatest if the patient is seriously undernourished.

Resistance.—A few cases have been met in which the daily injection of several hundred units of insulin was required to maintain control. Neither infection nor hyperthyroidism was responsible and the cause of the alarming phenomenon has not been discovered. Such a rare occurrence is to be borne in mind because in some cases it is transitory, so that after a few weeks or months, doses of ordinary magnitude are again effective.

Allergy.—The skin in rare cases may be sensitive to insulin so that annoying and often painful local swelling and redness occur at the site of hypodermic injections. It is sometimes possible to circumvent this by changing from the insulin of one manufacture to that of another, or desensitization is accomplished by methods such as are commonly employed in desensitizing. Severe cases of allergy with constitutional reactions are extremely rare.

Edema.—Subcutaneous edema may occur when patients who are severely emaciated are first treated with insulin. This is no cause for alarm and it disappears spontaneously as nutrition improves. If discomfort is caused the condition can be promptly remedied by restricting salt and treating with acid and mercurial diuretics.

Treatment of Acidosis.—The prompt recognition and early treatment of diabetic coma are life-saving, but care must be exercised in the diagnosis. A hasty decision to inject insulin may have serious consequences in coma of other than diabetic origin or in coma due to hypoglycemia.

Distinction of the coma of diabetic acidosis from the coma of hypoglycemia can be made, usually, on the signs evident on general examination. Time does not permit completing the examination of the blood before treatment is started and the presence of sugar in the urine is not always diagnostic. In acidosis the skin is dry, the cheeks are rosy, the lips are red, the breathing is hyperpneic (Kussmaul type), the breath smells strongly of acetone, the pulse is small and weak, and the eyeballs are soft. In hypoglycemia the skin is moist and pale, the lips are cyanotic, the breath is apneic, acetone is not detected, the pulse is full or even bounding, and the eyeballs are normal in consistence.

It sometimes happens that a patient in diabetic coma is overtreated with insulin and passes out of this coma, through a short period of consciousness, into the coma of hypoglycemia. Under these circumstances certain signs of diabetic coma, dry skin, soft eyeballs and acetone breath may persist.

The treatment of diabetic acidosis with or without actual coma is as follows:

Inject insulin subcutaneously; give 30 units at once; follow with injections of 5 to 20 units every one to three hours, depending on the condition of the urine.

Enforce absolute rest in bed; the constant supervision of nurses is necessary.

Maintain the body temperature by means of blankets and hot-water bottles. When diabetes is complicated by arteriosclerosis, especial care must be exercised to avoid burning the skin of the feet. It is better not to place hot-water bottles or other heating appliances near the feet.

Secure blood for determinations of blood sugar and carbon dioxide combining-power.

Wash the stomach with a warm 5 per cent solution of sodium bicarbonate. Leave 500 cc. of the solution in the stomach.

Wash the lower part of the bowel with an enema of warm soapsuds.

Administer 1000 cc. of fluids every six hours. Give this by mouth, or as warm physiologic solutions of sodium chloride by a retention enema. If the patient is severely dehydrated, give 1000 cc. of sterile physiologic sodium chloride solution subcutaneously.

If the patient is vomiting or is unable to retain the bicarbonate solution left in the stomach, or if the carbon dioxide combining power is below 20 per cent by volume, give by vein 300 to 500 cc. of a sterile 5 per cent solution of sodium bicarbonate prepared as follows: bring 500 cc. of freshly distilled water to boiling and boil three minutes; remove from flame and dissolve in it 25 grams of clean sodium bicarbonate. The bicarbonate solution must not be boiled. The injection should take at least thirty minutes.[1]

Inject digifolin subcutaneously; give 1 cc. every four hours for several doses, at least three or four. This is effective as a heart tonic and does not provoke nausea as easily as the oral administration of digitalis.

If complicating hyperthyroidism is suspected, give iodine by skin as follows: triple paint an area of skin 8 inches (20 cm.) square with tincture of iodine previously diluted with an equal volume of alcohol. This triple painting should utilize 3 cc. of the diluted tincture or about 0.15 gram of iodine. Repeat this triple painting every six hours, three times, using a different skin area each time. Later give iodine by mouth.

It is advisable to start administering small amounts of glucose soon after making the first injection of insulin. This serves as a "buffer" to the insulin and insures the presence of enough carbohydrate to control ketosis. A dose of 15 grams every three hours is adequate. When

---

[1] A more satisfactory neutralizing solution is Hartmann's solution of physiologic buffer salts dispensed in ampules by Eli Lilly and Company. The 10 cc. contents of each ampule is to be diluted twenty-five times with sterile distilled water; 2 ampules should be used, making 500 cc. of solution.

the patient can swallow, it may be given by mouth as orange juice (150 cc.); otherwise it should be incorporated in the retention enemas.

It is of vital importance for correct administration of insulin to make frequent examinations of the urine and blood. Unless urination is unimpeded the bladder must be catheterized and completely emptied once every three hours. Every specimen of urine obtained by catheter or by spontaneous voiding should be examined at once for sugar and aceto-acetic acid. It must be remembered that the effect of frequently repeated injections of insulin may be cumulative. It is safer, until the emergency is past, to leave traces of sugar in the urine as a safeguard against hypoglycemia rather than to attempt to suppress glycosuria completely. The certainty of treatment is greatly increased if the patient can be taken to hospital where facilities for examination of the blood are available, but no time should be lost in giving the first injection of insulin.

Treatment of Surgical Complications.—Surgical operation in the presence of diabetes was formerly attended with a rate of mortality so high as to be almost prohibitive, but today with commercial insulin available this is no longer true. It remains important, however, to maintain the strictest control of the metabolic condition, especially after an operation, and operation in the presence of diabetes should be attempted only by those who are experienced in the treatment of diabetes or are associated in this work with a physician with such experience. For a full consideration of this topic the reader is referred to the excellent monograph of McKitrick and Root. A word of warning on the score of the treatment of gangrene of the feet may be inserted here, namely, that with non-pulsating arteries and other evidence of impaired circulation in a foot, minor amputations of toes or portions of the foot are to be avoided. If healing does not occur with rest and control of the metabolic condition, or if for other reasons such as infection, amputation becomes necessary, this should be performed high, usually above the knee, with extraordinary precaution to avoid infecting the operative field and to obtain flaps with good circulation.

Treatment of Complicating Infectious Conditions.—Infections lower tolerance, increase insulin requirements, and themselves acquire increased virulence in the diabetic organism. Rigid control of the metabolic condition is thus made more difficult of accomplishment but increasingly important. The procedure here is much the same as in the treatment of diabetic acidosis, frequent tests of single specimens of urine, and 5 or 6 injections of insulin daily in such dosage as is indicated by repeated examinations of the urine.

General Treatment.—Regular habits as regards sleep, outdoor recreation, periodic visits to the dentist, the surgical removal of diseased teeth or tonsils and other measures of general hygiene should be given suitable consideration in all cases of diabetes. Because of the danger of diabetic gangrene, the care of the feet of elderly patients with evident arteriosclerosis must receive particular attention. Scrupulous cleanliness, moderate massage, and exercises of the Berger type are the essentials. Hot applications of all kinds and therapeutic application of roentgen-ray or radium are to be avoided. These extremities, like those of the patients with tabes dorsalis or syringomyelia, are often abnormally susceptible to burning and such injury may lead to infection and gangrene. By the same token every effort should be made to avoid abrasions of the feet due to the trimming of corns, the cutting of toe-nails or the rubbing of ill-fitting shoes.

It should be emphasized, in conclusion, that the criterion of successful treatment of diabetes is a normal state of physical and mental vigor. Well treated patients need not change their usual occupations. Children should be able to attend school and engage in ordinary sports and recreations. It is not enough merely to keep these patients alive. It is the duty of the physician to prevent diabetes from becoming a disability.

REFERENCES.

CAMPBELL, W. R., and MACLEOD, J. J. R.: Insulin, Medicine, 1924, **3**, 195.

GRAFE, E.: Die Krankheiten des Stoffwechsels und ihre Behandlung, Berlin, Julius Springer, 1931, 519 pp.

JOSLIN, E. P.: The Treatment of Diabetes Mellitus, 4th ed., Philadelphia, Lea & Febiger, 998 pp.

McKITTRICK, L. S., and ROOT, H. R.: Diabetic Surgery, Philadelphia, Lea & Febiger, 1928, 269 pp.

VON NOORDEN, C., and ISAAC, S.: Die Zuckerkrankheit und ihre Behandlung, Berlin, Julius Springer, 1931, 627 pp.

WARREN, SHIELDS: Pathology of Diabetes Mellitus, Philadelphia, Lea & Febiger, 1930, 212 pp.

WILDER, R. M.: A Primer for Diabetic Patients, 5th ed., Philadelphia, W. B. Saunders Company, 1934, 138 pp.

HYPERINSULINISM.

Definition.—Hyperinsulinism is a condition of irregular and excessive supply of the hormonal product of pancreatic island tissue, characterized by attacks of weakness, tremor and tachycardia, and followed in severe cases by delirium and loss of consciousness. These attacks are associated with abnormally low levels of blood sugar, and are promptly arrested by supplying carbohydrate food. The condition is the direct antithesis of diabetes mellitus.

Incidence and Pathology.—The disease has been recognized only recently and but few cases have been described. In the majority of them hypertrophy of island tissue has been found at operation or after death, usually in the form of adenoma; in some, surgical exploration has failed to reveal any abnormality, and it is therefore probable that histologically normal islet tissue may, under certain conditions, function excessively or irregularly.

Diagnosis.—The attacks have been mistaken for those of epilepsy, hysteria, or maniacal psychosis. Hyperinsulinism should be suspected if attacks are produced by fasting or strenuous physical exercise and if the symptoms are promptly arrested by administering sugar. The finding of a value for blood sugar below 60 mg. for each 100 cc. is supporting evidence, but differentiation is even then necessary because hypoglycemia may also occur in extensive disease of the liver and less commonly in certain other conditions.

Treatment.—Operative removal of an adenoma of the islands of the pancreas has resulted in cure. Resection of a part of the pancreas has been followed by some relief in cases wherein surgical exploration revealed a pancreas of normal appearance. Medical treatment is unsatisfactory. The obvious remedy is carbohydrate food in sufficient amounts and at the proper time to maintain the blood sugar at a normal level. In severe cases this is a complicated procedure which interferes with unbroken sleep and may fail to provide sufficient food to prevent attacks. Epinephrin hydrochloride, solution of pituitary, ephedrine and desiccated thyroid are of transitory benefit only.

REFERENCES.

WILDER, R. M., ALLAN, F. N., POWER, M. H., and ROBERTSON, H. E.: Carcinoma of the Islands of the Pancreas; Hyperinsulinism and Hypoglycemia, Jour. Am. Med. Assn., 1927, **89**, 348.
WILDER, R. M.: Hyperinsulinism, International Clinics, 1933 (June), **2**, 1.

ACIDOSIS.

Definition.—Acidosis is that condition of the fluids of the blood which is produced by the addition thereto of acid, or the withdrawal of base, to a degree sufficient to alter, beyond physiologic limits, the pH, the carbon dioxide tension, or the bicarbonate content of the plasma.

The notation pH is an abbreviated expression of hydrogen-ion concentration (reaction). Its value is the negative logarithm of hydrogen-ion concentration (grams of hydrogen ion contained in 1 liter). Thus, in the case of pure distilled water, the hydrogen-ion content of a liter is 1×10^{-7} and the pH is 7. The physiologic range of the pH of blood is from 7.35 to 7.45; the variations observed in disease are confined as a rule between 6.9 and 7.9. It is to be noted that increased acidity is indicated by a lower pH and *vice versa*. Thus 6.9 represents an extreme degree of acidosis, and 7.9 an extreme shift of reaction in the direction of more alkalinity.

A solution, like the fluid of the blood, which contains bicarbonates, hemoglobin and other proteins, phosphates or other weak acids and their salts, is buffered thereby so that relatively large amounts of acid or alkali can be added with a minimal change of pH. The ratio of the weakly dissociated acids to their bases is altered, however, by such additions, and hence, in the blood, the measurement of either the carbon dioxide tension (free carbonic acid) or the bicarbonate content, may reveal the presence of acidosis when the pH is still within normal range. On the other hand, acidosis due to excessive production or incomplete removal of carbon dioxide, as in pneumonia and other respiratory conditions, may cause a distinct shift of the pH in the direction of acidity without appreciable effect on the bicarbonate content.

The organism as a whole, in addition to its blood buffers, possesses a number of regulating mechanisms for preserving the normal reaction of its tissues. These function, for the most part, by causing excretion of more or less acid or base as occasion demands. Among them are included: (1) accelerated elimination of carbonic acid by the lungs by more vigorous respiration; (2) excretion of phosphates and sulphates, as monobasic salts in conditions of acidosis, or as dibasic salts when alkali is excessive; (3) the formation of ammonia by the kidneys, and its utilization, in acidosis, for combining with acids for excretion, thus sparing other bases, and (4) the formation of citric acid in alkalosis (Ostberg, Boothby).

Etiology.—Conditions leading to acidosis can be divided into additions of acid and withdrawal of base.

Additions of acid occur under the following circumstances: (1) ingestion of acid or acid salts (NH_4Cl), or their parenteral injection; (2) excessive muscular exertion, causing accumulation of lactic and carbonic acids; (3) carbohydrate starvation, diabetes mellitus, and the cyclic vomiting of childhood, causing accumulation of aceto-acetic and betahydroxybutyric acids; (4) nephritis resulting in retention of acid ions, chiefly phosphates and sulphates; possibly also the formation of hitherto unidentified organic acids; (5) pneumonia and other pulmonary affections, resulting in retention of carbonic acid and formation of unidentified organic acids, and (6) severe burns, anesthesia, infectious diseases, pregnancy and poisoning, causing the formation of unidentified acid metabolites.

Withdrawal of base occurs under the following conditions: (1) pancreatic fistula (experimental), and (2) diarrheal diseases, especially Asiatic cholera.

Diagnosis.—The more severe grades of acidosis are recognizable clinically by the symptom, hyperpnea. Air hunger is characteristic. The breathing is not only rapid, as in ordinary dyspnea, but deep, like that of a runner after a race. It was first described by Kussmaul and is often spoken of as Kussmaul breathing. Such other symptoms as headache, weakness, drowsiness and malaise are less diagnostic. Diabetic acidosis may be accompanied by severe abdominal pain, and thus may lead to the suspicion of appendicitis, cholecystitis or ruptured viscus. A considerably high leukocyte count may still further complicate the picture. Pains are also felt in the back and extremities. In the acidosis of diabetes, and that of carbohydrate starvation, the breath and excretions smell of acetone, but it should be emphasized that the milder degrees of formation of aceto-acetic and betahydroxybutyric acid can be compensated for by the formation and combination of ammonia and other regulatory means, so that no actual acidosis occurs. This condition of ketone accumulation with the pH and carbon dioxide content of the blood plasma remaining normal is designated by the term ketosis with compensated acidosis. It is possible even for ketosis to be associated with alkalosis (see Alkalosis, p. 1014).

Milder cases of acidosis, or early cases, can be recognized only by examination of the blood. Completely satisfactory information is obtained by a method such as that of Shock and Hastings, which gives, simultaneously, bicarbonate content, carbon dioxide tension and pH. If the character of the acidosis is desired, that is, knowledge as to whether one is dealing with retention of carbon dioxide or accumulation of fixed acids, one must determine at least two of these variables.

Less informative, but more convenient and clinically useful, especially in cases of diabetic acidosis, is measurement of the carbon dioxide combining power of the plasma by the method of Van Slyke.

Prognosis.—The prognosis largely depends on the underlying cause, although it should be recognized that severe acidosis is, in and of itself, an extremely serious condition which demands immediate treatment.

Treatment.—General measures include rest and warmth, support of the heart, and restoration of fluids and electrolytes. The latter is of extreme importance if dehydration is marked, as it usually is. Administration of alkali, as solution of sodium bicarbonate, may be life-saving when deficit of alkali exists, but caution must be exercised in determining the dose, for an excessive amount of bicarbonate may prove injurious. Sodium bicarbonate, 500 cc. of 5 per cent, may be given intravenously with safety if it is prepared without boiling. Bicarbonate is converted to the much more caustic carbonate by boiling (see treatment of diabetic acidosis and coma, p. 1008). Hartmann's solution of physiologic buffer salts (Eli Lilly & Co.) is recommended because it restores base without danger of overdosage. Any such infusion should be given very slowly to avoid overloading the heart.

Specific measures will depend on the cause of the condition. The use of insulin in diabetic acidosis has been considered in the section on Diabetes Mellitus. Oxygen, given by the tent method or by chamber, is indicated in respiratory conditions in which the hydrogen-ion concentration is increased without reduction of bicarbonate in the blood.

REFERENCES.

HARTMANN, A. F., and ELMAN, ROBERT: The Effects of Loss of Gastric and Pancreatic Secretions and the Methods for Restoration of Normal Conditions in the Body, Jour. Exper. Med., 1929, **50**, 387.

PETERS, J. P., and VAN SLYKE, D. D.: Quantitative Clinical Chemistry—Interpretations, Baltimore, The Williams & Wilkins Company, 1931. Vol. **1**, 1264 pp.

SHOCK, N. W., and HASTINGS, A. B.: A Micro-technique for the Determination of the Acid-base Balance of the Blood, Proc. Soc. Exper. Biol. and Med., 1929, **26**, 780.

ALKALOSIS.

Definition.—Alkalosis is that condition of the fluids of the blood which is produced by the addition thereto of base, or the withdrawal of acid, to a degree sufficient to alter, beyond physiologic limits, the pH, the carbon dioxide tension, or the bicarbonate content of the plasma.

Etiology.—The buffering systems of the blood, and the regulatory mechanism by which the normal reaction and the bicarbonate content of the blood are maintained, are considered under Acidosis (*v. s.*). Conditions leading to alkalosis are addition of base and withdrawal of acid.

Addition of base occurs when alkalies are ingested, such as sodium bicarbonate and others, in the treatment of peptic ulcer; in this case the bicarbonate content and the pH of the blood are both raised. Withdrawal of acid occurs under the following conditions: (1) hydrochloric acid is lost by persistent vomiting of gastric content, such as results from pyloric or high intestinal obstruction, or such as occurs, at times, from lesions of the brain, from toxemia, and in pregnancy. Under such circumstances both the bicarbonate content and the pH of the blood are raised. (2) Carbonic acid is lost excessively by over-ventilation of the lungs. This may be voluntary, hysterical, or result from a lesion of the brain which produces irritation of respiratory centers. In this case the carbon dioxide tension of the blood is decreased, the pH is elevated and the bicarbonate content is only slightly decreased.

Diagnosis.—The characteristic features of alkalosis are increased irritability, restlessness, excitability, paresthesia, tremor and convulsion. Chvostek's and Trousseau's signs are often present, and the response of the neuro-muscular apparatus to opening and closing of the electric current are those of tetany (Erb's sign). However, in mild cases, clinical evidence may be absent, so that the condition can be revealed only by examination of the blood. This manifests characteristic changes of pH, carbon dioxide and bicarbonate and in cases of loss of hydrochloric acid, lowered values for chlorides.

It should be emphasized that the clinical distinction between acidosis and alkalosis is not always easy; also, that mild grades of ketosis may coëxist with alkalosis.

Treatment.—Treatment depends on the underlying cause. If alkalies are being given as medication, this should be stopped. If hydrochloric acid has been lost by vomiting, and a deficit of chloride exists, physiologic salt solutions should be injected intravenously in an appropriate dosage of 1 or 2 liters. This supplies fluid as well as electrolyte. There seems to be some advantage in the empirical addition of glucose to such infusions. Hartmann's solution may also be used. In cases of overventilation and "blowing off" of carbonic acid, the patient must be told to breathe more slowly and less deeply. If his coöperation in this is impossible the dead space of the respiratory tract should be increased by applying a mask and causing rebreathing through a tube a foot or more long, or mixtures of carbon dioxide and oxygen should be given in the oxygen tent.

REFERENCES.

GAMBLE, J. L., and ROSS, S. G.: The Factors in the Dehydration Following Pyloric Obstruction, Jour. Clin. Invest., 1925, **1**, 403.

HARTMANN, A. F., and ELMAN, ROBERT: The Effects of Loss of Gastric and Pancreatic Secretions and the Methods for Restoration of Normal Conditions in the Body, Jour. Exper. Med., 1929, **50**, 387.

PETERS, J. P., and VAN SLYKE, D. D.: Quantitative Clinical Chemistry—Interpretations, Baltimore, The Williams & Wilkins Company, 1931. Vol. **2**, 1264 pp.

OBESITY.

Definition.—Obesity is a condition characterized by the accumulation and diffuse distribution of fat in excess of what is normal.

Etiology.—The conventional view that obesity represents a qualitative disturbance of metabolism is not borne out by the experience of the writer or by the investigations of Means, DuBois, and Newburgh. Except in cases of hypothyroidism, the basal metabolic rate of obese patients falls within the normal range; energy expended in the performance of measured amounts of work is not less than normal; the respiratory quotient, after a fast of fourteen or fifteen hours, is normal; the specific dynamic action of foods is sometimes depressed, but not regularly so, but the measurement of this phenomenon is attended with so many difficulties, and such wide variations occur with perfectly normal persons, that important inferences from the data obtained are unjustified; the urine contains no unusual metabolites, and its nitrogen partition and that of the blood plasma are normal; the blood fat is normal in amount and composition. In sum, there is usually nothing to suggest unusual economy in expenditure of energy or interference of any kind with oxidation. The question, then, why some persons grow stout on reputedly small amounts of food, whereas others, presumably larger eaters, remain thin, must be answered by negation of the inference that the former actually eat proportionately less. It is extremely easy for the person to be deceived as to how many calories he actually consumes, and the food requirement for maintenance varies from person to person, depending on age, height, weight, sex, activity and temperament, to a far greater extent than is commonly appreciated. The writer has never failed to observe loss of weight when control of diet was satisfactory and the calories supplied did not exceed the basal calorie requirement (obtained from the basal metabolic rate, calories each hour × 24).

Dysorexia.—If a causative abnormality is present in obesity, this is to be looked for in those centers of the central nervous system that determine appetite. Obese persons possess unusually good appetites, marked both by intensity of the feeling of hunger and delayed sensations of satiety. They develop, in consequence, habits of overeating (bulimia) which in turn create a vicious circle by furthering the desire for large meals.

Heredity.—The underlying disturbance of appetite, dysorexia (Umber), is often inherited. Obesity runs in families, and in this sense is a constitutional affection. Danforth described a strain of yellow mice in which the tendency to development of obesity was transmitted as a unit character.

Cerebral Lesions.—Evidence that control of appetite and thus of weight is regulated through nervous centers in the diencephalon is provided by experimental and clinical lesions of this region. Contrary to earlier views the hypophysis is usually not involved in obesity. Its complete removal is without effect on body weight, provided overlying structures of the brain are left uninjured, whereas lesions of the subthalamic region, which do not involve the pituitary body, provoke extreme gains in weight (Bailey and Bremer). Leschke reported that of 149 cases of adiposogenital dystrophy in which necropsy was performed, in only 21 was the abnormality limited to the pituitary body, and in the absence of more refined histologic examinations than have been available, it is doubtful whether participation of the diencephalon has ever been excluded with certainty. Injury to appetite-regulating centers of the diencephalon may result from tumors, cysts, hemorrhages, gummas, basal fractures, meningitis, or inflammatory lesions such as are formed by lethargic encephalitis. The resulting obesity is often enormous, and may develop rapidly in persons with no previous tendencies to gain in weight.

Hypothyroidism.—The only satisfactory evidence for primary involvement of the endocrine system, in the etiology of obesity, is that relating to the thyroid gland. Actual economy in expenditure of energy is evident in hypothyroidism and myxedema, and this usually, but not always, results in gain of weight. These cases are rare if the diagnosis is limited to patients with basal metabolic rates consistently below −20.

Symptoms.—In obesity from organic cerebral lesions, the principal symptoms are those of the lesion. They may include headache, bitemporal hemianopsia, transient glycosuria, polyuria (diabetes insipidus), and unusual somnolence. With simple or constitutional obesity some disturbance of water metabolism is frequently associated and somnolence is not uncommon. With thyrogenic obesity the symptoms of myxedema are more or less in evidence. Excessive weight, in all cases, may seriously embarrass the heart and cause edema of the legs and other evidence of circulatory failure. It is frequently accompanied by amenorrhea.

Diagnosis.—In the absence of edema or ascites, the diagnosis of obesity is readily made by comparison of the body weight to a standard for the given height, age and sex. The standards usually taken for reference are the tables of height, weight and age of the Medico-Actuarial Mortality Investigation of 1912. It should be recognized that the figures in these tables represent averages and are not to be regarded as optimal. A fair working rule is to consider as normal any deviation that does not exceed plus or minus 10 per cent.

Distinction of obesity into types is frequently attempted on the basis of the configuration of the body. Among the more significant of these are the Falstaffian or gluttony type, with large neck, protuberant abdomen, and thin buttocks; the thyrogenic type, with its characteristics of myxedema; the cerebral type with a fairly uniform distribution of fat and infantile characteristics, and the Fröhlich type, attributed, probably incorrectly, to pituitary insufficiency, and denoted by an intersexual or infantile habitus, absence of face and body hair, and atrophy of the external genitals. There appears to be little if any justification for establishment of a so-called pituitary type, supposedly characterized by special accumulation of fat at the pelvic girdle. The large majority of all cases of obesity are impossible to classify on this basis, and simple or constitutional obesity may imitate any one of the specific types. A distinction between exogenous and endogenous obesity is equally unsatisfactory.

Complications and Prognosis.—The actuarial studies of the life insurance companies have clearly demonstrated that life expectancy is decreased in rough proportionally to the degree of overweight. This is attributed to increased susceptibility to degenerative conditions, such as myocardial degeneration, hypertension, arteriosclerosis, nephritis and diabetes.

Treatment.—The treatment of lesions of the brain responsible for cerebral obesity is rarely successful. Cysts can be attacked by operation, tumors by roentgenotherapy and syphilitic affections by antisyphilitic measures. The treatment of hypothyroidism and myxedema is considered elsewhere (p. 821). The use of thyroid substance or extract in cases of obesity that are not clearly attributable to insufficiency of the thyroid gland is not to be recommended. Large doses are necessary and, as Means stated, they correct one evil by creating another. Dinitrophenol has been recommended recently. In doses of from 200 to 300 mg. it will raise the basal metabolic rate and thus promote weight loss. It does not cause the disagreeable symptoms encountered when preparations of thyroid are used in equally effective doses, but a feeling of being overheated is complained of by some patients, and not a few patients with idiosyncrasy react with urticaria and malaise. Whether the long-continued use of dinitrophenol is ever safe is highly doubtful, and certainly no patient should receive it unless constant supervision is maintained, with daily tests of the urine for urobilinogen. All the other drugs of reputed efficacy are either toxic or useless.

Strenuous physical exercise may be harmful, particularly when the intake of food is restricted; it is seldom effective otherwise. Mild exercise, massage and general hygienic measures are desirable. Chief reliance must be placed on dietetic management. The difficulties encountered in treating obesity fall into two categories: either the diet is insufficiently precise so that the patient's total consumption of calories is not actually limited, or it is so rigidly restricted as to be deficient in some essential factor or factors requisite for health. In the first case no weight loss occurs, in the second the resulting ill health necessitates the discontinuance of treatment. The portions of food must be measured as they are for the diabetic, and in planning the diet strict attention must be paid to the nutritional requirements for proteins, vitamins and minerals.

The author held the opinion in the past that patients should not be reduced at a rate greater than 2 pounds a week, having noted that when they lost faster than this they were easily fatigued and became irritable and nervous. But recently he has been following, with striking success, the procedure of Strang, McCluggage and Evans by which losses of weight of as much as 4 pounds weekly are obtained without discomfort or other evidence of injury. The guiding principle is to reduce the calories of the food to a minimum while providing supplementary salts and vitamins. This supplementation must not be neglected. The author has used a yeast vitamin tablet for vitamin B and has provided vitamins A and D in a concentrate of cod-liver oil or as halibut oil fortified with viosterol. On the assumption that the most important mineral deficiency in the diet is calcium, calcium phosphate is given in teaspoonful doses. Kalak water or Tyrode's solution without glucose are recommended to insure the adequacy of other minerals. Further details will be found in the author's Colver lecture on the "Treatment of Obesity." A sample diet which fully satisfies the requirements for an adequate supply of protein of satisfactory quality, together with what vitamin C is necessary, is given below.

WEIGHED REDUCTION DIET.

(To be supplemented as described in the text.)

Carbohydrate, 40 grams; Protein, 70 grams; Fat, 12 grams; (calories, 548.)

	Grams.
10 per cent Fruits	150
Orange } Best	
Grapefruit }	
5 per cent vegetable	125
(Have tomato or cabbage daily)	
Bread	10
Cottage cheese	75
(Made from skimmed milk)	
Milk, skimmed	200
Egg	1
Egg whites	2
Meat or fish from the following list	120

Meats and Fish Allowed.

(Meats must be cooked without added fat.)

Tenderloin steak, very lean
Round steak, very lean
Liver
Dried beef
Tripe, pickled
Roast veal, lean
Roast chicken, light meat
Roast turkey, light meat
Black bass
Cod steaks
Haddock
Smoked haddock
Halibut
Perch
Wall-eyed pike
Pickerel

Brook trout
Tuna fish, canned, not in oil
Crabs
Crabs, canned
Lobster
Lobster, canned
Shrimp, canned

Breakfast Menu.

Orange juice 50 grams $\frac{1}{4}$ glass
Egg   1 }
  and   } Poached
Egg whites 2 }
Bread 10 grams $\frac{1}{2}$ small thin slice
Coffee

Luncheon Menu.

Cold roast chicken 60 grams 1 average slice
String-beans 100 grams $\frac{1}{2}$ cup
Skimmed milk 200 grams 1 glass
Grapefruit 50 grams $\frac{1}{4}$ small size
Tea

Dinner Menu.

Bouillon, fat free 1 cup
Broiled tenderloin 60 grams 1 small lean tenderloin
Tomatoes 100 grams $\frac{1}{2}$ cup
Cottage cheese salad:
  Cottage cheese 75 grams $\frac{1}{3}$ cup
  Lettuce   25 grams $\frac{1}{8}$ head
  Mineral oil mayonnaise 1 tablespoonful
Fresh peach 50 grams $\frac{1}{4}$ cup

REFERENCES.

EVANS, F. A., and STRANG, J. M.: The Treatment of Obesity with Low Caloric Diets, Jour. Am. Med. Assn., 1931, **97**, 1063.

LESCHKE, ERICH: Stoffwechselkrankheiten, Dresden, T. Steinkopff, 1930, 130 pp.

McLESTER, J. S.: Nutrition and Diet in Health and Disease, 2d ed., Philadelphia, W. B. Saunders Company, 1931, 759 pp.

NEWBURGH, L. H.: The Cause of Obesity, Jour. Am. Med. Assn., 1931, **97**, 1659.

VON NOORDEN, CARL: Die Fettsucht, II. Aufl., Wien and Leipzig, 1910.

WILDER, R. M.: Colver Lecture: The Treatment of Obesity, International Clinics, 1933, **4**, 43d Series, 1.

LIPOMATOSIS.

Definition.—Conditions of abnormal deposition of fat, in which the adipose accumulations differ from those of ordinary obesity by being sharply localized or tumor-like, or possessing other unusual characteristics, are classified under lipomatosis.

Incidence.—Clinical Types.—The ordinary lipoma or fat tumor represents a very common abnormality, *lipomatosis simplex*. Such tumors occur singly or in numbers, are situated usually in the subcutaneous tissues, are nodular, soft, lobulated and encapsulated, are symptomless for the most part, but occasionally are tender or spontaneously painful, *lipomatosis dolorosa*. They vary in size from minute structures to huge masses, *lipomatosis gigantica*, and when very large may be associated with severe emaciation of the rest of the body, *lipomatosis atrophicans* (Günther). The forms other than lipomatosis simplex are rare. The fat of lipomas is less readily available for metabolism than that in the usual fat depots. The condition affects women more than men.

Related Conditions.—1. *Adenolipomatosis* (Fetthals), an extremely rare disorder, affects men more than women and is characterized by symmetrical accumulations of fat in the region of lymph nodes, especially of the cervical nodes, hence the name "fat neck." The fat in these deposits is not encapsulated, but accumulates in large, disfiguring masses which extend down over the shoulders and thorax. The lymphoid tissue is not involved.

2. Dercum's disease, *adiposis dolorosa*, is a special neurogenic form of lipomatosis, characterized by spontaneously painful and very tender symmetrical deposits of fat. It is seen almost exclusively in women, and occurs in asthenic persons with pronounced neurotic or psychopathic characteristics. Typical cases are extremely rare and, insofar as tenderness and pain are not infrequent in the deposits of fat of various types of lipomatosis, even in those of simple obesity, there is reason to question whether this characteristic alone entitles Dercum's disease to be regarded as a clinical entity. The histologic evidence of involvement of the central nervous system is inconclusive.

3. *Lipodystrophia progressiva*, an extremely rare disorder, affects chiefly women, begins in childhood and is characterized by disfiguring emaciation of the face, neck, arms and thorax, combined with grotesque obesity of the hips and legs. Its etiology is unknown; A. Simons considered segmental trophoneurosis.

Treatment.—Fat tumors may be removed by operation if their size or situation causes disfigurement or if they are otherwise troublesome. Dietetic treatment is usually a waste of effort, and endocrine preparations are useless. The treatment of lipodystrophia progressiva is particularly unsatisfactory, for persons affected gain weight rapidly when overnourished but put all the added fat into the already overweight lower half of the body.

Lipoatrophia Circumscripta.—This rare condition, which goes under the name of *cutis laxa* in the dermatologic literature, is regarded by Thannhauser as the clinical antithesis of lipomatosis. It is characterized by localized regions of atrophy which affects the subcutaneous fat, the corium and the epidermis. The skin of these regions is wrinkled and folded and can be pulled away from the underlying tissues like elastic rubber.

REFERENCES.

DERCUM, F. X.: Three Cases of a Hitherto Unclassified Affection Resembling in Its Grosser Aspects Obesity, but Associated with Special Nervous Symptoms; Adiposis Dolorosa, Am. Jour. Med. Sci., 1892, **104**, 521.

GÜNTHER, H.: Die Lipomatosis und ihre klinischen Formen, Jena, Fischer, 1920, 216 pp.

Pollak, F.: Beiträge zur Klinik und Pathogenese der progressiven Lipodystrophie, Ztschr. f. d. ges. Neurol. u. Psychiat., 1930, **127**, 415.

Thannhauser, S. J.: Lehrbuch des Stoffwechsels und der Stoffwechselkrankheiten, Munich, Bergmann, 1929, 741 pp.

DIABETES INSIPIDUS.

Definition.—Diabetes insipidus is a disorder of metabolism characterized by abnormal thirst, excessive excretion of urine and, in many cases, retention of chlorides.

History.—The disease was regarded by Galen as the same as diabetes mellitus and no distinction was drawn between the two until, at the close of the eighteenth century, Peter Frank noted the lack of sweetness of the urine in diabetes insipidus.

Incidence.—The disease is relatively rare. The diagnosis was made in only 98 cases in a period of ten years in the Mayo Clinic. It affects chiefly the young, but usually persists throughout life. More males than females are affected.

Etiology.—Heredity is important in some instances. A family is described by Weil, in which, in five generations, among 220 members, 35 were affected. The inherited disease begins early in life, but tends to mildness.

Organic lesions of the diencephalon which may precipitate secondary diabetes insipidus include fractures of the base of the skull, syphilitic or other forms of meningitis, encephalitis (a number of cases are reported as sequelæ of encephalitis lethargica), tumors, gummas, cysts, lymphomas and hemorrhage. Christian has described a syndrome, of which diabetes insipidus is a part, which results from multiple xanthomas of the cranium. Frequently, however, no definite etiology is discernible. Some cases occur as sequelæ of acute infections: scarlet fever, measles, rheumatic fever or influenza.

Pathology.—Anatomic interest in diabetes insipidus has centered, on the one hand, in the kidneys and cardiovascular system and, on the other, in the hypophysis and adjacent parts of the brain where regulation of water is presumed to be mediated. The kidneys are normal in uncomplicated cases in young persons; in older victims sclerotic changes may be found, but nothing that is characteristic. The same may be said for the heart and arteries. The diencephalon may be involved by gross lesions, tumors, cysts or inflammatory infiltrations, and in cases in which gross disturbances are absent, microscopic examination may reveal abnormality. The question whether the seat of the trouble is the pituitary gland or the overlying hypothalamus is still disputed, although the best of the more recent evidence favors the latter. A few cases of diabetes insipidus have resulted from local irritation of the vasomotor nerves to the kidneys by abdominal tumor or tuberculous peritonitis.

Symptoms.—The onset is usually insidious, but may be acute, following an injury to the brain, or following some infectious disease. The striking symptoms are polyuria and thirst. The urine passed in a day may equal, particularly in children, the weight of the body, and quantities as high as 10 or 15 liters are by no means uncommon. The

specific gravity of such urine is naturally very low; it seldom exceeds
1.005, but the significant feature is that it cannot be elevated appreciably by withholding fluids, and that attempts to reduce the intake
of water provoke agonizing thirst. The perspiration, on the other
hand, is not increased; in fact, the skin is abnormally dry. Constipation, headache and general malaise are accompaniments of the disease.
In cases in which there are gross lesions of the brain, one may expect
bitemporal amblyopia, optic atrophy, or severe headache. Obesity of
cerebral origin may accompany it, also acromegaly, gigantism or
infantilism. Transient glycosuria may be observed, but true diabetes
mellitus is extremely rare.

Cases are divided into two types, depending on the presence or
absence of retention of chloride: (1) the hyperchloremic (hypochlor-
uric), and (2) the hypochloremic (hyperchloruric or normochloruric).
In the former, administration by mouth of 10 or 20 grams of sodium
chloride causes striking elevation in the chloride of the blood. Pituitrin
causes suppression of the polyuria of the former, and is without effect
in the latter. This distinction may be of more theoretic than practical
interest.

Diagnosis.—When the urine exceeds 5 to 8 liters, is low in specific
gravity and free from sugar, the diagnosis is not in doubt, but mild
cases occur which are sometimes confused with polyuria of other origin.
The hyposthenuria of contracted kidney can be ruled out by absence
of other evidence of nephritis. The so-called primary types of polydipsia of neuropsychic (hysterical) origin are more difficult to exclude.
A "thirst test" gives valuable information. An appreciable loss of
weight during this test, with increasing values for blood chloride,
speaks strongly for diabetes insipidus.

Prognosis.—The prognosis, in the idiopathic cases, is not unfavorable; otherwise it depends entirely on the nature and rate of development of the cerebral lesion.

Treatment.—Regulation of the intake of salt is very helpful. A
salt-free diet is impractical for long periods, but limitation to 3 or
4 grams daily is reasonable and harmless. Some supervision of the
intake of protein, so that this will not exceed 1 gram for each kilogram
of body weight, is also advocated. Rigid restriction of intake of water
is out of the question, but some control of this is desirable, particularly
when the diagnosis does not definitely exclude a psychic element.

A spinal puncture should be made, primarily for diagnostic purposes, but also because the occasional case may be immediately and
sometimes permanently relieved by this procedure. Organic lesions
of the hypophysis or diencephalon may be attacked by operation, by
roentgen therapy or, if syphilis is present, by antisyphilitic treatment.

The majority of cases respond symptomatically to subcutaneous
injection of pituitrin, or to the constituent of this known as pitressin.
Thirst is at once arrested, the volume of urine diminishes, and its
specific gravity rises, although never higher than about 1.015. Also,
in the hyperchloremic cases, the percentage of blood chloride is diminished. This effect is exhausted usually in from six to twelve hours,
but repeated injections of 1 cc. of surgical pituitrin, two or three

times daily, can be given for months and years without ill effect. Satisfactory results are at times to be obtained when pituitrin is sprayed in the nose, also when posterior lobe powder is given by nasal insufflation as reported recently by Smith. Advantages of the powder treatment include ease of application, absence of intestinal and other side effects and reduction of cost. According to Zondek, a hormone *intermedin* is secreted by the pars intermedia of the hypophysis. Sulzberger considers this principle responsible for the antidiuretic effects of pituitary preparations.

REFERENCES.

BAILEY, P., and BREMBER, F.: Experimental Diabetes Insipidus, Arch. Int. Med., 1921, **28**, 773.
GRAFE, E.: Die Krankheiten des Stoffwechsels und ihre Behandlung, Berlin, Springer, 1931, 519 pp.
ROWNTREE, L. G.: Studies in Diabetes Insipidus, Jour. Am. Med. Assn., 1924, **83**, 399.
SMITH, F. M.: Diabetes Insipidus, Treatment by Intranasal Insufflation of Posterior Lobe Powder, Jour. Am. Med. Assn., 1934, **102**, 660.
VEIL, W. H.: Physiologie und Pathologie des Wasserhaushaltes, Ergebn. d. inn. Med. u. Kinderh., 1923, **23**, 648.

HEMOCHROMATOSIS.

Synonym.—Bronze diabetes.

Definition.—Hemochromatosis is a disorder of metabolism of pigment, which is characterized by deposits of iron-containing hemosiderin and other hemic pigments in the liver, spleen, pancreas and other organs, by bronzing of the skin from similar deposits, by cirrhosis of the liver, and diabetes.

Etiology.—Incidence.—Relatively few cases have been reported. The diagnosis was made in 27 cases in the Mayo Clinic in a period of ten years.

The cause of the disturbance is unknown. Mallory produced a similar disease experimentally by poisoning with copper, and obtained a history of exposure to copper in 16 of a series of 19 cases seen clinically. The iron which accumulates in the course of years may amount to as much as 40 grams, or ten times the normal iron content of the body. It is presumed that these deposits of iron injure parenchyma and provoke proliferation of connective tissue. Cirrhosis of the liver ultimately leads to portal obstruction and ascites; that of the pancreas to degeneration of islets and diabetes.

Pathology.—The liver is moderately enlarged, with hypertrophic cirrhosis. It is deep brown in color, as are also the pancreas, the spleen, and other organs, including the lungs. Histologic examination reveals heavy deposits of iron. This is largely contained in reticuloendothelial phagocytes, but also penetrates the parenchymatous cells.

Symptoms.—The outstanding features of the disease are a triad: enlarged cirrhotic liver, bronzed skin, and diabetes. Of the three, any one or two may be inconspicuous and overlooked. The diabetes is likely to develop late in the course of the disease, or to be very mild at first, and gradually increase in severity.

The onset is insidious. The first recognizable manifestation is often discoloration of the skin. This appears mainly on exposed parts, such as the face, neck and hands, but later affects the forearms, feet, legs and trunk. It gives a metallic, iron-brown appearance. The mucous membranes are usually not involved. The liver can be palpated for 3 or 4 cm. below the costal margin. Its edge is firm and likely to be fairly sharp. It is ordinarily not tender. The spleen often can be felt 2 or 3 cm. below the ribs. Glycosuria and hyperglycemia are usually conspicuous. In their absence a glucose tolerance test may reveal latent diabetes. Moderate secondary anemia is noted, but jaundice is absent. The signs of portal obstruction are terminal manifestations.

Diagnosis.—If the triad of symptoms (enlarged liver, bronzed skin, and diabetes) is fully developed, the diagnosis is made. Confirmatory evidence is obtained from a section of the skin (biopsy) after staining for hemosiderin with potassium ferrocyanide. Hemosiderin may also be identified in the urinary sediment (Rous). The melanosis of Addison's disease, the pigmentation of long-standing jaundice, and argyrosis are the principle conditions to be thought of in differential diagnosis.

Prognosis.—The disease runs a slow course, but by the time a diagnosis has been made a fatal outcome may be expected in a few months or one or two years. Exceptions occur; one of our patients has survived seven years since the appearance of symptoms. Death comes as a rule from hepatic insufficiency or from the complications of portal obstruction. The diabetes usually can be controlled successfully by the usual treatment, but resistance to insulin, in one case, made it impossible for us to prevent acidosis.

Treatment.—No specific treatment is known. Treatment is thus purely symptomatic. The diabetes is to be attended to by satisfactory diet and adequate insulin.

REFERENCES.

HALL, E. M., and MacKAY, E. M.: Experimental Hepatic Pigmentation and Cirrhosis. 1. Does Copper Poisoning Produce Pigmentation and Cirrhosis of the Liver? Am. Jour. Path., 1931, **7**, 327.

MALLORY, F. B.: Hemochromatosis and Chronic Poisoning with Copper, Arch. Int. Med., 1926, **37**, 336.

ROUS, PEYTON: Urinary Siderosis: Hemosiderin Granules in the Urine as an Aid in the Diagnosis of Pernicious Anemia, Hemochromatosis, and Other Diseases Causing Siderosis of the Kidney, Jour. Exper. Med., 1918, **28**, 645.

OCHRONOSIS.

Definition.—Ochronosis is a bluish-black pigmentation of cartilages, connective tissues and skin, which develops in the course of the metabolic disturbance known as alkaptonuria, and is also seen in chronic poisoning from phenol.

Incidence.—Oppenheimer and Kline in 1922 collected only 41 cases of ochronosis and few instances have come to notice lately.

Etiology.—Alkaptonuria is of great theoretical interest because of the insight it gives to the mechanism of deaminization and oxidation of the amino acids and for the suggestions it brings as to the origin of body pigments, particularly melanin. The urine, in alkaptonuria, contains homogentisic acid, an intermediate metabolite of tyrosin. This oxidizes in the air, forming a substance much like melanin which accounts both for the strong reducing power of urine containing it and for the black discoloration of such urine on standing or on addition of alkali.

Alkaptonuria is largely inherited. Umber describes a family in which 4 of 8 siblings were affected. It usually manifests itself in infancy by discoloration of the diapers. It may exist for years without ill effects; in some cases it is possibly always harmless, but in others certain cartilages and other tissues acquire an affinity for the abnormal metabolites and deposition of these leads to ochronosis.

Pathology.—The skin in ochronosis, particularly the skin of the axillæ, the scleræ and the cartilages of the nose and ears, develops a bluish-green coloration due to the deposit of derivatives of homogentisic acid. The cartilages of the joints are similarly affected. In the latter some irritation is produced by the foreign material, and proliferative osteo-arthritis results, that may be as debilitating and painful as any other form of arthritis. At necropsy, foci of pigmentation may be seen in the kidneys, the meninges, and the intima of the arteries. A condition very similar to this has also been found in cases of chronic poisoning from phenol. In a very few instances the urine has contained melanin rather than homogentisic acid.

Symptoms and Diagnosis.—A urine which reduces Benedict's solution when cold and turns black on standing or, more rapidly, when alkali is added, is diagnostic of alkaptonuria. Bluish-black pigmentation of the scleræ, the cartilages of the ear, and the axillary skin speaks for ochronosis. With such features alkaptonuric arthritis should be suspected if the joints are diseased.

Treatment.—The use of phenol or similar chemical as applications to the skin should be stopped. The diet ought to contain not over 0.50 gram of protein for each kilogram of body weight, and a part of this may be given in the form of gelatin, which contains only traces of tyrosin.

REFERENCES.

GRAFE, E.: Die Krankheiten des Stoffwechsels und ihre Behandlung, Berlin, Springer, 1931, 519 pp.

HOWARD, C. P., and MILLS, E. S.: Ochronosis, Oxford Med., 1932, **4**, 223.

OPPENHEIMER, B. S., and KLINE, B. S.: Ochronosis with a Study of an Additional Case, Arch. Int. Med., 1922, **29**, 732.

CHAPTER XXIII.

DISEASES DUE TO PHYSICAL AND TOXIC AGENTS.

By DAVID P. BARR, M.D.

DISEASES DUE TO PHYSICAL AGENTS.
Heat Exhaustion and Heat Stroke.
Caisson Disease.
Mountain Sickness.
Electric Shock.
Radio-active Substances.

THE INTOXICATIONS.
Alcoholism.
Opium Habit.
Cocainism.
Food Poisoning.
Botulism.
Milk Sickness.
Snake Venom Poisoning.

DISEASES DUE TO PHYSICAL AGENTS.

HEAT EXHAUSTION AND HEAT STROKE.

Introduction.—With wide fluctuations in the temperature of the environment the temperature of the human body is regulated within extremely narrow limits. Heat produced by oxidative processes is constantly lost from the surface by means of radiation and conduction and by evaporation of water from the skin and lungs. When the temperature of the environment equals or is greater than that of the body, no heat can be lost by radiation and conduction, and compensation is attempted by increasing vaporization of water through sweating and increased respiration. Haldane has shown that the storage of heat begins with less unfavorable conditions and that a man is unable to maintain his normal temperature when sitting in still, saturated air at 89° F. Under such circumstances there may be a gain of 1° F. per hour. In air saturated with water vapor at 94° F. the increase in body temperature is as much as 2°, and at 98° F., 4° per hour.

Sensitiveness to external heat varies greatly in different individuals and may be increased by a number of factors, such as fatigue, alcoholism and particularly by circulatory diseases. Continued exposure to heat sometimes seems to increase tolerance, but this may be explained at least in part by modified activity, increased muscular efficiency and lessened food intake. On the other hand, exposure to excessive heat gradually breaks down the mechanism for heat regulation and increases susceptibility.

Whenever environmental conditions or individual factors cause a retention of heat in the body, symptoms of greater or less severity become apparent.

Mild Heat Retention.—If with continued heat and damp atmosphere the body temperature rises 3° to 4° F., there is restlessness, headache, throbbing, dizziness, shortness of breath and rapidity of pulse-rate.

With the onset of these symptoms, sweating, which has been excessive, is diminished and micturition becomes more frequent.

Heat Exhaustion or Collapse.—In many cases the manifestations of mild heat retention become exaggerated and are accompanied by exhaustion, vertigo, dimness of vision and inability to walk or to make any effort. The pupils are dilated, the face becomes pale, the pulse weak and rapid. The skin often feels cold and clammy. Temperature by mouth may be normal, but the rectal temperature is usually moderately increased.

Heat Cramps.—These usually follow prolonged work in heated surroundings, such as the boiler or engine rooms of steamers. There is muscular twitching, followed by violent cramps of the muscles of the trunk and extremities. Spasms of the respiratory muscles are often sufficient to interfere with respiration. Nausea and vomiting may be prominent features. There is scantiness or suppression of urine, and demonstrable concentration of blood, signs which indicate dehydration and which might be expected when it is remembered that workers in extremely heated environments require 2, 3 or more quarts of water per hour.

Hyperpyrexia (Heat Stroke, Sunstroke, Insolation).—Extremely high temperature may develop suddenly in very heated chambers or in persons exposed to continued heat out of doors. Premonitory symptoms characteristic of heat retention, the most common of which is headache, may sometimes give warning of the attack. More often there is sudden collapse with rapid rise in body temperature. Unconsciousness or deep coma is occasionally preceded by a short period of delirium. The pupils, which are at first dilated, become contracted. The skin is dry and very hot. Petechial spots are not uncommon. The respiration is deep and labored, later irregular and of the Cheyne-Stokes type. The pulse is rapid, with rates of 160 to 180. There may be almost complete muscular relaxation and flaccidity, or twitchings and spasms may occur. Death is usually preceded by pulmonary edema.

Treatment.—The mortality from exhaustion, collapse and cramps is slight. The mildest forms require no therapy other than rest and removal to cool surroundings. With more severe symptoms correction of dehydration is the most important measure. Massage may be helpful in the symptomatic management of heat cramps. Cases of hyperpyrexia have a high mortality and much depends upon prompt treatment. Not only the height of the temperature but the interval during which it persists is important. Efforts must be instituted at once to lower the fever. The safest as well as the most effective means of reducing body temperature is to spray the patient with cool water and to evaporate the water rapidly with fans. Cool, wet sheets over which fans play may be substituted with good results. The circulation of the skin by which loss of heat by radiation depends must be maintained by constant rubbing. The older treatments by ice-packs and by ice-rubs are less effective and have certain disadvantages. The evaporation of 1 gram of water removes more than seven times as much heat as the melting of 1 gram of ice. Ice placed next to the skin, even under the conditions of heat stroke, may diminish the circulation of the skin and drive the blood to deeper portions of the body, causing interference with heat loss.   There is also danger that sudden changes in circulation may place extra strain on the heart and precipitate collapse.   In treatment the reduction in temperature should not be continued below 102° F. lest subnormal temperatures result.   Artificial respiration may be indicated in cases where muscular spasms of the diaphragm complicate the picture.   Since in any case of insolation dehydration may be an important factor, fluids should be given in abundance and, if they cannot be taken by mouth, should be administered by rectum, subcutaneously or intravenously.

Sequelæ.—Survival until the second day usually indicates recovery. A temperature of 102° or 103° F. may persist for several days, and in hot weather relapses sometimes occur.   The patient often remains excited, or may have delusions which require careful watching during convalescence.   Headaches which persist for many months and impairment of memory are not uncommon.   Recurrent attacks of muscle spasm have been reported, and there is in many cases a continued susceptibility to even moderate degrees of heat.

REFERENCES.

EDSALL, D. L.:   Two Cases of Violent but Transitory Myokymia and Myotonia Apparently Due to Excessive Hot Weather, Am. Jour. Med. Sci., 1904, **128**, 1003.

HALDANE, J. S.:   The Influence of High Air Temperatures, Jour. Hyg., 1905, **5**, 494.

STURGIS, C. C.:   The Effects of Heat, Oxford Med., 1926, **4**, 664 (1), New York, Oxford University Press.

CAISSON DISEASE.

Synonyms.—The Bends; Compressed air illness; Diver's palsy.

Definition.—The disease of caisson workers and divers caused by too rapid decompression following exposure to increased pressure.

History.—The history of diving and of caisson disease has been most attractively reviewed in Leonard Hill's monograph.   Physiologic studies of the effects of high pressure date from 1670, when Boyle experimented on animals under different air pressures and demonstrated the presence of gases in the blood. Hoppe-Seyler was able to demonstrate that bubbles of gas in blood could cause death in animals after rapid decompression, while von Leyden considered the bubbles in the white matter of the spinal cord as the cause of clinical paralysis. The classical studies of Paul Bert revealed the rôle of nitrogen in the causation of the symptoms.

Pathogenesis.—Since all of the air-containing cavities of the body are in communication with the exterior, changes in external pressure are immediately equalized and no direct mechanical effects are noted and no discomfort is apparent even at pressures of 6 to 7 atmospheres. It is true that occlusion of any communicating passage, such as the Eustachian tube, may lead to rupture of the ear drum and hemorrhage in the middle ear, but this is accidental and has no essential part in the clinical picture of caisson disease.

When the air in the environment is compressed the whole body comes into a new gaseous equilibrium.   According to Dalton's law gases are soluble in fluids according to their partial pressures.   At 4 atmospheres, therefore, the plasma leaving the lungs holds four times as much nitrogen as under normal atmospheric conditions. The tissues in turn become saturated at the new level at a rate which varies with the particular ability of the tissue to absorb the gas and with the adequacy of the circulation to bring nitrogen to the part. Fat, which absorbs about five times as much nitrogen as water, is saturated slowly. Ligaments, bones and the white matter of the spinal cord attain the new equilibrium more gradually because of a limited blood supply. Even with the increased circulation rate consequent upon manual work, several hours may elapse before the entire body is saturated at the new level.

When the pressure is again reduced the rate of desaturation is irregular and those parts which acquired nitrogen slowly tend to retain it. At the end of the period of decompression such tissues as fat may hold an amount of nitrogen which cannot be immediately dissolved in the blood. Bubbles may thus be formed either in the tissues or in the blood. These are seen most often in the venous blood, in fat deposits, in the synovial fluid of the joints and in the white matter of the brain and spinal cord. Air embolism in the pulmonary vessels is not infrequent.

Pressures to which divers and caisson workers expose themselves are usually measured in pounds or in terms of an atmosphere, which is approximately 15 pounds to the square inch. Pressure gauges record the amount by which the atmospheric pressure is exceeded. Ordinary caisson pressures for bridges and tunnels have not exceeded 30 to 35 pounds, although for the St. Louis Bridge across the Mississippi the gauge pressure of the chambers reached 48 pounds. Divers have descended, however, over 200 feet, where the extra pressure approximated 7 atmospheres.

The extent of damage in caisson disease does not depend upon the rate at which pressure is applied. The period required for compression is comparatively brief, depending chiefly upon the rapidity with which air-pressure can be equalized in the middle ear. The important factors are the degree of pressure, the total time the individual is exposed and the rate of decompression. In general the higher the pressure and the shorter the period of decompression the greater will be the risk. There is little or no danger at pressures less than 15 pounds above normal atmospheric conditions, no matter how rapidly the decompression is accomplished. Exposure for short intervals, even to extremely high pressures, is not followed by accidents. For this reason, naked deep-sea divers have little difficulty because they remain under water for only two or three minutes. In the caissons of the St. Louis Bridge Company no cases of bends occurred among many visitors, although of 352 employees, 12 were killed and 18 were seriously injured by caisson disease.

Symptoms.—The manifestations are extremely variable both because of the factors regulating the formation of nitrogen bubbles and because of their wide distribution. Commonly the onset of symptoms occurs from one to three hours after decompression. There is severe pain about one or more joints and in the muscles. In many cases the effects disappear in a few hours even without treatment. Somewhat less often there is severe abdominal pain associated with nausea and vomiting and with violent pains in the legs. These attacks are spoken of by the workmen as "the bends." There may be giddiness, or vertigo, and deafness from bubbles in the inner ear, or paralyses, usually in the legs, which appear suddenly and vary from weakness to complete loss of motion and sensation. Monoplegias and hemiplegias are rare. Keays found that 89 per cent of the patients observed during the building of the East River tunnels in New York showed pains in various parts of the body, 2 per cent symptoms referable to the nervous system. The fatalities amounted to 0.5 per cent of the total who presented symptoms. In these cases pains appear only a few minutes after decompression. The patient soon becomes unconscious and dyspneic. The temperature falls and the pulse becomes rapid and feeble. Examination may show bubbles of gas in the blood itself, with foam in the right heart.

Prophylaxis.—Rules have been formulated for the selection and care of caisson workers and divers. Obese individuals are believed to be especially susceptible. Exposure to pressures of 50 pounds for more than one or two hours has been considered hazardous. By far the most important of preventive measures, however, is properly conducted decompression. This may be conducted either by lowering pressure at a uniform rate until normal atmospheric conditions have been attained, or by the stage method, in which pressure is lowered immediately and rapidly to a previously determined safe level, at which it is held for an interval before further change of pressure. This method, which is less time-consuming than the gradual reduction, is based upon the discovery of J. S. Haldane that serious trouble is to be anticipated only when the pressure of the gas in the lungs falls below one-half that of the gas in the blood and tissues. When it is possible to use mixtures of helium and oxygen in caissons and deep-sea diving the risk of injury is less because the solubility coefficient of blood and tissues is less for helium than for nitrogen.

Treatment.—Relief from symptoms may be obtained by immediate recompression. Even cases with severe symptoms or with early paralytic manifestations may be saved if treatment is started at once. The need for prompt attention has led to the establishment of medical air locks and to rules that caisson workers shall sleep in the neighborhood of the caisson.

REFERENCES.

Du Bois, E. F.: Physiology of Respiration in Relationship to the Problems of Naval Medicine. VI. Deep Diving, U. S. Nav. Med. Bull., 1929, **27**, 311.
Hill, Leonard: Caisson Disease and the Physiology of Work in Compressed Air, London, Arnold, 1912.

MOUNTAIN SICKNESS.

Exposure to the atmospheric conditions of high altitudes and to lowered oxygen tensions from any cause produces symptoms which are included under the designation of mountain sickness, or anoxemia. The ill-effects are usually attributable to want of oxygen and have been most studied during ascents to high mountains, during balloon ascents or aëroplane flights, and in chambers especially devised to permit of variations in oxygen-pressure.

The rate at which oxygen-pressure is lowered is important. Sudden exposure to a considerable deprivation of oxygen, such as takes place in aviation, produces symptoms not unlike simple asphyxia, with cyanosis, muscular incoördination, intense irritability, grave disturbances in judgment, and unconsciousness. Some individuals faint with slight exposure. In others, unconsciousness is sometimes preceded by convulsions. There is a wide variation in the resistance of different people to altitude, some collapsing at 10,000 feet, while others are capable of resisting 20,000 feet for a short period. Few individuals fail to suffer some ill effects from ascents to more than 12,000 feet. It is believed that without the use of extra oxygen no flying is safe above 18,000 feet.

Effects become more gradually apparent during ascents of high mountains. Symptoms of headache, vertigo, mental dullness, abnormalities of vision are common. There may be also epistaxis, nausea, vomiting, cyanosis, dyspnea, palpitation and muscular weakness. With slight exertion, breathing becomes extremely labored. Hyperpnea produces diminished alveolar carbon dioxide tension and increases the excitability of the respiratory centers. There is a tendency to alkalosis, which is evident by a diminished excretion of acid and ammonia from the kidneys.

Patients with heart disease may be susceptible to moderate elevations, and symptoms such as precordial pain, breathlessness and irregularities in respiration may be greatly accentuated during exposure to altitudes.

Adaptation is accomplished by increased ability to absorb oxygen, dependent in part upon increased pulmonary ventilation and in part upon increase in the number of red cells and the amount of hemoglobin. In the highest habitable mountains the red blood counts of natives may average 8,000,000. Adaptation continues over a long period, but in a few days has progressed to the extent of diminishing the acute symptoms of mountain sickness.

Treatment consists entirely of oxygen inhalations and rest.

REFERENCES.

BARCROFT, J., BINGER, C. A., BOCK, A. V., and others: Observations Upon the Effect of High Altitude Upon the Physiological Processes of the Human Body, Phil. Trans. Roy Soc., London, 1923, B. 211, p. 351.

SCHNEIDER, E. C.: Physiological Effects of Altitude, Physiol. Rev., 1921, **1**, 631.

ELECTRIC SHOCK.

Serious or fatal injury from electricity may be caused by lightning and may follow contact with currents of high voltage or of voltages used in domestic lighting currents. When the common use of electrical apparatus is considered, it is remarkable that injury is not more frequent. In the statistics collected by Schereschewsky for the years from 1910 to 1920, less than 1 death per 100,000 was attributed to electricity. The deaths from lightning averaged about 1 in 200,000.

Death and Injury from Lightning.—Since a lightning flash may represent electrical force involving millions of volts and a current of thousands of amperes, it is not surprising that death is often instantaneous. In such cases there may be muscular rigidity which causes the victim to retain the attitude held immediately before the lightning stroke.

Possibly more than one-half of those who are struck by lightning recover. The most constant symptom is unconsciousness of variable duration. Respiration may cease temporarily and the breathing which is resumed spontaneously or through artificial respiration remains for some time irregular and stertorous. Collapse symptoms with cold extremities and small rapid pulse are not infrequent. There may be tremors or convulsions. Difficulty in swallowing and vomiting, conjunctivitis and photophobia are common. Burns, ecchymoses and lacerations may be found, particularly in the feet and legs.

High Tension Currents.—Contact with electrical currents of high voltage causes an instantaneous violent contraction of the muscles. There is a sudden leap followed by complete unconsciousness. When contact is made by the hands, the muscular spasm induced by the shock may cause the hands to freeze on the wire, making release difficult or impossible as long as the current is maintained. Death results from respiratory paralysis while the heart continues to beat vigorously, stopping only because of asphyxia. Burns at the site of contact are often extensive and range from singeing of the hair to carbonization of tissue. When the hands remain in contact with the current even the bones may be charred.

Low Tension Currents.—Lighting by incandescent lamps in the home is usually accomplished with low voltage, the standard varying from 110 to 120 volts. Although contacts with such tensions are frequent, accidents have been uncommon and there exists a general impression that no precautions are necessary. Under certain conditions, however, these voltages may become not only unsafe but an actual menace to life. While dry human skin has great electrical resistance, it is seldom completely dry, and when wet, either with copious perspiration or by contact with water, it offers a good conducting medium. Accidents have occurred not infrequently to people in bathtubs who have tried to apply electrical apparatus to themselves or who have attempted to move electric fans or heaters. When death occurs from low tension currents, it may be instantaneous with abrupt cessation of the heart-beat.

Causes of Death.—High tension currents kill by inhibiting the nerve centers, particularly the respiratory center. The heart remains unaffected. Low tension currents cause death by action on the heart. It is well known that auricular fibrillation may be produced in animals by passing a feeble alternating current through the auricular muscle. Ventricular fibrillation results when a current is passed through the ventricles and in larger animals causes immediate death. An electrical current flowing between moistened surfaces on the extremities will pass through the heart as well as other organs. Alternating current of low frequency offers, therefore, ideal conditions for the production of ventricular fibrillation and it is now believed that this is usually the cause of death. The same accidents may occur with direct current, but animals can stand from four to five times the voltage in continuous as in alternating current. Laboratory experiments with artificial lightning indicate that death is caused by a combination of cardiac and respiratory factors.

Treatment.—If the muscular spasm has not thrown the victim clear of the source of electricity, the most pressing need is to break the circuit. If the power cannot be shut off, attempts should be made to separate the individual from the source by a single quick motion. This may be attempted with a non-conductor, like wood or rubber. If the hands are used, they should be covered with a thick, dry, non-conducting material, such as a woolen garment. All moist or metallic substances should be avoided.

When the victim is conscious and the pulse and respiration are maintained, no special treatment is required. With loss of consciousness care must be taken to prevent interference with breathing, and preparations must be made to administer artificial respiration. If the breathing has stopped, artificial respiration by the Schaefer method should be instituted at once. In all cases in which the pulse is still perceptible there is a good chance for recovery. There is no practical means known at present to start again a heart which has undergone ventricular fibrillation.

REFERENCES.

SCHERESCHEWSKY, J. W.: The Effects of Electricity, Nelson Loose-leaf Living Medicine, New York, Nelson and Sons, 1920, **2**, 662.

WILLIAMS, H. B.: Hazard of Low Voltage Shocks, Jour. Am. Med. Assn., 1931, **97**, 156.

RADIO–ACTIVE SUBSTANCES.

The possibility of poisoning from radium and radium emanations has been emphasized recently by cases of poisoning which have occurred in connection with the luminous dial industry. Between the years of 1917 and 1924 a total of 800 girls were employed in a factory in New Jersey for the purpose of painting the dials of watches and clocks with luminous paint, which contained small amounts of radium and mesothorium. For precision in painting it was their custom to wet the brushes with their lips. Cases of poisoning have been studied by Martland, who found that they occurred only in those workers who had been employed for one or two years and that the symptoms did not become apparent until one to seven years after they had left the work. Symptoms were caused by the deposit of radio-active substances in the bones. These were found to give off emanations, 95 per cent of which were shown to be alpha rays. Symptoms in the early cases consisted of severe anemia, often of the aplastic type, leukopenia and destruction by necrosis of the lower or upper jaw or both. Certain chronic cases displayed an osteitis, more or less crippling, without anemia or osseous necrosis. In 18 patients whose deaths were attributed to work with radium paint, 5 developed osteogenic sarcoma.

REFERENCES.

MARTLAND, H. S.: Occupational Poisoning in Manufacture of Luminous Watch Dials, Jour. Am. Med. Assn., 1929, **92**, 466, 552.

———— The Occurrence of Malignancies in Radio-active Persons, Am. Jour. Cancer, 1931, **15**, 2435.

THE INTOXICATIONS.

ALCOHOLISM.

Ethyl alcohol, because of the great number of substances which undergo alcoholic fermentation and because of the pleasurable sensations which it may produce, is the most commonly used intoxicant and narcotic. In relatively small amounts alcohol diminishes the sensation of fatigue and induces joviality and a feeling of importance and increased ability. In larger doses it acts as a narcotic, causing temporary forgetfulness and sleep. There is no satisfactory proof that the moderate use of alcohol causes permanent damage, but in excess it is a poison which injures the parenchyma of internal organs and produces serious deterioration of mental and moral faculties. Continued use is dangerous because of habit formation and increased tolerance. Poisoning from alcoholic beverages is not always due to the alcohol itself but may be attributable in part to aldehydes, ethereal substances or contaminants.

Moderation has not been satisfactorily defined. It has been estimated that a daily limit for an average sedentary person may be 30 to 45 cc. of pure alcohol. The natural tolerance of individuals, however, varies widely and the relationship of tolerance to the toxic effects is almost entirely unknown.

Alcohol is absorbed rapidly and almost completely from the stomach and small intestines. It is oxidized in the body and can be used as a food, sparing the consumption of fat and carbohydrate. Relatively small portions escape in the breath and urine, the amount never exceeding one-tenth of the total and decreasing with habituation. The concentration of alcohol in the blood can be determined and varies with the original dose per kilogram of body weight. When the blood contains more than 0.1 per cent of alcohol there is definite inebriation and, with concentrations of 0.5 per cent, a possibility of fatal poisoning. The amount necessary to maintain a given concentration in the blood increases greatly with habituation, and an acquired tolerance to a daily consumption of 700 cc. of pure alcohol has been noted in chronic alcoholism.

Pathology.—In cases of chronic alcoholic poisoning degeneration of the parenchyma with increased connective tissues is frequently found. The cells of the heart muscle exhibit brown atrophy with fatty infiltration and fibroid replacement between muscle fibers. Arteriosclerosis, particularly of the aorta, the great vessels in the neck and the abdominal vessels, is often seen but is not certainly attributable to alcohol. In the liver there is evidence of parenchymatous degeneration, brown atrophy of cells, fatty infiltration and of the fibrous tissue replacement which characterizes cirrhosis. The spleen shows chronic fibrosis and congestion. There are also chronic fibrous changes in the pancreas and a chronic inflammation of the gastric mucosa. The kidneys are rarely normal in chronic alcoholism, but no definite lesion can be clearly associated with the intoxication.

Atrophy and fibrosis of the testicles and ovaries have been demonstrated. Stockard, by animal experiments, showed that in an animal, drunkenness at the time of mating causes definite injury of the germ cells, with abnormalities in the offspring which may be transmitted through more than one generation.

The membranes of the brain may be congested, with increased fluid in the arachnoid space, which is believed to be compensatory to a diminution in the size of the brain. Hemorrhagic internal pachymeningitis is not uncommon and may be responsible for fatal hemorrhages following trivial accidents. The microscopic appearance of nerve cells has been carefully studied, and changes in staining reactions are demonstrable, with degeneration of the cells of the cerebral cortex and of the ganglion cells of the anterior horns. Intense atheromatous degeneration of the vessels of the brain is frequently seen.

Symptoms.—Acute Alcoholic Intoxication.—When a large amount of alcohol is taken in a short period of time, the influence is chiefly apparent in the nervous system and consists of muscular incoördination and mental disturbances. The skin is flushed and the pulse is full. The pupils are dilated and the patient may become unconscious. Temperature regulation is interfered with and extremely low temperatures have been recorded. The respirations may be slow and deep and in extreme cases there may be circulatory collapse. The diagnosis of acute alcoholism is important and offers difficulties when alcohol has been taken or administered immediately before the onset of uremia, an attack of apoplexy, or an injury of the head. Fractured skulls have not infrequently remained undiagnosed with disastrous results, under the mistaken diagnosis of acute alcoholism.

Chronic Alcoholism.—The harmful effects of chronic alcoholism are numerous, and consist both in demonstrable organic damage and in changes and deterioration in mentality and personality. Many individuals whose nervous systems are extremely tolerant to large amounts of alcohol may suffer organic damage of the heart and liver. On the other hand, an intolerant nervous system may undergo serious degenerative changes without visible evidence of damage in other parts of the body. Deterioration in personality is probably the most constant accompaniment of chronic alcoholic intoxication. The influence of alcohol interferes with the association of ideas, with memory and with initiative. Reasoning and judgment are impaired. Emotional reactions are exaggerated. Laughter is easily induced and anger is aroused with slight provocation. Intentions remain good, but accomplishment is diminished. Partial consciousness of these shortcomings leads to excuses, self-justification and to lying, but also to a sense of inferiority and a deep resentment of criticism. There is often unjustifiable jealousy, extreme irritability and lack of consideration for others. At first these qualities are apparent only during and immediately following the period of alcoholic intoxication but later become permanent defects in character.

Delirium Tremens.—This particular manifestation of chronic alcoholism occurs most often when a severe illness, accident or shock follows a long period of alcoholic indulgence. Several years of previous chronic alcoholism are necessary for its development. Seldom seen in wine and beer drinkers, it is particularly liable to occur following continued ingestion of whisky and other strong liquors. Fractures of the arms, legs and skull, sunstroke and such infections as pneumonia and erysipelas are common predisposing causes. The onset occurs usually three to four days after a chronic toper has been suddenly deprived of alcohol. Actual delirium is preceded by many premonitory symptoms. There may be euphoria and a complete failure to realize any abnormalities. More often there is excitement and restlessness. Horrible dreams which lead to a feeling of dread and anxiety may at first be recognized as phantasies but are gradually replaced by definite hallucinations and delusions. Delirium disappears during the day to recur at night, and with treatment the whole condition may pass off in a few hours.

Persistence of the attack leads to serious illness. There is tinnitus simulating voices which are abusive, accusatory and persistent. The hallucinations are more often visual and may concern the occupation of the patient or consist in the appearance of household animals, or at other times snakes and monstrous unreal creatures. There is usually a lack of realization of the environment, a failure to recognize familiar objects or to remember past events. The patient may be quiet and absorbed or may shout and shriek with terror. Unless most carefully watched, he may do himself physical injury. Suicides during delirium have not been uncommon, although the absorbing character of the hallucinations usually prevents the patient from maturing any plans for self-destruction. A gross trembling, which has given to the condition its name, becomes more and more apparent, and both gait and arm movements become uncertain. The speech is tremulous. In violent attacks the temperature may rise without obvious infection. There is profuse sweating and the pulse may become rapid and weak. The tongue is heavily coated, the appetite disturbed and there is complete sleeplessness, which continues until the attack has ended.

The delirium usually lasts from five to ten days and ends abruptly with sleep, which may last from twelve to thirty hours. Upon awakening the hallucinations have disappeared and there is no longer excitement or fear. The mental processes, however, may remain impaired for many weeks.

When delirium tremens occurs in the course of an acute infection, the prognosis of the original disease is much worse. Pneumonia and erysipelas have an excessively high mortality in alcoholics.

Acute Hallucinosis.—This condition may be closely related to delirium tremens, although its manifestations and prognosis are quite different. It has also been called acute paranoia, or persecutory insanity. It tends to affect younger persons, is often accompanied by acute gastritis and by peripheral neuritis and may follow intense anger or fright. Unlike delirium tremens, hallucinations of hearing are more common than those of sight. Voices are heard coming from the floor, from the wall, accusing, insulting and infuriating the patient. Terror is evident and suicide extremely common. There is also a suspicion of people in attendance and a tendency to misinterpret therapeutic measures as efforts at poisoning. Tremor is not so evident, and orientation is usually maintained. The duration of the condition is usually from one to eight weeks. Recovery is not uncommon, but chronic delirium and Korsakoff's psychosis are frequent sequelæ.

Alcoholic Trance.—This form is noted in psychopathic individuals, in epileptics and following heat stroke and injuries to the skull. Orientation may be entirely lost. At times patients have behaved during the trance with great intelligence and at other times have committed serious crimes without recollection of any phase of their actions at a later time. The attacks are frequently repeated and may be induced by a single drink.

Wet Brain.—In chronic alcoholism, particularly following delirium or injury, there may occur a state of semi-coma, with low muttering delirium, pallor and almost complete immobility. The patient lies flat on his back with his head thrown back and his hands reaching up as in rope climbing. There is tremor and a mumbling, imperfect speech. Such patients are aroused with difficulty, show no interest in their surroundings, do not ask to be fed and in swallowing may inhale food into the trachea. There is usually a rapid pulse and a slightly increased temperature. Pneumonia, which frequently complicates the condition, is almost always fatal. The state may last for days. The legs and arms become stiff, the abdomen retracted and the eyelids closed. If recovery takes place, many weeks are required for convalescence and the mind may be permanently impaired.

Alcoholic Neuritis.—In steady drinkers, more often in women, a peripheral neuritis is not infrequent. The onset is gradual and is preceded by pains and tingling sensations in the extremities. Weakness and paralysis are apparent, first in the feet and legs, later in the hands and forearms. Since the extensor groups of muscles are more involved, foot-drop and wrist-drop are common. Sensory disturbance may be limited to numbness or there may be great pain. The muscles are sore and extremely tender when pressed. The feet and ankles are usually swollen and the gait is uncertain and often ataxic. Weeks or months are necessary for recovery, but the ultimate prognosis is not unfavorable. During recovery patients are apt to walk with a characteristic steppage gait, in which the feet are lifted high and flopped down to avoid the consequences of the foot-drop.

Korsakoff's Psychosis.—Peripheral neuritis is usually associated with moderate degeneration of the cortical cells of the cerebrum. Clinically, a combination of polyneuritis with chronic delirium and disturbed mentality is known as Korsakoff's syndrome or psychosis. This may start with a state like that of delirium tremens, in which the critical sleep fails to occur and in which the delirium changes to a psychosis. The patient may be excited, melancholic or anxious, but more often is jovial or silly. His attention is easily obtained but cannot be held. There is almost complete disorientation as to time and place. The retention of new impressions is defective and loss of memory of the recent past is combined with most extraordinary confabulation, in which imaginary occurrences and the hallucinations of delirium are interwoven to take the place of memory. The neuritis accompanying this condition affects both arms and legs with disturbances of motion and sensation. The cranial nerves may be involved. The pupils are unequal and contracted and may closely simulate the Argyll-Robertson pupil of tabes. There may be weakness of the eye muscles and ptosis.

Recovery is slow and is perhaps never complete. The personality remains permanently changed and there continues to be a lack of initiative, an emotional instability and a sensitivity to alcohol, small amounts of which may produce a recurrence of acute symptoms.

Dipsomania.—The influence of an alcoholic heredity plays a prominent rôle in this form of chronic alcoholism in which the craving for drink is periodic. During long intervals the victim may have no desire for alcohol. Then a single drink or some misfortune produces an irresistible craving for the narcotic effect of the drug. During the sprees drinking is usually continued until a state of utter forgetfulness has been attained. The hope of blotting out an unpleasant past or some particular sorrow, disgrace or disappointment may be the reason assigned for the individual episodes. It is now believed, however, that many cases express a phase of manic depressive insanity in which drinking is undertaken at the end of the period of exaltation.

Treatment.—Acute alcoholism rarely requires special therapeutic measures. If indulgence has been recent, the stomach should be washed out and, since the patient has usually been without food for some time, bland nourishment should be administered while the stomach tube is still in place.

Chronic alcoholism, when dependent upon a habit, is difficult to treat outside of an institution. When dependent upon heredity, recurrence of the habit is almost inevitable. In delirium tremens the patient must be confined to bed and watched continuously. Restraints should be sufficient but as gentle as possible to prevent struggling and exhaustion. Sodium bromide, in doses of 2 grams (30 grains), and chloral hydrate, in doses of 1 gram (15 grains), may exert a sedative effect. Paraldehyde, in amounts of 10 to 15 cc., is relatively safe and may be helpful in controlling the more violent manifestations of the delirium. Barbital, phenobarbital and other barbituric acid derivatives may be tried. During the summer months the extreme muscular activity and long duration of the condition may produce disturbance of heat regulation and result in heat stroke. Douches are required to control the temperature and when judiciously used sometimes exert a sedative effect. In the condition of wet brain recovery is aided by forcing the patient to sit up and by stimulating his attention.

Methyl Alcohol Poisoning.—Because of its use as an adulterant, poisoning by wood alcohol assumed added importance during prohibition. Unlike ethyl alcohol, it is not completely oxidized in the body but is converted into formic acid, which is the active toxic agent. Poisoning may occur from drinking, from rubbing the skin or from inhaling the fumes of methyl alcohol. Some persons show surprising idiosyncrasy and extremely small amounts have produced serious damage. The immediate effects are not unlike those of ethyl alcohol. Inebriation, however, is accompanied by intensely unpleasant symptoms: dizziness, nausea and vomiting, and abdominal pain, often with diarrhea. Dyspnea may become intense, and there is cyanosis which is not corrected by overventilation. Formic acid produces an acidosis with low carbon dioxide combining-power. There is intense thirst. Dimness of vision may not be immediately evident, but appears in a few hours and progresses to complete loss of light perception. In some cases restoration of vision appears after a few days, but is transient and followed by permanent blindness. *Treatment* consists of lavage of the stomach if the poisoning has been recent. Alkaline treatment by mouth and intravenously may control the acidosis but has little influence on the ultimate prognosis.

Ginger Paralysis (Jake Paralysis).—In 1930 several curious epidemics of peripheral neuritis occurred in the midwestern and southwestern parts of the United States. More recently there has been a similar outbreak in California. In all cases the symptoms followed drinking of adulterated fluid extract of Jamaica ginger, a preparation which had been adjudged non-potable and on which there were no sale restrictions. The attacks were surprising, since the ordinary official fluid extract of ginger produces no effects other than those of alcohol. Symptoms appeared from ten days to three weeks following ingestion of the drink. The clinical picture was that of a flaccid paralysis with bilateral foot-drop and wrist-drop. Smith and Elvove have shown that the neuritis is not due to alcohol or to any substance intrinsic in the Jamaica ginger but to an adulterant, a phenol ester having the pharmacologic properties of tri-ortho-cresyl-phosphate.

REFERENCES.

LAMBERT, A.: Intoxicants and Narcotics, Nelson Loose-leaf Living Medicine, New York, Nelson and Sons, 1920, **2**, 555.

SMITH, M. I., and ELVOVE, E.: Pharmacological and Chemical Studies of the Cause of So-called Ginger Paralysis, Pub. Health Rep., 1930, **45**, 1703.

——— Pharmacological Action of Certain Phenol Esters with Special Reference to the Etiology of So-called Ginger Paralysis, Pub. Health Rep., 1930, **45**, 2509.

OPIUM HABIT.

The habit of taking opium and opium derivatives (morphinism) may be acquired in several ways. In the Orient opium smoking is common. In large cities in the United States heroin addiction has in many instances been acquired almost as a social habit among the young. Continued pain, such as severe neuralgia, tabetic crises or colic may lead to habituation in others, and the carelessness of physicians in continuing the drug even in small doses during persistent pain has no doubt been responsible for many cases of addiction. In neurotic and emotionally unstable individuals the effects of the drug once experienced become a refuge from reality and a narcotic to produce forgetfulness of an unpleasant past or present.

Morphine may be taken by mouth or more often by hypodermic. Before heroin was withdrawn from the market and became so difficult to obtain, it was used widely by inhalation as well as by mouth. Codeine does not form a habit even when taken over long periods of time.

In sensitive individuals relatively small doses, 8 to 15 mg., of morphine sulphate, several times each day over two to three weeks, is sufficient to establish the habit. Tolerance is rapidly acquired, and the amount necessary to accomplish the desired effect constantly increases until huge amounts seem necessary. In some cases enormous doses are taken and tolerance for still greater amounts is established. Light found that patients receiving 1 gram per day were able to take 4 grams after four to five days without symptoms and without prolongation in the period when they were free from craving. A few individuals establish their dosage at 0.12 to 0.2 gram per day, a level which is not exceeded over long periods.

Symptoms.—Opium and morphine, unlike alcohol, produce no demonstrable lesions, but exert their effects entirely as functional poisons of the nervous system. Administration of the drug is often followed by euphoria, so intense and pleasant that few who have once experienced it can resist the desire for its return. Effects from ordinary dosage last from three to six hours and are followed by an almost complete return to normal conditions. With continued use, however, it is found that the usual therapeutic dose is no longer followed by the same pleasurable sensations and that with the disappearance of the initial effect there are disagreeable withdrawal symptoms, such as lassitude, nausea, moderate epigastric distress and mental depression. The obvious deleterious effects of the opium habit may be long delayed. Changes in character, selfishness, indifference to family responsibilities, slovenliness of dress and behavior may gradually make themselves apparent. There is restlessness, irritability, sudden unreasonable suspicion and anger. There may be periods of amnesia. Initiative is paralyzed so that the patient becomes more and more inactive. A feeling of remorse and inferiority leads to periods of bitter unhappiness and to ugly resentment against criticism and restraint. Sleep becomes fitful and hallucinations, both visual and auditory, may develop. The appetite is poor with frequent nausea and obstinate constipation. Itching is a prominent symptom.

The physical changes so often emphasized in descriptions of long-continued morphinism are avoidable by proper attention to nutrition. Many morphine addicts remain undetected for years. Light, in a recent study of 100 unselected cases, was unable to find any single sign or symptom entirely characteristic of morphine poisoning. Studies of vital capacity, of efficiency tests, of renal and hepatic function presented no abnormalities. On the other hand, there is in many cases emaciation, pallor and premature grayness. The pulse is slow with a low tension. Pupils are unequal and dilated except during the action of the drug, when they may be quite small. Deep reflexes may be absent and the soles of the feet often become so hyperesthetic as to interfere with walking. Unrestrained continuation of the habit with large doses leads to apathy, loss of appetite, profound emaciation and asthenia, in which the patient succumbs to accidental infection.

Prognosis.—Those who have acquired the habit in order to relieve severe pain are usually anxious to have treatment, coöperate well and are not likely to resume use of the drug if pain does not return. Those who have used opium as a defense or a narcotic undertake treatment reluctantly and return again and again to their habituation. Legal detention and enforced cures may not be sufficient for control.

Treatment.—The management of the opium habit usually demands institutional care. The patient should be isolated and in some cases kept in bed under strictest supervision for seven to ten days. There should be systematic, abundant feeding while the drug is gradually withdrawn. Ordinarily it is possible to reduce the dosage by one-half in twenty-four hours, and again by one-half during the second day. In each case, however, there is a minimum beyond which the dose cannot be rapidly reduced without profound suffering. The symptoms of withdrawal reach a maximum on the third day and consist of extreme restlessness, frequent yawning, muscular trembling, abdominal pain and pains in joints and muscles. Patients may become almost maniacal, frequently resort to violence and may stoop to any crime in order to obtain the drug. Physically there may be rapid loss of weight, concentration of the blood and marked leukocytosis, factors which can be largely controlled by adequate intake of fluid. The withdrawal symptoms disappear in ten to fourteen days. With their subsidence tolerance is lost, euphoria can be produced by small amounts of the drug, and doses formerly taken with slight effect may prove fatal.

Many drugs have been tried in the effort to hasten treatment and control the withdrawal symptoms. Codeine is the drug of choice. Lambert, in a recent comparison of the effects of various preparations, has advised the following treatment: The dosage of morphine habitually taken may be reduced one-tenth per day so that in ten days the withdrawal is complete. On the first day codeine is given in doses of 0.03 gram, every four hours. The dosage of codeine is increased as the morphine is withdrawn until on the fifth day 0.3 gram is given every four hours. This dosage is continued during the remainder of the period of withdrawal and for four days thereafter. The codeine administration is then rapidly tapered off for four or five days until no drug is being taken. With this treatment withdrawal symptoms are reduced to a minimum and consist only of moderate irritability and restlessness.

The breaking of habit is much easier than prevention of recurrence. In after-care, psychologic reëducation is essential but may not be sufficient in those who have sought the drug as an escape from reality and the humdrum of life.

COCAINISM.

Cocaine relieves fatigue, causes a sense of exhilaration and greatly increased muscular and mental strength. It induces voluble conversation which may be silly, rambling and without point. It is often taken by alcoholic and morphine addicts when the effects of their drugs begin to wear off. Following the stimulation of the drug there is restlessness, gross muscular tremors which at times may resemble large choreiform movements, and insomnia. Continuation of the habit leads to rapid moral deterioration. There is irritability and excite-

66

ment. The victim becomes suspicious, morose and exhibits unreasonable anxiety and dread. Hallucinations may be auditory, visual or tactile. Formication, or the sensation of insects crawling over or underneath the skin, is a frequent symptom. Persecutory delusions often make the victims extremely dangerous. To protect themselves from their persecutors they carry firearms, which they do not hesitate to use. Not infrequently true insanity develops. It is characterized by both hallucinations and delusions, and in many respects resembles alcoholic hallucinosis. Physically there is anemia, emaciation and extreme muscular flaccidity. *Treatment* is similar to that of morphine addiction. In general the habit is easier to break and it is usually possible to withdraw the drug at once. Recurrences are frequent.

REFERENCES.

LAMBERT, A.: Treatment of Drug Addiction, Jour. Am. Med. Assn., 1931, **96**, 825.

LIGHT, A. B.: Physiologic Aspects of Opium Addiction, Jour. Am. Med. Assn., 1931, **96**, 823.

FOOD POISONING.

Many injurious effects may be produced by the ingestion of food. Any poisonous substance can be introduced in food, either through accident or intent. Animal parasites as well as bacteria of such serious diseases as typhoid, diphtheria, scarlet fever, streptococcus sore throat and tuberculosis may contaminate food or drink. In many allergic and sensitive individuals foods which cause no difficulty in others may produce most distressing symptoms. Although the term of food poisoning could properly be applied to these conditions, it is usually reserved for several fairly well recognized clinical conditions: (1) food infection caused by members of the salmonella group of organisms; (2) food intoxication from the toxin of Clostridium botulinum; (3) poisons which occur naturally in a few foods.

"Ptomaine poisoning" is a confusing designation which in the past has been used almost as a synonym for food poisoning. Ptomaines are cleavage products of protein putrefaction and usually result from bacterial action. They have been under special suspicion because they react in some respects like vegetable alkaloids. It has not been demonstrated that these substances are active or poisonous in the body or that they are implicated in cases of food intoxication.

Food Infection.—Food infection is a condition usually caused by eating food which has been contaminated by Spirillum enteritidis and other members (Spirillum choleræ suis, Spirillum suipestifer, Spirillum aertrycke) of a group of bacteria which are Gram-negative and which occupy a position intermediate between the colon and typhoid bacilli. Other organisms, such as Bacillus proteus, Bacillus prodigiosus and even the Bacillus coli, have been, without convincing proof, considered as causes of food infection.

Epidemics usually occur during the summer and autumn, in those months when typhoid and dysentery are most prevalent. The outbreaks tend to be small, and those involving more than a few people are due to milk. The bacteria grow in the food before it is eaten.

Meat and meat products form the most frequent sources. Cattle and other food animals are susceptible to infection with the Gaertner bacillus, and meat from animals killed while suffering with diarrhea, local abscesses, puerperal sepsis and septicemia frequently carry the organism. Poisoning may be produced, however, by fresh foods which have been contaminated by extensive handling and allowed to stand for several hours. Human carriers of the organism are extremely uncommon, but rats and mice may carry Bacillus suipestifer and possibly Bacillus enteritidis. Contamination by the feces of these household pests may furnish the source of infection. The organisms of this group are not known to produce toxins, nor is their growth accompanied by any recognizable odor. Food is usually not altered in taste, smell or appearance and the presence of organisms can no more be noted than could that of typhoid, dysentery or cholera.

Recently several small outbreaks of food poisoning have been attributed to contamination with staphylococci, the evidence resting upon the demonstration of the organisms in food and upon the production of symptoms in human feeding experiments. Of 7 outbreaks studied by McBurney, 2 were traced to milk, 2 to cake, 1 to cheese, 1 to chicken gravy and 1 to chocolate eclairs.

Symptoms.—The incubation period varies from four to seventy-two hours, although usually it is between six and twelve hours. Several meals may be taken before the first symptoms appear and the food found in the stomach at the time of onset may not be that which caused the attack. The onset is usually abrupt, with headache, chills, and fever of 102° or 103° F. Gastro-intestinal symptoms are the most notable, and nausea and vomiting, abdominal pain, severe diarrhea, with tenesmus and frequent watery stools, are usual. There is prostration and sometimes nervousness, restlessness or abnormal drowsiness. The attack usually lasts only from twenty-four to forty-eight hours. The severity varies greatly in different epidemics. Symptoms may be insufficient to keep the patient from work, but rarely may be fulminant, with death in twenty-four hours. The average mortality of many epidemics has been only 1 or 2 per cent.

The symptoms resulting from contamination of food with staphylococci do not differ materially from those following infection by the salmonella group of organisms except in the relatively short incubation period which in McBurney's cases averaged about two to three hours.

Diagnosis.—Gross examination of food, even when it is recognized as the cause, furnishes no clue to the presence of organisms. Proof of infection rests in the demonstration of the bacteria in the food or, with severe cases, in the blood, urine, feces or viscera of the patient. The organisms may persist in the stools for a week or ten days following infection. Agglutination tests are seldom positive until six or eight days after the onset but are valuable diagnostic aids since positive reactions in low dilutions are seldom found in non-infected individuals.

Treatment.—If the patient is seen early, induction of vomiting or lavage with warm saline solution is indicated. Diarrhea is usually severe and sufficient to cause complete evacuation of the poison from the intestine without additional catharsis.   Bismuth subcarbonate, in doses of 1 to 2 grams, well stirred in water may be given frequently to allay irritation.   During the acute attack the diet should be limited to bland liquids and semi-solid foods.

Botulism (Allantiasis).—Botulism is a type of food poisoning caused by the toxins of the anaërobic saprophytic organism, Clostridium botulinum, a large Gram-positive bacillus which was discovered in 1894 by van Ermengen during an epidemic in Belgium.   There are three and possibly more types of the organism.   Like other anaërobes, its habitat is thought to be in the soil and in the intestinal canal.   It grows at room temperature or at 37° C.   The spores are destroyed by heat of 120° C. in six minutes but may resist boiling for five hours.

The bacillus produces a true soluble exotoxin which is unique in retaining its toxicity when taken by mouth.   It is produced by the bacillus only under anaërobic conditions, most abundantly at 37° C. It is not formed in brine containing over 6 per cent of sodium chloride and is readily destroyed by heating at 75° C. for ten minutes.   The toxin is extremely powerful, 0.000001 cc. being sufficient to kill a 250-gram guinea-pig in three or four days.   Tasting or nibbling badly infected food has not infrequently caused death in man.   The toxin injures especially the nervous system, but also causes dilatation, thrombosis and hemorrhages in blood-vessels.   Each strain of the organism elaborates a poison which produces a corresponding antitoxin.   All strains do not produce a potent toxin.

Clostridium botulinum grows in a great variety of protein-containing foods, both plant and animal.   Poisoning has occurred from infected sausage, ham, fish, corn, asparagus, beans and ripe olives.   It does not occur in fresh food and has appeared when food has undergone smoking, canning or pickling.   In the United States no commercially preserved food has been connected with any of the recognized cases of botulism since 1925.   Home-packed food has usually been responsible for poisoning because the methods of preserving are empiric and relatively unskilled, and the temperature may not be sufficient to kill the spores. In the United States the intoxication has usually been associated with plant foods, while in Europe meat, meat products and fish have been the most frequent causes.   Preserved food which contains botulinus toxin shows almost always some sign of spoilage, but if uncontaminated by other organisms reveals no special odor or taste.   To the expert a certain rancid odor present in cultures of the organism may be significant.

Botulism is relatively rare and has been more common in Europe than in America.   In 1931 Meyer found records in the United States of 191 outbreaks involving 625 people.   California, Washington and Colorado have furnished most of the cases.   In addition to the human disease, the organism is responsible for forage poisoning in horses, and limber neck in chickens and turkeys.

Symptoms.—The incubation period depends upon the amount and virulence of the toxin.   It is usually eighteen to thirty-six hours but may be four to six days.   Gastro-intestinal symptoms are by no means constant.   There may be at the onset considerable gastric distress with nausea, vomiting and diarrhea, which in a short time is followed by obstinate constipation with distention. The first symptoms in most cases are fatigue, headache, dizziness and muscular weakness, which are followed by the main features of the disease. There is dimness of vision, diplopia, ptosis, dilatation of the pupils, difficulty in articulation and in swallowing. The mucous membranes of the mouth and throat are dry and the tongue becomes coated and foul. Muscular weakness is progressive. There is incoördination, and in severe cases a complete flaccidity. A striking feature is the almost complete absence of sensory disturbance and of pain. Blindness may occur but the mind remains clear until a short time before death. The temperature remains low and is frequently subnormal. The pulse, which at first is slow in severe cases, becomes rapid. Death is most frequently due to respiratory paralysis.

Diagnosis.—The symptoms are usually sufficient for recognition of the condition. The mere presence of organisms does not permit positive diagnosis since the spores are frequently present in the soil. The toxin may be demonstrated by injection of the suspected food into susceptible animals.

Prognosis.—The duration of fatal cases may be as short as forty-eight hours or as long as four to eight days. Death has been recorded twenty-six days after the onset. A short incubation period indicates a severe intoxication which is apt to be fatal. The mortality has varied greatly with different epidemics and has been greater in outbreaks dependent on infected vegetables. In Meyer's 625 cases in the United States there were 411 deaths, a mortality of nearly 66 per cent. The average mortality in Germany, where meat and fish have usually been the infecting agents, has remained approximately 20 per cent.

Treatment.—Therapy is most unsatisfactory. In animals botulinus antitoxin will prevent the action of the toxin and will save susceptible individuals even after definite symptoms of poisoning have appeared. The experiments indicate that antitoxin should be helpful even after the development of symptoms. Since in the scattered outbreaks the diagnosis has seldom been made until after severe symptoms have developed and delay in obtaining serum has been unavoidable, satisfactory clinical trial of antitoxin has been extremely limited. Unless the type of organism is known, a polyvalent antitoxin should be employed. In cases showing early respiratory paralysis, artificial respiration should be thoroughly tried.

Milk Sickness (The Trembles).—Milk sickness is a malady of herbivorous animals, particularly in the western United States, transmissible to man, producing an acute non-febrile disease characterized by severe gastro-intestinal irritation, muscular weakness and pronounced nervous manifestations.

In man the disease is believed to occur only as a result of consuming the milk, milk products or flesh of cattle affected with "trembles." The intoxication appears to result from feeding on Eupatorium urticæfolium (white snakeroot) or Aplopappus heterophyllus (rayless goldenrod). The condition is much less frequent than formerly and occurs almost exclusively in newly settled areas.

Symptoms.—In man the onset is gradual, with anorexia, languor, muscular pains, headache and chilliness. After three or four days there are abdominal pain, great thirst, persistent nausea and vomiting, obstinate constipation and oliguria. Nervous symptoms are varied; some patients present excitement, delirium and convulsions; others have extreme somnolence which may go on to coma. The temperature is normal or subnormal, the pulse unduly rapid. The breath has a fetid, acetone odor, the tongue is enlarged and flabby, the blood-pressure is extremely low. Hypoglycemia and ketosis are said to occur. Acute cases may terminate fatally in four or five days; subacute or chronic types persist for many weeks. The mortality is high.

Diagnosis.—The diagnosis in man is suggested by the presence of trembles among animals in the vicinity. In children there may be confusion with poliomyelitis.

Treatment.—Absolute rest and measures to prevent dehydration and promote elimination are essential. An abundance of fluids given by all possible routes, a soft high-carbohydrate diet to combat acidosis, and stimulation to prevent cardiovascular collapse are recommended. If the symptoms are severe it is advisable to give glucose intravenously.

Natural Poisons in Food.—Many plants and a few animals produce poisonous substances. The mushroom, Amanita muscaria, has often been mistaken for the edible varieties. It contains the highly toxic alkaloid muscarine, the effects of which appear one hour after ingestion and consist of salivation, vomiting, diarrhea, with collapse and delirium. Other mushrooms contain a poison the symptoms of which may be delayed for several days. It produces degeneration of the liver and kidneys, and death from vomiting, diarrhea, jaundice and suppression of urine.

At the spawning season the roe of several fish has caused fatal intoxication. In the tropics natural poisons are found in several species of fish, notably in the varieties of Tetrodon in China and Japan. Fatal poisoning has followed the eating of mussels, an intoxication which has been attributed to a poison known as mytilotoxin. The symptoms are those of severe gastro-intestinal disturbance with paralyses. Fish are particularly liable to bacterial infection and many cases of intoxication attributed to natural poisons are more probably due to contamination.

Special poisons have been found in a number of grains and vegetables. *Ergotism* is the poisoning which results from the prolonged use of grain contaminated by the ergot fungus. Acute gastro-intestinal symptoms may be succeeded by trophic or gangrenous changes in the extremities or by nervous and convulsive manifestations. This condition has often been seen in Europe but is almost unknown in this country.

Poisoning has been frequently reported following the ingestion of sprouting potatoes. This is probably due to specific bacterial invasion rather than to the potatoes themselves. The poisonous principle, solanin, produces, in addition to gastro-intestinal symptoms, chills and fever, headache, prostration and in some cases jaundice and collapse.

REFERENCES.

BULGER, H. A., SMITH, F. M., and STEINMAYER, A.: Milk Sickness and the Metabolic Disturbances of White Snakeroot Poisoning, Jour. Am. Med. Assn., 1928, **91**, 1964 .

DICKSON, E. C.: Botulism, a Clinical and Experimental Study, Monographs of the Rockefeller Inst. for Med. Res., 1918, No. 8.

——————— The Epidemiology of Botulism, Pub. Health Bull., 1922, **127**, 1.

McBURNEY, R.: Food Poisoning Due to Staphylococci, Jour. Am. Med. Assn., 1933, **100**, 1999.

MEYER, K. F.: Newer Knowledge on Botulism and Mussel Poisoning, Am. Jour. Pub. Health, 1931, **21**, 762.

ROSENAU, M. J.: Preventive Medicine and Hygiene, 5th ed., D. Appleton & Co.

SAVAGE, W. G., and WHITE, P. B.: An Investigation of the Salmonella Group with Special Reference to Food Poisoning. Special Report Series 92. Medical Research Council Reports, London, 1925.

SNAKE VENOM POISONING.

Poisonous snakes are possessed of hollow teeth or fangs which connect with venom glands situated in the temporal regions of the head. Toxins are thus injected directly into the tissues, in a manner not unlike that of the hypodermic. Toxins are contained in the protein of venom and are of two kinds. One form, a hemotoxin, produces hemolysis of red blood cells, extravasation of blood, intense edema and widespread local destruction of tissue. The other form, a neurotoxin, causes delayed action on nerve centers and is characterized chiefly by paralysis of medullary respiratory centers. The two types of toxin are separable and each can exert its specific influence without the other. Most venoms contain both toxins but in different ratios. The vipers of tropical America possess a poison of potent hemolytic action. Symptoms occur rapidly with immediate swelling, local extravasation of blood, oozing of blood in the mouth, conjunctiva, stomach and bladder, with coma and death within six to twelve hours. In the cases which recover there is great local destruction of tissue. The venoms of North American rattlesnakes, the copperhead and the moccasin exert similar actions but less rapidly. The cobra secretes a neurotoxin. Local swelling is moderate and does not appear rapidly. The chief symptoms are difficulty in breathing, which progresses to respiratory paralysis. The venom of the coral snake, found in the southern portion of the United States, simulates that of the cobra. African vipers secrete both types of toxin, producing tissue destruction as well as neurotoxic actions.

Treatment.—Ligation and incision of the wound should be the first steps in the treatment of snake-bite. A tourniquet should be placed tightly above the wound and a deep incision made to include the area of the fang punctures. Suction should be exerted on the wound, preferably with an apparatus similar to a breast pump. The tourniquet must be slacked from time to time since it may be necessary to continue treatment for an hour or more. When local swelling occurs small cruciform incisions should be made in the swollen area. If kept moist with mild antiseptic solutions, these openings permit the escape of large amounts of serum, a most important consideration, if, as has been claimed, the serum contains traces of venom for several hours after the bite. Drainage can be greatly hastened by placing suction pumps over each incision.

Calmette was the first to produce antitoxin for snake-bites. By increasing injections of a mixture of cobra and viper venom, he immunized horses and produced a polyvalent serum. It was later found that immunization for each type of venom was more effective. With present methods it takes from six to eight months to immunize a horse so that it can withstand large amounts of venom. In North America the Antivenin Institute has established stations in various parts of the country. It produces a polyvalent serum for bites of rattlesnakes, moccasins and copperheads, the type of toxin of these three being sufficiently alike to render a single type of serum efficient. A dose of 10 cc. of the serum should be given at once, early injection being of great importance in preventing the hemotoxic effects of venom. This is given subcutaneously or, in cases where symptoms develop rapidly, may be administered intravenously. The dosage should be repeated at intervals until effects are satisfactory; 20 cc. may be enough for an adult. Since normal serum possesses some antitoxic power, children and slender individuals require more antitoxin than robust adults.

It is important to remember that serious symptoms of shock may follow the bite of a venomous snake. Fluids should be administered both by mouth and by hypodermoclysis or intravenous injection. Transfusion may be helpful both as a treatment of shocks and of a rapidly developing anemia. Preparations for transfusion should be made as early as possible both because collapse may develop in cases which at first appear mild and because the hemolytic action of the venom may later render grouping more difficult.

REFERENCES.

KELLAWAY, C. H.: Snake Venoms and Antitoxic Immunity, The Mathison Lectures, Med. Jour. Australia, 1931, **2**, 1.

NOGUCHI, HIDEYO: Snake Venoms; an Investigation of Venomous Snakes with Special Reference to the Phenomena of Their Venoms, Carnegie Institution of Washington, 1909.

CHAPTER XXIV.

DISEASES DUE TO CHEMICAL AGENTS.

By MAURICE C. PINCOFFS, M.D.

CARBON MONOXIDE POISONING.
LEAD POISONING.
ARSENIC POISONING.
  Acute Arsenic Poisoning.
  Chronic Arsenic Poisoning.

MERCURY POISONING.
  Acute Mercury Poisoning.
  Subacute Poisoning.
  Chronic Poisoning.
BENZENE POISONING.

CARBON MONOXIDE POISONING.

CARBON monoxide is a colorless and practically odorless gas, arising from incomplete oxidation of carboniferous matter. When inhaled it combines with hemoglobin, rendering the latter incapable of transporting oxygen, and thus leads to serious or fatal anoxemia. Carbon monoxide is today the most frequent cause of death from poisoning.

Sources of Carbon Monoxide Poisoning.—"Natural gas" does not contain carbon monoxide but manufactured illuminating gas is the commonest cause of carbon monoxide poisoning. The manufactured gas used in most American cities is a mixture of so-called coal gas (containing about 6 per cent carbon monoxide) and of water gas (40 per cent carbon monoxide). The mixture contains between 20 and 30 per cent of carbon monoxide. In addition, it may contain toxic amounts of benzene and toluene, as well as other hydrocarbons. A few accidental poisonings arise in the manufacture of illuminating gas, but the majority result from leakage or from imperfect combustion of the gas in the buildings where it is utilized. Leakage may come from faulty pipes or taps, but is more usually due to rubber connections which crack or loosen with age. Imperfect combustion results when the flame impinges on a cold surface, as in certain water heaters, or when there is insufficient air admixture to furnish the necessary oxygen. Suicidal deaths from illuminating gas are common.

Fatalities in small garages have become frequent, due to the high (7 per cent) concentration of carbon monoxide in motor exhaust gases. The chief source of industrial poisoning is the gas from blast furnaces in the steel industry which contains as high as 24 to 30 per cent of carbon monoxide. High concentrations are also found in mines after coal-dust explosions, or in connection with blasting. The smoke of burning buildings contains dangerous amounts. Charcoal braziers, coke-burning salamanders, lime kilns, brick kilns and in general all smouldering fires give rise to gases containing considerable percentages of carbon monoxide.

The Effects of Carbon Monoxide Inhalation.—Carbon monoxide is a non-irritant gas as well as an odorless one and its inhalation is therefore unaccompanied by any warning sensations from the nose, throat

1049

or deeper air passages.   Symptoms appear only as a result of the combination of the gas with hemoglobin.   Hemoglobin has an affinity for carbon monoxide 210 times stronger than its affinity for oxygen. Contaminated air containing $\frac{1}{210}$ (0.07 per cent) as much carbon monoxide as oxygen (20.9 per cent) would therefore, when inhaled, eventually result in the establishment of an equilibrium between the circulating hemoglobin and the two gases in which approximately one-half of the hemoglobin would be oxyhemoglobin and one-half carbon monoxide hemoglobin.   Incapacitating symptoms of anoxia would accompany this condition.   In fatal poisoning with higher concentrations of carbon monoxide practically complete saturation of the hemoglobin with this gas is only prevented by the cessation of respiration and circulation when about 80 per cent carbon monoxide hemoglobin has been formed.

The time required for a dangerous degree of anoxia to result from carbon monoxide inhalation depends upon the actual volume of carbon monoxide inhaled per minute.   It is estimated that 1 liter of this gas would be held in combination by all the hemoglobin in the average adult body.   In quiet breathing, about 5 liters of air are drawn into the lungs per minute.   If, as in the example given above, this inhaled air contained 0.07 per cent of carbon monoxide, the volume of the carbon monoxide inhaled in one minute would be only 3.5 cc.   In order to reach the predicted equilibrium in which 50 per cent of the hemoglobin would be saturated with carbon monoxide it would be necessary for 500 cc. of carbon monoxide to be inhaled and combined with the hemoglobin.   It is readily seen that this could only be accomplished by several hours' inhalation of the 0.07 per cent concentration of the gas.   On the other hand, if air were inhaled containing a very high concentration of carbon monoxide, for example 25 per cent, then the amount of this gas brought into the lungs in a minute (1.25 liters) would be sufficient to bring about a fatal degree of saturation of the hemoglobin within this period of time.

Exercise affects the speed of development of carbon monoxide poisoning by the marked increase of pulmonary ventilation it entails.   From 5 liters per minute, at rest, pulmonary ventilation may rise to 60 to 100 liters during violent exertion, with a corresponding increase in the volume of carbon monoxide inhaled, and a proportionately rapid saturation of the hemoglobin.   Moreover, in exertion the oxygen needs of the body are greatly increased so that the reduction in oxyhemoglobin is acutely felt.

It has been observed that anoxemia produced by carbon monoxide inhalation is more productive of symptoms than a similar degree of anoxemia due to other causes such as anemia.   This is apparently due to the fact that in the presence of carbon monoxide hemoglobin the oxyhemoglobin of the blood dissociates less readily.   The oxygen tension in the tissues is thereby reduced to a point as much as 50 per cent lower than it would be with a blood containing the same amount of oxyhemoglobin but free from carbon monoxide hemoglobin.   The actual tissue anoxia in carbon monoxide poisoning is, therefore, due to two factors: the reduction in the amount of oxyhemoglobin, and the abnormal reluctance of this oxyhemoglobin to yield its oxygen to the tissues. Argument still exists as to whether carbon monoxide in the blood may exert some direct toxic action upon the tissues, but the bulk of the evidence favors the view that its harmful effect is solely due to the anoxia it causes.

Tables 14 and 15 by Henderson and Haggard show in practical form the relation of carbon monoxide concentrations in both the air and the blood to the production of symptoms.

TABLE 14.—PHYSIOLOGIC RESPONSE TO VARIOUS CONCENTRATIONS OF CARBON MONOXIDE.[1]

	Parts of carbon monoxide per million parts of air.
Concentration allowable for an exposure of several hours	100
Concentration which can be inhaled for one hour without appreciable effect	400 to 500
Concentration causing a just appreciable effect after one hour of exposure	600 to 700
Concentration causing unpleasant but not dangerous symptoms after one hour of exposure	1000 to 1200
Dangerous concentration for exposure of one hour . .	1500 to 2000
Concentrations which are fatal in exposures of less than one hour	4000 and above

TABLE 15.—PERCENTAGE SATURATION OF THE BLOOD WITH CARBON MONOXIDE AND CORRESPONDING PHYSIOLOGIC EFFECTS.[2]

Per cent of hemoglobin in combination with carbon monoxide.	Physiologic effect.
10	No appreciable effect except shortness of breath on vigorous muscular exertion.
20	No appreciable effect in most cases except short wind, even on moderate exertion; slight headache in some cases.
30	Decided headache; irritable; easily fatigued; judgment disturbed.
40 to 50 . . .	Headache, confusion, collapse and fainting on exertion.
60 to 70 . . .	Unconsciousness; respiratory failure and death if exposure is long continued.
80	Rapidly fatal.
Over 80 . . .	Immediately fatal.

Pathology.—The skin shows red blotches and may show blebs and areas of superficial gangrene. The blood is bright cherry-red and flows freely. The serous membranes frequently show hemorrhagic areas. The lungs are congested and edematous. Areas of atelectasis may be observed. Bronchopneumonia is frequently found in those who have survived the initial poisoning for some days. The heart muscle often shows fatty changes. Areas of necrosis in the heart muscle have been described in some cases. The walls of the smaller vessels frequently exhibit marked degenerative changes, swelling of the intima, fatty changes in the media and frequently thrombosis. The liver and kidneys may likewise show fatty degeneration. The pathologic lesions in the central nervous system are highly

[1] Henderson, Y., Haggard, H. W., Teague, M. C., Prince, A. L., and Wunderlich, R. M.: Physiological Effects of Automobile Exhaust Gas, and Standards of Ventilation for Brief Exposures, Jour. Indus. Hyg., 1921, **3**, 79, 137.

[2] Henderson, Y., and Haggard, H. W.: Noxious Gases, The Chemical Catalog Company, New York, 1927, p. 108.

varied. The most constant finding is a bilateral symmetric necrosis of the globus pallidus. In addition a general engorgement of the cerebral vessels is present with petechial or larger hemorrhages both in the brain substance and in the meninges. Areas of cortical softening may be observed.

The interpretation of the pathologic reports on carbon monoxide poisoning is confused by the fact that in such poisoning in addition to carbon monoxide other gases may be inhaled (such as benzine in illuminating gas) whose toxic action may account for an undetermined part of the lesions described and especially of those in the central nervous system.

Symptoms.—The inhalation of very high concentrations of carbon monoxide results in immediate unconsciousness and death within the lapse of a few minutes. Such hyperacute cases of poisoning occur chiefly about blast furnaces or in mine explosions. If promptly rescued the unconscious patient usually recovers without sequelæ.

Where poisoning occurs more gradually warning symptoms are frequently noted. The commonest of these prodromes is throbbing pain in the temples. Tinnitus aurium, epigastric distress and nausea, weakness in the legs and mental confusion may also be experienced before unconsciousness develops. The mental confusion may interfere with attempts at escape.

If rescued early the patient may be merely stuporous. Restlessness, muscular incoördination, vomiting and incontinence of sphincters are common. The face is flushed, the respirations stertorous and the pulse full. After poisoning of longer duration the patient is found deeply comatose and relaxed. The skin is pale but frequently shows irregular red blotching. The respirations are rapid and shallow or may be intermittent and gasping. The pulse is weak and rapid. There is a leukocytosis of 10,000 to 15,000 and a trace of sugar may be found in the urine.

The stuporous patients usually show prompt improvement, though headache and slight mental dullness may persist for twenty-four hours and some weakness and tremor for several days.

The duration of coma is very variable. If pulmonary ventilation is adequately maintained the carbon monoxide will be eliminated from the blood within a few hours and consciousness may be restored within this period of time. However, cerebral injury due to the period of intense asphyxia (cerebral edema, hemorrhage, softening) may lead to the persistence of the comatose state. Death with hyperpyrexia of central origin is common in such cases. Pulmonary complications such as bronchopneumonia or pulmonary atelectasis are also prone to occur. Irregular pinkish wheals and large blebs may develop on the skin. In general, coma of more than twenty-four hours' duration has a serious prognosis.

The majority of patients who recover from carbon monoxide coma are free from after-effects. There are, however, serious sequelæ in some instances. Psychoses, dementia, amblyopia, paralyses and Parkinsonism have been described. In some cases the onset of these conditions is delayed for several weeks after the original poisoning.

Chronic carbon monoxide poisoning is said to occur in those repeatedly exposed over long periods to very minute concentrations of the gas. Compensatory polycythemia followed eventually by severe anemia has been described. Headache, dizziness, emotional instability, muscular weakness and abdominal pains may occur from this cause.

Diagnosis.—The diagnosis is usually made from the history of exposure to the gas and the condition of the patient. In the accident-room practice of large city hospitals, however, it is often necessary to have further confirmation of the cause of coma. The analysis of the blood should be carried out routinely because of the value from a diagnostic and therapeutic point of view of knowing the presence and percentage of carbon monoxide hemoglobin. Sayer and Yants' modification of the tannic acid test is the method most widely used in this country. Analyses of air from suspected localities may be carried out by the iodine pentoxide method.

Prognosis.—Gradual poisoning to the point of deep coma is more apt to result fatally than brief severe gassing short of instant death. The mortality of patients admitted comatose to general hospitals is about 20 per cent.

Prevention.—Conditions in the steel industry have much improved as a result of changes in the construction of blast furnaces, and through instruction of the workmen. Illuminating gas accidents and garage poisonings should be reduced by public education and by regular inspection. The industrial risks may be avoided to some extent by proper provision at danger spots of the mechanical carbon monoxide detectors, and the carbon monoxide gas masks for rescuers, perfected by the Chemical Warfare Service.

Treatment.—Prompt removal from the contaminated atmosphere and the maintenance of respiration are the immediate essentials. If on removal to fresh air the respiratory movements are found to have ceased, artificial respiration by the Schäfer prone pressure method should be started at once and coupled as soon as possible with the administration of oxygen containing 5 to 7 per cent carbon dioxide with the HH inhalator. When spontaneous breathing is well established the patient may be removed to the hospital where the administration of the oxygen and carbon dioxide mixture should be continued at intervals until the blood is freed from carbon monoxide.

The value of the high oxygen concentration consists in the acceleration of the reaction displacing the carbon monoxide from combination with hemoglobin, thus shortening the period of tissue asphyxia. The increased pulmonary ventilation resulting from the action of carbon dioxide acts powerfully in the same direction.

The intravenous injection of methylene blue solutions, as recently advocated, is at best an adjuvant measure which should not replace the use of the oxygen-carbon dioxide mixture. It is not without danger.

Other therapeutic measures of importance are warmth, sufficient fluids by available channels and, when necessary, circulatory stimulants. Frequent change of position and the stimulation of deep breathing and cough to avert atelectasis and pneumonia are important. In persistent coma increased intracranial pressure due to edema should be thought of, and if the spinal fluid pressure is found high hypertonic saline solution may be given, 50 cc. of 10 per cent salt solution in ten minutes.

Milder cases of gassing require chiefly absolute rest and warmth. It must be remembered that sudden collapse may come on if such patients undertake exertion requiring oxygen beyond the diminished oxygen-carrying capacity of their blood. Certain lay methods of resuscitation, such as walking the patient up and down, slapping and dousing with cold water, are useless and dangerous.

REFERENCES.

APFELBACH, G. L., revised by HAYHURST, E. R.: Carbon Monoxide Poisoning, Section 8, p. 369, in KOBER, G. M., and HAYHURST, E. R.: Industrial Health, Philadelphia, P. Blakiston's Son & Co., 1924.

DRINKER, C. K., and SHAUGHNESSY, T. J.: The Use of 7 Per Cent Carbon Dioxide and 93 Per Cent Oxygen in the Treatment of Carbon Monoxide Poisoning, Jour. Indust. Hyg., 1929, **9**, 301.

MACKAY, R. P.: Neurologic Changes Following Carbon Monoxide Poisoning, Jour. Am. Med. Assn., 1930, **94**, 1733.

PETERS, J. P., and VAN SLYKE, R. D.: Quantitative Clinical Chemistry, Baltimore, The Williams & Wilkins Company, 1931, p. 607.

SAYERS, R. R., YANT, W. P., and JONES, G. W.: The Pyrotannic Acid Method for the Quantitative Determination of Carbon Monoxide in Blood and Air, Washington, 1925, U. S. Bureau of Mines, Technical Paper 373.

LEAD POISONING.

The industrial use of lead antedates the Christian era, and lead poisoning was among the first recognized of the industrial diseases. Our knowledge of the clinical manifestations of lead poisoning dates chiefly from the treatise of Tanqueral des Planches (1839), in which this author gives descriptions of lead colic, paralyses, arthralgias and encephalopathies to which little has since been added. Much has been learned, however, concerning the mode of entrance into the body, the storage in the tissues and the elimination of the metal. As a result more intelligent industrial regulation of its use has begun to show an effect upon the incidence of the disease.

Incidence.—Plumbism is common among lead-miners working in shallow mines yielding the more toxic lead salts (carbonates, sulphates and oxides) and relatively uncommon among those employed in the deeper mines yielding poorly soluble lead sulphides. In the dry and dusty shallow mines the incidence is especially high, morbidity-rates as high as 27 per 100 having been observed.

The fumes and fine lead dust in plants for smelting and refining lead ores cause many cases of poisoning. The presence of lead in brass and in most zinc ores explains the occurrence of plumbism in zinc-smelting works and in brass foundries. The roasting of lead to form the oxides, the manufacture of white lead (basic lead carbonate), the casting and molding of lead, lead type founding, lead soldering and lead tempering have all been shown to be trades requiring careful control of the lead fume and dust hazards. Lead glazes and lead enamels are still widely used and occasion plumbism in pottery-workers and among makers of sanitary ware. The use of lead grids and of lead oxide paste in the making of storage batteries is an important source of poisoning. The highest incidence of industrial lead poisoning is among painters. Among 1108 deaths attributed to industrial lead poisoning, Hoffman found 841 among painters. The hazard in this trade is connected chiefly with the dry sand-papering of painted surfaces and the chipping and burning off of old paint. The modern method of spraying paint has added a new risk. The ingestion of lead with the food as a result of paint-contaminated hands and clothing is a lesser but real danger.

Non-industrial plumbism is not infrequent. In older communities houses still contain much lead water piping. It has been shown that at times the water may have sufficient plumbo-solvent properties to bring its lead content up to a dangerous level. The continued use of pills, ointments and pastes containing lead may cause acute symptoms of plumbism. Infants and young children may pick off and swallow scales of paint or enamel from their toys or cribs and be fatally poisoned. Women's cosmetics containing lead have also caused lead poisoning in infants. The storing of acid home-made wines in crocks with a lead glaze may add a dangerous amount of lead to these beverages.

Tetra-ethyl lead, which is used in gasoline to eliminate the knock, may induce lead poisoning if in the processes of manufacture or in its distribution the ethyl gasoline is spilled upon the skin, or sucked into the mouth in clearing gas lines, or the fumes of its combustion inhaled. Serious accidents occurred in the early days of its manufacture.

Absorption, Storage and Excretion.—Absorption of lead may occur through the skin, gastro-intestinal tract and the respiratory tract. Absorption through the intact skin is rarely a cause of poisoning. It is limited practically to such organic lead compounds as have fat-solvent properties. At present tetra-ethyl lead is the only widely distributed substance of this nature.

Ingestion of lead and absorption from the gastro-intestinal tract account for most of the non-industrial cases of plumbism. The action of the gastric juices increases the solubility of many of the less soluble lead salts, yet a large part of ingested lead is excreted without being absorbed. It is probable that the hydrogen sulphide of the lower digestive tract converts some of the soluble salts into the relatively insoluble lead sulphides. A further defensive mechanism lies in the ability of the liver to arrest the lead brought to it by the portal circulation and to re-excrete it in the bile.

Clinical experience with the dangers of lead dust and fumes points to absorption from the respiratory tract as the most frequent cause of industrial plumbism. Experimental work has confirmed the ready absorption of lead compounds both from the lungs and from the mucous membranes of the nose and throat. The absorption, indeed, is more complete than from the digestive tract and the absorbed lead enters at once into the general circulation.

Lead in the blood probably is carried in the form of a colloidal lead phosphate. Its distribution in the tissues depends to some extent upon the portal of entry. After ingestion of lead a higher percentage will be found in the liver than if the poisoning has been due to inhalation. It is in the bones, however, that almost all of the lead absorbed is eventually deposited in the form of tertiary lead phosphate. This ability of the skeletal tissues to remove lead from the circulation and to store it in a relatively insoluble form constitutes a protection to the more vulnerable tissues. There is evidence that the lead thus stored may be held in the bones for years. It has also been shown that variation in the reaction of the blood toward either the acid or the alkaline side may cause the solution and excretion of this stored lead. In many ways the deposition of lead in the bones and its removal from the bones parallels the similar behavior of calcium. A positive calcium balance has been shown to favor the deposition of lead and a negative calcium balance to aid in its solution. Sudden solution of stored lead is believed to account for "toxic episodes" in chronic lead poisoning. It is no doubt the circulating lead which affects the vulnerable tissues.

The excretion of lead is chiefly in the feces and to a lesser extent in the urine. The fecal content of lead during the course of lead poisoning is largely made up of ingested and unabsorbed lead; but it has been shown that there is also a true excretion of lead from the lining mucosa of the stomach and intestine as well as in the bile. The lead excreted in the urine, while smaller in amount, is of practical importance since its detection is proof that the patient has not only been exposed to lead but has absorbed lead into the blood stream.

The quantity of lead in the tissues at any one time is extremely small, usually less than 1 gram in the entire body. In the slow excretion of stored lead during recovery the quantities in the daily urine and stool are usually only fractions of a milligram.

The intake of lead necessary to produce acute or chronic forms of lead poisoning is not definitely known. In acute poisoning by ingestion of the soluble salts such as lead acetate, a single dose of as much as 25 grams has been survived. On the other hand, the ingestion of 1 cg. daily will produce acute symptoms in a few weeks. Legge has estimated that the inhalation daily of as little as 2 mg. of lead in dust or fumes could in the course of years produce chronic poisoning. In some of the dusty lead trades the amount inhaled may readily be several hundred milligrams daily. It is in such environments that the most acute and severe forms of industrial plumbism arise.

Pathology.—There is no single gross or microscopic lesion which is characteristic of lead poisoning with the exception of the "lead line" in the gums. In long-continued chronic lead poisoning the smaller arteries may show thickening of the media and periarteritis. Chronic interstitial nephritis, cirrhosis of the liver and gouty deposits are also frequently observed. Atrophy of the testicles is said to occur. In cases with palsy there is atrophy and fibrous infiltration of the muscles affected. The anterior horn cells and the peripheral nerves also show degenerative changes. Chronic fibrosis of the leptomeninges and a perivascular fibrosis in the brain substance have been observed in lead encephalopathy.

Symptoms.—*Acute Forms of Poisoning.*—The symptoms following the ingestion of a single large dose of a soluble lead salt are at first chiefly those due to the irritant action on the mucous membranes;

astringent metallic taste, vomiting, severe colic, diarrhea with dark bloody stools. In fatal cases these symptoms are followed after some hours by headache, muscular cramps, collapse and death.

In severe *subacute* cases such as those following exposure to high concentrations of lead dust, or occurring in infants after ingestion of lead the rapid development of an encephalopathy may be the first evidence of poisoning. In the industrial poisonings due to tetra-ethyl lead a period of restlessness and insomnia was followed by an acute maniacal state and death from exhaustion.

Chronic Poisoning.—Chronic plumbism is characterized by certain symptoms and signs indicative of the effects of circulating lead upon the tissues and by the intermittent appearance of more acute manifestations such as colic, arthralgia, paralyses or encephalopathy. Such so-called "toxic episodes" in lead poisoning may be recovered from only to recur upon renewed exposure. Cases of chronic lead poisoning are characterized moreover by a high incidence of degenerative lesions such as arteriosclerosis and contracted kidneys. Arterial hypertension is common. Many authors have also noted the frequent occurrence of gout.

The most common *symptoms* of chronic lead poisoning are fatigability, loss of weight, headaches, anorexia and constipation. These symptoms are too general in character to suggest lead poisoning unless there is known exposure. In a person exposed to lead, however, the development of such symptoms is of great significance. In women menstrual disturbances are frequent. Women lead-workers show a high incidence of sterility and miscarriages. The generative power in leaded males is less definitely affected, but the offspring are said to be frequently defective.

The important *signs* of chronic plumbism are pallor, the lead line in the gums, stippled red cells, anemia and weakness of the extensor muscles of the fingers and wrists. The face commonly shows a dirty gray pallor which suggests a higher degree of anemia than is found to exist.

The *lead line* occurs as a narrow black line near the margin of the gums. It is most pronounced opposite carious teeth. It is not on the surface and cannot be washed off. The insertion of white paper between the gum and the tooth shows that it lies in the gum. It is due to the deposition of lead sulphide granules in the connective tissue under the epithelium. When present the lead line is of great diagnostic value. A quite similar line, however, may occur in patients receiving injections of bismuth salts for syphilis. Moreover; the lead line is frequently absent in authentic cases of chronic plumbism.

Stippling of the red cells is a valuable sign. The basophilic granules of varying size are scattered throughout the body of the affected erythrocyte. They may be detected in the ordinary Wright stain but are best brought out by dilute Unna's alkaline methylene blue. The stippling is thought to be due to a degeneration of the reticulum of immature red cells. Similar stippled cells may be seen in scantier numbers in cases of arsenic poisoning, pernicious anemia and leukemia.

67

A count of over 7000 stippled cells to the cubic millimeter is, however, rarely found except in lead poisoning.

The destruction of red blood cells in lead poisoning, which leads to the throwing out of these immature and damaged stippled cells, is also evidenced by a mild secondary anemia (3,500,000 to 4,000,000 red cells) and by an increase of blood derived pigments in the plasma, the bile and the urine. Hematoporphyrin is frequently present in the urine.

Weakness of the extensor muscles of the fingers and wrists may often be demonstrated very early in the course of plumbism. It has been found a useful sign in the experience of industrial physicians who search for it as a part of the periodic examination of lead-workers.

Of the *acute episodes* which interrupt the course of chronic plumbism, *lead colic* is the most common. It may occur early in susceptible individuals or only after some years of slow lead absorption. It is seen occasionally in patients months after their exposure to lead has ceased, and in such instances is probably the result of mobilization of lead previously stored in the bones.

The onset of colic is usually preceded by a period of vague digestive unrest and of obstinate constipation. The blood pressure is usually elevated during the colic. When severe pain sets in it occurs in waves or paroxysms over the whole lower abdomen. The degree of prostration varies greatly. In severe cases there is every evidence of intense pain. The face is pale; the respirations hurried; the pulse slow and hard. The abdomen is retracted and tensely held. Between the paroxysms there is dull pain in the abdomen and often across the back. Vomiting is rare. The temperature is not elevated. There is frequently a moderate leukocytosis. Intestinal obstruction or acute perforative peritonitis may be simulated. There is, however, little abdominal tenderness and no true muscle spasm. In some instances abdominal pressure seems to give relief. The attack of colic lasts from a few days to a week.

The term *arthralgia* was used by Tanquerel to cover the pains, muscular cramps and paresthesias in the extremities that occur not infrequently as acute manifestations in chronic lead poisoning. The muscular cramps may be intense and may jump from one muscular group to another.

Lead paralysis is most common in the extensor muscles of the fingers and wrists, producing wrist- and finger-drop. Ankle-drop may also occur, due to paralysis of the peroneal muscles. The muscles of the shoulders are not infrequently affected and occasionally the eye muscles. There is a tendency for the paralysis to selectively involve muscles which subserve the same function and which are relatively overworked in the patient's occupation, whereas other muscles innervated by the same peripheral nerve may be spared. Recent work indicates that the primary lesion due to lead may be a degenerative myositis with secondary changes in the motor fibers and anterior horn cells supplying the affected muscles.

The onset of actual paralysis is usually preceded by weakness of the muscles and by tremor. Pain is not felt in the paralyzed limb and evidence of sensory impairment is not usually to be found. If exposure to lead is promptly discontinued recovery of function is usually complete within a few months. Repeated exposure may lead to progressive involvement of other muscle groups and to permanent paralysis.

Lead *encephalopathy* is a relatively infrequent but very important complication of lead poisoning. It is seen chiefly in infants and children and in those adults, especially women, who have been exposed to high concentrations of lead in dust and fumes. It may occur, however, after many years of exposure to smaller quantities of lead. The cerebral symptoms grouped under the term lead encephalopathy are extremely varied. The psychic disturbances include neurasthenic states, mild depressions, progressive dementia, and also attacks of acute mania and delirium terminating either in coma and death or in gradual and usually partial recovery. Convulsions are not infrequent as a part of the clinical picture of lead encephalopathy and may resemble both the grand mal and the petit mal attacks of idiopathic epilepsy. Cranial nerve palsies are described. Blindness may result from optic neuritis. The production of these varied symptoms is not clearly explained by our present knowledge of the pathology. In the more acute cases marked edema and swelling of the brain have been found with corresponding diminution of the size of the ventricular cavities. This is followed in later stages by brain atrophy with dilated ventricles and often with productive meningeal lesions. The spinal fluid is often under increased pressure and shows an increase of globulin and of lymphocytes (20 to 100). In chronic lead poisoning in older people cerebral symptoms may arise as a result of arterial hypertension and cerebral arteriosclerosis. Vascular spasm may play a part in the transient aphasias and amauroses of such cases. Cerebral hemorrhage is not unusual.

Diagnosis.—Lead poisoning should always be thought of as a possible cause of acute abdominal crises, lower motor neurone paralyses or acute maniacal states. In workers in lead trades, pallor, anorexia, headaches and nervousness should suggest lead intoxication. A positive diagnosis of lead poisoning cannot be made on the presence of lead in the stools, since lead may be ingested and excreted without absorption. The presence of a trace of lead in the urine indicates absorption but not necessarily the presence of sufficient lead in the blood stream to account for symptoms. The finding of lead in the excreta has nevertheless considerable diagnostic value as indicating exposure to lead. Unfortunately the analysis is technically difficult. Stippling of the red cells and the "lead line" are valuable signs and either one, taken together with characteristic symptoms such as colic or palsy, is sufficient for a positive diagnosis. In infants lead deposited in the bones can be detected roentgenologically as a dense band at the growing margins. It is most evident at the ends of the long bones and at the anterior ends of the ribs. Recently the spectroscopic determination of lead in small amounts of blood and of spinal fluid has been successfully used in diagnosis. Roughly quantitative results may be obtained.

Prognosis.—The debility, anemia, anorexia, constipation and nervousness of chronic lead poisoning disappear gradually after cessation of exposure. Acute lead colic usually lasts about a week. The prognosis in early cases of lead palsy is good but palsy of some duration is usually permanent in spite of removal from lead exposure. Severe forms of lead encephalopathy are frequently fatal or result in chronic psychoses.

Prevention.—The elimination of lead dust and fumes in manufacturing processes is being accomplished to an increasing extent by the substitution of wet for dry processes, by the enclosure of dust producing machinery and the free use of suction drafts. In the rubbing down of paint, sandpaper which can be moistened with oil should be used.

Working clothes should be kept separate from street clothes. Washing facilities should be ample. The instruction of workmen in the hazards of their trade is important. The contamination of food or tobacco with lead dust from the air, the hands, or the clothing should be guarded against. Periodic medical examination of lead-workers will lead to the detection of early symptoms and the removal of susceptible cases from exposure.

Treatment.—Patients showing symptoms and signs of chronic plumbism without such acute manifestations as colic or encephalopathy should, after removal from the lead hazard, be treated by methods designed to increase the elimination of lead from the body.

After cleansing of the bowel with magnesium sulphate to eliminate unabsorbed lead, potassium iodide may be given in doses of 0.2 gram (3 grains), three times daily, and the dosage gradually increased up to tolerance. The output of lead may be doubled by the use of this drug. The effectiveness of a low calcium diet in accelerating the excretion of lead has been demonstrated in recent years by Aub and his associates. The omission of milk and eggs from the diet and the inclusion of tomatoes, corn, potatoes, apples and bananas as the only vegetables and fruits are the chief features in this régime. Ammonium chloride (1 gram in a glass of water, ten times daily) may be used for its acid-forming properties, or alkalinization may be forwarded by giving 20 to 40 grams of sodium bicarbonate daily. It should be recalled that too rapid "deleading" has been known to precipitate attacks of colic or palsy, probably through the increased amount of lead dissolved from the bones and carried in the blood stream.

In the presence of acute symptoms such as colic, recent palsy or encephalopathy it may be assumed that the circulating lead is excessive in amount and that it will be reduced most rapidly by deposition in the bones. A positive calcium balance favors such deposition and may be established by giving large quantities of milk (1 to 2 quarts a day) together with calcium lactate (1 gram, four times a day). Prompt relief of colic may be obtained by the slow intravenous injection of 10 cc. of a sterile 5 per cent solution of calcium chloride. After acute symptoms have entirely subsided deleading measures may be cautiously instituted.

In the treatment of severe colic amyl nitrite is useful in alleviating the painful paroxysms. Atropine in large doses may also give relief. There is no contraindication to morphine, but its effect is uncertain.

Purgation is best withheld until the pain is subsiding. Enemas may be effectual.

In encephalopathy spinal puncture should be done and, if the pressure of the cerebrospinal fluid is high, the gradual withdrawal of 10 to 20 cc. of fluid may be beneficial. Recovery from palsy may be hastened by the use of the galvanic current and massage.

REFERENCES.

AUB, J. C., FAIRHALL, L. T., MINOT, A. S. and REZNIKOFF, P.: Lead Poisoning, Medicine, 1925, **4**, 1.
HAMILTON, ALICE: Industrial Poisons in the United States, New York, The Macmillan Company, 1925.
HOFFMAN, F. L.: Deaths from Lead Poisoning, U. S. Bureau of Labor Statistics, Bull. No. 426, February, 1927, p. 45.
OLIVER, T.: Lead Poisoning, London, H. K. Lewis, 1914.
SHIPLEY, P. G., SCOTT, T. F. McN., and BLUMBERG, H.: The Spectrographic Detection of Lead in the Blood as an Aid to the Clinical Diagnosis of Plumbism, Bull. Johns Hopkins Hospital, 1932, **51**, 327.
VOGT, E. C.: Roentgenologic Diagnosis of Lead Poisoning, Jour. Am. Med. Assn., 1932, **98**, 125.

ARSENIC POISONING.

Arsenic poisoning in the industries is not very frequent in this country. The medical use of arsenic and especially of the organic arsenicals in antisyphilitic treatment has greatly increased in recent years and has led to many instances of poisoning. Accidental, homicidal and suicidal arsenic poisonings are not very uncommon.

Acute Forms of Arsenic Poisoning.—The ingestion of white arsenic (arsenic trioxide), of Paris green (copper aceto-arsenite) and of rough on rats (arsenous oxide and barium carbonate) gives rise to the majority of accidental, homicidal and suicidal acute poisonings. In addition to the irritant action on the lining of the stomach and intestine, arsenic is absorbed and may be found after death in all the tissues. The largest amount is in the liver, in acute cases, but where death has been some time delayed arsenic will be found to have been retained longest in the bones and in the hair. The excretion of arsenic is in the feces, the urine and to some extent through the skin.

If the arsenic ingested is well diluted it will be tasteless and the gastric symptoms will be delayed for one-half hour or more. Severe abdominal cramps, persistent vomiting, often blood-stained, and intense diarrhea, with "rice-water" stools, then occur. Dehydration is rapid, with intense thirst, muscle cramps, oliguria, fall in blood pressure, coma and death in one to three days. In fulminant cases diarrhea may be less marked; early headache, spasmodic muscular contractions and stupor lead quickly to collapse and death. In the milder cases, after several days jaundice may develop, together with widespread skin eruptions of an urticarial type, and in some instances the more chronic effects of arsenic, such as pigmentation and peripheral neuritis, may follow.

The acute poisonings due to the intravenous injection of the arsphenamines in the treatment of syphilis are of a different clinical character. The immediate reaction at the time of injection, known as the "nitritoid crisis," and characterized by sudden flushing, precordial pain, dyspnea, cough, edema of the face and laryngeal stridor, is probably due more to physical changes in the blood as a result of the arsphena- mine solution than to the chemical properties of arsenic. This reac- tion is allayed by the immediate injection of epinephrin in full doses. Febrile reactions also occur, of a non-specific nature, which are explain- able by impurities in the water used. If the toxic acid solution of arsphenamine is injected without neutralization, immediate collapse and death may result. *Gastro-intestinal reactions* to arsphenamine include the common nausea and vomiting in the first hours and the more severe types, with continuous vomiting and diarrhea. *Jaundice* may appear some days after arsphenamine injection, due to a toxic hepatitis. In rare instances a fatal *acute yellow atrophy* develops. Urticarial and erythematous skin eruptions are observed. The repe- tition of arsphenamine injection in such cases may be followed by a generalized *exfoliative dermatitis* that is frequently fatal. *Hemorrhagic encephalitis* and an *aplastic type of anemia with purpura* are reported among the rarer serious sequelæ.

In industrial processes involving the action of acids upon metal, the nascent hydrogen formed will act upon any arsenic, present as an im- purity in either metal or acid, with the formation of hydrogen arsenide (AsH_3) gas which may cause acute poisoning. Storage batteries may evolve this gas and this has led to poisoning in submarines. Men entering empty metal acid tanks and stills have died of this cause. There have been fatalities in connection with commercial hydrogen generation for balloon-filling, and from reduction processes in dye works. The ore ferro-silicon, carried in the moist hold of vessels, has developed sufficient hydrogen arsenide fatally to poison members of the crew. Acute poisoning with hydrogen arsenide is characterized by marked prostration, with vertigo and headache; vomiting develops, with diar- rhea and later jaundice. There is evidence of intense hemolysis with rapid anemia, and very dark urine, containing hemoglobin, methemo- globin and hematin. An acute nephrosis with partial or complete suppression of urine has been noted. Acute pulmonary edema may occur.

Treatment.—In cases of poisoning due to the ingestion of arsenic, the stomach should be thoroughly lavaged and a saline cathartic administered. The official antidote for arsenic (ferri hydroxidum cum magnesii oxido) may be extemporaneously prepared by diluting 15 cc. of tincture ferri chloridi with 200 cc. of water and adding magnesium oxide in excess. Four to 6 ounces of this mixture may be administered three to four times in the first day, followed each time by a copious lavage of the stomach. The efficacy of this antidote is not clearly demonstrated. It is supposed to act by forming the less poisonous iron arsenates.

The dehydration should be actively combated by saline infusions and, if necessary, glucose solutions intravenously. Morphine and atropine may be needed for pain. Demulcents may allay some of the gastro-intestinal irritation.

In arsenic poisoning following the intravenous injection of organic arsenicals, or due to inhalation of hydrogen arsenide, the gastro-intestinal tract should be kept clear of excreted arsenic by saline purgatives and by daily colonic irrigation. For the severe anemia of hydrogen arsenide poisoning transfusion may be tried. If pulmonary edema threatens oxygen should be administered continuously.

In all forms of acute arsenic poisoning calcium thiosulphate should be given intravenously. One-half gram of chemically pure calcium thiosulphate is dissolved in 10 cc. of sterile distilled water. This dose may be repeated every twelve hours for the first two days and then given daily for five or more days.

Chronic Arsenic Poisoning.—Symptoms of chronic arsenic poisoning may occur as a sequela to those of acute poisoning due to a single large dose; more frequently, however, they follow the prolonged absorption of small quantities. The medicinal use of arsenic, the manufacture and utilization of sprays containing Paris green, of sheep dips containing arsenic, or of paper colored with arsenic pigments, and the accidental contamination of food or beverages with arsenic, have all occasioned chronic arsenic poisoning. Arsenic is usually present in small amounts in the sulphide ores of all heavy metals, so that arsenic fumes and dust are common about smelters and have frequently occasioned poisoning.

The chronic illness due to slow arsenic poisoning is often very obscure in nature unless its relation to arsenic exposure is discovered. At first the patient complains of weakness and anorexia, with intermittent nausea and vomiting of small amounts of mucus. Slight jaundice may be present. There is often a low fever. Hoarseness and naso-pharyngeal catarrh appear. Herpes is not uncommon. If the poisoning is due to dust or fumes containing arsenic, a slow necrosis of the cartilage of the nasal septum may occur. In such cases there is also inflammation of the eyelids and conjunctivæ; redness, swelling and ulceration of the skin of the scrotum, the groins and the axilla; and inflammation of the skin of hands and face. Such skin and mucous membrane lesions are less prominent when the arsenic is ingested. On the other hand, in this latter group generalized grayish pigmentation of the skin gradually develops, accompanied on the hands and feet by marked wart-like thickening of the epidermis. The palms and soles are first affected. The development of epithelioma from such areas of hyperkeratosis has been frequently observed.

In some cases of chronic arsenic poisoning marked sensory disturbances develop in the extremities, due to a peripheral neuritis. Paresthesias, in the form of tingling, burning, formication and pain on touch, are followed by a marked diminution in tactile acuity. The symptoms are usually more marked in the lower extremities. Motor paralysis is comparatively rare. Headache may accompany the development of neuritis. Optic atrophy has been observed. In very prolonged arsenic poisoning the patient may sink into a cachectic state and show evidence of mental deterioration.

Treatment.—The removal of the patient from contact with arsenic will usually result in a gradual disappearance of the symptoms. Elimination should be stimulated by the forcing of fluids and the use of mild saline cathartics. The intravenous injection of 10 cc. of a 5 per cent calcium thiosulphate solution every other day has appeared to hasten the clearing of the skin lesions. Pigmentation and hyperkeratosis may occasionally be permanent. Milder forms of neuritis have a good prognosis, but if motor paralysis is marked only partial recovery may be expected.

REFERENCES.

DUBREUILH, W.: Kératose arsénicale et cancer arsénical, Ann. d. dermat. et syph., 1910, 5th series, **1**, 65.

RAMBOUSEK, J.: Industrial Poisoning, translated by T. M. Legge, London, Arnold, 1913, p. 144.

STOKES, J. H.: Modern Clinical Syphilology, Philadelphia, W. B. Saunders Company, 1926, p. 281.

WEBSTER, R. W.: Legal Medicine and Toxicology, Philadelphia, W. B. Saunders Company, 1930, p. 479.

MERCURY POISONING.

The commonest form of mercury poisoning in this country is due to the ingestion of bichloride of mercury, usually with suicidal intent. A certain number of poisonings also arise as a result of the medicinal use of mercury compounds. Industrial poisoning is relatively common in quicksilver mines and in a limited number of trades.

Mercury may be absorbed through the digestive tract and, when in the form of vapor, through the lungs. Absoption may also occur through the skin and the vaginal mucous membrane. As in the case of arsenic and lead, mercury that is ingested is largely held at first in the liver and later is redistributed among the other tissues of the body. There is a considerable re-excretion of mercury in the bile. That the protection offered by the liver is not very great is shown, however, by the fact that mercury may be found in the urine in as brief a time as five minutes after ingestion of a large dose of a soluble salt. The excretion of mercury is chiefly through the digestive canal and especially through the colon. The saliva contains small amounts. The excretion through the kidneys is less considerable than that through the bowel.

Acute Forms of Mercury Poisoning.—Mercuric Chloride.—In the early period of antisepsis strong mercuric chloride solutions were employed freely for vaginal irrigations and for the irrigation of wounds. Many fatalities were reported. Since 1910 the number of suicidal deaths from bichloride has shown a marked increase, so that it is now the poison most commonly used for this purpose in this country.

The 0.5 gram (7½-grain) tablet, which is readily obtainable, is usually swallowed either whole or in pieces, and washed down with water. Occasionally the tablets are dissolved and the solution swallowed. The total dose taken is usually between 0.5 and 2 grams (7½ and 30 grains). As little as 0.1 gram (1½ grains) has caused death, and as much as 4 grams has been survived. As a rule, fatalities are rare unless more than 0.5 gram has been taken.

The chief determining factor is the length of time elapsing between ingestion of the drug and emptying of the stomach by vomiting or by lavage. Solutions of the drug are more fatal than gross particles. The presence of food in the stomach offers a measure of protection, but on the other hand may delay vomiting and postpone recourse to medical assistance until considerable amounts of the drug have passed beyond the stomach. Vomiting usually occurs within ten minutes after swallowing the bichloride tablets, but it may be delayed for several hours.

The character and the severity of the symptoms of poisoning vary greatly in different cases. There is usually an astringent metallic taste in the mouth, followed in a few minutes by upper abdominal pain and vomiting. If the stomach is effectively emptied by early vomiting, the ensuing symptoms may be very slight; slight intestinal unrest for a few hours, with perhaps one or two loose stools and no later evidence of renal damage. On the other hand, when the mercury is longer retained, repeated violent vomiting and retching up of blood-stained mucus and epithelial shreds may continue for hours, accompanied by severe abdominal pain and purging, with liquid bloody stools. Immediate anuria occurs. There is a sharp leukocytosis. With these marked gastro-intestinal symptoms there may be evidence of severe shock. Collapse and death may occur in the first forty-eight hours. The chief postmortem finding in such cases is the hemorrhagic and gangrenous gastritis. The kidneys show an early stage of nephrosis, there is cloudy swelling of the liver cells, and the mucosa of the colon is congested and edematous.

In a third group of cases the vomiting soon subsides and there is only a moderate number of mucous and bloody stools. After the first day the patient does not appear ill. The urine, however, is scant and heavily laden with albumin and casts; total anuria may occur. With the diminished output of urine the non-protein nitrogenous constituents of the blood rise rapidly day by day. There is usually a severe acidosis, as measured by the carbon dioxide combining power of the plasma. If vomiting and diarrhea have been severe the chlorides in the blood will be decreased. The blood pressure may show a moderate rise. Slight edema of the face is not uncommon. After a few days of anuria the patient becomes dull and toxic. Mercurial stomatitis appears, with a characteristic odor, salivation, swollen gums and shallow grayish ulcerations of the mucous membranes under the tongue and inside the cheeks. Weakness and stupor lead on to death. Convulsions do not occur.

Anuria frequently persists for only two or three days and with the reëstablishment of the renal output recovery may follow. The toxemia from ulcerative and gangrenous colitis and a severe stomatitis occasionally is fatal, in spite of increasing elimination by urine. The kidneys of cases dying after the first few days are large and soft. The cortex is pale and the cortical markings blurred. There is swelling and necrosis of the epithelium of the convoluted tubules, and to a lesser degree of the epithelium of Henle's loops. Calcium deposits are found in the degenerated epithelium and free in the lumen of the tubules. Early stages of regeneration of the epithelial lining of the tubules are observed after the first week.

Diagnosis.—In suicidal cases the history given by the patient is not always reliable. The gastric contents, the urine and the stools should be saved for analysis. For detection of mercury the electrolytic method of Booth and Schreiber is rapid and delicate.

Prognosis.—The dosage, the "emesis interval" and the thoroughness of treatment, all affect the prognosis in the individual case. Statistics show mortalities ranging between 6 and 42 per cent. In non-fatal cases there is almost always complete recovery from the nephrosis.

Treatment.—The details of the treatment of bichloride of mercury poisoning are discussed in the Section on Nephrosis, p. 541.

Subacute Poisoning.—The medicinal use of mercury compounds in the treatment of syphilis, exposure to vaporized mercury in quicksilver mines, the making of thermometers and barometers and the manufacture of the explosive fulminate of mercury, may all lead to a subacute form of poisoning. The outstanding symptom in these cases is mercurial stomatitis which may develop after from a few days up to several weeks of exposure. There is a metallic taste in the mouth and the teeth become sensitive to pressure. The gums look swollen and bluish. The tongue becomes flabby and edematous and grayish in color. The breath has a distinctive odor. The degree of ptyalism varies very much. It is usually not marked. In severe cases there is great difficulty in swallowing and in speech. The lips and cheeks are swollen, the cervical glands enlarged; the tongue and inner surfaces of the cheeks show areas covered with a grayish necrotic membrane. The odor is that of the fusiform bacillus infection, which is a common invader of the injured tissues. Rarely there is necrosis of the mandible. Such cases may also show mercurial tremor and the psychic symptoms which are more common in chronic poisoning.

Chronic Poisoning.—The chronic effects of mercury poisoning are rarely seen in this country except in the hatters' trade and in quicksilver miners. A tremor of a fine type, interrupted every few minutes by coarse shaking movements, appears in the hands first, but later affects the whole body, interfering with all coördinated effort. It is an intention tremor, increases with excitement and disappears in sleep. In addition to the tremor these patients suffer a remarkable change in personality, rendering them timid, shy and easily irritated. Pathologic somnolence may occur. Recovery is uncertain. Treatment, aside from avoidance of further exposure to mercury, is purely symptomatic.

REFERENCES.

HAMILTON, ALICE: Industrial Poisons in the United States, New York, The Macmillan Company, 1925, p. 234.

HASKELL, C. C., CARDER, J. R., and COFFINDAFFER, R. S.: The Value of Forcing Fluid in the Treatment of Mercuric Chloride Poisoning, Jour. Am. Med. Assn., 1923, **81**, 448.

LAMBERT, G. W., and PATTERSON, H. S.: Poisoning by Mercuric Chloride and Its Treatment, Arch. Int. Med., 1915, **16**, 865.

ROSENTHAL, S. M.: Mercury Poisoning, Jour. Am. Med. Assn., 1934, **102**, 1273.

WEISS, H. B.: Mercuric Chloride Poisoning, Arch. Int. Med., 1924, **33**, 224.

BENZENE POISONING.

Benzene, or benzol (C_6H_6), is produced commercially by the distillation of coal tar and is therefore a by-product of the illuminating gas and coke industries. Pure benzene is a volatile, colorless liquid, whose vapors are three times as heavy as air. Even high concentrations of benzene in air are non-irritant and not malodorous. Commercial benzene contains varying amounts of toluene, xylene and thiophene.

The limits of concentration within which benzene will produce acute or chronic poisoning by inhalation are not well established. In general, it may be said that fatal effects will be rapidly produced by concentrations of over 15,000 parts of benzene in 1,000,000 parts of air, while continued inhalation of as little as 200 parts in 1,000,000 may produce evidence of chronic poisoning. There is a wide variation in susceptibility. Young people, and in particular young women, tend to be more susceptible.

After absorption through the lungs, 15 to 30 per cent of the benzene is oxidized in the body to dioxybenzenes and phenols which after conjugation with glycuronic or sulphuric acids are slowly excreted by the kidneys. These retained oxidation products may be the chief toxic agents in benzene poisoning. The unoxidized benzene is readily eliminated through the lungs.

The industrial use of benzene is chiefly due to its solvent and to its rapid drying properties. The limitation of its use is largely because of its inflammability and the dangers of toxic effects.

It is employed on a large scale in the recovery of fats and oils by extraction processes, as a constituent of varnishes, shellacs and quick drying paints, and in many departments of the rubber, leather and sanitary can industries as a part of rubber cement. The diminished use of rubber cement containing benzene since the introduction of latex, a crude liquid form of rubber, for the same purposes has markedly reduced the incidence of benzene poisoning.

In the chemical industry benzene is used as the starting-point for the synthesis of many aniline dyes, of phenol and of the explosive, picric acid. Benzene is a constituent of many blended motor fuels. In all these industries benzene poisoning has occurred, but the majority of the reported cases has arisen as a result of the use of rubber cements and rubber liquid water-proofing preparations containing benzene, in warm and insufficiently ventilated rooms.

Acute benzene poisoning has occurred chiefly in the chemical industry in connection with the cleaning or repairing of vats, kettles and pipes which have contained benzene. The inhalation of high concentrations produces dizziness, incoördination and mental confusion, followed rapidly by unconsciousness and death. The symptoms may be progressive even after early removal to fresh air.

Chronic benzene poisoning is insidious in its onset. The prodromal symptoms are those of anemia: weakness, dizziness, palpitation and dyspnea on exertion. After several weeks or months more alarming symptoms set in rather abruptly.

Purpuric spots appear over the body, and spontaneous bleeding occurs from the nose, gums, throat, bowel and urinary tract. In women intractable metrorrhagia may occur. Death from profound anemia and exhaustion frequently follows the development of the bleeding tendency. In others, gradual improvement and eventual recovery have been observed. Removal of the patient from contact with benzene after the development of marked anemia does not always interrupt the progress of symptoms which may go on developing and lead to a fatal issue.

The effect of benzene is upon the circulating blood and upon the blood-forming tissues. There is an early reduction in the white blood cells to below 5000 and in the late stages counts of 1500 or less are not infrequent. This leukopenia is chiefly due to diminution in the polymorphonuclear white cells whose percentage in the differential count is often below 40. Later the platelets show a marked reduction and in severe cases practically disappear. The thrombocytopenia is related to the severe purpura of the late stages. The fall in the red cell counts and hemoglobin begins as a rule later than that in the white cells. The early stages of the anemia are due to injury to the marrow. Hemolysis is not a feature of the process. With the onset of bleeding, the red cell count falls more rapidly and frequently drops to 1,000,000 or less. Nucleated red cells are not seen and other immature forms are rare. The anemia is of an aplastic type. The pathology of reported cases has shown extensive damage to both the white and red bone-marrow.

Prevention.—Non-toxic substitutes for benzene should be employed when possible. Industrial processes in which benzene must be used should be safeguarded as far as possible by ventilation and suction drafts. Young girls, because of their susceptibility, should not work with benzene products. All employees coming in contact with benzene should have periodic blood examinations. The appearance of even moderate leukopenia or anemia should lead to their removal from contact with benzene.

Treatment.—Repeated transfusion of blood has been found the most effective measure in the severe cases with marked anemia and purpura.

PART IV.

DISEASES OF THE NERVOUS SYSTEM.

CHAPTER XXV.

DISEASES AND ABNORMALITIES OF THE MIND, INCLUDING THE NEUROSES.[1]

By EDWARD A. STRECKER, M.D.

THE PSYCHOSES.
  Paresis.
  Senile Psychoses.
  Psychoses with Cerebral Arterio-sclerosis.
  Epileptic Psychoses.
  Psychosis with Mental Deficiency.
  Psychoses with Cerebral Syphilis; Huntington's Chorea, Brain Tumor, Encephalitis, and Other Brain and Nervous Diseases; Traumatic Psychoses.

THE TOXIC PSYCHOSES.
  Exogenous Toxic Psychoses.
  Psychoses with Somatic Disease.
  Manic Depressive Psychoses.
  Involution Melancholia.
  Schizophrenia (Dementia Præcox)
  Constitutional Psychopathic Inferiority.
THE NEUROSES.
  Hysteria.
  Neurasthenia.
  Psychasthenia.
  Anxiety Neurosis.

THE PSYCHOSES.

Introduction.—The mode of presentation of the diseases of the mind to the physician and the medical student has become somewhat formalized. The praiseworthy effort to attain completion often results in unduly lengthy discussions and fails to place proper emphasis on those conditions that are commonly encountered in practice. After all, while a description of paranoia makes fascinating reading, it is so rare that the physician may go through a lifetime of practice without meeting a single instance. Much more important is a thorough understanding and appreciation of schizophrenia, which is, perhaps, the most common psychosis, or paresis, which in its early stages is vulnerable to intelligent therapeutic attack. Multiple personality in hysteria provides material for engrossing speculation, but much more practical for the doctor is the knowledge of the common neuroses and their everyday manifestations. It is the opinion of the author that *the neuroses and neurotic additions to organic disease constitute about 70 per cent of the practice of medicine.*

---

[1] The author acknowledges the courtesy of being permitted to quote from "Clinical Psychiatry," by Strecker and Ebaugh, 3d edition, P. Blakiston's Son & Co., 1931.

It is a grave mistake to isolate psychiatry.   It is part and parcel of internal medicine.   When one remembers that the human being is a *total organism*, with various physiologic and psychologic levels and that the whole organism must always be studied in reference to the environment, it is easy to appreciate that so-called mental symptoms are often only manifestations of causes which in other instances or even in the identical patient may produce fever, alteration in the pulse-rate and the like.   Thus, infection, fever, exhaustion, toxic agents like alcohol, drugs, certain metals and gases, the more chronic intoxications like lues and tuberculosis, metabolic deficiency and arteriosclerotic disturbances or endocrine imbalances, all have mental components or symptoms which are really not separable from physical phenomena. Conversely, that whole group of experiences ordinarily called "emotional" unquestionably influence the clinical pictures and even, to some extent, the course and outcome of organic disease, whether it be eczema or typhoid fever.   As a matter of fact, there is no dividing line between psychiatry and internal medicine.

Importance of Psychiatry.—It is unfair to burden the student with many statistics.   Perhaps the importance of psychiatry is sufficiently emphasized in the authorized statement that *more hospital beds are devoted to the care of the mentally afflicted than to all other classes of patients combined*.   It is a conservative estimate that 1 person out of 26 of the general population becomes mentally sick.   When one takes into consideration the many patients who never reach public hospitals and, further, the numerous psychopathologic borderline conditions such as psychoneuroses, which are often just as serious and disabling in their consequences as the psychoses, yet do not require institutional care, it becomes clear that mental disease constitutes a critical and far-reaching medical and economic problem.   It is obvious that only a small fraction of this great army of the mentally unfit comes to the specialist during the stage of incipiency when it is often possible to accomplish something constructive and to avert the calamity of chronicity.   Many individuals who are threatened with the spectre of insanity, but who are still struggling to live in the world of reality, are to be found in the consulting room of the busy general practitioner.   It is imperative that he at least be sufficiently informed about the bare outlines of psychiatry, so that he may be able to deal helpfully with such conditions.

General Considerations.—**Etiology.**—In the consideration of the individual psychoses the causal and determining agents will be stressed, but at this point a broader and more philosophic viewpoint may not be amiss.   In the final analysis, mental disease and, indeed, all disease, is due to the overthrowing of resistance.   Resistance against mental disease at any given point in the life history of an individual is determined by the sum total of his previous experiences (including ancestral assets and liabilities) and his reaction to them.   The vulnerability of this resistance is extremely variable not only from person to person, but also it varies during the life-cycle of the same individual, and, finally, it differs according to the amount of the particular resistance which may be developed against this or that specific threat to mental stability.

The resistance may be abruptly destroyed or it may be insidiously undermined. These simple diagrams may be illustrative (p. 1071).

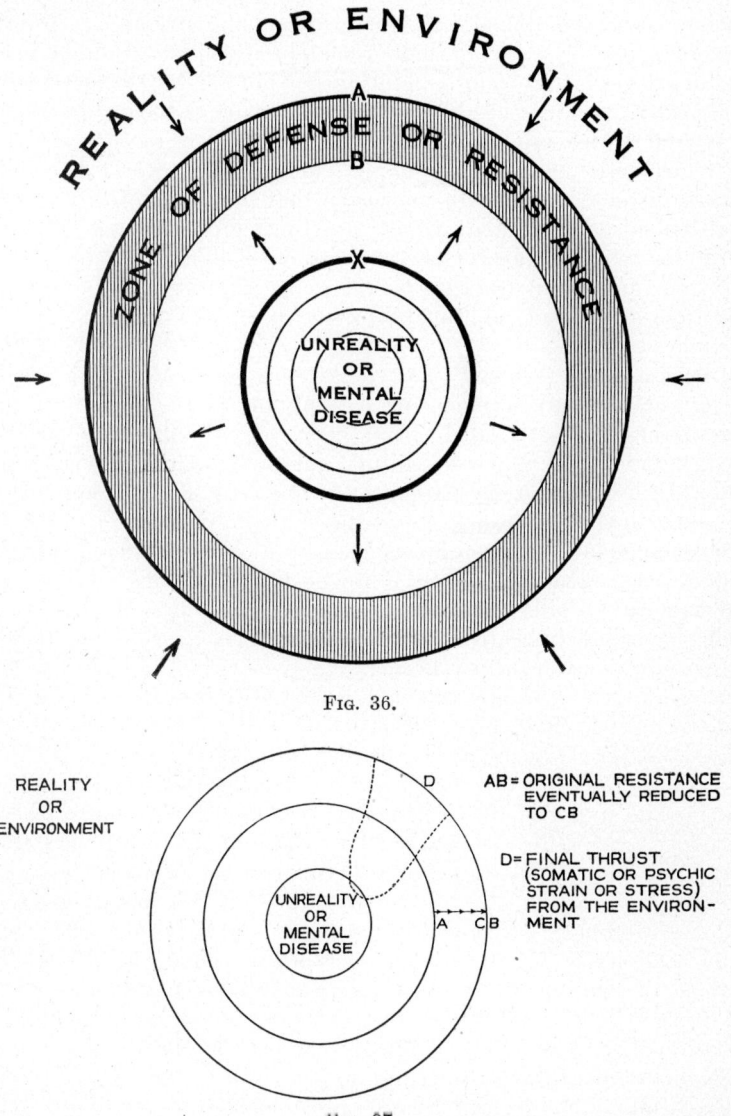

Fig. 36.

REALITY
OR
ENVIRONMENT

AB = ORIGINAL RESISTANCE
EVENTUALLY REDUCED
TO CB

D = FINAL THRUST
(SOMATIC OR PSYCHIC
STRAIN OR STRESS)
FROM THE ENVIRON-
MENT

Fig. 37.

Figs. 36 and 37.—In Fig. 36 a normal amount of resistance against mental disease is indicated by the line A–B. It is to be noted that this is in perfect contact with reality or environment at every point. Unreality or mental disease and its various degrees of severity is indicated by the inner circles. (From "Clinical Psychiatry," by Strecker and Ebaugh, Philadelphia, P. Blakiston's Son & Co., 1931.)

When the physician sees a patient who is mentally or "nervously" sick, he is witnessing the end-result of a serious disturbance of the normal relationship between that patient and his environment. It is easy to understand how this balance, representing normal mental health, may be upset not only by such physical agents as syphilis or arteriosclerosis of the brain, but also by the factors ordinarily denominated "emotional," as, for instance, the stress and strain of prolonged fear or worry, or, more remotely, by lack of training during childhood so that problems of adult life cannot be met.

Heredity.—Unquestionably, inheritance is influential in the genesis of mental disease but its influence must not be over-rated. It should be remembered that, in psychiatry, one must not expect Mendelian accuracy concerning heredity nor even that likelihood of transmission that attends such human defects as Huntington's chorea or family paralysis. At the present stage of its development psychiatry will derive greater profit from the biometrician, from clinical observation and from a study of environment, than from a rigid interpretation of the inheritance factor.

Diagnosis and Prognosis.—To type a psychosis or neurosis according to certain diagnostic formulæ and slavishly to prognose strictly according to the diagnostic label means little or nothing. In no field of medicine is it more important to take into account the personal equation; to consider first the patient and not be too much frightened by the name of the psychosis. For instance, schizophrenia may be hopelessly malignant, but in a given instance a careful review of the life history may reveal many hopeful prognostic indications.

Treatment.—Under each psychosis the chief lines of therapeutic endeavor will be indicated, but there should be some brief mention of: (*a*) prophylaxis and (*b*) psychotherapy.

Prevention.—Psychiatry abounds in opportunities for the institution of preventive measures. Every patient should be viewed from this angle. Never a case of paresis but that it should teach the importance of lessening the incidence of syphilis; never an instance of schizophrenia but that its study should yield safeguards applicable to the training of children; never a neurotic patient but whose life history should teach the prophylactic importance of a better contact between individual and environment.

Psychotherapy.—Psychotherapy is *not*, as popularly supposed, a kind of mental sleight-of-hand or miracle working that magically relieves patients of symptoms. It is the important therapeutic weapon of the psychiatrist. It is regrettable that it is not more generally employed in internal medicine. Psychotherapy has very broad limitations. It may be defined as an attempt to influence in the right direction the attitude of the patient, that is, to influence his attitude toward himself, toward his mental and physical processes and toward his environment. It is an effort to teach him to understand himself, his illness, and the cause or causes of his illness, whether this cause or these causes lie in his body, in his environment, or in the superficial or deeper layers of his mental life. Persuasion, suggestion, useful habit formation, self-understanding, strengthening of morale, are all valuable psychotherapeutic methods. Freudian psychoanalytic catharsis is a highly specialized technic that investigates the unconscious psyche (beyond the scope of the awareness of the patient) and, through the interpretation of the everyday behavior, free association and the dream life, seeks to give the patient enough self-knowledge so that he may sever the bonds of restricting fixations, become free of his symptoms and emotionally mature.

Classification.—In psychiatry, nosology faces even greater obstacles that it does in internal medicine. The body of information from which a classification scheme must be built is creditably large, but, unfortunately, it is not homogeneous. For instance, paresis in its etiology, pathology and symptoms is as clearly understood as is typhoid fever or tuberculosis, but, on the other hand, schizophrenia remains an unsolved riddle, yet it must be fitted into any list of mental diseases.

The accompanying grouping is based on a simple division into:

- (*a*) Organic.
- (*b*) Toxic.
- (*c*) Functional or psychogenic.

Certain psychoses are predominantly organic, that is, they present pathologic alterations in the structure of the brain; other psychoses are predominantly toxic, in other words, the symptoms are produced by bodily intoxication, either by poisons introduced into the body from without (for instance, alcohol), or by poisons created within the organism (uremia); finally, in some psychoses the important factors seem to be functional or psychogenic.

Naturally, such a classification is far from conclusive. As more knowledge is gained, unquestionably there will be shifting from the organic to the toxic group and *vice versa*. Even at this writing it is obvious that even in the most clear-cut organic psychosis (paresis) there are frequently toxic manifestations, while in the toxic reactions one often witnesses permanent structural alterations. Furthermore, the functional or psychogenic group as a whole will scarcely stand the test of time, since even now many interesting organic and toxic manifestations have been recorded. Finally, the student must always remember that the prepsychotic personality of the individual may color deeply the expression of any psychosis.

The psychoses that are starred will be described in some detail. Wherever reliable statistics are available percentage frequency is given.

A. Organic Psychoses.

1. Traumatic psychoses	0.3 per cent
*2. Senile psychoses	12.1 per cent
*3. Psychoses with cerebral arteriosclerosis	6.4 per cent
*4. General paralysis (paresis)	10.6 per cent
5. Psychosis with cerebral syphilis	
6. Psychoses with Huntington's chorea	
7. Psychosis with brain tumor	
8. Psychoses with other brain or nervous diseases. (Cerebral embolism, paralysis agitans, meningitis, tubercular or other forms, multiple sclerosis, tabes dorsalis, acute chorea, encephalitis lethargica, and other neurologic diseases.)	1.2 per cent
*9. Epileptic psychoses	2.7 per cent
10. Psychoses with mental deficiency	3.3 per cent

B. Toxic Psychoses.

*11. Alcoholic psychoses . . . .   2.2 per cent
     (This figure based on comparative admissions to the
     State hospitals in the United States in 1920. In
     1922–1923, of 4444 consecutive admissions to
     the Psychopathic Wards of the Philadelphia Hos-
     pital, 10.8 per cent had alcoholic psychoses.)
12. Psychoses due to drugs and other exogenous toxins .   1.1 per cent
13. Psychoses with pellagra . . . .   0.37 per cent
*14. Psychoses with other somatic diseases . . . .   2.81 per cent
     (Including delirium with infectious disease, post-
     fectious psychosis, exhaustion delirium, delir-
     ium of unknown origin, cardio-renal disease,
     diseases of the ductless glands, epidemic encepha-
     litis, other diseases or conditions.)
     The percentage figure is undoubtedly too low. It
     is based on admissions to public mental hospitals.
     The majority of these psychoses are encountered
     in general hospitals, in sanitoria, in private prac-
     tice, etc.

C. Functional (Psychogenic) Psychoses.

*15. Manic-depressive psychoses . . . .   16.0 per cent
*16. Involution melancholia . . . .   3.2 per cent
*17. Schizophrenia (dementia præcox) . . . . .   27.0 per cent
18. Paranoia or paranoid conditions . . . . . .   2.8 per cent
*19. Neuroses . . . .   2.1 per cent
     (This percentage figure gives no idea of the enor-
     mous frequency and importance of the neuroses.
     It is based on the number of neurotic patients
     admitted to public mental hospitals which con-
     stitutes only a small fraction of the total.)
20. Psychoses with psychopathic personality.

Examination and Symptoms.—The psychiatrist has no quick devices, reliable short-cuts and but few instruments of precision at his command. Perhaps this is the reason why psychiatry is such a fascinating subject. Master and student alike must utilize comprehensive and detailed history and conscientious examinations as a basis for sound and scientific opinion concerning diagnosis, prognostic possibilities and treatment.

To repeat the steps of history taking and physical examination is unnecessary. The student will find adequate guides in any standard text-book.[1]

It should be emphasized that the physical examination should be extremely thorough and the physician should not hesitate to utilize every reliable diagnostic procedure and laboratory aid. This is particularly true since, while specific organic findings are scarcely to be expected in the psychoses, yet there is frequently abundant pathology so that a thorough understanding of the body of each individual patient is needed if there is to be intelligent treatment.

Mental Examination.—A mental examination is a specialized but not at all a difficult undertaking. A few hints are worth consideration.

I. *Avoid rigidly formal examinations.* The patient is apt to become shy, frightened, suspicious and uncommunicative, and the examination itself degenerates into a cut-and-dried questionnaire.

II. *Encourage the patient to tell his story in his own words.* With a coöperative patient, this will produce a very satisfactory revelation of the mental life of the patient.

---

[1] The author uses the method outlined in "Clinical Psychiatry," by Strecker and Ebaugh, 3d edition, Chapter III, Philadelphia, P. Blakiston's Son & Co., 1931.

III. *Try to establish satisfactory contact with the patient.* The nearer the examination approaches a friendly discussion, the better will be the yield of information.

IV. *Let observation be complete.* Much of clinical value may be learned by observation, before direct questions are asked. This is, perhaps, particularly true of the so-called uncoöperative stage of a psychosis. Here the behavior often reveals valuable diagnostic and prognostic clues.

V. *The appreciation of the emotional reaction is highly important.* The appearance, posture, bearing and gestures of the patient, the amount and type of motor activity, the facial expression, etc., will usually furnish a more reliable index of the emotional status than answers to a great number of even very skillfully worded questions.

VI. *The examination should be reported carefully and completely.*

While formal routine mental examinations are to be deplored, yet the examination when completed should reveal information covering the following headings. Under each heading the reader will find a list of symptoms and signs, some of which he may expect to find, and by referring to the Glossary (p. 1107) he may gain some understanding of their meaning.

I. *Patient's Story.*

If the patient is willing to speak freely, the entire psychosis will be readily revealed.

II. *Attitude and General Behavior.*

Catalepsy	Mannerism
Catatonia	Mutism
Cerea flexibilitas	Negativism
Compulsive act	Obsession
Distractibility	Retardation
Echopraxia	Suggestibility
Impulsive act	Stupor

III. *Stream of Mental Activity and Speech.*

Dissociation	Neologism
Distractibility	Rambling
Echolalia	Retardation
Flight of ideas	Scattering
Garrulousness	Sound association
Incoherence	Stereotopy
Irrelevancy	Verbigeration
Mutism	Volubility

IV. *Emotional Reaction (Mood, Affect).*

By the careful observation of the patient and the asking of appropriate questions, an idea of the emotional reaction is gained. It is important to determine whether or not it is in keeping with the trend of thought.

IV. *Emotional Reaction (Mood, Affect).—(Continued).*

The psychotic patient may reverberate to any note in the emotional scale and here are listed only a few significant reactions:

Euphoric	Irritable
Exhilarated	Furious
Depressed	Silly
Anxious	Indifferent
Apprehensive	Dull
Suspicious	Apathetic
Perplexed	

The student should note also ambivalency, dementia and dissociation.

V. *Mental Trend.*

Autistic thinking	Ideas of reference
Delusions	Illusions
Hallucinations	Symbolizations

VI. *Sensorium, Mental Grasp and Capacity.*

Disorientation (disturbance of orientation).
Memory (both recent and remote).
Retention and recall.
Counting and calculation.
Reading and recall.
Writing.
Attention.
School, general and current knowledge.

VII. *Intelligence Rating.*

Use any of the standardized tests.

VIII. *Insight.*

The capacity of the patient to understand his psychosis and its symptoms. It is important to record the degree and character of the insight.

IX. *Psychologic Analysis.*

In selected cases the examinations may be extended to include free association, hypnosis and dream analysis.

Mental Mechanisms.—Psychiatry has passed beyond the descriptive phase. This phase reached its culmination in Emil Kraepelin whose descriptive observations were so accurate that they have become classical. But today, just as the internist is not content with hearing a curious sound which signifies aortic regurgitation, unless he can understand the mechanics of the sound, so likewise is the psychiatrist not satisfied with the knowledge of the fact that a patient has delusions or illusions, but he wants to know why in a given case the false beliefs or the sensory deceptions take this or that form. Such scientific curiosity has led to the present phase of interpretative psychiatry.

Interpretative psychiatry attempts to look beneath the surface of mental symptoms and discover their hidden meaning. For instance, why does a certain schizophrenic hallucinate so vividly and assert that everyone is calling him a sexual pervert? Why does another patient stand for hours with arms outstretched in the form of a cross? What is there in the hidden mental lives of these two patients which has determined the shaping of their mental symptoms? In an hysterical amnesia, what particular repressed experience is being concealed from conscious memory? In a psychasthenic fear, let us say, of feathers, is it the purpose of the phobia to keep from everyday thought an even more disagreeable and painful memory? And, if so, what is that memory? Is the given attack of acute mania, during which the patient is markedly exhilarated and seemingly without a care in the world, merely a pathologic compensation for conditions of life that the patient could no longer tolerate? The psychiatrist wishes to penetrate the concealed objective of these phenomena since the more he succeeds in unraveling their genesis, the greater are his chances of helping the patient.

The Organic Psychoses.

1. General paralysis (paresis).
2. Senile psychoses.
3. Psychoses with cerebral arteriosclerosis.
4. Epileptic psychoses.
5. Psychoses with mental deficiency.
6. Psychoses with cerebral syphilis, Huntington's chorea, brain tumor, encephalitis and other brain and nervous diseases.
7. Traumatic psychoses.

In this group we consider a group of psychoses in which, although there are wide symptomic variations, influenced by the previous make-up of the patient, yet the constant and dominant etiologic factor is the pathologic alteration in brain structure. The symptoms are deteriorative, and usually involve regression in the intellectual, emotional and ethical fields. In these psychoses there are generally definite physical and neurologic signs; the prognosis is poor but, often, the preventive opportunities are brilliant.

PARESIS.

Etiology.—The most notable example of an organic psychosis is paresis. As is well known, it is always due to invasion of the brain by the Treponema pallidum which may be demonstrated in the brain tissue.

Only a relatively small proportion of luetics become paretic, and, therefore, the nature of the secondary precipitating factor is an important and moot question. On the one hand, there must be considered a "nervous" strain of the specific organism; on the other, the effect of exogenous stress such as alcohol, head trauma and, indeed, a whole group of damaging physical and emotional agents. Since lues is more common in the male and, also, since it appears from ten to twenty years after the initial infection, paresis is obviously more frequent in men. It reaches its incidence peak in the fifth decade of life. Juvenile paresis appears before the twentieth year.

Pathology.—The picture is somewhat variable but typical findings are, *macroscopically,* a thickened pia arachnoid, especially in the fronto-parietal region, deepened sulci containing turbid fluid, small brain with shrunken convolutions, edema, dilated ventricles and granular ependymitis, particularly in the fourth ventricle, and, *microscopically,* sulcal infiltration with round cells (plasma cells and lymphocytes), dropping out of cortical ganglion cells, glial cell increase, rod cells, endothelial proliferation and vessel "collaring" by plasma cells and lymphocytes, degenerative changes in ganglion cells, cortical fiber atrophy, and by special technic *the presence of the treponema of syphilis.*

Symptoms and Diagnosis.—Artificial divisions of paresis into various stages are not justified by clinical experience. The diagnosis should scarcely ever be missed since it rests on a triad of findings, the serologic, the neurologic and the mental.

Of these three groups, the serologic is by far the most reliable and in fact is almost "fool proof" in its diagnostic incisiveness. This is particularly true in untreated patients.

Serologic Findings.—Blood and spinal fluid strongly positive; pleocytosis (lymphocytic); positive globulin; "steppage" gold curve.

Physical Neurologic Findings.—Somewhat less reliable diagnostically, but still strikingly important, are the physical neurologic signs. They usually begin insidiously, although careful examination is apt to discover several even in the early stages (a seizure may be an early phenomenon) and untreated patients progress rapidly to an emaciated, bedridden, helpless paralytic state.

Major physical neurologic signs: unequal, irregular, sluggish or Argyll-Robertson pupils; tendon reflexes, especially patellar, exaggerated; tremors: mouth, naso-labial folds, hands, tongue, entire body; speech: slurring and stumbling; apoplectic or epileptic convulsive seizures which leave only minor residuals.

Minor physical neurologic signs: *Early:* loss of weight, hypersomnia, insomnia, fatigability, digestive disturbances, impairment of vision, rheumatoid pains; loss of facial expression; transient eye-muscle pareses; tremulous handwriting; positive Romberg; shuffling, slouchy gait; inability to perform finer movements; absent knee-kicks (taboparesis); vasomotor and trophic: flushing, cyanosis, fainting, brief aphasias, bed-sores, failing nutrition.

Mental Findings.—Paresis, mentally, may simulate any psychosis and of the triad of findings—serologic, physical neurologic and mental—the mental are diagnostically far inferior. If they have any diagnostic conclusiveness at all, it is in the early and late stages of the disease. *Early* one may find with a fair degree of frequency a neurasthenic picture, irritability, slight changes in character and disposition, mental slowness, judgment defects, moral laxity and forgetfulness. In the final stages, a profound dementia, involving a loss of ethical, moral, emotional and intellectual life, which robs the patient of every faculty which distinguishes man from animal,

Due largely to the intrusion of prepsychotic personality traits, paresis at its height may mimic any psychosis but with fair constancy four chief types may be distinguished:

Expansive.—(10 to 25 per cent.) Extravagant, grandiose delusions concerning personal qualities and possessions and fantastic plans (strongest man in the world, all the gold and precious stones, a thousand wives, a million children, building interplanetary bridges, etc.), euphoria, periods of irritability, combativeness, motor activity.

Depressed.—(25 per cent.) Depression, horrible depressive somatic delusions (gullet or intestines stopped up, no stomach, intestines rotten, brain replaced by sawdust, blood-vessels made of glass, etc.).

Agitated.—(10 to 15 per cent.) Great psychomotor activity, principally motor, and clouding of consciousness.

Demented.—(40 per cent.) Rapidly increasing deterioration of all the faculties of the mind.

Prognosis.—Without treatment, a convulsive seizure, intercurrent disease as pneumonia, cystitis, bed-sores, choking, exhaustion and very occasionally suicide terminate life in about two years. Remissions which are much more frequent under treatment may last from a few days to one or even several years. The mental symptoms largely disappear, but significant neurologic and serologic signs are apt to remain.

Treatment.—Within the past fifteen years Wagner Jauregg and other workers have written a brilliant chapter in the therapy of paresis. Today it is scarcely justifiable to treat paresis with the arsenicals, excepting tryparsamide or when contraindications to fever treatment exist, and even then mercury or bismuth should be carefully considered. Indeed, there is a growing body of opinion that the arsenical treatment of lues even in the earlier stages hastens and increases the incidence of neurosyphilis.

The most useful therapeutic resources center around the induction of repeated fever by malaria, rat-bite fever or artificially by electricity. The author recommends the use of tertian malaria (Plasmodium vivax) inoculated into the patient from the malarial donor by the subcutaneous or intracutaneous injections of 2 to 3 cc. of citrated whole malarial blood. After an incubation period of three to twenty-one days, the patient is permitted to have about eight malarial paroxysms. Then termination is brought about by giving orally the bisulphate of quinine, 0.6 gram (10 grains), three times daily, until the blood has been free from the plasmodium for at least fourteen days. The chief contraindications are decompensating cardiac and aortic disease, rapidly progressing ("galloping") paresis, tabes with severe ataxia, juvenile paresis, primary optic atrophy, severe cachexia or such systemic diseases as diabetes, nephritis, hepatitis or tuberculosis.

SENILE PSYCHOSES.

Etiology.—Brain destruction conditioned by cerebral arteriosclerosis and other factors including old age and possibly by toxic and hereditarial influences. The greatest incidence is between the ages of sixty and seventy-five years.   Meggendorfer finds a familial tendency and believes that alcoholism favors early development.

Pathology.—Small brain, narrow convolutions, thick pia arachnoid, fluid-filled sulci, tortuous and sclerotic vessels and, microscopically, ganglion cell loss and atrophy, glial increase, thick, prominent vessels, cortical fat excess and in the cortex and basal ganglia the presence of typical senile plaques.

Symptoms.—The student may advantageously regard the senile psychoses from three symptomatic angles.   The first, psychologically at least, is closely connected with the restrictions and limitations of old age.   Here we may expect irritability, deterioration of normal emotional reactions, obstinacy, stubbornness, self-centering of interests, selfishness, outbreaks of temper, moral laxities or penuriousness.   The second is somewhat more closely connected with the brain pathology, and embraces defects of orientation, lessened mental capacity, defective attention, concentration and thinking, a tendency to reminisce and fabricate, and, finally, the keynote symptom upon which the other phenomena are to a certain extent dependent, namely, *the failure of recent memory*.   Far less important in the clinical picture are the symptoms that are in some degree at least influenced by the personality. Here, we may consider the following subdivisions:

(a) *Simple Deterioration.*—Defective retention and memory, reduced intellectual capacity, narrowed interests.   Often there is suspiciousness, irritability and restlessness, usually nocturnal.

(b) *Presbyophrenic Type.*—Marked memory and retention defect with complete disorientation.   The patient is mentally alert, attentive and able to grasp immediate impressions.   Forgetfulness leads to absurd contradictions and repetitions.   Prominent are suggestibility and fabrication.

(c) *Delirious and Confused Types.*—In the early stages there may be deep confusion or delirium.

(d) *Depressed and Agitated Types.*—Mental deterioration plus pronounced depression and persistent agitation.

(e) *Paranoid Types.*—Mental deterioration plus persecutory or expansive delusional trends.

(f) *Presenile Type (Alzheimer's Disease).*—Profound dementia occurring as early as the fortieth year, accompanied by aphasia, apraxia and often an irritable or anxious depressive mood.

Course and Prognosis.—There is apt to be a prodromal period of several months' duration, during which the patient is irritable, sleeps poorly, complains of malaise, muscular weakness and anorexia and becomes seclusive.   The patient wanders aimlessly about and may lose his way.   Then appear the typical defect and deterioration symptoms, involving all the intellectual, emotional and ethical faculties and notably the recent memory; the psychopathologic phenomena of old age and perhaps the type symptoms like presbyophrenia, delirium and confusion, depression and agitation or paranoid reactions.

The signs of senility and physical decay are obvious.

The course is essentially chronic and progressive and the outlook absolutely unfavorable.   Pneumonia, the "friend of the aged," may release the patient in a few years, or chronic colitis, cystitis or decubitus may close the scene.

Treatment.—Early recognition attains great importance in view of the fact that the senile dement is readily victimized by designing individuals and thus may bring disgrace to his family and waste his resources.

The patient should be protected from the consequences of his psychotic behavior. To be kept in mind are the liability of physical injury, of sexual offenses, or of disgraceful marriages. Pyromanic proclivities or simply memory losses may result in serious burns and loss of property. Suicide is frequent. An easily digested diet, warm clothing and measures against constipation must be provided. Insomnia may be controlled by mild hydrotherapy and simple hypnotics. Often a mental hospital is the wisest solution, not only for the patient but to relieve the distress of the family.

PSYCHOSES WITH CEREBRAL ARTERIOSCLEROSIS.

Finer differentiations between senile and arteriosclerotic psychoses which may be demonstrated at the autopsy table and under the eyepiece of the microscope usually fall by the wayside when subjected to the rougher and more practical test of clinical practice. Pathologically there are in the brain more areas of softening and not the typical finding of the senile brain—the senile plaque. Arteriosclerotic psychoses tend to begin earlier in life. Peripheral blood pressure helps little; it may be and often is low. Perhaps in the arteriosclerotic psychoses attacks of irritability and violent anger are more frequent and severe than in pathologic senility. A crude but fairly accurate clinical diagnostic guide is contained in the statement, "Refrain from a diagnosis of arteriosclerotic brain disease unless there is evidence of general (headache, dizziness, fainting attacks) or focal (aphasia, paralyses) brain damage."

EPILEPTIC PSYCHOSES.

Epilepsy, the historical and "sacred disease," is still a puzzle to science. Even the very questionable diagnosis of idiopathic epilepsy is certainly not permissible unless the epilepsies of gross brain disease (paresis, cerebral lues), toxic and infectious epilepsies (uremia, diabetes) and borderline condition epilepsies usually due to endocrine dysfunction are excluded.

Not every epileptic becomes definitely psychotic, and psychiatry is chiefly interested in the mental symptoms that occur in the course of epilepsy and in the personality of the epileptic.

Etiology and Pathology.—The actual cause of epilepsy remains hidden. Probably it revolves around those conditions which increase the sensitivity of the cortical platform to reaction. The stock is usually badly tainted and Gowers states that 76 per cent occurs before the age of twenty years. Various pathologic alterations in Ammon's horn, in the Pacchionian bodies or edemas have been described (Lennox, Cobb, Winkleman).   One also finds surface gliosis of the hemispheres, syphilis, arteriosclerosis, arrested development and toxic manifestations.   The difficulty is that, usually at autopsy, the picture is clouded by the result of the repeated terrific onslaughts of the seizures upon the brain.

Mental Symptoms.—There is scarcely a specific mental reaction in epilepsy and the diagnosis usually must wait upon the demonstration of the typical seizure or unquestioned petit mal.   Mentally, the traditional irritability may assume such proportions that it is really psychotic; epileptic dream or twilight states with considerable confusion; delirious confusion with an ecstatic hallucinatory delusional state or anxiety; "conscious delirium" (epileptic fugue state) which has considerable medico-legal import, since murder or sex crimes may be committed during the aimless journeys which the epileptic takes and of which he has not the slightest remembrance; epileptic furor states following seizures during which the patient becomes maniacal, homicidal, destructive and a dangerous menace to those about him; epileptic equivalent states in which a psychotic episode replaces the seizure; paranoid states in which the personality suspiciousness is carried to an extreme degree and, finally, not only grand mal epilepsy but also petit mal may terminate in profound dementia in which every faculty of the mind is extinguished.

While the epileptic may remain relatively normal mentally, yet his *personality* is almost always pathologic.   One must guard against the outcome of at least some of the following traits: egotism, conceit, emotional instability, hypochondriasis, sickly sentimentality in religion, inadaptability to environment, cruelty, laziness, irascibility, impulsiveness, excessive sexual tendencies, criminalism, violent impulses.

Course, Prognosis and Treatment.—Life is somewhat shortened, not only as a direct result of the damage of the disease, serious injuries, status epilepticus, secondary pneumonia, but also the epileptic is apt to be a sickly individual with various gastro-intestinal and skin disturbances.   The course is chronic and progressive.   The outlook is somewhat better in childhood.

Epilepsy constitutes a serious enough problem to stimulate legislative attention.   During the attack care should be exercised to protect the tongue, teeth and body from injury.   In every instance the patient constitutes an individual therapeutic challenge.   Foci of infection should be removed; rational surgical procedures should be carried out; endocrine dysfunction combated; lues and other systemic disease vigorously treated.   Practically in every patient it is necessary to prevent constipation, bring the nutritional and functional activity of the body up to *par* and help to select a suitable, non-dangerous and, if possible, out-door occupation.   Lennox and Cobb state that "anything that keeps the patient dehydrated, acidemic and oxygenated favorably influences the seizures."   A reduction of the fluid intake to at least 500 cc. daily, together with a lessening of salt intake and the use of Epsom salts has been advocated.   This method of treatment is still in the hypothetical and experimental stage.   Dietary measures, including salt-free and low-protein diets, are useful and starvation and the ketogenic diet are worth consideration. Bromides continuously and in large doses brutalize the patient. Probably the drug of choice is luminal, 0.1 gram (1½ grain) daily, omitting every seventh dose. With the appearance of definite mental symptoms, the protection of a suitable institution should be sought for the patient. Epileptics should be advised not to marry.

PSYCHOSIS WITH MENTAL DEFICIENCY.

Mental defect is not mental disease. Nevertheless, psychiatry is interested not only in the psychotic episodes of the feebleminded but in the problem of mental defect in itself. It is enormously important since there are about 500,000 mental defectives in the United States.

Etiology.—Inheritance is admittedly significant but scarcely the overwhelming cause it was once thought to be. Much weight must also be given to congenital syphilis, various congenital brain defects and arrests, birth injuries, acute infections, particularly meningitis, encephalitis, head trauma and endocrine defects.

Symptoms and Diagnosis.—The diagnosis of mental defect may be considered from two angles, namely, in the practical terms of life competition, and then, from the more hypothetical and also more scientific aspect of mental testing. According to the former, the idiot is not able to fend for himself even in the slightest degree and, indeed, has at best only an imperfectly developed instinct of self-preservation. The higher grades of imbecile may be laboriously taught to care for ordinary bodily needs, and, perhaps, to perform a few very simple, extremely routine tasks. The practical test of life very soon reveals the defect: Inability to learn the accepted performance of bodily functions, marked retardation in the time of walking and speaking, and, if not obvious in early life, then the criteria of home and school life which may be summed up in a significant backwardness in comparison to other children of the same age level. There may be even various physical marks, or so-called stigmata.

The moron is on a much higher plane intellectually and, under favorable supervised and standardized conditions, may become self-supporting in some routine occupation, but since the moron lacks average foresight, planning and judgment, he cannot compete under ordinary terms with his fellow-men.

By the criterion of the Binet and other standardized intelligence tests, an idiot has a mental age of three years or less, with an intelligence quotient (I. Q.) of less than 25; an imbecile has a mental age of from three to seven years and an I. Q. of 25 to 49; a moron, a mental age of seven to ten years, and an I. Q. of 50 to 74.

Mental defect must not be confused with mental retardation. This is of the utmost importance, since, if the cause of the mental retardation is discovered and adequately treated, the prognosis often becomes very hopeful. The retarding factor may be physical (anemia, parasitic infections, heart and kidney disease, adenoids, infected tonsils, hearing defects, eye-strain, tuberculosis, rickets); mental, in which some worry or conflict is engaging all the mental energy of the child, and environmental, in which there is some deleterious or destructive influence in the home.

Psychotic episodes in defectives are usually incomplete and poorly defined. Periods of confusion with hallucinosis or outbreaks of uncontrollable and unrelated motor activity are fair examples. The intelligence defect stands out prominently. When the symptoms are more elaborate and approximate more completely manic-depressive or schizophrenic syndromes, they should be considered as belonging to these groups. Much bad behavior and unhappiness results, because the defective child of fairly high grade may appreciate his limitations in comparison with other children. Conversely, normal siblings may be much damaged in their personality development by enforced association with a defective child.

Treatment.—Nowhere in psychiatry is there a better opportunity to drive home the teachings of prevention than in the problem of the mental defective. The awakening of the public to the grave dangers of inheritance either through feeblemindedness *per se* or through lues; close obstetrical attention to decreasing the birth-injury rate; adequate convalescence from the infections of childhood, and an intensive attack on the problem of infantile nutrition would measurably lower the statistical curve of mental deficiency.

At first glance, one might be led to suppose that treatment proper was solely an institutional question. Even were this necessary it could not be done, since it would be economically impossible to build enough institutions to house the defective population. Fortunately, this is unnecessary, since only 5 per cent of mental defectives have behavior disorders and delinquent tendencies, and of these only 2 per cent are serious (Fernald). This group should be placed in institutions, along with those who are very low grade or have serious physical handicaps. Much of the inevitable routine work of a highly standardized and industrialized civilization can be successfully done by the higher grades of mental defectives, providing there is a program of: (*a*) early recognition, classification and registration; (*b*) training especially in good-habit formation in scientifically conducted occupational schools; (*c*) supervision in the community; (*d*) further investigation into the nature and cause of mental deficiency.

PSYCHOSES WITH CEREBRAL SYPHILIS, HUNTINGTON'S CHOREA, BRAIN TUMOR, ENCEPHALITIS AND OTHER BRAIN AND NERVOUS DISEASES, TRAUMATIC PSYCHOSES.

In these psychoses the mental symptoms are not constant enough to be considered specific. The problem is largely a neurologic one as in the mental dullness of frontal lobe disease, or the hallucinosis in involvement of the occipital or temporal lobes or the dementia of Huntington's chorea.

Head trauma may produce a delirium, or a so-called traumatic constitution in which there is dispositional change, headache, fatigability, irritability, emotional instability and more rarely paranoid, hysteroid and epileptoid phenomena and, finally, a group of cases in which there is dementia.

Encephalitis, which is both organic and toxic, may in children, as a late result, condition extraordinarily bad behavior and even criminalism without any severe intellectual defect. These children are unquestionably sick and not merely "bad," and must be treated by careful and painstaking habit formation, usually away from home.

THE TOXIC PSYCHOSES.

Within the domain of the toxic psychoses is embraced a vast amount of clinical territory. Much of this is directly included in the province of the general practice. There is at once suggested a natural etiologic division: (*a*) into those psychoses primarily due to the ingestion of toxic agents into the body as in the instances of alcohol and opium; (*b*) those psychoses influenced by autointoxications within the body, as in any infectious disease, or in even more direct intoxications like uremia, in chronic infections like tuberculosis, in such deficiency disorders as pellagra, in decompensating heart disease, in the disturbances of metabolism occasioned by ductless gland dyscrasias. In the last analysis, *it is important to remember that every organic disease has its mental as well as its somatic components.* Generally speaking, the etiology of the toxic psychoses is usually clear whether it be on an exogenous or an endogenous basis; the physical findings are those of the disease in question with a fairly constant background of fever, leukocytosis and weight loss; and in the skin, kidneys, gastro-intestinal tract, and vasomotor and sympathetic systems, the usual accompaniments of fever or toxemia or both. The prognosis is good.

While the student must expect wide departure, particularly in degree, yet the mental paradigm of the toxic psychoses is *delirium*, which in its pure expression includes clouding of the consciousness, motor restlessness, hallucinosis, apprehension and emotional instability.

Even more important than the therapy of each individual toxic psychotic reaction are the highly important general principles of treatment: (1) a large intake of fluid by mouth and, if necessary, subcutaneous, colonic or intravenous administrations, excepting in instances where there is brain edema; (2) limitation of narcotics which are customarily used entirely too freely in the treatment of the toxic psychoses (in this connection it is suggested that the physician have in mind the toxicity and the elimination time of the hypnotic drugs he employs); (3) treatment of the usual accompanying constipation; (4) hydrotherapy; (5) free elimination; (6) removal of poisons and infections, including focal infection; (7) dietetic and tonic treatment; (8) protection of the patient against danger to himself and others.

Exogenous Toxic Psychoses.—Obviously not all the mental reactions caused by poisons which may be deliberately or accidentally taken into the body can be described. Even the list is formidable in its length.

The effect of *alcohol*, which is unquestionably toxic to the nerve system, furnishes a fair clinical example of the result of other serious poisons. It lessens motor activity, increases reflexes, diminishes physical strength, lowers the fatigue point, interferes with clarity of ideation, impairs judgment and work capacity, impairs memory and emotional stability and, finally, produces the debacle of complete intellectual, emotional and ethical deterioration.

Alcoholic poisoning may appear under the guise of *pathologic intoxication*, an acute mental disturbance marked by furious excitement with confusion, hallucinosis and subsequent amnesia; *delirium tremens*, a severe and often wild delirium with intense tremor, visual and auditory hallucinosis, insomnia, fever, rapid pulse, low blood pressure, weight loss, albuminuria; *Korsakoff's psychosis*, manifested either as a delirium or a non-delirious polyneuritis with retention defect and disorientation, fabrication, suggestibility, a tendency to misidentify persons, and hallucinosis; *acute and chronic hallucinosis*, the former showing an acute auditory hallucinosis with a fairly clear sensorium, marked fears and more or less systematized persecutory delusions, the latter being a persistence of the acute state but with a far less sharp emotional reaction; *acute and chronic paranoid types* marked by suspiciousness, misinterpretations, persecutory ideas, jealous trends and hallucinations, the chronic type being chiefly differentiated by failure to recover after withdrawal of alcohol; the various degrees of *alcoholic deterioration;* the mildest being ill-humor and irascibility, or a jovial, careless, flippant facetious mood; abusiveness to family; unreliability and tendency to prevarication; in some cases definite suspiciousness and jealousy; general lessening of efficiency and capacity for physical and mental work; moderate memory impairment.

The student must not be too ready to diagnose alcoholic psychosis. Alcoholism may be a symptom of paresis, manic-depressive, dementia præcox or epilepsy.

Opium and its derivatives, particularly *morphine*, are frequently the resort of the psychopath when faced with even the low hurdles of life. Their habitual use involves a profound deterioration of the ethics of the individual. This is strongly marked in his efforts to obtain the drug.

Cocaine is chiefly the drug of the underworld where it is often utilized by the criminal to "pep up" his courage for the commission of a crime, and also, to some extent, it is dabbled in by a certain irresponsible stratum of so-called "society." The prolonged use of either morphine or cocaine, as in the instance of alcohol, finally deteriorates the taker to a low intellectual, emotional and moral level.

The list of habit-forming drugs is long and includes not only *ether*, *chloroform, cannabis indica*, but even such milder hypnotics as *veronal*, *luminal*, the *bromides* and many others.

In the industries psychotic symptoms may be produced by *lead*, *arsenic, mercury* and the *gases*. In lead poisoning there is apt to be headache, restlessness, delirium, visual hallucinations, delusions of persecution, confusion and convulsive seizures. There is tremor, twitching of the facial muscles, inarticulate speech and insomnia. There may be wrist- and ankle-drop, atrophy of the hand muscles, steppage gait, and paresis or paraplegia of the legs.

Special Treatment.—In the toxic psychoses, prophylaxis is almost unlimited. Sensible explanatory scientific propaganda should lessen the incidence of psychotic reactions due to habit-forming drugs; protection and personal hygiene should make large inroads into the mental morbidity of the industrial poisons; proper diet, better control of infectious diseases and adequate periods of convalescence should reduce the mental pathology incident to metabolic deficiency and infectious diseases.

The therapy of any exogenous toxic psychosis may be summed up under withdrawal, free elimination, hydrotherapy, dietetic, toxic and reëducative measures. Emergency methods, such as spinal puncture in severe delirium tremens, must be kept in mind. The specific treatment of pellagra and other deficiency conditions and the industrial poisonings are a part of internal medicine. In the addictions the physician must insist on a sufficiently long period of control, not only to accomplish withdrawal of the drug, but chiefly to stiffen the morale of the patient. Excepting in the face of great asthenia or other dangerous complications, withdrawal should be abrupt, or at least very rapid. In morphinism, free purgation and hyoscine substitution are often used.

PSYCHOSES WITH SOMATIC DISEASE.

Probably the largest field for psychiatry in the practice of medicine is in the psychotic reactions coincident with the fever and toxemia of infectious diseases, with exhaustion, with metabolic and deficiency diseases, with cardio-renal disease and, in short, with every known pathologic condition. There is no dividing line. The patient with uncomplicated lobar pneumonia may in a few hours become delirious and consequently a problem in psychiatry. The patient who is convalescing from influenza may suddenly become depressed and suicidal. The patient with cardiac decompensation may rapidly become irritable, suspicious, confused and delusional. Every somatic disease has clinically a mental as well as a physical expression which are interrelated.

If the student keeps in mind the delirium paradigm—motor excitement, incoherence, hallucinosis, disorientation, deep confusion or at least some degree of clouding of consciousness, then the psychiatric diagnostic problem becomes surprisingly simple. Naturally variations in degree and departures will be encountered so that he may expect to find the framework of delirium filled in by such phenomena as convulsions, catatonia, stupor, fear, depression with suicidal attempts, euphoria, irritability, suspiciousness, delusional formation (usually transitory), dullness, apathy, coma or neurasthenic symptoms. Likewise, if the general therapeutic principles that have been stressed, together with the specific therapy of the basic disease, are kept in mind, then the problems of treatment are usually not difficult and the results are highly gratifying.

MANIC-DEPRESSIVE PSYCHOSES.

Definition.—A recoverable but persistently recurrent type of mental disease, second only to schizophrenia in importance and statistical frequency and marked by wide swings in mood and psychomotor reactions.

Etiology.—Unquestionably there are chemical, metabolic and organic factors at work in the genesis of this psychosis but they are still too little understood and too inconstant to be dignified into a specific etiologic rôle.   Many years ago Kraepelin indicated the distortion of personality—the prepsychotic makeup—when he observed that among those who developed frank manic-depressive reactions, 12.1 per cent cent had manifested previously a depressive makeup; 9 per cent, manic; 12.4 per cent were "irascible" and "nervous;" 3 to 4 per cent, cyclothymic.   More profitable etiologically than rigid neuropathologic interpretations is earnest attention to the "constitutional basis" which has its roots in heredity.   This basis has physical as well as psychologic components and in its pure type we may think of an individual of the pyknic type, heavy, broad and thick-set, who is an extrovert.

An extrovert is predominantly a man of action.   He "wastes" little time on reflective thinking, accomplishes much routine work and is often effective and executive.   He expresses himself readily and positively.   Concerning questions, issues, policies, beliefs he is apt to be very strongly *pro* or *con* but often his feelings are transitory.   His decisions are frequently of the "hair-trigger" type.   He is a loyal, enthusiastic friend and a bitter enemy but does not hold resentments for a long time and readily forgives.   He is energetic, cheerful and sociable.   This type of personality does not necessarily spell manic-depressive, but if the psychosis does occur it is often engrafted on similar dispositional traits.

As precipitating causes, one must consider psychogenic and somatic strain and stress and destructive influences traceable to faulty training and environment.   The psychosis is said to be more common among females and is apt to be manifested before the twenty-fifth year.

Symptoms.—Waiving strict scientific accuracy for the sake of clarity, the student will probably get a workable conception of clinical manic-depressive if he fixes his mind on the three functions which are chiefly affected—emotion (E), ideation (I), motor activity (M)—and pictures them either above or below a theoretical normal line according to the phase of mania or depression.   Thus, in classical or acute mania the emotions (affect, mood), the ideation (activity of thought) and the motor behavior all present themselves to the observer as definitely increased or raised well above a normal average, there being a more or less close agreement or parallelism between the individual unit symptoms.   Commonly the patient who is exhilarated or mercurial as to mood will likewise exhibit a corresponding degree of distractibility and flight of ideas as evidenced by speech, and also will be in a state of more or less marked physical or motor activity.   In acute melancholia the reverse is true.   This clinical point of view, usual parallelism between the unit symptoms and the chief degrees of severity of the psychosis are expressed in the following diagrams.

There are numerous mixed states in which the unit symptoms referred to emotion, thought and motor activity are not in accord.   The chief forms are represented in the diagram below by the simple expedient of transposing the unit symptoms above and below a normal level line. Thus, maniacal stupor clinically consists of emotional exaltation, slowing of thought and decreased motor activity.

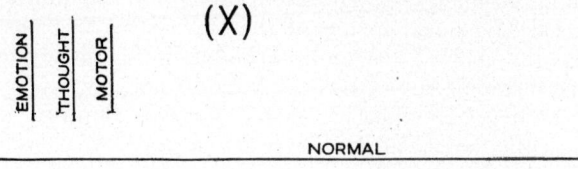

FIG. 38.—(From "Clinical Psychiatry," by Strecker and Ebaugh, 3d edition, Philadelphia, P. Blakiston's Son & Co., 1931.)

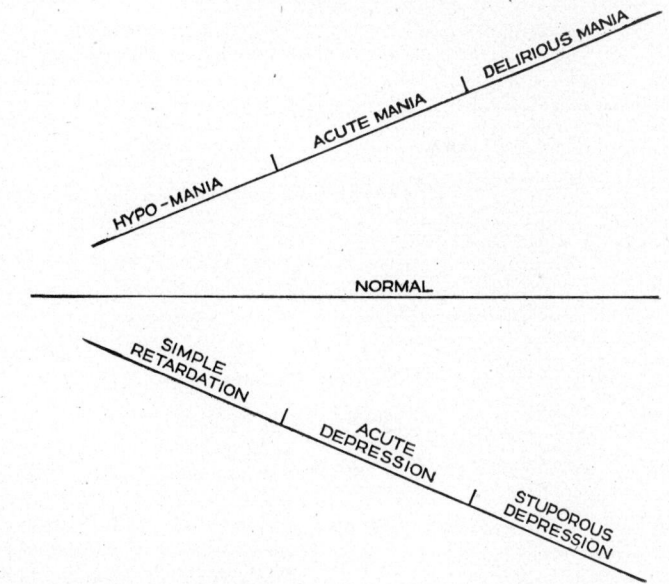

FIG. 39.—Illustrating variations in the intensity of the symptoms in manic-depressive psychosis. (From "Clinical Psychiatry," by Strecker and Ebaugh, 3d edition, Philadelphia, P. Blakiston's Son & Co., 1931.)

Since manic-depressive tends to recur throughout the life of the patient, one must expect many variations. Only a few are given:

Maniacal stupor	Agitated depression	Unproductive mania	Depressive mania	Depression with flight	Akinetic mania	
E	I M	E M	M	I	E I	
I M	E	I	E I	E M	M	Normal

(From "Clinical Psychiatry," by Strecker and Ebaugh, 3d edition, Philadelphia, P. Blakiston's Son & Co., 1931.)

69

Viewed from an objective *psychologic* platform, the patient in the manic phase of the psychosis is apparently without restraint and is seemingly unhampered by any counterbalance or inhibition in his emotional thought and motor expression; the melancholic seems bound in the chains of emotional depression, thought and motor retardation. This has led McDougal to regard the two contrasting phases of the diseases as the unchecked manifestation of the self-assertive and self-submissive instincts, respectively. A more total point of view might consider the depressive phase as a temporary withdrawal in the face of defeat in the management of ego, sex or (and) herd problems, and the manic phase, likewise a withdrawal and defeat which is psychologically camouflaged and prevented from reaching too clear a conscious realization by the unimpeded flow of energy in all directions, emotionally, ideationally and in the output of muscle energy.

Mental and Physical Symptoms.—In listed form the symptoms are given below, the more prominent ones being italicized:

TABLE 16

MENTAL.

Manic.	*Depressed.*
	Attitude and General Behavior.	
Euphoria, exhilaration and *rapid shift* of emotional range (irritability, impatience, anger, rage) to be noted in facies, posture, dress, general behavior.	*Depression* and *retardation.* In mixed and stuporous reactions one may encounter various catatonic reactions (catalepsy, cerea).
	Stream of Mental Activity and Speech.	
Distractibility, volubility, *flight of ideas*, rhyming, sound association.	*Poverty of thought, mutism.*
	Affect and Mood.	
All degrees of *euphoria, exhilaration,* irritability, *mercurial-like alterations of mood.*	Range from feelings of *inadequacy* and subjective lack of interest to *acute mental agony.* Suicidal attempts. Stupor.
	Mental Trend: Content of Thought.	
Inconstant, shifting, and often grandiose *delusions.*	More tenacious *delusions* of wrongdoing, self-accusation, hypochondriacal, somatic.

Paranoid trends, ideas of reference and influence, persecutory delusions—all may occur. Hallucinations rare, but do occur in very severe manic states and in stuporous phases. Illusions.   Illusions.

Sensorium, Mental Grasp and Capacity.

Excepting briefly or in severe grades of excitement, and depression, the sensorium, memory, attention, capacity, orientation, retention and recall, counting and calculation, reading and recall, school, general and current knowledge are not intrinsically disturbed. The manic patient is apt to cover page after page with hurried, lengthy, untidy, profusely capitalized, underscored and crudely illustrated communications.

Insight.

During the attack, especially in mania, insight is at best quite faulty though rarely completely absent.

Physical Summary.—The absence of a pathognomonic syndrome does not imply that organic morbidity is insignificant or absent. If the examination has been intensive and thorough *it will discover, in the majority of instances, somatic disturbances which are indirectly and perhaps even directly related to the psychosis* and which demand careful attention. In addition, the following phenomena have been reported by various observers.

1. *General.*—Disturbed sleep, impaired nutrition (in mania). These symptoms are intensified in hyperacute mania, and fever with delirium-like manifestations is often added. Insomnia, loss of weight, coated tongue, sallow skin, marked constipation (in depression).

2. *Body Systems.*—Overactive heart, increased output of urine, heightened metabolism (in mania). Cardiac activity weakened, decreased urine output, depressed metabolism. Gastric achylia is not uncommon (in depression).

3. *Subjective Sensations.*—Many varieties often associated with somatic delusions. In depression there are complaints of numbness, paresthesias, dizziness, ringing in ears.

4. *Neurologic.*—No constant findings but usually there are some disturbances. In high grades of mania there may be marked exaggeration of tendon reflexes and muscle tremor.

5. *Laboratory.*—While there are no specific criteria, there may be albuminuria and other pathologic urinary findings, diminished or absent hydrochloric acid, disturbances in blood chemistry. A high basal metabolic rate has been repeatedly reported. Recently, Torsten Sondén presented an exhaustive "Study of Somatic Conditions in Manic-depressive Psychosis." He finds a leukocytic increase in mania, especially at the beginning of the phase; in some cases a temperature and pulse-rate rise during mania and again particularly in its inception; a definite erythrocyte increase during the transition from normality to either excitement or depression and a fall under reverse conditions, *i. e.*, transition back to normality, and blood pressure is higher both in mania and in melancholia than in quiescence.

Prognosis.—Manic phases seem to be somewhat more common than depressions. Kraepelin stated that the first attack is a depression in 60 to 70 per cent of patients; two-thirds of the melancholias are followed by remission and one-third by mania and then a remission; when mania is the first manifestation two-thirds of the cases are likewise followed by remission. Recovery from the single attack is the rule and the duration of the illness ranges from a few days to several months or longer. Future attacks are often a repetition of the initial one, although the tendency is toward greater frequency and severity. The outlook seems to be better in proportion to the seriousness of the precipitating situation (so-called "reactive" types), the soundness of the heredity and the personality. It is somewhat doubtful if any valid index of prognosis can be taken from the psychotic content, though it has been stated that gross somatic and nihilistic delusions are unfavorable. Mental deterioration is exceptional and may usually be explained by the addition of a complicating factor, such as arteriosclerosis.

Treatment.—Given a strong constitutional basis, sensible *preventive* measures should be set into motion early in childhood and proper training should be followed by some effort to modify the more destructive conditions of life. In a large percentage of cases the attack itself must be dealt with in a suitable mental hospital or sanitarium. From the somatic aspect, each patient is a problem in internal medicine, and any pathologic finding—whether it be tuberculosis, heart or kidney, endocrine dysfunction, gastro-intestinal disturbance, colonic stasis or *actual* foci of infection—must be dealt with unhesitatingly and intensively. General measures of treatment are of the utmost importance. The nutrition should be kept at the highest possible point and in some cases nasal feeding is unavoidable; rest, and often rest in bed, particularly for depressed patients, is helpful, and hydrotherapy, including the prolonged neutral bath, is a valuable adjunct far superior to hypnotic overdrugging; the patient should be protected against the well-meant but usually harmful effect of many visitors. With kindness, sympathy, tact and firmness, the physician must manage the patient and attempt to direct his perverted energies into useful channels. If the patient is at all accessible he should be frequently encouraged to talk things over with the physician.

INVOLUTION MELANCHOLIA.

Involution melancholia is probably a mixed form of manic-depressive in which the motor retardation is often replaced by restlessness and agitation. It occurs more frequently in women than in men, the ratio being about 3 to 2; it appears during the fourth and fifth decades of life or even later; heredity is said to influence the development of about 60 per cent of cases and the little understood organic and psychic pathology of the climacteric is probably also determining.

The mood is depressed and apprehensive; there is usually some degree of motor overactivity which may mount to a veritable frenzy of agitated excitement; suicidal attempts are common; in about 10 per cent of patients there occur such catatonic phenomena as fixed attitudes, catalepsy, negativism, stereotypy, grimacing, mannerisms, automatic movements, food refusal, impulsive violence, resistiveness, destructiveness, violent scolding, unapproachability, mutism, retention of urine and feces; often there is poverty of thought with monotonous and repetitive speech; the delusional formation is apt to be along the line of depression, self-accusation, self-depreciation, with hypochondriacal and gross somatic ideas.

The organic morbidity is greater than in ordinary manic-depressive and one may expect to encounter evidences of precocious senility, insomnia, profound disturbance of nutrition, with anorexia and sometimes extreme weight loss; circulatory, pelvic and digestive symptoms, particularly constipation and a great variety of subjective sensations.

The course is quite protracted. After a prodromal period of about a year the psychosis may endure for two, three, four or even more years.

The prognosis is fairly good with a recovery-rate of from 23 to 40 per cent. About 25 to 32 per cent are said to dement. About 20 per cent die within two years and the death-rate by suicide and intercurrent disease is fairly high. The outlook is relatively unfavorable after the age of fifty-five years or in the presence of advanced senile changes.

It is generally considered that a rapid gain in weight and general physical improvement constitute hopeful signs.

Clinical Varieties.—The clinical picture with which the student should familiarize himself is *involutional melancholia*, with the syndrome of agitated depression. A great number of psychoses which occur at this age period have been split off from the main group. They cannot be separately described but their names will clearly indicate that a wide range of symptomatic expression may be encountered—involutional melancholia with retardation, melancholia vera of Farrar (prominence of self-accusatory ideas), anxiety presenilis of Farrar (anxiety referred principally to things outside the patient), depressio apathetica of Farrar, involutional paranoia of Kleist, involution paraphrenia of Serko, Seelert's paranoid psychoses in advanced years, presenile paraphrenia of Albrecht, late catatonia of Urstein. It is recommended that the time available be spent in an effort to formulate and possibly interpret the psychosis in the individual, rather than in hair-splitting attempts to force it into one or the other of the subdivisions.

SCHIZOPHRENIA (DEMENTIA PRÆCOX).

Etiology.—If manic-depressive is the psychosis of the extrovert, then schizophrenia is strikingly the psychosis of the introvert. The organic, toxic and endocrine implications of præcox have been investigated by Nissl, Mott, Josephy, Fünfgeld, Marcuse, Kitabayashi, Naito and others, but thus far the findings, while provocative, are still too inconstant to justify the assumption of a specific causal relationship. Perhaps our etiologic information is contained in the opening sentence of this paragraph.

Schizophrenia tends to develop in persons with the shut-in (Meyer), seclusive type of personality, often on the basis of mental conflicts, faulty habit formation and instinctive maladjustments, particularly along the lines of sex, extending back to early childhood and adolescence.

The physical habitus in its pure form is the leptic or light, relatively tall, slender type. The normal psychologic traits are those of the introvert.

The introvert is the antithesis of the extrovert. He is reserved, a deep thinker, disinclined to go into action. Thought is his powerful weapon. He is introspective and analytical. At his best he plans thoughtfully for the future and often confers immense benefits upon his fellow-men. At his worst he is an impractical theorist, visionary and dreamer. To the world he appears to be distant, gloomy, unfriendly and lacking in strong personal feelings.

The etiology of schizophrenia is so complex that in each individual patient there must be a careful evaluation of psychogenic, toxic and organic (often endocrine) elements. The psychosis frequently manifests itself early in life, the largest percentage of cases appearing before the age of twenty-five years. It is more frequent in males than in females; occurs earlier in males; is more prevalent in cities than in rural districts; is more common in the foreign population and more frequent in negroes than in whites.

Symptoms.—Psychologically, the foundation for the host of symptoms appears to be the withdrawal from reality and the dissociation between emotion (affect) and thought. The withdrawal is manifested in many schizophrenic reactions and, perhaps, reaches its height in catatonic stupor, during which the patient almost completely shuts himself off from contact with the environment. Schizophrenia means splitting or dissociation, and it, too, is strikingly illustrated in many of the psychotic reactions of the patients in which the emotional reaction apparently is at variance or very inadequate with the accessible content of thought. On such a foundation there is erected an elaborate structure of clinical symptoms. A summary based on a statistical study of many patients includes the following:

1. *General Behavior.*—Oddities of many types, silliness, incongruity, stereotypy, mannerisms, impulsive outbreaks, untidiness, marked mental inertia, rigidity and attitudinizing.

2. *Stream of Activity and Talk.*—Autistic thinking, dream-like ideas, feelings of being forced or of interference with the mind from the outside, physical and mythical influences. Incoherence, rambling, blocking, evasiveness, verbigeration, neologisms, echolalia, echopraxia, mutism, negativism, catatonia.

3. *Mood and Special Preoccupation.*—(a) Dissociation of affect, inadequate and incoördinate affect, ambivalence, apathy, indifference.

(b) *Trend Reactions, Topical Reactions, Projection.*—1. Persecutory ideas, feeling of mistreatment, food tampered with, poisoned, "doped."

2. Ideas of reference—feeling of being talked about, people pass remarks that "refer."

3. Ideas of influence—feeling of being hypnotized, under mental control, mental telepathy, mental spells, hypodermic injections, radio machines.

4. Hallucinations in various fields, auditory hallucinations, frequently of a religious pattern on the basis of overcompensation.

5. Bizarre somatic sensations and delusions—organs have been removed, brain has been removed, vagina has been stopped up, electric sensations over the body, electric wires connecting with the brain.

6. Overcompensation in the form of day-dreaming phantasies, being God, a saint, leader of a new religion.

7. Unintelligible and unexplainable activity.

In the *paranoid* type (25 per cent) delusions particularly of persecution or grandeur, often fairly well systematized, for a time at least, and hallucinations are prominent; in the *catatonic* type (10 per cent) there is negativism and conduct peculiarity with phases of stupor or excitement marked by impulsive, queer, stereotyped behavior and hallucinations; in *hebephrenia* (52 per cent) there is silliness, unexplained smiling, laughter, grimacing, mannerisms and peculiar and changeable ideas which have an absurd and grotesque content, and in the *simple* type (8 per cent) interest is at a low ebb, there is apathy and strange behavior and delusions and hallucinations are either abortive and fragmentary or absent entirely.

The field of *physical* symptomatology has been industriously tilled and, although a specific picture cannot be traced, many of the findings are strongly suggestive of underlying organic factors with an endocrine basis. If such a basis exists it is probably most clearly expressed in the physical habitus described as leptic or asthenic. The heart and vascular apparatus are often small. Vasomotor sympathetic phenomena such as cyanosis, localized sweating, edema, dilated pupils and increase in salivation are fairly common. Tuberculosis is rather frequent. In catatonic cases there is a tendency to show a low metabolic rate. Gastro-intestinal disturbances, undernutrition and extreme constipation are often observed. Kasanin reports high sustained sugar curve during stupor and Hertz finds shortening of the blood coagulation-time. Somewhat remarkable are the occasional marked improvements following accidental and severe acute infections.

Prognosis.—Variability in diagnostic standards and the difficulty of obtaining accurate information concerning mild, early and non-institutionalized patients render statistics misleading. Of the early and mild group probably one-fourth recover or at least attain a very satisfactory level of social readjustment. Of the more severe and outspoken symptomatically developed group, 7.4 per cent recovered and 40.9 per cent improved definitely in five years or less. Catatonic cases are somewhat more favorable.

Treatment.—The social and economic threat of schizophrenia is both quantitatively and qualitatively so grave that every intelligent preventive measure should be instituted. These aspects offer the most brilliant opportunities, particularly during the formative period of childhood. There is being delineated with more and more accuracy a personality pattern into which dementia præcox is so easily woven. This personality pattern has rather distinctive mental and even physical features, so that it is not difficult to identify. Children who present these characteristics should be made the target of intensive effort. Their innate difficulty is that they tend to shrink from the hard and somewhat crude facts of everyday life. This applies to the give and take of social relations, the economic measures of success, sex adaptation and, in fact, it involves almost every sphere.

There is great resistance against severing the bonds of dependency and this is, perhaps, particularly true in the complete accomplishment of heterosexual love. These children need to be socialized; they must be taught ease of social relationships; they must be guarded against misinformation about sex. One of the greatest dangers that confronts them is the tendency to compensate for the unpleasant facts of reality by the substitution of day-dreaming and phantasy. These children must be patiently taught the value of living in the world of reality. Many agencies are available and the home is the center. Here such a child must be able to find a pleasant and social atmosphere with every opportunity to "talk things over." He should be encouraged to play with other children. He should be taught to take part in group play and athletics. Boy and Girl Scouts, summer camps, and clubs are all helpful. Sex information should be on a high plane but the child should be given real knowledge and phantasy should be avoided. Too close emotional dependence on the mother or the father must be guarded against and there should be, instead of too much sickly sentimentality, more of the "pal" relationship. Jealousies and feelings of inferiority toward brothers and sisters ought to be prevented but not by a spoiling process. If parents and teachers will have in mind that the object to be accomplished is socialization and adaptation, then many cases of potential dementia præcox will never develop.

Once the psychosis has become definitely established, hospital or sanitarium care is indicated in a fairly large percentage of patients. The danger of suicide, panics, antisocial reactions to delusional beliefs, the disorganization of the home and its absence of proper treatment facilities, all prompt the utilization of proper institutional treatment. Here, certain troublesome symptoms may be readily handled.

Negativistic states and stupor: general hygiene and nursing care, ventilation, bathing, artificial feeding, change of scene. Excitement: adequate supervision and observation. Continuous baths and other types of sedative therapy such as packs. Apathy: useful occupation, games, entertainment.

Nevertheless a considerable proportion of patients who do not present urgent needs may be successfully managed in clinic and private practice. Each patient is a problem in internal medicine, and in addition to the treatment of any discovered organic pathology or endocrine deviation, there should be careful elimination, dietetic and tonic routine and removal of focal infection. Occupation is very valuable to prevent inactivity and stagnation and as a pathway back to reality. Whenever possible there should be the establishment of a satisfactory rapport with the patient, leading to frank explanation, a mutual estimate of personal assets and liabilities, and a careful search for a suitable niche in the environment. Many patients after a hospital residence adjust on a moderately good social and economic plane. There should be vocational supervision and follow-up of all discharged patients for a number of years.

CONSTITUTIONAL PSYCHOPATHIC INFERIORITY.

This is, at best, an unsatisfactory classification but, nevertheless, certain types of criminalism, emotional instability, inadequate personality, paranoid personality, pathologic lying and sexual psychopathy correspond rather closely to the conception which prompted the designation, constitutional psychopathic inferiority. There is an obvious defect consisting of an apparent constitutional lack of responsiveness to the social demands of honesty or truthfulness or decency or consideration for others, which incapacitates the patient from settling down to any permanent standardized activity. The individual is, therefore, emotionally unstable, is not to be depended upon, acts on impulses, shows poor judgment and is constantly led into unwise activities, the consequence of which he is able to realize intellectually, but not evaluate. Since one cannot explain or trace the abnormal behavior of these individuals to any definite disease or organic process, the conclusion is justifiable at present that there is always some constitutional lack of endowment in each case, and, for purposes of classification, the group is termed constitutional inferior, to which the word psychopathic is added to signify the marked instability and lack of the social responsiveness previously discussed. The social and educational problems of this class of patients, although very difficult, are of paramount importance. The relationship of this group to such problems as prostitution, venereal disease, vagrancy, delinquency, illegitimacy, alcoholism and drug addiction constitutes an active need for thorough research and the dissemination of knowledge throughout every community. The need for careful supervision and definite measures to safeguard society at large from these individuals should stimulate serious thinking by people in general. Kraepelin indicates the truth of this assertion when he shows that 54 per cent of the men and nearly one-third of the women in this group as a result of their moral deterioration come into contact with the courts on account of threats, assaults, quarrels and vagrancy.

It is probably fair to say that constitutional psychopathic inferiority represents a kind of feeblemindedness which involves all spheres save the intellectual one; that the inferior is like the low-grade defective in that *he fails to profit by experience.*

THE NEUROSES.

In the consideration of the neuroses, such an enormous clinical field is opened that it is extremely difficult to treat it briefly. One may only acknowledge without discussion the enormous debt which modern psychiatry owes to Binet, Janet, Babinski, Freud and the psycho-analytic school, Adolf Meyer and many others.

The neuroses may scarcely be considered even in brief presentation, without some reference to psychopathology, since the frequency of failure to diagnose and treat, and above all to understand, strikingly illustrate an outstanding and urgent need of a firm belief in the existence of a valid pathology which is not expressed in demonstrable structural damage. There is a point beyond which physical diagnostic efforts and therapy may become harmful and even pernicious. This is certainly so if they exclude a consideration of emotional factors; if they are intensively and solely directed at the correction of minor and conjectural physical defects, such as slight deviations of the nasal septum, on the assumption that a minor operation will cure a psycho-neurosis, or finally, if they are mistakenly focused on the physical expression of underlying emotional states.

Psychotherapy in its modern sense presupposes the acceptance of at least a minimum of psychopathologic doctrine. It is extremely difficult and hazardous to state what such a minimum implies. Many of the signs and symptoms familiar to the organic neurologist, for instance, sensations, have representations in the consciousness of his patient. In a sense, therefore, he studies minds, the content of which the subjects are clearly aware, and he studies and questions his patients chiefly from the standpoint of elucidating the findings obtained in his examination. The psychiatrist studies another mind, the content of which the patient does not clearly perceive, though the author is convinced that much of the content that is important in the therapy of the neuroses is nearer the threshold of consciousness than is commonly believed by psychoanalysts. Some of the rather far-flung boundaries of this mind described by several of the disciples of Freud seem to be more fantastic than real and, even if defensible along phylogenetic lines, it is unlikely that such theories are of material aid in the practical therapy of the psychoneuroses. Nevertheless, there is a not-conscious mind, the investigation of which is profitable to the psychiatrist, since it contains a record of what has happened to the person during his lifetime.

As in organic neurology a surface sign, for instance the eye-ground picture in tumor of the brain, may be a clue to an underlying and significant pathologic process, so may many so-called surface neurotic signs and symptoms and other less clear-cut phenomena strongly suggest a deeper psychopathologic condition. For convenience, "complex" may be used to denominate somewhat obscured material that is emotionally dynamic and persistent enough to demand expression in the every-day life of the person. Some of this complex material has been accumulated as a result of the reaction to psychically traumatizing experience and its subsequent repression. When such strong complexes lead to tendencies and desires not satisfactory to the self-criticism of the subject and usually not acceptable in the judgment of the majority of others, that is of the herd, there is apt to be conflict. Many psychoneurotic patients come to the psychiatrist at the stage when the respective demands of their ego, sex and herd complexes have become irreconcilable for them and their symptoms constitute a pathologic attempt to minimize or subdue the inner psychic conflict. Often the conflict is expressed in terms of physical symptoms and signs.

In the psychiatric attitude and approach, personality is the outstanding target for investigation and therapy. Not forgetting at all its hereditarial and somatic influences, one may state that it is the condensed record of the person's lifetime experiences and reactions thereto. It is highly important, therefore, to know what has gone into the making of the personality, and also to scrutinize it carefully for potential weapons that might be forged and shaped into weapons potent enough to be utilized in the attack on the real problems of life temporarily obscured by the neurosis. Inevitably, personality brings up the question of environment. In a given patient, no real psychiatric understanding can be won without appreciation of the tremendous part that has been played in the past, and the influence that is now being exerted, by environment, not only in its broad, material sense, but even in its most minute and personal implications. All this is simple and, perhaps, ridiculously elementary, but it may serve in a rudimentary way to emphasize the great importance of psychopathology to the practitioner of medicine.

A brief descriptive summary may be helpful in the symptomatologic survey of the neuroses.

HYSTERIA.

Somatic Symptoms.—*Sensory:* Hyperesthesias, hypoesthesias and anesthesias which are all non-explainable on any organic bases, narrowing of the visual fields, photophobia, blindness, hyperacousis, deafness, anosmia, loss of taste, headache. *Motor:* Paralyses of all varieties, flaccid or spastic and sometimes with contracture. Conclusive neurologic evidence of organic disease is wanting. All types of abnormal movements—clonic, choreiform, tremors—occur. Pathologic attitudes and gaits may be displayed. Every kind of vasomotor symptom may appear and muscular atrophy is not extremely uncommon. These manifestations are sometimes so striking that the French school of neurologists have attempted to differentiate such cases from true hysteria and have given them a separate grouping, halfway between organic and functional disease, under the name of "reflex paralyses." In addition to the symptoms, which mimic, usually in crude fashion, every syndrome resulting from organic nerve irritation or defect, there may be exhibited many unusual phenomena such as rhythmical movements of various parts of the body, head noddings, rotations and also bizarre attitudinizing. The classical, full-fledged convulsion is not usual, though abortive and partial convulsive seizures are seen fairly often. Perversion or loss of special function, aphonia or mutism, difficulty or inability of swallowing, "globus," vomiting, amenorrhea, anuria, constipation or diarrhea may be a part of the symptom-complex. So-called "anorexia nervosa," which is rare, may reduce the patient to such an extremity that he may fall an easy victim to some intercurrent disease, such as tuberculosis.

Mental Symptoms.—*Amnesia,* which is apparently a successful subconscious effort to keep something out of the field of consciousness. It may extend for a considerable period before and beyond a particular incident or experience. *Fugue:* A span of time for which the patient is amnesic, though during the fugue his actions are such that it seems to the observer that he must be conscious of his surroundings. *Double personality:* The fugue and the amnesic period probably have a content which is not acceptable to ordinary personal consciousness and, therefore, there is acquired a kind of new consciousness, constituting a second personality. *Hallucination:* It has been explained on the basis of partial failure in attempting to submerge a disagreeable complex, the remnant remaining as an hallucination. There may also be somnambulism, hysterical fits, deliriums, trances, stupor or dream states.

NEURASTHENIA.

General Symptoms.—*Fatigue:* Often present on slight exertion and may be curiously selective, in that it is chiefly manifested when the patient's interest is at low ebb. Loss of weight. Usually dependent on an appetite failure.

Local Symptoms.—*Alimentary:* Capricious appetite, anorexia, indigestion, distention, eructation, nausea, vomiting, constipation or diarrhea, mucous colitis. *Circulatory:* Varying degrees of cardiac discomfort, tachycardia, palpitation, pseudo-anginal sensations, heart irregularity. *Vasomotor:* Pallor, blushing, sweating, coldness, heat and numerous other phenomena. *Genito-urinary:* Impotence, nocturnal emissions, genito-urinary paresthesias, dysmenorrhea, dyspareunia, frequency of micturition, increased urinary output, "loose kidney." *Respiratory System:* Frequent "colds," shortness of breath, sometimes hastened respiratory rate with shallow breathing. *Nervous system:* Peculiar sensations in head and in fact in every portion of the body; feelings of swelling of scalp, band around head, bursting and stuffiness of head, headache, especially in occipital region, peculiar, uncomfortable or painful sensations in the abdomen, rectum or breasts. An almost universal complaint is backache. Giddiness and dizziness is common and insomnia is rarely absent. There may be photophobia, muscæ volitantes and eye-muscle fatigue, ear noises, intolerance of ordinary sounds. *Mental symptoms:* Inability to concentrate, uncertain memory, fear of insanity, awkwardness and self-consciousness in the presence of others, feelings of inferiority, irritability, depression, phobias, anxieties.

PSYCHASTHENIA.

Psychasthenia is marked by phobias, obsessions, morbid doubts, impulsions, feelings of insufficiency, nervous tension and anxiety. Episodes of marked depression and agitation may occur. There is no disturbance of consciousness or amnesia as in hysteria.

ANXIETY NEUROSIS.

A clinical type in which morbid anxiety or fear is the most prominent feature. A general nervous irritability (or excitability) is regularly associated with the anxious expectation or dread. In addition there are numerous physical symptoms which may be regarded as the bodily accompaniments of fear, particularly cardiac and vasomotor disturbances; the heart's action is increased, often there is irregularity and palpitation; there may be sweating, nausea, vomiting, diarrhea, suffocative feelings, dizziness, trembling, shaking, difficulty of locomotion. Fluctuations occur in the intensity of the symptoms, acute exacerbations constituting the "anxiety attack."

Psychogenetic Considerations.—The vast territory embraced by the neuroses is still too virginal to permit one to disregard a single possible determining factor. Organic aspects, a better evaluation of nerve fatigue, endocrine influence, all need additional rigid investigation. In each patient there is demanded a carefully scrutinizing physical survey and treatment of the discovered pathology, whether or not it be considered etiologic. It is nevertheless true that, at present at least, psychologic investigation and therapy are more fruitful.

Psychologically, hysteria is resultant upon repression and subsequent conversion. There is psychic trauma. Painful ideas, which for the particular individual are unacceptable to the conscious mind, are not given an emotional outlet, but are relegated or forced or *repressed* into the subconscious mind and become buried complexes. The said painful ideas, according to the Freudian school, have invariably a sexual content. Such repression often takes place during childhood. Later, these buried complexes are converted or rather the affect (emotion) with which they were associated is converted into a symbol which is objectively evident as an hysterical symptom.

In a non-Freudian sense an illustration may serve to clarify: After a sharp action during the World War, a soldier was left lying upon the field of battle. He feared to move because of the danger of an enemy sniper's bullet and for many hours he was compelled to remain rigidly quiet, surrounded by the dead and listening to the horrible cries and groans of dying. Later, he was led into an ambulance dressing-station totally deaf, although his hearing apparatus was physiologically intact. He was simply hysterically deaf and, furthermore, he was amnesic. He remembered the action and could recall being brought to the ambulance dressing-station but for the hours spent on the battlefield his mind was a complete blank.

What is the psychologic explanation? One may think of the horrors of war, fatigue and exposure as directly causative of this hysteria. They were not. Even the emotion-racking experience on the battlefield at most determined the time of the actual appearance of the hysteria. The dynamic mechanism, as always, was the conflict. In this instance, the conflict was between the instinct of self-preservation and contrasting and opposed self and soldierly ideals. Self-preservation triumphed, the conflict came to resolution and was converted into two disabling and protective symptoms—deafness and amnesia.

Hysteria is a large subject and only a few significant conceptions may be given: (1) Suggestion is an important factor. Babinski believed it alone served to explain hysteria. He felt that the symptoms were purely the result of suggestion and proposed for hysteria the designation "pithiatism." (2) The symptoms and signs of hysteria, unlike those of neurasthenia, tend to be total, such as deprivations of the special senses, paralyses and anesthesias. (3) The hysteric views his symptoms objectively; is less conscious of his personal problems or conflicts and is less emotionally tense than, for instance, the patient who has neurasthenia or an anxiety state. (4) Almost always the functional nature of the symptoms may be detected since they tend to exaggerate rather than simulate organic nerve or somatic disease, and there are many discrepancies in the clinical picture unexplainable on an organic basis. (5) Hysteria is a simple, naïve, childlike device and its mechanism is usually not too difficult to penetrate.

Neurasthenia and some of the anxiety states, too, are faulty responses—attempts to escape from the difficulties and conflicts of life. Freud stressed, as causative in neurasthenia, excessive masturbation in adult life and incompleteness of sex satisfaction. He stated that anxiety neuroses are more common in women and attributed them to coitus interruptus or ejaculatio præcox; in men to abstinence, frustrated sexual excitement, coitus interruptus or senile conditions. Nonsexual stresses may be operative. The mechanism consists in a "deviation of the somatic sexual excitement from the psychic and in the abnormal utilization of this excitement."

The physician must be on the alert to detect the neurasthenic complex which may be a precursor or accompaniment of serious organic disease, as, for instance, in paresis or brain tumor. Furthermore, he must constantly remember that neurasthenia does not exclude the presence of organic disease.

Neurasthenia develops much more gradually than hysteria. The fatigue that is such a prominent symptom is not, as is so often taught, the cause of neurasthenia. It is effect rather than cause and is the aftermath of a long battle of emotional cross-purposes. In the neurasthenic the circle of normal interests and activities rapidly diminishes and contracts so that eventually the attention is rigidly concentrated upon somatic sensations and reflexes such as the heart-beat, peristaltic movements of the stomach and intestines, muscle and joint movements, etc. In neurasthenia these sensations and reflexes impinge upon the consciousness and are extensively elaborated, while in normal health the individual is scarcely aware of their existence. It is true that in themselves they are unpleasant, uncomfortable and even painful, yet the center of psychologic attention has been shifted and the mind has escaped the even more difficult and unpleasant facing of problems and conflicts. Since the connection between the symptoms and the unsolved emotional problem is not open and direct in consciousness, the psychopathologic mechanism employed "saves the face" of the patient. Not only is the ego spared the humiliation of self-criticism, but social censure is avoided.

Some of the symptoms encountered in the evolution of neurasthenia and the anxiety states have their analogies in the condition of a frightened animal, let us say a cat frightened by a fierce dog. The cat is in the grip of fear. Physiologically, the emotion acts by putting its body in the most efficient state for fight or flight. The cat crouches, its skeletal muscles are tense, its hairs stand on end, the pupils are dilated, there is a hissing noise, the heart works rapidly, the blood flows quickly and its pressure is increased, breathing is quickened, movements of the stomach and intestines are reduced to a minimum, and there are numerous and important ductless gland reactions.

The human being is less often subjected to such acute and sthenic emotional crises but relatively the same effect is produced by less severe and more protracted emotional states resultant upon some serious life problem. There may be apprehension, anxiety, worry, shame, resentment, etc., and they, as in the instance of the cat, are likewise expressed in the finely adjusted physical organism. In the beginning the symptoms probably represent a fighting attempt to overcome the difficulty. Eventually, struggling and aggressiveness cease. The individual is defeated. He retires from the world of everyday normal distribution of interests and energies and engages in a close consideration of and an endless introspection into various residual sensations. The typical neurasthenic patient with his great variety of subjective somatic complaints has now been produced.

To illustrate, let us picture a quarrel between husband and wife.

The subject of contention is the third member of the household, the mother of the wife, a querulous, complaining and rather disturbing invalid, to whom, however, the daughter is devoted. For years husband and wife have quarreled about her presence in the home. The husband wants her to leave. The wife coaxes, threatens, gets into a violent temper, weeps. The husband goes to business. The wife for the hundredth time feels herself driven into a corner. Suddenly she is sick. There is the sensation of an aching band about her head, she is weak and tired, her muscles are sore, her heart seems to be racing along, she is nauseated and faint. She analyzes these sensations minutely. What dreadful illness is threatening her? Heart disease? Actually she is organically sound. The diagnosis is neurasthenia.

In the background of this case there are many years of worry. The conflict has been protracted and for this woman it has been very serious. On the one side of the balance, devotion to her mother and the dread of having her go to an institution; on the other, anxiety about her husband's love and the fear of losing him. The conflict produced friction and fatigue. The destructive emotional state began to be expressed by various physical sensations. At first they were only occasional and insignificant manifestations. Finally they became constant and alarming. They demand consideration and treatment and a pathologic escape from an apparently unsolvable problem has been made unconsciously available.

Psychasthenia was regarded by Janet as "a lowering of the psychological tension;" Meyer defines it as "a lowering of general interest and tendency to rumination over what is accessible to the patient in his memory, but is not squarely met, and where the normal reaction is replaced by rumination, substitution acts and panics;" Ross puts forward the suggestion that psychasthenia is a faulty response involving an effort to pretend that the conflict or difficulty does not exist.

In any event psychasthenia apparently utilizes the psychologic mechanism of displacement, substitution and symbolism.

As an example we may cite Ross' interesting case of psychasthenia in a man who was obsessed by a superstitious fear of the number 13. He remained in bed on the thirteenth day of the month; hopped over each thirteenth step; counted the syllables in conversations and felt a "shock" at the thirteenth or its multiples; would not walk in Oxford Circus because of a sign "Peter Robinson" containing thirteen letters and had numerous other disabling symptoms all associated with the number 13.

Modified analysis elicited that during his boyhood there had been an ignorant, superstitious serving maid in the home who had attempted sex relations with the boy. Subsequently he had been sent to a boarding school and had lived for some years in a rigid, religious atmosphere. The disgusting experience of childhood had passed beyond the ken of conscious awareness. The neurosis with the obsessive reaction to the number 13 had appeared in middle adult life.

We may assume originally a conscious union between the idea of sex experience and the unhappy emotions (disgust, fear, shame, remorse) called forth by the remembrance.   Soon the idea becomes too trouble-some, unpleasant and painful to be retained in consciousness where it must be constantly viewed.   By means of the psychologic mechanism of displacement, the union is severed and the repugnant idea is dropped into the unconscious.   This leaves free and unattached the emotion from which the idea has been detached.   The emotion is then attached to a concept in itself innocuous, in this case "13."   Thus, 13 becomes a substitute for and a symbol of the "forgotten" sex episode.   The second union is not altogether successful.   There is the tendency for the original idea to reappear, and whenever there is any danger that it may break through into consciousness, then there are manifested the frantic obsessive devices or symptoms related to the number 13.

Frequently psychasthenia may be retraced to childhood experiences. Not only sex experiences can be dynamic, but anything that induced a vivid and strong emotional reaction, that was never cleared up or explained and was finally repressed.

The following statistics derived from a study of 239 consecutive patients are worth consideration:

1. Psychoneurotic predisposition is determined to some extent by:

   (a) Unfavorable early home life (70 per cent of cases).
   (b) Constitutional predisposition (85 per cent of cases).
   (c) Chronic disease, sex conflicts, financial difficulties, restricted outlets and mental defect, play a leading part in from 3 to 12 per cent of all cases.

2. The most common precipitating factors in the psychoneuroses are:

   (a) Sex disturbances, including conflicts over masturbation, illicit intercourse, puberty and the menopause (22 per cent).
   (b) Accidents, with or without injury (13 per cent).
   (c) Marital crises (12 per cent).
   (d) Financial crises (11 per cent).
   (e) Operations (10 per cent).
   (f) Death or illness in the family (each 9 per cent).

3. The commonest physical findings are:

   (a) Operative scars (23 per cent).
   (b) Focal infections (9 per cent).
   (c) Physical defects, including developmental anomalies and operative amputations (9 per cent).

4. The commonest mental findings are:

   (a) Overconcern expressed regarding the symptoms complained of (89 per cent).
   (b) Anxiety (45 per cent).
   (c) Fears, including fear of disease, death, insanity (33 per cent).
   (d) Marked hypochondriacal trends (19 per cent).

5. The most frequent characteristics of prehospital treatment are:

    (*a*) The patient had been seen by many physicians in 34 per cent of the cases.

    (*b*) Operations were resorted to in 19 per cent.

    (*c*) Sedatives had been employed routinely in 15 per cent.

    (*d*) Quacks of various kinds had been consulted by the patient in 10 per cent.

The almost uniform occurrence of characteristic reactions in the history and clinical findings, together with the favorable results of active treatment instituted at relatively late periods in the course of these cases, lead us to the conclusion that many psychoneurotic conditions might be prevented by early recognition and proper management. The possible mental and emotional effects of diseases, accidents, operations and financial, sex and marital disturbances should be considered in the case of every patient consulting a physician.

Treatment.—General therapeutic indications are given since not only the particular neurosis, but the individuality of the patient and his setting in life will often determine modifications.

The history must be complete. In addition to the usual historical agenda it is important: (*a*) to let the patient "talk himself out;" (*b*) to obtain a clear picture of the social environmental relationship; (*c*) to study thoroughly the history of the neurosis as to its duration, major symptoms and the patient's ideas concerning causation; (*d*) to secure all available data concerning the previous makeup of the patient.

The next treatment step is the physical examination. There are at least three reasons why the physical examination should be thorough to the point of the employment of every useful diagnostic procedure, including the skill of the finished internist, instruments of precision, and the clinical laboratory. In the first place dynamic somatic pathology may be and often is uncovered; in the second place the examination in itself, if it is a searching one, has a beneficial effect on the patient, and in the third place it puts the psychiatrist in an advantageous and authoritative position for the future management of the case. Secure in the accurate knowledge he has acquired concerning the physical status, he will be able properly to weigh the numerous subjective phenomena which will present themselves.

The physician should now be able to answer for himself the following questions: What is the apparent genesis of the neurosis? What are the relative weights of the psychogenic, somatic and environmental social factors? Is the organic situation serious enough to indicate hospital or rest-house treatment? Is the psychogenic aspect of a type which should be analyzed? Will an analysis, other than a fairly superficial one, do more harm than good and had the physician better limit himself to simple explanation, persuasion and suggestion? Are the environmental social elements serious and destructive? Are they capable of correction?

Details of treatment which vary from patient to patient include hospital or rest-house care, rest in bed, scientific nursing, dietary control, massage, hydrotherapy, electrotherapy, occupational therapy, supervision of the patient's activities, including visitors, correspondence, reading, graduated exercise, tonic and in extreme conditions hypnotic medication. There must be correction of any *actual* organic pathology.

The principles of treatment for the neuroses as developed at Stockbridge by Riggs are as follows: The patient is given an opportunity to tell his story in detail. Next, there is a thorough physical and mental examination followed by a frank discussion with the patient concerning his difficulties and the reasons for his maladaptation. The patient is then informed of the plan of treatment and is given a daily schedule to meet his individual needs. It consists of exercise, diversion and rest. The keynote of the treatment is reëducation. It stresses the importance of dominating the emotions and of utilizing the intelligence to guide conduct. Efficiency is emphasized. The patient is impressed with the necessity of making clear-cut decisions at first in trivial, later in great matters. The proper use of the mind is described. The harmful effects of worry, unnecessary hurry, inattention and self-pity are elaborated. They are manifestations of inefficiency. The patient is instructed concerning rest, which is not synonymous with sleep and is chiefly the temporary and volitional abandonment of responsibility.

As a general guide toward rehabilitation the following steps are logical and helpful:

1. *Establishment of Rapport Between the Physician and the Patient.*— This rapport, to be effective, must be based on a certain amount of respect and confidence on the part of the patient. It is best furthered by a careful investigatory program instituted by the physician at the first interview.

2. *Aëration or Ventilation.*—Aëration or ventilation of the conflict material presented by the patient may be carried out by means of Freudian catharsis, by means of direct interviews, by means of discovering and probing for such material from outside sources, by hypnosis or by any other method. The important thing is that the patient is given an opportunity to discharge and bring out in the open all of those life experiences which have been causing him serious concern either consciously or unconsciously.

3. *Desensitization.*—Desensitization is the procedure wherein the patient is required to face frankly the traumatic and unpleasant experiences of his past. It is brought about, in the first place, by causing the patient to discuss at frequently repeated interviews the conflict material as elicited above. These interviews are repeated until the patient can review these experiences without excessive emotional concern.

4. *Reëducation.*—Reëducation is carried out in connection with all of the above procedures. It is essentially the development of clear insight on the part of the patient into the mechanism of his illness, the establishment of new habits of response (as in desensitization) and the formulation by him of an adequate industrial, social, recreational and activity program to ensure future stabilization.

5. In addition to the above, it is often advisable to desensitize the patient's family to his illness and reëducate them into new habits of response toward the patient.

6. All contributing physical factors are corrected as far as possible. Measures for their correction are instituted at the earliest possible interview and are utilized as psychotherapeutic aids.

GLOSSARY.

Affect—used synonymously with emotion or mood.

Ambivalency—every idea, impulse, action is presumed to have positive and negative values. Ambivalent conduct results from the conflict between these values which, of course, greatly interferes with and, in fact, may negate the performance of an action. Bleuler defines ambivalence as a "Specific schizophrenic characteristic, to accompany identical ideas or concepts at the same time with positive as well as negative feelings (*affective* ambivalence) to will and not to will at the same time the identical actions (ambivalence of the will) and to think the same thoughts at once negatively and positively (intellectual ambivalence)."

Amnesia—a loss of memory of any kind or extent.

Autistic Thinking—dream or phantasy thinking as contrasted to realistic thinking. It probably sets free subjective wishes which are unobtainable in practical life. An example would be the conducting of an imaginary love affair in the mind of the patient.

Catalepsy—a condition probably due to hypersuggestibility in which the limbs of a patient will remain in any position in which they are placed until they drop from muscular exhaustion.

Catatonia—literally—"I stretch tightly." Originally regarded as a muscular phenomenon, its meaning has been expanded to include many symptoms, such as certain types of violence, mutism, scolding spells, refusal of food, stereotopy. It occurs in many psychoses but is seen in its most typical manifestations in *dementia præcox*, either as catatonic stupor in which there may be mutism, absence of response to external stimuli, negativism, catalepsy, cerea, or catatonic excitement which to the observer appears as wholly purposeless activity.

Cerea Flexibilitas—a symptom often present in catalepsy in which the limbs may be moulded, almost, as if they were made of wax.

Compensation—an exaggeration of conscious trends serving as a defense against opposed unconscious wishes which are threatening to break into consciousness.

Complex—a system of ideas held together by strong emotional bond which has largely fallen into the unconscious, usually because it is not acceptable to the conscious mind.

Compulsive Act—an act, the performance of which seems to the patient to depend on a will which is not his own.

Conflict—interplay or struggle between unconscious and often frustrated desires and conscious trends. The conscious trends may be broadly viewed as the demands of civilization and society.

Delusion—a false belief which cannot be corrected by argument, persuasion or experience. Always more than a mere mistaken opinion, since it concerns a belief which is usually obviously and grossly erroneous. For instance, the delusion that the patient is Napoleon; or, again, is without a stomach or bowels, or is being conspired against by a powerful organization. Furthermore, the reasons given by the patient for the verity of the belief are not convincing or logical, except occasionally in true paranoia.

Dementia—a permanent loss of one or more of the mental faculties, as the deterioration of emotional life in unfavorable dementia præcox or the almost complete "loss" of mind observed in the last stages of paresis, senile dementia, epileptic dementia.

Disassociation—literally, without or lacking association or connection. For instance, to the observer the speech of the catatonic excitement of *præcox* seems without ideational connection, in contrast to the manic production in which a connection or association of ideas may usually be traced. Used also in psychiatry to indicate a failure of harmonious working; for instance, the incongruity or lack of agreement between the affect and thought content in dementia præcox. All express the mental operation which brings about a double personality, in which unpleasant material along with associated happenings is split off and forms a kind of separate consciousness.

Distractibility—unduly or abnormally responsive to distracting influences which may too readily interfere with and change the train of thought and action, as evidenced in the speech and behavior.

Double Personality—the formation of a second and separate personality. The individual is in some sense as if he were two persons, the two personalities functioning more or less independently and not communicating with each other. See Disassociation.

Echolalia—involuntary repetition of what is heard.

Echopraxia—involuntary imitation of what is done in the presence of the patient.

Euphoria—a feeling of well-being. Sometimes interpreted as a feeling of happiness.

Flight of Ideas—rapid changes in the direction of thought processes, as in mania, when the patient may never reach the completion of the goal idea because of the switching of the train of thought in response to external or internal stimuli.

Fugue—a state during which the patient for a certain period of time seemingly acts in a conscious way, perhaps travelling, buying food and in general comporting himself in a natural manner; yet, afterward he has no conscious remembrance for this period of time and his behavior during it.

Hallucination—a sensation or perception without an object. In an hallucination, for instance, the voices which are heard and the visions which are seen are purely imaginary; that is, they do not have a starting-point in sounds which are actually heard or sights which are actually seen.

Ideas of Reference—the interpretation by the patient of incidents and casual happenings in the environment as having a direct reference to him. For instance, a passer-by coughs and thereby conveys derision and insult.

Illusion—a misinterpreted sensation or perception. There is actual stimulation of one or more of the senses but the stimulus is grossly misinterpreted.

Impulsive Act—an act, the performance of which seems to the patient to depend on sudden, overwhelming impulses arising from within.

Introjection—subjectifying the objective or imputing to ourselves the motives of others. Also called identification.

Libido—appetite. Craving for satisfaction.

Mannerism—a stereotyped movement which seems to consist of a peculiar modification of an ordinary movement, as, walking in very straight lines or eating in a definite rhythm. There may be mannerisms of speech, as lisping, strange inflections, odd phrasing, repetitions.

Mutism—literally, without speech. Occurs in various psychoses. In depression it may be due to extreme retardation or to stupor. It may be negativistic when there is refusal to answer questions, although spontaneous speech exists.

Narcissism—love of self to the exclusion or incompleteness of heterosexual love.

Negativism—impulsive resistance to external stimuli such as requests or commands. For instance, in negativistic conduct the patient who is asked to stick out the tongue may press the teeth tightly together, or squeeze the eyelids together when an attempt is made to examine the pupils. It should not be confused with voluntary resistance or stubbornness.

Neologism—senseless expression. The expression of meaningless (to the listener) words, phrases or sentences.

Nosology—the science of the classification of disease.

Obsession—the domination of the patient by some thought or action, as in psychasthenia.

Orientation—clear comprehension of environment as to time, place and person. Absence of orientation is disorientation and may involve time, place or person.

Paranoid—resembling paranoia. The student must remember that as far as delusions are concerned the delusions of paranoid *præcox*, while they suggest the delusions of paranoia, nevertheless lack the consistency, logic and closely knit systematization of the latter.

Projection—objectifying the subjective or imputing to others motives which are really one's own motives.

Rationalization—an unconscious process of self-justification. An unwillingness to recognize real reasons.

Retardation—slowness and difficulty in thought, speech and motion.

Sublimation—the utilization of the energy of unobtainable wishes in order to erect a higher and usually more social goal.

Symbolization—letting one object represent something else. A Freudian mechanism which is said to operate principally in dreams, and which has for its object the representation of dream material in a form acceptable to the dreamer.

Transference—unconscious misidentification of external objects, usually persons, so that the patient may feel and behave toward them in a way which satisfies the experiences and impressions which refer to another (love or fixation) object.

Unconscious—the repository, not only of the previous experiences in the life of an individual but also of the historical past of the race (psychoanalytic sense).

Verbigeration—repetition for long periods of time and in a monotonous fashion of senseless expressions, sometimes only a single syllable or word. There may be manifestations of verbigeration in the writing of patients.

Volubility—excessive fluency of speech.

REFERENCES.

Association for Research in Nervous and Mental Diseases: Schizophrenia (Dementia Præcox), New York, Paul B. Hoeber, Inc., 1928.

BLEULERE: Text-book of Psychiatry, translated by Brill, Macmillan & Co., 1924.

HENDERSON, D. K., and GILLESPIE, R. D.: Text-book of Psychiatry, Oxford Med. Pub., Oxford University Press, 1927.

HOCH, AUGUST: Benign Stupors, New York, Macmillan Company.

JUNG, C. G.: The Psychology of Dementia Præcox, Nervous and Mental Diseases, Monograph Series No. 3.

MEYER, ADOLF: The Nature and Conception of Dementia Præcox, Jour. Abnorm. Psychol., December, 1910.

ROSS, T. A.: The Common Neuroses, New York, Longmans, Green & Co., 1923.

SONDÉN, TORSTEN: A Study of Somatic Conditions in Manic-depressive Psychosis, Upsala, 1927, Almquist & Wiksells Boktryckeri A.-B.

STRECKER, E. A., and APPEL, K. E.: Discovering Ourselves, New York, Macmillan Company, 1931.

STRECKER, E. A., and EBAUGH, F. G.: Clinical Psychiatry, 3d ed., Philadelphia, P. Blakiston's Son & Co., 1931.

CHAPTER XXVI.

ORGANIC DISEASES OF THE NERVOUS SYSTEM.

By GEORGE WILSON, M.D.

INTRODUCTION.
THE CRANIAL NERVES.
THE REFLEXES.
THE MOTOR SYSTEM.
  Gaits.
  Tremor.
SENSATION.
THE CEREBROSPINAL FLUID.
PREGNANCY AND THE PUERPERIUM.
NEUROLOGIC SYNDROMES.
NEUROSYPHILIS.
  General Paresis.
  Tabes Dorsalis.
THE SPINAL CORD.
  Tumors of the Cord.
  Tumors of the Spine.
  Subdural Abscess.
  Serous Meningitis.
  Tuberculous Spondylitis.
  Injuries.
  Hematomyelia.
  Amyotrophic Lateral Sclerosis.
  Progressive Spinal Muscular Atrophy.
  Combined Sclerosis.
  Syringomyelia.
  Myelitis.
  Hypertrophic Cervical Pachymeningitis.
  Friedreich's Ataxia.
  Diseases of the Blood-vessels.
  Herpes Zoster.
  Anterior Poliomyelitis.
  Multiple Sclerosis.

THE BRAIN
  Focal Signs.
  Aphasia.
  Disorders of Articulation.
  Diseases of the Blood-vessels.
  Subarachnoid Hemorrhage.
  Sinus Thrombosis.
  Cerebral Aneurysm.
  Tumors.
  Injuries.
DISORDERS OCCURRING AT BIRTH.
  Internal Hydrocephalus.
  Infantile Hemiplegia.
  Little's Disease.
  Amaurotic Family Idiocy.
BULBAR PALSY.
PSEUDOBULBAR PALSY.
MYASTHENIA GRAVIS.
PARALYSIS AGITANS.
SYDENHAM'S CHOREA.
HUNTINGTON'S CHOREA.
PROGRESSIVE LENTICULAR DEGENERATION.
EPIDEMIC ENCEPHALITIS.
EPILEPSY.
MIGRAINE.
PERIPHERAL NERVOUS SYSTEM.
  Neuritis of Various Types.
  The Neuralgias.
  Progressive Muscular Atrophy.
  Lesions of Nerves of Extremities.
THE MYOPATHIES.

Introduction.—In no branch of medicine is an accurate knowledge of the entire working of the body so necessary as it is in the study of nervous and mental diseases. Too much time is routinely spent in the teaching of nervous diseases in hopeless and incurable conditions, such as amyotrophic lateral sclerosis and syringomyelia, although an exact knowledge of how the symptoms and signs of such diseases are produced helps the student when he comes to make a diagnosis. For one to be properly equipped to diagnose and treat nervous diseases, he should have an adequate training in internal medicine and should have a good knowledge of the form and function of the nervous system. The nervous system is just as much a part of the field of general diagnosis as is the study of diseases of the chest. Infections, syphilis,

(1111)

tuberculosis, vascular disease and tumors, all affect the nervous system at times just as they affect other parts of the body.

The diagnosis of a nervous ailment frequently rests on accurate laboratory data, without which the diagnosis is obscure. On the other hand too much dependence should not be placed upon the laboratory and special forms of examinations, such as encephalography. The physician or student should preferably train himself to make as accurate a diagnosis as possible, without the many refinements of the present age, which may in time lead to a sort of machine-made diagnosis.

The history in a nervous case is often of more importance than a good examination. It should be taken carefully, in chronologic order and, as far as possible, in the patient's own words. He will, however, have to be led along in his story, but an effort should be made not to ask leading questions. This is in all events more important when one is dealing with a functional rather than an organic case. An idea of the patient's past life, his heredity, his mode of living, his recreations and vices, if any, is important. As the case unravels itself, questions will suggest themselves to the examiner. For example, a complaint of pain should always be elaborated upon; particularly its location, its reference if any, the type of pain, the presence of anything which aggravates it, such as moving or coughing, the time of day it occurs and, if present at night, whether it prevents sleep or awakens the individual. Functions of the sphincters, especially that of the bladder, should be carefully inquired into. Difficulties in the control of the urine which make their first appearance after the age of fifteen or twenty years, will quite often have to do with involvement of the central nervous system. If a local cause cannot be found for difficulty in the control of the bladder sphincter, it is usually nervous in origin. Direct questions should always be asked as to the presence of visual difficulties, such as dimness of vision or diplopia. Questions referable to the eighth nerve, that is, the presence or absence of tinnitus, vertigo and deafness should be inquired about. The history of the onset of an infection will often serve to make partially clear the type of lesion from which the patient suffers. Vascular accidents in the central nervous system produce sudden or apoplectiform onsets. A tumor growing in the brain or the cord may take some weeks or even years to produce the picture which the examiner sees, although it must not be overlooked that occasionally the onset in a case of spinal or brain tumor may apparently be sudden; a brain tumor growing slowly and producing few, if any, symptoms, may be the seat of a hemorrhage, and suddenly destroy a certain part of the brain. Because nerve fibers can function through a glioma, such a tumor may attain a large size before the symptoms are produced, or before a hemorrhage suddenly occurs into it. The progress of symptoms produced by an abscess is usually midway between a vascular accident and a tumor. The relation, if any, of a nervous condition to injury or an infection should be carefully inquired into. Many cases of chronic encephalitis were but mildly ill with the acute attack, which may have been entirely overlooked; questions, therefore, must be asked as to the occurrence of an illness characterized by double vision, lethargy or perhaps insomnia. The sequence of events is an extremely important part of the history; double vision occurring early in a history suggestive of brain tumor is of localizing importance, but if it occurs late it may be simply a manifestation of a general increase of pressure. The character of a headache, if complained of, should be closely scrutinized, and the index of suspicion of the examiner for such things as cerebral syphilis, brain tumor, sinus disease and eye strain should be high. If a spinal tumor is suspected the location of the original pain and the exact order of the development of symptoms is most necessary for a satisfactory diagnosis. The examiner should be alive to the possibility that pain, even though present in the abdomen or chest, may be due to an involvement of a spinal root, and that such a pain, because it is increased by coughing or sneezing, may simulate pleurisy. This pain is not, as a rule, developed or aggravated by deep breathing.

In obtaining the history of a patient suffering from convulsions it is important to inquire into aura, cry, whether or not he injures himself in falling, bites the tongue, loses control of the urine and sleeps after an attack. If there is a possibility that the case may be hysterical the symptoms should be put to the patient in a negative manner. She should be asked, "Of course, you never bite your tongue and never have a headache after a fit?" The same procedure should be followed when the abdomen or other parts are examined, not only by the student in neurology in search of knowledge, but by the surgeon. There can be no doubt but that many patients suffering from pain in the appendiceal region have it suggested to them by a surgeon who, poking his finger into McBurney's point, asks in a domineering tone, "That hurts you, doesn't it?" The history of a paresthetic phenomenon is sometimes a great aid in arriving at a diagnosis. Pernicious anemia is probably the commonest cause of numbness in the toes and and fingers coming on after the age of forty-five or fifty years. Questions should not be omitted pertaining to the general health of the patient. Symptoms referable to the lungs, heart and gastro-intestinal tract should be particularly inquired into. How the patient spends his spare time, if he has any, whether or not he has a hobby, whether he plays golf and whether or not he takes too keen delight in the pleasure of the table, may have a bearing on his condition and lead to a correct evaluation of the symptoms. A good history is one of the most important things which leads to a correct diagnosis. It was amazing to see Mills make rounds in the nervous wards at the Philadelphia General Hospital, to have a history recited to him and, if it was any good at all, to see him arrive at a diagnosis often without the necessity of examining the patient. By the time a good history is obtained, certain leads will be indicated as to the location of the lesion and the type of examination indicated. It is always wise, however, to have a definite examination routine, which should not be neglected in the early years of practice. For this reason some authorities believe that only by taking a history and recording the examination on a form will a complete and detailed result be obtained.

When the examination is made it should be done in a routine, systematic manner, and while there are many variations in the method of starting an examination, much will depend upon the circumstances under which the patient is seen as to the exact order in which various tests should be done. It is obvious that a patient seen in an office will be put through a little different routine than one seen in consultation in a hospital bed or at home. In like manner the examination of patients on ward service in hospitals will vary according to whether or not they are ambulatory. The mental state of the patient can often be well evaluated during the interview. His general emotional state, the orderliness with which he gives his history, his memory and the presence or absence of such things as depression, excitement and lethargy will be observed. If he is delirious or comatose the record of the case will have to be given by someone else.

After the mental status of the patient has been determined he should be weighed and his height taken. He should then be completely undressed and the examination carried out in the following manner:

Scheme for Neurologic Examination.

1. **Mental Functions.**—Intelligence, attention, emotional state, hallucinations, delusions, delirium, coma, stupor, insomnia; special tests such as Binet-Simon.

2. **Cranial Nerves.**—(a) Sense of smell in each nostril which should be preceded by the elimination of local disease in the nose. Sense of smell is tested by closing one nostril and having the patient smell with the other such things as vanilla, peppermint, whiskey or cloves. Ammonia or acetic acid should not be used because they irritate the fifth nerve.

   (b) Visual acuity; state of the fundi; visual fields.

   (c), (d), (e) Ocular movements and state of the lids; nystagmus; pupils for size, shape, regularity, reaction to direct and indirect light and to convergence; location in the iris.

   (f) Sensation in its distribution; lachrymal, corneal and conjunctival reflexes; action of the muscles of mastication.

   (g) Movement of the face, both voluntary and emotional; taste on the anterior two-thirds of the tongue.

   (h) Acuity of hearing; tinnitus; vertigo; special examinations such as Bárány, Weber, Rinne and Schwabach.

   (i), (j), (k), (l). Movements of the pharynx, larynx, sternocleido-mastoid, trapezius, of the tongue; taste, posterior third of the tongue; sensation in the pharynx and larynx; swallowing and pharyngeal reflex.

3. **Reflexes.**—(a) *Superficial.* Plantar, cremasteric, abdominal.

   (b) *Deep.* Patellar, Achilles, triceps, biceps, von Bechterew's, coracobrachialis, wrist.

   (c) *Organic.* Sphincter control, sexual potency, priapism.

4. **Motor Functions.**—(a) Convulsions, general or localized; details about fits.

   (b) Muscle power, whether paralyzed or weak, and the distribution of the involvement, such as hemiplegia, paraplegia and monoplegia. Test strength of hands with dynamometer and other joints against resistance.

(c) Type of paralysis, whether flaccid or spastic.

(d) Muscle atrophy or hypertrophy.

(e) Tremors or irregular movements, such as fibrillary tremors, athetosis, chorea, Parkinson's tremor, tics, finger-to-nose test, diadochokinesis, heel-to-knee test, station, gait, speech, right or left handedness, attitude posture.

5. **Trophic Functions.**—(a) Muscular atrophy; response of muscles to faradism and galvanism.

(b) State of skin: eruptions, ulcers, glossy skin, herpetic eruptions; bed sores; arthropathies; spontaneous or pathologic fractures.

6. **Sensory Functions.**—(a) Subjective symptoms such as pain, its type, location, radiation, frequency, conditions and posture relieving or aggravating it; paresthesia and dysesthesia.

(b) Headache, location, type, periodicity, conditions aggravating it, whether accompanied by nausea, vomiting or vertigo.

(c) Tenderness, hyperesthesia, and its location if present.

(d) Objective sensory tests for touch, pain, hot and cold, vibratory sense, stereognosis, sense of position, deep pressure pain, spot localization, graphesthesia, compass test; all abnormal sensory results should be charted. Objective sensory examination to be done when patient and examiner are not tired, irritable or disturbed, in a warm room preferably at the beginning of the examination.

7. **Vegetative Nervous System.**—(a) Cervical sympathetic, size of the pupil, enophthalmos, exophthalmos, narrowing of the palpebral fissure, flushing or sweating of the face, neck and upper extremities, the reaction of the pupil to cocaine.

(b) Raynaud's disease, neuralgia, angioneurotic edema, localized edema.

8. **Skeletal System.**—Depressions, enlargements, tumors, investigation of the joints, spinal column and mobility, scoliosis, kyphosis, tenderness.

9. **Complete Laboratory Data.**

THE CRANIAL NERVES.

First Nerve.—The olfactory nerve is sensory and its fibers are nonmyelinated. Loss of smell (anosmia) may be due to disease anywhere from the nose to the centers of the brain which are in the uncinate and hippocampal gyri.

It is extremely important to rule out local conditions in the nose before much significance is placed upon a loss of smell from a neurologic standpoint. If these local conditions have been ruled out, unilateral loss of smell may be seen from lesions at the base, such as syphilis, tumor, hemorrhage and fracture. In the uncinate group of fits, hallucinations of smell are common. Hallucinations of smell may also be found in mental illness, and perversion of this sense be discovered in psychoneurotics. Tests for smell should be made with volatile oils and not with such things as ammonia, which irritate the fifth nerve. The patient should be blindfolded during the test and each nostril tested separately.

Second Nerve.—Examination of the optic nerve is one of the most important parts of the neurologic examination. Vision may be tested roughly by asking the patient to count fingers at varying distances or it may be determined more accurately by means of Snellen's type. Changes in the visual fields can be roughly determined by the examiner bringing into the field of vision from all directions, his own hand, the fingers of which are either moving or still. In an aphasic or semi-stuporous patient this can be done by the so-called feeding test, that is, by bringing into the field of vision a spoon on which food has been placed. If the patient sees it he will usually open his mouth. The state of the optic nerve can be seen directly with the ophthalmoscope; optic atrophy, either primary or secondary, may be detected.

Neurons of the optic nerves arise in the ganglion cells of the retina, whence they pass in the optic nerve to the chiasm, where the fibers from the temporal half of the retina continue on the same side, whereas those from the nasal sides cross. The optic tract fibers then terminate in the primary optic centers, *i. e.*, external geniculate body, the pulvinar and the superior colliculus. The last neuron in the course of the tract then goes to the occipital pole, especially in the region of the calcarine fissure. There is no further crossing of the visual pathways, so that a lesion involving the optic tract anywhere behind the chiasm will produce lateral homonymous hemianopsia of some extent. The fibers for the reflex activity of the pupils run in the optic nerves and are both crossed and uncrossed. A lesion anterior to the chiasm results in impairment of vision or in blindness on the same side. A lesion at the chiasm, such as, for example, that which is seen in pituitary tumors, produces a bitemporal hemianopsia, due to paralysis of the nasal halves of the retinæ.

Binasal hemianopsia is a rare finding. It is due to bilateral lesions, usually a syphilitic exudate at the lateral aspects of the chiasm. Lesions in the optic tracts, in or anterior to the primary optic centers, may readily impair the pupillary reflex. Lesions posterior to the primary optic centers do not do so, being outside the reflex arc. The optic nerve may be implicated directly by tumor, syphilis, fracture, hemorrhage, aneurysm or meningitis. The nerve itself may be the seat of a glioma. Direct pressure on the nerve usually results in atrophy. If the nerve is involved behind the eyeball, the condition is called retrobulbar neuritis. If the nerve within the ball of the eye is the site of inflammation, it is spoken of as optic neuritis. There is no sharp line of demarcation between optic neuritis and choked disk or papilledema; most ophthalmologists, nevertheless, refer to the condition as optic neuritis, if the swelling is below the two diopters, and choking if the swelling is above. The changes in the eye-grounds which occur and which are of great importance from a neurologic point of view are atrophy, optic neuritis and choked disk. Optic atrophy is either primary or secondary. Primary atrophy is due to direct involvement of the nerve. It is usually bilateral and is a particularly common symptom in neurosyphilis, especially tabes, exogenous poisoning such as arsenic, lead, quinine, tobacco, carbon monoxide and, above all, alcohol. These poisons act by producing a retrobulbar neuritis which leads in time to optic atrophy. The infectious diseases probably frequently produce retrobulbar neuritis, and the optic nerves may also be involved in multiple neuritis. A large hemorrhage may produce optic atrophy, usually preceded by neuritis.

Inflammatory reactions or neoplastic conditions in or about the chiasm and suprasellar tumors often give rise to primary atrophy. In fact, the presence of optic neuritis or choked disk points decidedly away from lesions of the pituitary. There is a form of hereditary optic atrophy called Leber's disease, which usually appears before the age of twenty or twenty-five years. Like all hereditary diseases it is more common in the male, but is transmitted by the female.

Another type of hereditary optic atrophy is amaurotic family idiocy, described by Tay and Sachs, and is seen in Jewish children. The characteristic thing is a cherry-red spot seen at the macula. Spielmeyer has described another type of juvenile amaurotic idiocy.

Conditions in the optic tracts in or anterior to the primary optic centers may lead to primary optic atrophy inasmuch as the primary neuron is affected. Lesions posterior to these centers do not produce atrophy but do cause disturbance in the visual fields and may cause, by another mechanism, choked disk. A combination of optic atrophy on the side of the lesion and choked disk on the opposite side has been described in frontal lobe tumor.

Retrobulbar neuritis is often followed by optic atrophy, usually more marked on the temporal side of the disk. Some time elapses before the pallor is seen. The most characteristic visual field defect is bilateral central scotoma for red, blue and green. The visual affection is due to an interstitial neuritis of the papillomacular bundle. The eye symptoms of multiple sclerosis are frequently due to retrobulbar neuritis. Sphenoid and ethmoid diseases may produce either retrobulbar neuritis or neuritis. Optic neuritis may occur from any toxic or infectious cause such, for example, as kidney disease and diabetes. The disk may be raised somewhat and the differential diagnosis between neuritis and papilledema may be a difficult one.

Choked disks or papilledema has an etiology as yet unknown, but it is probably due to increased intracranial pressure, particularly in the ventricles. The choking of the nerve occurs at the optic foramen. Another theory as to the causation of the condition is that toxic products produce the inflammation. Choking is characterized by overfilling of the veins, contractions of the arteries, swelling and blurring of the disk and by haziness of the margins. Swelling of 4 to 6 diopters is not uncommon and it may be even higher. A high degree of choking of the disks is compatible with good or normal vision, but as a rule visual acuity is diminished. In most cases of choked disks, hemorrhages and exudates may be seen at the nerve head. Choked disk is usually bilateral but may be more marked on one side. The writer has seen unilateral choked disk of 4 and 6 diopters with blindness in the affected eye, in both instances sudden of onset, but which cleared up almost miraculously after the removal, in both cases, of badly diseased tonsils. At least 90 per cent of the patients suffering from choked disk have brain tumors. Syphilis, meningitis, ependymitis, sinus disease, anemia, infections and toxemias account for the remaining 10 per cent. Enlargement of the blind spot, contraction of visual fields, and interference with the pupillary response are common physical signs in choked disk. Each patient exhibiting choked disk should be considered as harboring a brain tumor until proved otherwise.

The exact determination of the state of the visual fields is of highest importance in the localizing of cerebral lesions. The fields should be plotted carefully and in a painstaking manner. It is often advisable to repeat the examination, particularly if the patient is dull or the examiner hurried. Furthermore, a change may occur as a natural result of the disease which may clinch the localization. Thus, due to a second study of the visual fields after a week, a patient with only slight defect in one temporal field at first, showed definite bitemporal defects, which aided greatly in localizing a large tumor at the base near the pituitary region. Lesions behind the chiasm furnish paralysis of the ipsilateral halves of the retinæ with, of course, homonymous hemianopsia on the opposite side.

Lesions deep in a temporal lobe may cause early quadrant anopsia on the opposite side. The student is referred to a text-book on ophthalmology for the technic of taking the visual fields.

Third Nerve.—The third nerve nucleus lies in the floor of the third ventricle near the upper part of the aqueduct of Sylvius. Fibers emerging from the nucleus go through the red nucleus and the substantia nigra and emerge between the peduncles. The nerve follows along the side of the sella in the outer wall of the cavernous sinus, and enters the orbital fissure to supply all the muscles of the eyeball, with the exception of the external rectus, superior oblique and the dilator of the pupil. The sphincter of the iris and ciliary muscles are supplied by the third nerve.

Fourth and Sixth Nerves.—The nucleus of the trochlear nerve lies behind the oculomotor. The course of the nerve is in the outer wall of the cavernous sinus. It supplies the superior oblique, whose function is to move the eyeball downward and outward. The nucleus of the *sixth* nerve is in the floor of the fourth ventricle in the lower part of the pons. The fibers cross the pons and after they emerge, run a long course over the temporal bone to the wall of the cavernous sinus. The nerve supplies the external rectus muscle which moves the eyeball outward.

While it is generally considered that the third, fourth and sixth cranial nerves are purely motor, it has been shown that part of their fibers are afferent, conveying impulses of kinetic sense from the extrinsic ocular muscles. Paralysis of any one of the ocular muscles will lead to double vision and a deviation of the eyeball. The diplopia is due to the fact that the image, instead of falling on each retina at the same place, strikes at different points because of the inequality of the muscles. Diplopia is present when both eyes are being used, although monocular diplopia, usually an hysterical phenomenon, may occur if a deformity of the cornea is present. If the third nerve is completely paralyzed, the upper lid droops because of the paralysis of the levator palpebræ superioris. Due to the unopposed action of the external rectus the eyeball is turned outward. The eyeball cannot be moved upward, downward or inward, although a slight downward and outward movement can be performed by the superior oblique muscle, which is supplied by the fourth nerve. The third nerve supplies the sphincter of the iris. Therefore, the pupil is wide, because of the unopposed action of the dilator which is supplied by the sympathetic. The pupil does not respond to light, nor does the eye attempt convergence. The third nerve may be completely paralyzed or partially affected. Paralysis of the fourth nerve results in involvement of the superior oblique muscle, which turns the eyeball downward and outward, and at the same time rotates the vertical meridian slightly inward at its lower end. It is extremely difficult to detect a paralysis of the superior oblique nerve, but it is usually determined by the diplopia which results when the patient attempts to look downward and outward. The false image stands lower than the true, and is especially likely to appear when the patient walks downstairs.

The sixth nerve supplies the external rectus and involvement of it produces paralysis of that muscle. The patient is unable to turn the eye outward beyond the midline. All other movements are normal. The diplopia is present when the eyes are directed toward the side of the paralyzed sixth nerve.

The Pupil.—The things to be noted about the pupil are the size, shape, equality, position and its reaction to light, to painful stimulation of the skin of the neck and to accommodation. Slight inequality (*anisocoria*) may occur in individuals free of disease and, if it is the only abnormality present, may be disregarded. If the inequality is considerable, and especially if accompanied by other signs, organic disease may be present. The pupils are abnormally large in poisoning by certain drugs such as the atropine group, alcohol and cocaine. *Mydriasis* may result from paralysis of the sphincter of the pupil or may be due to stimulation of the dilator. The pupils in blind eyes are usually dilated. *Myosis*, or abnormal smallness of the pupil, may occur from disease of the pons, in tabes and in cervical cord lesions, due to involvement of the cervical sympathetic. The pupils may also be contracted as the result of iritis and after excision of the Gasserian ganglion. Pilocarpin and opium contract the pupil.

The *shape of the pupil* should be carefully determined. Unequal and irregular pupils, if such local conditions as iritis, operative procedures and coloboma have been ruled out, are usually syphilitic in origin. The pupil may be ectopic. Occasionally such a condition indicates a lesion of the mid-brain. Testing of the pupillary reflex to light is an important part of a physical examination. Occasionally pupils will be found which react either to daylight or to an electric light, but not to both. Each eye should be tested separately because, if the light is thrown in both eyes at the same time, a pupil fixed to direct light might react consensually. The light reflex depends upon the integrity of the reflex arc. The fibers pass in the optic nerves to the mid-brain, and the efferent parts of the arc are made up of the third nerve and ciliary ganglion to the sphincter of the pupil.

At times a phenomenon known as *hippus* is found. This consists of a rhythmic contraction of the pupil. Loss of reaction of the pupil to light occurs in optic atrophy, involvement of the third nerve and affections of the ciliary ganglion. The loss of the direct reflex to light, with preservation of the contraction of the pupils in accommodation for near objects, is called the *Argyll-Robertson phenomenon* and is a sign extremely significant of neurosyphilis. It may, however, be seen in alcoholism, arteriosclerosis, multiple sclerosis and epidemic encephalitis, but is extremely uncommon in those conditions. An Argyll-Robertson pupil, as Spiller has pointed out, is not necessarily completely paralyzed to light at the beginning, but passes through different grades just as any other physical sign. For example, the knee-jerk is not suddenly lost in tabes, but gradually disappears. The reaction of the pupil to accommodation is the contraction of the pupil which is seen when the patient converges his eyes on a near object. The loss of the contraction to accommodation with preservation of the light reflex is occasionally seen in epidemic encephalitis and after diphtheria. The *paradoxical pupil*, when the pupil dilates instead of contracting on exposure to light, is seen in some cases of tabes, but in my experience not in such a number as Pilcz claims, who says it occurs in 40 per cent of the cases. The ciliospinal reflex, which is the reaction of the pupil to painful stimulation of the skin of the neck, thereby causing the pupil to dilate, is of value in estimating the state of the cervical sympathetic.

Nystagmus is a rhythmic tremor of the eyeballs, involuntary, bilateral and symmetrical. It may be present when the eyeballs are looking straight ahead, but is more likely to be developed when the patient looks upward, downward or laterally. What might be termed occupation nystagmus is seen in miners. It may be lateral, vertical or rotary, and is, in reality, a form of cerebellar ataxia. Nystagmus may be due to disease or stimulation of a labyrinth. It is produced in healthy individuals by syringing the ear with hot or cold water and thus may be used as a test for the functions of the eighth nerve. Nystagmus may occur from lesions of the mid-brain, pons and cerebellum and is frequently seen in such diseases as multiple sclerosis and Friedreich's ataxia. It is a fairly frequent finding in albinism, and myopic persons often have a type of it. Loss or disturbance of associated movements of the eyes upward or downward is an important localizing sign of disease of the anterior quadrigeminal bodies either directly or by pineal tumors. Loss of lateral associated movements, in which the eyes cannot be moved to one side, is due to a lesion in or near the sixth nerve nucleus or the posterior longitudinal bundle on the side of the paralysis; the failure of the opposite internal rectus to function properly is due to the loss of associated movements and not paralysis. *Conjugate deviation* is due to loss of power of turning both eyes toward the sides opposite the lesion, which is in or above the internal capsule. The movements that are not paralyzed draw the eyes toward the side of the lesion.

Fifth Nerve.—The trigeminal nerve is a mixed one. The motor root arises from its nucleus in the pons and supplies the muscles of mastication, the tensor tympani, tensor palati, mylohyoid and anterior belly of the digastric. The sensory fibers enter the pons and descend into the cervical cord, to the second or third segment. It is supposed that the fibers from the ophthalmic division descend farthest. The Gasserian ganglion lies in the middle fossa on the petrous portion of the temporal bone. The sensory root divides below the ganglion into three divisions. The *first*, or *ophthalmic division*, passes through the sphenoidal fissure into the orbit; it conveys sensation from the eyeball and lachrymal gland, the conjunctiva (except that of the lower lid), the skin of the forehead and scalp up to the vertex, the mesial part of the skin of the nose, and the mucous membrane of the upper part of the nasal cavity. It also contains efferent pupil-dilating fibers derived from the cervical sympathetic.

The *second*, or *superior maxillary division*, passes through the foramen rotundum to the infra-orbital canal; this branch is connected with Meckel's ganglion. The second branch of the fifth nerve conducts sensation from the skin to the upper lip, the side of the nose, and the adjacent parts of the cheek, the lower eyelid and part of the temple. It also innervates the conjunctiva of the lower lid, the upper teeth, the mucous membrane of the upper lip, the upper part of the cheek, upper jaw, hard palate, uvula, tonsil, naso-pharynx, middle ear and the lower part of the nasal cavity.

The *third*, or *inferior maxillary division*, contains, in addition to sensory fibers, the motor root. This division emerges through the foramen ovale. The sensory part of the nerve supplies the skin of the posterior part of the temple and the adjacent part of the pinna, the anterior and the upper wall of the external auditory meatus, part of the cheek, the lower lip and chin, the lower teeth and gums, part of the tongue, the floor of the mouth, the inner surface of the cheek and the salivary glands.

The taste fibers from the anterior two-thirds of the tongue are contained in a branch of the third division. They leave the lingual branch, course along the chorda tympani and reach the facial nerve in the Fallopian aqueduct. The taste fibers from the posterior third of the tongue are supplied by the glossopharyngeal nerve.

To test taste sensation the patient should protrude his tongue and keep it out until the test is completed. The tongue is tested in the anterior and posterior parts separately. Substances such as quinine, sugar and salt are used and are rubbed on the tongue. With his tongue out he should then be asked whether the substance is sweet, bitter or sour and he should communicate his opinion to the examiner by a nod of the head. Loss of taste is called *ageusia*. The important reflexes in the domain of the fifth nerve are the corneal, lachrymal and conjunctival. The *corneal reflex* is brought about by touching the cornea with a probe padded with cotton or with the head of a pin. Care should be

71

taken not to touch an eyelash or to bring the testing object over the pupil, because in either event the patient will blink. Both corneal reflexes are lost in anesthesia and coma. The sensory part of the arc is the fifth nerve and the motor part is the seventh. If the corneal reflex is lost from a lesion of the fifth nerve neither eye will blink. If the reflex is lost from a lesion of the seventh nerve the pain produced by the corneal contact will cause the other eye to blink. Loss of the corneal reflex is the earliest sign of involvement of the sensory part of the fifth nerve. The *conjunctival reflex* is taken in much the same way except the conjunctiva is touched rather than the cornea. The *lachrymal reflex* is tested by irritating the nasal mucous membrane with a probe padded with cotton. In the normal individual or in the hysteric whose fifth nerve is intact, a flow of tears will ensue. If the sensory branch of the fifth is implicated, tears will not form. If the motor root is paralyzed the temporal fossa is hollowed and the masseter wastes. When the patient is instructed to close his mouth the affected muscles do not harden under the examiner's fingers. When the patient opens the mouth, the jaw is pushed toward the paralyzed side. This occurs because the external pterygoid fails to draw the condyle forward on the affected side. Trophic disorders may occur on the side of a fifth nerve paralysis; the secretion of tears, of saliva, and of nasal mucus is diminished and thereby the functions of those parts are interfered with. The teeth may become loose on the side of the trophic lesion and fall out. Neuroparalytic keratitis may occur on the affected side. Facial hemiatrophy and hypertrophy are thought by some to be due to trophic lesions of the fifth nerve. Removal of the Gasserian ganglion has not been known to produce hypertrophy or atrophy of the face.

Seventh Nerve.—The facial nerve arises from a nucleus situated in the lower part of the pons, but some of its cells extend as high as the third nerve nucleus and others as low as the hypoglossal nucleus. The root of the facial nerve hooks around the nucleus of the sixth nerve. After it leaves the brain-stem it enters the internal auditory meatus, and thence to the Fallopian aqueduct. In the upper part of this canal the nerve traverses a swelling, the geniculate ganglia, which is joined by the sensory root or the nerve or Wrisberg. After giving off a branch to the stapedius it leaves the skull through the stylomastoid foramen. The main trunk of the nerve supplies all the muscles of the face with the exception of the levator palpebræ superioris, down to and including the platysma. The nerve contains the taste fibers of the chorda tympani. The facial transmits deep pressure pain. The nerve is frequently paralyzed by infections, exposure to cold, tumors of the parotid, middle ear disease, tumors in the angle and syphilis in the angle.

Eighth Nerve.—The auditory nerve is composed of the cochlear and vestibular portions. Paralysis of the cochlear portion of the nerve results in unilateral deafness. The cortical representation of the eighth nerve is in the temporal lobe, and the recognition and memory of words heard, in the first temporal convolution on the left. Involvement of the first temporal convolution will produce a condition known as *word deafness* in which, while the patient is able to hear the sound, the words are not recognized as such. The auditory nerve is frequently pressed upon by tumors, may be the seat of a toxic neuritis, and may be involved in syphilis at the base, in meningitis or by any acute infections, and it may be infiltrated in leukemia. A choking of the eighth nerves, comparable to the choking of the optic nerves, may be seen in cases of increased intracranial pressure. Hemorrhage or inflammatory reactions in the labyrinths may occur in any toxic or infectious state. In a patient suffering from diminution or loss of hearing, it is important to differentiate between nerve deafness and the deafness which arrives as a result of middle ear disease. The differential diagnosis is made by a careful neurologic examination and the use of Weber's, Rinne's and Schwabach's tests. Tumors of the eighth nerve are common. Involvement of the vestibular portion of the eighth nerve is exemplified by Ménière's disease or more properly Ménière's syndrome.

Syphilis, arteriosclerosis, and almost any infection or toxemia is capable of producing changes in the labyrinth. Two of the most pronounced cases seen by the writer were due to malaria. Acute involvement of the labyrinth produces vertigo, vomiting, disturbance of the equilibrium and of the gait and pronounced nystagmus. Any movement of the patient produces vertigo so intense that the patient may be thrown to the ground like a bolt. Tinnitus and impaired hearing, or even deafness are present, and usually remain after the other symptoms have disappeared. Diarrhea may also occur during an attack of acute labyrinthitis. Tumors in the angle, and syphilis of the base have always to be excluded when Ménière's syndrome presents itself. The acute attack may clear up, to be followed by signs of chronic labyrinthitis, which is also often due to middle ear disease. The symptoms may vary from tinnitus and slight deafness and vertigo, to dizziness so intense that the patient is thrown to the ground. The relief of these symptoms is very difficult. Intracranial section of the eighth nerve has been recommended. Ménière's syndrome is occasionally mistaken for epilepsy, but the dizziness, deafness and tinnitus unaccompanied by unconsciousness, although it is rarely present, should make the differentiation possible.

Ninth Nerve.—Involvement of the glossopharyngeal nerve rarely occurs by itself. If it should happen, the symptoms would be loss of taste over the posterior third of the tongue, dysphagia, loss of the pharyngeal reflexes and anesthesia in the upper portion of the pharynx.

Tenth Nerve.—Paralysis of the vagus nerve may be part of the symptom complex of bulbar palsy, tumors of the bulb, acute and chronic inflammations, syringomyelia and multiple sclerosis. The vagus nerve is occasionally acutely inflamed, especially after attacks of diphtheria. It is also involved, though infrequently, by poisons such as alcohol. After the nerve emerges from the bulb it may be involved by neoplasms, inflammatory reactions of the meninges, vascular disease, especially aneurysms, and disease of the base of the skull. It is occasionally injured during operations on the neck. The recurrent laryngeal branch of the nerve may be cut during an operation on the thyroid, and is frequently paralyzed by an aneurysm of the aorta, by dilatation of the left auricle such as occurs in mitral stenosis, and by neoplastic masses in the mediastinum. Paralysis of the tenth nerve produces unilateral paralysis of the palate, pharynx and larynx, which produces a nasal quality of the voice and dysphagia. The soft palate is immobile and is lower than normally, and the palatal and pharyngeal reflexes are absent. The homolateral cord is in the so-called cadaveric position, and fails to mobilate during phonation and respiration. The cardiac rate and rhythm are not altered and abdominal symptoms are usually absent. Bilateral recurrent paralysis is usually central in origin and causes complete loss of voice, respiration is difficult, stridor dyspnea is usually pronounced, and there is lack of closure of the glottis in coughing. Involvement of the tenth nerve is often associated with implication of the ninth, eleventh and twelfth.   ·

Eleventh Nerve.—The spinal accessory nerve is a motor one, consisting of two parts, the medullary and spinal. The bulbar part of the nerve is really part of the vagus. Fibers from the spinal part of the nerve arise in the anterior horn cells of the upper four or five cervical segments, ascend into the skull through the foramen magnum, unite with the bulbar fibers and then make their exit through the posterior lacerated foramen with the ninth and tenth nerves. The eleventh nerve supplies the sternomastoid and the trapezius. In general, it is affected by the same things which cause involvement of the ninth and tenth nerves and also by affections of the upper cervical cord. It is not infrequently cut during an operation on the neck for tuberculous glands. The paralysis of the nerve produces inability to turn the head toward the opposite side, and the head deviates to the affected side when the chin is forced downward against resistance. Involvement of the trapezius produces a low shoulder on the paralyzed side, alteration of the outline of the neck, shrugging of the shoulder is interfered with, and the scapula cannot be brought to the midline. The scapula is displaced down and out. The affected muscles are atrophic and show alterations to the electrical reactions.

Twelfth Nerve.—The hypoglossal nerve is a motor nerve supplying the muscles of the tongue. The nerve arises from the cells in the medulla. The nerve leaves the skull through the jugular foramen. It runs between the carotid artery and the jugular vein, then goes forward to supply the tongue. The tongue is usually involved in ordinary cases of hemiplegia, in which it deviates to the side of the paralysis, on protrusion. It does this because of the action of the uninvolved glossal muscle which pushes the tongue out and toward the opposite side. It is practically always involved in bulbar palsy and in vascular and inflammatory reactions in the bulb. Tumors of the bulb and the diseases of the spinal cord, especially amyotrophic lateral sclerosis and syringomyelia, may be complicated by involvement of the twelfth nucleus. Syphilis of the bulb or at the base of the brain may implicate the twelfth nerve. Nuclear disease, such as is produced by bulbar palsy, is practically always bilateral. Outside of the skull the nerve may be involved by malignant disease, trauma, disease or injury to the atlas, and aneurysm of the carotid artery. The affection of the nerve produces a paralysis of the tongue on the side of the lesion. The tongue appears wrinkled and atrophic, the electrical reactions are reversed and fibrillary tremors are usually pronounced, although they may be absent in peripheral involvement. If only one twelfth nerve is paralyzed, the ability to eat is not affected but, if the tongue is paralyzed on both sides, eating is indeed difficult and speech, which is also little affected by unilateral paralysis, is seriously involved.

THE REFLEXES.

The examination of the reflexes is a necessary part of each neurologic survey of an individual. One of the most important is the *plantar reflex* which, with the abdominal and cremasteric, make up the important superficial reflexes. To obtain the plantar reflex the patient should be lying down, the foot should be warm, externally rotated and grasped firmly at the ankle by one of the examiner's hands. The sole of the foot should then be stimulated at the junction of the outer and middle thirds, beginning at the heel and going forward. Practically any small object may be used, but the best is a pin. The least amount of stimulation necessary to bring about a response should be employed. If too light stimulation is used, no reaction whatsoever will be obtained. On the other hand, if the stimulation is too great, a mass of reflexes will occur from which nothing can be learned. In the person with an intact pyramidal system, the great toe flexes and the tensor fascia femoris contracts. If the pyramidal tract or the leg center in the cortex is affected by disease or injury, the great toe extends. The more slowly and more isolated the extension is, the more typical is the reflex. There may be other movements of the toes such as flexion, extension or fanning, but it is the movement of the great toe which makes the reflex. It is always pathologic, except in infants whose pyramidal tracts are not yet myelinated, and means interruption in some degree at least, to the functions of the pyramidal tract going to the extremity in which the reflex was obtained. The hamstring muscles usually contract as a part of the reflex. The abnormal plantar reflex, or Babinski sign, may occur after the cortical exhaustion of an epileptic fit, and it may also result from irritation of the motor fibers due for example, to the toxemia of uremia, diabetes or alcoholism. It is frequently necessary to attract the patient's attention while this reflex is being taken. Occasionally the reflex may be obtained when the skin of the heel is irritated, or by drawing a pin across the ball of the foot. There are many modifications of the Babinski reflex, all of which mean the same. The Babinski reflex has done a great deal to differentiate between organic and hysterical conditions. If disease exists in the reflex arc of the plantar reflex, due, for example, to loss of sensation or to a peripheral paralysis of flexion of the toes, the great toe will not flex but may even extend.

In the upper extremity a reflex comparable in its significance to the Babinski reflex, has been described by Trömner and by Hoffman. With the patient's forearm and hand midway between pronation and supination, the left hand of the examiner supports the forearm. and the nail of the middle finger is slightly stroked and flicked toward the palm. If the pyramidal tract is normal, the thumb does not move, if the pyramidal fibers to the hand are involved, the thumb is flexed and adducted.

The *abdominal reflexes* appear after the pyramidal tracts are medullated. They are normally present except in the obese, and in those whose abdominal walls are relaxed and atonic for any reason, the most important of which is pregnancy. The loss of the reflex is common in acute abdominal conditions. It is obtained by stroking the skin of the abdomen parallel with Poupart's ligament and the costal border. Any blunt object may be used but a pin produces better results. The reflexes are called the upper and lower, and the segments of the cord concerned are the eighth to the twelfth dorsal. The reflex consists of a dimpling or a pulling of the skin due to contraction of the abdominal recti muscles. In a healthy individual with normal abdominal walls, loss of reflex means an interruption in the reflex arc such as might occur, for instance, in anterior horn disease. It may also be due to involvement of the pyramidal tract and is, therefore, a frequent sign of hemiplegia. In the presence of other signs the absence of abdominal reflexes in a young individual is suggestive of multiple sclerosis. The abdominal reflexes are lost on the paralyzed side, if the pyramidal tract lesion is above the eighth dorsal segment.

The *cremasteric reflex* is obtained by stimulating the skin of the upper and inner side of the thigh, which produces an elevation of the testicle on that side. Its loss has the same significance as the abdominal reflex. The segments in the cord concerned with this reflex are the first and second lumbar. The *corneal reflex* is obtained by touching the cornea, usually with the head of a pin. The sensory part of the arc is in the fifth nerve, and the motor part is in the seventh. The result is a sharp closure of both eyes. The corneal sign is commonly taken during anesthesia and is used as an indication of the depth of the anesthesia. If the reflex is lost because of a lesion of the fifth nerve, neither eye blinks. If it is due to an involvement of the seventh nerve the eye on the opposite side will close. A loss of the corneal reflex is the earliest sign of involvement of the sensory part of the fifth nerve. Another test of the function of the fifth nerve is the *lachrymal reflex* which is tested by stimulating the mucous membrane of the nose with a probe wrapped in cotton. If the sensory arc is functioning there will be a flow of tears. This does not occur if the anesthesia is due to organic change in the fifth nerve.

The important *deep reflexes* (sometimes called tendon) are the patellar, Achilles, triceps and biceps. Complete relaxation of the muscles concerned in a reflex must be obtained, and the reflexes that are not obtainable while the patient is in bed, should, if possible, be tested when the patient is up before they are considered lost. Involvement of either the sensory or motor component of the arc will cause a diminution or disappearance of the reflex. Thus, lesions of the peripheral nerves, of the spinal roots, of the posterior columns, of the anterior horns, will cause a diminution or loss of the deep reflex at the level of the lesion. Involvement of the anterior horn cells of the cervical cord will not, of course, affect the reflexes of the lower extremities. A reflex may also be lost because of disease of the muscles as in muscular dystrophy, where the reflex disappears with the muscle. The deep reflexes are exaggerated in disease of the pyramidal tracts, in functional nervous disorders, especially hysteria, as a rule in joint disease, after exercise and in irritation of the nervous system from the excessive use of tea, coffee and alcohol. It is only in disease of the pyramidal tract, however, that the Babinski sign occurs. A generalized increase in the deep reflexes without Babinski's sign or ankle clonus is not of nearly as much importance as the diminution, loss or inequality of the reflexes.

The *biceps reflex* is obtained by tapping the biceps tendon. The *triceps reflex* is obtained by striking the triceps tendon.

The best position in which to obtain the *patellar reflex* is to have the patient sitting in a chair with the feet flat on the floor. The patellar tendon should then be located, one of the examiner's hands placed on the thigh while the other wields the hammer which should strike the tendon a sharp, quick blow. If the reflex is difficult to obtain or is diminished, it may be brought out by reinforcement. In the case of the patellar reflex this may be done by having the patient squeeze his hands at the count of three, or better yet, by having him press downward with the ball of his foot as the patellar tendon is tapped. The *Achilles reflex* is obtained by having the patient kneel on a chair with the feet hanging over the seat, or by having him rest his hands on a desk or chair while flexing one leg off the floor. The examiner supports the foot at the ankle and taps the tendon of Achilles. A jar may be misinterpreted as a reflex. *Ankle clonus*, which is frequently seen in pyramidal tract disease, and which consists of a rhythmic contraction of the soleus muscle, is obtained by having the knee moderately flexed. The examiner then sharply extends the foot, exerting pressure on its ball. A pseudoclonus may occasionally be found in hysteria. The *vegetative reflexes* (vesical, rectal, genital and uterine) are due, in most part, to contraction of involuntary muscles; their centers are in the sacral cord, below the third sacral segment, and in the sympathetic nervous system. The *cilio-spinal reflex*, which is brought out by pinching the skin of the neck, consists in a dilation of the pupil on the ipsolateral side, and is due to stimulation of the cervical sympathetic. Pressure backward on the eyeballs produces the *oculo-cardiac reflex* by which the rate of the pulse is slowed. This maneuver has been tried in cases of tachycardia. The segments with which the important deep reflexes are concerned are as follows:

Biceps, fifth cervical.

Triceps, sixth cervical.

Patellar, second to fourth lumbar.

Achilles, fifth lumbar, first and second sacral segment.

THE MOTOR SYSTEM.

Involvement of the motor system produces one of the most distressing results of disease to a patient, namely, loss of or impaired power. He will usually indicate where the weakness or paralysis exists. All of the muscles should be tested against resistance and the power of the hands should be determined with a dynamometer. An apparent loss of power may occur in hysteria, especially compensation hysteria, and power may be weak in the presence of muscles apparently splendidly developed, such as occurs, for example, in pseudohypertrophic muscular dystrophy. To examine properly the muscular system, the individual muscles should be observed and palpated. It should be recorded whether or not the muscles are normal, flabby or atrophic. The muscles may be atrophic from: lesions of the peripheral motor nerve, anterior root, anterior horn cells, from a disease of the muscles themselves (such as dystrophy), from bone and joint disease and from wounds of an extremity, which produce the so-called muscular reflex atrophy, and rarely from a cerebral lesion. Atrophy of muscles rarely occurs from a cerebral lesion, implicating the parietal cortex; the atrophy is on the contralateral side to the lesion, is not severe and must be differentiated from wasting produced by disuse and ankylosis of joints. Lesions of the motor peripheral nerve produce a flaccid, atrophic paralysis with loss of reaction to faradism and equalization or reversal of the polar reactions in galvanism. The deep reflexes in the distribution of the paralysis are lost or decreased. Fibrillary tremors occur in the atrophic muscles if the lesion is in the anterior horn cells; rarely does an involvement of the peripheral nerve produce this phenomenon. Fibrillary movements of the muscles are of great significance if they occur with other signs of organic disease. It is a common symptom in the tongue in bulbar palsy and in muscles wasted from anterior horn disease.

Fibrillary tremors or muscle quivering are seen in neurasthenic, poorly nourished individuals and in those who take tea, coffee, alcohol or tobacco to excess. In such instances the tremors are especially common in the deltoid, biceps, the large muscles of the thighs and of the eyelids. Anterior horn symptoms always occur at the level of a lesion. The atrophy which occurs in bone or joint disease is usually limited to a segment of the extremity involved, but it may implicate the entire extremity. If a joint is involved acutely, the muscles about it may waste as rapidly or more so than they do in lesions of the motor nerves or anterior horn cells. The neighborhood deep reflex is increased but Babinski's sign, fibrillary tremors and reactions of degeneration do not occur. If the joint disease is bilateral and produces reflex atrophy, the case may be mistaken for amyotrophic lateral sclerosis. A lesion of the anterior root will simulate closely that due to involvement of the anterior horn, with one important exception; fibrillary tremors are not present.

Paralysis means a loss of power due either to functional or organic interruption in any part of the motor path and including the muscle itself. *Paresis* means a weakness. The two are often used rather loosely. The term paralysis is employed when partial loss of power is meant.

Paralysis of a mixed nerve will produce both motor and sensory loss. Multiple neuritis is an involvement of many of the mixed nerves, and is commonly due to alcoholism and other intoxications such as lead, arsenic, infectious diseases, especially diphtheria, and produces, at a certain stage, a lower motor neuron type of paralysis, involving especially the extensors of the fingers, hands, feet and toes. The paralysis is usually preceded by a paresthetic phenomenon, likely to be localized in the feet and prone to be of a burning, stinging variety. To recapitulate, a lower motor neuron disease producing flaccid palsy of muscles supplied by the nerve, anterior root or anterior horn cells and later atrophy, develops. The neighboring deep reflex is lost and the response to faradism is absent. Galvanism response is slow and with a reversal of the polar reactions. Fibrillary tremors occur in anterior horn disease but not, as a rule, in disease of the peripheral nerves.

The tone of an extremity weakened or paralyzed by involvement of the voluntary motor pathway anywhere in its course from the motor cortex to the lower part of the cord, is increased. The paralysis or weakness which occurs is below the level of the lesion; if this is above the decussation in the bulb, the paresis is on the contralateral side. Below the decussation the weakness which ensues is on the side of and below the lesion. If both pyramidal tracts are involved above the decussation, the condition is referred to as *diplegia*. A lesion in an internal capsule produces weakness or paralysis of the opposite side, face, arm and leg. A complete lesion of the spinal cord in the cervical cord will produce *tetraplegia* or, as it is called by some, *quadriplegia*. Implication of both pyramidal tracts of the spinal cord below the second dorsal will produce a *crural paraplegia*. Paralysis of both upper extremities from a cord lesion is referred to as a *brachial paraplegia* and, though rare, may occur, for example, from acute anterior poliomyelitis or from occlusion of the anterior spinal artery.

Paralysis of one extremity, called *monoplegia*, is the result of a cerebral, spinal or peripheral lesion, or of hysteria. If part of an extremity is paralyzed, the result of a cerebral lesion, it has been called by Spiller, *segmental monoplegia*. In pyramidal tract disease, particularly in cortical involvement, movements and not muscles are paralyzed. The deep reflexes are increased and various types of clonus may be elicited, such as ankle, patellar or wrist clonus. The plantar reflex is of the extensor or Babinski type. The muscles do not become atrophic from upper motor neuron palsy, but may be seen in such a condition if ankylosis of a joint or arthritis occurs, on the paralytic side. In this case the atrophy is due to joint disease and not to the pyramidal tract affection. The muscles react normally to electricity. In progressive pyramidal tract involvement with total paralysis, seen especially in cases in which the cord has been injured or is pressed upon from without, for example by Pott's disease or a tumor, the reflexes of defense or spinal automatism may occur. Thus, in a totally paralyzed extremity, even in one in which sensation may be completely abolished, sharply flexing the toe (*Sinkler's phenomenon*) or irritating the extremity up to a level corresponding to the height of the lesion, especially the foot, the paralyzed extremity may be sharply withdrawn. That is, the foot and toe are extended and the knee and hip flexed. This may be mistaken for a voluntary movement, especially if the idea is entertained that the patient is hysterical. It is a bad prognostic omen, unless the cause can be removed, and is not a sign of returning power.

If the pyramidal tract fibers to an extremity are completely obliterated, such as occurs, for example, in the destruction of the spinal cord from injury or disease, there is a flaccid paralysis of the extremity below the lesion with a loss of the deep reflexes and a plantar reflex of the flexor type, or the plantar reflex may be absent, the so-called *Bastian's law*, which is seen in its most typical form in paralysis coming on suddenly as the result of injury. It may, however, be due to disease.

Paralysis may be crossed, that is part of the paralysis on one side of the body and part on the other, due to a single lesion; for example, a lesion in the right cerebral peduncle will produce a third nerve palsy on the side of the lesion and implication of the face, arm and leg on the opposite side: *Weber's syndrome*. If, in addition, there is a tremor of the weak or paralyzed side of the body, it is referred to as *Benedikt's syndrome;* the third nerve fibers, the pyramidal tract and the red nucleus are implicated. A lesion in the pons at the level of the facial nucleus will bring about facial paralysis of the peripheral type on the side of the lesion, and of the arm and leg on the contralateral side: the *Millard-Gubler syndrome*. A crossed sensory paralysis may occur in occlusion of the posterior inferior cerebellar artery with a loss of pain, heat and cold on the side of the face corresponding to the lesion and on the opposite side of the body. In arriving at the diagnosis of a crossed paralysis, due to a single lesion, the history of the attack must be perfectly clear. Thus, in a case seen by the writer at the Philadelphia General Hospital, a patient recently admitted with hemiplegia developed a few days later a peripheral palsy on the opposite side of the face, which was an ordinary Bell's palsy. If the history were unknown the location of the lesion causing the facial paralysis in this case would have been misplaced. In another case a patient had a left hemiplegia due to softening in the right capsular region, and a few months later, he developed an oculomotor palsy on the right side as a result of basilar syphilis.

The increased tone in pyramidal tract disease is supposed to be due to release of the cortical inhibition. Increased tone, even rigidity, may be seen in lesions of the extra-pyramidal system which is phylogenetically older than the pyramidal system. The most intense rigidity which the writer has ever seen was in a case of bilateral lenticular degeneration, due to carbon monoxide poisoning; all of the joints, including the jaws, were so stiff that it was impossible to move them. Despite the intense rigidity in such cases, Babinski's sign is not present. If the increased tone, however, is accompanied by an irregular movement such as chorea or athetosis, extension of the great toe may occur coincidently as the foot is stimulated. The extra-pyramidal system, when involved, produces in addition to rigidity some type of irregular movements, as choreiform movements and athetosis. Paralysis agitans has its most characteristic pathologic finding in this pathway. In the latter disease the rigidity is of the cog-wheel variety, and automatic movements, such as blinking and the swinging of the arms in walking, are lost.

A combination of upper and lower motor neuron disease may occur in the same individual; thus, disease or injury to the cervical cord may produce paralysis of the anterior horn cells with resulting signs at the level of the lesion. Implication of the pyramidal tracts at the same time will produce a spastic paralysis below; this is not an uncommon finding in syringomyelia. Involvement of the lumbosacral cord will cause a flaccid, atrophic paralysis at the level of the lesion. Disease of the muscles themselves, such as occurs in progressive muscular dystrophy, produces weakness and ultimately paralysis of the affected parts. The nervous system is intact in this disease. There are no sensory losses, and the reflexes and electrical reactions disappear with the muscles. Certain muscles, especially the deltoids and those of the calves, may be the site of pseudohypertrophy.

Involvement of the cerebellum or its tracts does not produce disturbance of sensation, but causes *incoördination*. The function of the cerebellum is motor, to assemble and make even and smooth voluntary motor impulses. This makes for a *synergic movement*. If this element is lacking, the movement becomes jerky, ataxic and asynergic. The movements are not synchronized and occur separately, disjointedly instead of in one uniform result. Attempting the finger-to-nose test he overshoots the mark, producing a symptom called *hypermetria*. If a vertical line is drawn on a sheet of paper and the patient tries to draw a series of horizontal lines to the vertical line, he overshoots or undershoots the mark. The *rebound phenomenon of Holmes* is elicited in the following manner: if an attempt is made by the examiner to extend the forearm against resistance the force is suddenly discontinued, the hand rebounds unchecked against the shoulder. Another characteristic symptom of cerebellar disease is *adiadochokinesis*, which means a loss of the ability rapidly to perform a movement which calls into play antagonistic groups of muscles. Thus, supination and pronation of the hands, slapping the palms and extensor surfaces down on the knee each time, is an easy way to elicit this symptom which is rightly done by a normal person. The cerebellar case, on the other hand, does it in an incoördinate way. Cerebellar catalepsy is a rare symptom. It should be emphasized that there is no loss of sensation and no loss of power in the sense that it occurs in upper or lower motor neuron disease.

Cerebellar fits, originally described by Hughlings Jackson, are tonic in type and, in reality, the picture of decerebrate rigidity is produced. Cerebellar fits, due to involvement of the vermis, are bilateral, those due to involvement of one of the cerebellar lobes are unilateral and on the side of the lesion.

Gaits.—Although all disturbances of gaits are not due to involvement of the motor system, they will be discussed under that heading.

In testing a patient's gait he should be told to walk across the room, preferably in a straight line and to turn sharply and walk back. In spastic crural paraplegia the lower extremities are moved stiffly, the steps are short, the toes are scraped along. If there is pronounced adductor spasm, the so-called scissor gait occurs, in which the feet are alternately placed, one in front of the other. This gait may also be seen in bilateral cerebral lesions. In a spastic gait occurring in paraplegia the soles of the shoes at the toe are worn off long before the rest of the shoes, and the uppers are scuffed at the toes due to catching those parts in going upstairs. In the hemiplegic gait the lower extremity on the affected side is swung from the hip, the joints are flexed little or not at all, and the anterior part of the foot is scraped on the ground. In addition, the upper extremity is held in a characteristic attitude. The steppage, or high-stepping, gait is that which occurs in a patient suffering from foot-drop, due especially to lesions of the anterior horns or the peripheral nerves, and occurring in its best illustration in multiple neuritis and poliomyelitis. A lesion of one popliteal nerve may produce a unilateral steppage gait. In the steppage gait, the extensors of the toes and feet being paralyzed, the patient must raise the knees high to make the toes and feet clear the ground and, as the feet come down, it makes a flip-flop sound, due to the striking of the anterior part of the foot first and the heel second. The gait of muscular dystrophy produces the duck or waddling gait, quite similar to that seen in double congenital dislocation of the hips. In this gait the feet are more widely separated than normally and a distinct lordosis occurs. The ataxic gait, frequently incorrectly referred to as the tabetic gait, is seen in tabes dorsalis, in some patients with multiple neuritis, and in any condition which involves the posterior columns, such as the combined sclerosis of pernicious anemia. The patient's walking base is widened, he lifts the feet jerkingly and suddenly throws them too wide and too high, and then stamps the heels to the ground. An ataxic gait can be told not only by sight, but also by hearing, since he makes a very characteristic stamping noise as he walks. To reënforce his faulty position sense, his eyes are glued to the ground, He has difficulty in walking a straight line, and in proceeding with the eyes shut, in the dark or backwards. When the pyramidal tracts and posterior columns are both involved in the same patient, for example, in the combined sclerosis of pernicious anemia, the gait assumes an element of both spasticity and ataxia. A reeling or drunken gait is significant of cerebellar disease, and if the cerebellar involvement is unilateral the patient has a tendency to veer toward the side of the lesion.

The variety of gait frequently seen in elderly people with multiple areas of cerebral softening is the gait of "little steps" in which the patient takes short, quick steps, often with evidence of spasticity on one or both sides. Patients suffering from marked chorea, either Sydenham's or Huntington's but especially the latter, have a peculiar bizarre gait, which is caused by the irregularly appearing choreiform movements in the muscles of the lower extremities, the pelvic girdles and the trunk. This causes the patient to sway or pitch now to one side, now to the other, or perhaps forward. The gait and also the posture of Parkinson's disease is characteristic. The upper extremities are flexed at the elbows, wrists, arms and hands which are held in the writing position. The trunk and neck are flexed. Often as he arises from a chair and before he is started in walking, he takes involuntary steps laterally or backward. When he is fairly well advanced in the disease he then shows the shuffling, festinating gait which is so significant of the illness. As he walks, the gait becomes faster and faster, until finally he has to grasp hold of something so that he may stop and rest. No matter how marked the festination it is unusual for a case of paralysis agitans to fall.

In testing the gait much can be learned, not only from the manner in which the patient walks, but also from the ease and facility with which he turns, because, in turning, the first disturbance in gait may be seen. The gaits of hysteria are many and varied. *Astasia-abasia* is used to describe that symptom of hysteria in which a patient capable of moving the lower extremities can neither stand nor walk. In hysterical hemiplegia the affected foot is pushed or dragged along, and rigidity of the joints or scraping of the foot along the floor is not found as it is in organic hemiplegia. In a case of compensation hysteria the patient appeared as though he had springs in both feet, and popped up and down like a Jack-in-a-box. Hysterical disturbances of gait may be grafted upon an organic disease. A case of hysterical disturbance of gait can often, by suggestion, be made to walk much better backward than forward, whereas all organic gaits are made worse by walking backward.

Involvement of the middle lobe or vermis produces in the gait a tendency to fall forward or backward, and often the asynergia of the trunk muscles is so great that it is impossible for the patient to walk at all. In 2 cases of cerebellar agenesis at the Philadelphia General Hospital, the patients cannot stand without support and cannot walk in the ordinary way at all. They get along, however, by walking on all fours.

Involuntary and irregular movements occurring in diseases of the various parts of the nervous system, especially those involving the basal ganglia, such as paralysis agitans, progressive lenticular degeneration, athetosis, chorea and spasmodic torticollis, probably all have the pathologic processes at fault in these structures. *Myoclonus* is a shot-like contraction of the muscles occurring at regular or irregular intervals, and varying from two or three a minute to one almost every second. This was a common symptom in epidemic encephalitis involving especially the abdominal muscles, although the muscles of the extremities were occasionally affected. *Hiccough* is a myoclonic contraction of the diaphragm due to excitation of the inspiratory center. Hiccoughing is a common symptom in encephalitis, but may be a result of other toxemias or reflexly from visceral disturbances.

Tremor.—By the word tremor is meant an involuntary rhythmic movement of a part of the body, which is the result of the contraction of muscle groups. Tremors may be simple, in which only a single muscle group is involved, may be compound where there are several groups affected, may be rhythmic or non-rhythmic, rapid or slow, and may be increased or diminished by action. Tremors, like all other involuntary movements, stop during sleep. Tremors may be toxic in origin, for example, those due to exophthalmic goiter, alcohol, tobacco, tea and coffee. Emotional excitement, especially fear, may produce a generalized simple tremor. Senile tremor may resemble closely that of Parkinson's disease, but usually occurs bilaterally from the onset, and without the rigidity of Parkinson's disease. This tremor is usually not affected or increased by action. A senile tremor also affects the head and face more than the ordinary paralysis agitans tremor. In some individuals a tremor of the head, speech and upper extremities seems to be hereditary. In a young medical man recently examined by the writer there was a tremor of this sort, which appeared at the age of eighteen years and which also had appeared at this time in his father and his grandfather. Tremors of the head accompanied by nystagmus may occur in poorly nourished, rachitic children.

SENSATION.

To test for sensation, special instruments and methods of precision may be used, but ordinarily complicated instruments are not needed. Much may be learned about the sensory condition of a patient with no other instrument than a pin, and even test-tubes of hot and cold water may be needless luxuries. The most trying part of a neurologic examination is that which has to do with sensation, and it is imperative that both the examiner and the patient be free of fatigue and irritation. The best time to do a sensory examination is early in the morning. Outside distractions should be prevented, the room in which the examination is made should be warm, interruptions should not be allowed and the patient himself should be warm, relaxed and in the recumbent position. To diagnose and to localize lesions the result of faulty sensation, it is necessary to understand the pathways by which the sensory tracts ascend. Most of the peripheral nerves are mixed, and involvement of them produces, in addition to paralysis, loss of sensation which will, of course, correspond to the distribution of the particular nerve involved. If all of the nerves of an extremity are involved, the sensory loss is always most marked in the distal segment of the extremity and all forms of sensation are involved. It is rarely that a dissociation sensory loss occurs from a lesion of a peripheral nerve, but such a thing occasionally occurs in postdiphtheritic multiple neuritis. In this condition, however, there is a possibility that the posterior columns of the cord may be affected. The sensory fibers pass into the posterior roots and thence to the cord. Involvement of a posterior root produces irritative sensory phenomena in the distribution of that particular root. This is in the nature of a pain, usually of the sharp, cutting type so common in tabes dorsalis. The pain is increased by sneezing, coughing or jarring and, if it occurs in the chest, it is often mistaken for pleurisy or angina. If it is in the abdomen, it is frequently thought to be appendicitis, or some other acute abdominal condition and, if it occurs in an extremity, it is called neuritis, rheumatism or sciatica. As the root becomes more involved, a loss of sensation occurs. The form of sensation lost earliest and most frequently is *pain*, so that in time the patient has an area in which he has a great deal of pain, but in which pain sense itself is diminished, delayed or lost. The painful areas referred to the skin, due to posterior root involvement, may be small and of the so-called "spot" variety, which are common in tabes dorsalis. When the root enters the spinal cord, the fibers relaying sensation from the muscles, tendons, joints and bones, all the so-called gnostic sensations enter the posterior columns and ascend uncrossed to the gracilis and cuneate nuclei, on the ipsolateral side of the medulla. Shortly afterward, the fibers cross the midline in the internal arcuate fibers, thus forming the sensory decussation of the fillet. They then pass through the crus to the optic thalamus, where the fibers are again separated, most of them end in the thalamus, and some continue to the postrolandic area.

Deep pressure pain is obtained by pressing on an area until the patient complains of pain or discomfort. *Touch* in ordinary practice can be tested with the examiner's finger, but it should be stroked as lightly as possible on the area to be tested; a wisp of cotton, a camel-hair brush or a feather may also be used. *Heat* and *cold* are usually tested by test-tubes filled with hot or cold water, and the tubes applied in an irregular manner to the skin. In all sensory examinations the patient should be blindfolded or should not be permitted to see what is going on. Without the test-tubes the patient may be tested for hot and cold by blowing hot or cold on the area. The sense of position, or joint or posture sense, is tested by moving passively a joint into various positions. The part being moved should be grasped laterally. For example, if the sense of position is being tested in the toe, it should not be pushed upward or downward, but should be grasped on either side and pulled in the desired direction. This is important because a patient may have disturbance in the sense of position but, if other forms of sensibility are normal, he will be able to appreciate that his toe is pushed upward or downward. When the member being tested is placed in a position, the patient is then asked to describe the position in which it has been placed.

Bone or osseous sense is tested by means of a tuning fork, 128 C, which, having been sent into vibration, is placed upon a bone. The normal patient says he feels a thrill, whereas the one with loss of bone sense feels nothing. *Stereognosis* or stereognostic perception is the ability of an individual to recognize an object placed in the hand, by appreciation of its weight, size, shape, temperature or texture. Loss of stereognostic perception may occasionally be due to a peripheral nerve lesion, but is more often the result of involvement of the parietal cortex, the optic thalamus or the posterior columns of the cord. While it is commonly taught that touch sense ascends in part uncrossed in the posterior columns, lesions of the posterior columns which produce complete loss of position and vibratory sensation do not cause a loss of touch. This is a common finding, for example, in the combined sclerosis of pernicious anemia. The ability of a person to determine the exact location of a spot which is touched goes closely with the position sense and is lost in a lesion of the parietal cortex. The fibers for temperature and pain cross through the central part of the cord almost immediately, and ascend on the opposite side in the spinothalamic tract. They ultimately reach the thalamus and are redistributed for discrimination to the cortex. Cortical lesions will rarely produce much disturbance of pain, heat and cold sensations, whereas a lesion of the thalamus does cause a severe diminution or loss of these forms of sensation. Most of the fibers for light touch and deep pressure cross the cord immediately and ascend to the thalamus anterior to the spinothalamic tract. The loss of sensation which one sees in a cortical lesion, that is, involvement of the parietal lobe, has more to do with the so-called gnostic sensation than the vital ones. Thus pain, heat and cold are little affected, if at all, but stereognostic perception, sense of position, spot localization, the discrimination of the two points of a compass are involved. *Vibratory sense* is not usually affected in cortical lesions. *Dissociation sensory loss* occurs in syringo-myelia where the lesion is usually in the central part of the cord. A single lesion in this location will involve the fibers of pain, heat and cold, which have entered by way of the posterior roots and are crossing. The singling out of the functions of the posterior columns is seen in its most typical form in the combined sclerosis of pernicious anemia, in which condition position and vibration sensations are lost, and pain, heat, cold and touch are normal. Little is needed to make a good sensory examination except a knowledge of the location of the sensory tracts. If pain sense is normal, heat and cold are likely to be so. If position sense is normal, vibratory sense will likely be so, and if neither pain nor position senses are impaired, it will be unlikely that touch, spot localization or stereognostic perception will be. Pain, heat and cold sensations have been called the vital sensations. The ability of the individual to tell correctly numbers drawn on his skin by the examiner's finger, has been designated by Spiller as *graphesthesia;* it goes with the gnostic sensibilities.

It is always important to differentiate between hysteria and organic disease. This is so in ordinary civilian practice, but is particularly important in times of war, and in dealing with the individual who is trying to collect compensation or damages for injuries. It is obvious that the diagnosis of any functional nervous disorder should never be made until all possibility of organic disease has been ruled out. It is, therefore, highly imperative that a knowledge of organic disease be acquired by the individual who limits his practice to functional dis-orders, otherwise confusion will be sure to exist.

Sensory loss in hysteria never corresponds to known anatomic dis-tributions, and the sensory loss is often bizarre and unusual. The form of sensation most frequently lost in hysteria is pain. This loss occurs only after the patient has been examined by one or more physicians. The part of the body which shows a loss of sensation will also often show loss of power or paralysis. An extremity which presents a com-plete loss of power and sensation can have such findings, if due to organic disease, only from a lesion of the peripheral nerves which go to that extremity. If such were the case, the extremity would show atrophy, loss of reflexes and reactions of degeneration, findings which never occur in hysteria. The writer recently saw a case of hysteria with complete loss of power and of sensation in an upper extremity for an attor-ney for the plaintiff. The original diagnosis of injury to the brachial plexus had been made by a physician for an insurance company. On this diagnosis she had collected sick and accident insurance for eighteen months. Paralysis of one side of the body, if organic, may be accompanied by loss of all forms of sensation, if the optic thalamus and internal capsule are involved, but in such cases the deep reflexes will be increased, ankle clonus and Babinski sign will be present, and the abdominal reflexes lost on the side contralateral to the lesion. Paralysis of one side of the body with loss of sensation due to hysteria will show no alteration of the reflexes, neither deep nor superficial. All forms of sensation are usually not affected, and there often is deafness and blindness on the affected side.

The deep reflexes are never lost in hysteria, but they may be hyperactive or exaggerated. The superficial reflexes are normal, and a pseudo ankle clonus may be present. The pupillary reflex is not affected and the eye-grounds are normal. Visual defects in hysteria, however, are common, especially the loss of panoramic vision or the occurrence of the so-called tubular vision. Sudden loss of vision may occur in hysteria, but may also be seen in certain toxic states such as nephritis, in brain tumors and in multiple sclerosis. The history of the illness will aid greatly in differentiating these forms of amaurosis. Hysterical deafness may be detected by ear tests and also by the following reflex: if a sudden noise is made beside a person whose hearing is normal, the eyes blink. If he is deaf from an organic cause no blinking would occur, but if the deafness is due to hysteria, the reflex arc being still intact, the eyes will blink. Casual conversation about an hysterically deaf person held in his presence may later on be repeated by him.

Paralysis of a part of the body due to hysteria is never similar to that seen in organic disease. The reflexes are not altered, the muscles are not atrophic, the sensory loss is not according to anatomic distributions. It must not be overlooked that hysteria may complicate an organic affection. A patient who has had an organic paralysis may recover, but an hysterical paralysis may ensue and prolong the illness. Many cases of hysteria or functional nervous disorders are found in organic affections outside the nervous system, especially in persons who are frightened by the physician and a bad prognosis given. Atrophy of muscles, fibrillary tremors, reactions of degeneration, pathologic reflexes, fixed pupils, optic atrophy, sensory loss according to known anatomic distributions and fever do not occur in hysteria.

Roentgenologic Studies.—In recent years mechanical measures have been used extensively to aid in the diagnosis and the location of lesions, especially tumors of the brain and spinal cord. Dandy introduced the injection of air directly into the ventricles as a diagnostic procedure; following this the practice of introducing air into the subarachnoid space by way of lumbar puncture was recommended; these procedures are called ventriculography and encephalography. If a brain tumor is undoubtedly present and cannot be accurately localized, ventriculography may be performed, if a tumor is suspected encephalography may be cautiously performed. The procedure in doing an encephalogram is to remove 5 to 15 cc. of fluid and to inject a corresponding amount of air. This is repeated until from 100 to 150 cc. of fluid have been removed and replaced with air. Removal of such a large amount of fluid is a risky thing in brain tumors and should not be done routinely. Some surgeons insist on an immediate operation after a ventriculo-gram, whereas others wait from one to five days. Both of these diagnostic measures are not without danger, and death sometimes results from them. Many of the patients are greatly shocked by either a ventriculogram or encephalogram.

To aid in the location of a spinal subarachnoid block such as is produced by a neoplasm, lipiodol may be injected into the cisterna magna. Normally this heavy oil would fall to the lowest part of the cord, but if a block exists the descent of the oil is arrested and can be demonstrated by roentgen-ray. Occasionally the oil may slip by a block, and sometimes it is apparently arrested in its descent when no block exists. If it is not removed it may remain in the spinal canal for years and occasionally may produce signs of root irritation, especially of the lower spinal roots.

Mechanical aids will be used in frequency in indirect proportion to the doctor's knowledge of neurology.

Cerebrospinal Fluid.—The cerebrospinal fluid is secreted in the ventricles of the brain by the ependymal cells overlying the choroid plexuses. The fluid starting within the lateral ventricles passes through them and escapes by the foramen of Monro into the third ventricle, thence through the aqueduct of Sylvius into the fourth ventricle, whence it escapes into the subarachnoid space by the foramina of Magendie and Luschka. The fluid then passes forward beneath the medulla, pons and mid-brain to the cisterna interpeduncularis, and then over the lateral and anterior aspects of the brain. From the cisterna magna the fluid also goes downward around the spinal cord in the subarachnoid space. Most of the absorption of the fluid takes place through the subarachnoid spaces. There is probably an upward current of spinal fluid from the cord toward the brain. The amount of spinal fluid present in the normal individual varies greatly but the average is 140 to 150 cc. I have seen, in preparing for encephalography, as much as 225 cc. of fluid withdrawn from a person who had no gross lesion of the brain. Spinal fluid is commonly withdrawn for examination between the third and fourth lumbar vertebræ. The cord normally ends not lower than the interspace between the first and second lumbar vertebræ, and usually ends at the lower border of the first lumbar. The injection of a needle, therefore, between the third and fourth vertebræ will not damage the spinal cord. The fluid may also be withdrawn between the fourth and fifth lumbar vertebræ or by puncture of the cisterna magna. The examination of the spinal fluid was first done in 1891 by Quincke. With the patient lying on his side, preferably on the left, a line drawn between the highest points of the iliac crests intersects the spine at the fourth lumbar vertebra. The patient should recline on the left side, the spine sharply flexed and the chin approximated as close to the knees as possible. The bed on which he lies should be rigid so that sagging of the trunk does not occur. It is possible and often easier to do a lumbar puncture with the patient sitting on a stool with the trunk flexed. This should be done, however, only if difficulty is encountered in obtaining fluid in the other way. The entire procedure should be done under aseptic precautions, and it is advisable for the operator to wear gloves and a sterile gown, although thousands of lumbar punctures have been done and will be done without these precautions.

Cerebrospinal fluid may be obtained by puncture of the cisterna magna or the lateral ventricles, the latter, of course, being done in the adult after a button of bone has been removed from the skull. A cisterna puncture should be performed only after practice on a cadaver, and it is indicated only as a means of introducing serum into the meninges and as a means of proving that a block exists. It is performed too freely in some hospitals. It is not without danger. The writer has seen at least 3 brains removed from patients who had this procedure done, and in one the puncture had caused a severe basilar hemorrhage.

Technic.—The skin is sterilized in the ordinary surgical manner, and the skin and subcutaneous tissue should be anesthetized with a 1 to 2 per cent solution of novocaine, 5 to 10 cc. usually being required. After a few minutes the needle, which should be of medium bore (usually of the length of 8 cm.), is inserted. For a baby a needle 4 cm. is long enough. The needle should be inserted a little to the outside of the midline and pushed obliquely inward and upward between the laminæ. As the needle pierces the dura a slight "give" is felt, which indicates, as a rule, that the needle is in the subarachnoid space. If the needle is off the line, bone may be encountered and the subarachnoid space will not be entered; the needle should be withdrawn to the skin and reinserted. If great difficulty is encountered, another interspace may be tried, or the puncture done with the patient sitting up. Not infrequently the patient complains of pain in one of the lower extremities, which means that a root has been struck by the needle. The failure to obtain fluid (a dry tap) in the vast majority of cases means that the operator has not reached the subarachnoid space, but occasionally, in purulent meningitis or in cases of complete block, the fluid will run with difficulty. The pressure should always be taken before any fluid is withdrawn, the normal pressure with the patient recumbent being 6 to 8 mm. of mercury and between 100 and 200 mm. of water. If, in the absence of meningitis, the pressure is high enough to warrant the suspicion of a brain tumor if that suspicion has not already been entertained, very little if any fluid should be withdrawn. The amount of fluid necessary for a complete examination is from 10 to 15 cc.

Before any fluid is withdrawn in spinal cord cases, in order to determine whether or not a spinal subarachnoid block exists, jugular compression should be done. This is the *Queckenstedt test* devised in 1916. In the normal individual when the jugular veins are compressed with the spinal manometer in place, the pressure in the spinal manometer rises promptly and, on the release of pressure on the jugulars, falls suddenly. If, however, there is a block in the subarachnoid space above the puncture, the pressure rises little or not at all on jugular compression, and falls slowly and in a step-ladder fashion. The conditions which may cause a block are spinal tumors, diseases and injuries of the vertebræ such as Pott's disease, extradural abscess, inflammatory conditions in the meninges, especially acute purulent meningitis, adhesions and serous meningitis. Syringomyelia occasionally produces a block, either partial or complete. If a complete subarachnoid block exists, two chambers for the spinal fluid are formed, and the fluid below the block undergoes definite changes. The protein content is increased, supposedly due to venous transudation. This is the Nonne syndrome. If, in addition, the fluid is yellowish and coagulates shortly after it is withdrawn, it is called the Froin syndrome. These syndromes are both part of the same processes. The spinal fluid in these instances does not contain an excess of cells. The point of block may be determined mechanically by the injection of 1 cc. of lipiodol into the cisterna magna with the patient sitting. The oil will fall to the point of block and can be seen by means of the roentgen-ray. The oil may also be injected into the lumbar space and, with the patient in the Trendelenburg position, it stops at the lowest end of the block. In tumors of the cauda equina the Nonne-Froin syndrome may be found in fluid removed above the tumor. If possible, however, a puncture should be made both above and below. In thrombosis of the lateral sinus the Ayer-Toby modification of the Queckenstedt test may give valuable information. Under such a condition, compression of the jugular vein on the side of the lesion does not cause a rise of the fluid in the manometer, whereas compression on the normal side causes an elevation. Ayer says the test is more reliable in sinus thrombosis on the right side than on the left.

Laboratory Examinations.—Normal spinal fluid is colorless, alkaline, with a specific gravity of 1.006 to 1.008; it contains sodium chloride in the percentage of normal saline; albumin, 0.025 to 0.05 per cent; urea, 0.02 to 0.05 per cent, and glucose, 0.4 to 0.6 per cent. It contains no organisms but may, on microscopic examination, show an occasional lymphocyte. Some believe that any lymphocytes in the spinal fluid represent an abnormal condition, but any number up to 10 may be considered normal or nearly so.

Tests which should be done on the spinal fluid are those for total protein, globulin, cells with their differentiation, quantitative sugar, Wassermann and colloidal-gold test. If evidence points to the possibility of meningitis, a smear of the spinal fluid should be made and studied and the fluid should be cultured. A turbid fluid may be due to the presence of bacteria or cells. Although the cell count may be greatly increased in neurosyphilis, the spinal fluid is usually clear and colorless. If meningitis exists the fluid will be turbid or perhaps purulent. If a clot forms on standing, fibrin is present and is pathologic. A yellowish fluid (xanthochromia) may be due to a hemorrhage, which has occurred in the subarachnoid space, especially in the cranium, some days before the fluid was withdrawn. The fluid may be actually bloody, due to blood in the subarachnoid space, caused, for example, by spontaneous subarachnoid bleeding, traumatic subarachnoid bleeding or rupture of a cerebral hemorrhage into the ventricles with escape into the subarachnoid space. It may also be due to faulty technic. Many bloody fluids due to subarachnoid bleeding are considered to be caused by incorrect technic. If the fluid is bloody from injury to a vessel at the site of the puncture, the fluid should be collected into 2 to 5 test-tubes. It will be seen that the fluid in the various tubes will become clear as more fluid is withdrawn, while fluid discolored by the presence of blood in the subarachnoid space will be uniformly bloody. Evidence of hemolysis may also be seen if the blood comes from the subarachnoid space. The blood in the subarachnoid space acts as an irritant to the meninges, therefore the white cells will be in excess. If the spine is tapped daily, bloody spinal fluid due to subarachnoid hemorrhage will gradually become less and less bloody and within a week or ten days will be clear but yellow. In another week or ten days the fluid will become normal. Extradural bleeding does not cause a discoloration of the spinal fluid. Cells, if present, should be counted and their type determined. An increase in cells is present in anything which causes an inflammatory reaction in the subarachnoid space, such as neurosyphilis and meningitis. The type of cells in neurosyphilis and tuberculous meningitis is lymphocytic and in the purulent type of meningitis is polymorphonuclear. The number of cells in neurosyphilis may vary from 10 to 2000, a count of 20 to 100 being common. Occasionally tumor cells may be found in the spinal fluid. An increase of cells is called pleocytosis. The cells are frequently increased in epidemic encephalitis and in acute anterior poliomyelitis, where the cells are first of the polymorphonuclear variety and then become lymphocytic. Eosinophilia of the spinal fluid usually means parasitic involvement of the central nervous system. When the fluid is withdrawn for diagnostic purposes in cases where meningitis or encephalitis is suspected, quantitative tests for sugar should always be done. In meningitis of any type except syphilitic, the amount of sugar in the spinal fluid is diminished or absent, whereas in epidemic encephalitis, a disease which was frequently confused with meningitis, the amount of sugar in the spinal fluid is often increased. The sugar in the fluid is normal in acute anterior poliomyelitis, brain tumor, neurosyphilis and in the chronic degenerative diseases of the nervous system. It is increased in diabetes. The chlorides in the spinal fluid are reduced in the various forms of meningitis.

Colloidal-gold Test.—In 1912 Lange described this test, and subsequently the gum mastic and benzoin tests were devised. Certain changes occur in the precipitation of the reagents which are read by the number of the tube affected and which, when plotted, are referred to as curves. A curve high to the left with fives and fours predominating has been called the paretic curve, because it was thought to be diagnostic of general paresis. It may occur, however, in almost any form of neurosyphilis, in meningitis and in multiple sclerosis. The presence of a paretic curve in the spinal fluid with other evidence of syphilis, such as increased cell count, increased globulin and positive Wassermann, is practically diagnostic of neurosyphilis, but cases with all of these findings are not necessarily general paresis, but may be due to other forms of neurosyphilis. If the diagnosis of general paresis is made only on the laboratory findings without due consideration of the clinical symptoms and history of the case, many cases will be diagnosed incorrectly. If the curve is high in the middle, it has been referred to as the tabetic or meningitic curve, and is frequently seen in neurosyphilis and meningitis. Such a curve may also be seen in multiple sclerosis and in some organic affections of the nervous system, especially acute inflammatory disease. In a patient who has not been receiving treatment for syphilis, a change in the colloidal-gold test unaccompanied by a positive Wassermann points away from rather than toward syphilis as the diagnosis. Yet, many times such a colloidal-gold curve, under the conditions mentioned, is considered enough on which to base the diagnosis of neurosyphilis. In a series of cases which Winkelman and the writer examined pathologically at the Philadelphia General Hospital, cases so diagnosed proved to be such conditions as arteriosclerosis, cerebral neoplasm, pellagra, alcoholic psychosis and encephalitis.

The spinal Wassermann is an extremely important part of the examination of the spinal fluid and should be performed with varying dilutions of the fluid from 0.05 to 1 cc. Ninety to 95 per cent of tabetics will show positive Wassermann of the fluid before treatment. The more acute forms of meningovascular syphilis will usually show a higher percentage of positive reactions, and the untreated case of general paresis will show a positive reaction even when small amounts of the fluid are used in 98 to 100 per cent of cases. It is indeed a rare case of general paresis which has a negative Wassermann of the spinal fluid before treatment. If the neurosyphilis happens to be a vascular type of the disease, for example, hemiplegia or occlusion of an artery in any part of the central nervous system, a Wassermann reaction of the fluid may be negative.

The estimation of the amount of *protein in the spinal fluid* is important. The normal content is 20 to 40 mg. per 100 cc. The amount of protein in the spinal fluid is increased in fluid obtained below a block, and it may also be increased in cerebral neoplasm, especially subtentorial ones. Testing for globulin, which is especially increased in various phases of neurosyphilis, may be carried out by the methods recommended by Noguchi, Nonne-Appelt or Pandy.

Inoculation of guinea-pigs with fluid obtained from cases suspected of having tuberculous meningitis may be performed, but the results will usually be obtained after the patient has recovered or died. It is difficult to find the tubercle bacillus in cases of tuberculous meningitis. On one occasion, in a case which the writer had diagnosed tuberculous meningitis, the laboratory reported "myriads of tubercle bacilli," but when the patient died she had sarcomatosis of the meninges!

The value of information obtained from a lumbar puncture cannot be overestimated. In view of the great frequency with which neurosyphilis is associated with a negative blood Wassermann, it is imperative that every patient showing organic involvement of the nervous system have an examination made of the spinal fluid. The only exception to this rule should be those cases in which the possibility of a brain tumor exists, and then it is safe to perform a lumbar puncture in order to estimate the pressure. If this is high, no fluid need be withdrawn. There are many cases of vascular disease and of inflammatory reaction of the brain that are confused with tumor, and low spinal pressure may be of great importance in helping to clear the diagnosis. In patients obviously suffering from a brain tumor—that is, having such symptoms as headache, vomiting, and choking of the disks—a lumbar puncture is not needed for diagnostic purposes, but where the disks are normal and the symptoms and signs are non-conclusive it is advisable. In the presence of signs of meningitis and fever, a spinal puncture with the withdrawal of fluid may sometimes cause the spread of infection to the meninges, if such does not already exist. The great frequency of general paresis, and the many ways in which it may act, makes it imperative that the spinal fluid be examined in every mental case and also in every patient suffering from what seems to be a psychoneurosis. In arriving at the diagnosis of a patient in coma, an examination of the spinal fluid is as necessary and urgent as an investigation of the urine and blood.

The withdrawal of the spinal fluid may be blamed for accidents which are coincidental. A few patients with cerebral neoplasm in the posterior fossa die suddenly, yet, if a lumbar puncture has been done in such a case, it is always blamed for the death. A patient whom the writer examined and who had signs of cerebral syphilis, was given a note to enter a hospital the following day for the purpose of an examination of the spinal fluid. That night, before his admission to the hospital, he had an attack of cerebral thrombosis which would certainly have been attributed to the spinal puncture had it occurred twenty-four hours later.

To avoid a lumbar puncture headache, a narrow gauge needle should be used and the patient should be kept in bed with the head low for twenty-four hours. Lumbar punctures are frequently performed in physicians' offices and no harm results, as a rule. Occasionally, however, a patient may collapse on the way home, especially if he has had increased intracranial pressure. If a large needle is used a tear may be made in the dura, which permits a seepage of fluid for some days. If the headache does occur it may last from a day to three or four weeks. The headache is often accompanied by a pain in the neck between the shoulders, dizziness and even vomiting. Fluid should be given freely to a patient suffering from lumbar puncture headache, and 1 cc. of obstetrical pituitrin given hypodermically may relieve the distress.

PATHOLOGIC STATES OF THE NERVOUS SYSTEM OCCURRING DURING PREGNANCY AND THE PUERPERIUM.

Any one of the ills to which woman is heir may occur during pregnancy or the puerperium and in many instances have no relation to these states, except by coincidence. However, if a woman has any unusual illness during a pregnancy, it is usually attributed to that condition. I have seen a number of brain tumors entirely unsuspected in the course of pregnancy. The symptoms resulting from these tumors, namely, headache and vomiting, were thought to be due to a toxemia.

The convulsions which occur during pregnancy may be the result of toxic states induced by that condition, or they may be the first manifestation of epilepsy. Hysteria may be the cause of fits during pregnancy, although one would suppose that the uterus was firmly anchored and could not wander. Many of the numerous causes of increased intracranial pressure, such as tumors and abscesses, may also begin during pregnancy and produce convulsions.

Hemiplegia, while an infrequent complication of pregnancy, has been the subject of numerous articles. It usually occurs in the last half of the pregnancy and has been frequently reported as occurring during the puerperium, coming on one or two weeks after child-birth. The pathology of this form of hemiplegia is obscure, although most of the cases are due to thrombosis or embolism; certainly few patients die, which would be the case if the condition were due to hemorrhage. Some of these cases may be due to a toxic factor producing encephalitis more or less limited to the motor cortex. If syphilis was present in the individual, the added strain of pregnancy and delivery might readily produce thrombosis of a diseased cerebral vessel. If infection is present in a case of hemiplegia occurring during pregnancy or puerperium, the possibility of an abscess or of encephalitis should be considered. Aphasia may come on, and is probably due to the same cause that produces hemiplegia, the only difference being that the lesion is a smaller one.

The diagnosis of brain tumor in the course of pregnancy is a difficult one, and fortunately one which is not frequently encountered. There may exist in pregnancy a type of toxemia producing choked disks, vomiting and the other signs suggestive of increased intracranial pressure. The question as to who makes the diagnosis of choking of the disks is an important one, because an ophthalmologist, accustomed to seeing choked disks in cases of brain tumor, can usually differentiate between the involvement of the nerve due to increased intracranial pressure and that due to a toxemia. Where a doubt exists as to the presence of a brain tumor in pregnancy, it is always wise to wait rather than to rush in with a surgical procedure.

During the years when epidemic encephalitis was extremely prevalent, it occurred not infrequently during pregnancy. Epidemic encephalitis, if occurring during a pregnancy, is frequently mistaken for toxemia or for a brain tumor. The choreiform type of encephalitis may be mistaken for chorea occurring during pregnancy. The most difficult differentiation is between epidemic encephalitis and toxemia. Careful and repeated laboratory examinations, including that of the spinal fluid, may be necessary. The occurrence of an ocular or of other cranial nerve palsies points directly toward encephalitis as the diagnosis. The effects on children born of patients suffering with epidemic encephalitis are not yet known. Bassoe found no lesions in the nervous system or viscera of a seven-month fetus dying *in utero*. Jorge found that a fetus in a case of his had had the disease transmitted to it. It is likely that the effects on the fetus are similar to those which occur in many infectious diseases. The mortality of encephalitis is increased if it complicates pregnancy. The effect of pregnancy on chronic encephalitis is usually to increase the signs of cerebral involvement. In fact, pregnancy may precipitate the appearance of a Parkinsonian syndrome.

Choreiform movements which occur during pregnancy may be due to chorea, encephalitis or hysteria. The majority of cases appear in the first six months and are greatest in women under the age of twenty-five years. The mortality in this type of chorea is supposed to be high and has been estimated from 15 to 20 per cent. This naturally raises the question as to whether or not pregnancy should be terminated.

Whether or not the chorea which occurs during pregnancy is a distinct disease, or whether it is simply Sydenham's chorea occurring during the course of pregnancy, has not been settled. The chorea of pregnancy is likely to be more severe than Sydenham's chorea, and the mortality-rate is much higher. Such conditions, however, might be due to the complicating conditions of pregnancy. Just as there is no mental disease peculiar to pregnancy and the puerperium, it is likely that there is no chorea peculiar to these states. But if hysteria and encephalitis have been ruled out, the instances of chorea are of Sydenham's type.

Peripheral multiple neuritis may be a complication of pregnancy or the puerperium. Cases of this complication seen by the writer during pregnancy, and occurring in women who were not alcoholic, were due to infections.

Involvement of the optic nerve is usually of the toxic type secondary to kidney involvement. Real choking of the disks, however, may be seen as the result either of toxemia or of brain tumor. Disturbance of vision of various types may occur, the most dramatic of which is sudden blindness. Occasionally retrobulbar neuritis may be seen in pregnancy. The presence of sinus disease, other sources of toxemia besides pregnancy, and hysteria should be considered. Fink reported a case of postpuerperal amaurosis in a woman who lost 1200 cc. of blood following delivery. Changes in the visual fields, especially on the temporal sides, may be a frequent finding in pregnancy and are due to the enlargement of the pituitary gland which, according to Shaffer, may increase to two or three times its normal size. Paralysis of the motor cranial nerves is extremely rare in pregnancy and the puerperium. Involvement of the spinal cord may occur at any time during pregnancy or the puerperium and may be the result of toxemia, infection, or of the severe strain of delivery. Most authorities believe that, while some of the forms of myelitis or paralysis due to spinal cord disease which occur during pregnancy are secondary to such things as syphilis or disease of the vertebræ, the extraordinary exertion and strain incident to delivery may produce changes in the vessels or spinal cord. Myelitis has been known to occur in three successive pregnancies in the same woman. The extent of the paralysis and the type of it will depend upon the level and the part of the spinal cord involved.

NEUROLOGIC SYNDROMES.

Certain syndromes which will frequently be referred to under the name of the individuals who first described them are given below. Elsewhere through this section a full description of the syndrome will not be given, but will be referred to as, for example, "Horner's syndrome."

Brown-Séquard's Syndrome.—This classic picture was described by Brown-Séquard and is due to a unilateral lesion on the cord. Clinically it is due to injury such as those inflicted by stab or bullet wounds, by disease, especially syphilis, and by spinal tumors. If one-half of the cord at a distinct level is absolutely destroyed, the symptoms will be as follows: paralysis of the spastic type with pyramidal tract and posterior column signs on the side of the lesion and below it; and anterior horn symptoms at the level of the lesion. There will also be disturbance in all forms of sensation at the level of the lesion. On the opposite side and below there will be loss of pain, heat and cold and, in some cases, of touch and deep pressure. In disease it is rare to see a complete hemisection of the spinal cord, and one is more likely to observe a loss of pain, heat and cold opposite to the lesion and below it, and pyramidal tract signs on the same side and below.

Horner's Syndrome.—This is a paralysis of the cervical sympathetic and results in the following symptoms: enophthalmos, which is due to paralysis of the non-striated orbital muscle of Müller; myosis—the cervical sympathetic dilates the pupil and, if this function is paralyzed, the constrictor supplied through the third nerve functions unopposed and produces a small pupil. The pupil does not dilate normally when shaded but contracts quickly to light and in convergence. Pseudoptosis is due to paralysis of the non-striated part of the levator palpebræ, and also to the fact that, as the eyeball is retracted, the lids come closer together. Vasomotor signs may also occur and the intraocular tension is diminished on the affected side. Instillation of 2 per cent cocaine solution fails to dilate the pupil. Furthermore, stimulation of the side of the neck on which the paralysis exists does not produce dilatation of the pupil which it normally should do. This is the ciliospinal reflex. The disturbance of sweat secretion may be brought out by injection of pilocarpin. Cervical sympathic paralysis may occur from lesions of the medulla, such as syringobulbia, and occlusion of the posterior-inferior cerebellar artery, by lesions within the cord and also by involvement of the eighth cervical or first thoracic root, especially the latter, and the ascending fibers of the cervical sympathetic in the neck. The latter are frequently injured in operations of the neck.

Klumpke's Paralysis.—A paralysis of the lower roots of the brachial plexus which is due to lesions which involve the nerves derived from the seventh and eighth cervical and the first dorsal roots. The roots may be torn, as for example, by a dislocated shoulder or efforts at reduction. It is due to efforts at delivery, especially breech births, and also to any condition such as cervical rib, tumor, syphilis or injury, which might impair the function of the roots. In addition to Horner's syndrome, which is present if the sympathetic rami are injured, the small muscles of the hand and the flexors of the forearm are paralyzed. Sensory disturbances are usually present and are limited to the ulnar side of the hand and forearm.

Landry's Paralysis.—*Acute ascending paralysis* is a syndrome and not a disease. Most instances of it are due to poliomyelitis, disseminated encephalomyelitis and acute infectious polyneuronitis, with cranial nerve symptoms. The symptoms begin with flaccid paralysis of the feet and ascend rapidly, and finally involve the bulb. As a rule it produces death in three or four to ten days. The paralysis is a flaccid one with loss of deep reflexes. Sensation, as a rule, is not involved, neither are the sphincters. Atrophy is not seen, because it does not have time to take place. When the bulb is affected certain cranial nerve palsies may take place, and death occurs from respiratory failure. The treatment is supportive and the patient usually must be placed in a respirator.

Ménière's Syndrome.—Due to an affection of the semicircular canals and the auditory nerve, the three symptoms which make up this syndrome are deafness, dizziness and tinnitus. Nausea, vomiting and sweating are secondary symptoms. The condition may be ushered in with epileptiform suddenness or may be a slowly progressive affair, depending upon the etiologic factor at fault. An attack may come on suddenly, with vertigo so severe that the patient drops as though struck. He may be momentarily unconscious so that the diagnosis of epilepsy is considered. Due to the intense dizziness he becomes nauseated, vomits and breaks out in a cold perspiration and occasionally has diarrhea. He is afraid to move because of dizziness, which he fears may be increased by movement. The acute attack may last from a few minutes to a few days. The frequency of the attacks varies greatly.

The pathology of the syndrome is obscure. Ménière describes it as a hemorrhagic effusion in the inner ear. It has been suggested by Cheatle that the phenomena are analogous in some respects to glaucoma and may possibly be due to a sudden rise of tension in the endolymph or perilymph. Toxemias and intoxications, syphilis and occasionally tumor in the angle may produce the symptoms of Ménière's syndrome. The writer has seen it in a most marked form in malaria.

The treatment must be directed to the cause. Intracranial section of the eighth nerve has been suggested in those cases in which total deafness is present and intense vertigo still persists. Bromide and luminal may cut down the frequency and severity of the attacks while investigation as to the cause is under way.

Laurence-Biedl Syndrome.—This is a state in which Fröhlich's syndrome is associated with other hereditary and congenital defects, such as retinitis pigmentosa, mental deficiency and polydactylism. The name Laurence-Biedl syndrome was first suggested by Solis-Cohen and Weiss.

NEUROSYPHILIS.

Introduction.—Syphilis of the nervous system, or neurosyphilis, embraces all the conditions of the nervous mechanism and their membranes, which are due to the infecting agent of syphilis. This includes, of course, diseases of the blood-vessels of the brain and cord, produced by syphilis. Spirochæta pallida rarely, if ever, affects the peripheral nervous system. The symptoms of syphilis of the nervous system usually manifest themselves from five to fifteen years after the initial lesion. However, neurosyphilis may occur while the patient has the secondary rash, and may be delayed thirty to forty-five years; vascular neurosyphilis in particular may occur in the first years of the infection. The effect of the spirochetal involvement of the nervous system is widespread, and while the location of the syphilitic process in a particularly vital spot may lead to disabling symptoms, examination of other parts of the cord and brain in such a patient will reveal the fact that the disease has not been entirely localized. One of the commonest manifestations of neurosyphilis is tabes dorsalis; in this disease the pathology which accounts for the disabling symptoms in the lower extremities exists in the lumbo-sacral part of the cord, yet a considerable syphilitic process may, and usually does, exist at the base of the brain in addition. Why certain people with syphilis never develop disease of the nervous system is not known, but it is probably linked with the laws of immunity. Certain of the older writers, Lloyd in particular, thought that the use of arsenicals, such as neoarsphenamine, before the patient had had an opportunity to produce immunity, predisposed to neurosyphilis. Before the discovery of Spirochæta pallida and the specific tests for syphilis in the blood and spinal fluid it was common to speak about neurosyphilis as being metasyphilitic or parasyphilitic. These latter terms are no longer employed. There is some evidence, but not entirely proved, that there may be a special neurotrophic strain of spirochetes with a predilection for the nervous system. Conjugal neurosyphilis, which is not infrequent, lends strength to the theory that a special strain of spirochetes exists. Others believe that the occurrence of neurosyphilis depends upon the constitution of the individual. Some believe that, given a patient with syphilis, overwork, worry and especially the excessive use of alcohol predispose to the occurrence of neurosyphilis. It is certainly true that alcohol and syphilis do not mix well, and the excessive use of the drug is a common point in the history of neurosyphilis. The frequency of the various types of syphilis has been reviewed by Mattauschek and Pilcz, who found that in a group of over 4000 syphilitic Austrian army officers, 4.8 per cent developed paresis, 2.7 per cent tabes dorsalis and 3.2 per cent other forms of neurosyphilis. It has been estimated that 10 to 15 per cent of the patients in the hospitals for the mentally ill are there because of paresis or dementia caused by syphilis. This, more than any other point, shows the tremendous economic problem involved by neurosyphilis.

Types of Neurosyphilis.—Neurosyphilis is divided into the meningeal, parenchymatous, vascular, and meningovascular types. An isolated gumma or syphiloma is a rare form of neurosyphilis, although gummatous meningitis is common. The syphilitic meningitis may occur at any part of the cerebrospinal axis, but is particularly common in the region of the optic chiasm, in the interpeduncular space and in the cerebellopontine angle. It also occurs in the spinal cord, especially on the dorsal aspect. The meninges are infiltrated with round and plasma cells. The parts of the central nervous system beneath the involved meninges show evidence of inflammatory reaction; in such cases the process may be referred to as meningoencephalitis and meningomyelitis. Hypertrophic pachymeningitis is usually found in the cervical cord, consists of great thickening of the dura and is usually, but not always, due to syphilis. This process leads to rim degeneration of the cord, atrophy of the roots and involvement of the vessels which nourish the cord. As a result, cavitation in the central parts of the cord often occurs.

The two forms of neurosyphilis which are examples of the parenchymatous type are general paresis and tabes dorsalis. Pathologically, general paresis is a syphilitic meningoencephalitis characterized by a fibrous thickening and infiltration of the meninges with round cells of the lymphocytic and plasma type, the infiltration being particularly limited to the deeper pial layers. In the cortex the findings are a breaking up of the architecture independent of the vascular supply, perivascular infiltration with cells identical with those of the pia, the occurrence of rod cells in great number, and new vessel formation. By means of the newer staining methods it is possible to detect the increase of iron and enormous numbers of so-called Hortega and Cajal cells of the glial type. A certain percentage of cases, probably not over 15, have sclerosis of the posterior columns of the cord and the usual syphilitic meningitis, producing the clinical picture that is commonly called taboparesis. Remissions, either spontaneous or as a result of therapeutic measures, may bring about decided improvement in the pathologic picture. Tabes is an affection of the posterior roots, posterior ganglia and the meninges covering the dorsal aspect of the cord, with secondary changes in the posterior columns. Whether the lesion is primarily in the roots or the meninges has not been settled satisfactorily. Occasionally in tabes the anterior roots and the anterior horn cells may be involved. Basilar meningitis usually exists in tabes and accounts for the cranial nerve symptoms.

In vascular syphilis the syphilitic process is found in the bloodvessels, more particularly in the arteries. The muscular and elastic fibers are infiltrated with lymphocytes. The walls of the vessels, especially the intima, are ultimately involved, with the formation of a thrombus in the vessels. An artery may also be the site of an aneurysm although syphilis is not a common cause of aneurysm of the cerebral vessels. If an artery is completely thrombosed or if it ruptures as the result of aneurysm, cerebral softening or cerebral hemorrhage results.

The relation of trauma to syphilis of the nervous system is an important one. Trauma, of course, cannot produce neurosyphilis but it can bring out its symptoms or aggravate them. The question of relationship between trauma and syphilis has a very direct medico-legal significance.

GENERAL PARESIS.

Synonyms.—General paralysis of the insane; Paretic dementia.

Introduction.—Among the various forms of mental disease there is none which may start in such a variety of ways and exhibit such a protean symptomatology as general paresis. It has been known for a long time that the initial symptoms of paresis are often similar to those of the psychoneuroses; the onset may also be with excitement, depression or a paranoid trend. Recently Bunker has reviewed the record of 74 paretics, interviewed their relatives, and found that some of them showed psychic abnormalities for at least four years before the mental breakdown occurred. Irritability, "nervousness," brady-phrenia and other common neuropsychiatric complaints were among some of the frequent early symptoms in Bunker's cases. How often is the significance of such symptoms overlooked!

It goes without saying, therefore, that long before the old conception of paresis, namely, delusions of grandeur and dementia occurs, there must be prodromal symptoms which may antedate the acute mental upset by years.

Paresis is such a common mental disease, making up 10 to 20 per cent of those in mental hospitals, and may masquerade under such different guises that it should always be thought of in any psychiatric disturbance occurring between the ages of twenty-five and seventy years; furthermore, juvenile paresis is common enough in the psychoses of childhood.

From a diagnostic standpoint, too much stress has been laid upon the grandiose form of paresis and too little upon the other and more common ways in which the disease asserts itself. Once general paresis is in full bloom with changes in character, delusions of grandeur, physical signs and mental deterioration, a tyro can, or at least should, make the diagnosis with facility.

Symptoms.—All the psychoneurotic manifestations should be considered as potentially due to paresis. This is particularly so if these symptoms have come on in a male between the ages of twenty-five and forty years without a history of previous attacks. Of course the psychoneurotic who has had his symptoms for many years should not be under suspicion, although he may develop paresis if he acquires syphilis after the onset of symptoms. The direct mental symptoms which initiate syphilis may be those of excitement or depression; the patient may simulate manic-depressive insanity in either phase. Ideas of grandeur, especially in regard to strength and wealth, are common, but many diagnoses of paresis will be missed early if the physician waits for the appearance of ideas of grandeur. Memory is impaired and judgment is affected in all lines. This leads the paretic into difficulties, especially in regard to alcohol and sex. He becomes loose in his manner of dress and in his talk. Because of lack of attention and loss of memory he loses interest in, or ruins, his business; he forgets important appointments. He often orders or buys an unwarranted amount of materials. For example, a baker doing a small business ordered 27 delivery trucks to take care of the enormous increase in his business which he thought was about to occur. While the paretic is usually happy and euphoric he is also given to outbursts of temper, and is frequently unmanageable. While not usually suspicious the paretic may become extremely paranoid. He rarely attempts suicide, but may become assaultive, especially if his aims are interfered with. Some of the cases will pursue a course which runs into a state of simple dementia with mental dilapidation.

Signs.—The physical signs of paresis are important and many of them are found in most cases. The speech is of a tremulous, slurred, dysarthric variety, and is made much worse if the patient drinks alcohol. Test phrases such as "Methodist Episcopal Hospital," "The Royal Riding Artillery Brigade" and "Peter Piper picked a peck of pickled peppers" are said with difficulty. The lips, tongue and fingers show a distinct simple tremor. The face has more or less of a masked expression. The pupils are of Argyll-Robertson type, and may show every characteristic of syphilis. Many cases of what might be considered early paresis will not show changes in the pupils and, if possible, the diagnosis should be made before they occur and before the presence of delusions of grandeur. To wait for symptoms and signs of this sort to occur is comparable to waiting on the sidelines until cavitation occurs in tuberculosis. Ocular palsies and optic atrophy may be seen but are not as common as they are in other forms of neurosyphilis. All of the deep reflexes, because of cortical involvement, are increased but it is rare that ankle clonus or Babinski's sign appears. The handwriting shows a tremor, is carelessly done, and letters, words and even sentences may be left out when the patient writes from dictation. If the posterior columns are affected, Romberg's sign and a loss of the deep reflexes may be detected. Attacks of hemiplegia, monoplegia, aphasia, status epilepticus and partial continuous epilepsy may occur in the course of paresis. The paralytic phenomena may disappear as quickly as they appeared. Many of the patients become bedfast, emaciated, develop infections in the urinary system, have bedsores and finally die of pneumonia, tuberculosis or status epilepticus.

Laboratory Findings.—Examinations of the blood and spinal fluid are of great aid in the diagnosis of paresis. In the untreated cases, practically 100 per cent will have a positive spinal fluid Wassermann. Cells may vary, in a series of cases of ours from 1 to 400, the average being 31. Almost every untreated case will show an alteration in the colloidal-gold curve, such as 5555543521; fives and fours should predominate in the reading of the first 4 to 6 tubes. The globulin is increased. It must be remembered that cases of diffuse neurosyphilis, non-paretic in type, can produce in the spinal fluid changes almost exactly similar to those of paresis. The finding, therefore, of a 4 plus Wassermann, an increase in the cells, and a colloidal-gold curve of the paretic curve in the spinal fluid is not enough on which to say, ex-cathedra, "general paresis." The blood Wassermann is positive in 90 to 95 per cent of the cases. Some of the foreign writers say that

American syphilologists cure many cases of non-paretic cerebral syphilis which they diagnose incorrectly as general paresis. On the other hand, if a case is suspected to be one of general paresis, has not received anti-syphilitic treatment and the blood and spinal fluid are negative for syphilis, such an individual will usually be proved to have a brain tumor, arteriosclerosis, chronic alcoholism, pernicious anemia or pellagra. Multiple sclerosis frequently shows an alteration of the colloidal-gold curve at some stage of the paretic type, but the Wassermann of the blood and the fluid are negative and there is no increase of cells.

Before the advent of fever therapy the *prognosis* in paresis was very bad, practically all cases dying within three to five years. Since fever therapy and tryparsamide have been used, about 50 per cent of the cases do well, and the span of life of the remaining is increased.

The *diagnosis* of paresis should be made as early as possible. The frequency of the disease and the various ways in which it may begin make it imperative that every psychotic individual be examined physically and from the laboratory standpoint for syphilis. Chronic alcoholism, drug poisoning by such things as barbital, frontal tumors, pellagra, arteriosclerosis and multiple sclerosis are all at times mistaken for general paresis. Occasionally the mental symptoms produced by pernicious anemia are similar to those of paresis. It is in such instances that the laboratory is of great aid in ruling out the presence of syphilis. Diffuse neurosyphilis, especially that characterized by bilateral lesions either of softening or of gumma, may produce a group of symptoms and laboratory findings that are almost indistinguishable from those of general paresis. Hallucinations as a rule do not occur in paresis unless the patient is in addition an alcoholic. Sometimes a case of dementia precox, especially one of the paranoid type, acquires syphilis and later develops neurosyphilis; in such conditions hallucinations may be present.

Treatment.—The important considerations in the handling of a case of paresis are the protection of the patient, the treatment of the underlying condition, and the appointment of a guardian to handle his affairs and money. Properly to protect the patient from injury, he should be institutionalized in a hospital for mental patients; this will usually mean commitment proceedings. An occasional case may be treated in a general hospital. Steps should be taken, immediately after the diagnosis is certain, to have the patient's affairs controlled by a guardian; this will usually have to be done by a court proceeding. It is rare for a paretic to voluntarily give the power of attorney to anyone.

The most important therapeutic procedures in the treatment of the disease are fever therapy and tryparsamide, before the use of which results were uniformly unfavorable. Swift-Ellis treatment and the injection of salvarsanized serum into the cerebrospinal fluid spaces of the brain are, in my opinion, not only worthless but dangerous. The use of fever therapy was first begun by Wagner von Jauregg, who used malaria. The contraindications to the use of fever are tuberculosis, serious heart diseases, nephritis and severe anemia. The consent of a relative or friend should be obtained just as in a major operation. The type of malaria to be used should be tertian or quartan and should be of a proved benign type. Before the patient is injected, it should be determined that he has no idiosyncrasy for quinine. Two or 3 cc. of blood should be removed from the patient known to have malaria, preferably during a chill, and the blood injected into the subject either subcutaneously, intramuscularly or intravenously. The intravenous way usually shortens the incubation period. Most patients have their initial rise of temperature six or seven days after the inoculation, but the advent of malaria may be delayed two or three weeks. The patient should be in a room thoroughly screened while he has malaria. During the course of the malaria he should not have arsenic, quinine, aspirin or phenacetin. He should be permitted to have from 8 to 16 elevations of temperature, which often occur every day, even though the variety of malaria used is the tertian. Distinct chills are often absent. Careful watch should be kept on the patient, his blood counted and the urine examined daily and the state of circulation investigated frequently. Rapidly progressing anemia, high continued elevation of temperature and cardiac weakness call for the termination of the fever. Generally speaking, the more elevations of temperature the better will be the result. The malaria may recur and, if it does, it is wise to let the patient have a few more elevations of temperature if he is in good condition. Other means of inducing fever may be tried; a satisfactory way, and by some considered better than the use of malaria, is to employ typhoid vaccine intravenously. The initial dose is 50,000,000 organisms; depending on the result, the dose should be increased 25 to 50 per cent. The reaction desired is a temperature of 102° to 104° F. for from two to four hours. If one injection does not produce the desired result the next one may then be doubled. On the other hand, if too great a reaction is produced, the next dose should not be increased. Typhoid vaccine can be given when desirable and the reaction more or less controlled. On the other hand, an obstreperous paretic may not permit the injection of typhoid vaccine, whereas if he has been given malaria he has no recourse. Rat-bite fever, relapsing fever and diathermy may also be used to produce fever.

After the fever therapy is completed the patient should not be given any anti-syphilitic drugs for two to four weeks, and this is particularly so in regard to the use of arsenic. The use of fever undoubtedly produces changes in the nature of the cloudy swelling in important organs, such as the liver and kidneys, and if an added burden is thrown on these structures they may collapse. The drug of choice is tryparsamide, but before it is given the eye-grounds and fields should be carefully examined. The patient should be questioned before every injection in a non-suggestive way as to whether he has any disturbance of vision in the way of dazzling lights or dots, or dimness of vision. If he has, the use of the drug should be discontinued. If the optic nerves are healthy the chances of injuring them with tryparsamide are small. In a series of 700 cases receiving 20,000 injections at the Philadelphia General Hospital the writer has not seen visual disaster result if the eyes were reported normal, but I have seen blindness occur in cases which had optic atrophy or neuritis before tryparsamide was used.

73

The dose is 3 grams given in 15 to 20 cc. of distilled sterile water intravenously weekly for eight weeks. A rest period of two to four weeks should then be given, followed by another course of tryparsamide. The total number of injections will depend upon the improvement of the patient. Iodides, mercury and bismuth should also be given at this stage. I have never seen any benefit occur from the use of other arsenicals, the use of which frequently renders the blood and spinal fluid negative, but the patient goes down-hill. The opposite condition occurs after the use of tryparsamide and fever. The fever probably has a sterilizing effect on the spirochetes. It is certain that fever due to any cause will produce the same result as malaria which, therefore, must have no particular merit in itself. Hot baths for the production of fever have been tried and have been found beneficial.

TABES DORSALIS.

Synonyms.—Locomotor ataxia; Posterior spinal sclerosis.

Symptoms.—Tabes dorsalis is always due to syphilis, but there is a pseudotabes, usually due to multiple neuritis with loss of deep sensation and caused by such conditions as diabetes and diphtheria, and may be mistaken for real tabes. As a rule, five to fifteen years elapse after syphilis has been acquired before the symptoms of tabes ensue. However, the writer has seen a case of tabes dorsalis bedridden because of ataxia fourteen months after the initial lesion. The question is often asked in examinations, "What are the early symptoms and signs of tabes?" This is an unfair question because any of the symptoms and signs may be the earliest. However, in a large group of cases certain symptoms appear more frequently than others. Probably the commonest early symptom is pain, which usually appears in the lower extremities, in the buttocks and about the abdomen. The pain of tabes may occur in the chest, in the upper extremities or in the distribution of the fifth nerve. It has been described as a boring, lancinating pain, and patients have said that the pain feels as though it were produced by a knife stuck into the flesh and turned around. It comes out of a clear sky and may last for a few moments, hours or days. If the symmetrical roots are involved, the patient has a *girdle sensation*. Occasionally pressure on the painful area will relieve the pain, but not infrequently the area is as tender as though the patient had multiple neuritis. The pains have a tendency to occur in spots; the patient describes these spots as though they contained a thousand toothaches and could be covered with a dime or quarter. The pain is mistaken for neuritis, arthritis, phlebitis, acute abdominal conditions, pleurisy, angina pectoris and hysteria.

The next important group of symptoms are those referable to the functions of the conus. Most common of these is the *disturbance in the control of the bladder*, resulting in retention of urine, incontinence and difficulty in passing it. Any of these symptoms appearing in an adult for the first time should arouse suspicion of syphilis of the nervous system. Loss of control of the rectal sphincter is occasionally seen, but more often constipation occurs. Diminished or lost libido is also a symptom frequently complained of, and is due to involvement of the lowest part of the cord. Symptoms referable to *the cranial nerves* are next in importance. Diplopia, dimness of vision, deafness, bilateral facial palsy, in fact any of the cranial nerves may be involved by the syphilitic meningitis which is so common at the base in cases of tabes dorsalis. *Gastric crises* and other forms of crises are frequent and are seen in their worst form in the patients who have lancinating pains. The usual form of crisis is a gastric one which, like a lancinating pain, may strike with lightning rapidity. It is characterized by extreme pain in the abdomen and vomiting. It may last for hours, or days and cause marked reduction in weight and severe dehydration of the patient. The extremes of crises may vary from a mild affair to one which makes life unbearable. The exact manner in which a crisis is produced is not known. It is also needless to say that this is the type of patient who is subjected to exploratory laparotomies. Gastric and intestinal studies in these cases are normal. Crises referable to the intestines, rectum, larynx and vision may be observed. Paresthesias in the feet and especially along the ulnar borders of the hands and forearms may be early symptoms.

Ataxia is not an early symptom of tabes and is due to changes in the posterior columns. It is most noticeable to the patient when he walks in the dark or with his eyes closed. *Trophic conditions* may be the first to be observed by the patient but, as a rule, are late in appearing. The commonest trophic disorders are perforating ulcers, found on the soles, and Charcot joints which usually affect the hips, knees and ankles. The lumbo-sacral spine is not an infrequent site for Charcot joints.

Physical Signs.—When the patient is examined the following signs may be detected in the order of their importance and onset: (1) loss of the deep reflexes, especially the Achilles and the patellar. The biceps and triceps are not involved early, unless the patient has cervical tabes; (2) pupillary abnormalities consisting of inequality, irregularity, eccentricity, sluggishness and finally a loss of the light reflex with a preservation of the reaction of the pupils to accommodation (*Argyll-Robertson phenomenon*); (3) cranial nerve signs including palsies, deafness and optic atrophy; (4) disturbance of pain sense in the areas in which the patient has pain; this form of sensation is disturbed earliest in tabes, much before vibration and position; (5) ataxia of station and gait, and ataxia in the upper extremities; and (6) trophic disorders, especially Charcot joints and perforating ulcers.

The deep reflexes are lost because of interruption of the reflex arc. While the patellar reflexes are usually the ones tested, it is of equal importance to determine the Achilles reflexes. The skin reflexes are not altered unless there be a distinct loss of sensation in the distribution of the reflexes. The same pupillary signs may occur in tabes as in other forms of syphilis. They may vary in size from pin-point to wide dilatation; the inequality may be slight but the patient may have one pin-point and one widely dilated pupil. The pupils are usually irregular, react sluggishly to light and, as the disease progresses, lose their reaction. The reaction to accommodation is preserved early, but in an advanced case of tabes the pupils may be fixed. Occasionally the so-called paradoxical reaction occurs, in which the pupils dilate instead of reacting to light.

Any of the motor cranial nerves may be implicated but those which are commonly affected are the third and sixth. Bilateral seventh nerve palsy, especially if it is accompanied by bilateral eighth nerve symptoms, is usually due to syphilis. Optic atrophy in some degree is a frequent sign if it is looked for.

The common loss of sensation in tabes dorsalis is for pain. If the patient is seen early enough and tested for sensation it will usually be found that all forms of sensation are preserved except pain sense, which is diminished, retarded or lost in the area in which the patient complains of pain. When ataxia becomes evident, position and vibration senses are disturbed.

Ataxia is present in station and is called the *Romberg sign.* The patient standing with his feet together and with his eyes closed will sway abnormally if his sense of position is involved, and this is what finally happens in the tabetic. His gait is ataxic for the same reason; he throws the feet far, brings the heels down in a stamping manner, the feet are likely to be more widely separated than usual and the knees are hyperextended, because of hypotonia and relaxation of the joints and tendons. Early ataxia in gait may be brought out by having the patient walk a "chalk line," by having him walk with his eyes closed or by walking backward. The patient himself complains that he walks poorly in the dark. The test for ataxia in the upper extremities is the finger-to-nose test and in this the patient with involvement of the cervical cord cannot accurately place his index finger on the tip of his nose with the eyes closed.

The joint most frequently the site of a Charcot joint (arthropathy) is the knee. It is a painless swelling with proliferation and the destruction of cartilage, capsule and bone surface and the formation of a new bone. Quite often the joint is the site of an effusion. If the joint affected is the knee, the patella is likely to be greatly increased in width. Spontaneous fractures of the bones may occur, particularly in the neighborhood of the Charcot joint. Charcot joints rarely become infected. In a patient of Spiller's at the Philadelphia General Hospital a man had Charcot joints in both elbows and both became infected. Perforating ulcers usually occur on the soles of the feet. They are deep, painless affairs and difficult to cure. Localized atrophy of the muscles occasionally occurs in tabes. A more common symptom is for the muscular system to become generally soft, flabby and underdeveloped. It is rare that one sees a fat tabetic.

Cystoscopic examinations will reveal a "cord" bladder.

Laboratory Findings.—The spinal fluid Wassermann is positive in 90 to 95 per cent of the untreated cases. The blood Wassermann is positive in approximately 50 per cent of the untreated cases. The cells of the spinal fluid are increased and may vary in number from 10 to 200 or 300, with an average of 30 to 75. The colloidal-gold curve test shows an alteration to the left and in the middle, such as 1223100000. Occasionally in tabes a stronger colloidal-gold reaction may be found, even of the paretic type.

The *diagnosis* of tabes should be made before many physical signs present themselves. Pain, bladder disturbance and cranial nerve symptoms point directly to syphilis of the nervous system, most likely tabes, as the diagnosis which should be made before ataxia occurs. Tabes may be confused with the pseudotabetic form of multiple neuritis and with the combined sclerosis of pernicious anemia. The juvenile type or tabes which is due to congenital syphilis may be confused with Friedreich's ataxia or with a cerebellar tumor. The course of the disease is usually slowly progressive, but there are some cases which run a rapid course and become bedfast or chairfast but then live on for years.

Treatment.—The treatment of tabes should not consist of blind intravenous and intramuscular injection of arsenicals and mercurials to the exclusion of the treatment of the patient as well as the disease. He should be placed in the best possible general health, his diet and mode of living made ideal, alcohol, tobacco and excesses of all sorts forbidden, and plenty of sunshine, fresh air and rest prescribed. He should not be permitted to take long walks, to work until he is exhausted or to become fatigued. Massage and reëducation of the ataxic extremities greatly benefits the tabetic. Attacks of pain and crises may be relieved by analgesic drugs, perhaps even morphine, although the danger of addiction is great. The signs once manifested rarely disappear under treatment. The writer has never seen optic atrophy become less or a Charcot joint smaller under the most vigorous treatment. The cranial nerve palsies, especially the ocular ones, may clear up. Section of the posterior roots, cordotomy and fever therapy are usually not well borne by the tabetic. He frequently develops severe gastro-intestinal or urinary symptoms after such treatment. It is questionable whether tryparsamide should be used in tabes, because of the frequency of optic atrophy in that disease. Spinal drainage may be advised and some report good results. The introduction of salvarsanized serum into the spinal canal, in my experience, has given only bad results as far as the patient is concerned, and sleepless nights to myself. The specific treatment of the disease should be limited to mercury and iodides, arsphenamine and neo-arsphenamine in proper doses. A cure is difficult to obtain but an arrest of the disease may be brought about. Iodides and mercury should be prescribed for two to four weeks before arsenic is used, in order to avoid the Herxheimer reaction. Some patients who go to dispensaries for the treatment of syphilis have received 100 or more injections of arsenicals and, the writer is afraid, suffer as much from the cure as from the disease itself. Forced drainage of the cerebrospinal fluid has been recommended in syphilis of the nervous system, as well as in other infection of the brain and cord.

Other Forms of Neurosyphilis.—In addition to paresis and tabes dorsalis, syphilis may produce meningomyelitis, myelitis, Brown-Séquard's paralysis, meningoencephalitis, bilateral cerebral lesions, especially gummas and endarteritis, and hemiplegia due to vascular syphilis. Occasionally syphilis of the spinal cord produces the so-called combined tabes which consists of the symptoms of tabes plus pyramidal tract signs. In meningomyelitis or myelitis due to syphilis the patient may have signs of mild involvement of all of the tracts in the cord up to a given level or he may have a sudden paraplegia occur due to vascular occlusion. If one excludes poliomyelitis and injury to the vertebræ and cord, it is probably true that the commonest cause of paralysis of the lower extremities due to spinal cord disease is syphilis-producing meningomyelitis. In meningoencephalitis the patient has headaches, stupor and perhaps convulsions; he will have signs referable to the area involved. Hemiplegia caused by syphilis is usually due to vascular disease in the region of the internal capsule. Vascular syphilis affecting the nervous system comes on earlier than other forms of neurosyphilis. Given a patient with organic disease of the nervous system or with symptoms suggestive of a psychoneurosis, it is highly important to examine both the blood and the spinal fluid for evidence of syphilis. In the untreated case of syphilis of the nervous system, positive results of some variety will usually be found. It should be remembered that if the patient has received a course of treatment the blood and spinal fluid may be negative but pathologic evidence of syphilis may be found at autopsy. In vascular neurosyphilis the spinal fluid may be, and often is, negative. The diagnosis of paresis should never be made in an untreated case if the spinal fluid and blood are negative.

THE SPINAL CORD.

COMPRESSION OF THE SPINAL CORD.

The cord may be compressed by disease of the vertebræ such as tuberculosis and malignancy, by fractures and dislocations of the spine, by tumors either within or without the cord, by abscesses, by erosion of the vertebræ due to an aneurysm, by inflammatory reactions, by Hodgkin's disease and by leukemia. In view of the fact that practically all of the conducting pathways between the brain and the parts below are in the spinal cord, definite changes in motion and in the control of the sphincters result. Segmental or radicular motor and sensory manifestations will often help in locating the site of the lesion.

TUMORS OF THE SPINAL CORD.

Tumors of the cord may be intramedullary or extramedullary and the latter type may be either subdural or extradural. Intramedullary tumors are usually gliomas. The ordinary subdural tumor grows from the pia and the arachnoid, the spinal root or the dura. The extradural tumor grows between the vertebræ and the dura. While all varieties of neoplasms occur in or about the spinal cord, the commonest spinal cord tumors are endotheliomas and fibromas. They are usually benign and encapsulated. An extramedullary tumor, occurring intradurally, is the usual finding. The size of the tumor varies greatly. The tumor frequently makes a nest for itself not only in the cord, but also in the vertebræ. It displaces the cord, and signs of compression are practically always seen.

Tumors are more common in the dorsal and lower cervical cord than elsewhere. The *symptoms* usually are slow in onset and, as a rule, sudden paralysis does not occur. Unless the neoplasm is growing from the anterior and antero-lateral surface, which is not common, the earliest symptom is pain. Most tumors originate from the lateral or postero-lateral aspects of the cord and involve a posterior root early in the history. The pain is usually unilateral and, as the tumor enlarges, may be bilateral. It follows a root zone and, if it occurs about the trunk or abdomen, it may be interpreted as a unilateral girdle sensation. The pain is increased by sneezing, jarring or coughing and is of a sharp stabbing nature. Intramedullary tumors do not give rise to radicular pain, but may produce central pain. Occasionally tenderness to percussion and rigidity of the spine occur at the site of the tumor. The symptoms and physical signs will vary greatly, depending upon the location of the lesion. The common type of tumor growing from the postero-lateral aspect of the cord will produce pain of a radicular type, followed by hyperesthesia and loss of sensation in the distribution of the root or roots which are affected. If the tumor is far enough anterior to involve the anterior horns, signs of compression of these structures will be noted at the level of the tumor. As the tumor presses against the cord, a Brown-Séquard paralysis which may not be entirely complete occurs. Bilateral pyramidal tract symptoms may be seen, and later on signs of interruption of all the pathways in the spinal cord may come on. If the tumor lies directly over the posterior columns, as it did in a case of the writer's of spinal lipoma, the functions of the posterior columns and of the pyramidal tracts are severely interfered with. If the tumor lies on the anterior aspect of the cord a syringomyelic loss of sensation may occur below the level of the tumor. Difficulty in the control of the sphincters appears as the spinal cord compression progresses. Reflexes of defense are seen in cases that have severe or complete paralysis. Signs of a subarachnoid block, most important in the diagnosis of a spinal cord tumor, are present. The Nonne-Froin syndrome, so marked that the fluid may coagulate spontaneously after withdrawal, is further evidence of spinal block. The cells in the spinal fluid are not usually increased, although tumor cells occasionally are found. Sometimes, as has been shown by Ayer, xanthochromic fluid may be found above a tumor. The colloidal-gold curve frequently shows an alteration in the middle zone. The roentgenogram may aid in the diagnosis and also in the location of the tumor by showing bone atrophy at its site. Lipiodol may be used as an aid in localization.

Intramedullary tumors are usually without pain except, and that rarely, of a burning type. The *symptoms* are likely to be bilateral and symmetrical and very often of a syringomyelic type. Before any suspected spinal cord tumor is operated upon, malignancy throughout the body should be ruled out, careful roentgen-ray studies made of the spine, search made for syphilis both by clinical and laboratory examinations, and the possibility of localized subdural infections ruled out.

The differential *diagnosis* is to be made from diseases of the vertebræ, various conditions which produce degeneration in the spinal cord, such as syphilis, multiple sclerosis, the combined sclerosis of anemia, pachymeningitis and subdural abscess.

The correct *localization* is the *sine qua non* of successful surgery. A tumor involving the *cauda equina* will bring about signs and symptoms according to the roots affected. Pain is a common and distressing symptom. Paralysis, when it occurs, is of the flaccid type. Loss of control of the sphincters and impotence takes place. Sensation, pain first and then other forms, is lost in the distribution of the roots diseased. *Tumors of the conus* (the four lowest segments of the cord, *i. e.*, S., 3, 4, 5, and coccygeal, 1) resemble symptomatically those of the cauda, with the following exceptions: (1) lesions of the conus usually produce symmetrical, of the cauda, non-symmetrical symptoms and signs; (2) saddle anesthesia is more common in lesions of the conus; (3) sphincter involvement and loss of libido occur more often in lesions of the conus; (4) fibrillations occur in conus disease; (5) dissociation loss of sensation in conus involvement; and (6) paralysis of the lower extremities and alteration of the patellar and Achilles reflexes do not happen as long as the lesion is confined to the conus; those signs are common in lesions of the cauda equina.

Cervical cord tumors often produce rigidity of the neck, spinal hemiplegia and ultimately tetraplegia. At the level of a cervical tumor, severe pain, atrophy, loss of the deep reflexes, Horner's syndrome or Klumpke's syndrome may be found. C. 4 adjoins T. 3 at the second rib so that a sharp transmission from the loss of sensation to normal may occur if a tumor involves the lower cervical cord.

Localization of the tumor will be made upon: (1) the area in which the early pain of root irritation occurred; (2) the sensory level and whether it is segmental or root; (3) the extent of the motor paralysis; (4) the presence of localized atrophy; (5) the loss of the triceps on one side or of one of the abdominals; and inequality of the reflexes, or reflex alteration.

Careful, repeated sensory examination with comparison of the results with sensory charts will help most in the localization. Tumors are usually localized too low.

The *treatment* is surgical. Brilliant results may be had if operation is not postponed until secondary changes have taken place in the spinal cord.

TUMORS OF THE SPINE.

Any form of malignancy, including myeloma, may involve the vertebral column, but carcinoma and sarcoma are those which mostly do so. Carcinoma of the spine is always metastatic in origin. In the writer's experience it most frequently arises from a primary lesion in the prostate, rectum or breast, although carcinoma anywhere in the body may metastasize to the spine. It may occur at any time in the history of carcinoma and he has seen a number of cases, especially of the prostate, where the primary growth had not been discovered before death. Sarcoma and osteosarcoma may arise in the vertebral column from a neighborhood primary growth. Carcinoma, of course, is more common after forty-five or fifty years of age, whereas sarcoma may be seen early in life.

In a case studied by the writer the man developed a sudden paralysis of motion with a sensory level at the second rib due to a sarcomatous condition of the upper dorsal vertebræ. This came on about thirteen months after the removal of a sarcoma from the left thumb, where no evidence of recurrence existed.

The process usually involves two or more vertebræ. In fact, in carcinoma all of the vertebræ may be diseased. The roots are infiltrated as they pass to and from the cord. The meninges are involved and finally the cord itself may be the seat of an actual carcinomatous growth. Just as interference with the blood supply in Pott's disease may produce sudden paralysis, so also may a spinal stroke occur in cases of carcinoma when the blood supply is interfered with (Spiller and others). An important thing to appreciate is that after a primary growth has been successfully removed, metastasis to the spine may occur. In one of the writer's patients the interval was eight years. Acute angulation of the spine does not, as a rule, occur, and the exquisite tenderness seen in cases of Pott's disease is not common. Pain is the most frequent and most terrible feature of this disease. At first it is of a root nature, the location of which depends upon the vertebra first affected. Any jarring of the bed of the patient or rough handling of the lower extremities may produce excruciating pain. This condition is sometimes called paraplegia dolorosa. As the disease progresses, symptoms similar to Pott's disease are found. The roentgenogram will aid greatly in the diagnosis but it is true here, as in Pott's disease, that roentgen-ray pictures made of the spine early in the disease may fail to show metastasis.

Myeloma, leukemia and Hodgkin's disease may involve the spinal cord directly or through metastasis to the vertebræ.

Treatment of malignancy of the vertebræ is ineffectual. The patient should be kept under the influence of narcotics, or a cordotomy should be done. This was first suggested by Spiller, first carried out by Martin and refined by Frazier; it will often give relief from the pain unless fresh metastasis occurs above the level of the cordotomy. Deep roentgen-ray therapy or radium may be tried, but are usually of no value except to relieve pain.

SUBDURAL ABSCESS OF THE SPINAL CORD.

Occasionally, in the course of abscess formation anywhere in the body, but more frequently secondary to boils on the back or on the neck, a collection of pus or inflammatory material may localize in the subdural space. This usually occurs in the mid-dorsal region, for the anatomic reasons pointed out by Dandy. The writer has seen pus from an empyema burrow along a rib and ultimately produce an extradural abscess; in another case osteomyelitis of the seventh and eighth ribs on the left side was followed by paraplegia due to an extra-dural abscess. The most constant early symptom is backache, followed by root pains, and then more or less slowly progressing pressure on the spinal cord with signs of block. The case mentioned above as being secondary to an empyema had a complete spinal block and died about one hour after a lumbar puncture had been done. If the nature of the illness is recognized, operation should be done with a fair chance of success, unless there already happens to be other infections throughout the body.

CIRCUMSCRIBED SEROUS MENINGITIS.

This condition, which is usually confused with spinal cord tumor, is a circumscribed collection of fluid in the meninges. The symptoms are indefinite and are usually those due to compression of the cord which, if long continued, may lead to secondary degeneration. It may come on as the result of meningitis. Backache, root pain, weakness in the lower extremities and symptoms of a mild compression usually complete the picture.

The treatment is surgical evacuation of the fluid.

TUBERCULOUS SPONDYLITIS (CARIES OF THE SPINE, POTT'S DISEASE).

Tuberculosis of the spine usually begins in the bodies of the vertebræ, occasionally in the joints or the ligaments, and very rarely in the arches and processes. The disease progresses rather slowly to caseation and necrosis. The cord is not usually involved by deformity of the vertebræ or by the bone disease, but by an extradural collection of the tuberculous pus. The dura becomes greatly thickened but is rarely ruptured. It is also unusual for a tuberculoma to be seen in the spinal cord of a patient suffering from Pott's disease. As the vertebræ become more diseased, a knuckling occurs at the site of the lesion. The abscess which results from the tuberculous caries may point in the retropharyngeal space, in the region of the psoas muscle or posteriorly. While tuberculous caries may be primary, it is practically always secondary to tuberculosis elsewhere in the body. It occurs most frequently in the dorsal region, and while most common in children, it is frequently seen in adults. At the site of compression the cord may be swollen, but is usually compressed. In a case of long standing, secondary degeneration occurs in the cord.

The first *symptom* is localized pain in the diseased vertebra. Pain, which is usually of a dull type, is increased by any movement, but especially by jarring, sneezing or coughing. Rather early in the course of the disease the spine is held rigid by reflex action. Tenderness on percussion will be found or, if the head is sharply depressed, pain will occur at the diseased vertebræ. Spinal deformity in the nature of a kyphosis may occur at any time in the disease, although, unless the vertebræ collapse, kyphosis is a late symptom. When the roots are affected, sharp, shooting radicular pains of a type seen in any condition affecting a posterior root occurs. These pains may be unilateral or bilateral and, if sensation is tested in these painful areas, some loss of sensation will be found, especially for pain. The site of the radicular pains will naturally depend upon the level of the lesion. The girdle sensation may occur at the site of the lesion. Involvement of the anterior roots will cause atrophy, flaccid palsy and a loss of the deep reflexes in their distribution. As the cord is pressed upon by the cold abscess, signs of a spastic paralysis occur below the level of the lesion. Sensory symptoms also come on and, if the disease is unchecked, all forms of sensation and of motion are lost below the lesion. Due to the involvement of the antero-lateral tracts, a loss of pain, heat and cold may be the first sensory lack. Sphincter disturbance, trophic and vasomotor signs, bed sores and urinary infections are seen. The onset is usually slow, taking weeks or months to develop but occasionally, if the vertebra suddenly gives way, or if the blood supply is interfered with by compression, the signs may be acute in their manifestation. If the lumbo-sacral region is the site of caries, a flaccid palsy occurs in the lower extremities with excruciating pain. If the cervical spine is involved, flaccid paralysis in the upper extremities and a spastic paralysis below may be noted. If a high cervical Pott's disease is present, all four extremities may be very weak and spastic, and respiratory disturbances and bulbar symptoms may also be manifested as the upper vertebræ are diseased. Reflexes of defense and involuntary jerkings of the lower extremities are common physical signs when the cord is markedly compressed. These signs practically always indicate severe involvement. Fever is present or absent, depending on the presence of complications or of tuberculosis elsewhere in the body. About one-half of the cases die. Those with involvement of the dorsal vertebræ have the best chance of a good outcome. While the paralysis may clear up, some cases suffer permanent loss of power even though the tuberculous process heals. The hunchback usually represents a healed Pott's disease.

The spinal fluid is frequently xanthochromic and may coagulate spontaneously. Signs of a subarachnoid block are usually present. Roentgenograms will usually be characteristic, but, in the writer's experience, the pictures are often negative for evidence of the disease in its early stages. It is imperative, therefore, not to permit one negative roentgenogram to keep one permanently away from the diagnosis of Pott's disease. Malignancy of the spine, tumors of the cord, spondylitis, spinal syphilis, aneurysm and hysteria are to be considered in the diagnosis. In a case of A. A. Stevens' which the writer saw at the Philadelphia General Hospital, hysterical paraplegia occurred early in the history of the case of Pott's disease, in which the roentgen-rays of the spine were negative at first. The hysterical paraplegia was cured, but in the course of five weeks the patient slowly became paralyzed in the lower extremities with signs of pyramidal tract involvement. If every patient showing paralysis of spinal origin were subjected to careful roentgen-ray studies of the spine, spinal puncture for evidence of syphilis and block, and careful repeated neurologic examinations, only a rare case would be a diagnostic problem.

The *treatment* of this condition is primarily that of tuberculosis. Orthopedic operations are sometimes indicated and the writer has seen some brilliant results come from them. Extension and immobilization of the spine are necessary. An air-bed or water-bed, careful nursing, especially for the prevention of bed sores, are important. The evacuation of an abscess is indicated if present. Even after paralysis has lasted some months complete recovery may occur.

INJURIES TO THE SPINAL CORD.

The spinal cord may be injured by fracture, dislocation, fracture-dislocation, stab wounds, bullet wounds, concussion or by hemorrhage into the cord as a result of trauma, the vertebræ escaping damage.

As in skull fracture and cerebral implication, injury is of importance in direct relation to the amount of cord damage done. Fracture of the vertebral body without displacement, and fractures or tears of the vertebral processes, while they may produce disability and discomfort, do not so much concern us here as does direct injury to the cord produced by injury. The symptoms which come on as a result of fracture or fracture-dislocation, gunshot wounds and stab wounds will vary with the location of the injury. If the lesion is high, bulbar symptoms may be seen. In a case which the writer recently saw the man had distinct nystagmus, vomiting and a slow pulse, in addition to mild symptoms referable to the lower extremities; the seventh cervical vertebra was fractured. Root pains and the signs of a spinal cord compression which may vary from slight involvement to complete loss of all functions below the level of the injury may be seen. Occasionally a Brown-Séquard syndrome may make up the picture. Reflexes of defense may be detected. If the cord is completely destroyed at a certain level a flaccid palsy with loss of all reflexes below may be seen (Bastian's law). If a patient with a complete lesion of the cord does not die from shock or injury within the first week or two, the lower end of the cord regains a certain amount of automatic function, including that of the bladder. The reflexes may become extremely active below the lesion, and the slightest stimulation below it may produce a series of mass reflexes, occasionally with evacuation of the bladder. In a woman, whose case was reported by Harte and Stewart, and later presented to the Philadelphia Neurological Society by Cadwalader, it was thought that some return of function had occurred after the spinal cord, which had been severed, was sewed together. Cadwalader was of the opinion that the case represented an instance of an automatic spinal cord with pronounced reflexes of defense.

HEMATOMYELIA.

Hemorrhage into the spinal cord is practically always the result of trauma. It usually involves the gray matter, and most often that about the central canal. It is important to appreciate that hematomyelia may occur without injury to the vertebræ. One or more segments may be involved by the hemorrhage, the location of which depends upon the site of the injury, although the cervical region seems to be most susceptible to trauma. While the trauma which causes it is usually direct, the writer has seen two instances of cervical hematomyelia due to a blow on the head. In one case an orderly at the Philadelphia General Hospital was struck squarely on the top of the head by a falling window screen. He was dazed by the blow and in a few hours was totally paralyzed from the neck down. Autopsy, a few weeks later, revealed hematomyelia. Another patient was riding in an automobile, and was bounced upward against the support of the roof of the car and developed symptoms of hematomyelia. He recovered. Hematomyelia may also be caused by a fall on the buttocks, or by landing on the feet after a fall of considerable distance.

The *symptoms* of hematomyelia are usually sudden in onset and are rarely delayed more than a few hours. The extent of the paralysis will depend on the site of the hemorrhage. At the level of the lesion there is loss of pain, heat and cold and, if the hemorrhage has extended into the anterior horn cells, signs of involvement of those parts. Pyramidal tract signs usually occur below the level of the lesion, due either to the extension of the hemorrhage or to edema of the cord. Sphincter disturbances occur at this stage and trophic and vasomotor signs may also be seen. Signs of a complete transverse lesion may exist.

Sudden death may occur if the lesion is a high one. Some cases may recover completely, but some of them show residual conditions which are found at the point of greatest involvement of the spinal cord. The symptoms due to edema of the cord clear up, but those due to hemorrhage are slow in disappearing and some of the symptoms may persist. Syringomyelia may develop in a person who has been the victim of hematomyelia.

The *diagnosis* in hematomyelia is made by the history of injury, the absence of vertebral injury and the signs and symptoms enumerated above.

The *treatment* of injuries to the cord should be conservative. If the spinal cord has been injured by fracture or a fracture dislocation, it is unlikely that the surgical removal of the vertebra will bring about the recovery of the individual. Operation in the stage of shock is absolutely contraindicated; it certainly hastens the death of a number of these patients. The writer's experience is that operation does no good and that whatever improvement, if any, occurs cannot be traced to surgical intervention. If operation is not performed upon such cases many of them make excellent recoveries. If operation is done in the early stages before the patient has recovered from shock, death may result. In a case of the writer's on the wards of the Philadelphia General Hospital a man became paralyzed in all four extremities after falling downstairs. The vertebræ were not injured and a diagnosis of hematomyelia was made. A complete block was present and, because of this, it was thought by some that an operation was indicated. However, a conservative plan of treatment was carried out and the man was discharged from the hospital six months later with almost complete recovery. Competent nursing, an air-bed or water-bed, the avoidance of catheterization as long as possible, and careful regulation of the gastro-intestinal tract are important things in the care of these patients. Fresh air and sunshine, the prevention of deformity, passive movements, especially to the large joints, light general massage, and extreme care of the skin will aid greatly the chances of recovery.

AMYOTROPHIC LATERAL SCLEROSIS.

Amyotrophic lateral sclerosis is a relatively rare disease involving the motor system. The pyramidal tracts, the anterior horn cells of the cord and sometimes the nuclei of the seventh, ninth, tenth and twelfth cranial nerves are affected. The usual case begins with involvement of the anterior horn cells and the pyramidal tracts in the lower cervical and upper dorsal cord. The cause of the disease is unknown except that a congenital weakness of the parts affected is supposed to exist. Recent attempts have been made to consider the disease as an infectious or toxic one. Occasionally a patient who has had acute anterior poliomyelitis may later develop amyotrophic lateral sclerosis. The writer saw a soldier with such a picture; apparently the condition was due to excessive use of the motor system during training.

Symptoms.—The age of onset is usually between thirty and fifty years, although the disease may occasionally be seen in childhood.

The motor fibers have been involved in the pons, peduncles, and occasionally even the cells of the motor cortex are affected. The signs of the anterior horn disease are usually the first symptoms to occur, and these are exhibited in the hands, with a gradual progression upward so that the forearms, arms, shoulder girdles and neck muscles may become atrophic. At the same time or shortly afterward pyramidal tract signs appear in the lower extremities; the reflexes may also be increased in the upper extremities, as long as there are cells remaining in the anterior horns to transmit the reflexes. Claw-hand results and the patient may ultimately be paralyzed in all four extremities. When the cranial nerve nuclei are affected by the disease the signs of bulbar palsy ensue. Pain is uncommon but a tired sensation may be noted in the muscles undergoing or about to undergo atrophy.

The *prognosis* is bad, most cases succumbing under three years. The onset of a bulbar palsy always hastens the end which may be due in such cases to choking secondary to the lodging of a piece of food in the trachea or to an aspiration pneumonia.

The *differential diagnosis* is to be made from spinal syphilis, which may simulate very closely amyotrophic sclerosis, progressive spinal muscular atrophy, atrophy produced by arthritis, syringomyelia and cervical Pott's disease. Syphilis may produce a meningomyelitis in the lower cervical region; pain, sphincter disturbance, pupillary changes and the laboratory tests will keep the diagnosis clear. In progressive spinal muscular atrophy the reflexes are lost, bulbar palsy is later in making its appearance and the disease is more slowly progressive. Arthritis by producing atrophy of the muscles and exaggeration of the deep reflexes may lead to an erroneous diagnosis. The absence of definite pyramidal tract signs, of fibrillary tremors which are rare in joint atrophy and of the reactions of degeneration in conjunction with the presence of signs of arthritis will help in the differentiation. Syringomyelia may be differentiated by its slow progress and by the sensory loss. Diseases of the vertebræ, especially cervical Pott's disease, should cause no difficulty in the diagnosis if the spine is always examined in cases exhibiting symptoms referable to all four extremities.

The *treatment* is ineffectual. Careful nursing, selection of food which can be easily swallowed and the avoidance of overexertion are important. Stimulating drugs, such as strychnine, usually do more harm than good.

PROGRESSIVE SPINAL MUSCULAR ATROPHY.

This disease, which is rare, begins in middle life, although there is a familial form which may be seen in infancy or childhood. The anterior horn cells of the spinal cord are involved and, just as in amyotrophic lateral sclerosis, the nuclei of the seventh, ninth and twelfth cranial nerves may be affected. The process, which begins insidiously, is slowly progressive, affects the lower cervical and upper dorsal cord first, from which it spreads both upward and downward.

The *symptoms* are those of anterior horn disease, which may in time be present throughout the extremities, the trunk and in the muscles supplied by the cranial nerve nuclei mentioned above. Whereas amyotrophic sclerosis usually destroys in less than three years, sufferers from progressive spinal muscular atrophy may live five to twenty years. A patient who has suffered for years from progressive spinal muscular atrophy may develop pyramidal tract signs, thus producing the picture of amyotrophic lateral sclerosis.

Syringomyelia is *differentiated* by the presence of the dissociation sensory loss; disease of the meninges and of the vertebræ, by pain, objective sensory disturbance, spinal block and by evidence of vertebral disease or of syphilis. Multiple neuritis produces pain, sensory disturbance and the history of alcoholism is usually obtained.

The *treatment* is essentially that of amyotrophic lateral sclerosis. Massage to the involved muscles and perhaps mild faradism serve to keep up the tone of the atrophic muscles.

COMBINED SCLEROSIS DUE TO PERNICIOUS ANEMIA
(POSTERO-LATERAL SCLEROSIS).

The cord changes which occur in primary anemia commence in the posterior columns and in the pyramidal tracts; both are involved at approximately the same time, although disease of either one may slightly antedate the other. Severe secondary anemia and occasionally cachexia from any cause may produce a similar picture. While the exact cause of the degeneration of the spinal cord is not known, it is likely that the *etiologic factor* which produces pernicious anemia causes the cord changes. The writer has seen, however, a case of combined sclerosis occurring in severe secondary anemia, the result of a bleeding papilloma of the stomach, and also a case due to pronounced cachexia occurring in an unrecognized pansinusitis. The spinal cords of both cases showed a condition exactly similar to that seen in pernicious anemia. It is unlikely that the anemia causes changes in the cord, because of the fact that one occasionally sees combined sclerosis before any change whatsoever has occurred in the blood. The cord implication may take place during a remission of the blood picture. As the disease progresses the entire white matter of the cord may be involved. The disease is much more frequent than multiple sclerosis, amyotrophic lateral sclerosis, syringomyelia and chronic progressive spinal muscular atrophy.

Symptoms.—The symptomatology varies somewhat, according to the parts of the cord diseased. In the usual run of cases the following is the order in which the symptoms occur: Paresthesias in the fingers and toes are an extremely common early symptom, although the paresthesias may be limited either to the hands or the feet. While pain is uncommon, the involuntary jerking of the lower extremities, which frequently occur, may produce pain by the overaction of the muscles. The gait becomes involved and is of the ataxic type with an element of spasticity in it. The involvement of the pyramidal tracts produces a spastic weakness below the level of the pathology with the ordinary signs of such disease. If the sclerotic patches in the posterior columns are pronounced and occur at the level of the reflex arc, that particular reflex may be abolished even though the voluntary motor system be affected. For example, if a patient had marked sclerosis of the posterior columns from the second to fourth lumbar segments, the knee-jerks might readily be diminished or lost, due to cutting of the arc. So long as the sclerosis of the posterior columns is confined to the dorsal cord a spastic weakness will usually be seen in the lower extremities. Sphincter disturbances and a girdle sensation may occur, but if they do it is usually late in the course of the disease. The results of physical examination of the nervous system in the typical case, not far advanced, will show pyramidal tract signs, loss of the forms of sensation carried upward by the long fibers in the posterior columns, *i. e.*, sense of position, of vibration and of tactile discrimination. This may occasionally occur in other conditions, but is very characteristic of the combined sclerosis of pernicious anemia. If the cervical cord is involved, ataxia in the finger-to-nose test, astereognosis and the other posterior column symptoms may be seen in the upper extremities. Pupillary disturbances and ocular palsies practically never occur. The optic nerves are not usually affected, although occasionally optic neuritis may be seen in pernicious anemia.

Mental symptoms not infrequently appear; the patients are often garrulous, disorientated, their memory fails and depression and delusions may be seen. In a case on the writer's psychopathic service at the Philadelphia General Hospital a confusional psychosis existed for six weeks before changes occurred in the blood. The patient never developed cord signs. It is important to know that the mental symptoms and the spinal cord changes may occur before the anemia or during a remission. The patient should be examined thoroughly from a general medical standpoint for the signs and symptoms of pernicious anemia if he presents on neurologic examination pyramidal tract and posterior column signs. Before the advent of liver therapy the outlook was usually bad and the patient lived not more than three years. Now the expectation of life is much greater, and some of the nervous symptoms may be brought under control and the patient's life accordingly prolonged and physical signs of cord involvement actually disappear.

The *differential diagnosis* is to be made from tabes, postero-lateral sclerosis of syphilis, pellagra, multiple sclerosis and tumor of the cord. The singling out of the posterior and lateral columns without producing pain, pupillary and ocular disturbances, the negative tests for syphilis, the absence of a spinal block and the Nonne-Froin syndrome and the presence of achylorhydria and anemia should keep the diagnostician in the fairway of correct conclusions.

The *treatment* is that of pernicious anemia. Careful nursing, the prevention of bed sores by cleanliness, the use of an air-bed or water-bed and the prevention of infection of the genito-urinary system are important points to be considered. Light massage and plenty of fresh air and sunshine are adjuncts in the treatment of this condition.

SYRINGOMYELIA.

The term signifies an abnormal cavity in the spinal cord which is usually due to congenital anomaly of development affecting the central canal. Spinal gliosis produces the picture of syringomyelia because cavities are produced by the new growth, especially in the central part of the cord. Hematomyelia and hypertrophic cervical pachymeningitis may also lead to cavitation within the cord and produce symptoms somewhat similar to those of syringomyelia. The level of the cord usually affected first is the lower cervical and upper dorsal.

Symptoms.—The early symptoms of syringomyelia are usually referable to the hands, and consist of a loss of pain, heat and cold, and atrophy in those parts. However, if the cavity involves the upper or the mid-cervical region, signs and symptoms will be found at the level of the involvement. Sensory symptoms in the nature of paresthesias, aching pains and even actual pain may occur. Due to a loss of pain sensation the patient frequently burns himself without experiencing discomfort and may have pathologic fractures without pain. If the cavity spreads longitudinally, the loss of sensation in the upper extremities becomes greater and will ultimately involve them entirely, and later implicate part of the trunk. If the descending root of the fifth nerve is implicated, the loss of pain, heat and cold may occur in the face. Trophic disorders such as arthropathies, painless felons, pathologic fractures and bone necrosis, spontaneous amputation of the tips of the fingers, and thickening of the fingers are seen. Hemiatrophy of the face may occur, and is most likely due to sympathetic involvement. Scoliosis and kyphoscoliosis in the cervical and dorsal regions are usually found. If the cavity spreads high enough to involve the bulb, signs of bulbar palsy due to syringobulbia may exist. If the cavity spreads transversely the pyramidal tracts are implicated and

74

signs of this involvement are found below the level of the lesion. Certain congenital deformities such as spina bifida, hydrocephalus, and cervical ribs may be seen. A patient of the writer's with syringomyelia had choked disks of 6 diopters. The only thing to account for the swelling of the disks on microscopic examination of the brain was ependymitis.

The *differential diagnosis* should not be difficult if one remembers that anterior horn symptoms occur in the upper extremities, pyramidal tract symptoms in the lower extremities and a dissociation loss of sensation, *i.e.*, a loss of pain, heat and cold at the level of the cavity. The prognosis for cure is bad, but for life is good, some cases living from twenty-five to fifty years.

There is no drug which has any merit in the *treatment* of syringomyelia. Radium and roentgen-ray have been used with some success. Recently operative treatment for this has been recommended. The cord is exposed and an opening made into the cavity. The writer has seen 2 cases who have been operated upon with far from satisfactory results.

MYELITIS.

The spinal cord may be the seat of inflammation, which arises in certain infectious diseases, any one of which may be at fault. Disseminated encephalomyelitis may have as part of its pathology a myelitis of varying intensity. Pressure on the cord from without, as by a tumor or disease of the bones, may produce changes in the cord, which may also be due, but rarely so, to poisoning such as lead. Probably the commonest cause of myelitis and meningomyelitis is syphilis. The process is often most intense at a definite level, which may be in any part of the cord, but more commonly in the dorsal region. Secondary degeneration takes place upward and downward. Closure of the vessels, especially in the syphilitic type, is extremely common, and the same thing probably occurs in the form of myelitis, which develops in the course of labor. Trauma is not a cause of myelitis, except in so far as it produces hemorrhage into the cord (*v.* hematomyelia).

The process may involve an entire section of the cord, when it is referred to as transverse myelitis. The inflammatory areas may be present in patches and be of a diffuse nature, or they may be limited to one side of the cord and produce a Brown-Séquard paralysis. While the inflammatory reaction in poliomyelitis is most intense in the anterior horn cells, there is some reaction in the meninges and in the white matter. The cord, on gross examination, is softened, shrunken and at times firmer than usual. The spinal cord, removed from rapidly fatal cases, is of almost a putty consistency. The vessels are the seat of round-cell infiltration. The ganglion cells are distorted and swollen, as are also the myelin sheaths and the axis cylinders. Fatty degeneration ensues and there is an accumulation of glia cells. Microscopic examination shows descending and ascending degeneration of a secondary nature. The meninges are frequently considerably involved, especially in the syphilitic type.

Symptoms.—These will vary according to the location of the lesion and its severity. During or shortly after an acute infection the patient may develop pain in his back, often accompanied by a girdle sensation. If the disease is localized to one or two segments, pain, except at the level of the lesion, is not a common symptom, but paresthesias frequently exist below the inflammatory reaction. The involvement of the pyramidal tracts will produce the most alarming symptom, as far as the patient is concerned, and these signs usually run true to form. Just as the deep reflexes are occasionally lost on the side paralyzed in apoplexy, so the deep reflexes may be lost in myelitis early in the history of the case, but they later usually become exaggerated. The Babinski sign, ankle clonus and perhaps patellar clonus soon become positive. If the posterior columns are involved there will be a loss of sense of position, vibration and tactile discrimination, and disease of the anterolateral tracts will result in loss of pain, heat and cold. All reflexes at the level of the lesion will be abolished. Disturbances of functions of the sphincters is extremely common; the usual history is that there is first retention and then incontinence of urine. Due to the difficulty in the control of the bladder, infection of the urinary tract occurs many times, complicates the case and lessens the possibility of recovery. While there may be incontinence of feces, most cases have marked constipation from the start. Occasionally priapism is a symptom, especially in lesions of the cervical cord. The writer has seen it in a syphilitic involvement of the lower cord. Trophic disorders, such as loss of sweat secretion, rarely increase of sweat, various vasomotor phenomena, bed sores, occurring especially over the heels and the sacrum, are common symptoms. Involuntary jerkings of the lower extremities with reflexes of defense (Sinkler's toe phenomenon) are frequently seen in severe forms of myelitis, and are sometimes mistaken for return of power. The recoverability of the patient depends in a large measure upon the prevention of bladder infection and bed sores. Many cases do extremely well. In the spring of 1917 the writer saw a healthy, robust man, aged twenty-six years, who developed a transverse myelitis, with loss of motion and all forms of sensation below the sixth dorsal segment. The condition had come on during an attack of acute tonsillitis. He walked at the end of three months, and was passed by the draft board in the spring of 1918. The writer has seen many cases make no improvement and remain bedfast. Extreme degrees of flexion may occur after the paralysis has existed for some months.

The writer has seen at least 3 cases of complete transverse lesions of the cord, following the use of Swift-Ellis treatment, in patients with neurosyphilis, 1 with tabes and 2 with meningomyelitis of mild degree.

The *diagnosis* is made by the history, and a more or less rapidly occurring paralysis of motion and sensation below a definite level, accompanied by paralysis of the sphincters. Multiple sclerosis occasionally has a sudden onset, and the writer has seen a patient who became suddenly paralyzed in the lower extremities as the first symptom of that disease. The history of injury will serve to differentiate myelitis from hematomyelia. Tumors and Pott's disease are diagnosed by the history, roentgen-ray, Queckenstedt test and the examination. Multiple neuritis, presenting as it does an atrophic, peripheral type of paralysis, should cause no trouble in diagnosis. The virus of poliomyelitis, while occasionally producing a transverse lesion, practically always shows a picture depicting anterior horn involvement.

The *treatment* is largely symptomatic. The patient should be placed in bed and an air-mattress or water-mattress used. Extreme care should be taken of the skin, which should be bathed often with alcohol and powdered with a mild antiseptic. Frequent change of position to prevent constant pressure on one particular point is imperative. The fact that the patient is incontinent of urine makes the nursing job an extremely arduous one, inasmuch as the bed linen should be changed whenever it is soiled. Catheterization should be postponed as long as possible. Daily irrigation of the bladder with a mild antiseptic may be necessary. A daily enema will usually be necessary and occasionally a laxative should be given. The lower extremities should be protected with a cradle and a good position at the large joints maintained, if necessary, with splints. Daily passive movements to the large joints is also indicated. Urinary antiseptics may be tried. The one which the writer has found most beneficial in this stage is pyridium, the dose of which is 2 grains (0.12 gram), three or four times daily. Hydrotherapy and physiotherapy are of service when the patient begins to recover and will serve to relieve the spasticity in the lower extremities.

HYPERTROPHIC CERVICAL PACHYMENINGITIS.

As the name indicates, this is a thickening of the membranes, especially the dura, which may readily be twelve times the normal thickness. The enlargement of the dura is dense and causes the meninges to adhere to each other as well as to the roots and the spinal cord. The cord is compressed and later on may be the seat of a rim degeneration, secondary degeneration and even cavitation. While the lower part of the cervical cord is most frequently involved, the process may extend to include the entire cord and even the medulla and pons. The exact etiologic factor is not known, but in cases of the writer's at the Philadelphia General Hospital the commonest conditions found at autopsy were syphilis and tuberculosis. One case started as cerebrospinal meningitis, was thought to be tuberculous and the tubercle bacillus was found in the spinal fluid. The man was treated with intraspinal injections of magnesium sulphate and recovered sufficiently to leave the hospital. He returned, however, in a few weeks with the symptoms of cervical pachymeningitis which was found at necropsy.

The earliest *symptom* is pain, of a root nature, which occurs at the level of the lesion. This is followed by compression of the anterior roots or disease of the anterior horn cells, which produces atrophic paralysis at the level. In view of the fact that the lower cervical cord is more frequently affected, the foregoing symptoms are first seen in the upper extremities, especially the hands. Horner's syndrome may occur from involvement of the eighth cervical and first dorsal roots.

As the condition progresses, the signs of compression of the cord occur with interruption of the functions of the sensory paths and of the pyramidal system. Disturbance of the sphincters is also seen.

If the process is syphilitic in origin other signs of neurosyphilis may be present. Spinal tumor, syringomyelia and caries of the spine will have to be differentiated.

If the condition is due to syphilis, *treatment* along that line is necessary. If this etiologic factor is not found there is no medical remedy which has any merit. Mills thought that operation was indicated and advised making a slit in the dura for the purpose of decompression.

FRIEDREICH'S ATAXIA.

Family or hereditary ataxia is a chronic, progressive, hereditary, degenerative, rare disease of the nervous system beginning, as a rule, before the age of ten or twelve years, more common in males and affecting chiefly the posterior columns, spino-cerebellar tracts and the pyramidal tracts, and associated at times with an atrophy or agenesis of the cerebellum. The *symptoms* are ataxia in all four extremities, loss of the deep reflexes, although they may occasionally be exaggerated with Babinski's sign, dysarthria often of the scanning type, nystagmus and ataxia in station and gait. Club-foot, pes cavus, Friedreich's toe which consists of extension of the first phalanx of the great toe with flexion of the second to a right angle, and scoliosis make up the physical deformities. Occult spinal bifida may also be seen. If the disease is of long standing, atrophy due to disease of the anterior horn cells may occur in the upper extremities. This happened to a brother and sister affected with the disease on the wards of the Philadelphia General Hospital. The so-called Marie's hereditary cerebellar ataxia resembles Friedreich's ataxia in many ways, except that it occurs after twenty or thirty years and is not so likely to be associated with physical defects. A few years ago the writer presented before the Philadelphia Neurological Society homologous twins, Jews, whose symptoms came on at the age of thirty-two years and progressed in an exact manner to the present. Two other cases on his service at the Philadelphia General Hospital came on at the age of thirty-two and thirty-eight years. These 4 patients all had marked generalized ataxia, greatly increased reflexes without Babinski's sign or nystagmus, and all had dysarthria. None of them had skeletal deformities or optic atrophy. In one, who was subjected somewhat callously by the writer to an encephalogram, the collection of air in the region of the cerebellum led us to believe that that organ was atrophic.

The greatest trouble in *differential diagnosis* will be with juvenile tabes which will show the characteristic pupillary state and areflexia, laboratory signs of syphilis and the absence of skeletal deformities, although Charcot's joints and trophic ulcers may be seen. Multiple sclerosis may be mistaken for Friedreich's ataxia, although the former is very rare in childhood.

Treatment of Friedreich's ataxia and Marie's hereditary cerebellar ataxia is unavailing. Marriage of members of families in which

Friedreich's disease is known to exist should be advised against. In the cases of Marie's ataxia seen by the writer, in only one instance was there a familial history.

DISEASE OF THE BLOOD-VESSELS OF THE SPINAL CORD.

Two anterior spinal arteries are derived from the two vertebrals and unite, shortly after their origin, to form the anterior median spinal artery which terminates at the level of the fifth cervical segment. Below this point the anterior spinal artery, which descends in the ventro-median sulcus, is formed by the confluence of the lateral spinal arteries which take their origin from several sources, such as the vertebral and ascending cervicals; in the thorax from the intercostal arteries; in the lumbar region from the lumbar arteries; in the pelvis from the sacral arteries. The anterior spinal artery supplies the anterior horns, the central canal and Clarke's columns. The two posterior spinal arteries, which are derived from the vertebrals, run downward along the posterior aspect of the cord and close to the posterior roots. These arteries are reinforced by small ones which enter the vertebral canal along the posterior roots so as to form a peripheral system of arteries called the vasocorona, which encompasses the spinal cord. From this surrounding arterial system arterioles dip into the spinal cord, supplying the white matter and the posterior cornua, with the exception of Clarke's columns. Undoubtedly, the anterior spinal artery supplies the white matter on the anterior surface of the cord. Either of the arterial systems of the spinal cord, posterior or anterior, may be occluded as a result of the disease which is most frequently syphilis. The free flow of blood through the vessels may also be interfered with because of tumors, either benign or malignant, especially the latter, which involve them. It is also likely that the sudden paralysis which sometimes takes place in Pott's disease or carcinoma of the spine may be due to interference with the vascular supply. In Spiller's case of occlusion of the anterior spinal artery, the first reported with necropsy, the occlusion occurred at the level of the eighth cervical and the first thoracic segment. The anterior horns were softened at this region as high as the fourth cervical segment. The lesions implicated the anterior horns, the anterior part of the cord in advance of the crossed pyramidal tracts and the most anterior part of the posterior columns. The most outstanding symptoms, therefore, will be referable to the parts of the cord involved. Sometimes, however, pyramidal tract signs are seen below the level of the lesion and there may be dissociation sensory loss (A. Ornsteen). The arteries in the posterior aspect of the cord are more frequently involved than those of the anterior. The usual cause is syphilis.

HERPES ZOSTER (ZONA OR SHINGLES).

Herpes zoster is an affection of the sensory spinal or cranial ganglia. There are two types of herpes zoster, in one a primary infectious process which may even occur in epidemics, and the other due to secondary involvement of the ganglia by such conditions as syphilis, tumor or perhaps by acute infectious disease. Some evidence exists to show that herpes zoster is caused by transmissible virus, and that it may be related to chickenpox. It is also thought by some that there is a relation between herpes zoster, acute anterior poliomyelitis and epidemic encephalitis. A case recently seen developed shingles ten days after sleeping in the same room with a patient who had recently developed a herpes zoster. In brief, it may be due to anything which can affect a sensory ganglion, which is frequently the site of hemorrhage and destruction. Secondary degeneration may occur both in the peripheral nerve and in the dorsal root. Some have called herpes zoster, acute posterior poliomyelitis.

If the condition is due to an acute infection the *symptoms* may be of a general nature, such as fever, headache and malaise. The first symptom is pain, which is of a definite root nature, and in the root distribution. In many cases it is sharp and unbearable. If the patient is examined at this stage it will be seen that there is hyperesthesia and perhaps a loss of pain sense in the distribution of the root affected. From a few hours to a few days after the onset of pain the skin throughout the entire course or a part of the course of the nerve becomes red and the site of vesicles. The skin disturbance lasts a few days, although if infection occurs the skin lesions may not clear up for two or three weeks. Scarring and pigmentation, especially the latter, may appear and persist. After the eruption has taken place pain may subside, but, on the other hand, the pain may persist. This is especially so when the herpes involves the face or if it occurs in an elderly person. While any part of the body may be affected, herpes zoster most usually implicates the chest. Geniculate ganglion herpes occurs in the ear and is usually accompanied by Bell's palsy. The disease is practically always unilateral and recurrences are rare. Corneal ulceration with secondary infection may occur in herpes of the ophthalmic division of the fifth nerve. As an evidence of meningeal reaction, lymphocytosis of the spinal fluid is seen. The prognosis is good but intractable neuralgic pain may be an uncomfortable sequence.

In considering the *treatment* it is important to find the cause for the condition. The possibilities of spinal tumor, Pott's disease and neurosyphilis should be considered and eliminated. Locally, alcohol saturated with boric acid and frequently applied to the vesicles will cause them to dry up. Drugs, such as acetylsalicylic acid, acetphenetidin and perhaps even codein or morphine may be necessary to relieve the pain. In patients in whom the pain persists for some weeks or months it may be necessary to section the root involved or to inject it with alcohol.

ACUTE ANTERIOR POLIOMYELITIS.

Synonyms.—Infantile spinal paralysis; Heine-Medin disease.

Acute anterior poliomyelitis is an infectious disease with a special tendency to involve the nervous system. The pathologic process involves the anterior horns of the cord, the meninges, the cranial motor nuclei and occasionally the white matter of the cord and brain.

The *cause* of the disease is a filterable virus, although some think that a coccus of one kind or another is responsible. This latter belief is based chiefly on the finding of organisms in culture media, although it is believed by many investigators that the organisms so found are contaminators. The exact period of incubation is not known, but it is probably under two weeks.

The chief *pathologic change* consists of hyperemia, edema and slight hemorrhage, with considerable perivascular infiltration in the anterior horn cells, which are swollen and show chromatolysis with marked neuronophagia. The cells ultimately disappear and are replaced by glia cells. The motor roots, nerves and muscles also become atrophic after the acute stage has subsided.

In addition to changes in the nervous system, hyperplasia of the lymphoid tissue throughout the body, enlargement of the spleen and changes in the liver and kidneys in the nature of cloudy swelling occur.

The disease is probably contagious, although the exact mode of transmission is not kown. Some investigators think the agent of the disease enters through the naso-pharynx. The possibility that the virus may be transmitted by an insect or through the food has not been entirely eliminated. Once the virus has gained access to the naso-pharynx it spreads to the central nervous system, probably by way of the lymphatics.

While the disease is especially common in the late summer and autumn, it occurs endemically throughout the rest of the year. It involves the sexes about equally and is most common in children under the age of twelve years. In many epidemics, however, a large number of cases occurred in adults. The disease was first placed upon a firm basis by Heine in 1840. It is especially common in Norway and Sweden, northern Europe, Australia and in the United States. While multiple cases in a household do occur, it is rare, and this, of course, points away from a high degree of contagiousness.

Symptoms.—The disease is ushered in with a mild degree of fever, usually below 101° or 102° F. but which may go as high as 104° F. Headache, loss of appetite, anorexia, constipation, vomiting, diarrhea, irritability, drowsiness and pain in the back and legs may be present. Occasionally convulsions occur early in the course of the disease, but probably mean no more than the occurrence of convulsions at the onset of the other acute infectious processes. Pronounced pain may be present on handling the extremities. In a case in which pain is a common symptom it may be due to meningeal irritation or to the fatigue produced by the paralyzed extremity lying in one position for a considerable time. In other cases a mild degree of multiple neuritis may exist. The general symptoms and the fever may be so slight as to escape notice and frequently, especially in hospital and dispensary cases, the mother of the child had not been aware that more than a slight indisposition was present.

Much has been written recently concerning the symptoms which occur in the so-called preparalytic phase of the disease. The preparalytic signs as given by Ayer are as follows: fever, headache, rigidity of the neck, tremor of the lips and hands, and perhaps coarse twitching during sleep, apathy, vomiting, retention of urine for twelve to twenty-four hours, constipation and sweating. Ayer states that in the bulbar type the preparalytic period is not constant. In some papers, when the histories of the so-called preparalytic cases are carefully reviewed, it is quite evident that many of the cases have no relation to poliomyelitis. On the other hand, in a series of 116 patients in which a diagnosis of preparalytic state was made by one observer, 71 subsequently were reported to have developed some degree of paralysis. It certainly must be true that there are many cases of acute anterior poliomyelitis that are extremely mild and that never develop paralysis either with or without prophylactic serum injection.

While any part of the spinal cord may be involved in the ordinary type of the disease, the lumbo-sacral region is most frequently affected and usually in an irregular manner. The paralysis, which is a flaccid one, will depend upon the anterior horn segments involved and will be in the distribution of those segments. The muscles of the abdomen, the back and even those of the neck may be paralyzed to the exclusion of others. Certain writers believe that the commonest cause of scoliosis is poliomyelitis, which, having involved the dorsal region of the cord with subsequent atrophy of the muscles of the spine, allows that structure to sag. An entire extremity or a part of it may be paralyzed and the involvement may be so irregular as to produce a paralysis of an upper and the opposite lower extremity. Some years ago the writer saw a colored man, who apparently had widespread involvement of the anterior horn cells limited to one side and extending from the upper cervical to the lower lumbar region. The paralysis is accompanied by a loss of the deep and superficial reflexes in the domain of the segments involved, and after a week or two there is loss of contractibility of the muscles to faradism and galvanism, and in severe cases complete reactions to degeneration. As a rule, the height of the paralysis is reached within seventy-two hours of the onset. In many cases, especially infants, the exact date of paralysis is not known. Some of the cases described under the heading of Landry's paralysis are in reality instances of poliomyelitis. Involvement of the bulb or of the ocular nuclei may occur either as distinct types of the disease or as part of the general picture. The involvement of the lower cranial nuclei is referred to as polioencephalitis inferior of Wernicke and, if the ocular motor nuclei are involved, it is spoken of as polioencephalitis superior of Wernicke. The virus of poliomyelitis can also affect the motor cortex, producing hemiplegia of the spastic type. To this condition the term of polioencephalitis is applied. The involvement of the cranial nerves will produce paralysis in the distribution of the nuclei affected. Kernig's sign, stiff neck and pain on manipulation of the paralyzed extremity are common physical findings. Tenderness on percussion over the side of the pathologic process may be found. Cerebellar symptoms, due either to involvement of the cerebellum or of the cerebellar peduncles, may occasionally be encountered. Those cases with involvement of the bulb not infrequently die suddenly. Loss of sensation does not occur, and disturbance of the sphincters, except for retention of urine in the first few hours, is a rare finding. Trophic lesions and bed sores are extremely uncommon complications, although the skin of the paralyzed extremity may be cool, mottled and show disturbance of sweat secretion.

The leukocytes in the blood are usually increased, the number varying from a slight advance to 15,000 or 20,000. The spinal fluid is usually under increased pressure, is clear, shows excessive globulin and has a normal percentage of sugar. A mild alteration of the colloidal-gold curve, chiefly in the middle zone, may be seen. The cells are definitely increased from 10 to a few hundred. Though the granular leukocytes predominate in the early stage of the disease, they quickly give way to lymphocytes.

Diagnosis.—Once the disease is in full bloom, but little diagnostic difficulty will be encountered. In times of an epidemic all illnesses characterized by fever, headache and gastro-intestinal symptoms should be regarded with suspicion as possible cases of poliomyelitis, but other conditions should be also considered. Pott's disease, hip disease, meningitis of any type, epidemic encephalitis and infantile scurvy are often mistaken for acute anterior poliomyelitis. The so-called "pink" disease may also be wrongly diagnosed poliomyelitis. The writer recently saw a case of trichinosis labeled infantile paralysis. Occasionally during epidemics of infantile paralysis, instances of widespread involvement of the white matter of the cord may be seen, and the picture of myelitis rather than poliomyelitis results. It is a wonder this does not happen more frequently, because in many sections of the spinal cord from cases of infantile paralysis there is microscopic evidence of involvement of the white matter in a mild degree and even of the posterior columns.

Prognosis.—The prognosis varies in different epidemics, the mortality being from 5 to 25 per cent. The most unfavorable cases are those with bulbar symptoms. After the acute symptoms have subsided, the remaining picture is that of anterior horn disease: a flaccid, atrophic paralysis, loss of deep reflexes in the distribution of the segments involved, fibrillary tremors and changes in electrical reactions. The paralysis may clear up rapidly, or the other extreme may be encountered and no improvement take place. It is impossible to say in a given case how much improvement will take place, but it is important "to keep the flag flying" and to be optimistic as to the amount of recovery possible. At one time, in the Episcopal Hospital, there were 2 cases of infantile paralysis admitted about the same time; one with total paralysis of all four extremities, marked respiratory difficulty and dysphagia. This child made a complete recovery except that the deep reflexes did not return. The other child had a paralysis of one lower extremity, was never seriously sick and yet there was practically no return of power at all. Deformities and contractures are prone to occur, especially if the paralyzed extremity is not properly handled during the first few weeks of the illness. The improvement may keep up for as long as two years. As in any paralysis of the peripheral nerve or anterior horn type, the early return of normal reactions to galvanism or faradism is a good prognostic omen.

Treatment.—If the diagnosis is certain the patient should be put to bed and isolated, even though the direct mode of transmission of the disease is not known, and the ordinary sterilization of secretions and excretions carried out. Lumbar puncture has not only a diagnostic but a therapeutic value. Removal of the spinal fluid is especially indicated in those patients who have signs of meningitis and pain in the back and extremities. There is no specific for the disease. Antisera from cultures of various types of streptococci are without merit.

Serum Treatment.—In 1910 Levaditi and Landsteiner, Flexner and Lewis and others demonstrated the possibility of serum treatment. These workers also found that twenty-four hours after an intradural injection of a fatal dose of virus, 10 cc. of immune serum given intraspinally likewise protected the monkey from paralysis, but injections given later than twenty-four hours were not so successful in aborting the process. These experimental results were utilized as a basis of serum therapy in man. Immune serum is obtained from individuals who have recovered from the disease. The serum is carefully separated, inactivated and to it should be added a preservative; 100 cc. of clear serum can usually be obtained from 250 cc. of blood. It is extremely important that the possibility of the donor being syphilitic should be thoroughly ruled out. Serum is given intraspinally by the gravity method. The amount usually given is 10 to 25 cc., depending upon the age and weight of the patient. The serum should be repeated in eighteen to twenty-four hours, if improvement does not take place in the case. It should be remembered that the first lumbar puncture with the introduction of serum will cause a considerable meningeal reaction so that the examination of the second spinal fluid will not give a clear index as to the activity of the disease. Third and fourth doses of the serum are usually unnecessary as the child, according to Ayer, is usually better or paralyzed. Ayer believes serum is contraindicated in bulbar types of paralysis. Intravenous use of serum is recommended by some and disapproved by others, 10 to 100 cc. may be employed in this manner.

The use of convalescent human serum intramuscularly, or subcutaneously, to the amount of 10 to 20 cc. has been recommended as a means of producing immunity. In the cases in which the writer has seen immune serum used, no results were obtained which he had not seen equalled in cases receiving no specific treatment at all or, at the most, simply lumbar puncture. He has seen an aggravation of the paralysis occur shortly after immune serum was injected into the spinal canal; this may have been due to the natural course of the disease. On the other hand, there have been many papers written recently strongly advocating the use of human serum, especially in the preparalytic stage, and figures are given to prove that paralysis was present. However, he is certain from reading the histories of these cases that, if poliomyelitis did exist in them, it was probably of the abortive type, and the disease would have disappeared without producing paralysis. Due to the widespread advocacy of the use of immune serum, he feels confident that it has been employed in many cases in which poliomyelitis did not exist and that, personally, he has seen a number of instances of such. If the respiratory paralysis threatens or ensues, the patient should be placed in a respirator.

During the acute stage it is most important to protect the paralyzed muscles and extremities. Various splints and appliances should be used to prevent contractures occurring in the muscles. It is also important to move passively the large joints of the extremities which are paralyzed, two or three times daily, although many believe that nothing of this sort should be done within the first four to six weeks. Orthopedists recommend that no passive movement or massage be employed for the first three months. Under no circumstances should the paralyzed extremity be massaged as long as it is the seat of pain on manipulation. At the end of six or eight weeks massage and more active passive movement should be instituted, unless the patient has pain, and earlier if he does not. These forms of physiotherapy should be employed daily, but only for a few minutes at the start, and then the amount of time devoted to them gradually increased. All treatment to the paralyzed limbs should be gentle, and the vigorous manhandling type of massage should not be countenanced. Electric treatments should also be employed daily or every other day. After the acute stage has subsided, care should still be employed to prevent the occurrence of deformities. It is often necessary to use supports and braces. Roentgen-ray therapy and diathermy have been employed by some over the level of the cord involved. It is important to keep up treatment for at least two years before considering orthopedic procedure for the relief of deformities and paralysis. If spontaneous recovery is taking place the child should not be allowed to use the recovering part too freely.

MULTIPLE SCLEROSIS.

Synonyms.—Disseminated sclerosis; Insular sclerosis.

This is a chronic disease of the central nervous system, although it may run an acute or subacute course. The cause of the disease is not known, although it is perhaps due to a toxic or an infectious agent. From time to time an organism is found which is thought to be the cause of multiple sclerosis, but further investigations do not confirm it. Some believe that multiple sclerosis may be a deficiency disease. Heredity and syphilis take no part in the production of multiple sclerosis, although multiple areas of syphilis in the central nervous system may simulate it. It may follow after an acute infectious disease. Apparently in some cases it has been precipitated by pregnancy. Trauma produces a condition which simulates multiple sclerosis, but trauma probably has nothing to do with the onset of the disease.

The age at onset is usually between twenty and forty years. In cases occurring in children, especially in more than one member of a family, it should be considered with suspicion as probably being a familial disease of the extrapyramidal system.

Pathologically the disease is characterized by numerous patches of sclerosis scattered through the central nervous system. The sclerotic patches are characterized by a degeneration of the myelin sheaths and a preservation of the axis cylinders, which, however, are affected later. The optic nerves are involved, usually in the nature of a retrobulbar neuritis. The irregularity and the number of the sclerotic patches frequently makes for peculiar and bizarre symptoms. The white matter of the central nervous system is much more affected than the gray, which is not seriously involved. The pyramidal tracts, due to their great length, are practically always caught by sclerotic patches. The cerebellum is not usually affected.

Symptoms.—The onset of the disease, while usually insidious, may be apoplectic. The writer has seen sudden blindness, hemiplegia, crural paraplegia and an ocular palsy come on abruptly and clear up; the subsequent course of these cases proved them to be multiple sclerosis. The preservation of the axis cylinders accounts for the return of power. The history in the ordinary case is usually first of numbness, parasthesia and weakness in the lower extremities, followed by ataxia and tremor in the upper extremities, ocular disturbance and involvement of speech. The ocular signs are dimness of vision, blindness, nystagmus or perhaps a palsy of an ocular nerve. The classical *triad of Charcot*, namely tremor, scanning speech and nystagmus, were at one time considered the chief symptoms in multiple sclerosis. The writer would be extremely hesitant in diagnosing multiple sclerosis without the presence of pyramidal tract signs. While sensory disturbances may be present, one would expect to see such changes more often than they occur. The type of sensory loss will depend upon the exact location of the sclerotic patch responsible for it. The tremor which is called an intention or action tremor is made worse by movement. While it is usually best brought out in the finger-to-nose test, any voluntary action on the part of the patient may throw not only the particular part in action, but also the entire body. The disturbance of speech, dysarthric in nature, is probably produced in the same way as the tremor. While it is sometimes of a scanning nature it may simulate the speech of general paresis. Nystagmus, which may be lateral, vertical or rotary or all three, is usually due to a patch of sclerosis in the medulla or pons. The vision may be disturbed in multiple sclerosis long before changes of the fields or eyegrounds. If, however, a careful investigation is kept on the latter, pallor of the disks, especially of a bitemporal nature, will be found. Impairment of the fields, particularly central scotomas for color, is often present and may occur in the absence of changes in the disks. Ocular palsies are not as prominent as pallor of the disks and nystagmus. The abdominal reflexes, due to involvement of the pyramidal tracts, disappear. The symptoms of pseudobulbar palsy, especially the emotional disturbance, and a general euphoric trend may be seen.

A definite psychosis is occasionally seen in multiple sclerosis, and while it may take on the picture of a depression, it is more often characterized by euphoria, excitement and delusions. If the patient with multiple sclerosis lives long enough, he may present the picture of complete dementia. The blood Wassermann is negative, the spinal fluid, as a rule, shows a normal cell count, normal globulin content and a negative Wassermann. The colloidal-gold curve commonly demonstrates an alteration of the paretic type or perhaps the curve is high in the middle. The frequency of the disease, which is slightly more common in males, is disputed. Spiller says it is rare in this country, except possibly in New York, where the foreign population is so large.

Remissions are common in the disease, especially those which begin acutely. The duration is from one to twenty-five years, the average being about ten. A remission may last from a few months to years. The longest which the writer has seen was in a man who developed a hemiplegia which lasted nine months; he then was entirely well for six years when the classical symptoms of multiple sclerosis came on.

Practically every patient suffering from multiple sclerosis becomes chair- or bed-ridden in a few years, although, as in every disease, there are cases which run a benign course.

Diagnosis.—The conditions which may be confused with multiple sclerosis are disseminated neurosyphilis, arteriosclerosis, the combined sclerosis seen in pernicious anemia, Friedreich's ataxia, tumors of the cerebellum and the cerebellopontile angle, tumors of the cord, hysteria, multiple areas of softening, or diseased areas the result of trauma and pseudosclerosis. While some of these conditions undoubtedly will cause confusion at times, mistakes in diagnosis can be kept to a minimum. The signs, symptoms and laboratory findings of neurosyphilis, the blood picture and the gastric analysis in pernicious anemia, signs and symptoms of a tumor, should keep the record clear as far as these conditions are concerned. Because of a remission which may apparently be brought about by psychotherapy, the diagnosis of hysteria is frequently made. A careful examination with the elicitation of signs such as nystagmus and Babinski's sign, which are always due to an organic involvement of the central nervous system, should avoid the hysterical pitfall. In the so-called acute multiple sclerosis a differential diagnosis is extremely hard to make between that form of disease and disseminated encephalomyelitis (Spiller). The mere fact that acute involvement of the nervous system of an apparent inflammatory type clears up does not rule out the possibility that the case may be one of multiple sclerosis. Recently the writer had 2 cases, one still under his care at the Philadelphia General Hospital, of injury to the nervous system simulating multiple sclerosis. One of these cases had been so diagnosed, but at autopsy multiple microscopic lesions were found in the brain, which were probably the result of hemorrhage.

Treatment.—There is no specific for the disease. Arsenicals, germanin, fever therapy, mercury, iodides, bismuth have all been tried without result. The writer has seen a number of cases recently in which infected sinuses were present, but despite clearing them up surgically the disease continued. The patient should be placed in the best possible health, foci of infection removed and freedom from work and worry instituted. Massage and hydrotherapy to keep the muscles and skin in good condition should greatly aid the patient. Later on, as the patient becomes chair- or bed-ridden, careful nursing is required.

THE BRAIN.

FOCAL SIGNS DUE TO LOCALIZED CEREBRAL LESIONS.

Lesions of the *frontal lobe* produce, as a rule, definite changes in the intellectual capacity of the individual. Irritability, loss of memory, undue jocosity, and disorientation in space and position may characterize disease of the frontal lobe. Weakness of the contralateral side of the face may be the only physical sign detected, but it must be interpreted with care inasmuch as many normal persons cannot move both sides of the face equally well. In blinking, the eye on the affected side of the face may close just a little later than its fellow. Lesions at the base of the frontal lobe, especially tumors, may cause diminution or loss of smell, and may also, by pressure on an optic nerve, produce primary optic atrophy on the side of the lesion and choked disk on the opposite side. Lesions of the lower part of the third left prefrontal in a right-handed person will cause motor aphasia. Two patients with hemorrhage over both frontal lobes presented a mental picture similar to Korsakoff's psychosis. The attention is often difficult to obtain and hold. Inattention to the sphincters leads to frequent soiling of the person.

Lesions, especially tumors of the *corpus callosum*, are characterized chiefly by pronounced mental symptoms, due to interference with the association tracts. Memory is defective, speech difficult or impossible and apraxia a common symptom. The mental symptoms are often mistaken for senile dementia or paresis. Patients frequently do not respond to questioning and look blankly at the examiner. A patient with a tumor in the cerebellopontile angle, with secondary atrophy of the corpus callosum, made no effort whatsoever to eat and would have starved to death had he not been fed by the nurse. This man was not paralyzed in any of the extremities. Paralysis or weakness of the extremities may occur, but usually mean extension of the lesion into the motor parts. Cranial nerve symptoms are not present.

The upper part of the *motor cortex* governs movement of the lower part, that is, the toes and foot, of the opposite side of the body. The lowest part of the left motor cortex is in close relation to Broca's area. The center for the lower extremity is supplied by a branch of the anterior cerebral artery, and the rest of the motor cortex by a branch from the middle cerebral artery. An occlusion of the artery supplying the foot and leg centers may produce a monoplegia on the opposite side with the usual signs of pyramidal tract disease. In one case of this sort considerable edema was present, and because of this a diagnosis of phlebitis was considered. Involvement of the motor cortex will produce weakness and finally paralysis of the opposite side of the body, and if the lesion is an irritative one, Jacksonian epilepsy or partial continuous epilepsy may be present on the weakened side. A slowly progressive hemiplegia is quite characteristic of a new growth, a slow hemorrhage or cerebral abscess. Early in the stage of a gradually growing lesion segmental cerebral monoplegia may occur. This is a term used by Spiller to denote a weakness or paralysis of a part of one extremity. Sensory loss does not occur in a lesion which is pre-Rolandic. Subcortical lesions produce a progressive hemiplegia and, in some cases, focal epilepsy. Irritation of the motor cortex, instead of causing frank Jacksonian epilepsy, may produce twitching movements on the opposite side.

Lesions of the *right temporal lobe,* which is in the present state of our knowledge a silent area, are difficult to recognize, and it is only after neighboring structures are involved, that localizing signs can be detected. Lesions deep in the temporal lobe may involve the optic radiation, causing thereby defects in the visual fields of the opposite side, defects which are in the early stage of the condition of a quadrantic nature. Later on hemianopsia is produced.

Lesions involving the *uncinate region* are characterized by peculiar epileptiform seizures. The aura of the seizure is often referred to smell or taste and is frequently, although not always, an unpleasant one. The patient then passes into a peculiar dreamy state and this is followed by tasting or chewing movements. If the visual fibers have been implicated crude visual hallucinations may occur in these attacks which may end in a generalized fit. Lesions of the posterior part of the first and second temporal convolutions on the left in a right-handed person will produce word deafness and jargon or sensory aphasia.

Implication of the *postcentral gyrus* and *parietal lobe* is characterized chiefly by loss of sense of position, point discrimination and localization, and a disturbance of stereognostic perception. The other forms of sensation such as pain, touch, heat and cold are little, if at all, affected. Implication of the *left supramarginal gyrus* may produce apraxia, and of the *left angular gyrus,* word and letter blindness (alexia). If a lesion of this area, such as tumor, grows forward, motor symptoms may be produced; if downward into the subcortical region, the visual fibers may be involved and temporal lobe symptoms also brought about.

Occipital Lobe.—The chief localizing symptom here produced is homonymous hemianopsia in the contralateral visual fields. Irritation of the visual cortex or of the optic radiations may produce visual hallucinations which are crude and often ill-defined.

Implication of the *optic thalamus* produces disturbance or loss of all forms of sensation on the opposite side of the body, accompanied by dysesthetic phenomena. For example, if a piece of ice or a very hot test-tube is placed on the hand of the affected side, the patient cannot appreciate them as cold or hot, but says that it produces a nasty, disgreeable, painful sensation. Deep pressure and scratching with a pin will often produce the same unpleasant sensation. While not pathognomonic of lesions of the optic thalamus, such symptoms are extremely suggestive. Spontaneous disagreeable and painful sensations may occur on the contralateral side. If the *pulvinar* is involved, hemianopsia on the opposite side may occur. Mild lesions of the thalamus may not produce the devastating signs mentioned.

Lesions of the *corpus striatum* produce various types of involuntary movements and rigidity. If the internal capsule is not involved by lesions of the optic thalamus and corpus striatum pyramidal tract signs will not be present on the opposite side.

Involvement of the anterior part of the *internal capsule* produces hemiplegia on the contralateral side. Monoplegia is rarely, if ever, produced by a lesion in this locality. Implication of the posterior part of the internal capsule produces sensory loss and hemianopsia on the opposite side.

Corpora Quadrigemina.—This locality contains functions which are chiefly visual and auditory. The superior corpora quadrigemina have to do with vision, and the inferior, with hearing. The pupils are often dilated and fixed. Paralysis of upward gaze and signs of ocular palsies, especially of the third nerve, are common. Deficiencies of hearing may occur if the inferior colliculi are implicated. Extension of the lesion to the red nucleus and superior cerebellar peduncles produces tremor and ataxia.

Pineal Body.—Lesions of this structure, which are usually tumors, produce in effect the same symptoms as those of the corpora quadrigemina. In addition to the signs enumerated above, pubertas præcox may occur. Tumors of the corpora quadrigemina and of the pineal body cause internal hydrocephalus and choked disk early.

Cerebral Peduncle (Crus Cerebri).—A lesion of the anterior portion of this structure produces one of the typical forms of crossed hemiplegia, namely, third nerve paralysis on the side of the lesion, and the face, arm and leg on the opposite side. This is Weber's syndrome. If, in addition, the dorsal part of the peduncle is involved, tremor and ataxia occur in the opposite limbs. The tremor simulates to some degree that of paralysis agitans, but usually is not decreased on voluntary effort. The ataxia and tremor in such a case are due to implication of the red nucleus. This symptom complex is referred to as Benedikt's syndrome.

Pons.—The type of crossed paralysis found in lesions of the pons is for the fifth, sixth and seventh nerves to be paralyzed on the side of the lesion and the extremities on the opposite side. The common type of paralysis is for the seventh nerve on the ipsolateral side of the body to be involved, and the extremities on the contralateral side. This is Millard-Gubler type of crossed paralysis. The sixth nerve may be implicated in a Millard-Gubler paralysis. Gliomas of the pons may assume great size before definite symptoms are produced. Tumors of the pons do not usually cause choked disk.

Medulla.—Alternating hemiplegia and cranial nerve paralysis may occur from lesions of the medulla. Lesions implicating both pyramidal tracts will produce symptoms of such involvement below the level of the lesion. Occlusion of the posterior inferior cerebellar artery cause softening in the dorso-lateral portion of the medulla, with involvement of the descending root of the fifth nerve and the spinothalamic tract,

75

which causes a crossed sensory paralysis—face on the side of the lesion and extremities and trunk on the opposite.   In addition, certain cranial nerves, especially the ninth and tenth, may be involved.

Cerebellum.—The usual lesion in this structure is a tumor.   The symptoms produced are ipsolateral and consist of asynergia, hypotonia and weakness, which is not, however, of pyramidal tract origin, but is due to the decreased muscle tone.   Alteration in the finger-to-nose test, the Holmes rebound phenomenon, a widened base of support and nystagmus occur in cerebellar lesions.   The gait is ataxic and reeling, is not affected by closure of the eyes, and the patient has a tendency to deviate to the side of the involvement.   The reflexes are reduced or lost and asthenia may be so pronounced as to simulate paralysis. Involvement of the cerebellar peduncles may also produce cerebellar symptoms.

Cerebellopontile Angle.—This is a common location for neoplasms and inflammatory reactions, especially syphilis.   The common tumor is one growing from the sheath of the eighth nerve, producing in effect Ménière's syndrome, that is, dizziness, deafness and tinnitus.   Other cranial nerves, especially the fifth and seventh, may be implicated. When the fifth is involved, symptoms simulating trigeminal neuralgia may occur, but are differentiated by the sensory loss on the affected side.   The seventh nerve may be paralyzed, but irritation of it may produce facial hemispasm or fits of twitching comparable to Jacksonian epilepsy.   Cerebellar symptoms and signs of increased intracranial pressure then ensue.

Pituitary Gland (Hypophysis).—The gland may be the seat of atrophy or enlargement, but the common lesion is a neoplasm, which produces bitemporal hemianopsia.   This, however, may be preceded by minor visual field defects.   Choked disk in pituitary tumor is most uncommon but primary optic atrophy is frequently seen, due to direct pressure on the chiasm.   Fröhlich's syndrome may occur.   Roentgen-ray evidence of involvement of the sella may be found.

APHASIA.

Stewart defines aphasia as impairment or loss of speech, due to the loss of memory for those signs, vocal or written, by means of which we exchange ideas with our fellow-men.   The cortical centers which have to do with speech are on the left side of the brain in a right-handed individual and on the right side in a left-handed individual.   There are three important cortical areas concerned with speech, namely, the lower part of the third left prefrontal, which is the area for motor speech or Broca's area, the posterior part of the first and second temporal convolutions, which has to do with word hearing and sensory speech and is sometimes called Wernicke's zone, and the angular gyrus in which are stored images for words, letters, figures and signs.   Exact and precise localization of important functions in the cortex is denied by some, especially Marie.

Motor aphasia is caused by a lesion of Broca's area.   Because of the proximity of the face, tongue and hand centers to Broca's area, lesions of the latter will often implicate cortical motor centers and produce segmental cerebral monoplegia. In motor aphasia the patient has lost the power, partially or completely, to express himself in spoken words. The extent of the aphasia will vary with the severity of the lesion. He may have slight difficulty with speech or, if the lesion is extensive, speech may be entirely lost. If the disturbance of speech is slight and mistakes are made, the patient usually recognizes them. While the patient may be speechless, he is practically never wordless, but has a recurring utterance which he will use either spontaneously or in reply to questions. Expressions of some of the patients at the Philadelphia General Hospital who had recurrent utterances were as follows: "anyone any," "I know, I know, I know," "all right" "oh, pshaw," and "oh boy, oh boy." Another man named Tommy Kane could say nothing but his name which he would repeat over and over in a sing-song voice. Tommy Kane could also carry the tune of a song, due probably to an intact singing center? The ability to write may be, and usually is, preserved in motor aphasia, although the patient may have to learn to write with the left hand. The power of pantomime is also preserved in motor aphasia. In hysterical loss of speech the patient, as a rule, cannot say any words at all and other evidence of hysteria will be present. Furthermore, during the second stage of etherization the hysteric with loss of speech will talk. The motor acts of speech are stored up in Broca's area, and perhaps in the immediately adjacent parts of the brain.

Involvement of Wernicke's zone or the posterior part of the first and second temporal convolutions on the left produces sensory aphasia, also called jargon aphasia and Wernicke's aphasia. Implication of this particular part of the cortex produces word deafness. The patient is unable to understand perfectly what is said to him, although his hearing is normal. The words are as strange to him as though they were part of a foreign language; he cannot obey commands. In a pronounced type of word deafness he will be unable to follow a simple request, such as "put your right hand on top of your head." On the other hand, the word deafness may be so slight that the patient fails only when given a number of commands at once, as, for example, "walk over to the door, open it, take off your coat and shake hands with me." He must not be shown what to do. He is often unable to name a common object such as a knife or handkerchief which is shown him, although he may be able to use the object perfectly well. Because of his word deafness he is unable to write from dictation or to appreciate mistakes in speaking which he makes. Unlike the motor aphasic who suffers from a paucity of words, the sensory aphasic has plenty of words which he uses in a jargon. Lesions in the word-hearing center are frequently complicated by cuts in the visual fields, due to involvement of the optic radiation.

Visual aphasia (word blindness—alexia) is due to a lesion of the left angular gyrus and produces a condition in which the patient can see words, letters and symbols but cannot interpret them. Here again it is as though he were gazing at a page written in a foreign language. Visual aphasia may vary from slight interruption to a complete loss of ability to name letters and words. He cannot copy sentences. Defects of the visual fields and parietal lobe symptoms may occur on the opposite side, if the lesion extends beyond the angular gyrus. Involvement of all functions which go to make up speech produces *global aphasia.*

Apraxia is the inability to perform simple movements with the extremities when those parts show no loss of power or sensation, and the individual himself no intellectual loss. Apraxia may be either sensory or motor. Lesions anterior to the Rolandic area produce motor apraxia and those behind sensory apraxia. A common test for apraxia is to give the patient a box of matches and a cigarette and tell him to smoke. He will often put the match in his mouth and strike the cigarette. Apraxia is more often produced by lesions of the left hemisphere than those of the right. Lesions of the corpus callosum and frontal lobes, especially, produce apraxia.

The testamentory capacity of patients suffering from various forms of aphasia is often brought up. The uncomplicated cases of motor aphasia will usually have testamentory capacity and a disposing mind. By talking with such an individual his will and desire can be appreciated. On the other hand, it is impossible to communicate sufficiently with the patient suffering from sensory aphasia to know what disposition of his property he might want made, and there is a question if wills made by such patients should be allowed to stand, especially if they are unjust and unreasonable.

DISORDERS OF ARTICULATION.

Articulation has nothing to do with cortical functions but is a function of the bulb and its peripheral mechanisms. A patient with advanced bulbar palsy or pseudobulbar palsy may be unable to put forth a single word, yet he is not speechless. Difficulty in articulation is spoken of as dysarthria and is common, for example, in pseudobulbar palsy. If the disturbance of articulation is advanced it may render the patient unable to say a word or make a sound. This is called *anarthria.* Involvement of articulation may be due to lesions of the cranial nerves or their nuclei, which have to do with speech, to supranuclear involvement, as in pseudobulbar palsy, or to incoördination of the muscles of the lips, tongue, palate, pharynx and larynx. A slurred type of speech is common in alcoholism and paresis. Sometimes the speech of multiple sclerosis may be slurred and simulate that of general paresis. Tremor or involuntary movements affecting the movements of articulation may produce *dysarthria.* In paralysis agitans the voice is monotonous and often has a festinating character. The most common type of speech disturbance is stammering. This is most frequently found in males who are usually above the average intelligence and are frequently of a psychasthenic makeup. *Stammering* is an incoördination between the vocal and oral mechanisms of speech, and the stammerer frequently sticks on an initial consonant or syllable. Stammering is usually increased by excitement, and for the most part disappears when the stammerer sings. Most stammerers acquire certain tricks which aid them to overcome their speech defect; they most commonly make certain grimaces or quick tic-like movements of the body or the extremities. These are often not unlike the tic movements which the psychasthenic shows. When stammering appears it should be treated by exercise and speech-training. While the child may "grow out of it," he will certainly do so more quickly if he has the proper training.

Hysteria may produce certain disturbances in articulation in which the voice may be entirely lost or the patient can speak only in a whisper. *Hysterical mutism* may or may not be accompanied by paralysis, and the patient can always write.

DISEASES OF THE BLOOD-VESSELS OF THE BRAIN.

Etiology.—The commonest condition affecting the blood-vessels of the brain is arteriosclerosis, which may be part of the generalized disease, or it may be limited rather sharply to the vessels of the brain. Vessels which are diseased by arteriosclerosis may rupture, causing a cerebral hemorrhage; they may thrombose, causing secondary softening beyond the point of the lesion; or the cerebral vessels may be the site of aneurysms. On the other hand, a cerebral vessel may be plugged up with an embolus, or it may be implicated by aneurysm produced by the lodging of microörganisms in its wall with subsequent weakness and dilatation. Any vessel of the brain may be the site of vascular insult; but the lenticulo-striate artery is so frequently involved that it has been called the artery of cerebral apoplexy. The result of occlusion of this vessel, or of the middle cerebral, produces the commonest condition seen as the result of vascular injury, namely, *hemiplegia*. The ordinary type of hemiplegia is more frequent in men, and usually occurs after the age of forty or forty-five years. If a "stroke" occurs before forty it is imperative that such things as syphilis, embolism, brain abscess, cerebral tumor and encephalitis be ruled out as the causative factor. The causes of cerebral arteriosclerosis are those of arteriosclerosis in general.

The usual location of hemorrhage or softening is in the region of the internal capsule. The size of a hemorrhage may vary greatly, from a small lesion to a large one, which may involve a great part of the cerebral hemisphere, and which may ultimately rupture into the ventricles. If the patient dies shortly after a cerebral hemorrhage has occurred, the lesion will have the appearance of freshly coagulated blood; later it goes through various color changes, and a cyst or cavity remains. The apoplectic seizure may be initiated by injury, may come on as the result of severe muscle exertion, such as the exertion of paroxysmal coughing, as occur in whooping cough, straining at stool, during coitus, parturition or any severe muscular effort. Many cases of apoplexy occur in patients with low blood pressure. The *apoplectic seizure* may be preceded by certain premonitory symptoms, such as numbness on the side of the body about to be paralyzed, headache, dizziness, vomiting, convulsions or confusion. Many patients have been conscious for months or years that they are the victims of high blood pressure and kidney disease; but, on the other hand, others feel in normal health.   Physical overexertion and anxiety may apparently produce a cerebral attack in middle age, and in supposedly healthy individuals.

Symptoms.—Immediately after a vessel has been damaged the patient usually becomes comatose, although occasionally consciousness is completely retained.   In a patient who has a cerebral hemorrhage the onset is more rapid and the coma deeper than in a patient with thrombosis.   The case of cerebral hemorrhage is hard hit from the start, the breathing stertorous and, at times, of the Cheyne-Stokes type.   The face is flushed; the pupils may be small, normal or dilated, and are frequently unequal.   The corneal reflexes are abolished; the individual is shocked; all the extremities are likely to be flaccid; the deep reflexes, especially on the side of the paralysis, may be destroyed. The plantar reflex will practically always be of the extensor type on the paralyzed side, even though the deep reflexes are lost.   Despite the fact that all the extremities are flaccid and drop helplessly to the side when they are lifted from the bed, those on the paralyzed side are much more toneless than those on the other.   In the stage of shock, swallowing is impossible and the control of the sphincters is lost. Some degree of fever occurs a few hours after the onset, and a steadily rising temperature is a bad sign.   Later on, the presence of fever may be due to pneumonia.   If the urine be examined it will frequently be found to contain evidence of nephritis or of diabetes; however, sugar may be found in the urine as the result of cerebral lesion alone.   If the hemorrhage ruptures into the ventricles the patient becomes extremely ill, signs of meningitis may occur and also convulsions or shivering movements.   The picture of decerebrate rigidity may present itself in patients with hemorrhage into the ventricles.   Pyramidal tract signs are bilateral.   Pronounced respiratory difficulties ensue; the pulse, slow at first, becomes rapid; the temperature may become subnormal or high, and the patient dies, as a rule, within two to seven days.   Lumbar puncture reveals a bloody fluid.

The onset in cerebral thrombosis is usually not so abrupt; premonitory symptoms are more commonly seen, the patient is not so severely shocked; stupor, if present, is not so deep as in hemorrhage.   Furthermore, partial paralysis may exist a number of hours, even a week or more before becoming complete.   This is especially so when the Sylvian artery is thrombosed.

The *optic nerves* will usually show arteriosclerosis and rarely, indeed, signs of neuritis or of choking.   It is the experience of the writer that those cases of hemiplegia associated with optic neuritis or choked disks are usually due to cerebral neoplasm with acute onset.   A conjugate deviation of the eyes, usually toward the side of the cerebral lesion, may be seen.   Most cases of cerebral hemorrhage die.   Sudden death, such a frequent happening in cardiac disease, does not take place from a cerebral hemorrhage no matter how large it may be, but the case usually lingers on for days or weeks.   A patient with cerebral thrombosis has a much better chance to survive.   If he does, he will then present the picture of a hemiplegia, that is, paralysis or weakness of one side of the body with contractures and the signs of pyramidal tract disease.

Sensation is not affected in the ordinary case of hemiplegia, although it may be, if the thalamus or the posterior limb of the capsule is involved. Pain on the paralyzed side is due to thalamic irritation or to joint disease which is especially likely to occur in the shoulder. Early in the history of the case the patient's *speech* will be dysarthric, or even absent. If the left cortex has been involved speech may be greatly affected, and either motor or sensory aphasia or both exist.

Many patients suffering from cerebral vascular disease die within a few weeks; others recover enough power on the affected side to permit their getting up and around. The lower extremity recovers more power than the upper, and the proximal segments of the upper extremity regain more strength than the distal ones; in fact, the ordinary case of hemiplegia who survives regains very little, if any, power in the hand and wrist. In walking, the hemiplegic patient swings the entire lower extremity on the affected side, from the hip; the knee is held rigidly and the toe is scraped along the floor. The arm is slightly abducted, the elbow usually flexed to a right angle, the hand is pronated and bent and the fingers are flexed. Often the hand on the paralyzed side is carried across the lower part of the abdomen, although occasionally it is held in extension at the side. *Contractures* will occur unless attention is directed to their prevention. If the paralysis remains a flaccid one, the patient will not, as a rule, recover function. Continuation of the flaccid palsy on the paralyzed side usually means pronounced involvement of the sensory pathways or the parietal lobe. Atrophy may occur on the paralyzed side and may be due to the cerebral lesion, to inactivity and to ankylosis. *Electrical reactions* remain normal. In a lesion of the thalamus or posterior limb of the capsule all forms of sensation may be seriously affected, hemianopsia may occur and the paralyzed or weak limbs may be the site of disagreeable sensations or actual pain. Pain on the paralyzed side may be produced, especially in a lesion of the thalamus, by testing the patient for sensation; thus, the application of a piece of ice, an extremely hot test-tube or deep pressure on the paralyzed side, or scratching it with a pin may provoke an abnormal response, which has been referred to as *dysesthesia*. While this is characteristic of disease of the thalamus, it may occur from irritation, to the sensory pathways in other parts of the central nervous system.

Trophic disorders may occur on the paralyzed side in the joints, skin or nails and muscular atrophy may be due to trophic disturbances or to joint disease. Occasionally one sees hemiplegia which, after a few hours' duration, clears up suddenly. This is supposed to be due to a spasm of the cerebral vessel similar to that which occurs in the lower extremities in cases of intermittent claudication.

If the carotid artery is thrombosed before it gives off the ophthalmic artery, a syndrome described by Cadwalader and others may be found, namely, blindness on the side of the lesion and a hemiplegia on the opposite side.

Even in the most favorable case a certain amount of reduction in the *mental faculties* of the individual ensues. If the lesion has been a large one, and especially if bilateral changes caused by arteriosclerosis are present, various grades of dementia may be found. Vascular disease involving the pons or medulla may occur. These usually produce a crossed paralysis. Thus, involvement of the pons at the level of the seventh nerve will bring about a peripheral type of paralysis of the face on the side of the lesion and of the extremities on the opposite side. This is the *Millard-Gubler syndrome.* Occlusion of the posterior inferior cerebellar artery produces a crossed paralysis for sensation, pain, heat and cold being lost in the distribution of the fifth nerve on the side of the lesion and on the opposite side of the body. Loss of pain, heat and cold is due to involvement of the descending root of the fifth nerve and the spinothalamic tract. Quite often in occlusion of the posterior inferior cerebellar artery, other cranial nerves, particularly the ninth and tenth, may be involved on the side of the lesion. Hemorrhage into the pons sometimes occurs in brain abscess or tumor or in other conditions producing increased pressure, and frequently causes sudden death.

Occlusion of the branch of the anterior cerebral artery supplying the foot and leg center will cause a *monoplegia* of the lower extremity on the opposite side to the lesion. Occlusion of the Sylvian artery is not an infrequent occurrence, and if the left Sylvian artery be involved, a devastating group of symptoms ensues because of implication of the special centers located on the left side of the brain. Any one of the branches or the Sylvian artery may become affected without involvement of the entire artery; motor aphasia, sensory aphasia, alexia, parietal lobe symptoms or paralysis may ensue without the production of symptoms referable to the entire cortex supplied by the artery.

In considering the *differential diagnosis* of apoplexy, it is necessary to consider all of the things which may produce stupor or coma. One of the most important papers on the relative frequency of the various forms of coma was written by Bissell and Le Count who analyzed the records of 200 patients, admitted to the Cook County Hospital in coma, who died and on whom autopsies were performed. Of the 200 cases 85 were skull fractures, 53 apoplexy, 12 uremia, 10 lobar pneumonia, 8 meningitis and 6 diabetic coma. The rest were due to scattered causes. There is no doubt of the frequency with which *uremia* is overdiagnosed. A great tendency exists to label a patient, unconscious, with paralysis of one side and with albumin and casts in the urine, as a uremic hemiplegic. As a matter of fact, such cases are most often due to cerebral hemorrhage. *Injuries to the head*, especially those cases who suffer cerebral hemorrhage without fracture, can usually be differentiated by the history. *Diabetic coma* can be determined by the analysis of the blood and urine, but it must be remembered that cerebral lesions may produce glycosuria. The diagnosis between *apoplexy* and *postepileptic stupor* can be made in some cases by the record, by the absence of paralysis, although the plantar reflex may be of the extensor type due to cortical exhaustion after a fit. Furthermore, scars will be found upon the face and tongue of the epileptic and he may have the facies peculiar to those people. In some cases an exhaustion paralysis occurs after a series of epileptic fits, especially if they are unilateral. On the other hand, an epileptic may rupture a cerebral vessel (either intra- or extra-cerebral) during a spasm and a hemiplegia result. *Hysterical hemi-plegia* is differentiated in that there are no abnormal reflexes; loss of sensation often exists on the paralyzed side; hearing and vision may be affected on the paralyzed side; other symptoms suggestive of hysteria may be detected. Alcoholic coma can be diagnosed by the history of the individual, the usual absence of pathologic reflexes and of paralysis and the tendency toward delirium and restlessness. Because of the ease with which such *drugs* as barbital and luminal are obtained, patients are not infrequently seen in coma produced by the overuse of those drugs. In the absence of the history, therefore, the diagnosis is difficult. Hematoporphyrin in the urine may give an important clue in patients comatose from such drugs as veronal. *Hyperinsulinism* may produce coma and be accompanied by bilateral pyramidal tract signs. The diagnosis is made on the low sugar content of the blood. Hypoglycemia brought about by other causes may also cause stupor. The writer has seen it in extensive carcinoma of the liver and in a suprasellar tumor. Spontaneous *subarachnoid hemor-rhage* may induce stupor, and, because of the presence of blood in the spinal fluid, may be confused with cerebral hemorrhage with rupture into the ventricles. However, in the latter, the patient is always much sicker than in the former, is more deeply stuporous and will show more extensive paralysis. A patient suffering from a *brain tumor* may have a hemiplegia of apoplectic suddenness due to a hemor-rhage into the tumor. The possibility of brain tumor is often not thought of in such cases, but examination of the eye grounds and estimation of the spinal pressure will help in the diagnosis.

Treatment.—The most important thing under this heading is pro-phylaxis. For this, the reader is referred to the article on arterio-sclerosis. In the acute attack the patient must necessarily be put to bed; the head should be slightly elevated. Olive oil or a simple enema should be given immediately, and if the blood pressure is high vene-section may be practised, especially in those cases in which hemorrhage is suspected. The amount of blood withdrawn should not be over 200 or 300 cc. Owing to the frequency with which hypostatic pneu-monia develops, the patient should be kept off his back and on the paralyzed side as much as possible. The position should be changed frequently. An air-mattress or water-mattress should be used to pre-vent the occurrence of trophic sores. An ice-bag to the head, sedatives for great restlessness and absolute cleanliness of the skin are important considerations in the treatment. If swallowing is either impaired or impossible, great care should be used in giving the patient food or liquids by mouth. For the first two or three days it is better to give liquids by rectum or with a nasal tube, rather than to run the risk of having the patient aspirate it into the lungs. The treatment in the main is symptomatic. The mildest case should be kept in bed at least three weeks.

If the patient survives to become a hemiplegic the paralyzed limb should be given massage and passive movement. These forms of physiotherapy should be employed early in the case, certainly by the end of the first week. Otherwise the tendency toward contractures and joint changes will be great. Electricity is of some service but does most good by acting on the mind of the patient—he feels that something is being done for him. Occasionally orthopedic operations, such as tenotomy, may be employed. Aphasia, if present, may improve spontaneously, but it is usually necessary to attempt to reëducate the individual.

SPONTANEOUS SUBARACHNOID HEMORRHAGE.

This condition is much more frequent than it is commonly thought to be. For it to occur, some weakened blood-vessel wall, either congenital or acquired, must undoubtedly be present. The causes of weakness of the meningeal vessels are syphilis, acute infections, especially meningitis and acute rheumatic fever, and infectious emboli. Syphilis is not nearly so common an etiologic factor as it is in aneurysm of the aorta. Trauma frequently produces subarachnoid hemorrhage if the vessels are normal and it may break an already weakened one. Arteriosclerosis of the meningeal vessels may also be a factor.

Symptoms.—The onset of a subarachnoid hemorrhage is, as a rule, sudden. In a series of 15 cases which McIver and the writer reported the onset was abrupt in all and was occasionally preceded by severe muscular effort. Dizziness and headache are frequent symptoms, and then the individual becomes stuporous or delirious. The neck becomes stiff, and Kernig's sign is nearly always present. The pupils may be of any size, and occasionally one or more cranial nerves is affected. A complete hemiplegia, such as seen in intracerebral hemorrhage, is not present, although there may be weakness on one side of the body, usually more marked in the face and upper extremity. The tendon reflexes vary greatly; they may be increased or in some cases decreased. The pathologic Babinski toe sign is sometimes seen on one side or both. If the patient is not completely stuporous he will probably complain of a severe headache, associated perhaps with vomiting. Tenderness upon pressure may, now and then, be noted on the side of the hemorrhage. The eye grounds may reveal swelling and, if the retinal vessels are choked, hemorrhage may occur. The pulse and respiration may be slow or rapid, depending upon the intracranial pressure and shock, and a moderate rise of temperature frequently exists. Glycosuria and hyperglycemia have been found at times and may lead to an erroneous diagnosis of diabetic coma. The spinal fluid is bloody and the pressure increased; days after the onset the fluid is yellow.

Diagnosis.—The diagnosis of spontaneous subarachnoid hemorrhage is not considered often enough as a possibility in a patient with a stupor. Meningitis, encephalitis, uremia, diabetic coma and intracerebral hemorrhage with rupture into the ventricles were the diagnoses most frequently made. The outlook in most cases of subarachnoid hemorrhage is good.

Treatment.—Spinal drainage, limitation of the fluids to 500 to 1000 cc. in twenty-four hours, a moderate dose of magnesium sulphate, by mouth or rectum, and an intravenous injection of dextrose will decrease the intracranial pressure and bring about an improvement in the patient's condition. Intravenous injections of a blood coagulant will also tend to limit the bleeding. If the patient is allowed to drift along the increased intracranial pressure will frequently lead to death. If complete recovery does not take place permanent disability may result, due to such complications as epilepsy, mental retardation and motor weakness.

SINUS THROMBOSIS.

The various sinuses of the brain may be occluded either as the result of infection or as a terminal state in such conditions as tuberculosis, paresis, cardiac disease and after any long-standing debilitating disease. The type of sinus thrombosis produced by infections is frequently complicated by meningitis or brain abscess, and also by extradural collections of pus. The sinus most frequently involved is the lateral sinus which is affected secondarily to disease of the ear. The cavernous sinus may be implicated by infections about the face, especially those on the upper lip and about the tip of the nose. The common cause of thrombosis of the superior longitudinal sinus is long-standing illness.

The sinus thrombosis may be localized or may be very extensive, especially in the type produced by infections. The walls of the sinus may be eroded, and death occur suddenly from hemorrhage. The color and state of the thrombus will depend upon the age and its cause. Cerebral hemorrhage may occur, especially when the superior longitudinal sinus is thrombosed, because the brain cannot properly be drained of blood, and hyperemia and bleeding ensue.

Symptoms.—Symptoms of occlusion of the superior longitudinal sinus are as follows: signs of increased intracranial pressure are present, often accompanied by paralysis, which is due, as a rule, to cortical bleeding. Convulsions may also occur. These may be generalized or Jacksonian. In one patient the fits were Jacksonian, involving one side of the body at a time; as the convulsive movements ceased on one side they began on the other. Signs of meningitis may be present.

Thrombosis of the cavernous sinus produces swelling of the eyelids on the affected side, swelling at the root of the nose, exophthalmos and, as a rule, paralysis of all the ocular nerves on that side. Visual disturbances are common, and there may be choking of the disk. Implication of the ophthalmic division of the fifth nerve may cause pain in its distribution. The opposite cavernous sinus may be involved secondarily. Thrombosis of the sigmoid or the lateral sinus may produce a swelling at the upper part of the jugular vein, which may be palpated. Swelling in the mastoid region, signs of meningitis and occasionally paralysis of the lower cranial nerves on the affected side may be discovered. A modification of the Queckenstedt test, the Toby-Ayer test, may produce valuable evidence in lateral sinus thrombosis. In this test the pressure on the jugular vein on the normal side causes a rise in the spinal pressure, whereas if the jugular vein is thrombosed there will be no rise. Occasionally in cases of infections of the ear the so-called *Gradenigo syndrome* may be present. The chief symptom of this is a paralysis of the sixth nerve on the side of the lesion and occasionally symptoms indicative of implication of the sensory fifth. These symptoms are due to an aseptic meningitis which may quickly disappear; however, there is always cause for alarm in the possibility of meningitis or abscess.

Signs of meningitis make it imperative to perform a lumbar puncture. Only enough fluid should be withdrawn, however, to determine the color and transparency, to count the cells and make a smear for organisms. The withdrawal of a large amount of fluid may aid in production of meningitis. The fluid may contain an excess of cells and no organisms. On the other hand, there may be signs of an infecting agent present.

The outlook in cases of sinus thrombosis is bad, especially when the superior longitudinal or the cavernous sinus is affected. Sepsis, pyemia and meningitis are causes of death in the majority of cases of involvement of the cavernous and lateral sinuses.

There is no successful *treatment* for thrombosis of the superior longitudinal sinus. Ligation of the facial vein should be employed as a prophylaxis against the involvement of the cavernous sinus. Operative treatment in cases of lateral sinus thrombosis offers the patient hope and cure. Brain abscess will have to be treated surgically, if it occurs, and meningitis will be treated accordingly.

CEREBRAL ANEURYSM.

Infectious emboli lodging in the walls of the cerebral vessels may, by causing later on a weakness of the wall at that point, produce aneurysms which, however, may also be due to arteriosclerosis. While syphilis is the great cause of aneurysms of the aorta, it is not such a prominent factor in producing those of cerebral vessels. The arteries at the base of the brain are more frequently involved and aneurysms are likely to be multiple. They are usually small but occasionally attain a fairly large size before rupturing. The parts of the brain in the immediate vicinity of a cerebral aneurysm will undergo a pressure atrophy. Trauma may play a rôle in the production of a cerebral aneurysm and it is certain that sufficient trauma can cause the rupture of a cerebral aneurysm already present.

Before the rupture occurs the disease may produce such *symptoms* as headache, often referred to the side on which the aneurysm exists, and vomiting and dizziness. A murmur may be heard over the skull. This may be localized or over a widespread area. A murmur may also be heard over the skull in rickets, hydrocephalus, hyperthyroidism and occasionally over a neoplasm. General signs of increased pressure are rarely found. If an aneurysm ruptures, which it may do either spontaneously or as a result of trauma or severe muscular effort, a massive hemorrhage may occur if the entire coat of the vessel is perforated, or slow bleeding may take place into the subarachnoid space. If the aneurysm is near the ventricular system and ruptures into it, signs of intraventricular hemorrhage will exist. On the other hand, oozing from an aneurysm of moderate size or the rupture of an aneurysm of small size may produce the syndrome of subarachnoid bleeding. In the case reported by Winkelman and the writer, an aneurysm at the base involving the vertebral artery, hemorrhage occurred into the pons, although the aneurysm itself did not rupture. Aneurysm of the large vessels of the brain other than those at the base will produce symptoms referable to the parts of the brain involved. The optic and olfactory nerves may be pressed upon by an aneurysm of the anterior cerebral artery, and an aneurysm of the internal carotid may affect the ocular nerves in addition to the optic and olfactory and even occasionally the fifth. If the aneurysm perforates into the cavernous sinus, pulsating exophthalmos may occur. The pulsation of an aneurysm, as in the case of the aorta, may erode bone and cause pressure atrophy.

The *diagnosis* of cerebral aneurysm is extremely difficult and is rarely made during life. In a patient suffering from subarachnoid bleeding, non-traumatic in origin, it is fair to assume the hemorrhage has been due to the rupture of a small aneurysm. The outlook is bad in cases of cerebral aneurysm, especially if the one which is present involves a large vessel. In cases of ordinary subarachnoid hemorrhage the prospects are good. The treatment, in general, is that of subarachnoid hemorrhage and of cerebral hemorrhage.

BRAIN TUMORS.

The brain may be the seat of primary and secondary neoplasms. Of the ones affecting the brain primarily, those most frequently seen are gliomata, endotheliomata and sarcomata. Of neoplasms involving the brain secondarily the most common is carcinoma. Infectious new growths, such as abscess, tuberculomata and gummata, are observed.

Pathology.—The most common brain tumor is a *glioma,* and it accounts for 40 to 50 per cent of all intracranial neoplasms. It appears as a grayish or reddish infiltrating growth, the color depending upon the vascularity of the tissue and whether or not the growth has been a seat of hemorrhage. Circumscribed and occasionally cystic and encapsulated gliomas may be seen. The usual types of glioma are spongioblastoma, astrocytoma and medulloblastoma. The former is usually seen in middle life, occurs in the hemispheres, is malignant and attains large size. An astrocytoma is more benign, has a tendency to become cystic and may involve the cerebrum or cerebellum. A medulloblastoma is a rapidly growing neoplasm which often spreads through the subarachnoid space, and occurs most frequently in the mid-line of the cerebellum in children. This type of tumor can be held in check by radiation. Gliomata occur most frequently in the hemispheres, are usually single and are frequently the site of degeneration and hemorrhage. They grow slowly, and it is possible for the nerve fibers to function through a gliomatous tumor for a considerable period before the function of the fiber is destroyed.

Endothelioma (fibroblastoma, meningioma) usually arises from the arachnoid or dura, and may occasionally become calcified, when it is called a psammoma. Fibroblastomata produce hyperostosis of the cranium, or occasionally thinning or even erosion of the bone. Often, quite a "bossing" of the skull occurs. Acoustic fibromata are benign circumscribed growths, usually growing from the dural sheath of the eighth nerve. It may occur as bilateral angle tumors. Gardner reported a large series of angle tumors occurring in one family. *Tuberculoma* may be single or multiple, usually the latter, and is secondary to tuberculosis elsewhere in the body. It usually has a connective tissue capsule and frequently central caseation occurs. Rarely the tubercle becomes calcified and does not produce symptoms. A diffuse tuberculous meningitis is a common end-result of a tuberculoma. They are probably more predominant in children, grow slowly and are seen most frequently in the cerebellum, pons and cortex.

Gummata are rare and usually multiple. Gummatous meningoencephalitis is common, but an isolated gumma of the brain is not. A gumma is soft and gelatinous at first, and later on may become fairly firm.

Adenomata occur in the pituitary gland and are extremely important in relation to acromegaly and Fröhlich's syndrome.

Sarcomata are either primary or secondary and single or multiple. They usually grow from the meninges into the brain and may be encapsulated or invasive. Most sarcomata are hard. They may be secondary from sarcomata elsewhere in the body. *Other tumors*, such as cholesteatoma, dermoid cysts and teratomata, are rare.

Carcinoma is practically always secondary in the brain, grows rapidly, is usually multiple and is quite vascular. The presence of carcinoma anywhere in the body should always be ruled out before operating upon a brain tumor suspect. This is especially important when a person is above the age of forty years.

Angiomata arise from the blood-vessels of the meninges and may be associated with birthmarks on the scalp or face. Angiomata are especially likely to be seen in the precentral region. *Lindau's disease* consists of angioma of the brain and angiomatosis of the retina.

The *cause* of brain tumors is in the same maze of uncertainty as tumors elsewhere in the body. Their relation to trauma is a most important one, especially from a medico-legal aspect. Endotheliomata are undoubtedly sometimes due to trauma. The general symptoms of a brain tumor may be abruptly brought on by head injury, but it is extremely doubtful if the tumor itself can be produced by trauma.

Symptoms.—The expressions of brain tumors are both general and focal. The most constant symptom is headache and, while it may be occasionally absent, it practically always occurs sometime in the history of the case. Severe *headache*, especially if associated with dizziness and vomiting, should always arouse suspicion of a cerebral neoplasm. The headache is usually generalized, but may be located either in the occipital or frontal regions when it may be associated with local tenderness. This is especially seen over dural tumors. Headache is due to stretching of the dura. *Choked disk* or papillo-edema is an extremely characteristic symptom of brain tumor and occurs in approximately 75 per cent of cerebral neoplasms. On the other hand, the presence of choked disk indicates a brain tumor in at least 90 per cent of the cases. If a patient, therefore, presents papilloedema, the chances are about 10 to 1 that he has brain tumor, and the burden of the proof is on him who propounds another diagnosis. Choked disk is most frequently seen in a tumor which causes increased ventricular pressure, and is an extremely common sign in tumors in the posterior fossa. It is usually bilateral, but frequently is more pronounced on one side. It is possible to have a high degree of choking disk without much change in vision, although, as a rule, the condition leads to changes in the visual fields, impairment of vision, which may go on to blindness, and secondary optic atrophy. Blindness may occur suddenly. Choked disk is extremely uncommon in tumors of the pituitary which produce, as a rule, optic atrophy. *Vomiting* may occur at any time, and is a particularly common symptom in the tumors of the posterior fossa; it is due to irritation of the centers in the medulla. Vomiting is not, as a rule, associated with with nausea, it has no relation to meals and may or may not be of the projectile type. Hiccoughing is a rare symptom. *Dizziness* as a symptom of brain tumor is frequently due to neoplasm in the posterior fossa and those which involve the vestibulbar pathways. Sudden change of position may induce vertigo, especially if the tumor is in the fourth ventricle.

While *convulsions* may occur at any time in the history of a neoplasm, they are infrequent. On the other hand, the occurrence of convulsive seizures after the age of twenty-five or thirty years should arouse the suspicion of a brain tumor. Attacks simulating petit mal, loss of consciousness and status epilepticus may sometimes be seen in brain tumors. Jacksonian fits and partial continuous epilepsy are of focal rather than general significance. Disturbance in the rhythm of the pulse and respiration occur, most frequently due to tumors in the posterior fossa and are due to medullary compression. The pulse becomes slow and the respiratory rate is decreased; even Cheyne-Stokes breathing may be seen. Sudden respiratory failure is a fairly common cause of death in brain tumor, and in such cases the heart may continue to beat for some time after respiration has ceased. Mental changes may occasionally be classified under the general symptoms of brain tumor but, if stupor and drowsiness are excepted, mental changes are more frequently focal symptoms. In a recent brain tumor of the left frontal lobe the man was slightly disoriented and aphasic; in addition, he would get out of bed, walk to the corner of the ward in a casual manner and urinate. To evacuate his bowels, he always went to the bathroom. The facial expression, especially of the patient who has a high degree of choked disk or a tumor of the corpus callosum, may be characteristic.

Alteration of the temperature, which may be either subnormal or increased, is a rare symptom of a brain tumor. Glycosuria and diabetes insipidus are focal rather than general symptoms.

Localizing Symptoms.—It is important to record the symptoms and signs in the order of their development. The earlier a symptom or sign appears, the more important it is from a focal standpoint. Late appearing symptoms have to be largely discounted. For example, the occurrence of a sixth nerve palsy early in the history of a brain tumor may have some importance as a focalizing sign, but if it occurs late it may be and usually is due to general increase of intracranial pressure. Sometimes a posterior fossa tumor produces symptoms referable to the frontal lobes, and the exact reverse may occur. It is not infrequent that well-marked general symptoms of a brain tumor exist, and few, if any, focalizing signs are seen. The onset of the general and localizing symptoms in a brain tumor are usually insidious, but occasionally they may occur with epileptiform suddenness. Winkelman and the writer reported a series of cases, chiefly from the wards of the Philadelphia General Hospital, illustrating this point. Acute alcoholism and injury to the head often serve as the precipitating factor. It is likely that the cases of hemiplegia supposedly due to vascular disease, and associated with choked disk, are instances of brain tumors with sudden onset. When the physician is confronted with a patient suffering with headache, dizziness, choked disk and perhaps some localizing signs, a systematic investigation of the patient along the following lines should be instituted: A careful and painstaking history of the case with the date of onset and the order of the occurrence of the symptoms should be obtained. A complete and exhaustive physical examination including not only neurologic and mental, but of the body as a whole, should be made. For example, in a person suspected of having a brain tumor it is important to know whether or not he has a carcinoma, tuberculosis or syphilis, and it is also necessary to be certain that the individual does not have nephritis or malignant hypertension. The possibility of sinus disease, producing as it sometimes does headache, optic neuritis and perhaps double vision, should be looked into. The presence of pus anywhere in the body, but especially about the head, is of vital importance when the possibility of brain tumor is under discussion. The characteristic distribution of the headache in migraine with its periodicity, family history and distinctive symptoms should keep the diagnostician straight, but in a patient with migraine who exhibits paralytic phenomena, such as temporary hemiplegia, monoplegia or hemianopsia, a diagnosis of brain tumor may be persisted in, even to the point of operation. During the years in which epidemic encephalitis was common, mistakes were frequent in both directions. Patients proved at operation or necropsy to have brain tumors were frequently carried along for weeks or months with a diagnosis of encephalitis, largely because of the presence of stupor.

The existence of choked disks is extremely important both from the positive and negative standpoint. It occurs in at least 75 per cent of brain tumors and, if present, usually indicates a neoplasm. Choking of the disk is an extremely important negative sign if the diagnosis of encephalitis or of tumor of the pituitary region are considered. Choking is an extremely uncommon finding in both of these conditions.

Papillo-edema may occur in sinus thrombosis, sinusitis and meningitis. An expert ophthalmologist can usually distinguish between the eye-ground changes of a tumor and those which occur in uremia, malignant hypertension and toxemias in general. Unilateral choked disk may sometimes be seen on the side of a brain tumor. On the other hand, it may be due to focal infection. Choking of the disk may occasionally be seen without the general symptoms of a brain tumor. In a case which was seen by the writer some years ago the disks were swollen to 6 diopters with impairment of vision; other symptoms, except fatigue and slight headache, were absent. This man made a complete recovery, but no reason was found for the choking. Careful studies of the visual fields often give valuable information and should never be neglected.

Diagnosis.—The term "pseudotumor" is often used when a patient has been operated upon and no tumor found. Instead of "pseudo-tumor" it should be called "pseudodiagnosis." Two patients with inflammatory reactions involving the seventh and eight nerves were given Bárány tests and the findings were reported as conclusive of a tumor in the angle. It was indeed difficult to save these patients from operation, yet both of them made complete recovery without surgical intervention. Had they been operated upon and nothing found, the condition might have been classified as "pseudotumor." A slowly progressive hemiplegia due to thrombosis of the middle artery, especially that part in the Sylvian fissure, may prove troublesome in differentiating it from a brain tumor.

The history and the absence of focal signs of a brain tumor should help in the diagnosis. Neurosyphilis should always be considered and ruled out before the patient is subjected to operation for brain tumor. General paresis, especially, should be eliminated. Occasionally a brain tumor may develop in a syphilitic, who has positive laboratory findings in the blood and spinal fluid. If such a patient does not improve after a reasonable amount of antisyphilitic therapy, the possibility of a non-specific tumor or a gumma, which cannot be dissolved by treatment, should be made and operation advised. Hydrocephalus, either acute or chronic, may produce symptoms closely resembling those of a brain tumor. However, the history and the usual absence of focal signs will help to clear up the diagnosis. If a case of multiple sclerosis begins abruptly, especially with visual changes, optic neuritis and signs which might be focalizing ones, such as Jacksonian epilepsy, it may be mistaken for and operated upon for brain tumor.

Roentgen Diagnosis.—Roentgen-ray plates of the skull, if read by an expert constantly seeing tumor cases, will often give important information. E. P. Pendergrass, of the University of Pennsylvania, has kindly written the following:

"The roentgen examination of the head is becoming increasingly more valuable in the diagnosis of tumors of the vault and of the brain. Tumors of the vault can be easily demonstrated by the changes that occur in the bones that make up the skull, such as fibroblastomas and osteomas. Bone disease, such as syphilis, tuberculosis and fibrosing osteitis, is also easily demonstrable, and the appearance of these

76

diseases is usually very easily differentiated. In diagnosing intracranial lesions, there are two groups: sellar and intrasellar. One can diagnose a pituitary tumor in approximately 97 per cent of the cases, and possibly the percentage may be increased when there is a correlation of clinical and roentgenologic findings. The diagnosis of an extrasellar tumor is somewhat more difficult, and depends upon several factors: (1) Calcification within the tumor is seen in some gliomas and endotheliomas, and there may occur calcification of suprasellar tumors such as Rathke's pouch tumor and in tuberculoma. (2) The changes in the dorsum sellæ are due to a blocking of the ventricular system, such as occurs in tumors involving the pineal, the angle, fourth ventricle and cerebellum. In fact, anything that will block the ventricular system will show an atrophy of the dorsum sellæ. Another valuable sign is the displacement of the pineal body. This may be of localizing evidence. It is almost impossible to diagnose frontal lobe tumors by roentgen-ray examination unless there is a displacement of the pineal body or some other procedure such as encephalography or ventriculography is used."

The injection of air into the ventricles, as introduced by Dandy, is a decided help in some cases. This is done by removal of a small button of bone in the occipital region, the withdrawal of some ventricular fluid and injection of air. Part of the ventricular system may be obliterated, distorted or the system may present alteration in its size and shape. This procedure, which is not without danger, should be done only after a careful neurologic examination has failed to reveal conclusive focalizing signs, and an operation should be done immediately after the plates have been read, but only if they show signs of focal value. Examination of the fluid removed by ventricular tap often gives valuable information. *Encephalography* is a risky procedure in a brain tumor suspect, and should under no circumstances be done if the pressure is above 16 mm. of mercury.

Lumbar Puncture.—Whether or not this should be done in patients suffering from cerebral neoplasm is a disputed point. It is not as dangerous as some writers contend. If the spinal tap is done carefully, a small needle used and no fluid withdrawn if the pressure is above 16 mm. of mercury, practically no danger will occur to the patient. The great risk in this procedure is in tumors in the posterior fossa. Quite a few of these patients succumb suddenly, due to respiratory failure. If a lumbar puncture had been done upon such a patient this would have been blamed for the death. Under no circumstances should a large amount of fluid be taken out if the spinal pressure is elevated, but enough can be removed so that the important laboratory examinations on the fluid may be performed. In a patient suspected of having a tumor and without choking, an examination of the spinal fluid is indicated, not only for pressure but also for syphilis.

The Bárány tests are of great value in localizing tumors in the cerebellopontile angle or in saying that a tumor does not exist in that region. Otherwise little help is obtained from these tests.

Treatment.—The treatment of brain tumors is surgical. Brilliant results may be obtained, although most cases do poorly. Roentgen-ray treatment is of value in a small group. Dehydration, by the limiting of fluid intake to 500 cc. in twenty-four hours, the intravenous injection of 50 cc. of 50 per cent glucose and the use of magnesium sulphate by mouth or rectum, is frequently indicated in cases of brain tumors who go into stupor or collapse before operation can be performed.

INJURIES OF THE BRAIN.

In the analysis of a patient suffering from head injury, it is important to know the following:

1. The length of the period of unconsciousness.
2. Whether paralysis or other localized cerebral symptoms existed.
3. Whether there was bleeding or escape of cerebrospinal fluid from the orifices, especially the ears.
4. Evidence by roentgen-ray of fracture of the skull.
5. Was the spinal fluid bloody?
6. Were there convulsions?
7. Proved post-traumatic dislocation or distortion of the ventricles.

A blow to the head may be followed by a fracture of the skull, injury to the brain or the meninges, cerebral blood-vessels or the cranial nerves. Injury to the brain, vessels or cranial nerves, especially the vessels, may occur in the absence of definite fracture of the skull and the blow producing such injuries may be slight. On the other hand, many patients suffer from fracture of the skull with little or no involvement of the brain. A blow producing fracture of the skull or injury to the brain may be direct or indirect, and is usually followed by at least momentary loss of consciousness which may, however, be very deep and lasting. The varieties of fractures are similar to those seen elsewhere in the body, although the commonest kind of fracture is the simple, linear type; depressed and comminuted ones are infrequently seen. A blow on one side of the head may occasionally produce a fracture on the other side (contrecoup). Fracture of the skull due to bullets or shrapnel wounds will vary according to the size of the missile and its velocity. In many cases it is likely to cause more or less splintering of the bone. The blow to the head, with or without fracture, may also produce *concussion*. In many instances of concussion, a simple molecular alteration in the cerebral cells occurs, but it is probably true that most cases of concussion are accompanied by actual microscopic changes in the cells with secondary degeneration. The vessels of the brain may be torn and extensive injury and laceration of the brain may be seen. A depressed bone may produce symptoms, as may also a collection of blood and the edema which follows a cerebral commotion. Either or both tables of the bone may be fractured, although the inner one is more usually involved. Numerous hemorrhages may be seen scattered through the brain of a person who has died from concussion. Evidence of local injury to the skull may be present in the form of contusion or laceration, and ecchymoses are common about the eyes and the mastoid region. Those which occur in the latter area are called Battle's sign, which may not appear for a number of hours. Bleeding from the orifices of the head usually means fracture at the base, and cerebrospinal fluid may escape as the result of such injuries. In the presence of a compound or comminuted fracture, or a fracture at the base of the skull with escape of blood or spinal fluid from the mouth, nose or ears, infection of the meninges or actual brain abscess is more likely to occur, but such infection may also come on after a simpler fracture. The best illustration of a simple concussion of the ·brain is the knock-out punch given to a prize-fighter, the period of unconsciousness lasting but a few seconds; on emerging from unconsciousness the patient may suffer from headache, dizziness and vomiting. The headache may be occipital, frontal or generalized and is often referred to the neck.

Vertigo ranks second to headache in frequency as a symptom after cerebral concussion, and is often accompanied by nausea and vomiting. The patient is irritable, lacks concentration, complains of poor memory, insomnia and lack of energy and inability to work, most of these symptoms being especially common in litigation cases, and those who were injured at work and strive to receive compensation. It must always be remembered, however, that even a slight blow on the head may be followed by small hemorrhages scattered through the brain. The duration of the symptoms following concussion varies greatly and one of the factors which has important bearing on the length of symptoms is the question of litigation. After the acute stage has been passed, headache, dizziness and fatigue are commonly complained of, and the importance of them is difficult to evaluate. Investigation by means of the Bárány tests in those cases complaining of dizziness occasionally shows evidence interpreted as being due to interference in the function of the vestibular fibers, although the importance of such a finding is discounted by many. Amnesia for the accident and for the events immediately preceding and following it is common.

The *prognosis* in simple concussion of the brain is good; one of the most important things on which to base the prognosis is the length of the period of unconsciousness. Cases may be cured only to relapse, especially if legal complications occur. A patient of the writer's at the Episcopal Hospital, who suffered a severe concussion with stupor for one hour, recovered completely in three weeks, having been kept isolated completely during that time. She was discharged from the hospital without a complaint, consulted a lawyer of questionable reputation, and within a week had headache and dizziness. The desire to get well is an important consideration in a head injury case.

Fracture of the skull is accompanied by some degree of unconsciousness in practically every case, although the length of unconsciousness may vary from a few minutes to hours or days, and the patient may remain in a stupor until he dies. There is usually a swelling at the site of injury and later about the eyes or mastoid region. Fracture of the base is especially likely to be accompanied by injury to the cranial nerves, especially the sixth, seventh and eighth; a general increase of intracranial pressure will produce swelling of the optic nerves. The pupils are usually unequal with a dilated pupil on the side of the cerebral injury, although they may be small and fixed to light. If a hemorrhage occurs it compresses the brain, or if the latter has been contused and is edematous, stupor may be profound, the pulse slow and the respiratory rate slow and often of the Cheyne-Stokes variety. Focal signs will depend upon the presence of a depressed fracture, collections of blood over the cortex or injury to the brain itself. As the patient regains consciousness he is confused, amnesic, delirious or even psychotic. On two occasions the writer has seen a picture of Korsakoff's psychosis following severe injury to the brain. While mental symptoms are, of course, frequently due to the injury, a careful history of the patient's habits as regards alcohol should be obtained, because in many instances the mental symptoms are more pronounced and prolonged due to the alcoholic tendencies of the individual. The possibility of cerebral syphilis in one of its forms being brought out or aggravated by a head injury should also be borne in mind. Not infrequently a man works successfully and intelligently up to the time of his injury, from which he passes immediately into the stage of general paresis. Brain tumors may be present and produce no symptoms before a head injury and afterward produce marked signs, which may be confused with those due to the trauma. If the fracture has gone through a sinus, or if the dura has been ruptured, pneumocephalus may be found on roentgen-ray examination. Lumbar puncture, which should always be done in a case of head injury, will often reveal a bloody fluid and sometimes increased pressure. When the patient recovers, the same symptoms that are found after a concussion are complained of but usually in a more marked degree and, as in cerebral concussion, the duration of these symptoms frequently has a direct relationship to the presence or absence of litigation. The mental symptoms that are seen after a fracture of the skull consist of loss of memory, fatigability, loss of inhibition and of attention and change in personality. Mental symptoms of a hysterical nature are occasionally seen. Severe injuries to the brain are followed by epilepsy in a certain percentage of cases, which has been estimated from 5 to 36. Seven to 10 per cent would probably be nearer the truth. The epileptic attacks may be localized or focal in type, and while the first fit may occur during the stage of acute injury, it may be delayed a number of years. Injury to the motor cortex naturally produces more instances of post-traumatic epilepsy than injury to other parts of the brain, but implication of parts remote from the motor cortex may be succeeded by convulsions.

Epidural hemorrhage or *subarachnoid hemorrhages* may occur from a head trauma with or without fracture. Bleeding may come on as a result of rupture of the middle meningeal artery or vein, or may be due to a tearing of the sinus. Just as a fracture of the skull may be produced by a blow on the opposite side, so also may a traumatic hemorrhage of the brain occur on the side opposite to that to which the force was applied. The frequency of epidural hemorrhage, due to bleeding from the middle meningeal supply, has been greatly overestimated, but the importance of recognizing the syndrome producing it is extremely necessary. The typical history is as follows: A patient receives a blow on the head which produces momentary unconsciousness, he recovers and may even resume his work or participate in a football game and then, after a period which varies from a few minutes to weeks and in which the individual is gradually accumulating blood over the cortex, he becomes dull, stuporous and unconscious, with signs of increased intracranial pressure, although the latter may be absent. In fact, the spinal pressure may be actually lower than normal. Weakness develops on the side opposite to the hemorrhage, is progressive and is frequently accompanied by twitching or convulsions. The pulse and respirations are slow, and the respirations may be of the Cheyne-Stokes type. Signs of pyramidal tract disease are present on the paralyzed side, although, if the parietal cortex is involved, the deep reflexes may be lost. Signs of meningitis are not usually present, although if bleeding also occurred at the base, the neck may be stiff.

In the *diagnosis* the history is most important. In subarachnoid bleeding, which may be confused with epidural hemorrhage, the spinal fluid is bloody, whereas in the latter it is colorless although it may be of a yellowish tinge. The treatment of the vast majority of head injuries is medical, the great exception is rupture of the middle meningeal artery where prompt and efficient surgery is life saving. Complete rest, an ice-bag to the head, sedatives if the patient is restless or delirious, a continuous but if maniacal excitement exist, a daily lumbar puncture if bloody spinal fluid is present, limitation of fluid to 750 to 1000 cc. in twenty-four hours and magnesium sulphate by mouth or rectum is the line usually pursued by the writer. Physical restraint may be necessary.

Chronic subdural hematoma is a collection of blood between the dura and the arachnoid membranes, as a rule over the convexity of the cerebral hemisphere. The blow to the head responsible for the condition may be severe or extremely trivial. The latent period between the receipt of the blow and the appearance of symptoms may vary from hours to months, and, according to some, more than a year. In some cases the lesion is bilateral. In addition to trauma, it may occur in such conditions as general paresis, in hemorrhagic diathesis and in infections, but in these cases it is likely that a forgotten blow may have been the real cause of the bleeding. The inner surface of the dura is thickened either locally, or more or less extensively. Evidence exists of inflammation as well as of hemorrhage. A combination of hemorrhage and inflammation leads in time to marked thickening of the inner layer of the dura with adherence to the arachnoid. The contents of the hemorrhagic cysts vary from a thin yellowish-brown fluid to a firm clot. External hydrocephalus will be pronounced. The onset of *symptoms* may be apoplectiform or insidious. Mental symptoms consisting of dullness, irritability and delirium are common, and headache, vomiting and convulsions are frequently seen. The convulsions may be either focal or general. Stupor, followed by pronounced coma with slow pulse and respiratory rate or Cheyne-Stokes breathing, may occur. Signs of meningitis, hemiplegia or monoplegia, and papillo-edema are seen in some cases. The hemiplegia may be present on the side of the lesion, due to pressure on the opposite crus.

Automatic states and amnesia, disturbances of speech and of vision may be present if the hemorrhage involves other specialized areas. Fracture of the skull may or may not be determined by roentgen-ray.

The *spinal fluid* shows, as a rule, increased pressure, may be bloody or simply xanthochromic. The deep reflexes are frequently unequal, usually increased, but if the parietal cortex is involved they may be absent on the contralateral side. Cranial nerve symptoms are usually discovered if hemorrhage has occurred at the base. There may be localized tenderness to percussion of the skull. The *diagnosis* is not easy; strict attention should be paid to a patient with head symptoms, who has suffered a cranial trauma in the weeks preceding the onset of his illness, with the thought that cerebral hemorrhage may have happened. Coma may deepen or disappear in remissions. The *treatment* of the condition is surgical, especially in traumatic cases.

DISORDERS OF THE CENTRAL NERVOUS SYSTEM OCCURRING AT BIRTH.

Injury to the central nervous system during birth is common and accounts for a large percentage of the deaths of babies. Blood found in the spinal fluid of babies immediately after birth usually means injury, and bloody spinal fluid has been found in the new-born in a large percentage of cases. This does not necessarily imply that the obstetrician is in any way at fault. The usual cause is disproportion between the baby and the birth canal. Injury to the central nervous system during birth is a common cause of infantile hemiplegia, cerebral diplegia, the various grades of feeblemindedness and epilepsy. Though injuries to the cord are less frequently seen, they may occur in breech deliveries or in babies on whom version was practised. Another reason for injury to the brain at birth is prolonged labor with asphyxiation.

The *symptoms* of injury at birth will, of course, depend upon the location of the injured part. The lesions most frequently involve the basal regions with the resulting symptoms of tremor, rigidity and athetosis. In these cases a diagnosis of cerebral diplegia is frequently made. If the pyramidal system has been involved on one or both sides, symptoms of such involvement will be found. A hemorrhage may occur only on one side and, in such a case, will produce infantile hemiplegia. The fact that the child has hemiplegia is often not recognized until it should be sitting up or walking. Convulsions are especially likely to occur in children who have had a cerebral injury. Many children who have suffered from diffuse cerebral hemorrhage without exact localizing signs are found to be late in walking and talking, and show arrested cerebral development. On the other hand, a child who has had hemiplegia, the result of an injury at birth, may show little or no mental deficiency. Implication of the spinal cord as the result of birth injury is not nearly so common as cerebral injury, and is more often due to obstetrical interference. The cord may be completely ruptured or may be the seat of partial disintegration. If the involvement is high death as a rule results quickly. Children born prematurely may show symptoms which are confused with birth injury. The child born prematurely is a bad risk and may show signs of lack of cerebral development, and is usually late in walking and talking. The pyramidal tracts are late in developing and may never develop fully below the mid-dorsal region. This will result in spastic paraplegia. Infection occurring in the first few weeks of life may produce inflammatory reactions in the central nervous system which are thought to be traumatic.

The *diagnosis* is difficult and much depends upon a proper history. The duration of labor, whether or not the child cried promptly after birth or gave evidence of asphyxiation, are all extremely important considerations. The occurrence of an acute infection of any description in the first few weeks of life is also important. Of equal significance is the health of the mother during pregnancy, especially the consideration as to whether or not she had a severe infectious disease. Certain neurologic conditions occurring early in life, such as hydrocephalus, microcephalus, spinal bifida, various forms of muscular atrophy occurring in children, hereditary ataxia must be differentiated from birth injuries. Children born in a long and difficult labor, especially if instruments were used, should be subjected to careful physical examination from the neurologic standpoint. In many instances a lumbar puncture may be necessary to aid in the diagnosis.

If an intracerebral hemorrhage exists it must be *treated* along those lines. If, however, blood is found in the spinal fluid and the examination does not indicate that the hemorrhage has occurred into the brain, the patient should be treated as one of subarachnoid bleeding. Decompressive operations should be resorted to only as a last resort, and will usually be unavailing. However, if signs exist pointing to a localized hemorrhage, surgery should be given a chance. Occasionally a baby who has an extracerebral hematoma will develop enlargement of head simulating hydrocephalus; operation is indicated in such cases. If the child survives to the age of three or four years or beyond he will often be found to be a case for speech-training and frequently will have to be sent to a special school, depending upon the amount of intellectual damage done. If infantile hemiplegia results, various orthopedic operations may assist the child in making the greatest use of the power which exists but is unavailable because of contractures. On the other hand, the writer has seen cases of this sort subjected to many operations without any result whatsoever.

Internal Hydrocephalus.—Internal hydrocephalus is a condition in which there is an increase in the amount of fluid within the ventricles of the brain, usually with an enlargement of the ventricles. Spinal fluid is formed in large part by the choroid plexuses in the lateral ventricles. The fluid passes through the foramen of Monro, through the third ventricle, goes through the aqueduct of Sylvius to the fourth ventricle, and escapes to the subarachnoid space through the foramina of Magendie and Luschka. Some of the fluid flows upward over the hemispheres to the cortex, where a large part of it is absorbed, especially through the arachnoid villi and the venous sinuses. The fluid does not connect directly with any vessel wall or with the lymphatics. Part of the fluid may be absorbed by osmosis into the veins and some of it may pass directly through the capillaries of the pia arachnoid. The total amount of fluid under normal conditions varies from 100 to 200 cc. The fluid probably has metabolic functions, undoubtedly draining off waste products from the brain. It also acts as a water cushion to the central nervous system. An unusual rate of production or an interference with the outward flow leads to the condition which is called hydrocephalus.

The usual cause of hydrocephalus is a block somewhere along the closed sac in which the fluid circulates. The usual location of the block is in the region of the fourth ventricle. In this case all of the ventricles are enlarged. If the escape of the fluid is interfered with at the arachnoid villi, there is free circulation through the ventricles, but the fluid cannot be absorbed through the sinuses. This produces both internal and external hydrocephalus. The cause of internal hydrocephalus, which is the common variety, is the interference with the free flow of fluid, and may be due to a congenital anomaly, tumor, infection or injury. The common infection is meningitis, which causes adhesions around the foramina of Magendie and Luschka, and prevents the escape of fluid from these orifices. In such cases it is difficult to obtain spinal fluid by lumbar puncture. Tumors in the posterior fossa frequently produce internal hydrocephalus, as may also tumors in or close to the ventricular system. Injuries producing bleeding in the subarachnoid space, particularly at birth, may lead to adhesions and the formation of an obstructive type of hydrocephalus. Congenital syphilis, children of tuberculous parents, rickets and heredity, at times play a rôle in the production of hydrocephalus.

The *symptoms* of hydrocephalus are usually present in some degree at birth, which may be difficult or impossible, because of the size of the head. The head, which normally has a circumference of 35 to 40 cm. at birth, may show two or three times that in hydrocephalus. The skull is round, the frontal end is prominent, the sutures are separated and the fontanels are wide open and often pulsate. The scalp is thin, and the patient has little or no hair. The face, in contrast to the skull, seems small and triangular. The sclera are visible, and the eyes are widely separated. The child is a poor specimen physically, may be hemiplegic or paraplegic, and, if it learns to walk at all, it does late. Convulsions and optic atrophy are common. Various grades of retarded mentality are found, from the rare case which is almost normal, to low-grade idiots. These patients are extremely susceptible to infections, and, as a rule, die early in life. Hydrocephalus is often associated with other peculiarities of development, such as spinal bifida or encephalocele.

The *diagnosis* should offer little difficulty. The injection of dyes may be used to determine whether the hydrocephalus is communicating or obstructive. The dye is injected into one of the lateral ventricles. If the hydrocephalus is of the communicating type, it will be recovered by the lumbar puncture. If there is no recovery of the fluid from the lumbar tap, there is an obstruction somewhere in the ventricular system. If hydrocephalus occurs after the sutures are closed, signs of increased intracranial pressure ensue. These cases are practically always due to meningitis or tumor, although occasionally fracture of the base with subarachnoid bleeding may block the escape of fluid.

The *treatment* of hydrocephalus usually produces no satisfactory results. Most of the procedures recommended to date are palliative. If syphilis is present antiluetic treatment should be pushed.

Infantile Hemiplegia.—As a result of trauma or asphyxiation during birth or due to encephalitis, the result of infections of practically any variety, or to an embolism, an infant may become hemiplegic. This will make the child slow in walking and talking, and a candidate for epilepsy. If the hemiplegia is on the right side, speech, if present, may be lost but may be regained or reappear probably by the training of the centers on the opposite side of the brain. If the hemiplegia is produced by encephalitis occurring in the cortex, Jacksonian epilepsy or partial continuous epilepsy may be present. If hemiplegia develops in an infant the limbs on the paralyzed side do not develop and are smaller and shorter than their fellows, and there is a marked tendency toward contractures at the wrist, fingers and ankle. In this type of case orthopedic operations may do considerable good, although these procedures are certainly not underdone.

Little's Disease.—In infants born prematurely and sometimes in twins, the pyramidal tracts fail to develop properly beyond the mid-dorsal region. As a result spastic paraplegia with signs of pyramidal tract disease exists. The upper extremities may be involved but not to the extent of the lower. In other cases the upper extremities escape entirely and the mentality of the child may be normal. In some instances there is a general arrest of cerebral development, the mentality of the child is greatly affected, and the speech may be restricted or absent. Convulsions occasionally occur. While children suffering from this condition are late in walking, they may develop a fair gait.

The atmosphere concerning the various types of paralysis that occur in infants is somewhat clouded. The factors at fault are premature birth, difficult and prolonged labor, especially instrumental ones, and asphyxiation. Acute infectious disease of the mother during pregnancy may account for changes in the central nervous system of the fetus and acute infections of the child in the first few weeks of life may produce encephalitis, which subsequently leads to various types of paralysis. Convulsions occurring early in life may be followed by a cerebral hemorrhage. Epilepsy, various grades of mental retardation, speech defects, ocular palsies and irregular movements, especially athetosis, are common complications. Occasionally the cerebellum seems to be particularly involved.

Tay-Sach's Disease.—Amaurotic family idiocy (Tay-Sach's disease) is a combination of blindness from hereditary optic atrophy and idiocy from arrested cerebral development. A child who appears normal at birth shows the foregoing symptoms usually in the first year of life. It practically always occurs in Jewish children. Gradual signs of cerebral diplegia occur with nystagmus, diminution of vision followed by blindness. The course of the condition is rapid, the child usually dying before the age of six years. One of the most characteristic things in the examination of the patient is a cherry-red spot seen at the macula. This is due to atrophy of the retina, which permits the choroid to shine through.

Bulbar Palsy.—This relatively rare condition of unknown etiology comes on, as a rule, after or during the fifth decade. The pathologic changes consist of degeneration of the nuclei of the seventh, ninth, tenth and twelfth cranial nerves. The upper parts of the seventh nerve nuclei occasionally, and at times the motor fifth, are implicated. Bulbar palsy is frequently a part of the picture of amyotrophic lateral sclerosis and progressive spinal muscular atrophy. The *symptoms* are difficulty in speaking, swallowing, chewing and phonation, coming on gradually. The speech develops a nasal twang. The labials and linguals are with difficulty pronounced, and the speech gradually becomes worse and worse, so that in time anarthria results. The same thing takes place as far as swallowing is concerned, so that in time food may regurgitate through the nose or lodge in the larynx. A progressive atrophy occurs in the muscles of the lips, tongue, larynx and also in those of mastication. All the signs of anterior horn disease occur in the atrophic muscles. Attacks of involuntary emotionalism, usually weeping, while not as common as in pseudobulbar palsy, may occur.

The *diagnosis* is to be made from acute bulbar palsy, which is usually due to a vascular accident, encephalitis or myasthenia gravis, which is, in reality, bulbar palsy without anatomical findings, pseudobulbar palsy and tumors of the bulb.

There is no successful *treatment* and the patient usually succumbs within two years of the onset.

Pseudobulbar Palsy.—Strictly speaking, this is not a disease but is a syndrome depending upon bilateral cerebral lesions involving the upper motor neurons. These lesions are usually the result of vascular disease with resulting softening, but in the so-called extrapyramidal type the lesions are in the basal ganglia. Anyone of the numerous processes which may produce bilateral lesions in the brain may be the etiologic fault, thus arteriosclerosis, syphilis, chronic encephalitis, multiple sclerosis and multiple emboli may be the cause of pseudobulbar palsy.

The movements which are controlled bilaterally from the cortex are not markedly involved by a unilateral lesion; thus in the ordinary type of hemiplegia, swallowing and chewing are little affected and usually only early in the illness. In bilateral lesions, however, these functions are interfered with. Lesions in the region of the lenticular nuclei are especially likely to produce disturbance of swallowing and chewing, centers for which are supposed to exist in the basal ganglia. In a pseudobulbar palsy the lesions are above the nuclei, and the symptoms of anterior horn disease seen in bulbar palsy are lacking. In pseudobulbar palsy the patient has a spastic involvement of the muscles supplied by the bulb.

The history of the onset is most important. It is discovered that the patient has had at least two apoplectic attacks, one involving each side of the body, and it is frequently true that one of the attacks was mild. In some of the patients the hemiplegia lasts only a short time. After bilateral lesions have occurred the patient develops difficulty in chewing, swallowing and talking. Difficulty in chewing and swallowing may be so pronounced that the patient has trouble in obtaining enough nourishment. He frequently chokes, and food may regurgitate through the nose. The difficulty in speech may vary from a mild dysarthria to anarthria. Attacks of involuntary emotionalism are common and the patient may have uncontrollable laughter or crying without cause. Anything which plays upon the emotions of the individual may serve to bring further involuntary laughter or crying; especially is this so of the latter.

Signs of pyramidal tract disease may be present on both sides of the body and the gait may be characteristic of cerebrospinal arteriosclerosis, namely, the gait of little steps; it may be spastic on one or both sides. In pseudobulbar palsy one may also see *symptoms* referable to any part of the brain. These symptoms will, of course, depend upon the location of the pathologic lesions. Disturbance in the control of the sphincters may also be present and is usually due to involvement of the basal ganglia. In striatal pseudobulbar palsy signs of basal ganglia disease are present.

The *diagnosis* of pseudobulbar palsy is usually easy and is made on the history, the involuntary emotionalism, difficulty in chewing and swallowing and talking, without the signs of nuclear disease. On two occasions the writer has seen pseudobulbar palsy with attacks of involuntary weeping mistaken for manic-depressive insanity in the depressed phase.

The *outlook* in cases of pseudobulbar palsy is poor. The most fortunate thing from the standpoint of the patient is a history of syphilis and in such cases improvement may occur. Some of these patients choke to death or develop pneumonia, due to the difficulty in swallowing, so that special care is necessary as far as feeding is concerned.

Myasthenia Gravis.—*Asthenic bulbar paralysis,* also referred to as *bulbar palsy without anatomic findings,* is rather an uncommon disease of the muscular system and is without changes in the nervous apparatus. The endocrine system may be at fault. The muscles most frequently affected are those of the eyes, face and tongue, throat and neck, although all the muscles of the body may be involved, and sudden death, probably from involvement of the myocardium, has been reported. The muscles may be infiltrated with round cells and an enlarged thymus may be found.

The most important *symptom* of myasthenia gravis is weakness followed by paralysis of the muscles, brought on by use. As mentioned before, the muscles most usually affected are those of the eyes, resulting in diplopia; of the lips, tongue, pharynx and jaw resulting in dysarthria, dysphagia and difficulty in chewing, and of the muscles of the neck, resulting in difficulty in holding the head erect. To bring the symptoms out, it is only necessary to have the patient perform some given muscular effort a number of times. When the muscles become fatigued movement is no longer possible. The same thing, in a way, is accomplished by stimulating the muscles with faradic current. After a number of stimulations the muscle reacts feebly and finally fails to respond; after a rest the excitability returns. The disease is more frequently seen between the ages of twenty and fifty years; females are more involved than males. Remissions are common. The disease is not a common one. Sensory loss, atrophy, fibrillations and the reversal of the electrical reactions do not occur. The outlook is bad for recovery.

The *diagnosis* is to be made from bulbar palsy, encephalitis, tumors of the bulb, cerebral syphilis and tumors of the corpora quadrigemina. There is no successful *treatment* of the disease. The patient should be placed at rest and fatigue avoided. The diet should be soft and liquid. Tonics, ephedrine sulphate, glycine, pilocarpine and epinephrine are recommended.

PARALYSIS AGITANS.

Synonyms.—Parkinson's disease; Shaking palsy.

Definition.—Paralysis agitans is a chronic, slowly progressive disorder, characterized by tremor and rigidity and due to changes in the extrapyramidal motor system.

A definite *etiologic factor* has never been found, although the Parkinsonian syndrome is extremely common after epidemic encephalitis and is due in such cases to inflammatory changes the result of infection. It may be that many of the cases that we consider ordinary paralysis agitans are, in reality, due to infections causing encephalitis years before the onset of the symptoms of paralysis agitans. This is particularly true in the juvenile types of the disease. Although hereditary and familial forms have been reported, they must be extremely uncommon. Men are affected much more frequently than women, and the disease usually appears after the age of forty-five years. Emotions and injuries have been mentioned as etiologic factors. In the latter case it is likely small hemorrhages occur in the basal ganglia. Syphilis probably plays very little, if any, rôle in the production of paralysis agitans. Large tumors in the frontal areas of the brain may produce Parkinsonism. The underlying *pathology* of paralysis agitans is an affection of the corpus striatum with degeneration of the large motor cells.

Symptoms.—These appear insidiously and little change may take place for weeks or months. In the early stage of the disease the tremor, which is usually the first symptom to be noticed, may disappear for a short time. The tremor, as a rule, first appears in an upper extremity and practically always in the hand or fingers. It is rhythmical, may be either fine or coarse and vibrations range from four to seven a second. In the early stages it may be limited to one finger or thumb, then gradually spreads to involve the entire upper extremity, the lower extremity of the same side, and then usually goes through the same procedure on the other side of the body; it may, however, remain unilateral for a number of months. The tremor is present during rest and ceases or diminishes during an action. An occasional patient can control the tremor voluntarily; but in such a case, as in a tic, the tremor may then be exaggerated temporarily. The characteristic tremor is the pill-rolling one, but flexion and extension of the wrist and fingers or pronation and supination of the forearm are common without a definite pill-rolling element. The tremor involves the head, jaw and occasionally the tongue. Like practically all irregular movements, it disappears during sleep. The tremor may be imparted to the handwriting, and the tremor plus rigidity produce a progressive smallness of the handwriting, which is characteristic of the disease.

Objective Signs.—Although there are types of paralysis agitans in which rigidity is marked and the tremor slight or absent, the rigidity usually follows the tremor. This is the so-called *paralysis agitans sine agitatione.* When the extremities are passively moved a wax-like resistance occurs, the cogwheel symptom. Rigidity of the face causes the masked expression; the bodily attitude is that of the position of and old, bent man, the trunk flexed, head flexed and slight flexion of the upper extremities and at the knees. The hand may assume various positions, the flipper hand being not uncommon. The thumb may be held in the palm of the hand and the fingers flexed over it. Because of the rigidity, all voluntary movement is slowly initiated and slowly carried out. Change of position is difficult and often impossible. The common maneuver in getting up is for the nurse to grasp both hands of the patient and slowly pull him to a standing position. A common complaint among cases of paralysis agitans is their inability to turn over in bed; many of them if they desire to change their position must get out of bed and then reënter it. The winking reflex is usually affected. An involuntary step backward or to either side as the patient arises from a sitting position is a common symptom and may be among the earliest. These signs are referred to as retropulsion and lateropulsion. The most characteristic thing as the patient walks is the loss of the automatic swinging movements of the arms; the foot drags and shuffles. Another characteristic of the gait, usually not seen until the disease has advanced, is *festination.* In this condition the patient starts off slowly and then the rate of progression becomes more rapid until he is running and the body is bent forward. Although it would seem as though he must fall, he rarely does so. He stops himself by grasping hold of a person or an object in his path.

The various emotions are rarely transmitted to the facial expression, although a wan, ghost-like smile occasionally occurs. Anger or displeasure may cause flushing of the face. The loss of movement which occurs is not a paralysis in the ordinary sense of the word, but is more an inhibition of motion due to rigidity, which may become so pronounced that the patient has practically no voluntary movement left except in the eyes. Reflex acts, such as swallowing, are not affected, if at all, until late in the disease, and the sphincters usually remain intact. Speech, often a monotone, may develop a sort of festination and, as the disease progresses, the patient may become completely anarthric. The deep reflexes are normal or slightly hyperactive, but if much rigidity is present they may be difficult to obtain. The superficial reflexes are normal. Babinski's sign does not occur in the ordinary case of paralysis agitans.

Sensation, objectively tested, is not involved. Pain is not an infrequent symptom in paralysis agitans, especially in the upper extremities. A burning sensation is not uncommon, and flushing and excessive sweating are frequently seen. Patients with paralysis agitans often stand the cold much better than the hot weather and some of them are much better when they wear light clothing. Salivation, a common symptom in the Parkinsonism due to epidemic encephalitis, is not so frequently seen in the ordinary type of the disease. The mentality of a patient suffering from paralysis agitans is not altered, although they are often fussy, irritable and unreasonable. They are more subject to depression than the normal person, and also more likely to develop a real psychosis, which is usually of a depressive, suspicious nature.

Diagnosis.—In the early stage of the disease, however, when the tremor is slight, neuralgic pains present and nothing found to account for them, the patient suffering from Parkinsonism may be thought to be psychoneurotic. The tremor of paralysis agitans will disappear on the paralyzed side if the patient has an attack of cerebral thrombosis. The tremor of senility will probably offer the greatest difficulty in differentiation. This tremor affects chiefly the head and upper extremities and is increased during action. The so-called rabbit tremor or jaw tremor is more characteristic in the senile case. Multiple sclerosis and other forms of irregular movement such as chorea and athetosis should not be difficult to differentiate. It is often difficult to say whether a patient suffering from paralysis agitans is a victim of the old-fashioned disease or whether he has Parkinsonism due to chronic encephalitis. The distinction will be particularly difficult in those cases of chronic encephalitis where there is no history of an acute infection.

The *prognosis* in paralysis agitans is unfavorable for recovery. The outlook for life is good, the patient often living from five to twenty years. The duration depends largely upon the age of onset.

Treatment.—No known treatment is curative; however, much can be done to help the patient and to relieve his suffering. He should be placed in the best possible state of general health, he should have pleasant surroundings and the people with whom he comes in contact should be agreeable, kindly and optimistic. He should avoid excitement and excessive physical exertion. Hydrotherapy, mild massage, passive movement and exercises within reason are indicated. Some times mild electricity seems to improve the sufferer from paralysis agitans, largely because of its psychic effect. From the drug standpoint a combination of bromide and hyoscine does most to relieve the tremor. The dose of these drugs should be small at first and gradually increased. In some cases tincture of stramonium has a beneficial effect upon the tremor. Sleeplessness, pain and distress in the extremities caused by tremor and rigidity call for the use of hypnotics and analgesics. In the advanced case of paralysis agitans who suffers intensely it is as justifiable to prescribe opium in some form as it is to do so for cancer. The use of such drugs as tobacco, coffee, tea and alcohol are capable of producing tremor and should be forbidden.

SYDENHAM'S CHOREA.

Synonyms.—St. Vitus's dance; Acute chorea.

For years Sydenham's chorea was thought to be a functional nervous disorder, but it is now considered an infectious disease closely allied to rheumatism. It is probable that a non-hemolytic streptococcus is the causative factor of the disease and that its toxins produce encephalitis. It has no relation to epidemic encephalitis, which, however, has a choreiform type. A mental shock or trauma sometimes seems to bring on the disease, certainly they exaggerate the condition if already present. The disease has a tendency to be complicated by endocarditis, polyarthritis and tonsillitis. The pathology of Sydenham's chorea is not on a firm basis, although it is assumed that changes in the corpus striatum are responsible for the choreiform movements. In a patient who died of acute chorea, reported by Winkelman and the writer, no characteristic changes were found in the brain, although other writers had reported changes in the striatum. The brain may be hyperemic and occasionally, if a case is complicated by endocarditis, emboli may occur. Eosinophilia is frequently found.

The disease is one which occurs particularly between the ages of five and fifteen years, and girls are more susceptible than boys. The disease is more frequent in February and March and in October and November. Heredity has nothing to do with the onset of the acute chorea, and hereditary chorea and Sydenham's chorea have no relation as far as etiology is concerned. It is more common in races which are temperamental, and also is seen more frequently in children who are in a low state of general health. Pregnancy predisposes to Sydenham's chorea, and relapses of chorea are especially common during pregnancy. The first pregnancy is more likely to be complicated by chorea than later ones.

Symptoms.—The disease usually appears gradually. The child is out of sorts and suffers from headache, anorexia and a general slowing up. The temperature may be slightly elevated during the early stages of chorea. The choreiform movements may be localized to one side of the body or to one extremity or they may be generalized. The movements are slow and purposeless, never rhythmical and, as far as rapidity is concerned, are midway between athetosis and tic. Like practically all spontaneous movements they cease during sleep, though in some cases they may be so severe as to prevent sleep. Any movement which the patient attempts will be affected if the part used is choreic. Throughout the disease, for example, the patient suffering with acute chorea has difficulty in feeding himself and frequently drops dishes. The child has a tendency in performing an act to overdo it. At first, one side may be affected more than the other, and in rare cases chorea may be confined to one side, but, as a rule, both sides of the body are irregularly affected as the disease progresses.

Involvement of the muscles of speech is common and in severe cases the speech is extremely dysarthric. When the choreiform movements affect the face, grimacing results and involvement of the tongue produces disturbance of speech and chewing. Due to the irregular movements and the incoördination which results, weakness of the affected extremities may be present and may be so pronounced as to produce the so-called paralytic type of the disease. While pyramidal tract signs may be seen, they certainly are extremely rare. It is quite common in any form of chorea for the great toe to extend as a manifestation of chorea; if the plantar surface is stimulated just as this choreiform movement occurs, the patient may be thought to have a Babinski sign. Inasmuch as the state of the deep reflexes varies, there is nothing characteristic about them. Excitement and fatigue increase the movements. The pupils and ocular nerves, electrical reactions and sensation are normal. Pain may occur in the extremities, especially if the movements are severe or if the individual has arthritis. The patient suffering from Sydenham's chorea is irritable, dull and shows a general reduction in his mental faculties. A toxic exhaustive psychosis may ensue, with excitement, visual and auditory hallucinations and delusions. Cases of chorea complicating pregnancy are especially liable to develop mental symptoms. Evidence of tonsillitis, arthritis and endocarditis may be found. The average duration of the disease is two or three months, the extremes being six weeks to eight months.

The greatest mistake in *diagnosis* is in calling cases of tic or habit spasm, chorea. The tic or habit spasm is quick, apparently purposeful, usually limited to certain groups of muscles and does not vary from week to week. They are especially likely to involve the face, head or shoulders. Choreiform and choreo-athetoid movements may occur in the acute stage of epidemic encephalitis, or may be a manifestation of chronic encephalitis. The movements appear much more rapidly in encephalitis; as a rule they are more marked and are accompanied by other signs, especially ocular palsies. Hysteria may be mistaken for chorea, especially in pregnancy. The irregular movements which occur in hysteria are usually not distinctly choreiform, but are more tic-like in character. Furthermore, the patient usually responds quickly to isolation and psychotherapy.

The *prognosis* for recovery is excellent, an occasional case dies and rarely does one become chronic. The writer has seen but one death from ordinary chorea. The death-rate in chorea complicated by pregnancy has been estimated as high as 20 per cent; that seems to the writer to be too high. If endocarditis occurs, signs of that affection will persist.

Treatment.—The most important consideration is rest in bed, which should be continued until the movements have disappeared. The patient should be placed in the sunniest and best-ventilated room in the house and visitors excluded. Stimulating games and reading should not be permitted. In view of the fact that many of the children are underweight and undernourished, a high-caloric diet and one rich in greens and fruit should be ordered. Hydrotherapy, especially

77

a continuous warm tub if available, decreases the choreiform movements as do also warm packs or an ordinary warm bath. The drugs which the writer has found most efficacious are bromides, salicylates and Fowler's solution, all of which may be given in one prescription, and in doses appropriate to the age and weight of the patient. Barbituric preparations may be used for their hypnotic and sedative effects. Various specific sera, such as Small's, have been advised in chorea and a non-specific protein therapy, such as typhoid vaccine, has been recommended. The writer has seen a few excellent results in which the course of the disease was apparently cut short by the injection of typhoid vaccine. Nirvanol (phenylethylhydantoin) has been used; it is supposed to have an antirheumatic value and it does produce fever. The use of various arsenicals intravenously has been recommended, but he believes the arsenical effect can be obtained quickly enough if the drug is given by mouth. The modern tendency of course is to give drugs intravenously, and the writer is afraid that this tendency sometimes is not a good thing for the patient. Particular attention should be paid to the general health of the patient; he should be given plenty of fresh air and sunshine, bad teeth and tonsils should be removed, and other infections such as pyelitis cleared up. If endocarditis has occurred the child should be kept in bed for a longer period of time. In cases with tachycardia an ice-bag should be applied over the heart. After the movements have ceased the child may be gotten out of bed, but haste should be made slowly, by easy stages, permitting him to go down stairs and then out of the house. It will usually not be necessary to employ physiotherapy, although occasionally massage may be beneficial. Stimulating physiotherapeutic treatment, such as electricity, should not be used.

HUNTINGTON'S CHOREA.

Hereditary chorea begins about the age of thirty-five or forty years, usually involves more than one member of a family, and the history of its occurrence in the family may date back many years. On the other hand, occasional cases of Huntington's chorea are seen in which the family occurrence of the disease is absent. The main facts on which the diagnosis is based are heredity, choreiform movements and dementia. The choreiform movement, as a rule, begins in one hand or in the face, and then gradually spreads to involve the entire body. The irregular movements do not differ from those of Sydenham's chorea. When the disease is far advanced it is necessary to confine the patient to a wheel chair or bed, because the violence of the movements causes falls and injuries. Movements of the face produce grimacing, and those of the trunk, pelvis and lower extremities produce a bizarre, disordered gait, the patient dipping and swaying forward, backward and to either side. Mentally the patient deteriorates and, if he lives long enough, suffers from complete dementia.

In the early stages he may show ideas of persecution, and get into legal difficulties because of poor judgment and loss of memory. As in most hereditary diseases, males are affected more than females. In a family in which this disease exists there may be instances of chorea without dementia, mental disease without chorea and some instances in which neither distinct mental disease nor chorea is found, but, who, however, are queer and eccentric.

Huntington's chorea has no relation to Sydenham's chorea and rheumatic infections. The underlying *pathology* of Huntington's chorea is an atrophy of the motor cells of the corpus striatum and also atrophy of the frontal cortex. At times changes suggestive of encephalitis are found in the brain. The disease is progressive, incurable and may last from one to fifteen years or more. Huntington's chorea may be confused with other forms of chorea produced by changes in the basal ganglia.

The *treatment* is ineffectual but for a time the chorea may be controlled by sedatives such as bromide, hyoscine and stramonium. It is practically always necessary in time to institutionalize the patient. Marriage of members of families in which the disease exists should be advised against.

PROGRESSIVE LENTICULAR DEGENERATION.

A description of progressive lenticular degeneration by Wilson, in 1912, focussed attention on the basal ganglia. Wilson's disease is a familial condition appearing, as a rule, before the age of thirty years and complicated by a hob-nail cirrhosis of the liver. It is characterized by a slow, rhythmic tremor of the extremities, usually of the paralysis agitans type, although occasionally choreiform or athetoid movements are seen. The tremor, unlike that of paralysis agitans, is increased by action. The extremities and face are hypertonic, the hypertonicity of the muscles of the face producing a spastic smile. Involuntary emotionalism, especially of laughter, is commonly seen. Because of the hypertonicity of the extremities, contractures develop. The deep reflexes are usually hyperactive, but positive signs of pyramidal tract disease are lacking. True paralysis is not present, but the scope of movement is greatly limited because of tremor and rigidity. The pupils, cranial nerves, abdominal reflexes and sensation are normal. The involvement of the muscles of speech and swallowing produce dysarthria and dysphagia. The disease is progressive, incurable and fatal, as a rule, under ten years.

In addition to hob-nail cirrhosis of the liver, *postmortem examination* reveals degeneration of the lenticular nuclei, most marked in the putamina and to a less degree in the globus pallidus. The degeneration sometimes ends in cavitation.

Pseudosclerosis.—The syndrome of pseudosclerosis is similar in many respects to Wilson's disease, and, by many, Wilson's disease and pseudosclerosis are considered varieties of the same condition. Cirrhosis of the liver is found in both, although more frequently in Wilson's disease. Enlargement of the spleen is sometimes found in pseudosclerosis. Tremor, especially an intention tremor, is commonly seen in pseudosclerosis and rigidity is usually absent. In pseudosclerosis a peculiar greenish discoloration of the corneal margins is frequently observed. This has been called the Kayser-Fleisher ring or Fleisher-Strümpell ring. The speech and type of tremor may suggest multiple sclerosis but nystagmus, optic atrophy, pyramidal tract signs and alteration of the colloidal-gold curve test are absent.

EPIDEMIC ENCEPHALITIS.

The condition which we now commonly refer to as epidemic encephalitis was first described by von Economo, under the title of *lethargic encephalitis*. There is much in medical history to indicate that the disease has been prevalent in the past and has been described under various titles. After its appearance in Europe, in 1917, the disease spread over the entire world. The first cases in the United States occurred toward the end of 1918 and the early part of 1919. The first great epidemic of encephalitis came after the severe and widespread epidemic of influenza. The type of the disease varied in different years. It is not contagious in the ordinary sense of the word, and, while more than one case has occurred in a family, even this is uncommon. The writer has never seen a case develop in a hospital ward, either among other patients or among the doctors and nurses handling cases of epidemic encephalitis.

Pathogenesis.—The cause of the disease is supposed to be a filterable virus. Strauss and Loewe have isolated a virus from the nose, throat and brain of patients who have had encephalitis and have transmitted the disease to animals. Rosenow believes that encephalitis is due to a streptococcus. To date there is no proof as to the exact cause of the disease. Whether there is a relation between encephalitis and influenza or encephalitis and poliomyelitis and epidemic meningitis is not known. There is much evidence to associate herpes febrilis and encephalitis and also, perhaps, chickenpox. The infection probably enters through the naso-pharynx and the incubation period is about ten days.

Pathology.—The brunt of the disease is borne by the region of the aqueduct of Sylvius, the basal ganglia, the pons and medulla and substantia nigra. While the cortex and spinal cord may be involved, the disease has a predilection for the parts mentioned. The meninges usually show a mild to moderate inflammatory reaction. *Grossly* the brain may appear normal except for a general congested appearance. *Microscopically* the chief feature is a perivascular infiltration with lymph or round cells. In some cases small hemorrhages, and occasionally a large one, are found. In the subacute and chronic cases of encephalitis changes are found, especially in the corpus striatum, thalamus, in the hypothalamic structures and in the substantia nigra. Changes in other parts of the nervous system may be discovered, but are uncommon. In a young adult the residual conditions were characteristic of change and signs of anterior poliomyelitis involving the lumbo-sacral cord on one side. The ganglion cells show alteration of an acute and chronic nature and lymphocytic infiltration around the vessels may be observed. The vessel walls often show degeneration and pseudocalcareous deposits.

Symptoms.—The disease involves the sexes about equally, and, while it occurs at any age, young adults are more frequently involved. Many types of the disease have been described as far as symptomatology is concerned, and the various types mean nothing more nor less than that different parts of the nervous system are affected by the virus. While it is true that the regions of the aqueduct are most frequently affected, other parts of the central nervous system do not escape, and many bizarre and irregular types of disease are prevalent. Furthermore, the symptomatology varies in different years. The most common symptoms are headache, lethargy and diplopia. The temperature is elevated, as a rule, but does not often go above 101° to 102° F. The lethargy varies from a slight stupor to a profound coma. Quite often, even in the deepest stupor, the patient may be aroused. He will then carry out a command or two and drop back to sleep. The ocular palsies present in the disease are due to the inflammatory reactions in or near the nuclei of these nerves. The ocular palsies either persist or clear up, and other cranial nuclei may be involved, especially the seventh. Therefore, a bilateral facial palsy, giving an expressionless appearance to the face, is seen. An acute bulbar palsy is occasionally a manifestation of epidemic encephalitis. There is no other disease of which the writer is aware which produces an irregular succession of cranial nerve paralyses in the course of a few hours or a few days, and quite often, as a fresh involvement occurs, the muscles first involved clear up. Neck rigidity and Kernig's sign are frequently seen in the acute stage of epidemic encephalitis and, in the first two or three years in which the disease became prevalent, often led to the erroneous diagnosis of meningitis, especially tuberculous. Involvement of the bulb produces dangerous symptoms, often with irregularity of the pulse and respiration, and is a common cause of death which may occur suddenly. Catatonia occasionally is seen. Early in the history of the disease this symptom leads to mistakes in diagnosis, which are usually hysteria or dementia præcox. The deep reflexes are frequently unaltered, and Babinski's sign a great rarity. Involvement of the sphincters does not usually occur, but incontinence of urine is occasionally seen, probably due to the stupor of the patient. Impairment of accommodation and loss of pupillary reaction are frequently seen in the acute stage. A paralysis agitans syndrome, coming on acutely, is occasionally encountered. Radicular pains, myoclonic movements in various parts of the body, especially in the abdominal muscles, are common symptoms. In some patients, particularly in children, insomnia rather than lethargy occurs, and a reversal of the sleep formula is seen. Hiccough was a prominent symptom in one or two years in which the disease appeared. The leukocytes in the blood are, for the most part, slightly to moderately increased. The number of cells in the spinal fluid varies in different years. In some cases the count is practically normal and others it goes as high as 400. Thirty to 40 cells is a common finding. The cells are usually lymphocytes. The most important finding in the spinal fluid is the increase in the sugar content. The globulin is also increased and not infrequently an alteration in the colloidal-gold curve in the middle zone is found. The urine often shows signs of nephritis which is in a few cases a contributing cause of death. Delirium, excitement, maniacal states and one suggestive of Korsakoff's psychosis may be seen. While herpes is a common symptom in certain acute diseases such as pneumonia, meningitis and malaria, it is an uncommon complication of epidemic encephalitis. Slight optic neuritis may be seen. There are undoubtedly many mild and abortive types of the disease, just as there are of acute anterior poliomyelitis.

Diagnosis.—In view of the signs of meningitis, the most common mistake in diagnosis is in assuming that tuberculous or some other form of meningitis is present. The greatest help in differentiating these two conditions is in the examination of the spinal fluid. In meningitis the sugar content is reduced or absent, whereas in epidemic encephalitis it is present and very often increased. The chloride content of the spinal fluid is also greatly reduced in meningitis and the cell count is greater than in encephalitis. While cranial nerve palsies occur in meningitis, it is not usually the succession of cranial palsies which occur in encephalitis. Finding the tubercle bacilli in the spinal fluid will clear up the diagnosis. Other forms of meningitis, especially the meningococcic type, may be differentiated by examination of the spinal fluid.

It is often extremely difficult to distinguish between acute multiple sclerosis and acute disseminated encephalomyelitis from epidemic encephalitis; in fact, some instances of acute disseminated encephalomyelitis may be due to the virus of encephalitis. The presence of definite pyramidal tract signs will usually point to these conditions rather than to epidemic encephalitis. Neurosyphilis, especially if producing lethargy and cranial nerve palsies, often presents a problem in differential diagnosis. Occasionally a patient under treatment for neurosyphilis develops epidemic encephalitis. The history of the case and examination of the blood and spinal fluid will aid greatly in the differential diagnosis. Cerebral neoplasm often presents difficulties in differential diagnosis. A careful history of the case, the evaluation of the symptoms found, and the appreciation that choked disk is usually due to a brain tumor and practically never occurs in encephalitis, should help to keep the diagnosis clear. Uremia and diabetes can usually be distinguished by a complete survey of the case. Encephalitis occurring in the course of acute infections, especially in children, may produce obstacles in diagnosis.

Prognosis.—The mortality varies in different years from 5 to 25 per cent. The duration of the acute symptoms varies from a few hours to a number of months. The longer the patient has remained ill at the onset, the more likelihood there is that he will develop evidence of chronic encephalitis. This is not, however, a constant rule. The most foreboding thing that happens in the course of the illness is signs of bulbar paralysis, frequently resulting in sudden death. Many cases never make a complete recovery, but immediately develop signs of Parkinsonism or other evidences of chronic encephalitis. Depending on the predominance of symptoms, types of the diseases are classified as lethargic, hyperkinetic, myostatic, meningitic, psychotic, bulbar, myelitic and neuritic.

The percentage of cases which develop signs of *chronic encephalitis* is high. The commonest syndrome of chronic encephalitis is a Parkinson one, which may begin during the acute illness or which may not appear for years afterward. The paralysis agitans syndrome is occasionally without tremor which, if present, may be exaggerated rather than diminished by voluntary effort. Champing movements of the jaws, salivation, an oily skin, which in many cases becomes a seborrheic eczema, are frequently seen. Various types of irregular movement, such as chorea, athetosis, facial tic or spasms, are occasionally symptoms of the chronic stage of the disease. The pupils not infrequently are irregular, unequal and either dilated or contracted. Loss of accommodation and at times an Argyll-Robertson pupil may be observed. So-called oculogyric crises, in which the eyeballs become fixed in one position for a few minutes to hours, are very disturbing symptoms in the chronic stage. Tachypnea with signs of hyperventilation are rare manifestations of chronic encephalitis. Behavior disorders and reversal of the sleep formula are known sequels, especially in children. Narcolepsy, in many instances, is due to chronic encephalitis. Symptoms very suggestive of a psychoneurosis frequently exist for months or years before the patient develops signs, which make it possible to say that the disease is definitely organic and of an encephalitic nature.

Treatment.—There is no specific in the treatment of this disease, which is largely symptomatic. Expert nursing is perhaps the most valuable aid which we have, and careful attention to feeding, to the hygiene of the mouth, frequent change of position and watchful care of the skin are important points in the nursing of epidemic encephalitis. Acute bulbar palsy may make it necessary to tube-feed the individual and to place him in a respirator. A lumbar puncture is often indispensable for the diagnosis, but it is of doubtful value as far as treatment is concerned, and, in fact, it may tend to spread the infection. In the psychotic cases and in those who show irritability and insomnia, sedatives may be necessary. Fixation abscess, injections of the various arsenicals, non-specific protein therapy, iodides intravenously, in fact every known form of treatment has been tried in the acute stage of the disease, but as far as the writer's experience goes, without any result whatever. In the chronic stage hyoscine hydrobromide in ordinary doses has an alleviating effect upon the tremor and rigidity. Tincture of stramonium seems to be more effective than hyoscine in many cases. The writer has used fever, produced either by malaria, typhoid vaccine or Coley's fluid, in some cases of chronic encephalitis, but have obtained no results worthy of note. However, he has knowledge of 2 cases of chronic encephalitis at the Philadelphia General Hospital who developed typhoid fever, and both of them were improved. Mild massage and hydrotherapy, if the patient can afford them, relieve the symptoms temporarily and make the patient feel as though something were being done for him. Many of the patients, especially those showing pronounced rigidity and tremors and the children showing behavior disorders, will have to be hospitalized.

EPILEPSY.

By the term epilepsy is meant a loss of consciousness which may be momentary, called *petit mal*, or which may be prolonged for minutes or more and be accompanied by a convulsion. Furthermore, certain mental states such as amnesia, automatism or periods of excitement may take the place of the fit. While there is a tendency to discard the use of the terms idiopathic and essential in considering epilepsy, and while it is true that the use of these terms may block progress in our knowledge of the disease, it is nevertheless a fact that there is an extremely large group of individuals who have fits and who suffer from mental deterioration for which no cause can be found. Furthermore, in the so-called idiopathic type of the disease, very little indeed has been found in the brain to account for the attacks. Involvement of the cornu ammonis occurs frequently, but is probably a result of the disease, and not the cause of it. Occasionally, one finds thickening of the pia, and an excessive collection of fluid over the cortex. The ventricles may be dilated and drawn to one side. Occasionally evidence of an attack of encephalitis may be found, but this is not common. The cerebrospinal fluid shows no alteration and the pressure is normal or low.

Etiology.—Most cases of epilepsy develop before the age of twenty-five years, and a large percentage appear before the age of six years or before puberty. Convulsions occurring after twenty-five or thirty years of age should always cause a vigorous search to be made for evidence of gross intracranial disease, evidence of old injury to the brain or for various toxemias such as arise from diabetes and nephritis, and alcohol should be considered as the possible cause. Epilepsy may occur late in life on an arteriosclerotic basis, and is referred to as *epilepsia tarda*. The most important etiologic factor is heredity, which, in some series, may be as high as 50 per cent. Heredity may not be direct, but may be passed on as an evidence of instability. The incidence of epilepsy due to congenital syphilis or defects produced by syphilis in the parents is probably much greater than is generally supposed. The percentage of epileptic children who show positive blood or spinal fluid findings of syphilis is probably not more than 1 per cent. Convulsions, of course, may occur in individuals who have congenital syphilis either of the paretic or meningoencephalitic type. Alcoholism in the parents, particularly if the child is conceived during a debauch, is supposed to account for a number of epileptics. Difficult or prolonged labor, especially with instrumentation, is probably an important etiologic factor in the production of convulsions. At least 10, and perhaps as high as 20 per cent of normal babies have blood in the spinal fluid after birth, and this may later serve as a predisposing factor in the production of convulsions. Convulsants will act much more quickly and effectively if an injury to the brain has been produced first. In certain cases of prolonged labor with asphyxiation changes may occur in the cortical cells, which may later on be a cause of epilepsy. The influence of a severe fright in the production of convulsions is probably not great, but the writer has seen a few cases in which the history at least indicated that the first fit occurred after a severe fright. Convulsions frequently occur in susceptible children in the early stage of infectious diseases, especially scarlet fever, and an infectious disease may produce changes in the brain which later on predispose the individual to convulsions. An occasional case of epidemic encephalitis develops epilepsy as a sequela.

The importance of the so-called reflex epilepsy has been greatly over-estimated, and it is unlikely that abnormal or diseased conditions of the eyes, ears, teeth, gastro-intestinal disease or a scar on an extremity or disease of the genital organs can produce epilepsy although, if present, they may tend to make the patient worse. A few patients suffering from intestinal parasites undoubtedly have convulsions which are probably not reflex, but due to the toxemia produced by the infestation, and while the removal of the worms may cause a cessation of the fits, they may not be entirely arrested. In considering the possible reflex cause of the convulsive seizures it is wise to keep an open mind about it and to correct any defect or disease found in the patient.

Various intoxicants may produce convulsions, the commonest one being alcohol. There are quite a few people who have fits when they indulge excessively in alcohol and as long as they refrain from use of this drug they do not have convulsions. Repeated attacks of delirium tremens may produce changes in the meninges and cortex of sufficient degree to cause recurring spasms. In France, where absinthe drinking is common, the so-called absinthe epilepsy is frequently seen. Epileptics are not usually alcoholic, but if an epileptic does take alcohol either moderately or to excess he will have a greater number of convulsions than if he refrained from the use of the drug. The occurrence of seizures during pregnancy, while often attributed to a toxemia as the result of that state, is quite often due to epilepsy. Epileptiform seizures of some description may occur after severe head injury. The percentage of cases, however, which develop a convulsive state is not great, probably about 7 per cent. It has been proved experimentally that in animals who have been subjected to head trauma, convulsants such as absinthe or camphor will more readily cause fits. This is an important point from a medico-legal standpoint as well as from other considerations. Scarring of the brain, with distortion of the ventricular system, especially with the pulling of the ventricle toward the side of the lesion, occurs. In the histories of epileptics it is common to see scarlet fever, diphtheria or other infections given as the cause of the first convulsion. Gross organic disease of the brain, such as tumor, syphilis, abscess and vascular disease, sometimes cause fits, especially if the person is predisposed by heredity. Generalized convulsions, however, are not common in gross organic disease of the brain except paresis.

Chronic poisonings by such metals as lead, heart-block (Stokes-Adams syndrome) and tetany may all produce convulsions, as will also hypoglycemia and the excessive use of insulin. The occurrence of spasms during infancy, from any cause whatsoever, is frequently the forerunner of epilepsy later in life.

While it is readily seen, therefore, that there are numerous factors which must be considered in arriving at a diagnosis in a patient who has convulsions, it is quite true that there are many patients in whom no cause for the fits can be found. The name epilepsy may not sound well, and may produce terror in the heart of the patient, but it should be retained as a diagnosis until our knowledge is much farther advanced than it is at the present time.

While Jacksonian fits are frequently due to organic disease of the brain such as a tumor or syphilis, many idiopathic epileptics have what has been referred to by some as an inside Jacksonian affair. Some authorities agree that the commonest single cause of Jacksonian epilepsy is idiopathic epilepsy. This accounts for the frequency with which epileptics are trephined. The history shows that the fit often begins on one side and may even be localized there for some time before spreading to the other. In the absence of general signs of increased pressure or definite localizing signs, Jacksonian epilepsy in itself is not sufficient evidence on which to open the head of a patient. Various toxemias, especially alcoholism, may also produce Jacksonian fits.

Symptoms.—The vast majority of epileptic seizures come under the heading of *petit mal* or *grand mal*. The attack of petit mal or minor epilepsy is characterized by a sudden loss of consciousness which occurs without warning, without a convulsion and without the patient falling to the ground, and the whole affair lasts but a few seconds. The minor attacks may come on at any time and often escape notice of the family. As a rule, the patient suddenly stops what he is doing, stares straight ahead, the face becomes pale and there may be a slight movement of the tongue and lips or eyes, and more rarely of an extremity; the patient may yawn, make chewing or swallowing movements, and then frequently rubs his face and the fit is over. The patient often refers to these attacks as "bilious" or "dizzy spells." The epileptic may have an enormous number of attacks of petit mal in one month. Petit mal attacks may occur without major fits, but as a rule are associated with them. The patient suffering from major attacks may have them disappear under treatment only to be replaced by minor spells.

Pyknolepsy is a type of minor epilepsy characterized by the great number of attacks and by the extremely transient period of unconsciousness or semiconsciousness of no more than a few seconds without convulsive movements or falling. It is thought by some that major fits do not occur after such attacks but the writer has seen it happen. The ordinary anti-epileptic remedies have little, if any, effect on attacks of pyknolepsy.

Whether or not *narcolepsy* is a variety of epilepsy is a disputed point. It is a condition in which an irresistible tendency to sleep occurs, the sleep apparently being natural. It is likely to occur during any monotonous activity, for example, a recent secretary of the writer's would fall asleep during the monotony of typing. The narcoleptic frequently under emotion, especially laughter, has extreme weakness of the legs, which give way and he sinks to the ground powerless, but usually conscious. Narcolepsy may follow epidemic encephalitis.

Ephedrine sulphate by mouth in moderate doses daily has given some results in the treatment of narcolepsy.

The grand or major attack in epilepsy is the most dramatic part of the disease, and is often preceded by a change in disposition of the patient, or by vertigo. As a rule, however, it begins suddenly with unconsciousness. In about one-half the cases it is preceded by a warning or *aura*, which is a subjective sensation referable to various parts of the body or special senses. One of the commonest of the auræ is that referable to the epigastrium. The patient says he has a peculiar feeling in the pit of the stomach, which ascends to the head, and when it reaches the eyes he becomes unconscious. He may have a visual aura which may resemble the scintillating scotomata of migraine. He may see animals, bright lights or something which appears in the distance, which rushes toward him producing unconsciousness when it strikes him. Sometimes the aura is referable to an extremity or one side of the body, and consists of a paresthesia or dysesthesia. The aura may consist of tinnitus which seems to begin in the distance and rapidly approaches the person. The next step in the fit is a *cry*, or guttural noise, which occurs in a large percentage of cases. The cry is often loud and piercing and rather terrifying to the listener. If standing, the epileptic *falls* and frequently injures himself. Many epileptics pitch suddenly forward or backward, and as a result this type of case has many injuries and scars on the face. In the tonic phase of the *fit* the entire body becomes rigid in extension. If the tongue or cheek is caught between the jaws, as they are closed, it may be severely bitten. The patient may assume an attitude of opisthotonos, and occasionally one of decerebrate rigidity. The pupils will contract, then dilate and become fixed to light; the muscles of respiration being fixed in the tonic phase, respiration is impossible, and the patient becomes cyanotic. The *tonic phase* lasts from a few seconds to a minute or two, and is followed by the *clonic stage*, which lasts from a few seconds to four or five minutes. The head jerks violently, the muscles of the extremities are vigorously contracted and relaxed, and are the seat of electric-like movements. The contraction of the muscles of mastication causes a frothy saliva to exude from the mouth and, if the tongue, lips or cheeks have been bitten, the saliva is blood-tinged. Dislocation of joints, especially the shoulder, is not infrequently produced in this phase. The facial muscles twitch, the eyeballs roll around and respiration is noisy. The pupillary reflexes remain lost in this phase, and the deep reflexes are obtained with difficulty. The pulse is small and rapid, and the blood pressure, which may be slightly elevated at first, drops during the spasm. The Babinski reflex may frequently be obtained after the convulsion. Hemorrhages may occur in various parts of the body, especially into the brain and conjunctivæ. An occasional convulsive movement may persist for some minutes after the severity of the fit has subsided. The epileptic usually sleeps after an attack; the period of sleep may vary from a few minutes to a number of hours. Quite often after an attack and either before or after the stupor, the patient performs purposeless automatic acts in which he attempts to undress or fumbles with his clothes. When the patient recovers consciousness he practically always complains of headache, which may last for hours. Vomiting is an occasional symptom after a fit. As a rule, there is complete amnesia for a major spell, and this period may last a number of days, during which the patient may wander away and perform automatic deeds. Owing to the severity of the muscular contractures, the epileptic usually has muscular soreness after a fit. The temperature is slightly elevated and the patient passes considerable urine after a spell and it often contains albumin and casts which are not found on subsequent examinations but which may give rise to confusion in the diagnosis. Relaxation of the sphincters, especially the urinary sphincter, occurs either during the tonic or clonic stage. It does not occur in all attacks but is a symptom at some time in the history of most epileptics.

In an attack of the so-called running epilepsy, or *epilepsia procursiva*, the patient suddenly begins to run, usually forward, and at the end of a few seconds' running he may become confused or may fall and have a fit. Many gradations of epileptic fits occur between the attack of petit mal and the grand seizure. Some become unconscious and pitch forward and that is the entire attack; others fall and have a few convulsive movements and the attack is over. Some have what they themselves call the "jerks," in which violent muscle spasms occur, often of sufficient severity to throw the patient to the ground, and as a rule without unconsciousness. These muscle spasms are accompanied by considerable pain.

The disposition of an epileptic is always trying. He is non-coöperative, quarrelsome and pugnacious, given to attacks of depression, is suspicious, hypersensitive and many have violent tempers. He is frequently loquacious and will talk unceasingly, often in a monotonous tone, of his complaints. Many of them are pathologic liars and most are egotistic. His memory is poor and he tends to become asocial. Mental deterioration practically always ensues and in the end his mental dilapidation may be complete. Mental disturbances may occur before or after a seizure, or the so-called *psychic equivalent* may be the manifestation of a fit. Fortunately, the psychic equivalent is rarely seen, but in it the patient may develop a homocidal mania in which he may kill one or a number of people. Murders committed in this phase are often extremely brutal. After any variety of attack, the patient may be violent, confused or delirious. He also frequently suffers from delusions and hallucinations, especially the latter, and the symptoms frequently are of a religious nature. For the maniacal phase after a fit the patient is usually amnesic. This condition may last from a few hours to weeks. Occasionally an automatic state may be a substitute for a fit. Among 100 epileptics at the Pennsylvania Epileptic Hospital and Colony Farm, there are always from 10 to 20 who have to be placed in what is called the recovery room after a fit because they are quarrelsome, destructive, may commit criminal acts, and often wander away.

Epilepsy is occasionally used as a defense for crime, but all epileptics who commit crimes are not irresponsible. It might truthfully be said, however, from a medical standpoint, that in most instances an epileptic has reduced responsibility.

Status epilepticus is one of the most severe manifestations of epilepsy and a frequent cause of death. In status, which consists of a series of convulsions without consciousness being regained between attacks, the patient may have from two to hundreds of seizures. There are some epileptics who apparently have their fits only in series and who may then go some time without having any major attacks. After status, stupor becomes deep, the temperature rises to 103° to 106° F. or higher, the breathing becomes noisy and occasionally Cheyne-Stokes, the heart action may become irregular, and edema of the lungs ensues and frequently causes death. Trophic sores are common in some epileptics who have status. Occasionally status epilepticus is limited to one side of the body, when the term *status hemiepilepticus* is applied. Occasionally after a convulsion or particularly after a series of convulsions an exhaustion paralysis of one side may occur.

In *epilepsia partialis continua* the attacks are limited, as a rule, to an extremity or a part of an extremity, or to the face and tongue. This condition is usually due to gross organic disease of the brain, such as syphilis, tumor or encephalitis, but may occur in idiopathic epilepsy. The attacks of epilepsy may be diurnal, nocturnal or both.

The frequency of the fits varies greatly from one every few months to numerous fits daily. The fortunate epileptic is he who has only an occasional major attack, and that at night. The individual who has petit mal spells is likely to have numerous ones. The epileptic who is most disabled is the one who has numerous attacks of petit mal.

Diagnosis.—In arriving at the diagnosis of epilepsy, which can be satisfactorily done in the vast majority of cases by the history, it is sometimes necessary to observe a convulsion, especially if the question of hysteria enters into the picture. Hysterical convulsions, which are most uncommon in this country, are the opposite of the epileptic ones. They occur during the daytime, the typical aura and cry are absent, the patient practically never injures himself, the tongue is not bitten, the sphincters do not relax, and the tonic and clonic phases of the ordinary epilepsy are lacking. The pupils react to light, the conjunctival reflex is preserved and the Babinski sign is never seen. The patient does not sleep after an hysterical fit, does not vomit and, the atmosphere being cleared by an attack, usually feels better. Strong suggestion may stop the attack, which also will cease if the patient is left alone. While the term hystero-epilepsy is not accepted, some epileptics have hysterical fits as well. An important consideration in the differential diagnosis arises in the cases of epilepsy who have Jacksonian fits and who are frequently trephined. The history of long-continued fits, the epileptic makeup of the patient and the absence of localizing signs such as paralysis or alteration of the reflexes should make the surgeon forego his fishing expedition. The later in life the first attack of epilepsy begins, the more thorough should be the search for conditions capable of producing convulsions, especially a cerebral neoplasm which may exist for years without localizing signs. Paresis, alcoholism, cerebral trauma and toxemias, such as produced by nephritis and diabetes, should be considered. Convulsions occurring during pregnancy are, of course, frequently due to a toxemia, but, on the other hand, they are also frequently due to epilepsy. The convulsions of strychnine poisoning, tetanus and tetany should be easily differentiated. Narcolepsy, the so-called Gelineau syndrome, may be sometimes confused with attacks of petit mal with which it may be closely related. The confused state with a fear of fainting, complained of by many psychoneurotics, may also be mistaken for minor epilepsy. In the differential diagnosis of epilepsy and hysteria it is well to remember that in epilepsy the thumb is frequently clenched under the fingers; this sign does not occur in hysteria.

The relation of infantile convulsions to epilepsy is an important one. Acute infections, teething and gastro-intestinal conditions may be associated with convulsions. It shows that the infant has an unstable central nervous system. Although every patient who has infantile convulsions does not become an epileptic, many of them do.

Prognosis.—The prognosis in epilepsy is poor as regards cure and while the outlook for life is good, the disease does cut short the span. The percentage cured of attacks is small and probably falls between 5 and 10. If the first seizure occurs late in life the outlook is better than if it had happened early. A patient with one or two fits a year will naturally respond more favorably than one who has daily attacks. Bad heredity also affects the prognosis, as does also the history of status epilepticus.

Treatment.—While the treatment of epilepsy offers poor results as far as cure is concerned, sufficient and prompt treatment does reduce the number and severity of the fits in a large percentage. Before any treatment is instituted, a most thorough physical survey of the patient should be made and obvious defects and deficiencies corrected. While it is true that even the most painstaking search for an etiologic factor may produce nothing of importance, many conditions may be found which can be remedied and the patient given improved general health as a result. In the individual suffering from convulsions, such conditions as brain tumor, cerebral syphilis, nephritis, diabetes, residual of a head injury, cardiac disease, anemia, in brief, every condition which is known occasionally to produce convulsions, should be considered and ruled out. It is only by attacking the problem in this way that unfortunate errors in diagnosis can be avoided.

The *prophylaxis* of epilepsy should begin before conception; marriage of the epileptic, feebleminded, insane and the syphilitic should be advised against. Prevention of injuries at birth, and their proper treatment, if present, are important. The nervous, high-strung child, especially he who has had infantile convulsions or such diseases which may be closely allied to epilepsy, such as night terrors, sleep walking, nocturnal enuresis, or the child who has had severe head injury with unconsciousness, should be closely observed by the medical attendant and kept in good general health. The history of infantile convulsions should call for close observation of the development of the child, who should be treated as a potential epileptic. If a child has a convulsion which has no relation to an acute infectious disease, head trauma or other obvious cause, treatment should be instituted immediately to cut down the tendency which all such individuals have to develop recurring attacks of unconsciousness with convulsions. It must be borne in mind that there are many epileptics who, having had a few convulsions before the age of six years, may have no further attacks until puberty or later. Any treatment in such cases may acquire a reputation which it does not deserve. While acute infections, pregnancy and surgical operations frequently initiate convulsions, in some cases they seem to produce remissions. There is no one line of treatment which is successful in all patients. We certainly are not in a position to speak of the *cure* of epilepsy.

Nothing can be done to cut short an attack once it has begun, although certain patients feel that sometimes they may abort an attack by various maneuvers, such as tightly squeezing the extremity in which the aura appears. In the attack itself the chief concern should be to prevent injury. Some object should be inserted between the teeth to prevent biting of the tongue, lips and cheek, such as a spoon or tongue depressor padded with cotton and a bandage. A pillow should be placed under the head or the head supported to prevent its being knocked against the floor. Sometimes an extremity must be supported, because in the severe clonic stage it may be injured by hitting the floor or surrounding objects. After the convulsion is over the patient should be watched and prevented from doing automatic acts which are dangerous to himself or others, and to see that he does not wander away. The epileptic should be allowed to sleep out the fit and no effort should be made to hasten his recovery from the postepileptic stupor.

The subject of the epileptics' employment is an important one, although at the present time with workmen's compensation laws, it is practically impossible for a known epileptic to keep a job. He should never be allowed to continue at work which is obviously hazardous, such as working around machinery, driving an automobile, any job which takes him off the ground, railway work, in fact anything which might prove to be injurious to himself and others, if he had an attack. Swimming should not be permitted. Work is an excellent thing, but excessive fatigue should be avoided. Life in the country, either on a farm or in a colony for the treatment of epileptics, is the ideal thing for most of these unfortunate people. Stimulants, which in themselves can cause convulsions and general nervousness, should be prohibited. Such things as alcohol, tobacco, coffee and tea would fall in this group. Rigid care of the gastro-intestinal tract, daily bathing, fresh air and sunshine are all extremely important adjuncts in the treatment of epilepsy.

In the past, many different varieties of diets have been recommended for the epileptic. The salt-free diet was especially in vogue when the bromides were the favorite drug in the treatment of the disease, and this diet aided the action of the bromides by producing an increased tolerance for the drug. A purine-free diet and excessive carbohydrates have also been recommended. Starvation was tried in the last decade, but if this form of treatment has any merit, it was probably due to the acidosis which it produced. Acidosis also may be brought about by prescribing a ketogenic diet, by the administration of acids and acid-forming salts. Cobb and Lennox attributed the beneficial results of acidosis in epilepsy to chemical changes in the nerve cells which rendered them less liable to explosions. Dehydration, brought about largely by limiting the fluid intake, has been recommended by some. The ketogenic diet, starvation and dehydration are more likely to cause beneficial results in children in whom remissions are common without any method of treatment. The good obtained from these methods of treatment in adults is meager. For the past two years the writer has had about 24 adult epileptics on alternating periods of dehydration and what might be called hydration, on the one hand limiting the fluid intake from 300 to 1000 cc. in twenty-four hours, and, on the other hand having the patient take from 2000 to 4000 cc. in twenty-four hours. The diet, the method of living and drug therapy in these cases were not altered, and, after a number of months of treatment, he could see that no benefit accrued to the individual while he was on a restricted amount of fluid. Some of the patients had their best months while they were taking over 2 quarts of liquid in twenty-four hours. In his experience the best results are obtained by giving a diet low in carbohydrates with an excessive amount of fat and the elimination of things from the diet that are obviously indigestible. The cooking should be simple and devoid of extra seasoning, it should be rich in vitamins and highly nutritious. One of the most difficult things to control in an epileptic is the amount of food which he eats. He should have the heavy meal in the middle of the day and should under-eat rather than over-eat. A daily evacuation of the bowels is imperative, and laxatives or one of the mineral oils should be prescribed if there is a tendency toward constipation. Each ten days or two weeks the intestinal tract should be cleaned out with a moderate dose of magnesium sulphate.

The drugs which have been recommended for the treatment of epilepsy are countless, and only those which have given the best results will be mentioned. The drug most in vogue at the present time is phenobarbital, which probably acts by producing an inhibition reaction on the motor cortex. The dose of luminal will vary with the age and weight of the patient, but for the ordinary young adult, $\frac{1}{2}$ to 3 grains (0.03 to 0.2 gm.) may be prescribed daily. If more than 1 grain is given in the day, it should be in divided doses. If given to excess, it will produce mental dullness, slurred speech, pronounced lethargy and occasionally a rash which simulates scarlet fever. If luminal is used in the treatment of epilepsy, it should not be suddenly withdrawn because status epilepticus may ensue. Some have advised that sodium luminal be given intravenously in doses of 3 to 5 grains (0.2 to 0.3 gm.) each day, or as often as indicated as a substitute for luminal by mouth. If only one dose of luminal is given a day, it is more convenient for the patient to take it at bedtime. Until the advent of luminal the remedy most prescribed was bromide, which acts by a direct effect upon the cortex, the excitability of which is diminished.

The dose of bromide prescribed, and any one of the salts may be used, will vary with the age and weight of the patient; 5 to 30 grains (0.3 to 2 gm.) or more may be prescribed, three or four times daily. It should be combined with Fowler's solution which is supposed to prevent the occurrence of acne. In certain cases, especially those complicated with vasomotor instability, a combination of bromides and atropine, or atropine alone, seems to bring about improvement. The general effect of bromide must be carefully observed in the treatment of epilepsy. Best results are often obtained by a combination of luminal and bromide, giving the bromide salt in the daytime and the luminal on retiring. Curiously enough, in 2 or 3 patients with unusually low blood pressure, the longest freedom from attacks was obtained by the use of large doses of strychnine. Various glandular extracts, particularly thyroid, have been prescribed, especially by the French. Paraldehyde occasionally does more good than either luminal or bromide and may be used in doses of 20 to 60 minims (1 to 4 cc.), two or three times daily.

Operations on the brains of epileptics produce few, if any, good results. Many patients who have convulsive attacks which begin in one extremity or on one side of the body have had trephine operations performed because of this fact, and the result is practically always disappointing and, in the writer's opinion, not worth the effort. A patient who has had epileptic fits for many years, beginning on one side of the body or in one extremity, and without definite localizing signs between attacks, should not be operated upon, but, if localizing signs do exist a surgical procedure should not be deferred. Excision of part of the motor cortex has been tried unsuccessfully. In the post-traumatic type of epilepsy with scarring of the brain, the excision of the scar has been advised and improvement reported. This reminds one very much of the abdominal operations for the relief of adhesions, which usually produce nothing more than more adhesions. Operations on the body, other than the head, have been resorted to on numerous occasions. Any organ of the body which is diseased should be corrected by surgery, if that is possible, but it is most unwise to permit the surgeon to perform exploratory operations on epileptics, many of whom have had ovaries removed, the large gut extirpated, appendectomy performed for the purpose of permitting free irrigation of the colon, and other equally futile operations. We laugh at the efforts of the ancients who treated epilepsy by cauterizing the scalp, if necessary right down to the skull, but some of the treatments to which epileptics have been subjected in the last thirty years are equally ridiculous.

The treatment of an attack of status is a difficult one. Epsom salts should be administered, if necessary by a nasal tube, and 3 ounces given in 6 ounces of water, by rectum. The use of sodium luminal intravenously in doses of 5 to 10 grains (0.3 to 0.6 gm.) should be employed, and if the attacks still persist, a lumbar puncture may be performed, and sodium luminal in doses up to 5 grains (0.3 gm.) given intraspinally. Chloral and bromides, by rectum, have been recommended in the treatment of status, but the depressing effect of chloral

78

is great and it should be watched for. It is interesting to observe that in many cases of severe status an extreme degree of dehydration ensues, yet the convulsions continue. Venesection has been advised, but, in the writer's opinion, should never be done in the case of ordinary epilepsy. The patient in status must be carefully watched for signs of pulmonary edema and heart failure, and if either one of these complications occur appropriate treatment should be instituted. It is occasionally necessary to give inhalations of chloroform or ether to stop status epilepticus. During an attack of status trophic sores on the heels and buttocks not infrequently occur, and to prevent this the patient's bed should be cleaned frequently and padded, and the back bathed with alcohol and powdered often. There are many epileptics who have a confusional or delusional episode not only after an attack of status, but even after a single fit, and it is necessary to confine such a patient rather closely to a room in which the windows are protected, dangerous objects removed and the door locked.

The psychotherapeutic treatment of an epileptic has an important place. He should be encouraged and a continued effort made to get him to coöperate in his treatment. In many cases the best results are obtained by placing the patient in an institution where he develops a routine and a method of living that is best suited to his disease. Life in an institution will also give him an opportunity to pursue an outdoor occupation and to participate in games. The epileptic needs a kindly, sympathetic but firm attitude adopted toward him. They are extremely difficult and contrary people to live with.

MIGRAINE.

Synonyms.—Sick headache; Hemicrania.

Migraine is a periodic headache limited to one side of the head, and accompanied by certain eye symptoms and vomiting. The attack often terminates in sleep.

The most important factor in the *etiology* of migraine is heredity. There is a close relationship between migraine and epilepsy; some believe that a person suffering from migraine is more likely to produce epileptic children than an epileptic. This is questionable. Attacks of migraine may cease and be replaced by epilepsy, or attacks of the two diseases may alternate. Evidence exists that migraine may be an anaphylactic phenomenon. Certain foods have been known to precipitate an attack of migraine in which eosinophilia may also occur. Indiscretions in diet, worry and exhaustion may serve to initiate an attack. Various endocrine abnormalities have been cited as the etiologic factor in migraine, but the case has not been proven. There is more in favor of the pituitary gland being responsible than other glandular structures. The frequency of ophthalmic symptoms has been used as evidence in favor of the pituitary origin of the disease. Other facts, such as the relation of migraine to menstruation, with its occasional disappearance during pregnancy or lactation or at the menopause, have been used to support the theory that the ductless glands are at fault. A theory as to the causation of the attacks is that vascular spasms occur, probably secondary to sympathetic instability. Attacks of hemiplegia, of aphasia and of hemianopsia during the attack of migraine lend strength to this theory. Some consider migraine a sensory form of epilepsy. The condition is about twice as common in females as in males.

Symptoms.—The attack of migraine is usually ushered in by a general ill-feeling, drowsiness, slight pain in the head and dizziness. These symptoms may last for a number of hours, and are followed by a severe headache, which is limited to one side of the head in the attack, although it may be frontal or occipital in location. Some patients have the pain on the same side in all attacks and in others the locality may vary. It is an unbearable, excruciating type of headache and frequently gives the patient thoughts of suicide. Sometimes the head is tender to touch. The headache lasts from a few hours to two or three days and is practically always accompanied by vomiting. After the acute headache subsides a dull one may be present for a few hours. There is a distinct periodicity to the attacks, which have a tendency to occur at the menstrual periods in women. The headache is aggravated by noise, light and confusion, and the patient suffering from a migrainous headache prefers to be alone. Visual disturbances are frequent. Hemianopsia may occur and be accompanied by dazzling lights, bright dots or zig-zagging phenomena in the blind fields. In some patients the hemianopsia precedes the headache and can be regarded as an aura. While the hemianopsia practically always clears up, occasionally it becomes permanent. Temporary paralysis of an ocular nerve, especially the third, sometimes occurs and after lasting a few weeks or rarely longer, passes away. Hemiplegia or hemiparesis, parasthesia or dysesthesia limited to one side of the body, and aphasia may complicate an attack of migraine. Psychotic episodes resembling very much those seen after an epileptic fit, such as confusion, maniacal outbreaks and an hallucinatory state are rare happenings, but give an added similarity to certain manifestations of epilepsy and migraine. Gastro-intestinal symptoms in the nature of persistent vomiting and even diarrhea have been described. The frequency of the attacks vary from one or two a month to about the same number a year. They have a tendency to disappear at the menopause.

The *diagnosis* of migraine is usually simple, especially when the visual phenomena accompany it. A case of migraine complicated with a paralytic phenomenon may be mistaken for a tumor or a vascular accident. After a patient has had migraine for many years, is advanced in years and arteriosclerotic, it may be difficult to differentiate between a paralytic state due to hemicrania and vascular disease. Sinus disease, syphilis, trigeminal and especially atypical forms of neuralgia and headache due to eye strain have occasionally to be differentiated. Headaches of psychogenic origin may be confused with migraine. The course of migraine is not easily altered. While the patient is free from pain between headaches, they are likely to recur until the time of the menopause, and in many patients persist throughout life.

Treatment.—In the management of a case of migraine, as in epilepsy, the initial step should be to place the patient in the best possible condition of general health, and diseased conditions in any part of the body should be corrected. The avoidance of both mental and physical fatigue, a definite number of hours' sleep nightly, and regularity in the habits of life are essential. In the attack itself, as in epilepsy, very little if anything can be done to abort it. Hypodermics of morphine may do so, but the danger of creating a habit is great, and the use of this drug should be avoided. The patient himself will withdraw to his room and remain as quiet as he can until the attack subsides. Some authorities recommend the use of calcium lactate, in doses of 20 to 50 grains (1.5 to 4 gm.), by mouth, as the prodromal symptoms of a headache appear, and it is thought that this drug may abort the attack. The use of luminal in much the same way as it is prescribed in epilepsy may be advised between headaches, and it frequently reduces the number and severity of the attacks. If any evidence of anaphylaxis can be found, a lead for treatment may be obtained in that way. Miller and Roulston advised the injection of 0.5 to 2 cc. of a 5 per cent solution of peptone, the first injection being 0.5 cc. and the dose increased to the maximum of 2 cc. The injections are first given twice weekly, and then, if an effect is produced upon the headaches, the injections are given weekly. Endocrine therapy has been tried. Abnormal conditions in the gastro-intestinal tract should be corrected and the diet should consist of simple, easily digestible foods.

THE PERIPHERAL NERVOUS SYSTEM.

NEURITIS.

General Discussion.—If one excludes Bell's palsy and multiple neuritis, there are not many instances of real neuritis left. Joint disease, affections of the posterior roots due to syphilis, spinal tumors, vertebral tumors and growths along the course of the nerves will account for most of the things which have been diagnosed neuritis.

Etiology.—The causes of neuritis are trauma, pressure as from crutches, tight bandages or casts and pressure from tumors; intoxication by alcohol, lead and arsenic, and infectious diseases, any of which may produce neuritis. However, diphtheria, sepsis, influenza and scarlet fever are most usually at fault. Chronic focal infection often is an added etiologic factor in cases of multiple neuritis due, for example, to alcohol. Beriberi is due to a deficiency of vitamin B in the diet. It is likely in alcoholic multiple neuritis, in addition to the intoxication by alcohol and focal infection, that deficiency in food may play a rôle.

Pathology.—If a peripheral nerve is diseased or injured, the nerve beyond the point of involvement undergoes definite changes of a pathologic nature; sometimes the nerve proximal to the site of injury degenerates, even as high as the anterior horns. This affects the physiologic and anatomic continuity of the nerves, and the symptoms which result will be expressed in those terms. The amount of involvement of the points distal to the nerve diseased will depend upon the extent of the inflammatory process. All axis cylinders, with the exception of the sympathetic and olfactory nerves, are covered by myelin sheaths, and the sheath of Schwann forms the external membrane of the nerve fiber. The nerve fibers are held together in small bundles by endoneurium. Several of these bundles are united into larger ones by perineurium and the entire peripheral nerve is surrounded by epineurium. Lymph spaces are continuous with subarachnoid spaces of the brain and spinal cord, run in the perineurium and the endoneurium. When a nerve is involved for any reason whatsoever, the myelin sheath breaks up into lecithin bodies and fat droplets. The cells of the sheath of Schwann proliferate and the axis cylinder splits and becomes fragmented. These processes ultimately result in scarring and the formation of connective tissue.

Symptoms.—These vary, depending upon the nerve involved. Most nerves are mixed, containing both motor and sensory fibers, so that in practically every case of neuritis there is a disturbance of both motion and sensation. The greatest discomfort which the patient has is due to the involvement of the sensory part of the nerve, producing pain and paresthesias which may be characterized by the patient as burning, pins and needles, tingling or a sensation of bugs crawling over the skin. Sometimes, especially if the median or sciatic nerve is involved, intense burning pain ensues, and to this condition the term causalgia has been given. Movement intensifies the pain, and tenderness occurs if the nerve is pressed upon.

Objective Signs.—In such cases there will be found some disturbance of sensation, which is found in the peripheral distribution of the nerve involved and which fades out as the sensory examination approaches the trunk. All forms of sensation are involved, touch probably more than the others. Hyperesthesia and hyperalgesia may be seen in certain areas of the nerve. If the nerve involved is a mixed nerve, disturbances of power will occur in the muscles supplied by the nerve. This varies from barely perceptible weakness to complete paralysis. As a rule, the extensor muscles are more affected by neuritis than the flexors. The muscles supplied by the affected nerve become atrophic, flaccid and, if a deep reflex is present in the domain of the nerve affected, it is lost. In addition, the affected nerves show the reactions of degeneration or the loss of contractility to faradism. Fibrillations may occur in multiple neuritis, but are uncommon, and if present, usually denote anterior horn changes. Trophic and vasomotor disturbances may be seen and are due to implication of the sympathetic and trophic fibers present in the peripheral nerve. The skin is often tense, shiny, cold and blue. Desquamation, occurrence of trophic sores and of trophic conditions of the nails and an increase or loss of sweat may be seen. Contractures of the muscles and joints, are frequently seen in cases of neuritis, especially multiple neuritis, and occur most distinctly in those cases that are not properly treated.

Diagnosis.—The diagnosis of neuritis should be made only after a careful diagnostic survey of the individual. Joint disease simulates neuritis by producing pain, limitation of motion and wasting of the muscles, and should be considered, especially if the pain is confined to one extremity or part of one extremity. Arthritis of the shoulder or hip, and bursitis in these regions are frequently labelled neuritis in the early course of the illness. The reflex activity is increased in arthritis, and sensory loss and reactions of degeneration do not occur. Any affection which involves the posterior roots of the spinal cord is frequently called neuritis or neuralgia. Such things as spinal syphilis, spinal tumors, and disease of the vertebræ are misdiagnosed early and late. Tumors along the course of the nerve, especially pelvic sarcomas, are frequently called sciatica. Occasionally the person suffering from continuous pain, for example, from that due to disease of the optic thalamus or irritation of the central pathways, may be diagnosed neuritis. Pressure of a cervical rib on the brachial plexus is sometimes considered as a neuritis arising in the nerve itself. While on theoretical grounds the reflexes may sometimes be increased early in cases of neuritis, it is unwise to diagnose neuritis if the deep reflexes are present, active or increased.

Multiple Neuritis (Polyneuritis).—One of the commonest forms of neuritis is multiple neuritis which is due, in the vast majority of instances, probably 90 per cent, to chronic alcoholism. The amount of alcohol necessary to produce neuritis varies with the individual, just as the amount of alcohol needed to bring about intoxication depends upon the person. Some individuals, especially women, whose nervous systems are especially susceptible to alcohol, may develop signs of multiple neuritis after what might be considered moderate drinking. Thus, a woman who takes a patent medicine containing 15 to 25 per cent of alcohol may develop signs of neuritis after indulging in a few bottles. The writer has seen a few men suffering from multiple neuritis who averaged 1 quart of liquor a day for five to twenty years before developing signs of neuritis.

The earliest *symptom*, as a rule, occurs in the feet and is a paresthesia which may be of any description. One of the commonest and most characteristic symptoms is a burning sensation in the toes and feet, so intense that the patient often places his feet in cold water, even on a cake of ice, to control the painful sensation. Another common habit of the patient suffering from alcoholic multiple neuritis is to keep his feet uncovered at night because the warmth produced by blankets increases the burning feeling. The paresthesias gradually ascend the feet and legs and about this time involve the fingers and hands. Tenderness on pressure over the nerves, the pressure of shoes and of the feet on the ground when the patient attempts to walk are unbearable. The tenderness of the feet is best elicited by squeezing the feet; this produces pressure on the nerves as they are passing between the metatarsal bones. Weakness and ultimately paralysis of the muscles come on, usually more marked in the extensors, but finally involving all the muscles. The toe- and foot-drop and the finger- and wrist-drop are the earliest paralyses seen, but if the patient continues to use alcohol, if he has a focal infection or if an acute infection should attack him he may lose power in all four extremities.

The deep reflexes in the arcs of the affected nerves become diminished and then lost. The paralysis, which is a flaccid one, is accompanied by atrophy, changes in electrical reactions and trophic disorders. All forms of sensation become impaired in a case of any severity. The loss of sensation occurs first in the distal portions of the extremities and even in severe cases may not be found above the ankles and the wrists. If the patient can still walk when first seen and has paralysis, he will usually show a _steppage gait_ which is due to double foot- and toe-drop. Occasionally in the so-called pseudotabes type of multiple neuritis the gait may be ataxic. Sphincter disturbances do not occur as a rule. If the patient suffers from a mental condition the reflexes, due to pyramidal tract irritation, may exist throughout the course of the illness, may even be exaggerated and may return much earlier than is usually seen after multiple neuritis. Cranial nerve symptoms, with the exception of involvement of the optic nerves, are uncommon in alcoholic multiple neuritis but occur more frequently in polyneuritis due to infections. In alcoholic multiple neuritis any of the forms of mental disease due to alcoholism may be seen. But there is one, namely, _Korsakoff's psychosis_, characterized by confusion, disorientation, marked loss of memory and confabulation, which is most commonly noticed. Korsakoff's psychosis may occasionally be due to other toxemias, to infections, and the writer has seen the syndrome after head injury. The consumption of an unusual amount of liquor in a chronic alcoholic, the use of liquor full of deleterious products, the occurrence of acute infections, exposure, excessive drinking with restriction in the amount of food ingested, may all serve to bring out and accentuate early symptoms of multiple neuritis. It may take some months for the individual to reach the height of the illness. If properly handled, most cases will recover but some will do so incompletely.

The most important thing in the _treatment_ of a case of alcoholic multiple neuritis is to have the patient discontinue the use of the drug, which in most instances can be done immediately. Unless the patient is hospitalized there is a great chance that he will continue to obtain alcohol. A high caloric diet rich in vitamins, plenty of fresh air and sunshine are extremely important in the management of these cases. The patient should be immediately placed in the best health possible and all foci of infection removed. If foci of infection are permitted to remain, they may be a sufficient drag on the patient to prevent a good recovery. An air-bed or water-bed should be used and a cradle should be placed over the lower extremities to keep the weight of the bedclothes off those parts. If actual paralysis exists, splints should be applied and the extremities affected placed in a neutral position. This is extremely important, because if foot- and wrist-drop are permitted to exist for some time changes take place in the muscles and tendons which may result in contracture, so that the patient will find after he has recovered from multiple neuritis that he cannot walk because of contractures at the ankles or knees. Drugs are often necessary for the relief of pain and paresthesias, but care should be taken that the patient should not be given an opportunity to develop a new habit.   Opium and its derivatives should be used only after everything else has been tried and failed.   A combination of bromides and salicylates will often serve to quiet the patient and to relieve him of pain.   If insomnia is present, as it often will be early in the treatment, such drugs as barbital and luminal may be tried.   The gastro-intestinal tract should be carefully regulated, if possible, with the milder laxatives.   The use of tonics must be carefully considered before they are employed.   Such things as arsenic, mercury and tryparsamide should not be used.

The consideration of local treatment is important.   Baking and physiotherapeutic measures which produce heat will often increase the pain if employed early in the course of the illness.   As the pain and paresthesias diminish, light gentle massage to the affected parts should be employed every day and mild electrical treatments, either galvanic or faradic, should be used three or four times a week.   It is highly important that the joints in the distribution of the paralysis be passively moved every day and that the tendons about them be lightly manipulated.   If contractures have developed an effort should be made to overcome them by stretching, passive movement and by deep massage.   If all of these are of no avail, tenotomy may have to be done. Even after paralysis of all four extremities has persisted for six to twelve months, a fair to perfect recovery is possible.

Lead Multiple Neuritis.—This is more of a neuronitis than a neuritis because the anterior horn cells of the cord are often affected.   Not infrequently the brain is also affected, giving rise to the so-called lead encephalopathy.   The multiple neuritis of lead is essentially a motor one, and sensory symptoms, if present at all, are extremely mild. The ordinary signs of lead poisoning are usually present for some time before those of neuritis develop.   The condition usually begins in the upper extremities and is practically always bilateral.   The first sign of paralysis is in the extensors of the hand and forearm, and gradually the entire extremity is involved.   The supinator longus muscle usually escapes, and this fact is considered as evidence that the condition is due more to cord disease than to implication of peripheral nerves.   Atrophy and reactions of degeneration occur, but fibrillations do not.   If the disease progresses the peroneal group of muscles is affected in the lower extremities.

Lead encephalopathy may be characterized by maniacal excitement, stupor, delirium, convulsions or focal signs.   In a patient suffering from lead encephalopathy the result of working in the manufacturing of tetraethyl lead, a high fever with signs indicative of encephalitis occurred.

General signs of lead poisoning exist.   The treatment is that of plumbism, neuritis and the cerebral state if present.

Postdiphtheritic Multiple Neuritis.—The type of palsy occurring after diphtheria most frequently seen is limited to the uvula, palate and ciliary muscles.   The symptoms are difficulty in swallowing, regurgitation of fluids through the nose and paralysis of accommodation.   Some of the other cranial nerves may be paralyzed, but as a rule are not.   The paralysis may occur in the course of the diphtheria or may be postponed for days, weeks, a month or more; the paralysis varies from little to much. It is supposed that the infection involves the nerves directly at first but later becomes generalized. Paralysis of a part of an extremity may occur if the diphtheritic infection has taken place in that region.

If the polyneuritis of diphtheria becomes generalized, the symptoms due to involvement of the nerves affected will appear. As a rule, pain is not a common symptom, but the other signs such as loss of reflexes and of sensation, foot-drop and steppage gait occur. The gait may be ataxic. In a series of cases which the writer reported some years ago the loss of sensation was exactly similar to that which occurs in the cord disease commonly seen in pernicious anemia: loss of position and vibratory sensations. The outlook is good. Involvement of the cranial nerves, however, is a dangerous thing and sudden death may occur from heart failure, or the patient may choke to death on a piece of food which lodges in the larynx. Aspiration pneumonia is also the cause of some fatal results. Possibly the rôle of antitoxin is an important one in the causation of palsies. S. B. Hadden and the writer recently reported a number of cases of brachial plexus and other forms of neuritis which came on after the prophylactic use of sera, especially antitetanus. We considered this an anaphylactic reaction and it is probably more common than is suspected.

The *treatment* of diphtheritic multiple neuritis is along the same general lines as mentioned for other forms of multiple neuritis. It is important, however, that the throat and tonsils be cultured to make certain that the patient does not have a chronic infection from the Klebs-Loeffler bacillus.

Arsenical Multiple Neuritis.—Arsenical multiple neuritis presents no outstanding features except that it is usually very painful. Certain skin manifestations such as pigmentation, exfoliating dermatitis, herpes and keratoses on the palms and soles of the feet may be seen. Arsenical multiple neuritis is not infrequently due to the use of drugs in a therapeutic way and may follow the use of Fowler's solution and arsenic trioxide and various arsenicals used for intravenous therapy. The writer has seen a case of arsenical multiple neuritis develop in a man who was being slowly poisoned by his wife. Arsenic as the possible factor in a case of multiple neuritis should always be thought of.

The *treatment* does not vary from that of other forms of the disease.

Diabetic Multiple Neuritis.—The *symptoms* here may be due to involvement of the peripheral nerves or to changes in the cord. The lower extremities are especially involved and the affection is frequently of the tabetic type. Alcohol sometimes plays a contributing rôle in this condition.

Other conditions may produce multiple neuritis, such as carbon monoxide poisoning, beriberi, leprosy and so-called pink disease, or *erythredema polyneuritis*. It has also been called *acrodynia*. The latter condition is usually seen in children, and is frequently accompanied by insomnia, restlessness and swelling and redness of the fingers and toes and possibly also trophic conditions, even gangrene. The pink disease is probably an infectious or deficiency one.

Polyneuronitis.—Any infection may produce multiple neuritis, but there is one with a special tendency to involve the peripheral nervous system and to produce in addition paralysis of certain of the cranial nerves, especially the seventh. While this has been described under the heading of multiple neuritis, the central nervous system is frequently involved so that the condition should more properly be referred to as a *neuronitis*, a term first suggested by C. K. Mills. The condition was especially prevalent among the troops during the World War, but had been seen in civilian practice before the war and after it.

Signs of involvement of the nervous system come on a few days or a week or two after an infection, which usually involves the upper respiratory system, and the progress of the paralysis sometimes suggests very strongly the syndrome known as Landry's paralysis. The *symptoms* resemble those seen in multiple neuritis, but cranial nerve involvement, especially of the seventh nerve, is a common additional sign. Bulbar symptoms frequently are seen and may produce sudden death. In one of a series of cases which Robertson and the writer reported, a sinus infection seemed to be the etiologic factor. The condition has been described under a number of names, due to the fact that in different epidemics the distribution of the paralysis varies. As is mentioned above, one of the commonest physical findings is the bilateral seventh nerve paralysis. The treatment is symptomatic.

Sciatica.—While real sciatica does exist, the diagnosis of this condition is frequently made without sufficient basis, and if patients on whom the diagnosis is made are observed over a long period, it will often be found that some condition other than primary inflammation of the nerve exists. Disease of the spinal roots, especially syphilis, tumors of the cord, disease and tumors of the vertebra, pressure on the nerve anywhere along its course, such as tumors in the pelvis, are conditions which are frequently mislabelled sciatica. Furthermore, many cases of arthritis limited to the hip are called sciatica some time in the course of the illness. Varicose veins or adhesions along the course of the nerve may be responsible for sciatic symptoms. Whether to call the condition sciatica or sciatic neuralgia is a question not entirely settled, but it is likely that most of the cases of real sciatica have changes in the nerve.

Sciatica is more frequently seen in males, who are usually past middle age. It frequently is observed after infectious diseases or may be due to chronic focal infection, especially in the prostate. It also is supposed to occur in gout, rheumatism and diabetes. The writer has seen a number of cases follow exposure to cold. It may occur after the intragluteal injection of medicine for the treatment of syphilis or malaria, when the nerve has been injured directly or by an abscess. It may come on after a heavy lifting or a marked muscular exertion, especially in people not used to such. True sciatica is usually unilateral. If double sciatica exists it is imperative to rule out the conditions mentioned above, such as syphilis and tumor of the spinal cord. It may be an occupational disease such as that which occurs in a locomotive engineer where the condition is due to pressure on the nerve due to prolonged sitting.

Symptoms.—Usually slow in onset, but in certain infectious cases and in those due to stretching of the nerve during a physical exertion, the signs may come on abruptly. Pain begins, as a rule, in the buttock and follows the course of the nerve down the back of the thigh, calf, heel and to the foot. It is important, as in any patient who complains of pain, to have the individual trace or locate without suggestion the site of the pain. While the pain is usually constant, it may be paroxysmal, and like most pains is worse at night. Coughing, sneezing, jarring and motion aggravate the pain, which is usually sharp but may be dull. The patient tries to prevent pain by keeping the extremity flexed at the ankle and the hip, and if he is in bed he holds the extremity flexed at the knee and abducted. He is likely to stand on the healthy extremity, the gluteal fold is low on the affected side and a scoliosis is usually seen with the convexity toward the diseased area. Anything which stretches the nerve, such as bending forward to touch the floor with the fingers, or testing for Lasègue's sign, which is done in the same manner as Kernig's sign, makes the patient cry out with pain. Tender points may exist along the course of the nerve. Paralysis and sensory loss are uncommon, but the latter especially may occur in the distribution of the nerve. The knee-jerk is not affected; in fact, due to the tenseness of the patient, it may be slightly exaggerated. The Achilles reflex, which is in the domain of the sciatic nerve, is diminished or lost. Muscular atrophy and changes in electrical reactions do not occur except in very rare cases. Trophic and vasomotor signs may be seen.

Most patients will recover, although the condition may be very resistant to treatment and persist for months. From a prognostic standpoint much depends upon the general health of the patient.

As far as the *differential diagnosis* is concerned, a condition should be called sciatica only as a last resort. Careful investigation of the pelvis, of the rectum, of the spine, particular search for evidence of syphilis and of spinal cord tumors, careful survey of the patient for focal infections and for evidence of arthritis, especially of the hip and sacro-iliac joint, elimination of flat feet and of arterial disease should be gone into before the diagnosis of sciatica is made.

The most important element in the *treatment* is rest. A combination of bromide and salicylate will quiet the patient and relieve the pain. In view of the fact that the condition may be prolonged, opium and its derivatives should not be used. Heat, either dry or wet, usually gives the patient considerable relief, and diathermy over the nerve is sometimes of considerable value. The writer has seen a number of patients greatly relieved by counterirritation or by the use of dry or wet cups along the course of the nerve. Massage, galvanism and faradism are of no value. If the pain is very severe, 5 to 10 cc. of a 1 per cent solution of novocaine may be injected epidurally in the sacral canal, and followed in a few minutes by the injection of 50 cc. of normal sterile saline. Direct injection into the nerve sheath of normal saline or alcohol and stretching of the nerve have been used but usually with poor results. The less stretching and injection done, the happier the patient and doctor both are. In some cases exposure of the nerve and freeing it of adhesions have benefited the patient.

Peripheral Facial Paralysis (Bell's Palsy, Prosoplegia).—This is probably the commonest type of peripheral neuritis. It is much more frequently seen in the spring and fall and is usually due to exposure and chilling of the face. It is likely that, when exposure seems to be the cause, an infection really is at fault. A facial palsy may be seen in the course of any infectious disease, in ear infection, in tumors of the parotid, tumors in the cerebellopontile angle, syphilis in the cerebellopontile angle and direct trauma to the nerve. It is occasionally the result of operations on the parotid or on the ear. Tetanus, especially when the wound of entrance is about the face, may produce facial paralysis. Facial diplegia is usually due to neurosyphilis at the base, to polyneuronitis and to encephalitis. Occasionally facial diplegia is seen in myasthenia gravis and muscular dystrophy. The weakness of the face which occurs in bulbar palsy is only for the lower half. A lesion in the pons at the level of the seventh nucleus will produce facial paralysis of the peripheral type, but signs indicative of pontile rather than peripheral disease will be present.

Symptoms.—The symptoms which result from a peripheral facial paralysis are constituted by paralysis of the muscles on one side, which is flattened, the corner of the mouth droops and the face may seem drawn to the normal side. The wrinkles and folds normally present on the affected side will be smoothed out either in part or entirely, the eye cannot be closed and the palpebral fissure is wider than normal. Voluntary movement on the affected side is impaired and this may vary from slight weakness to total paralysis. The patient has difficulty in chewing because food has a tendency to collect between the gums and the cheek. He frequently drools at first and has slight difficulty in speaking. Because the blinking reflex is lost tears often flow from the eye on the affected side. The loss of reflexes is due to involvement of the motor part of the arc. If the chorda tympani is involved there is a disturbance of taste on the side of the lesion on the anterior two-thirds of the tongue. Occasionally herpes of the internal auditory meatus and the auricle with pain in these parts may be a part of the picture and has been written about especially by Hunt, as a syndrome of the geniculate ganglion. In this there is deep-seated pain in the ear and the mastoid region and occasionally lymphocytosis of the cerebrospinal fluid. Occasionally the eighth nerve is involved. Sensation is not affected in the ordinary type of Bell's palsy. In bilateral paralysis of the face the facies are masked and chewing and talking are interfered with. Tears and saliva frequently roll down the face. In ten days to two weeks after the onset of paralysis, changes in the electrical reactions may occur. These changes may vary from slight reduction in contractility to faradism to complete reactions of degeneration.

One of the exhibitions of idiopathic Bell's palsy to which but little attention has been paid in the past is the often profound mental depression associated with the nerve lesion. This is out of all proportion to the severity or gravity of the disturbance. For some reason or another these patients are frequently a high-strung, nervous type of individuals. The very obvious alterations in the appearance of the face makes them self-conscious and introspective. The difficulties in speech add to their sensitivity, and the drooling of saliva makes them further aware of their abnormal condition and of their, to them, unhappy state.

Diagnosis.—The most important consideration in the diagnosis of Bell's palsy is to differentiate it from a paralysis of the face of central origin which is usually a part of the picture of hemiplegia. In this condition only the lower part of the face is involved. The tongue, because of simultaneous involvement of the muscle moving it on protrusion, deviates to the paralyzed side. Electrical reactions are not affected. The muscles may move well during emotionalism. Furthermore, in hemiplegia the rest of the same side of the body will be affected.

When the eighth nerve is paralyzed in conjunction with the seventh, due to an acute inflammatory reaction, the diagnosis of a tumor in the angle has occasionally been made. The most important things in this connection are the history at the onset and, instead of rushing into an operation, careful judicial watching of the patient. In bilateral facial paralysis, syphilis, polyneuronitis and encephalitis should be considered from a diagnostic standpoint. If syphilis is to blame, involvement of the eighth nerve may also be seen.

Prognosis.—The prognosis in facial paralysis naturally depends upon the cause. If it is the ordinary type, due to exposure, the chances for a complete recovery are good. The most valuable aid in prognosis is the reaction of the nerve to electricity two weeks after the onset. The milder the changes to faradism or galvanism, the better is the prognosis. Mild cases will do well in three to six weeks, whereas severe cases may last from three months to one year. If the nerve has been cut during an operation or if involved by a parotid tumor, the outlook is not good. Many cases will recover with contractures, especially those who are treated too vigorously by local measures. Associated movements may be seen on the side of the face which has recovered partially from a Bell's palsy, for example, when a patient winks the eye on the affected side the angle of the mouth draws up, and *vice versa*. It is supposed that the reason for this is some of the fibers destined for the upper part of the face and some from the lower grow to the wrong destination. Years after a Bell palsy has cleared up facial spasm may be noted on the affected side.

Treatment.—This consists in protection of the patient against exposure and drafts in the early stages and the application of a blister or some form of counterirritation to the point of exit of the nerve. Because Bell's palsy is in many instances an infectious process, it is usually wise to have the patient rest in bed for a few days at the onset. The eye should be protected with a patch and washed out frequently with warm boric acid. After the patient has been permitted to be up and around he should protect the paralyzed side against drafts and winds. Small to moderate doses of sodium salicylate and sodium iodide should be given as soon as the patient is seen, and continued for two or four weeks. He should be told to support the paralyzed side with the hand; if there is much drooping on the weakened side, this may be strapped up with adhesive. This is on the theory that any pull or drag should always be removed from the paralyzed muscles, especially if the paralysis is a peripheral one. Ten days to two weeks after the onset of paralysis electrical treatment should be initiated on alternate days. If faradism produces a response, that type of electricity should be used; if it does not, galvanism should be employed. On the alternate days mild gentle massage will aid in recovery. As soon as voluntary movement begins to return the number of local treatments should be reduced, and when fair movement has been established all local treatment should be stopped. Treatment should be persisted in for at least six months after the onset, and even after six months of paralysis some cases may make a good recovery. Anastomosis of the central end of the hypoglossus or of the spinal accessory with the distal slump of the facial has been tried. Anastomosis with the spinal accessory has been discarded, and anastomosis with the hypoglossal is not, as a rule, successful.

Facial Hemispasm.—This condition may involve either the entire distribution of the nerve or one of its branches. The movements are painless and resemble those produced by electrical stimulation of the nerve. It occasionally occurs without any detectable cause, but may be a symptom of pressure on the nerve as, for example, by a tumor in the angle. It has been known to follow years after an ordinary Bell palsy, and the writer has seen it come on a few months after a shrapnel wound of the face which had partially paralyzed the nerve. In another case it was due to a small thrombotic lesion in the facial cortical center. He has also seen partial continuous epilepsy limited to the face resemble very much a case of hemispasm of the face.

With the foregoing symptoms in mind, careful search should be made in the distribution of the seventh and eighth nerves for evidence of disease. Some of the cases of facial tic are psychogenic in origin. The frequency of the facial movements may vary from an occasional spasm to almost constant twitching of the face.

Treatment should depend on the cause; if none is discoverable psychotherapeutic procedures, injection of the nerve with alcohol or partial section of it may be tried.

Progressive Facial Hemiatrophy.—This is a condition which usually begins before puberty, is more common in females and more frequently involves the left side of the face, although Archambault denies the latter. The atrophy is first noted in the skin, usually at the external angle of the orbit, or at the angle of the mouth, and then gradually spreads until it involves the entire side of the face. The skin becomes thin, fat disappears and later on the underlying muscles and bones become atrophic, but actual paralysis and reactions of degeneration do not occur. The corresponding side of the tongue, even of the soft palate, may become atrophic. Changes in the hair and of the sweat secretion on the side of the face involved may be found. There is neither loss of sensation nor disturbance of taste. The cause of this condition is unknown, although in Mendel's case neuritis of the fifth nerve was found, along with changes in the spinal nucleus of the fifth nerve. In another case, interstitial neuritis of the Gasserian ganglion and the parts distal to it was discovered. However, removal of the Gasserian ganglion or avulsion of the roots does not produce facial hemiatrophy. If facial hemiatrophy occurs in syringomyelia the typical dissociation loss of sensation will be found. The condition has been attributed to trauma and may have an important medico-legal aspect. In a recent case the parents of a child were awarded a substantial verdict because the jury believed injury to the face resulted in a pronounced form of facial hemiatrophy.

Facial Hemihypertrophy.—Facial hemihypertrophy is an extremely rare condition in which the soft tissue and the bones on one side of the face hypertrophy. This may occasionally be found associated with enlargement of one entire side of the body.

NEURALGIA.

General Discussion.—Neuralgia is usually a symptom and not a disease. It consists in paroxysmal attacks of pain in the course of the sensory nerve. It might be some time before the organic nature of the condition is suspected, but such things as root involvement, toxemias or pressure of an aneurysm will be found. If the neuralgic condition is hysterical in origin, it should properly be called psychalgia. Certain infections, especially malaria, have an important rôle in the production of pain in the course of a nerve. The most common form of neuralgia is trigeminal (tic douloureux or trifacial neuralgia).

Trigeminal Neuralgia.—Trifacial neuralgia (tic douloureux) is most frequently seen in patients in middle or advanced life. Its cause is not known. It is apparently not hereditary, but a family history of such things as migraine, epilepsy and anxiety neurosis may be obtainable, as they are, however, in many histories. The pain is in the distribution of the fifth nerve. If confronted with a patient suffering from pain in the face, either in one or all of the branches of the fifth nerve, it is important to rule out things which may either by pressure or reflexly cause pain in the area of the trigeminal nerve. Tumors in the angle, tumors of the Gasserian ganglion, diseases of the teeth or the sinuses, basilar syphilis and general toxemias or infections, especially malaria, should be considered. The real *cause* of the condition is not known, and it is unlikely that there is much pathologic involvement of the sensory roots because of the absence of sensory changes.

Symptoms.—The pain will obviously be in the distribution of the branch involved, but it may spread to the entire supply of the trigeminal nerve. Occasionally the pain is bilateral. The pain occurs suddenly, is excruciating, burning and violent. It may last a few seconds or minutes and occurs paroxysmally. After a number of attacks in the course of days, the pain may subside and disappear for weeks or months. During an attack the patient holds the face and head in a set manner, because opening the mouth, talking, chewing, or swallowing may bring on an attack of pain. Washing the face or exposure to cold may also bring on an attack. Flushing of the skin, and an abnormal flow of tears or saliva and local sweating may be seen. Tic-like movements of the face, smacking of the lips and movements of the jaw may occur. The tender points, or *trigger zones*, so called because irritation of them may bring on an attack, are found along the course of the nerve. The symptoms are usually more marked in the daytime. The patient will usually continue to have pain, unless operated upon or the nerve injected.

Diagnosis.—The diagnosis is made chiefly from the conditions mentioned in the foregoing remarks; however, the so-called Meckel's ganglion, Sluder's neuralgia, glossopharyngeal neuralgia, migraine and hysteria should also be considered. The presence of sensory findings will rule out organic affections of the ganglion and of the roots of the nerve. The pain of Sluder's neuralgia is not limited to the fifth nerve, and has a tendency to radiate to the shoulder; the importance and frequency of this has been greatly overestimated. In glossopharyngeal neuralgia the pain radiates from the pharynx to the side of the neck and to the ear. The tonsil may act as a trigger zone, thus swallowing may bring on an attack.

Treatment.—The medical treatment of trigeminal neuralgia is usually without result unless there is something specific to attack, such as syphilis or malaria, and in such cases the individual does not have real trifacial neuralgia. Heat, especially diathermy, may produce considerable relief. Many drugs were formerly employed, but, as a rule, none of them produce any permanent result.

The patient usually has to submit either to injection of the branches of the nerves or ganglion with 80 to 90 per cent alcohol or to avulsion of the sensory root. The injection with alcohol is often first chosen by the patient, and it is also an important diagnostic procedure in distinguishing between trigeminal neuralgia and the atypical ones. Avulsion of the sensory roots was first suggested by Spiller, and refinements of the operation have been perfected by neurosurgeons, especially Frazier. The mortality following the operation is less than 1 per cent, and it results in few postoperative complications, of which facial paralysis, trophic disorders and deafness are the commonest. Loss of sensation, of course, occurs in the distribution of the fifth nerve. The operation is curative.

Glossopharyngeal Neuralgia.—The paroxysmal pain of this condition is similar to that seen in tic douloureux, except for the distribution. The pain radiates from the pharynx to the side of the neck and to the ear. The pharynx and tonsil often act as a trigger zone and, as a result, swallowing frequently causes a paroxysm of pain. Yawning may bring on a paroxysm. The cause is unknown. The differential diagnosis is to be made especially from trigeminal neuralgia. Injection of the fifth nerve with alcohol will not produce a loss of pain, if the condition is due to glossopharyngeal neuralgia. Alcohol injection of the glossopharyngeal is hazardous, because of the danger of injecting the vagus. Avulsion of the root is curative and should be done intracranially. The other types of neuralgia, such as occipital, brachial, intercostal and that of the lumbo-sacral regions usually have an organic basis behind them and will not be discussed here.

Coccygodynia.—Neuralgia of the coccygeal nerves, or coccygodynia, in which the pain is referred to the tip of the coccyx, which is tender, is usually hysterical. It comes on after trauma or childbirth and is aggravated by walking or sitting. The proper treatment is psychotherapy. Removal of the coccyx does not cure the condition unless it does so by its psychotherapeutic element.

NEUROTIC PROGRESSIVE MUSCULAR ATROPHY.

Synonyms.—Peroneal muscular atrophy; Charcot-Marie-Tooth muscular atrophy.

This disease, an hereditary degenerative type, is more common in males, and may affect several members of one family. Pathologic changes have been found in the peripheral nerves, posterior columns and anterior horns and roots. The age of onset is usually before twenty-five or thirty years. It frequently comes on in childhood or early adult life, although the onset may be delayed to twenty-five or thirty years. The atrophy begins in the distal portions of the lower extremities, and even in long-standing cases there may be little or no involvement of the thighs. The earliest paralysis usually occurs in the peroneal group, producing foot-drop with its characteristic steppage gait. Various deformities of the feet may ensue. The legs become extremely atrophic and present signs of vasomotor instability. The reflexes disappear, mild sensory disturbances, especially in the distal portions of the extremities, and a varying decrease of the reactions to electrical current are found. The upper extremities are involved, as a rule, months or years after the symptoms have appeared in the lower extremities, although the writer has seen one case where the symptoms came on at the same time. The symptoms in the upper extremities are usually confined to the parts below the elbows.

The *treatment* is symptomatic. Massage, electrical treatment, orthopedic appliances and operations will improve the patient's condition.

LESIONS OF THE PERIPHERAL NERVES OF THE EXTREMITIES.

A complete understanding of the results of paralysis of the peripheral nerves can be had only by careful study of the anatomy of the nerve, the muscles which it supplies and the areas of the skin which it serves with sensation.

Ulnar Nerve.—The ulnar nerve is derived from the inner cord of the brachial plexus and from a root standpoint, from the eighth cervical and first dorsal roots, most of whose fibers go to form the nerve. The nerve supplies the two inner heads of the flexor profundus digitorum, the adductors of the thumb, the inner head of the flexor brevis pollicis and the muscles of the hypothenar eminence, the inner two lumbricales and all of the interossei. The sensory part of the nerve supplies the palmar and dorsal surface of the little and the inner half

79

of the ring finger, and the inner side of the palm, and back of the hand to a short distance above the wrist. The nerve may be injured by direct trauma or by pressure, such as, for example, pressure exerted on the deep branch of the ulnar in the palm, or the pressure of leaning the elbows on a desk or chair. The nerve may be involved in a lesion of the brachial plexus, dislocation of a shoulder or elbow, by pressure of splints, fractures in or about the elbow, which later give rise to excessive callus formation. The latter condition may cause an ulnar paralysis months or years after the primary injury. Leprosy has a special tendency to involve the ulnar nerve. If the injury is high, flexion of the hand is weak and it is turned toward the radial side. Extension of the distal phalanges and flexion of the proximal ones are impaired or lost, so that claw-hand (*main en griffe*) is formed, due to unopposed action of the radial nerve. Adduction of the fingers is impaired; adduction of the thumb is lost. The muscles supplied by the nerve waste. This is especially noticeable in the hypothenar eminence, in the palm and the interosseous spaces which become hollowed out. Sensory loss corresponds to the anatomic distribution of the nerve and in mild cases is usually greater for touch than for any other form of sensation. Pain and paresthetic phenomena may be severe, and vasomotor and trophic changes may cause distressing complications.

The Median Nerve.—The median nerve is made up by the outer and inner cords of the brachial plexus, the fibers of the nerve being derived from the sixth, seventh and eighth cervical and first dorsal roots. It supplies the pronator quadratus and the pronator radii teres, the flexor carpi radialis, the flexor sublimis, the two outer heads of the flexor profundus digitorum, the abductor and opponens of the thumb, the flexor longus and part of the flexor brevis pollicis, and the two outer lumbricales.

The sensory part of the nerve supplies the outer part of the palm from the middle of the ring finger to the thumb. On the dorsal aspect of the hand the nerve supplies the last two phalanges of the index, middle and radial half of the ring fingers. The median is especially rich in trophic and vasomotor fibers. The nerve may be affected anywhere along its course; for example, by dislocation of the shoulder, by bullet or stab wounds, and it may be involved as a part of a general multiple neuritis. Depending on the level at which the nerve is involved, the extent of the paralysis varies. Ordinarily implication of the nerve produces weakness of flexion at the wrist, and flexion at the distal phalanges of the middle and index fingers, especially the latter, are greatly disturbed. The thumb is adducted and extended and the terminal phalanx of the thumb cannot be flexed. The thumb cannot be brought to touch the tips of the fingers. The thenar eminence and the pulps of the middle and index fingers and thumb become atrophic. Sensory loss is, as a rule, as great as the distribution of the nerve. Involvement of the median nerve usually produces a severe amount of burning pain, which was designated by Mitchell as *causalgia*. It is a burning, boring, intractable pain which makes life unbearable.

The nails in the distribution of the nerve become dry, brittle and furrowed and the skin tense and glossy.

Musculospiral Nerve (Radial Nerve).—This nerve is derived from the posterior cord of the brachial plexus and is made up mainly of fibers from the sixth and seventh cervical roots. It supplies the triceps, the anconeus, the brachioradialis, the extensors of the forearm and the long extensors of the fingers and thumb. The cutaneous distribution of the nerve varies. The posterior aspects of the hand not supplied by the median and ulnar are innervated by the radial. This is approximately the radial half of the dorsal aspect of the hand, dorsal aspect of the thumb, of the index finger to the first phalanx and the radial half of the middle finger to the first phalanx. The musculospiral nerve is frequently injured, especially by pressure in the axilla from a crutch, during deep sleep, especially a drunken one, in which the weight of the head rests on the humerus and presses against the nerve, and by fracture of the humerus. It can also, of course, be injured by bullet wounds or stab wounds. The commonest cause is pressure on the nerve by drunken sleep, the so-called Saturday night paralysis. Lead produces a double musculospiral paralysis in which the supinator longus muscles are spared. The paralysis which results from musculospiral palsy will depend upon the height of the injury to the nerve; for example, if it is injured in the axilla, there is paralysis in the entire distribution of the nerve, including the triceps. The usual location of the involvement which is in the arm spares the triceps. There is paralysis of the extensors of the hand, thumb and fingers, the proximal phalanges of the latter being involved. The rest of the finger extension is done by the non-paralyzed interosseous muscles. The forearm is pronated, the wrist drops and the thumb is adducted, flexed and opposed. The hand grip is weak if the patient attempts to grasp an object with the wrist dropped, but if the hand is supinated the grasp will be good. The sensory loss is not nearly so extensive as the distribution of the nerve, and, in many cases, practically no sensory loss occurs.

Long Thoracic Nerve.—This nerve is a motor one, and is derived from the fifth, sixth and seventh cervical roots and supplies the serratus magnus. Its chief function is fixation of the scapula and to aid in the abduction of the arm above the horizontal plane. It may be paralyzed from injury, carrying heavy weights on the shoulder and from inflammatory reactions. The inferior angle of the scapula stands away from the chest and, on elevating the arm, the scapula becomes winged. Weakness is encountered in raising the arm above the horizontal plane. The lifting ability of the patient is diminished. Pain is not usually present and the prognosis for recovery is fair.

Circumflex Nerve.—This nerve is derived from the fifth and sixth cervical roots and supplies the deltoid and teres minor. The function of the nerve is to elevate and abduct the arm to a right angle, above which the arm is carried by the serratus magnus and trapezius. The sensory branch of the nerve supplies an oval space over the deltoid muscle. Paralysis of the nerve is caused by direct injury, by fractures or dislocations implicating the nerve, by pressure or by infections and toxemias. If the nerve is completely involved, the shoulder joint is relaxed, the deltoid atrophic and the arm cannot be abducted. Changes in electrical reactions occur. Due to involvement of the teres minor outward, rotation of the arm is interfered with. Pain is frequently severe and a loss of sensation occurs in the distribution of the nerve. In arriving at a diagnosis local conditions of the shoulder must be considered and ruled out.

External Popliteal.—This is the external division of the sciatic, and supplies the antero-external muscles of the leg, the extensor longus digitorum, the extensor proprius pollicis, the tibialis anticus, the peroneus brevis and the peroneus longus. It innervates the skin on the dorsal surface of the first metatarsal and big toe, the antero-external surface of the leg and the dorsum of the foot, including the dorsum of the great toe, first, second and third toes up to the second phalanges. This nerve is frequently involved by direct injury, especially as it winds around the head of the fibula, where it is susceptible to the pressure of a cast, to direct blows and to disease involving the upper part of the fibula. It may be paralyzed as the result of occupation when the nerve is frequently squeezed, for example, in hardwood floor polishers and people who work in gardens and frequently bend the knees. Lead involves the nerve bilaterally. It is also occasionally injured in the pelvis during difficult labors. Involvement of the nerve produces paralysis of the extensors of the foot and of the extensors of the proximal phalanges of the toes, and impairment of eversion. Foot-drop, pes equinovarus and occasionally flat-foot result. Steppage gait on the affected side appears. Contractures due to unopposed muscles may set in. Pain, trophic and vasomotor changes are unusual and the cutaneous sensory loss is less than the supply of the nerve itself.

Treatment.—This will depend in a large measure upon the cause. If there is evidence that the nerve has been directly injured by bullet wounds, stab wounds or fracture or by pressure of the fragments of bone, it should be investigated surgically as soon as possible, although many patients with peripheral nerve injury complicated by complete paralysis of the nerve may make a total recovery without operation. Some choose to wait six to twelve weeks before surgical interference. If the nerve has been involved by pressure or infections or toxic cause, surgical intervention is usually not indicated. A splint or appliance should be made to support the muscles paralyzed; for example, in a paralysis of the external popliteal, a light brace should be applied to overcome the foot-drop; in a case of musculospiral paralysis, the hand and forearm should be placed on a cocked-up splint. Massage should be given daily or at least three times a week and faradism or galvanism applied to the affected nerve three times a week. The outlook in pressure cases is usually good, although the individual nerve may take from three to six months to recover. Various orthopedic operations may produce more useful extremities if the nerve paralysis does not recover.

THE MYOPATHIES.

PROGRESSIVE MUSCULAR DYSTROPHY.

This disease is strictly limited to the muscles. The causes, other than familial tendency to the disease, are not known, although there is some evidence that the endocrine system and perhaps the liver may have a rôle in the production of muscular dystrophy. The nervous system, both central and peripheral, is intact. The muscle fibers show atrophy, though occasionally a true hypertrophy may be seen. The wasted fibers are replaced by fibrous tissue and fat, producing myosclerosis. Pseudohypertrophy occurs in a form of the disease, especially implicating the deltoids and muscles of the calf. The muscles, apparently enlarged, have a hard, non-elastic feel. The age of onset is usually before ten years, but it may be delayed as late as twenty-five years, and cases have been reported even up to forty years of age. The amount of creatinine excreted daily is lower the greater the incapacity of the patient. A diminished tolerance for creatine exists, which bears some relation to the severity of the symptoms.

Symptoms.—The muscles involved are those of the trunk, the shoulder girdles, pelvic girdles, arms and thighs. The muscles below the elbows and below the knees may be affected early, but this is contrary to the rule and serves as one of the chief differential points between muscular dystrophy and the atrophies of the spinal origin. The face, while implicated in many cases, is not as a rule first involved. Due to involvement of the muscles of the hip and of the spine, the gait is of the so-called duck or waddling type and resembles, to a degree, that seen in double congenital dislocation of the hips. Weakness of the muscles of the spine causes distinct lordosis and great difficulty when the patient attempts to arise from a sitting position on the floor. The manner in which a patient with muscular dystrophy arises from the floor (he climbs up himself) is one of the most characteristic things in the disease, but may be seen in any patient who has weakness of the back and gluteal muscles from other causes. The involvement of the muscles of the shoulder girdles and the arms produces loose shoulders and winged scapulæ. As the muscles waste, their movements become weaker and gradually disappear. The same thing holds good for the deep reflexes. Sensation is normal and fibrillations are not seen. While the electrical reactions diminish and finally disappear, there are no reactions of degeneration. Some of the muscles may appear unusually large. This is due to replacement of the muscle with fat or connective tissue; in some cases actual hypertrophy of the muscle occurs. Such a muscle is harder than usual, and yet may be weak to the point of paralysis. If the face is involved the so-called myopathic facies is seen. Wrinkles are absent, the folds are flattened out, tapir mouth ensues and the palpebral fissures are widened. All these symptoms are due to weakness in the distribution of the seventh nerves. The smile is a transverse one. The muscles are involved bilaterally and more or less symmetrically. Tonic preservation may occur in the muscles of the hands. The heart muscle has been involved in some cases. Contractures and ankylosis frequently occur, especially in patients who have very little attention paid to them in the line of physiotherapy. Some of the cases of dystrophy become freaks in the side-shows of circuses. It is rare to have involvement of the tongue, ocular and jaw muscles.

The course of the disease is gradually progressive; victims suffering from it are quite likely to be carried off by acute infections, but many live twenty to forty years after the onset. In some the disease progresses so very slowly that it appears to be arrested.

If it be borne in mind that the disease occurs early in life, chiefly in males, that the proximal segments of the limbs are affected, power, reflexes and electrical reactions gradually disappear, that there are no changes in sensation and that fibrillary tremors are unknown, there should be no difficulty in the diagnosis.

There is no specific *treatment*. Massage and passive movements to the joints may prevent the occurrence of deformities. Feeding with pituitary and thyroid extract may be of service. Injection of suprarenal extract has been tried. In the last few years the use of glycine or glutamic acid has been attended with some success. Improvement in metabolism occurs. The average increases in creatine and in creatinine excretions are considerable under this therapy for a few weeks when there is a return to the former levels.

BIBLIOGRAPHY.

BAILEY, PERCIVAL, and CUSHING, HARVEY: A Classification of the Tumors of the Glioma Group on a Histogenetic Basis with a Correlated Study of Prognosis, Philadelphia, J. B. Lippincott Company, 1926.

BUZZARD, E. F., and GREENFIELD, J. G.: Pathology of the Nervous System, New York, Paul B. Hoeber, 1922.

CADWALADER, W. B.: The Sudden Onset of Paralysis in Pott's Disease Without Deformity of the Vertebræ, Am. Jour. Med. Sci., 1911, 141, 546.

GOWERS, W. R.: The Border-land of Epilepsy, Philadelphia, P. Blakiston's Son & Co., 1907.

HADDEN, S. B., and WILSON, GEORGE: Neuritis and Multiple Neuritis Following Serum Therapy, Jour. Am. Med. Assn., 1932, 98, 123.

JELLIFE, S. E., and WHITE, W. A.: Diseases of the Nervous System, Philadelphia, Lea & Febiger, 1929.

McIVER, JOSEPH, and WILSON, GEORGE: On the Postero-lateral Sclerosis Seen in Cases of Severe Anemia, Pa. Med. Jour., 1921, 25, 189.

———— Spontaneous Subarachnoid Hemorrhage, Jour. Am. Med. Assn., 1929, 93, 89.

OPPENHEIM, H.: Text Book of Nervous Diseases, Edinburgh, The Darien Press, 1911.

ORNSTEEN, A. M.: Thrombosis of the Anterior Artery, Am. Jour. Med. Sci., 1931, 181, 654.

PENDERGRASS, Clinic of DR. EUGENE P.: Value of and Indications for Encephalography and Ventriculology with Discussion of the Technique, from Dept. of Roentgenology, Hospital of University of Pennsylvania.

PURVES-STEWART, JAMES: Diagnosis of Nervous Diseases, New York, E. B. Treat & Co., 1924.

SPILLER, W. G.: Encephalomyelitis Disseminata, Arch. Neurol. and Psych., 1919, 22, 547.

———— The Relation of the Myopathies, Brain, 1913, 36, 75.

———— The Subacute Form of Multiple Sclerosis, Arch. Neurol. and Psych., 1919, 1, 219.

SPILLER, W. G., and FRAZIER, C. H.: The Division of the Sensory Root of the Trigeminus for the Relief of Tic Douloureux, University of Pennsylvania contribution to William Pepper Laboratory, Philadelphia, 1902, p. 12.

TURNER, ALDREN: Epilepsy, London, Macmillan & Co., 1907

WEED, L. H.: Cerebrospinal Fluid, Physiol. Rev., 1922, 2, 171.

WILSON, GEORGE: The Diagnostic Significance of Jacksonian Epilepsy, Jour. Am. Med. Assn., 1921, 76, 842.

WILSON, S. A. K.: Modern Problems in Neurology, New York, William Wood & Co., 1929.

INDEX.

A

ABDOMEN, rigidity of, in acute peritonitis, 684
tenderness of, in acute peritonitis, 685
Abortion in undulant fever, 60
Abscess of liver, 667
of lung, 729
of kidney, 558
of spleen, 896
peritoneal, 685
subdural, 1161
subphrenic, 685
Achilles reflex, 1127
in sciatica, 1243
Achondroplasia, 920
Acidosis, 1012
buffer salts in, 1014
causes of, 1013
diabetic, treatment of, 1008
hyperpnea in, 1013
leukocyte count in, 1013
Acrodynia, 1241
Acromegaly, 845
body development in, 846
facies of, 846
in pregnancy, 846
operation in, 846
roentgen-ray in, 846
sella turcica in, 846
Actinomycosis, 353
of lung, 777
Adams-Stokes syndrome, 435
Addis count in nephrosis, 544
in urine, 506
Addison's disease, 837
asthenia in, 838
course of, 837
crises in, 837
hypotension in, 838
incidence of, 837
pigmentation in, 838
cause of, 839
substitution therapy in, 840
Adenitis in scarlet fever, 317
Adenolipomatosis, 1020
Adenoma, toxic, of thyroid, 814
Adiposis dolorosa, 1020
Adrenal cortex, function of, 836
hyperfunction of, 841
tumors of, 841
sex changes in, 841
glands, disorders of, 835
medulla, function of, 835
hyperfunction of, 840
tumors of, 841
blood pressure in, 841
Adrenals, hemorrhage into, 842
Aëdes ægypti mosquito, 176
albopictus mosquito, 181

Aërophagia, 592
Affect, definition of, 1107
Ageusia, 1121
Agglutination reaction in bacillary dysentery, 47
in cholera, 110
in glanders, 106
in tularemia, 81
in typhoid fever, 32
in undulant fever, 59
Weil-Felix, 194
Agranulocytosis, 887
leukocyte count in, 887
nucleic acid in, 887
primary, 886
secondary, 886
throat in, 887
Ainhum, 350
Akamushi disease, 202
Alastrim, 169
Albuminuria, 509
in streptococcal sore throat, 125
in yellow fever, 178
orthostatic, 509
source of, 509
sport, 509
Alcoholism, 1034, 1086
absorption in, 1034
acute, 1035
blood concentration in, 1034
chronic, 1035
delirium tremens in, 1035
dipsomania, 1038
hallucinosis, acute, in, 1036
Korsakoff's psychosis in, 1037
neuritis in, 1037
trance in, 1037
wet-brain in, 1037
Aleukemic leukemia, 884
Alexia, 1184, 1187
Algid cholera, 109
malaria, 265
Alimentary tract, diseases of, 565
Alkalosis, 1014
causes of, 1014
hydrochloric acid in, 1015
signs of, 1015
Alkaptonuria. *See* Ochronosis, 1024
Allantiasis, 1044
Allergy, 959
allergen in, 961
anaphylaxis and, 902
bacterial, 965
constitutional reactions in, 967
diseases of, 959
eye test in, 966
hereditary, 960
immunology of, 962
in tuberculosis, 737
induced, 959
patch test in, 966

(1255)

Allergy, pathologic, 960
  reactions, types of, 962
physical, 462
physiologic, 959
precipitins in, 963
skin tests in, 966
spontaneous, 960
tests, interpretation of, 966
types of reaction in, 964
  delayed, 964
  immediate, 964
Alzheimer's disease, 1080
Amaurotic family idiocy, 1210
Ambivalency, definition of, 1107
Amebiasis, 232
acute, 235
anayodin in, 239
carriers of, 234
  symptoms in, 235
chiniofon in,. 239
chronic, 236
complement-fixation test in, 237
diagnostic points differentiating Endamœba, 238
diet in, 241
distribution of, 232
emetin in, 240
Endamœba histolytica in, 233
liver abscess in, 236
stools in, 235
Amebic colitis, 232
dysentery, 232
enteritis, 232
Amenorrhea, 853
Amnesia in epilepsy, 1224
Amyotrophic sclerosis, 1166
  signs in, 1166
Anacidity, gastric, 589
Anarthria, 1188
in bulbar palsy, 1211
Ancylostoma braziliense, 279
duodenale, 279
Ancylostomiasis, 279
Ancylostoma duodenale in, stages
  of, 280
carbon tetrachloride in, 281
eosinophilia in, 281
prevention of, 282
tetrachlorethylene in, 281
Anemia, 856
Addisonian, 863
aplastic, 870
  after arsphenamine, 1062
  blood count in, 870
  in benzene poisoning, 1068
  petechiæ, 870
chronic microcytic, 859
  secondary, 859
due to blood loss, 859
  cancer, 860
  infection, 860
idiopathic microcytic, 861
  dysphagia in, 861
  iron in, 862
  koilonychia in, 861
  Plummer-Vinson syndrome
    in, 861
  transfusions in, 862
in diseases of ductless glands, 860

Anemia in plumbism, 1058
macrocytic, in sprue, 956
mechanism of production in, 856
pernicious, 863. *See* Pernicious anemia
progressive, 863
sickle-cell, 873
  leg ulcers in, 873
  sickling in, 873
splenic, 890
  hemorrhage in, 891
  roentgen-ray in, 891
  spleen in, 891
  splenectomy in, 891
  stages of, 891
Anesthesia in leprosy, 67
Aneurysm, 487
arteriovenous, 487, 497
basilar, 490
classification of, 487
congenital, 487
dysphagia in, 489
false, 487
headaches in, 490
hemoptysis in, 489
mycotic, 487
of cerebral vessels, 1196
operation in, 491
roentgen-ray in, 490
syphilis and, 488
thoracic, 489
tracheal tug in, 490
vertebral, 490
vessels affected by, 489
vocal-cord paralysis in, 489
Angiomata of brain, 1198
Angioneurotic edema, 982
Angina, agranulocytic, 886
pectoris, 380
  incidence of, 381
  mechanism of, 381
  pains in, 382
  physical findings in, 383
  surgical treatment of, 385
Vincent's, 569
  organisms of, 570
  stomatitis in, 570
Anhydremia, 930
Animal inoculation in undulant fever, 61
Animals and glanders, 104
Anisocoria, 1119
Anopheline mosquitoes, 260
Anoxemia, 1030
Anoxia in carbon monoxide poisoning,
  1050
Anthracomucin, 88
Anthracosis, 712
Anthrax, 87
cause of death in, 88
death-rate in, 90
edema in, 89
gastro-intestinal, 90
immune serum in, 91
incidence of, 89
leükocyte count in, 90
mode of transmission of, 88
prevention of, 91
pulmonary, 89
Antimony in kala-azar, 247

Anti-sera in coccal infections, 116
Antitoxin for snake-bite, 1048
    in botulism, 1045
    in diphtheria, 313
    in scarlet fever, 320
    in tetanus, 74
Antivenin, 1048
Aorta, coarctation of, 397, 492
    cause of death in, 492
    collateral circulation in, 492
Aortic valve disease, 415
    insufficiency, 416
        effects on heart, 416
        electrocardiogram in, 419
        physical findings in, 417
        vascular phenomena in, 418
    stenosis, blood pressure in, 420
        electrocardiogram in, 420
        physical findings in, 420
Aortitis, syphilitic, 392
Aphasia, 1186
    global, 1188
    motor, 1187
    sensory, 1187
    visual, 1187
    Wernicke's, 1187
Aphthæ tropicæ, 953
Aphthous fever, 188
Aplastic anemia, 870
Apoplexy, 1189
Appendicitis, acute, 638
    bacteriology of, 639
    leukocyte count in, 640
    operation in, 640
    suppurative pylephlebitis in, 640
    tenderness in, 639
Apraxia, 1188
Arachnida, 302
Arachnogastria, 665
Argyll-Robertson pupil, 1120
    in paresis, 1151
    in tabes, 1155
Arrhythmia, sinus, 433
Arsenic poisoning, 1061
    chronic, 1063
        hyperkeratosis in, 1063
        neuritis in, 1063
Arsenical polyneuritis, 1241
Arsphenamine in anthrax, 91
    in syphilis, 225
    poisoning, 1061
        anemia in, 1062
        encephalitis in, 1062
        exfoliative dermatitis in, 1062
        jaundice in, 1062
        nitritoid crisis in, 1061
Arterial disease, classification of, 456
    occlusion, embolic, 486
    phenomena in aortic insufficiency, 418
Arteries, functional disturbances of, 457
    generalized forms, 462

Arteries, functional disturbances of,
    Raynaud's disease, 457
    vasoconstricting disturbances of, 457
    vasodilating disturbances of, 460
Arteriography, 499
Arteriosclerosis, 493
    cardiac, 497
    cerebral, 497
    generalized, 493
        cause of death in, 496
        classification of, 493
        expressions of, 496
        incidence of, 493
        physiologic pathology, 495
    in diabetes, 1003
    localized, 481
    pulmonary, 716
    renal, 497
    with thrombosis, 481
Arteriosclerotic heart disease, 375
    congestive failure in, 377
    coronary arteries in, 375
    electrocardiographic findings in, 379
    irregularities in, 377
    physical findings in, 378
Arteriovenous fistula, 497
    arteriography in, 499
    Branham's sign in, 499
    incidence of, 498
    pathologic physiology of, 498
Arteritis, 491
Arthritis, 904
    acute, 919
    chronic, 904
        syphilitic, 918
    classification of, 907
    deformans, 908
        bones in, 912
        climate in, 915
        focal infection in, 908
        joints in, 911
        pathogenesis of, 909
        shock therapy in, 915
        vaccines in, 915
    degenerative, 916
    gonorrheal, 917
    in acute chorea, 1217
    in dysentery, 46
    in undulant fever, 60
    infectious, 908
    metabolic, 918
    non-suppurative, 908
    pneumococcal, 136
    rheumatoid, 908
Arthropods involved in disease, 302
Articulation, disorders of, 1188
Artificial respiration in carbon monoxide poisoning, 1053
Asbestosis, 712
    cause of, 714
Ascariasis, 283
Ascaris lumbricoides, 283
Aschoff body in rheumatic fever, 338
Ascites in cirrhosis of liver, 666
Astasia-abasia, 1133
Asthenia in Addison's disease, 838

Asthenia in myasthenia gravis, 1212
  neurocirculatory, 428
    tachycardia in, 428
    tolerance to exercise, 428
    tremor in, 429
Asthma, 968
  and autonomic system, 970
  cardiac, 362
  Charcot-Leyden crystals in, 971
  Curschmann's spirals in, 971
  dyspnea in, cause of, 969
  epinephrin in, 972
  excitants of, 969
  infective, treatment of, 973
  leukocyte count in, 971
  lungs in, 970
  sputum in, 971
  tests of, 972
  thymic, 855
Atabrine in malaria, 272
Ataxia, Friedreich's, 1173
  hereditary, 1173
  in tabes, 1155
Atelectasis, pulmonary, 699
  bronchial occlusion in, 700
  classification of, 699
  massive, 700
  roentgen-ray in, 702
  signs of, 702
Atheromatosis, 493
Atherosclerosis, 493
Auricular fibrillation, 444
  circus movement in, 444
  digitalis in, 446
  electrocardiogram in, 445
  in mitral stenosis, 412
  in thyrotoxic heart disease, 395
  mechanism of, 444
  mitral stenosis and, 444
  paroxysmal, 444
  flutter, 442
Auriculo-ventricular bundle, 430
  node, 430
Austin Flint murmur, 413, 418
Autacoids, 806
Autistic thinking, definition of, 1107
Automatism in epilepsy, 1224
Autonomic system in asthma, 970
Avitaminoses, 929
  latent, 933
Ayerza syndrome, 717
Azotemia in uremia, 519

B

Babinski reflex, 1125
Bacillary dysentery, 43
  agglutination reaction in, 47
  atypical, 46
  carriers in, 48
  chronic, 50
  death-rate in, 48
  distribution of, 45
  pain in, 45
  stools in, 47
  treatment of, specific, 49
Bacillus anthracis, 87

Bacillus anthracis, spores of, 88
  comma, 107
  diphtheriæ, 309
  dysenteriæ, 43
  mallei, 104
Bacteriemia in anthrax, 90
  in erysipelas, 128
  in plague, 85
  in pneumonia, 144
  in typhoid fever, 33
  in undulant fever, 60
  staphylococcal, 118
  streptococcal, 126
    complications of, 126
    mortality of, 126
Bacteriophage in cholera, 107
Bacterium pneumosintes, 93
Balantidial dysentery, 273
Balantidiasis, 273
  Balantidium coli in, 274
  distribution of, 273
Bang's disease, 51
Banti's disease, 890
Bárány test in cerebellopontile tumors, 1202.
Barlow's disease, 940
Basal metabolic rate in cretinism, 825
  in exophthalmic goiter, 817
  in leukemia, 882
  in myxedema, 822
  in polycythemia vera, 892
  in thyroid disease, 812
Basedow's disease, 815
Bastian's law, 1130
Battle's sign, 1203
B.C.G. vaccine in tuberculosis, 774
Bell's palsy, 1244
Bence-Jones albumose, 922
Bends, the, 1028
Benedikt's syndrome, 1130
Benzene poisoning, 1067
  acute, 1067
  chronic, 1067
    anemia in, 1068
    leukopenia in, 1068
    petechiæ in, 1068
Beriberi, 936
  dry, 938
    heart changes in, 938
    neuritis in, 938
  electrocardiography in, 938
  incidence of, 936
  infantile, 940
  prevention of, 939
  Vedder's signs in, 939
  vitamin B and, 936
  wet, 938
    edema in, 938
    neuritis in, 938
Beurger's disease, 483
Bile ducts, congenital obliteration of, 679
  diseases of, 672
  stenosis of, 679
Bilharziasis, 299
Biliary colic, 676
Bilirubinuria in cirrhosis of liver, 665
Birth injuries to nervous system, 1207
Bismuth in syphilis, 225
"Black death," 85. *See* Plague

Black-water fever, 266
Bladder, decompression of, 557
Blastomycosis, 353
Blood chemistry in parathyroidectomy,
831
in tetany,·832
count in malaria, 261
in pernicious anemia, 866
in typhoid fever, 32
diseases of, 856
incidence of, 856
symptoms of, 857
fat in diabetes mellitus, 999
in carbon monoxide poisoning, 1053
in myxedema, 824
platelets in thrombocytopenic purpura, 876
pressure, high, 463
in aortic insufficiency, 418
stenosis, 420
in pulsus alternans, 447
low, 479
normal, 462
sugar in diabetes mellitus, 998
Blood-urea clearance test of kidney function, 522
Blood-vessels, cerebral, 1189
apoplexy in, 1189
hemorrhage, 1189, 1190
Cheyne-Stokes breathing
in, 1190
thrombosis, 1190
diseases of, 455
Blue baby, 398
Bone changes in rickets, 946
complications of typhoid fever, 32
Bones, carcinoma of, 922
congenital defects of, 920
diseases of, 920
in Hand-Christian syndrome, 902
in syphilis, 216
neoplasms of, 922
non-congenital defects of, 921
sarcoma of, 922
Botulism, 1044
antitoxin in, 1045
diarrhea in, 1045
eye signs in, 1045
organism of, 1044
Bowel, paralysis, 637
Bradycardia in heart block, 436
sinus, 432
Brain, disorders of, 1183
focal signs in, 1183
injuries of, 1203
Battle's sign in, 1203
concussion in, 1203
headache in, 1204
vertigo in, 1204
tumors of, 1197
choked disk in, 1198
convulsions in, 1199
encephalography in, 1202
headache in, 1198
localizing signs in, 1200
lumbar puncture in, 1202
operation in, 1202
pathologic types of, 1197
roentgen diagnosis in, 1201

Brain, disorders of, vomiting in, 1199
Branham's sign in arteriovenous fistula,
499
Breathing, mechanism of, 688
Bright's disease, 525
albuminuria in, 552
arteriosclerotic, 550
hypertension in, 550
degenerative, 539
nocturia in, 551
retinal lesions in, 553
uremia in, 552
Brill's disease, 190
Broadbent's sign, 407
Bronchi, foreign bodies in, 728
bronchoscopy in, 728
roentgen-ray in, 728
Bronchiectasis, 717
hemoptysis in, 719
lipiodol in, 720
operation in, 721
prevention of, 721
production of, 717
roentgen-ray in, 720
signs of, 719
sputum in, 719
Bronchitis, acute, 725
chronic, 726
peri-, 727
Bronchopneumonia, 129
collapse of lung in, 131
death-rate in, 129
empyema in, 131
in measles, 327
interstitial, 130
pneumothorax in, 131
prevention of, 132
sputum in, 131
streptococcal, 130
Brown-Séquard's syndrome, 1146
Brucella melitensis, 52
Brucelliasis, 51
Bubo in plague, 84
Buboes in glanders, 104
Bubonic plague, 82. *See* Plague
Buccal-pharyngeal structures, neoplasms
of, 572
syphilis of, 571
Buffer salts in acidosis, 1014
Bugs, hemophagous, in disease, 306
Bulbar palsy, 1211
Bursæ, diseases of, 919
Bursitis and neuritis, 1239
sub-deltoid, 919

C

CABOT'S ring forms, 866
Cachexia hypophyseopriva, 847
strumipriva, 821
Caisson disease, 1028
air pressure in, 1029
Dalton's law, 1028
decompression in, 1030
genesis of, 1028
prevention of, 1030
"the bends" in, 1030
Calcium in diet, 932

Calcium in lead poisoning, 1060
  in migraine, 1236
  in tetany, 832
Calculi, pancreatic, 683
  renal, 557
Cancer of bones, 922
  of brain, 1198
  of colon, 646
    laboratory examinations in, 647
    leukocyte count in, 647
    metastasis in, 646
    roentgen-ray in, 647
  of esophagus, 581
  of gall-bladder, 674
  of larynx, 724
  of liver, 669
    primary, 671
    secondary, 669
  of lung, 782
  of mediastinum, 799
  of pancreas, 681
  of peritoneum, 687
  of pleura, 785
  of rectum, 653
  of small intestine, 645
  of spine, 1160
  of stomach, 617
  of thyroid gland, 827
Cancrum oris in kala-azar, 246
  in measles, 327
Capillary pressure, 456
  pulse, 418
Carbohydrate action on pneumococcus, 134
Carbon monoxide poisoning, 1049
    artificial respiration in, 1053
    blood analysis in, 1053
    carbon dioxide inhalation in, 1053
    coma in, 1052
    effects of, 1049
    leukocyte count in, 1052
    prevention of, 1053
    sources of, 1049
  tetrachloride in uncinariasis, 281
Carcinoma of lung, 782
    hemoptysis in, 783
    histogenesis of, 782
    pleural effusions in, 784
    roentgen-ray in, 784
    sputum in, 783
Cardiac complications of hypertension, 474
  irregularities in arteriosclerotic heart disease, 377
  mechanism, normal, 430
  neuroses, 427
  pacemaker, 431
  rate, normal, 431
Cardiacos negros, 717
Carotene, 933
Carotid arteries, pulsating, 492
Carpopedal spasm in tetany, 832
Carriers in amebiasis, 235
  in scarlet fever, 315
  in typhoid fever, treatment of, 41
Casoni reaction, 292
Casts, renal failure, 507

Casts, varieties of, 507
Cataract, diabetic, 1003
Catatonia, definition of, 1107
Catatonic schizophrenia, 1094
Causalgia, 1250
Cell count of spinal fluid, 1141
Cellulitis, pelvic, 126
Cephalin in hemophilia, 879
Cerea flexibilitas, definition of, 1107
Cerebellar fits, 1131
  involvement, signs of, 1131
Cerebellopontile angle, lesions of, 1186
Cerebellum, lesions of, 1186
Cerebral aneurysm, 1196
  hemorrhage in hypertension, 474
  peduncle, lesions of, 1185
Cerebrospinal fever, 148
    bacteriology of, 149
    cause of death in, 154
    clinical forms of, 152
    epidemiology of, 150
    incidence of, 148
    Kernig's sign in, 152
    leukocyte count in, 151
    lumbar puncture in, 153
    pathogenesis of, 150
    serum therapy in, 153
    skin in, 152
    spinal fluid in, 151
  fluid, 1138. See Spinal fluid
Cervical cord, tumors of, 1160
  rib and neuritis, 1238
Cestode infections, 290
Chagas disease, 254
  forms of, 255
  Schizotrypanum cruzi, 255
Chalicosis, 712
Chancre, clinical appearance of, 211
  of lip, 571
  of oral cavity, 571
  pathology of, 208
Charbon, 87
Charcot joint in syphilis, 219
  in tabes, 1155
  triad in multiple sclerosis, 1181
Chaulmoogra oil in leprosy, 69
Chemical agents, diseases due to, 1049
Chest, barrel-shaped, 706
Cheyne-Stokes' breathing, 362
Chickenpox, 329
Chilblain, 462
Chilomastigiasis, 242
Chlorosis, 872
  blood in, 872
  iron in, 873
Choked disk in brain tumor, 1116, 1198
  in second nerve lesions, 1116
Cholangitis, 672
  leukocyte count in, 673
Cholecystitis, acute, 673
    leukocyte count in, 673
    operation in, 673
  and gall stones, 677
  chronic, 674
    operation in, 674
  in typhoid fever, 31
Cholecystography, 677
Cholelithiasis, 675
  and cholecystitis, 677

Cholelithiasis, biliary colic in, 676
 clinical syndrome of, 676
 diet in, 678
 genesis of, 675
 incidence of, 675
 operation in, 679
 reflex symptoms of, 676
 roentgen-ray in, 677
Cholemia, 666
Cholera, 107
 algid, 109
 ambulatory, 108
 cholerine, 108
 clinical forms of, 108
 death-rate in, 111
 gravis, 109
 hypertonic saline solution in, 111
 leukocyte count in, 109
 prevention of, 110
 skin lesions in, 110
 toxins in, 108
 transmission of, 107
 vaccination in, 111
 vibrio, 107
Cholerine, 108
Chondrodystrophia, 920
 hereditary, deforming, 920
Chorea, acute, 1216
 Huntington's, 1218
 heredity in, 1218
 mentality in, 1218
 Sydenham's, 1316
 arthritis in, 1217
 body movements in, 1216
 death-rate in, 1217
 dysarthria in, 1217
 endocarditis in, 1217
 nirvanol in, 1218
 serum in, 1218
 streptococcus in, 1216
 tonsillitis in, 1217
Chvostek's sign in tetany, 832
Circumflex nerve, lesions of, 1251
 shoulder-joint in, 1251
Circus movement, 444
Cirrhosis of liver, 663
Climacteric arthritis, 917
Climate in arthritis deformans, 915
 in tuberculosis, 767
Clonorchis sinensis, 296
Clonus, ankle, 1127
Clostridium tetani, 70
Clubbing of fingers, 699
 in bronchiectasis, 719
 in congenital heart disease, 398
Coarctation of aorta, 397
Cocainism, 1041, 1086
 formication in, 1042
 hallucinations in, 1042
Coccal diseases, 113
 leukocyte count in, 116
 local signs of, 115
 symptoms of, 115
Cocci, transmission of, 115
Coccidiosis, 256
Coccygodynia, 1249
Cochin-China diarrhea, 953
Coin test in pneumothorax, 796
Cold, common, 185

Cold, common, droplet infection in, 185
Colic, biliary, 676
 lead, 1058
Colitis, ulcerative, 641
 bacteriology of, 641
 diarrhea in, 642
 diet in, 642
 leukocyte count in, 642
 proctoscopy in, 642
 roentgen-ray in, 642
Collapse therapy in pulmonary tuberculosis, 770
Colles' law, 222
Colloidal-gold curve in spinal fluid, 1141
 in tabes, 1156
Colon bacillus infections, 41
 cystitis, 42
 pyelitis, 42
 septicemia, 42
 congenital dilatation of, 651
Complex, definition of, 1107
Compressed air illness, 1028
Concentration test of kidney function,
 524
Concretio cordis, 406
Concussion, cerebral, 1203
Condylomata lata, 209
Conflict, definition of, 1107
Congenital heart disease, 396
 physical findings in, 398
 polycythemia in, 398
 syphilis, early manifestations of, 221
 pathology of, 210
Constipation, 628
 atonic, 629
 diet in, 630
 enemas in, 631
 roentgen-ray in, 630
 spastic, 629
Contacts in cerebrospinal fever, 149
Contagious diseases, differentiation of,
 319
Continued fever, 17
Conus, tumors of, 1160
Convalescence in brain tumor, 1199
 in epilepsy, 1227
 in influenza, 97
Cord changes in pernicious anemia, 865
Cornea in pseudosclerosis, 1219
Coronary artery disease, 380
 occlusion, 386
 coronary arteries in, 386
 death-rate in, 390
 dyspnea in, 388
 electrocardiography in, 389
 leukocyte count in, 387
 pain in, 387
 shock in, 388
Corpora quadrigemina, lesions of, 1185
Corpus callosum, lesions of, 1183
 striatum, lesions of, 1185
Corrigan pulse, 418
Coryza, acute, 185, 722
 allergic, 974
 perennial, 978
 seasonal, 975
Cough in pulmonary disease, 694
 significance of, 695
 types of, 696

Cowpox, 170
Creatinine clearance test of kidney function, 522
"Creeping eruption," 282
Cretinism, 825
  body build in, 825
  dwarfism in, 825
  incidence of, 825
  juvenile, 826
  mentality in, 825
  thyroid in, 826
  voice in, 825
Crises, gastric, in tabes, 1155
  in Addison's disease, 837
  of thyrotoxicosis, 817
Crisis in pneumonia, 144
  oculogyric, in encephalitis, 1223
Crustacea, 302
Currents, high tension, 1032
  low tension, 1032
Cushing's syndrome, 850
Cutaneous tests of smallpox, 168
Cyanosis in cholera, 109
  in congenital heart disease, 398
  in influenza, 96
  in pericarditis, 404
  in pulmonary disease, 698
Cylindruria, 507
Cystitis, colon bacillus, 42
Cysts of pancreas, 682
Cytotropism, 160

D

Dalton's law, 1028
Dark-field examination for spirochetes, 212
Decompression in caisson disease, 1030
Deficiency diseases, 929
Dehydration in brain tumor, 1203
  in cholera, 109
Delhi boil, 248
Delirium tremens, 1035
Delusion, definition of, 1108
Dementia, definition of, 1108
  in pellagra, 952
  paretic, 1150
  præcox, 1093
Dengue, 180
  epidemiology of, 181
  leukocyte count in, 182
  skin in, 182
  stages of, 181
Dental disease, clinical aspects of, 568
Dercum's disease, 1020
Dermatitis, exfoliative, after arsphenamine, 1062
Dermatomyositis, 923
Desensitization in serum therapy, 147
Dextrocardia, 396
Diabetes, bronze, 1023
  insipidus, 1021
    diencephalon in, 1021
    heredity in, 1021
    pituitrin in, 1022
    polyuria in, 1022
    types of, 1022
  mellitus, 992

Diabetes mellitus, acidosis in, 1002
  arterial disease in, 1003
  azoturia in, 996
  blood fat in, 999
    sugar in, 998
  course of, 100
  diet in, maintenance, 1006
    observation, 1004
    qualitative, 1005
  D/N ratio in, 996
  eye affections in, 1003
  glucose tolerance in, 995
  glycosuria in, 1001
  heredity in, 993
  hyperglycemia in, 995, 1001
  hypophysis in, 994
  incidence of, 992
  infectious diseases in, 993
  insulin in, 999
  ketogenesis in, 997
  ketone bodies in, 998
  ketosis in, 998
  obesity in, 993
  pancreas in, 994
  polyuria in, 1001
  renal threshold in, 998
  respiratory quotient in, 996
  skin infections in, 1002
  thyroid in, 994
  tolerance tests in, 999
  total metabolism in, 996
  treatment of acidosis, 1008
    of infectious conditions, 1010
    of surgical complications, 1010
  tuberculosis in, 1002
  xanthelasma, 1001
  xanthosis in, 1001
Diabetic polyneuritis, 1241
Diaphragm, descent of, 803
  diseases of, 801
  dysfunction of, 802
  function of, 802
  elevation of, 802
  hernias of, 803
    . false, 803
    genuine, 803
    roentgen-ray in, 803
Diaphragmitis, 804
Diarrhea, 631
  causes of, 632
  classification of, 632
  Cochin-China, 953
  diet in, 634
  in cholera, 108
  laboratory examination in, 633
  pain in, 633
  proctoscopy, 633
  roentgen-ray in, 633
Dick test, 320
Diet in amebiasis, 241
  in arthritis deformans, 916
  in beriberi, 940
  in cholelithiasis, 678
  in cirrhosis of liver, 666
  in congestive failure, 450
  in constipation, 630
  in diabetes mellitus, 1004

Diet in diarrhea, 634
  in epilepsy, 1082, 1231
  in gastric ulcer, 614
  in gout, 991
  in hemorrhagic nephritis, 537
  in hypertension, 469, 476
  in indigestion, 595
  in infectious jaundice, 662
  in intestinal neuroses, 625
  in multiple neuritis, 1239
  in nephrosis, 546
  in obesity, 1018
  in pellagra, 953
  in pernicious anemia, 868
  in pneumonia, 147
  in pulmonary tuberculosis, 766
  in scurvy, 944
  in sprue, 957
  in typhoid fever, 38
  in ulcerative colitis, 642
  mineral elements, 931
  normal, 929
  protein requirements, 931
  vitamins, 932
Digitalis in auricular fibrillation, 446
  in congestive heart failure, 451
  intoxication, 451
Dilution test of kidney function, 524
Dinitrophenol in obesity, 1018
Diphtheria, 309
  antitoxin in, 313
  Bacillus diphtheriæ, 309
  faucial, 310
  immunization, active, 312
    passive, 312
  laryngeal, 310
  membrane in, 309
  nasal, 310
  paralysis, post-diphtheritic, 311
  prevention of, 312
  Schick test, 312
  serum reactions, 314
  types of, 310
Diphtheritic myocarditis, 425
  post-, polyneuritis, 1240
Diphyllobothriasis, 293
  blood count in, 293
Diphyllobothrium latum, 293
  sparganum, 294
Dipsomania, 1038
  heredity in, 1038
Dipylidiiasis, 293
Dissociation, definition of, 1108
Distomiasis, 294
  intestinal, 295
  liver in, 296
  pulmonary, 297
  stools in, 295
Diver's palsy, 1028
Diverticula of intestine, 651
    multiple, acquired, 651
  of stomach, 624
Diverticulitis, 651
Diverticulosis, 651
Donder's pressure, 794
Double personality, definition of, 1108
Droplet infection in influenza, 94
    in meningitis, 150
Ductus arteriosus, patent, 397

Duodenal stasis, chronic, 651
  ulcer, 600
Duodenum, dilated, 651
Duroziez sign, 418
Dwarfism, achondroplasic, 920
  hypophyseal, 848
  in cretinism, 825
  in pituitary disease, 845
Dysarthria, 1188
  in acute chorea, 1217
Dysentery, amebic, 232
  bacillary, 43
  bacilli, 43
  balantidial, 273
Dysphagia in aneurysm, 489
  in esophageal spasm, 578
  in microcytic anemia, 861
Dyspnea in asthma, 969
  in coronary occlusion, 388
  in emphysema, 705
  in heart disease, 361
  in pulmonary disease, 697
  paroxysmal, 362
Dystrophia adiposogenitalis, 849
Dystrophy, progressive muscular, 1252
    electrical reactions in, 1253
    gait in, 1253
    muscles in, 1253

E

Echinococcosis, 291
  granulosus, 291
Echolalia, definition of, 1108
Echopraxia, definition of, 1108
Eczema, 983
Edema, acute pulmonary, 362
  angioneurotic, 982
  in Bright's disease, 510
    oncotic pressure and, 510
    pathologic physiology of, 510
    sodium in, 512
  in nephrosis, 544
Effort syndrome, 428
Eighth nerve, lesions of, 1122
  Meniéré's syndrome, 1123
  word deafness in, 1123
Electric shock, 1031
  artificial respiration in, 1033
  cause of death in, 1032
  high tension currents in, 1032
  lightning, 1031
  low tension currents, 1032
Electrocardiogram in aortic insufficiency, 419
  in aortic stenosis, 420
  in arteriosclerotic heart disease, 379
  in auricular fibrillation, 445
  in beriberi, 938
  in coronary occlusion, 389
  in heart block, 436
  in mitral stenosis, 412
  in myocarditis, 426
  in premature contractions, 438
  in rheumatic heart disease, 368
  in thyrotoxic heart disease, 395
  normal, 431

Eleventh nerve, lesions of, 1124
Embolectomy, 487
Emboli in rheumatic heart disease, 368
    in subacute bacterial endocarditis,
        373
Emetin in amebiasis, 240
Emphysema, 703
    barrel-shaped chest in, 706
    cyanosis in, 705
    dyspnea in, 705
    functional pathology of, 705
    incidence of, 703
    interstitial, 707
    of mediastinum, 801
    roentgen-ray in, 706
    signs of, 706
Empyema, 791
    in bronchopneumonia, 131
    in pneumonia, 144
    influenzal, treatment of, 103
    of gall-bladder, 677
    of mediastinum, 800
    operation in, 792
    organisms in, 791
    roentgen-ray in, 792
    signs of, 792
    streptococcal, 132
        operation in, 133
        thoracentesis in, 133
        thoracotomy in, 133
Encephalitis, chronic, 1223
    crises, oculogyric, 1223
    narcolepsy in, 1223
    Parkinson syndrome in, 1223
    epidemic, 1220
        abortive cases of, 1222
        and influenza, 1220
        bulbar palsy in, 1222
        catatonia in, 1221
        death-rate in, 1222
        herpes and, 1220
        hiccough in, 1221
        in pregnancy, 1144
        lethargy in, 1221
        leukocyte count in, 1221
        ocular palsies in, 1221
        spinal fluid in, 1221
        types of, 1223
        virus in, 1220
    in varicella, 331
    lethargica, 1220
    postinfluenzal, 99
    vaccination in, 172
Encephalography, 1137
Encephalopathy, hypertensive, 516
    in plumbism, 1059, 1240
Endamebiasis, 232
Endamœba histolytica, 233
    pathogenesis of, 233
    transmission of, 233
Endocarditis, bacterial, 371
    acute, 371
    subacute, 372
        blood count in, 374
        signs of, 373
        Streptococcus viridans in,
            372
        valvular lesion of, 372
    in acute chorea, 1217

Endocarditis, staphylococcal, 118
Endocrine glands, diseases of, 806
        general discussion of, 806
Enterobius vermicularis, 285
Enteroptosis, 651
Eosinophilia, 979
    in ancylostomiasis, 281
    in asthma, 969
    in hay-fever, 979
    in trichinosis, 288
Epidemics in influenza, 94
Epidemiology of infectious diseases, 20
Epilepsia, partialis continua, 1229
    procursiva, 1228
    tarda, 1224
Epilepsy, 1081, 1224
    "absinthe," 1225
    amnesia in, 1228
    aura in, 1227
    barbitals in, 1232
    causes of, 1224
    cry in, 1227
    diet in, 1082, 1231
        acidosis and, 1232
    disposition in, 1228
    employment in, 1231
    fall in, 1227
    fit in, 1227
        clonic stage, 1227
        tonic phase, 1227
    fugue state in, 1082
    Gelineau syndrome in, 1230
    grand mal in, 1226
    head injuries and, 1225
    heredity in, 1081, 1224
    Jacksonian fits and, 1226
    marriage in, 1230
    mental symptoms in, 1082
    narcolepsy in, 1226
    operations in, 1233
    personality in, 1082
    petit mal in, 1224
    prevention of, 1230
    psychic equivalent of, 1228
    pyknolepsy in, 1226
    reflex, 1225
    running, 1228
    status epilepticus, 1229
        hemiepilepticus, 1229
Epinephrin, action of, 835
    sympathectomy in, 836
Epiphysis, 854
Epithelioma of oral cavity, 572
Erb's sign in tetany, 832
Ergotism, 1046
Erysipelas, 127
    bacteriemia in, 128
    leukocyte count in, 128
    pathogenesis of, 127
    serum in, 129
    skin reaction in, 128
Erythema infectiosum, 334
    multiforma, 341
Erythredema polyneuritis, 1241
Erythremia, 891
Erythrocytes, resistance of, 872
Erythromelalgia, 460
Eschatin, 836
Esophagus, 576

Esophagus, **cancer of,** 581
    metastases in, 581
    operation in, 582
    roentgen-ray in, 582
  congenital malformations of, 576
  diverticula of, 576
  foreign bodies in, 576
  mediastinal abscess in, 581
  peptic ulcer of, 577
  spasm of, 577
    dysphagia in, 578
    roentgen-ray in, 578
  stricture of, 577
Espundia, 244
  Leishmania braziliensis, 250
Eunuchism, female, 852
  male, 854
Eventration of diaphragm, 803
Exanthema subitum, 334
External popliteal nerve, lesions of, 1252
    foot-drop in, 1252
Extrovert, the, 1088
Eye involvement in facial paralysis, 1244
  reactions in syphilis, 213
  signs in botulism, 1045
    in exophthalmic goiter, 816
    in pituitary disease, 845
  tests of smallpox, 169

F

F**ACIAL** hemiatrophy, progressive, 1246
    skin in, 1246
  hemihypertrophy, 1247
  hemispasm, 1246
  paralysis, peripheral, 1244
    causes of, 1244
    electric reactions in, 1245
    eye care in, 1245
    facial expression in, 1244
    mental depression in, 1244
    operation in, 1246
    pain in, 1244
Facies, hepatic, 665
  Hippocratic, 684
  in facial paralysis, 1244
  in paralysis agitans, 1214
Farcy, 103
Fasciola hepatica, 296
Fasciolopsis buski, 295
Fat, blood, 999
Faucial diphtheria, 310
Febricula, 349
Fever, acute rheumatic, 336
  aphthous, 188
  black, 244
  black-water, 266
  deer-fly, 76
  dum-dum, 244
  ephemeral, 349
  glandular, 345
  jail, 190
  Japanese River, 202
  malarial, 257
  miliary, 349
  pappataci, 183
  phlebotomies, 183
  rabbit, 76
  80

Fever, rat-bite, 229
  relapsing, 229
  Rocky Mountain spotted, 197
  sand-fly, 183
  ship, 190
  spotted, 190
    camp, 190
  therapy in neurosyphilis, 1152
    in paresis, 1079
  "three day," 95
  trench, 200
  types of, 17
Fibroses, pulmonary, clinical, 708
    occupational, 708
Fibrositis, 926
Fifth disease, 334
  nerve, lesions of, 1121
    ageusia in, 1121
    conjunctiva reflex, 1122
    corneal reflex, 1121
    lacrymal reflex, 1122
Filaria, Bancroft's, 289
Filariasis, 288
  blood examination in, 290
  Filariidæ (family), 288
Filatow-Duke disease, 334
First nerve, lesions of, 1115
    anosmia in, 1115
Fits, cerebellar, 1131
Flavine in pellagra, 950
Fleas in disease, 305
Fleisher-Strümpell ring, 1220
Flies in disease, 304
    blood-sucking, 304
Fluke infections, 294
Flutter, auricular, 442
    paroxysmal, 443
Focal infections, 120, 568
  in lung disease, 722
  infected teeth in, 122
  non-specific treatment of, 122
  tonsils in, 122, 575
  vaccines in, 122
Food poisoning, 1042
  causes of, 1042
  diarrhea in, 1043
  infection in, 1042
Foot-and-mouth diseases, 188
Foot-drop in external popliteal neuritis, 1252
  in polyneuritis, 1238
  in progressive muscular atrophy, 1249
Fourth disease, 334
  nerve, lesions of, 1118
Fragility of bones in scurvy, 942
Frambœsia, 228
Friction rub in pericarditis, 401
Friedreich's ataxia, 1173
  signs of, 1173
Fröhlich's syndrome, 849
    amenorrhea in, 849
    genitalia in, 849
    obesity in, 849
    sugar tolerance in, 849
Frontal lobe, lesions of, 1183
Fugue, definition of, 1108
Fungus diseases (non-bacterial), 352
    internal, 354

Fungus disease (non-bacterial), of gastro-intestinal tract, 356
of genito-urinary system, 356
of nervous system, 356
of skeleton, 353
of skin, 353
of respiratory tract, 354

G

GAIT, 1132
ataxic, 1132
festinating, 1133
hemiplegic, 1132
in multiple neuritis, 1239
in muscular dystrophy, 1253
in paralysis agitans, 1214
reeling, 1132
scissor, 1132
spastic, 1132
steppage, 1132
testing for, 1133
waddling, 1132
Gall-bladder, 672
cancer of, 674
diseases of, 672
visualization of, 674
Gall stones, 675
Gametocytes, 259
Ganglionectomy in thrombo-angiitis obliterans, 486
Ganglionitis, infectious, 461
Gangosa, 351
Gangrene of lung, 734
pre-senile, 483
senile, 481
Gas poisoning, 1049
Gastric analysis, 586
in pernicious anemia, 866
ulcer, 600
causes of, 601
diet in, 614
frequency of, 600
gastric analysis in, 603
hemorrhage in, treatment of, 615
malignant changes in, 611
management of, 612
marginal, 617
operation in, 616
perforation in, 609
treatment of, 616
roentgen-ray in, 603
with hemorrhage, 605
with indigestion, 602
with pyloric obstruction, 606
alkalosis in, 608
treatment of, 616
urine in, 607
visible peristalsis in, 607
Gastritis, 598
acute, 598
chronic, 599
gastric analysis in, 599
Gastro-intestinal anthrax, 89

Gastro-intestinal influenza, 97
Gaucher's disease, 900
Gentian violet in strongyloidosis, 287
Giardiasis, 242
Gigantism, 847
in pituitary disease, 845
Ginger paralysis, 1039
Girdle sensation in tabes, 1154
Gland puncture in trypanosomiasis, 253
Glanders, 103
agglutination reaction in, 106
buboes in, 104
chronic, 105
death-rate in, 106
forms of, 104
incidence of, 103
laboratory procedures in, 105
prevention of, 106
skin lesions, 104
transmission of, 104
Glands, endocrine, diseases of, 806
Glandular fever, 345
tularemia, 79
Glioma, 1197
types of, 1197
Globulin in spinal fluid, 1142
Glomerulonephritis, diffuse, 526
acute, 528
chronic, 529
focal, 530
Glossitis in pellagra, 951
in pernicious anemia, 865
Glucose in heart disease, 426
in spinal fluid, 1141
Goiter, 811
adenomatous, 814
diffuse, toxic, 815
endemic, 812
course of disease, 813
incidence of, 812
iodine and, 812
prevention of, 813
exophthalmic, 815
basal metabolism in, 817
course of, 816
crises in, 817
eye signs in, 816
iodine response in, 817
operation in, 818
sequels of, 819
signs in, 816
intrathoracic, 815
lingual, 829
nodular, 814
course of disease, 814
operation in, 815
thyrotoxicosis in, 814
sporadic colloid, 814
Gonads, female, disorders of, 851
hormones of, 851
hyperfunction of, 852
hypofunction of, 852
male, disorders of, 853
hyperfunction of, 854
hypofunction of, 854
Gonococcal infections, 154
Gonococcus, 155
Gonorrheal rheumatism, 155
Gout, 985

Gout, alcohol in, 987
  arteriosclerosis in, 989
  big toe in, 988
  diet in, 991
  heredity in, 986
  hypertension in, 989
  incidence of, 985
  joint changes in, 988
  lead and, 987
  leukocyte count in, 988
  meat in, 987
  prevention of, 990
  purine metabolism in, 986
  roentgen-ray in, 990
  tophus in, 988
  uric acid in, 986
Graham Steell murmur, 419, 423
Grand mal, 1226
Graphesthesia, 1136
Graves' disease, 815
Grippe, 92. *See* Influenza
"Ground itch," 280
Guinea-worm, 289
Gull's disease, 821
Gumma of brain, 1198
  pathology of, 209
Gummata of oral cavity, 572
Gyrus, lesions of, 1184

H

HAIR in syphilis, 213
Hallucination, definition of, 1108
Hallucinosis, acute, in alcoholism, 1036
Hand-Christian syndrome, 902, 922
  bones in, 902
  diabetes insipidus in, 902
  exophthalmos in, 902
Hay-fever, 974
  asthma in, 976
  eye changes in, 976
  incidence of, 975
  infection in, 976
  multiple allergies in, 976
  pollens in, 975
  prevention of, 977
  skin tests of, 976
Headache in brain tumor, 1198
  in lumbar puncture, 1143
  in migraine, 1235
  indurative, 925
  sick, 1234
Heart beat, disorders of, 430
  block, 434
    auriculo-ventricular, 434
    bundle-branch, 437
    complete, 435
    electrocardiogram in, 436
    partial, 435
    sino-auricular, 434
  conduction, disturbances of, 434
  diseases of, 359
    chronic valvular, 408
      valves involved in, 409
    congenital, 396
    etiologic classification of, 359
    hypertensive, 375
    rheumatic, 365

Heart, diseases of, syphilitic, 391
  thyrotoxic, 394
  failure, congestive, diet in, 450
    theophyllin in, 449
    treatment of, 448
  functional disorders of, 427
  in myxedema, 824
  in pneumonia, 142
  in rheumatic fever, 339
  in syphilis, 216
  in thyrotoxicosis, 820
  irritable, 428
  premature contraction of, 437
    electrocardiogram in, 438
    quinidine in, 440
Heartburn, 592
Heat cramps, 930, 1027
  exhaustion, 1027
  retention, 1026
  sequels of, 1028
  stroke, 1027
Hebephrenia, 1094
Heberden's nodes, 917
Heine-Medin disease, 1175
Helminthic diseases, 278
Hematoma, chronic, subdural, 1206
  signs of, 1206
  spinal fluid in, 1207
Hematomyelia, 1164
  operation in, 1165
  signs in, 1165
Hematuria, 507
  endemic, 299
Hemiatrophy, progressive, facial, 1246
Hemicrania, 1234
Hemihypertrophy, facial, 1247
Hemiplegia, 1189
  hysterical, 1193
  in pregnancy, 1144
  infantile, 1210
Hemispasm, facial, 1246
Hemochromatosis, 1023
  glycosuria in, 1024
  liver in, 1023
  skin in, 1024
Hemoglobinuria, 508
Hemolytic jaundice, chronic, 871
  blood count in, 871
  fragility of erythrocytes in, 872
  hemolysis in, 871
  reticulocyte count in, 872
  splenomegaly, 871
Hemophilia, 878
  blood in, 879
  cephalin in, 879
  hemorrhages in, 879
  transfusion in, 880
Hemophilus influenzæ, 92
Hemoptysis in aneurysm, 489
  in mitral stenosis, 411
  in pulmonary disease, 697
    causes of, 697
  in tuberculosis, 751
Hemorrhage, cerebral, 1190
  epidural, 1205
  from gastric varices, 666
  gastric, treatment of, 615
  in hemophilia, 879

Hemorrhage in jaundice, 658
  in leukemia, 885
  in plague, 84
  in scurvy, 942
  in splenic anemia, 891
  in typhoid fever, 30
        treatment of, 39
  into spinal cord, 1164
  subarachnoid, spontaneous, 1194
Hemorrhagic smallpox, 167
Hemorrhoids, 654
  in cirrhosis of liver, 665
  proctoscopic examination in, 655
Hepatitis, acute, 659
        laboratory tests in, 660
  chronic, 663
  non-suppurative, 658
  subacute, 663
  suppurative, 667
Heredity in allergy, 960
  in diabetes insipidus, 1021
    mellitus, 993
  in dipsomania, 1038
  in epilepsy, 1081, 1224
  in Friedreich's ataxia, 1173
  in gout, 986
  in Huntington's chorea, 1218
  in hypertension, 468
  in lenticular degeneration, 1219
  in migraine, 1234
  in obesity, 1016
  in ochronosis, 1025
  in progressive muscular atrophy,
    1249
  in psychoses, 1072
Hernia of diaphragm, 803
Herpes in pneumonia, 141
  zoster, 1174
        and varicella, 330
        and virus infection, 1175
        skin lesions in, 1175
Heterophyes heterophyes, 296
Hexylresorcinol, 282
Hiccough, 1133
Hippocratic facies, 684
Hippus, 1120
Hirschsprung's disease, 629
Histamine test, 587
Histiocytosis, lipoid, 901
Hodgkin's disease, 888
        abdominal, 889
        biopsy in, 889
        fever in, 889
        glandular enlargement in, 889
        leukocyte count in, 890
        pruritus in, 889
        roentgen-ray in, 890
Holmes phenomenon, 1131
Homeostasis, 836
Hormones, female sex, 808
  growth, of pituitary, 843
  of anterior pituitary, 843
  of endocrine glands, 806
  of posterior pituitary, 844
  ovarian, 851
  sex, of pituitary, 843
Horner's syndrome, 1146
        after sympathectomy, 460
Housemaid's knee, 919

Howell-Jolly bodies, 866
Huntington's chorea, 1218
Hutchinson teeth in congenital syphilis,
  221
Hydatid cyst, 291
  disease of lung, 780
  thrill, 292
Hydrarthrosis, intermittent, 918
Hydrocephalus, internal, 1208
        cause of, 1209
        dissociated lesions with, 1209
        head in, 1209
        spinal puncture in, 1209
Hydronephrosis, 555
        pyelography, intravenous, in, 556
        urethral obstruction in, 556
Hydrophobia, 172
Hydropneumothorax, 794
Hydrops of gall-bladder, 677
Hydrothorax, 794
Hymenolepiasis, 292
Hymenolepis diminuta, 292
        nana, 292
Hyperacidity, gastric, 589
Hyperavitaminosis, 935
Hypergonadism, male, 854
Hyperglycemia in diabetes mellitus, 1001
Hyperinsulinism, 850, 1011
        operation in, 1012
        pancreatic adenoma and, 1011
Hypermetria, 1131
Hyperparathyroidism, 833
        bone changes in, 834
        kidney changes in, 834
Hyperpiesia, 463
Hyperpnea in acidosis, 1013
Hyperpyrexia, 1027
Hypersecretion, gastric, 588
Hypertension, 463, 479
        arteries in, 472
        arteriolar pressure in, 471
        benign, 466
        cerebral hemorrhage in, 474
        classification of, 465
        constitutional characteristics in, 479
        diet in, 469, 476
        essential, 465
        experimental, 466
        eye grounds in, 473
        heart in, 474
        heredity in, 468
        in arteriosclerotic Bright's disease,
          550
        in Bright's disease, 512
              habitus in, 513
              renal tumors and, 513
              retinitis in, 514
        in diabetes mellitus, 1003
        in hemorrhagic nephritis, 533
        in nephrosis, 544
        incidence of, 464
        infections in, 470
        intermittent, 467
        kidney in, 475
        malignant, 466
              eye changes in, 468
        menopausal, 467
        operative risks in, 476
        paroxysmal, 467

Hypertension, postural, 480
  with syncope, 480
  pregnancy in, 470
  primary, 466, 479
    stages of, 466
  remittent, 467
  retinitis of, 473
  secondary, 466, 480
  surgical treatment of, 478
  sympathetic system in, 470
  types of, 479
Hypertonic saline solution in cholera, 111
Hypertrophic pyloric stenosis, congenital, 624
Hypoacidity, gastric, 589
Hypocapnia, 694
Hypoglycemia in Addison's disease, 839
  in hyperinsulinism, 1011
Hypogonadism, female, 852
  male, 854
Hypometabolism following exophthalmic goiter, 820
  without myxedema, 829
Hypophamine, 844
Hypophysis, 842. *See* Pituitary gland
Hyposecretion, gastric, 588
Hyposthenuria, 552
Hypotension in Addison's disease, 838
Hypothyroidism, congenital, 825
Hypoxemia, 693
Hysteria, 1099
  mental symptoms in, 1099
  motor signs in, 1099
  reflex paralyses in, 1099
  sensory symptoms in, 1099

I

ICTERUS, 656
  index, 658
    in pernicious anemia, 867
Idiocy, amaurotic, 1210
Idiopathic microcytic anemia, 861
Idiot, 1083
Ileus, paralytic, 638
Illusion, definition of, 1109
Immunity, 14
  acquired, 14
  natural, 14
Immunization, active, in scarlet fever, 320
Inclusion bodies, 160
Indigestion, 591
  causes of, 593
  diet in, 595
  symptoms of, frequency of, 592
    mechanism of, 592
Infantilism, genital, in Frölich's syndrome, 849
  sexual, 854
Infection, focal, 120, 568
  massive, 15
  mode of, 15
  wound, 125
Infections in hypertension, 470
  of upper respiratory tract, 721
Infectious cold, 185
  diseases, diagnosis of, 18
    effect of, on other conditions, 20

Infectious diseases, epidemiology of, 20
  hypersensitivity in, 18
  incidence of, 21
  mechanism of recovery from, 16
  prevention of, 19
  symptoms of, 16
  treatment of, 19
Influenza, 92
  and common cold, 100
  and tuberculosis, 99
  cause of, 94
  death-rate in, 100
  droplet infection in, 94
  duration of epidemic, 95
  encephalitis in, 99
  facies in, 96
  gastro-intestinal, 97
  incidence of, 95
  leukocyte count in, 100
  lung abscess in, 99
  nervous, 97
  pneumonia in, 98
    treatment of, 102
  pregnancy in, 99
  prevention of, 101
  relapses in, 97
  temperature in, 96
  vaccination in, 101
Insecta, 302
Insects in disease, 304
  blood-sucking, 304
  nettling, 307
Insolation, 1027
Insulin, 1000
  shock, 1000
  therapy, 1007
    allergy in, 1008
    edema in, 1008
    reaction to, 1007
    resistance to, 1008
  unit of, 1000
Intelligence quotient, 1083
Interauricular septum defect, 397
Intermittent fever, 17
Interstitial emphysema, 707
  pneumonia, 130
Intestinal flagellate infestations, 242
  obstruction, 634
    causes of, 635
    leukocyte count in, 637
    operation in, 638
    pain in, 636
    roentgen-ray in, 637
    toxemia in, 635
  perforation in typhoid fever, 30
  polyps, 645
Intestine, anomalies of, 651
  cancer of, 645
  deformities of, 651
  disorders of, 624
  diverticula of, 651
  indigestion, 625
  neuroses of, 625
  obstruction of, 634
    large bowel, 636
    small bowel, 636
  polyps of, 645
  small, cancer of, 645
  stasis in, 625

Intestine, **tuberculosis of,** 644
   roentgen-ray in, 644
   sites of, 644
   stool examination in, 644
   tumors of, 645
Intoxication, water, 930
Intoxications, 1034
Intraventricular septum defect, 397
Introjection, definition of, 1109
Introvert, the, 1093
Iodine in diet, 931
   in goiter, 931
   response in exophthalmic goiter, 817
Iron in diet, 932
   in secondary anemia, 862
Isosthenuria, 552

J

JACKSONIAN epilepsy, 1226
Jackson's veil, 651
Jaundice, 656
   catarrhal, 347, 660
   chronic, acholuric, 871
     familial, 871
   hemolytic, 871
   epidemic, 230, 347
   hemorrhage in, 658
   icterus index in, 658
   in arsphenamine poisoning, 1062
   in pneumonia, 142
   in yellow fever, 178
   infectious, 347, 660
     course of, 662
     diet in, 662
     leukocyte count in, 661
   mechanism of production, 656
   pulse in, 658
   regurgitation, 657
   skin in, 658
   spirochetal, 230
   urobilinuria, 657
   Van den Bergh reaction in, 658
   Weil's disease, 230
Joint changes in gout, 988
   fluid in gonorrheal rheumatism, 156
Joints, Charcot's, 918
   chronic septic, 918
   diseases of, 904
   trophic, 918

K

Kala-azar, 244
   antimony in, 247
   cancrum oris in, 246
   Leishmania donovani in, 244
   prevention of, 247
   spleen in, 245
   vector of, 244
Kayser-Fleisher ring, 1220
Keratitis, interstitial, syphilitic, 222
Kernig's sign, 152
   in poliomyelitis, 1177
Ketatonic phenomena in involution melancholia, 1082
Ketosis in diabetes mellitus, 998
Kidney, abscess of, 558
   bacterial infections of, 558

Kidney, bacterial infections of, colon
    bacillus in, 558
   chronic passive congestion of, 554
     albuminuria in, 554
     pain in, 555
   function, tests of, 521
   infarcts of, 553
   tuberculosis of, 562
   tumors of, 563
Kidneys in pneumonia, 142
   in yellow fever, 177
   polycystic, 563
   symptomatology and pathologic
     physiology of, 505
Klumpke's paralysis, 1146
Koch phenomenon, 737
Koilonychia, 861
Koplik spots, 326
Korsakoff's syndrome, 1037
   in polyneuritis, alcoholic, 1239
Kupffer's cells, 899
Kussmaul breathing in acidosis, 1002

L

LAMBERT treatment of mercurial poisoning, 541
Landry's paralysis, 1147
Lane's kinks, 651
"Larva migrans," 282
Laryngeal diphtheria, 310
Laryngitis, acute, 722
   chronic, 723
   tuberculous, 723
Larynx, cancer of, 724
   edema of, 723
   syphilis of, 724
Lasègue's sign in sciatica, 1243
Laurence-Biedl syndrome, 1147
Lead, absorption of, 1055
   colic, 1058
   encephalopathy, 1059
   excretion of, 1055
   line, 1057
   neuritis, 1240
   paralysis, 1058
   poisoning, 1054
     acute, 1056
     anemia in, 1058
     arthralgia in, 1058
     calcium in, 1060
     causes of, 1054
     chronic, 1057
     colic in, 1058
     de-leading in, 1060
     encephalopathy in, 1059, 1086
     incidence of, 1054
     industrial hazards of, 1055
     lead line in, 1057
     paralysis in, 1058
     prevention of, 1060
     roentgen-ray in, 1059
     spinal puncture in, 1061
     sterility in, 1057
     stippling of red cells in, 1057
   storage of, 1055
Leber's disease, 1117
Leishmania braziliensis, 250

Leishmania, donovani, 244
Leishmaniasis, 243
  American, 249
  Brazilian, 249
  cutaneous, 248
  muco-cutaneous, 249
  vector in, 248
Lenticular degeneration, progressive,
    1219
    heredity in, 1219
    liver cirrhosis in, 1219
    tremor in, 1219
Lepra cells, 66
Leprosy, 64
  anesthetic type, 67
  cutaneous type, 67
  incidence of, 64
  location of bacilli, 68
Leukanemia, 880
Leukemia, 880
  acute, 884
    blood in, 885
    hemorrhages in, 885
  chronic lymphatic, 882
    leukocyte count in, 883
    lymphocyte count in, 883
    spleen in, 883
  myelogenous, 881
    basal metabolic rate in, 882
    leukocyte count in, 882
    myelocytes in, 882
    spleen in, 882
  classification of, 881
  roentgen-ray in, 883
  transfusions in, 884
Leukocyte count in abscess of liver, 668
  in acidosis, 1013
  in acute tonsillitis, 573
  in agranulocytosis, 887
  in appendicitis, 640
  in asthma, 971
  in benzene poisoning, 1068
  in cancer of colon, 647
  in carbon monoxide poisoning,
    1052
  in cerebrospinal fever, 151
  in cholangitis, 673
  in cholecystitis, 673
  in cholera, 109
  in chronic lymphatic leukemia,
    883
    myelogenous leukemia, 882
  in coronary occlusion, 389
  in dengue, 182
  in dysentery, 47
  in epidemic encephalitis, 1221
  in erysipelas, 128
  in gonorrheal rheumatism, 156
  in gout, 988
  in Hodgkin's disease, 890
  in infectious jaundice, 348, 661
  in influenza, 100
  in intestinal obstruction, 637
  in measles, 327
  in mercurial nephrosis, 540
    poisoning, 1065
  in Niemann-Pick's disease, 901
  in opium poisoning, 1041
  in pappataci fever, 184

Leucocyte count in pernicious anemia,
    866
  in pertussis, 323
  in plague, 85
  in pneumonia, 144
  in poliomyelitis, 1178
  in polycythemia vera, 892
  in pulmonary tuberculosis, 757
  in pyelonephritis, 560
  in rabies, 174
  in rheumatic fever, 342
  in Rocky Mountain spotted
    fever, 199
  in rubella, 335
  in scarlet fever, 316
  in scurvy, 943
  in serum sickness, 981
  in smallpox, 168
  in sprue, 956
  in streptococcal sore throat, 125
  in subacute bacterial endocardi-
    tis, 374
  in tetanus, 72
  in thrombocytopenic purpura,
    876
  in trench fever, 201
  in trichinosis, 288
  in tularemia, 80
  in typhoid fever, 32
  in typhus fever, 194
  in ulcerative colitis, 642
  in undulant fever, 59
  in uremia, 517
  in yellow fever, 178
Leukocytes, "stab," 116
Leukocythemia, 880
Leukocytosis in coccal diseases, 116
Leukopenia, 348
Libido, definition of, 1109
  in pituitary disease, 845
Lice in disease, 306
    Pediculus humanus, 306
    Phthirus pubis, 306
Lightning, injury from, 1031
Lindau's disease, 1198
Lipiodol in bronchiectasis, 720
Lipoatrophia circumscripta, 1020
Lipodystrophia progressiva, 1020
Lipoidal nephrosis, 541
Lipomatosis, 1019
  atrophicans, 1020
  dolorosa, 1020
  gigantica, 1020
  simplex, 1019
Little's disease, 1210
Liver, abscess of, 667
    in amebiasis, 236
    leukocyte count in, 668
    roentgen-ray in, 668
    solitary, 667
  cancer of, 669
    anomalies of form, 671
    of position, 671
    metastases from, 670
  cirrhosis of, 663
    alcoholic, 663
    ascites in, 666
    atrophic, 663
    biliary, 664

Liver, cirrhosis of, classification of, 663
  collateral circulation in, 664
  diet in, 666
  Hanot's, 664
  hematemesis in, 664
  hemorrhage in, 666
  in pseudosclerosis, 1219
  infectious, 663
  laboratory tests in, 665
  melena in, 664
  pigment in, 663
  skin in, 665
  syphilitic, 663
  toxic, 663
  with lenticular degeneration, 1219
  disorders of, 655
  divisions of, 655
  laboratory tests in, 656
  roentgen-ray in, 656
  extract in pernicious anemia, 868
  tumors of, 669
Loa-loa, 288
Lobar pneumonia, 137
Lobstein's disease, 921
Locomotor ataxia, 1154
  system, diseases of, 904
Long thoracic nerve, lesions of, 1251
Ludwig's angina, 125
Lues, 204
Lugol's solution in thyrotoxic heart disease, 396
Lumbago, 924
Lumbar puncture, 1139. See Spinal puncture
Lung, abscess of, 729
  bronchoscopy in, 732
  course of, 731
  operation, 733
  postural drainage in, 732
  roentgen-ray in, 731
  signs of, 730
  sputum in, 734
  cirrhosis of, 710
  collapse of, 699
  in bronchopneumonia, 131
  cystic disease of, 717
  gangrene of, 734
  hydatid disease of, 780
  mycotic diseases of, 777
  non-tuberculous basal infection of, 727
  syphilis of, 775
  congenital, 775
  roentgen-ray in, 776
  tumors of, 781
  benign, 781
  carcinoma, 782
  hemoptysis in, 783
  roentgen-ray in, 784
  malignant, 782
Lutein, 851
Lymphadenopathy in tularemia, 78
Lymphadenosis, benign, 349
Lymphatic vessels, diseases of, 502
Lymphedema, 502
Lymphoblastoma, 888
  of stomach, 623
Lymphocytosis in pertussis, 323

Lymphoma, malignant, 888
Lyssa, 172

M

MACROCYTES in pernicious anemia, 866
  in sprue, 956
Main en griffe, 1250
Malaria, 257
  algid, 265
  atabrine in, 272
  blood count in, 261
  cachexia, 267
  carriers, treatment of, 271
  distribution of, 257
  estivo-autumnal, 264
  latent, 266
  mosquitoes transmitting, 260
  pernicious, 265
  plasmochin in, 271
  plasmodia of, 258
  morphology of, 259
  prevention of, 269
  quartan, 263
  quinine in, 270
  relapses in, 267
  spleen in, 267
  therapy in paresis, 1079
  tertian, 262
Malarial fevers, 257
Malignant pustule, 87
Malleus, 103
Malta fever, 51
Manic-depressive psychosis, 1087
  constitutional makeup in, 1088
  extrovertism in, 1088
  laboratory findings in, 1091
  mental symptoms in, 1090
  physical expressions in, 1090
  prevention of, 1091
Mantoux test in tuberculosis, 757
Marriage and syphilis, 227
  in epilepsy, 1230
Measles, 325
  atypical forms of, 327
  bronchopneumonia and, 327
  convalescent serum in, 328
  German, 334
  Koplik spots, 326
  leukocyte count in, 327
  prevention of, 328
  rash of, 326
Median nerve, lesions of, 1250
  causalgia and, 1250
  sensation in, 1250
Mediastinitis, acute, 800
  chronic, 800
Mediastinum, diseases of, 797
  D'Espine's sign in, 798
  roentgen-ray in, 798
  emphysema of, 801
  empyema of, 800
  inflammatory processes of, 800
  syphilis of, 801
  tumors of, 799
  benign, 799
  malignant, 799
Mediterranean fever, 51
Medulla, lesions of, 1185

Melancholia, clinical varieties of, 1093
  involution, 1092
    ketatonic phenomena in, 1092
Ménière's disease, 1147
  deafness in, 1147
  dizziness in, 1147
  tinnitus in, 1147
Meningitis, circumscribed serous, 1162
  epidemic, 148
  meningococcal, 148
  pneumococcal, 136
Meningococcus, 149
  types of, 149
Menopause, 852
Mental deficiency, idiocy in, 1083
  intelligence quotient in, 1083
  moronity in, 1083
  psychotic episodes of, 1083
    with psychosis, 1083
  examination, 1074
    mechanisms of, 1076
Mentality in cretinism, 825
Mercurial nephrosis, 540
Mercury in syphilis, 225
  poisoning, 1064
    acute, 1064
    anuria in, 1065
    blood chemistry in, 1065
    chronic, 1066
    diarrhea in, 1065
    stomatitis in, 1065
    subacute, 1066
    urine in, 1065
Merozoites, 259
Metabolism, diseases of, 984
  purine, in gout, 986
Metaphyllin in congestive failure, 452
Metazoal diseases, 276
Methyl alcohol poisoning, 1038
    blindness in, 1039
    formic acid in, 1038
Microcytic anemia, idiopathic, 861
Microörganisms, 14
  selective localization of, 16
  toxins of, 15
  virulence of, 14
Migraine, 1234
  allergy in, 1234
  calcium in, 1236
  gastric symptoms in, 1235
  headache in, 1235
  heredity in, 1234
  peptone in, 1236
  visual disturbances in, 1235
Milk sickness, 1045
Millard-Gubler syndrome, 1130
Milroy's disease, 502
Mineral elements in diet, 931
Mites in disease, 302
  species of, 303
Mitral valve disease, 409
    Austin Flint murmur in, 413
    electrocardiogram in, 412
    hemoptysis in, 411
    infarction in, 411
    insufficiency, 414
      physical findings in, 414

Mitral valve disease, physical findings in, 411
  pulmonary congestion in, 413
  roentgenologic findings in, 412
  stenosis, 411, 419
Mobile cecum, 651
Mold disease of lung, 779
Monilia psilosis in sprue, 953
Monocytic leukemia, 885
Mononucleosis, infectious, 345
  blood count in, 346
  enlargement of spleen in, 346
  mononucleosis in, 346
Morbilli, 325
Morbus coxæ senilis, 916
Moron, 1083
Morphine in myxedema, 824
Morphinism, 1039
Mosquito and filariasis, 289
Mosquitoes, anopheline, 260
  in disease, 305
    Anophelini, 305
    Culicini, 035
Motor cortex, lesions of, 1183
  system, lesion of, 1127
    adiadochokinesis, 1131
    atrophy in, 1128
    diplegia in, 1129
    fibrillary tremors in, 1128
    incoördination in, 1131
    monoplegia in, 1129
      segmental, 1129
    paralysis in, 1128
    paraplegia in, 1129
    paresis in, 1128
    quadriplegia in, 1129
    syndrome of, 1130
    synergic movement in, 1131
    tetraplegia in, 1129
Mountain sickness, 1030
  cerebral symptoms in, 1031
  polycythemia in, 1031
Mouth, pharynx and tonsils, 565
  relation to systemic disease, 567
Mucous membranes in syphilis, 213
  patches of mouth, 571
Mumps, 232
  oöphoritis, 333
  orchitis in, 333
  prevention of, 333
  susceptibility to, 332
Murmurs, functional, 423
Muscarine, 1046
Muscles, diseases of, 923, 1252
Muscular atrophy, progressive neurotic, 1249
    Charcot-Marie-Tooth, 1249
    foot-drop in, 1249
    heredity in, 1249
    peroneal, 1249
    reflexes in, 1249
    spinal, 1167
  dystrophy, progressive, 1252
Musculospiral nerve, lesions of, 1257
  paralysis in, 1257

Mutism, hysterical, 1189
Myalgia, 924
Myasthenia gravis, 1212
Mycetoma, 354
    Madura foot, 354
Mydriasis, 1119
Myelitis, 1170
    bladder in, 1171
    causes of, 1170
    priapism in, 1171
    reflexes in, 1171
    signs of, 1171
    transverse, 1170
    trophic disorders in, 1171
Myelocytes in leukemia, 882
Myeloma, 922
    Bence-Jones albumose in, 922
Myiasis-producing insects in disease, 306
Myocarditis, 424
    diphtheritic, 425
    electrocardiogram in, 426
    glucose in, 426
    in typhoid fever, 31
    tachycardia in, 425
Myocardium, diseases of, 424
    fatty degeneration of, 427
        infiltration of, 426
Myoclonus, 1133
Myopathies, the, 1252
Myosis, 1119
Myositis, 923
    dermato-, 923
    fibrosa, 923
    ossificans, 923
        progressiva, 923
    trapezius, 925
    traumatic fibrosa, 923
Myrapoda, 302
Myxedema, 821
    after thyroidectomy, 820
    basal metabolism in, 822
    blood in, 824
    habitus in, 825
    heart in, 824
    in uremia, 518
    infantile, 825
    morphine in, 824
    psyche in, 824
    response to thyroid in, 823
    tongue in, 822

N

Narcissism, definition of, 1109
Narcolepsy, 1226
    in chronic encephalitis, 1223
Nasal diphtheria, 310
Nausea, 592
Negativism, definition of, 1109
Negri bodies, 173
Neologism, definition of, 1109
Nephritis, 525
    hemorrhagic, 526
        and pregnancy, 527
        arteries in, 530
        blood changes in, 532
        cause of, 527
        diet in, 537

Nephritis, hemorrhagic, exacerbations
    of, 532
    function tests in, 535
    hypertension in, 533
    prevention of, 536
    stages of, 531
    terminal stage of, 534
    urine examination in, 536
    vascular changes in, 533
    in scarlet fever, 317
    postdiphtheritic, 311
Nephrocalcinosis, 834
Nephrolithiasis, 557
    hematuria in, 558
    pyuria in, 558
Nephrosclerosis, 550
Nephrosis, 539
    amyloid, 546
        tuberculosis and, 546
    chronic, 541
        contracted kidney in, 543
        diet in, 546
        fatty changes in, 543
        hypertension in, 544
        serum protein in, 544
        syphilis in, 542
        tetany in, 544
        tuberculosis in, 542
    larval, 539
    lipoidal, 541
    mercurial, 540
        anuria in, 540
        blood chemistry in, 540
        Lambert treatment of, 541
        leukocyte count in, 540
    necrotizing, 540
    of pregnancy, 548
        clinical groups of, 548
        eclampsia in, 549
Nerve, circumflex, 1251
    long thoracic, lesions of, 1251
    median, lesions of, 1250
    musculospiral, lesions of, 1251
    olfactory, 1115
    radial, lesions of, 1251
    ulnar, lesions of, 1249
Nerves, cranial, lesions of, 1115
    peripheral, lesions of, 1249
Nervous influenza, 97
    system, birth injuries to, 1207
                operation in, 1208
                spinal fluid in, 1208
    diseases of, 1111
    in pneumonia, 142
    organic diseases of, 1111
        history in, 1112
    peripheral, 1236
Neuralgia, glossopharyngeal, 1248
    Sluder's, 1248
    trigeminal, 1247
        alcoholic injections in, 1248
        causes of, 1247
        operation in, 1248
        pain in, 1247
        trigger zones in, 1248
Neurasthenia, 1099
    fatigue in, 1099
    symptom complexes of, 1099
Neuritis, 1236

Neuritis, alcoholic, 1037
  and joint disease, 1238
  bursitis and, 1238
  causalgia in, 1237
  causes of, 1236
  cervical rib and, 1238
  in acidosis, 1002
  multiple, 1238
    acrodynia, 1241
    alcohol and, 128
    arsenical, 1241
      skin in, 1241
    causes of, 1238
    diet in, 1239
    erythredema, 1241
    foot-drop in, 1238
    gait in, 1239
    in pregnancy, 1145
    lead, 1240
    postdiphtheritic, 1240
      vibratory loss in, 1241
    psychosis in, 1239
    reflexes in, 1239
    sensation in, 1238
    tenderness in, 1238
    wrist-drop in, 1238
  pain in, 1237
  sensation in, 1237
  signs of, 1237
  steppage gait in, 1037
Neurologic examination, scheme for, 1114
  syndromes, 1146
Neuronitis, 1242
Neurorecurrence in syphilis, 214
Neuroses, 1097
  anxiety, 1100
  cardiac, 427
  characteristics of, 1105
  development of, 1102
  Freudian theory of, 1101
  history in, 1105
  intestinal, 625
    diet in, 628
    irritable bowel and, 626
    mucous colitis, 626
    roentgen-ray in, 627
    stool examination in, 627
  management of, 1106
  mental findings in, 1104
  personality in, 1098
  physical findings in, 1104
  precipitating factors in, 1104
  psychogenetic considerations of, 1101
  psychoneurotic predisposition to, 1104
Neurosyphilis, 1148
  asymptomatic, 218
  arsphenamine and, 1148
  general paresis, 1150
  incidence of, 1148
  meningeal, 1148
  meningovascular, 1148
  miscellaneous forms of, 1157
  parenchymatous, 1148
  tabes dorsalis, 1154
  types of, 1148
  vascular, 1148

Neutropenia, idiopathic, malignant, 886
Niemann-Pick's disease, 901
  leukocyte count in, 901
Night-blindness, 933
Ninth nerve, lesions of, 1123
  dysphagia in, 1123
Nitritoid crises, 227, 1061
Nitroglycerin in angina pectoris, 385
Nodules, subcutaneous, in rheumatic fever, 341
Normal diet, 929
Nutrition, diseases of, 929
Nyctalopia, 933
Nystagmus, 1120
  in multiple sclerosis, 1181

                    O

Obesity, 1015
  cerebral lesions in, 1016
  diet in, 1018
  dinitrophenol in, 1018
  dysorexia in, 1016
  heredity in, 1016
  hypothyroidism in, 1017
  in diabetes mellitus, 993
  in Fröhlich's syndrome, 849
  in hypertension, 469
  types of, 1017
Occipital lobe, lesions of, 1184
Occlusion, coronary, 386
Ochronosis, 1024
  alkaptonuria and, 1024
  heredity and, 1025
  skin in, 1025
  urine in, 1025
Oculoglandular tularemia, 79
Oöphoritis in mumps, 333
Operation in acromegaly, 847
  in acute cholecystitis, 673
  in aneurysm, 491
  in appendicitis, 640
  in arteriovenous fistula, 499
  in birth injuries, 1208
  in brain tumor, 1201
  in bronchiectasis, 721
  in cancer of thyroid, 827
  in cholelithiasis, 679
  in chronic cholecystitis, 674
  in diabetes mellitus, 1010
  in empyema, 792
  in epilepsy, 1233
  in exophthalmic goiter, 818
  in facial paralysis, 1246
  in gastric cancer, 620
    ulcer, 616
  in general peritonitis, 685
  in glossopharyngeal neuralgia, 1248
  in hematomyelia, 1165
  in hyperinsulinism, 1012
  in hypertension, 476, 478
  in intestinal obstruction, 638
  in lung abscess, 733
  in neuralgia, 1248
  in nodular goiter, 815
  in pulmonary fibrosis, 712
    tuberculosis, 773
      apicolysis, 772
      phrenicotomy, 772

Operation in pulmonary tuberculosis, thoracoplasty, 772
  in sciatica, 1243
  in splenic anemia, 891
  in thrombocytopenic purpura, 877
  in ulcerative colitis, 643
Opisthotonos in tetanus, 72
Opium habit, 1039, 1086
  euphoria in, 1040
  itching in, 1040
  Lambert treatment in, 1041
  leukocyte count in, 1041
  signs of, 1040
  tolerance in, 1040
Optic nerve involvement in pregnancy, 1145
  thalmus, lesions of, 1184
Oral cavity, neoplasms of, 572
Orchitis in mumps, 333
  in undulant fever, 60
Oriental sore, 248
Osler's disease, 891
Osteo-arthritis, 916
  climacteric, 917
Osteogenesis imperfecta, 921
Osteogenic sarcoma, 922
Osteitis deformans, 922
  fibrosa cystica, 921
    generalisata, 833
Osteomalacia, 921
Osteopsathyrosis, 921
Otitis media in measles, 327
  in scarlet fever, 317
  pneumococcal, 136
Ovarian hormones, 851
  therapy in hemophilia, 880
Oxycephaly, 921
Oxygen inhalations in influenza, 102
  in pneumonia, 147
Oxytocin, 844
Oxyuriasis, 285
  Oxyuris vermicularis, 285

P

PACHYMENINGITIS, hypertrophic, cervical, 1172
  causes of, 1172
Paget's disease, 922
Pain, cardiac, 363
  in angina pectoris, 382
  in coronary occlusion, 387
  in facial paralysis, 1244
  in pericarditis, 403
  in sciatica, 1243
  in trigeminal neuralgia, 1247
  renal, 555
Palpitation in heart disease, 363
Palsy, Bell's, 1244
  bulbar, 1211
  pseudo-bulbar, 1211
  shaking, 1213
Pancreas, calculi in, 683
  cancer of, 681
  cysts of, 682
  diseases of, 679
  hormone of, 850
Pancreatitis, acute, 680

Pancreatitis, acute, fat necrosis in, 680
  chronic, 681
    fat necrosis in, 681
Panniculitis, 927
Pappataci fever, 183
  epidemiology of, 183
  leukocyte count in, 184
Paragonimus westermani, 297
Paralysis agitans, 1213
  anarthria in, 1214
  and encephalitis, 1213
  causes of, 1213
  facies in, 1214
  festination in, 1214
  gait in, 1214
  sine agitatione, 1214
  tremor in, 1213
  asthenic, bulbar, 1212
  bowel, 637
  general, of insane, 1150
  ginger, 1039
  in poliomyelitis, 1177
  jake, 1039
  lead, 1058
  post-diphtheritic, 311
  "Saturday night," 1251
Paranoia, acute, 1036
Paranoid schizophrenia, 1094
Paraplegia dolorosa, 1161
Parasthesia in neuritis, 1238
Parathyroid glands, disorders of, 831
  functions of, 831
Parathyroidectomy changes in, 831
Parathyroidism, hyper-, 833
  hypo-, 831
Paratyphoid bacillus infections, 41
Paresis, general, 1077, 1150
  expression of, 1150
  fever therapy in, 1079, 1152
    methods, 1153
  incidence of, 1150
  laboratory examinations in, 1151
    cell count in, 1151
    globulin in, 1151
    Wassermann reaction in, 1151
  in syphilis, 1077
  mental findings in, 1078
  neurologic findings in, 1078
  signs of, 1151
  spinal fluid findings in, 1078
  Swift-Ellis treatment in, 1152
  tryparmaside in, 1153
  types of, 1079
Paretic dementia, 1150
Parietal lobe, lesions of, 1184
Parkinson's disease, 1213
Parotiditis, 332
Parotitis, epidemic, 332
  in uremia, 519
Paroxysmal tachycardia, 440
Parry's disease, 815
Pasteur treatment in rabies, 175
Pasteurella pestis, 82
  tularensis, 76
Pastia's sign, 318
Pellagra, 949
  dementia in, 952

Pellagra, diarrhea in, 951
  diet in, 953
  flavine in, 950
  glossitis in, 951
  incidence of, 949
  nervous system in, 952
  prevention of, 952
  sine eruptione, 952
  skin in, 951
  vitamin B₂ in, 950
  vitamin G in, 950
Pepsin, gastric, 590
Periarteritis nodosa, 591
Peribronchitis, 727
Pericarditis, 400
  acute, 400
    fibrinous, 401
      friction rub in, 401
      pain in, 401
    chronic adhesive, 406
      ascites in, 407
    roentgenology in, 407
    signs of, 403
      roentgenologic, 404
      thoracentesis, 406
    uremic, 519
    with effusion, 402
Pericardium, adherent, 406
Perinephritic abscess, 559
Peripheral nerves, lesions of, 1249
Peritoneum, cancer of, 687
  rectal shelf in, 687
  diseases of, 683
  tumors of, 687
Peritonitis, acute general, 683
    facies in, 684
    incidence of, 684
    operation in, 685
  chronic adhesive, 686
    ascites in, 686
  localized, acute, 685
    chronic, 685
Pernicious anemia, 863
    addisin in, 869
    blood in, 866
    cause of, 864
    cell measurements in, 867
    cord changes in, 865
    diet in, 868
    gastric analysis in, 866
    glossitis in, 865
    hemic murmur in, 865
    hyperbilirubinemia in, 867
    icterus index in, 867
    incidence of, 863
    leukocyte count in, 866
    liver in, 868
    macrocytes in, 867
    reticulocyte response in, 868
    tongue in, 865
    ventriculin in, 868
  malaria, 265
Pertussis, 322
  age and, 323
  bronchopneumonia in, 323
  leukocyte count in, 323
  prevention of, 324
  vaccines in, 325
Petechiæ in benzene poisoning, 1068

Petechiæ in cerebrospinal fever, 152
  in plague, 84
  in Rocky Mountain spotted fever, 198
  in smallpox, 169
  in typhus fever, 192
Petit mal, 1224
  manifestations of, 1224
Phenolsulphonephthalein test of kidney function, 525
Phlebotomus fever, 183
  flies, 184
Phosphorus in diet, 932
Physical agents, diseases due to, 1026
Pick's disease, 406, 666
Pigmentation in Addison's disease, 838
Pineal body, disorders of, 855
    lesions of, 1185
    tumors of, 855
"Pistol-shot" sound, 418
Pithiatism, 1101
Pitocen, 844
Pitressin, 844
Pituitary gland, anterior lobe hormone, 843
    disorders, 842
    lesions of, 1186
    posterior lobe hormone, 844
Plague, 82
  bacteriemia in, 85
  carriers of, 83
  forms of, 85
  bubonic, 85
  pneumonic, 85
  immune serum in, 87
  leukocyte count in, 85
Plasmochin in malaria, 271
Plasmodia, differentiation of, 269
  life cycles of, 258
  of malaria, 258
Pleura, cancer of, 785
  diseases of, 786
Pleural pressure in atelectasis, 702
Pleurisy, 786
  chronic, 792
  chylous, 790
  diaphragmatic, 793
  encysted, 793
  fibrinous, 786
    friction rub in, 787
    roentgen-ray in, 787
  hemorrhagic, 791
  in rheumatic fever, 340
  interlobar, 793
  localized, 793
  mediastinal, 793
  purulent, 791
  serofibrinous, 787
    fluid in, 789
      aspiration of, 789
    roentgen-ray in, 788
    signs in, 787
Plumbism, 1054
Pneumococcal infection, 133
    anti-serum, 135
    epidemiology of, 135
    immunology of, 135
Pneumococci, 133
  distribution of, 135

Pneumococci, types of, 134
　　typing of, 145
Pneumoconiosis, 712
　　course of, 715
　　prevention of, 716
　　roentgen-ray in, 714
　　signs of, 714
　　stages of, 713
Pneumonia, chronic, organizing, 710
　　in erysipelas, 128
　　in plague, 84
　　in typhoid fever, 32
　　influenzal, 98
　　lobar, 137
　　　　bacteriemia in, 144
　　　　circulation in, 142
　　　　diet in, 147
　　　　distribution of, 137
　　　　empyema in, 144
　　　　endocarditis in, 145
　　　　epidemiology of, 140
　　　　experimental, 139
　　　　fever in, 143
　　　　frequency of, 137
　　　　heart in, 142
　　　　incidence of, 138
　　　　　　season, 138
　　　　kidneys in, 142
　　　　leukocyte count in, 144
　　　　nervous system in, 142
　　　　oxygen in, 147
　　　　pathogenesis of, 139
　　　　pathologic stages of, 140
　　　　pericarditis in, 145
　　　　respiratory system in, 142
　　　　serum therapy in, 146
　　　　skin in, 141
　　　　sputum in, 143
　　　　unfavorable signs of, 146
　　lobular, 129. *See* Bronchopneu-
　　　　monia
　　staphylococcal, 118
　　　　roentgen-ray in, 119
　　　　treatment of, 119
　　streptococcal, 98
Pneumonitis, interstitial, 710
Pneumothorax, 794
　　artificial, in tuberculosis, 771
　　causes of, 794
　　Donder's pressure in, 794
　　roentgen-ray in, 796
　　signs of, 796
　　　　coin test in, 796
　　　　succussion splash, 796
Podagra, 985
Poisoning, arsenic, 1061
　　arsphenamine, 1061
　　benzene, 1067
　　food, 1042
　　lead, 1054
　　mercury, 1064
　　methyl alcohol, 1038
　　mushroom, 1046
　　snake venom, 1047
Poisons in food, natural, 1046
Polioencephalitis, inferior, 1177
　　superior, 1177
Poliomyelitis, acute anterior, 1175
　　　　cord changes in, 1176

Poliomyelitis, acute anterior, incidence
　　of, 1176
　　leukocyte count in, 1178
　　orthopedic treatment of,
　　　　1180
　　paralysis in, 1177
　　pre-paralytic signs of, 1176
　　serum treatment of, 1179
　　spinal fluid in, 1178
　　virus of, 1176
Pollens in hay-fever, 975
Pollinosis, 975
Polycythemia in mountain sickness, 1031
　　in congenital heart disease, 398
　　in pulmonary disease, 699
　　vera, 891
　　　　basal metabolism in, 892
　　　　blood count in, 892
　　　　headaches in, 892
　　　　leukocyte count in, 892
　　　　phenylhydrazine in, 893
　　　　roentgen-ray in, 892
Polydipsia in hyperparathyroidism, 834
Polyglandular syndrome, 808
Polymyositis hemorrhagica, 923
Polyneuritis, 1238
Polyposis, gastric, 623
Polyps, intestinal, 645
Polyserositis, 686
Polyuria in acromegaly, 846
　　in hyperparathyroidism, 834
　　in pituitary disease, 845
Pons, lesions of, 1185
Posterior spinal sclerosis, 1154
Postural hypotension, 480
Pott's disease, 1162
Precordial pain, 363
Pregnancy in acromegaly, 846
　　in Addison's disease, 839
　　in hypertension, 470
　　in syphilis, 227
　　nervous disorders in, 1143
　　thyroid problems of, 830
Presbyophrenic psychosis, 1080
Price-Jones curve, 867
Progestin, 851
Prognathism in acromegaly, 846
Projection, definition of, 1109
Prolan A, 843
　　B, 843
Prosoplegia, 1244
Protein requirements of diet, 901
　　complete, 931
　　reduction of, 931
Proteinuria, 508
Protozoal diseases, 232
Pseudohermaphroditism in hyperfunc-
　　tion of adrenal, 841
Pseudoleukemia, 888
Pseudosclerosis, 1219
　　corneal change in, 1219
　　liver and, 1219
Psilosis, 953
Psittacosis, 186
　　bronchopneumonia in, 187
　　parrots and, 186
　　prevention of, 187
Psychasthenia, 1100
Psychic equivalent in epilepsy, 1228

Psychoanalysis, 1072
Psychopathic inferiority, constitutional, 1096
Psychoses, 1069
  causes of, 1070
  classification of, 1073
  epileptic, 1081
  functional, 1074
  heredity in, 1072
  incidence of, 1070
  manic-depressive, 1087
  organic, 1073
  prevention of, 1072
  senile, 1079
    types of, 1080
  toxic, 1074, 1085
  traumatic, 1084
  with brain disease, 1084
  with cerebral arteriosclerosis, 1081
  with mental deficiency, 1083
  with nervous disease, 1084
  with somatic disease, 1087
  with syphilis, 1084
Psychotherapy, 1072
Ptosis of stomach, 624
Puberty, precocious, 852
Puerperium, nervous disorders in, 1143
Pulmonary arteriosclerosis, 716
  anthrax, 89
  congestion in mitral stenosis, 413
  disease, functional pathology of, 688
  fibrosis, 708
    causes of, 709
    operation in, 712
    roentgen-ray in, 711
    signs in, 711
    types of, pathologic, 710
  gas exchange, 692
  hypertrophic osteoarthropathy, 917
  stenosis, 399
    congenital, 397
  valve disease, 422
    insufficiency, 423
Pulse, Corrigan, 418
  water-hammer, 418
Pulsus alternans, 447
  blood pressure, in, 447
Pupil, 1119
  Argyll-Robertson, 1120
  hippus in, 1120
  inequality of, 1119
  nystagmus in, 1120
  paradoxical, 1120
  shape of, 1119
Purkinje system, 431
Purpura, allergic, 878
  Henoch's, 878
  non-thrombocytopenic, 878
  primary, 875
    classification of, 874
    ecchymoses in, 874
    petechiæ in, 874
  Schönlein's, 878
  thrombocytopenic, 875
    blood in, 876
    leukocyte count in, 876
    platelet count in, 876
    splenectomy in, 877
    tourniquet test in, 876

Purpura, thrombocytopenic, transfusion in, 877
Pustule, malignant, 87
  of anthrax, 89
Pyelitis, 559
  colon bacillus, 42
  defloration, 560
Pyelography, intravenous, 556
Pyelonephritis, 559
  chronic, 561
  leukocyte count in, 560
Pyelonephrosis, 555
Pyknolepsy, 1226
Pyopneumothorax, 794

Q

Queckenstedt test, 1139
Quinidine in auricular fibrillation, 447
  in paroxysmal tachycardia, 441
  in premature contractions, 440
Quinine in malaria, 270

R

Rabies, 172
  epidemiology of, 173
  leukocyte count in, 174
  Negri bodies in, 173
  specific therapy of, 175
  stages of, 173
Radial nerve, lesions of, 1251
Radioactive substances, 1033
Radium, poisoning from, 1033
Râles redux, 143
Rash. *See* Skin
Rat-bite fever, 229
Rationalization, definition of, 1109
Rats in plague, 83
  destruction of, in plague, 86
Raynaud's disease, 457
  disturbed physiology in, 458
  extremities in, 459
  sympathectomy in, 460
Recurrent fever, 229
Rectum, cancer of, 653
  disorders of, 652
  infections of, 652
  polyps of, 653
  syphilis of, 653
  tuberculosis of, 653
  tumors of, 653
Reflex, abdominal, 1126
  Achilles, 1127
    in sciatica, 1243
  ankle clonus, 1127
  Babinski, 1125
  biceps, 1127
  conjunctiva, 1122
  corneal, 1121
  cremasteric, 1126
  deep, 1126
  in epilepsy, 1225
  in multiple neuritis, 1239
  in myelitis, 1171
  in progressive muscular atrophy, 1249
  in tabes dorsalis, 1150

Reflex, lacrymal, 1122
  patellar, 1127
  plantar, 1125
  tendon, 1126
  triceps, 1127
  vegetative, 1127
    ciliospinal, 1127
    oculo-cardiac, 1127
Relapsing fever, 229
    Spironema obermeieri, 229
      recurrentis, 229
Remittent fever, 17
Renal calculi, 557
  carbuncle, 559
  complications of hypertension, 475
  function, tests of, 521
    blood-urea clearance, 523
    concentration, 524
    creatinine clearance, 522
    dilutin, 524
    phenolsulphonthalein, 525
  pain, 555
  threshold in diabetes mellitus, 998
Respiratory quotient in diabetes mellitus, 996
  system in pneumonia, 142
  tract, diseases of, 688
Reticulocyte count in pernicious anemia, 868
Reticulo-endothelial system, diseases of, 899
Reticulo-endotheliosis, 900
Reticulosis, aleukemic, 900
Retinal lesions in nephrosclerosis, 553
Retinitis angiospastica, 514
  cotton-wool exudate in, 514
  hypertensive, 468, 514
Rheumatic fever, 336
  Aschoff body in, 338
  death-rate in, 342
  heart changes in, 339
  hemolytic streptococci in, 337
  in children, 341
  incidence of, 336
  leukocyte count in, 342
  nephritis in, 341
  pleurisy in, 340
  salicylates in, 342
  skin eruptions in, 341
  subcutaneous nodules in, 341
  heart disease, 365
    course of, 369
    electrocardiographic findings in, 368
    incidence of, 365
    prevention of, 369
    signs of, 367
    valvular lesions in, 366
Rheumatism, acute articular, 336
  chronic, 905
  gonorrheal, 155, 917
    joint fluid in, 156
    leukocyte count in, 156
  muscular, 924
Rhinitis, hyperplastic, 979
  infective, 979
  vasomotor, 975
"Rice-water" stools in cholera, 108

Rickets, 944
  and vitamin D, 944
  blood chemistry in, 948
  body build in, 947
  bone changes in, 946
  calcium-phosphorus ratio in, 945
  ergosterol in, 946
  Harrison's groove in, 947
  incidence of, 944
  roentgen-ray in, 948
  rosary in, 947
  sunlight in, 945
  viosterol in, 948
Rickettsia, characteristics of, 190
  prowazeki, 191
Rickettsiæ, diseases due to, 190
Riedel's struma, 828
Risus sardonicus, 72
Rocky Mountain spotted fever, 197
    death-rate in, 199
    eastern type of, 197
    eruption of, 198
    leukocyte count in, 199
    prevention of, 199
    Rickettsia in, 197
    splenomegaly in, 197
    temperature curve in, 198
    vectors of, 197
    western type of, 197
Roentgen-ray in abscess of liver, 668
  in acromegaly, 846
  in aneurysm, 490
  in atelectasis, 702
  in bone disease. *See* Specific diseases
  in brain disease, 1137
    tumors, 1201
  in bronchial foreign bodies, 728
  in bronchiectasis, 720
  in cancer of colon, 647
    of esophagus, 582
    of lung, 784
  in cholelithiasis, 677
  in constipation, 630
  in diaphragmatic hernia, 803
  in diarrhea, 633
  in diseases of thyroid gland, 812
  in emphysema, 706
  in empyema, 792
  in esophageal spasm, 578
  in exophthalmic goiter, 818
    sequels of, 819
  in fibrinous pleurisy, 787
  in fracture of skull, 1205
  in gastric cancer, 619
    disorders, 590
    ulcer, 603
  in gout, 990
  in Hodgkin's disease, 890
  in intestinal neuroses, 627
    obstruction, 637
    tuberculosis, 644
  in lead poisoning, 1059
  in leukemia, 883
  in liver disorders, 656
  in lung abscess, 731
  in mediastinal disease, 798
  in mitral stenosis, 412
  in pericarditis, 407

Roentgen-ray in pneumoconiosis, 714
  in pneumonia, 145
  in pneumothorax, 796
  in polycythemia vera, 892
  in pulmonary fibrosis, 711
    tuberculosis, 753
  in rickets, 948
  in scurvy, 943
  in serofibrinous pleurisy, 788
  in spinal cord disease, 1137
    tumors, 1159
  in splenic anemia, 891
  in syphilis of lung, 776
  in syringomyelia, 1170
  in thymus enlargements, 855
  in tuberculous spondylitis, 1163
  in ulcerative colitis, 642
Romberg's sign in paresis, 1151
  in tabes, 1156
Rosary in rickets, 947
Rose spots, 30
Roseola infantum, 334
Rubella, 334
  adenopathy in, 335
  atypical forms of, 335
  leukocyte count in, 335
  susceptibility to, 335
Rubeola, 325
Rumple-Leeds sign, 318

S

SACRO-ILIAC arthritis in sciatica, 1243
  strain, 924
Saint Vitus' dance, 1216
Salicylates in rheumatic fever, 343
Salmonella paratyphosus, 41. *See* Paratyphoid infections
  Schottmülleri, 41. *See* Paratyphoid
    infections
Salyrgan in pericarditis, 408
Sand-fly fever, 183
Sarcosporidiosis, 273
Scarlatina, 314
Scarlet fever, 314
  arthritis in, 317
  carriers in, 315
  convalescent serum in, 319
  desquamation in, 316
  Dick test in, 318
  immunization in, active, 320
    passive, 320
  leukocyte count in, 316
  nephritis in, 317
  otitis media in, 317
  prevention of, 318
  rash of, 316
  Schultz-Charlton test in, 318
  sore throat in, 316
  susceptibility to, 315
  tongue of, 316
  urine in, 316
Schick test, 312
Schistosoma hæmatobium, 298
  japonicum, 298
  mansoni, 298
Schistosomiasis, 298
  dermatitis in, 301

Schistosomiasis, eosinophilia in, 300
  intestinal, 300
  vesicle, 299
Schizogony, 258
Schizonts, 258
Schizophrenia, 1093
  clinical expressions of, 1094
  etiology of, 1093
  habitus in, 1093
  invertism in, 1093
  physical signs in, 1094
  prevention of, 1095
  social relations in, 1095
  types of, 1094
Schultz-Charlton phenomena, 318
Sciatica, 1242
  causes of, 1242
  Lasègue's sign in, 1243
  operation in, 1243
  pain in, 1243
  reflex, Achilles, in, 1243
  sacro-iliac arthritis and, 1243
Sclerosis, amyotrophic, lateral, 1166
  combined, 1167
    and pernicious anemia, 1167
    postero-lateral, 1167
    signs of, 1167
  disseminated, 1180
  insular, 1180
  multiple, 1180
    cause of, 1180
  posterior spinal, 1154
Scorbutus, 940
Scorpions in disease, 304
Scurvy, 940
  deprivation period of, 941
  diet in, 944
  fragility of bones in, 942
  hemorrhages in, 942
  incidence of, 941
  infantile, 940, 942
  latent, infantile, 943
  leukocyte count in, 943
  prevention of, 944
  roentgen-ray in, 943
  sclerosis in, 942
  vitamin C and, 941
Second nerve, lesions of, 1116
    binasal hemianopsia in,
      1116
    bitemporal hemianopsia in,
      1116
    choked disk in, 1116
    optic atrophy in, 1117
      etiology of, 1117
      hereditary, 1117
    neuritis in, 1116
    papilledema in, 1117
    vision testing in, 1116
Secretin, 807
Segmental monoplegia, 1129
Sella turcica in acromegaly, 846
Sensation, deep pressure pain, 1135
  dissociation loss of, 1136
  disturbances of, 1134
  graphesthesia, 1136
  in neuritis, 1237
  stereognosis in, 1135
  testing of, 1134

Sensation, vibratory, 1135
Septic sore throat, 573
Septicemia, colon bacillus in, 42
    in coccal infections, 118
    streptococcal, 126
Serologic reactions in syphilis, 214
Serum, albumin-globulin ratio in nephro-
        sis, 511, 544
    convalescent, in measles, 328
    immune, in anthrax, 91
        in plague, 87
    in acute chorea, 1218
    reactions, 314
    shock, 981
        pathogenesis of, 981
        prevention of, 981
    sickness, 980
        epinephrin in, 981
        immunology of, 980
        leukocyte count in, 981
    treatment of bacillary dysentery, 49
        of cerebrospinal fever, 153
        of diphtheria, 313
        of erysipelas, 129
        of pneumonia, 146
        of poliomyelitis, 1179
        of scarlet fever, 320
        of streptococcal infections, 123
Seventh nerve, lesions of, 1122
Sexual precocity in pituitary disease, 845
Shiga bacilli, 43. *See* Bacillary dysentery
Shingles, 1174
Shock, electric, 1031
    in coronary occlusion, 388
    serum, 981
    therapy, 122
        in arthritis deformans, 915
Siderans, cholera, 110
Siderosis, 712
Silicosis, 712
Simmonds' disease, 847
Sinkler's phenomenon, 1129
Sinus arrhythmia, 433
    bradycardia, 432
    tachycardia, 432
    thrombosis, 1195
        Gradingo syndrome in, 1196
        signs of, 1195
Sixth nerve, lesions of, 1118
Skin in arsenical neuritis, 1241
    in cerebrospinal fever, 152
    in cirrhosis of liver, 665
    in dengue, 182
    in erysipelas, 128
    in hemochromatosis, 1024
    in herpes zoster, 1175
    in jaundice, 658
    in measles, 326
    in ochronosis, 1025
    in pellagra, 951
    in pneumonia, 141
    in rheumatic fever, 341
    in rubella, 335
    in scarlet fever, 316
    in smallpox, 166
    in syphilis, 212, 215
    in typhus fever, 193
    infections in diabetes mellitus, 1002
    tests in allergy, 966

Skin tests in hay-fever, 976
    in undulant fever, 61
Skull, fracture of, 1204
    lumbar puncture in, 1205
    roentgen-ray in, 1205
    signs of, 1205
Sleeping sickness, African, 251
Smallpox, 163
    diagnostic tests of, 168
    droplet infection in, 164
    epidemiology of, 164
    immunity in, 164
    inclusion bodies in, 164
    leukocyte count in, 168
    modification by vaccination, 169
    prevention of, 170
    skin in, 166
    stages of, 165
    vaccination in, 171
Snake-bite, 1047
Snake-venom poisoning, 1047
        hematoxin in, 1047
        neurotoxin in, 1047
Snuffles in congenital syphilis, 221
Sodium chloride in diet, 931
        loss in Addison's disease, 837
Sodoku, 229
"Sonne" dysentery bacilli, 46
Sore throat in scarlet fever, 316
    streptococcal, 124
Sparganosis, 294
Specific therapy of rabies, 175
Speech, disorders of, 1188
    scanty, in multiple sclerosis, 1181
Spiders in disease, 304
Spinal cord, blood-vessels, disease of,
        1174
    compression of, 1158
    disorders of, 1158
    injuries to, 1164
    subdural abscess of, 1161
    tumors of, 1158
        cervical, 1160
        conus, 1160
        intramedullary, 1159
        localization of, 1159
        roentgen-ray in, 1159
        symptoms of, 1159
    fluid, 1138
        cell count of, 1141
        colloidal-gold test, 1141
        examination in paresis, 1151
        gross examination of, 1140
        in cerebrospinal fever, 151
        in epidemic encephalitis, 1221
        in hematoma, 1207
        in multiple sclerosis, 1182
        in poliomyelitis, 1178
        in tabes dorsalis, 1156
        in tetanus, 72
        in trypanosomiasis, 252
        in tuberculous spondylitis, 1163
        laboratory examination of, 1140
        method of obtaining, 1139
        protein in, 1142
        sugar test of, 1141
        Wassermann in, 1142
        xanthochromia in, 1140
    muscular atrophy, progressive, 1167

Spinal paralysis, infantile, 1175
  puncture, 1139
    in brain tumor, 1202
    in cerebrospinal fever, 153
    in fracture of skull, 1205
    in hydrocephalus, 1209
    in lead encephalopathy, 1061
    in subarachnoid hemorrhage,
      1205
    Queckenstedt test in, 1139
    technic of, 1139
Spine, carcinoma of, 1160
  caries of, 1162
  fracture of, 1164
  poker, 919
  tumors of, 1160
Spirillum infections, in food poisoning,
  1042
Spirochætosis icterohæmorrhagica, 230
Spirochetes, diseases due to, 204
  varieties of, 204
Spironema obermeieri, 229
  recurrentis, 229
Spleen abscess of, 896
  ague-cake, 267
  amyloid of, 896
  anomalies of, 895
  atrophy of, 895
  congestion of, 896
  cysts of, 898
  diseases of, 894
  enlargement of, in tularemia, 78
  enlargements of, 894
  floating, 895
  in chronic lymphatic leukemia, 882
    myelogenous leukemia, 882
  in kala-azar, 245
  in malaria, 267
  in splenic anemia, 890
  infarction of, 896
  malaria of, 898
  movable, 895
  syphilis of, 897
  torsion of, 896
  tuberculosis of, 897
  tumors of, 898
Splenectomy, 896
  in cysts, 898
  in Gaucher's disease, 901
  in purpura, 877
  in thrombosis, 897
  in torsion, 896
Splenic vein, thrombosis of, 897
Splenomegaly, chronic infectious, 897
  cirrhotic, 897
  diagnosis of, 894
  hemolytic, 871
  siderotic, 898
Spondylitis deformans, 911, 919
  hypertrophic, 917
  tuberculous, 1162
    kyphosis in, 1162
    roentgen-ray in, 1163
    spinal fluid in, 1163
Sporogony, 259
Sporotrichosis, 354
Spotted fever, 190
Sprue, 953
  asthenia in, 955

Sprue, blood picture in, 956
  diet in, 957
  gastric contents in, 956
  incidence of, 953
  leukocyte count in, 956
  liver extract in, 957
  macrocytic anemia in, 956
  Monilia psilosis, 953
  stool in, 955
  tetany in, 955
  tongue in, 955
  vitamin B₂ and, 954
Sputum in asthma, 971
  in bronchiectasis, 719
  in bronchopneumonia, 131
  in gangrene of lung, 734
  in influenza, 99
  in lung abscess, 730
  in pneumonia, 143
  in pulmonary disease, 696
    characteristics of, 697
    significance of, 696
    tuberculosis, 751
Stammering, 1188
Status epilepticus, 1229
  thymicolymphaticus, 855
Steppage gait in polyneuritis, 1239
Stereognosis, 1135
Stippling of red cells in plumbism, 1057
Stokes-Adams syndrome, 435
Stomach, anomalies of, 624
  cancer of, 617
    incidence of, 617
    laboratory examination in, 619
    operation in, 620
    roentgen-ray in, 619
    site of lesion, 618
  deformities of, 624
  disorders of, 583
    classification of, 583
    diagnosis of, 585
      gastric analysis in, 586
      history in, 585
  displacements of, 624
  diverticula of, 624
  foreign bodies in, 624
  hour-glass, 624
  ptosis of, 624
  syphilis of, 623
  tumors of, 623
    benign, 623
Stomatitis, epidemic, 188
  mercurial, 1065
Stools in cholera, 110
Streptococcal infections, 117
  bacteriology of, 119
  distribution of, 117
  pathogenesis of, 117
  sore throat, 124
  septicemia, 126
Streptococcus, anhemolytic, 119
  hemolytic infections, 122
    bacteriology of, 122
    distribution of, 120
    epidemiology of, 123
    immunology of, 163
    in erysipelas, 127
    in rheumatic fever, 337
    pathogenesis of, 123

Streptococcus, hemolytic infections, recovery from, 123
    non-hemolytic, 119
        pathogenesis of, 120
    viridans, 119
Streptothricosis, 777
Strongyloides stercoralis, 286
Strongyloidosis, 286
    Strongyloides stercoralis, 286
Strophanthin in congestive heart failure, 451
Struma, 812. *See* Goiter
Subarachnoid hemorrhage, 1205
        spinal puncture in, 1206
        spontaneous, 1194
            causes of, 1194
            hyperglycemia in, 1194
            Kernig's sign in, 1194
            spinal drainage in, 1195
Subdural abscess, 1161
Sugar, blood, 998
Sulphoxylate, sodium formaldehyde, 541
Sunstroke, 1027
Sweating sickness, 349
Swift-Ellis treatment in neurosyphilis, 1152
Sydenham's chorea, 1216
Symbolization, definition of, 1109
Sympathectomy in Raynaud's disease, 460
Sympathetic nervous system and epinephrin, 836
Sympathin, 807
Symptoms, general, of heart disease, 364
Syndrome, Adams-Stokes, 435
    Ayerza, 717
    Benedikt's, 1130
    Brown-Séquard's, 1146
    Cushing's, 850
    effort, 428
    Fröhlich's, 849
    Gelineau, 1230
    Gradenigo, 1196
    Hand-Christian, 902
    Horner's, 460, 1146
    Klumpke's, 1146
    Korsakoff's, 1037
    Landry's, 1147
    Laurence-Biedl, 1147
    Ménière's, 1147
    Millard-Gubler, 1130
    neurologic, 1146
    None-Froin, 1159
    Parkinson, 1223
    Plummer-Vinson, 861
    polyglandular, 808
    Weber's, 1130
Synergic movement, 1131
Syphilis, 204
    and aneurysm, 488
    and marriage, 227
    and nephrosis, 542
    bone involvement in, 210
    buboes in, 212
    central nervous system in, 214
    chancre in, 208
        appearance of, 211
    condylomata lata in, 209

Syphilis, congenital lesions of, 210
    early, 221
    course of, 206
    cutaneous lesions of, 212
    dark-field examination in, 212
    eye reactions in, 213
    gumma, 209
    hair in, 213
    immunity in, 222
    in paresis, 1077
    in utero, 206
    incidence of, 205
    joint reactions in, 213
    late manifestations of, 215
        bone, 215
        cardiac, 216
        central nervous, 217
        cutaneous, 215
        optic nerve in, 219
        spinal fluid in, 217
        testes in, 220
        viscera in, 220
    of joints, 918
    of larynx, 724
    of liver, 668
    of lung, 775
    of mediastinum, 801
    of mouth, 571
    of nervous system, 1148. *See* also Neurosyphilis
    of pharynx, 571
    of rectum, 653
    of spleen, 897
    of stomach, 623
    of thyroid gland, 828
    prevention of, 223
    reinfection in, 222
    secondary stage lesions, 209
    serologic reactions in, 214
    superinfection in, 222
    tertiary lesions of, 209
    treatment of early, 225
        late, 226
        in pregnancy, 227
        reactions in, 227
    Treponema pallidum in, 205
Syphilitic heart disease, 391
        aorta in, 391
        dyspnea in, 392
        objective signs in, 392
        Wassermann reaction in, 393
Syringomyelia, 1169
    roentgen-ray in, 1170
    signs of, 1169

T

Tabardillo, 190
Tabes dorsalis, 1154
    Argyll-Robertson pupil in, 1155
    arsenic in, 1157
    ataxia in, 1155
    bladder disturbances in, 1154
    Charcot joint in, 1155
    cord bladder in, 1156
    cranial nerves in, 1155
    early symptoms of, 1154

Tabes dorsalis, gastric crises in, 1155
  girdle sensation in, 1154
  libido in, 1154
  rectal disturbances in, 1154
  reflexes in, 1150
  Romberg's sign in, 1156
  spinal fluid in, 1156
  trophic changes in, 1155
Tâche cérébrale in cerebrospinal fever, 152
Tachycardia, paroxysmal, 440
  sinus, 432
Tænia saginata, 290
  solium, 290
Tapeworm infections, 290
Tay-Sach's disease, 1210
Temperature curves in virus diseases, 161
Temporal lobe, lesions of, 1184
Teniasis, 290
  stool examination in, 291
Tennis elbow, 919
Tenth nerve, lesions of, 1123
Test meal in gastric analysis, 586
Testes in syphilis, 220
Testicle, tumors of, 854
Tetanus, 69
  antitoxin in, 75
  death-rate in, 73
  incidence of, 71
  leukocyte count in, 72
  local, 72
  prevention of, 74
  specific therapy in, 75
Tetany, parathyroid, 831
  calcium in, 832
  Chvostek's sign in, 832
  corpopedal spasm, 832
  Erb's sign in, 832
  in nephrosis, 544
  in sprue, 955
  stridor in, 832
  Trousseau's sign in, 832
Tetrachlorethylene in uncinariasis, 281
Tetralogy of Fallot, 397
Theobromin in angina pectoris, 385
  in congestive failure, 452
Therapy, non-specific, in coccal infections, 117
Third nerve, lesions of, 1118
Thoracentesis in empyema, 133
  in pericarditis, 406
Thoracotomy in empyema, 133
Thrill, cardiac, in mitral stenosis, 411
  hydatid, 292
  in goiter, 816
Thrombo-angiitis obliterans, 483
  surgical measures in, 486
  tobacco in, 484
  vascular signs in, 485
Thrombo-arteriosclerosis obliterans, 481
  arteriography in, 482
  classification of, 481
  organic extracts in, 483
Thrombocytopenia in benzene poisoning, 1068
Thrombophilia, 486
Thrombophlebitis, 500
  causes of, 500
  roentgen therapy in, 501

Thrombosis, cerebral, 1190
  dysesthesia in, 1191
  monoplegia, 1192
  sinus, 1195
  trophic disorders in, 1191
  simple, 486
Thrush, 354
Thymic asthma, 855
Thymus, disorders of, 855
  enlargement, roentgen-ray in, 855
  tumors of, 855
Thyroid and nephrosis, 542
  gland, aberrant, 829
  cancer of, 827
  developmental anomalies of, 828
  diseases of, 809
    basal metabolism in, 812
    classification of, 811
    roentgen-ray in, 812
  function of, 809
  hyperfunction of, symptoms of, 810
  hypofunction of, symptoms of, 810
  in cretinism, 826
  in myxedema, 823
  malignant disease of, 827
  operation of, 827
  heart disease, 820
Thyroidectomy in thyrotoxic heart disease, 396
  subtotal, 820
Thyroiditis, acute, 828
  chronic, 828
  ligneous, 828
Thyrotoxic heart disease, 394
  auricular fibrillation in, 395
  incidence of, 394
  Lugol's solution in, 396
  signs of, 395
  thyroidectomy in, 396
Thyrotoxicosis, 817
  and pregnancy, 830
  in heart disease, 394
Thyroxin, 809
Tic douloureux, 1247
Ticks in disease, 302
Tobacco in thrombo-angiitis obliterans, 484
Tongue in myxedema, 822
  in pellegra, 951
  in pernicious anemia, 865
  in sprue, 955
Tonsillitis, acute, 572
  exudate in, 573
  leukocyte count in, 573
  prevention of, 574
  chronic, 574
  tonsillectomy in, 575
  follicular, 572
Tonsils as foci of infection, 575
  tuberculosis of, 575
Toxic adenoma of thyroid, 814
  psychoses, causes of, 1085
  delirium in, 1085
  exogenous, 1085
  causes of, 1086

Toxic psychoses, general principles of treatment in, 1085
Tracheal tug in aneurysm, 490
Tracheitis, 725
Trance, alcoholic, 1037
Transference, definition of, 1110
Transfusion in hemophilia, 879
in purpura, 877
in secondary anemia, 862
Trapezius myositis, 925
Trematode infections, 294
Trembles, the, 1045
Tremor, 1133
in lenticular degeneration, 1219
in multiple sclerosis, 1181
in paralysis agitans, 1213
types of, 1133
Trench fever, 200
febrile types of, 201
leukocyte count in, 201
mouth in, 569
prevention of, 202
vector of, 200
Treponema morsus muris, 229
pallidum, 205
pertenue, 228
Trichinella spiralis, 287
Trichinosis, 287
eosinophilia in, 288
leukocyte count in, 288
prevention of, 288
Trichinella spiralis, 287
Trichocephaliasis, 283
Trichomoniasis, 242
Trichuriasis, 283
Tricuspid valve disease, 421
insufficiency, 421
physical findings in, 421
stenosis, 422
Trismus in tetanus, 72
Trophozoites, 258
Trousseau's sign in tetany, 832
Trypanosoma gambiense, 252
rhodesiense, 252
Schizotrypanum cruzi, 254
Trypanosomiases, 251
African, 251
Brazilian, 254
Tryparsamide in neurosyphilis, 1153
in trypanosomiasis, 253
Tsutsugamushi disease, 202
adenopathy in, 203
eruption of, 203
vector of, 202
Tubercle bacillus, 734
R- and S-forms of, 735
virulence of, 735
Tuberculin in pulmonary tuberculosis, 757
Tuberculosis, allergy in, 737
in diabetes mellitus, 1002
of intestine, 644
of larynx, 723
of rectum, 653
of spine, 1162
of spleen, 897
of thyroid gland, 828
pulmonary, 734

Tuberculosis, pulmonary and silicosis, 749, 761
aspects, clinical, 750
B.C.G. in prevention of, 774
calcification in, 741
caseation in, 741
cavities in, 749
classification of comparative condition, 765
of lesions, 764
of symptoms, 764
climate in, 767
clinico-pathologic forms of, 743
hematogenous, 745
phthsic, 747, 760
primary, 744
transitional, 746
collapse therapy in, 770
complement-fixation test in, 757
concurrent diseases in, 736
cough in, 754
course, clinical, 750
diet in, 766
etiology of, 736
examination in, 754
fibrosis in, 741
focal symptoms of, 751
hemoptysis in, 751
heredity in, 736
hoarseness in, 752
leukocyte count in, 757
Mantoux test in, 757
pleural effusion in, 752
pneumothorax in, 771
roentgen-ray in, 753
sputum in, 751
examination in, 756
symptoms, general, 752
tubercle formation in, 740
tuberculin in, 757
relation of, to influenza, 99
Tuberculous infection, 734
evolution in body, 738
specific predisposing factors in, 737
transmission of, 735
Tularemia, 76
agglutination reaction in, 81
distribution of, 77
forms of, 79
in animals, 77
incidence of, 77
prevention of, 81
skin lesions in, 80
Tumors, acute splenic, 896
of adrenal cortex, 841
medulla, 841
of bowel, 645
of brain, 1197
of liver, 669
of lung, 781
of mediastinum, 799
benign, 799
malignant, 799
of peritoneum, 687
of pineal body, 855
of rectum, 653
of spinal cord, 1158
of spine, 1160

Tumors of spleen, 898
  of testicle, 854
  of thymus, 855
Twelfth nerve, lesions of, 1124
Typhoid fever, 23
  bacillus, 23
    carriers of, 24
    distribution of, in body, 24
    mode of conveyance of, 24
  bacteriemia, 33
  blood count in, 32
  diet in, 38
  expression of, 28
  immunization in, 36
  in infants, 27
  in vaccinated individuals, 26
  incidence of, 25
  mortality in, 34
  pathogenesis of, 23
  prophylaxis of, 35
  pulse in, 30
  rose spots in, 30
  temperature curve in, 29
  varieties of, 26
  Widal reaction in, 32
Typhoidal tularemia, 79
Typhus fever, 190
  agglutination reaction in, 194
  death-rate of, 195
  delirium in, 194
  eruption of, 193
  gangrene in, 192
  leukocyte count in, 194
  lice and, 191
  petechiæ in, 192
  prevention of, 196
  Rickettsia prowazeki, 191
  spinal fluid in, 194
  temperature curve in, 193

U

ULCER, duodenal, 600
  gastric, 600
  gastro-jejunal, 617
Ulceroglandular tularemia, 79
Ulnar nerve, lesions of, 1249
  claw hand in, 1250
  sensation in, 1250
  wasting in, 1250
Uncinate region, lesions of, 1184
Undulant fever, 51
  abortion in, 60
  agglutination reaction in, 59
  animal inoculation in, 61
  arthritis in, 60
  clinical varieties of, 55
  duration of, 62
  epidemiology of, in cattle, 55
  incidence of, 53
  infection, mode of, 52
    source of, 52
  leukocyte count in, 59
  mortality of, 63
  orchitis in, 60
  skin test in, 61
  special signs of, 58
  spleen in, 53

Undulant fever, temperature in, 56
  vaccination in, 64
Uremia, 515
  acidosis in, 517, 520
  anemia in, 520
  azotemia in, 519
  blood chemistry in, 519
    pressure in, 517
  chronic, 518
  convulsive seizures in, 516
  eclamptic, 516
  encephalopathy, hypertensive, 516
  epileptiform, 516
  false, 516
  Kernig's sign in, 517
  Kussmaul breathing in, 518
  leukocyte count in, 517
  lumbar puncture in, 518
  management of, 537
  monoplegia in, 517
  myœdema in, 518
  optic disk in, 518
  parotitis in, 519
  pericarditis in, 519
Uric acid in gout, 986
Urinary passage, bacterial infections of, 558
  tract, diseases of, 505
Urine, 506
  Addis count in, 506
  albumin in, 508
  blood count in, 507
  casts in, 507
  fibrin in, 508
  hemoglobin in, 508
Urobilinuria, 657
Urticaria, 982
Uterine bleeding, functional, 853

V

VACCINATION against cholera, 111
  typhoid fever, 36
    methods of, 36
    results of, 36
  in influenza, 101
  in smallpox, 171
    complications of, 172
    indications for, 172
    method of, 171
  in undulant fever, 64
Vaccine, Haffkine's, 87
  in cholera, 111
Vaccines in arthritis deformans, 915
  in focal infection, 122
Vaccinia, 171. *See* Vaccination
Valvular heart disease, chronic, 408
Van den Bergh reaction, 658
  in pernicious anemia, 867
  in yellow fever, 179
Vaquez's disease, 891
Varicella, 329
  and herpes zoster, 330
  prevention of, 331
  rash in, 330
  susceptibility to, 330
Variola, 163
Varioloid, 169

Vasopressin, 844
Vector of trench fever, 200
Vectors of typhus fever, 191
Vedder's signs in beriberi, 939
Veins, diseases of, 499
    structure of, 456
    thrombosis of, in typhoid fever, 31
Venesection in congestive failure, 452
Ventriculin in pernicious anemia, 868
Ventriculography, 1137
Verbigeration, definition of, 1110
Vesicating insects, 307
Vibratory sensation, 1135
Vibrio, cholera, 107
Vincent's angina, 569
Viosterol, 948
Virilism in hyperfunction of adrenal, 841
Virus, 159
    cytotropism in, 160
    diseases, 159
        criteria for classification of, 162
        epidemiology of, 161
        general discussion of, 159
        temperature curve in, 161
    filterability of, 159
    filterable, in influenza, 93
    inclusion bodies of, 160
Visceral reactions in syphilis, 220
Vitamin A, 933
        carotene in, 933
        deficiency of, 933
        epithelial changes in, 933
        sterility in, 933
    B, 934, 936
        digestive disturbances in, 934
        nerve changes in, 934
    C, 934, 941
        ascorbic acid in, 934
        deficiency of, 934
    D, 934
        deficiency of, 934
        excess of, 935
        infantile tetany in, 935
        osteomalacia in, 935
        viosterol in, 934
    E, 935
        sterility and, 935
    G, 935
        black tongue and, 935
        pellagra and, 935
        pernicious anemia and, 935
        sprue and, 935
Vitamins, 932
    nomenclature of, 932

Von Recklinghausen's disease, 921
    tetany in, 921

W

Wassermann reaction in syphilis, 214
    in syphilitic heart disease, 393
    in yaws, 229
Water, 930
    hammer pulse, 418
Weber's syndrome, 1130
Weil-Felix agglutination reaction, 194
Werlhof's disease, 875
Wet brain, 1037
Whooping cough, 322
Widal reaction in typhoid fever, 32
Widow, black, 304
Wilson's disease, 1219
Woolsorter's disease, 87
Wound infection, 125
Wrist-drop in plumbism, 1058
    in polyneuritis, 1238

X

Xanthochromia, 1140
Xanthomatosis, 902
Xerophthalmia, 933

Y

Yaws, 228
    stages of, 228
    transmission of, 228
    Treponema pertenue, 228
Yeast diseases of lung, 779
Yellow fever, 176
    death-rate in, 179
    epidemiology of, 176
    jaundice in, 178
    leukocyte count in, 179
    mosquito and, 177
    prevention of, 180
    stages of, 178
    urine in, 178

Z

Zona, 1174